ENCYCLOPEDIA OF
BIOETHICS

ENCYCLOPEDIA OF
BIOETHICS

REVISED EDITION

Warren Thomas Reich

EDITOR IN CHIEF

Georgetown University

Volume 3

MACMILLAN LIBRARY REFERENCE USA

SIMON & SCHUSTER MACMILLAN

NEW YORK

SIMON & SCHUSTER AND PRENTICE HALL INTERNATIONAL

LONDON   MEXICO CITY   NEW DELHI   SINGAPORE   SYDNEY   TORONTO

Simon & Schuster Macmillan
866 Third Avenue, New York, NY 10022

PRINTED IN THE UNITED STATES OF AMERICA

printing number
 2 3 4 5 6 7 8 9 10

LIBRARY OF CONGRESS CATALOG-IN-PUBLICATION DATA

Encyclopedia of bioethics / Warren T. Reich, editor in chief. — Rev.
   ed.
     p. cm.
     Includes bibliographical references and index.
     ISBN 0-02-897355-0 (set)
     1. Bioethics—Encyclopedias.   2. Medical ethics—Encyclopedias.
   I. Reich, Warren T.
   QH332.E52   1995
   174'.2'03—dc20   94-38743
                                                         CIP

Lines from the poem "The Scarred Girl" by James Dickey, quoted in the entry on "Interpretation," originally appeared in *Poems, 1957–1967,* © 1978 by James Dickey, Wesleyan University Press, and have been reprinted here by permission of the University Press of New England.

The paper used in this publication meets the minimum requirements of American National Standard for Information Sciences—Permanence of Paper for Printed Library Materials, ANSI Z39.48-1984.

I

IATROGENIC ILLNESS
AND INJURY

"Iatrogenic" derives from the Greek roots *iatros* (physician) and *genic* (produced or generated by). "Iatrogenic illness and injury" thus are adverse effects produced by a physician in a patient. However, "iatrogenesis" may also refer to harmful effects caused by patterns of practice among physicians, by health-care institutions, and by nonphysician health professionals. The adverse effects in the patient include physical and psychological harms resulting from negligence as well as nonnegligent mishaps. Some discussions of iatrogenesis may also more widely include anticipated risks, complications, and side effects of treatment.

Authors have identified historical periods in which medicine was more or less iatrogenic to patients. It is commonly noted that prior to the development of germ theory, medical care was at least as likely to harm as to help a patient. The insights and efficacy of twentieth-century medicine, however, have brought no end to iatrogenesis and, in fact, have offered new opportunities for its appearance. Famous examples include the harm caused by physicians in the Nazi concentration camps, by the U.S. Public Health Service in the Tuskegee syphilis trials, by thalidomide, by psychosurgery, and by diethylstilbestrol (DES).

These cases of severe harm were pivotal to the development of modern biomedical ethics. In 1947 the trial of the Nazi physicians yielded the Nuremberg Code, governing research with human subjects. Outrage over the Tuskegee trials helped motivate passage of the National Research Act of 1974, which created institutional review boards (IRBs) as part of a system to protect human subjects in research. Both scandals contributed to the sense that medical ethics should not be determined only by physicians, but required public debate, value judgments, and oversight. To a great extent, key iatrogenic events gave birth to modern bioethics.

Concern about iatrogenesis has varied over time. Paul Starr (1982) has identified the 1960s and 1970s as a time when medicine's efficacy was doubted and its capacity for harm decried. Ivan Illich's *Medical Nemesis* (1976) condemned an "epidemic" of iatrogenesis, physician-inflicted injuries ("clinical iatrogenesis"), harm from medical bureaucracies ("social iatrogenesis"), and broad cultural changes produced by the medical enterprise ("cultural iatrogenesis"). Other writers found medicine especially iatrogenic to women (e.g., Corea, 1977). The Tuskegee trials and other events have provoked investigation of medical harm to African-Americans and other historically disadvantaged groups (e.g., King, 1992).

Empirical research on iatrogenesis beginning in the late 1970s fueled further concern. A California study showed medical injury in 4.65 percent of hospital admissions (Mills, 1978); a New York study showed a rate of 3.7 percent (Leape et al., 1991). Research showed that iatrogenesis was common (Leape et al., 1991, p. 380) and "a major source of morbidity and mortality for hospitalized patients" (Bedell et al., 1991, p. 2815). Researchers also explored the association of iatrogenesis with lack of health insurance and other patient characteristics (e.g., Burstin et al., 1992).

Finally, the HIV (human immunodeficiency virus) epidemic has provoked concern over the possibility of seropositive physicians and other health-care workers infecting patients (e.g., Gostin, 1989, 1990). Despite analysis indicating that such HIV transmission is extremely rare, controversy has erupted over what steps, if any, should be taken to prevent it. Further debate has surrounded the possibility of harm caused by health-care professionals suffering from AIDS (acquired immunodeficiency syndrome)-related dementia. The outbreak of drug-resistant tuberculosis associated with the HIV epidemic has added to this cluster of concerns over iatrogenesis through transmission of disease or through disease-related error.

Ethically, the major questions raised by iatrogenesis are what the category should include; what moral judgments should be made about different kinds of iatrogenesis; and what compensatory and other steps should be taken in response.

Identifying iatrogenesis

Dealing with these ethical questions requires differentiating types of iatrogenesis. Intentional harm, negligent injury, and predicted side effects are unlikely to prompt the same moral assessment. Barry Furrow and colleagues (1991) have identified a spectrum of events causing injury. *Willful or reckless events* would include intentional deviation from professional norms without good reason. The surgeon who knowingly uses poor technique, or who operates while under the influence of alcohol, or who sexually abuses a patient would cause harm in this category. *Negligent acts* would be those falling below accepted standards of practice. Thus a physician who errs because of poor training, a lapse in technique, or inattentiveness would be acting negligently.

Samuel Gorovitz and Alasdair MacIntyre (1975) argue that the customary view of medical fallibility attributes all error either to the failure of the physician to act in keeping with medical norms or to the limits of medical knowledge at any given time. In recognizing this, they add another category to the spectrum identified above, all of which involves deviation from norms: Physicians may cause harm because of *medical ignorance.* Medical science may not yet recognize a group of patients who will react adversely to a certain drug, or the only currently accepted treatment for a given condition may produce negative side effects. Nearly every medical procedure carries the risk of negative consequences. Physicians practicing state-of-the-art medicine may still cause harm to patients.

Gorovitz and MacIntyre add a further category of events causing harm. These are errors resulting from *in-dividual patient variation.* The physician cannot know everything about an individual patient; thus, the physician's predictive ability is constrained. Science and medicine equip the physician with reasonable expectations based on empirical research. The individual case, however, may deviate from the rule. A usually safe vaccine, for example, may nonetheless produce harm in a particular patient. Most generalizations in medicine are probabilistic. Thus, a physician may recognize that a treatment will produce harm in a certain percentage of cases but may not be able to recognize in advance that a particular patient is one of those cases.

One can therefore distinguish three kinds of harm: harm from an intentional or negligent failure to observe professional norms; harm from conformity to professional norms that reflect the current limits of knowledge in medicine; and harm from the difficulty of applying normative generalizations to individual patients. All three kinds of harm can be physical or psychological, as suggested above. They can also result from acts or from omissions, such as the decision not to hospitalize, give a certain drug, run a diagnostic test, or perform a procedure.

There are additional categories of phenomena that may produce harm beyond those suggested by Furrow and Gorovitz and MacIntyre. One is the *absence of agreed professional norms.* A class of clinical events may escape attention and not be the subject of professional norms until it is recognized that those events cause harm. The absence of professional norms may result from ignorance or from the emergence of a new disease-producing entity. It could also theoretically result from a deliberate decision not to generate norms. For example, generating norms in a particular arena might be seen as contrary to physician or hospital interests, or the relevant research might be difficult or costly.

Another category of phenomena that may cause harm is conformity to *professional norms that incorporate bias against certain groups.* Here the defect in the norm results, not from the limits of medical knowledge at any one time, but from the limits of social tolerance and insight at any one time. The Tuskegee trials, for example, have been seen as testimony to the racism in medicine at that time rather than as a deviation from nonracist norms (King, 1992). Authors writing on gender have often found bias against women built into the medical norms of any particular period (e.g., Corea, 1977). There is ample cause to worry about and investigate other types of bias built into medical norms, including bias against the elderly, the poor, and the uninsured.

A further category of phenomena that may produce harm moves the focus from individual physicians and the norms of the profession to the *acts or omissions of health-care institutions.* It can be argued that the modern health-care institution has the responsibility to look for patterns of iatrogenesis, to set up feedback and research mechanisms to alert physicians to such patterns, and to take institutional steps to prevent and minimize such harm. Epidemiological research on patterns of iatrogenesis (e.g., Tancredi and Bovbjerg, 1992) suggests just such duties. The institution that fails to attend to iatrogenesis in these ways is itself producing harm through the omission.

Moral evaluation

The central evaluative question is when blame should attach to iatrogenesis. Because "iatrogenesis" refers to harm inflicted on the patient, the central moral mandate at issue is the physician's duty to avoid harm. As Tom Beauchamp and James Childress (1994) note, that duty has been associated with the often cited maxim *primum non nocere*, "above all, do no harm."

The fundamental injunction to avoid harm poses an obvious problem: Since iatrogenesis involves causing harm, does all iatrogenesis violate the duty of nonmaleficence and warrant moral blame? It seems too sweeping to condemn the physician for the limits of state-of-the-art medicine diligently applied, for example. It also seems too indiscriminate to censure unintended errors and intentional harm to the same degree. Moreover, some harm, such as amputation, may be necessary to achieve the patient's treatment goals.

All of this shows that one must distinguish types of iatrogenesis for purposes of moral evaluation. First, some iatrogenesis results from the physician's intentional, reckless, or negligent failure to act in keeping with professional standards. Such action violates the physician's professional obligation of due care. Physicians are properly held morally accountable for acting in accordance with professional standards, and patients rely on them to do so. Thus, the physician whose actions fall below professional standards, thereby causing harm, is blameworthy.

Much is packed, however, into the notion of due care. A physician may exercise due care, yet harm the patient nonetheless. When the harm is necessary to achieve the patient's treatment goal, the harm is justified. It is worth noting, though, that a separate wrong would be committed if the physician failed to inform the patient in advance of the risks of such harm and to obtain the patient's consent. That wrong would not be morally excused by achievement of the treatment goal.

Just as following the standard of due care will justify some harms, so the principle of double effect is often said to excuse still others. The principle applies to harm caused in pursuit of a good goal, but only under the following circumstances: The harm-causing action cannot be intrinsically wrong; the actor must intend the good goal and not the harm; the harm cannot be a necessary means to achieve the goal; and the good effects must outweigh the bad (Beauchamp and Childress, 1994).

Laying aside the justification of due care and the excuse of double effect, when blameworthy violations of professional standards do occur, the degree of blame will vary. The surgeon who intentionally inflicts grave injury on a patient, contrary to professional standards, will be held more culpable than the one who negligently inflicts a minor harm. Thus, the actor's intent and the extent of the injury caused will bear on the degree of blame.

So far we have morally evaluated only the categories of iatrogenesis differentiated by Furrow and colleagues (1991). Gorovitz and MacIntyre's account of error due to individual patient variation is more difficult to analyze. When such errors are caused by a failure to assess the patient with due care, they will be covered by the notions of willfulness, recklessness, and negligence, considered above. But that still leaves a category of error without individual fault. Even when the physician is observing professional standards, application of such standards will result in some harm in some individual cases.

Here moral blame seems hard to justify. Physicians cannot be held to a standard of omniscience and blamed for what they neither know nor control. Albert Jonsen (1977), however, suggests a limit on this exoneration, in finding that "do no harm" requires risk–benefit and detriment–benefit assessments. Thus, the expected risk and threatened detriment to each patient must be justified by the expected benefit, even if the physician cannot know with certainty whether this patient will suffer the risks at all. In addition, here again failure to disclose to the patient predictable risk and to obtain consent may be a separate and quite blameworthy harm. The physician may also be held to standards that would require vigilance with respect to individual cases and the minimization of harm.

The additional categories of iatrogenesis suggested above pose more novel questions. If there are no agreed professional norms, physicians cannot violate them. Yet physicians may nonetheless retain general nonprofessional duties of due care. Moreover, they may have a responsibility to remain alert to the emergence of new problems and to be socially responsive, so that they can help spot areas requiring the development of professional norms and engage in constructive deliberation over the content of norms proposed.

Iatrogenesis caused by observing professional norms that incorporate bias is particularly troublesome; such harm has been done repeatedly. Again, the physician's culpability cannot rest directly on violation of professional norms; the problem is that the physician is observing them. Culpability rests on other grounds. First, physicians do not stop being human beings by virtue of their professional status. Following professional norms that cause unjustified harm and violate general non-professional duties of nonmaleficence can be held blameworthy. Second, one can argue that biased professional norms are actually defective, no justified norms at all, and so provide no true warrant for the infliction of any harm. Third, there are now so many clear examples of professional norms (not merely medical ones) incorporating bias, that one could argue physicians have a duty to scrutinize the profession's norms for bias and to refrain from translating such bias into action.

Finally, iatrogenesis due in part to institutional failings raises an important set of questions about institutional culpability. Full exploration of this vital topic, including whether institutions can constitute moral agents and shoulder organizational responsibility, is beyond the scope of this entry. One could argue, however, that standards of due care for health-care institutions include duties to monitor and minimize iatrogenesis. The institution that fails to observe such standards may be deemed worthy of censure.

Responding to iatrogenesis

Iatrogenesis may warrant three general categories of response: compensation (through malpractice litigation or otherwise), research, and prevention. By far the longest controversy has concerned the first of these. In the United States, compensation has been attempted largely through malpractice litigation. This mechanism, however, fails to compensate in many cases of iatrogenic harm. Malpractice is defined as violation of professional norms that causes injury. As explained above, however, some categories of iatrogenesis do not involve violation of such norms. Moreover, research has suggested that only a fraction of harm caused by negligent violation of professional norms is successfully compensated by the malpractice system (e.g., Localio et al., 1991).

In response to these problems, some have advocated shifting to a system of no-fault compensation for iatrogenic harm. This would broaden the group of patients receiving compensation. Depending on how such a system was financed, it would also alter the group paying the costs of iatrogenesis. Thus arguments about whether to make this shift raise questions of compensatory and distributive justice.

Responding to iatrogenesis through research is less problematic morally, though there may be practical obstacles to good epidemiological research on iatrogenesis. Now that substantial rates of iatrogenesis have been documented, however, the duty of nonmaleficence seems to mandate research to identify patterns and suggest ways to minimize harm.

Prevention would seem to be equally mandated. Concern about possible HIV transmission from physician to patient, however, has raised the question of how far preventive steps should go. Given an extremely small statistical risk of transmission, what steps, if any, should be taken? Larry Gostin (1989, 1990) and others have examined this question in detail, exploring the tension between preventing harm to patients and protecting the privacy and employment rights of health professionals. Gostin has argued that HIV-positive professionals should report their serostatus to their employer and personal physician under conditions of confidentiality, should be monitored for conditions impairing performance such as dementia, and should refrain from performing seriously invasive procedures (which are more specifically defined), while health-care facilities should provide support and compensation.

Further issues

Research on iatrogenesis will continue to deepen understanding of the kinds of harms inflicted upon patients. That research must examine iatrogenesis both in treatment and in the course of clinical experiments. Research on iatrogenesis provides the starting point for moral and legal debate, not only by demonstrating empirical patterns but also by developing an analytic sophistication that may suggest new categories of iatrogenic behavior.

Harm to patients in the course of health care and human experimentation is a grave concern. It can also be tremendously unnerving for patients, their health professionals, and those conducting the experiments. A pivotal task for modern bioethics has been to reveal and to morally evaluate such harm. This gives analysis of iatrogenesis a central role in any discussion of bioethics.

Susan M. Wolf

Directly related to this entry are the entries Injury and Injury Control; Medical Malpractice; Harm; Risk; Hospital, *article on* contemporary ethical problems; *and* Conflict of Interest. *For a further discussion of topics mentioned in this entry, see the entries* AIDS; Eugenics, *article on* historical aspects; Feminism; Impaired Professionals; Psychiatry, Abuses of; Psychosurgery; Race and Racism; Research, Unethical; *and* Sexual Ethics and Professional Standards. *Other relevant material may be found under the entries* Double Effect; Information Disclosure; Informed Consent, *article on* clinical aspects of consent in health care; Law and Bioethics; Medical Codes and Oaths; *and* Professional-Patient Relationship, *article on* ethical issues.

Bibliography

Apfel, Robert J., and Fisher, Susan M. 1984. *To Do No Harm: DES and the Dilemmas of Modern Medicine.* New Haven, Conn.: Yale University Press.

BEAUCHAMP, TOM L., and CHILDRESS, JAMES F. 1994. "The Concept of Nonmaleficence." In their *Principles of Biomedical Ethics*, 4th ed., pp. 190–211. New York: Oxford University Press.

BEDELL, SUSANNE E.; DEITZ, DAVID C.; LEEMAN, DAVID; and DELBANCO, THOMAS L. 1991. "Incidence and Characteristics of Preventable Iatrogenic Cardiac Arrests." *Journal of the American Medical Association* 265, no. 21:2815–2820.

BOSK, CHARLES L. 1979. *Forgive and Remember: Managing Medical Failure*. Chicago: University of Chicago Press.

BRENNAN, TROYEN A. 1991. "Physicians and Quality of Medical Care." In his *Just Doctoring: Medical Ethics in the Liberal State*, pp. 121–146. Berkeley: University of California Press.

BRENNAN, TROYEN A.; HEBERT, LIESI E.; LAIRD, NAN M.; LAWTHERS, ANN.; THORPE, KENNETH E.; LEAPE, LUCIAN L.; LOCALIO, A. RUSSELL; LIPSITZ, STUART R.; NEWHOUSE, JOSEPH P.; WEILER, PAUL C.; and HIATT, HOWARD H. 1991. "Hospital Characteristics Associated with Adverse Events and Substandard Care." *Journal of the American Medical Association* 265:3265–3269.

BRENNAN, TROYEN A.; LEAPE, LUCIAN L.; LAIRD, NAN M.; HEBERT, LIESI; LOCALIO, A. RUSSELL; LAWTHERS, ANN G.; NEWHOUSE, JOSEPH P.; WEILER, PAUL C.; and HIATT, HOWARD H. 1991. "Incidence of Adverse Effects and Negligence in Hospitalized Patients: Results of the Harvard Medical Practice Study I." *New England Journal of Medicine* 324, no. 6:370–376.

BURSTIN, HELEN R.; LIPSITZ, STUART R.; and BRENNAN, TROYEN A. 1992. "Socioeconomic Status and Risk for Substandard Medical Care." *Journal of the American Medical Association* 268, no. 17:2383–2387.

COREA, GENA. 1977. *The Hidden Malpractice: How American Medicine Treats Women as Patients and Professionals*. New York: William Morrow.

DUTTON, DIANA B.; PRESTON, THOMAS A.; and PFUND, NANCY E. 1988. *Worse Than the Disease: Pitfalls of Medical Progress*. New York: Cambridge University Press.

FURROW, BARRY R.; JOHNSON, SANDRA H.; JOST, TIMOTHY S.; and SCHWARTZ, ROBERT L. 1991. "The Problem of Medical Error." In *Liability and Quality Issues in Health Care*, pp. 24–39. Edited by Barry R. Furrow. St. Paul, Minn.: West.

GOROVITZ, SAMUEL, and MACINTYRE, ALASDAIR. 1975. "Toward a Theory of Medical Fallibility." *Hastings Center Report* 5, no. 6:13–23.

GOSTIN, LARRY. 1989. "HIV-Infected Physicians and the Practice of Seriously Invasive Procedures." *Hastings Center Report* 19, no. 1:32–39.

———. 1990. "The HIV-Infected Health Care Professional: Public Policy, Discrimination, and Patient Safety." *Law, Medicine and Health Care* 18, no. 4:303–310.

ILLICH, IVAN. 1976. *Medical Nemesis: The Expropriation of Health*. New York: Pantheon.

JONSEN, ALBERT R. 1977. "Do No Harm: Axiom of Medical Ethics." In *Philosophical Medical Ethics: Its Nature and Significance*, pp. 27–41. Edited by Stuart F. Spicker and H. Tristram Engelhardt, Jr. Dordrecht, Netherlands: D. Reidel.

KING, PATRICIA A. 1992. "Twenty Years After: The Legacy of the Tuskegee Syphilis Study: The Dangers of Difference." *Hastings Center Report* 22, no. 6:35–38.

LEAPE, LUCIAN L.; BRENNAN, TROYEN A.; LAIRD, NAN; LAWTHERS, ANN G.; LOCALIO, A. RUSSELL; BARNES, BENJAMIN A.; HEBERT, LIESI; NEWHOUSE, JOSEPH P.; WEILER, PAUL C.; and HIATT, HOWARD. 1991. "The Nature of Adverse Events in Hospitalized Patients: Results of the Harvard Medical Practice Study II." *New England Journal of Medicine* 324, no. 6:377–384.

LOCALIO, A. RUSSELL; LAWTHERS, ANN G.; BRENNAN, TROYEN A.; LAIRD, NAN M.; HEBERT, LIESI E.; PETERSON, LYNN M.; NEWHOUSE, JOSEPH P.; WEILER, PAUL C.; and HIATT, HOWARD H. 1991. "Relation Between Malpractice Claims and Adverse Events Due to Negligence: Results of the Harvard Medical Practice Study III." *New England Journal of Medicine* 325, no. 4:245–251.

MILLS, DON HARPER. 1978. "Medical Insurance Feasibility Study: A Technical Summary." *Western Journal of Medicine* 128, no. 4:360–365.

ROBIN, EUGENE D. 1984. *Matters of Life & Death: Risks vs. Benefits of Medical Care*. New York: W. H. Freeman.

STARR, PAUL. 1982. *The Social Transformation of American Medicine*. New York: Basic Books.

STEEL, KNIGHT; GERTMAN, PAUL M.; CRESCENZI, CAROLINE; and ANDERSON, JENNIFER. 1981. "Iatrogenic Illness on a General Medical Service at a University Hospital." *New England Journal of Medicine* 304, no. 11:638–642.

TANCREDI, LAURENCE R., and BOVBJERG, RANDALL R. 1992. "Advancing the Epidemiology of Injury and Methods of Quality Control: ACEs as an Outcomes-Based System for Quality Improvement." *QRB: Quality Review Bulletin* 18, no. 6:201–209.

WEILER, PAUL C.; HIATT, HOWARD H.; NEWHOUSE, JOSEPH P.; JOHNSON, WILLIAM G.; BRENNAN, TROYEN A.; and LEAPE, LUCIAN L., eds. 1993. *A Measure of Malpractice: Medical Injury, Malpractice Litigation, and Patient Compensation*. Cambridge, Mass.: Harvard University Press.

ICELAND

See MEDICAL ETHICS, HISTORY OF, *section on* EUROPE. *subsection on* CONTEMPORARY PERIOD, *article on* NORDIC COUNTRIES.

ILLNESS

See HEALTH AND DISEASE; MENTAL HEALTH; *and* MENTAL ILLNESS.

IMPAIRED PROFESSIONALS

Impairment is a widespread problem of professional life. Attorneys, airline pilots, doctors, nurses, and all other professionals are susceptible to becoming impaired (Morrow, 1984). The impaired professional creates legal and ethical difficulties for himself or herself, and can cause harm to others as well. For these reasons, the impaired professional merits serious attention (Morreim, 1993).

Defining the problem

In common usage, the word "impair" connotes the worsening or deterioration of a person or thing. An impairment diminishes the value or excellence of an individual or item. Stress, for example, may impair the integrity of an individual; metal fatigue may impair the quality of an aircraft. In each instance, we mean that the person or thing has deteriorated significantly enough to endanger his, her, or its capacity to function adequately.

When impairment refers to a professional, its meaning becomes more technical and restrictive. Because professions are self-regulating and resist external oversight, professionals largely determine what impairment means for them. Things that might impair an individual in the eyes of the lay community might not be defined as such within the professional community (Freidson, 1970; Rueschemeyer, 1986; Abbott, 1988).

Typically, the impaired professional is one whose ability to function in his or her professional capacity has deteriorated because of a physical or mental difficulty. Impairing conditions traditionally have included drug dependency, alcohol dependency, illness, and disability (physical as well as mental). The American Medical Association, for example, defines the impaired physician as one "unable to practice medicine with reasonable skill and safety to patients because of physical or mental illness, including deteriorations through the aging process or loss of motor skill, or excessive use or abuse of drugs including alcohol" (La Puma and Schiedermayer, 1994, p. 91). A professional may also be regarded as impaired if his or her abilities are significantly compromised as the result of stress or other factors (Nelson and Jennings, 1992).

While impairment raises concerns about an individual's professional competence, being impaired is not necessarily the same as being incompetent. An incompetent professional lacks the minimally acceptable levels of knowledge and skills needed to practice within a field. Such a person may once have been competent, as in the case of the individual who has passed the requisite qualifying examinations but who has failed to maintain his or her knowledge and skills. One can be incompetent without being impaired.

Impairment's implications

The impaired professional poses a serious problem to himself or herself and to others. The existence of an impairment may adversely affect the professional's relationships with colleagues, with patients and their families, and with the professional's institution or workplace. It can affect a professional's relationship with friends and family. An impairment can also affect a professional's relationship with him or herself, as when the impaired professional engages in self-destructive behavior.

Impairment is a grave problem to those who seek professional assistance. The public expects professionals to help, an expectation created by the profession's representations that its members are competent and look out for the public's interests, presumably including the protection of the public against impaired practitioners. The public's expectations are compounded by its vulnerability in dealing with professionals. Members of the public seldom possess the expertise needed to evaluate the quality of services being provided to them. Their potential vulnerability becomes even more significant when other factors (e.g., being sick or injured, being in an unfamiliar setting, or being a member of a different socioeconomic class) make it difficult for a layperson to question a professional's assistance. Given the vulnerabilities and expectations of the public, it is fair to say that people have a right to expect competent help from an unimpaired professional.

If severe, unrecognized and unattended professional impairment can spell disaster. The impaired professional can cause severe harm, even death, to others. This can give rise to legal liability for the professional, for colleagues and coworkers, and for the institution in which the impaired professional works (Curran, 1984).

The persistence of impairment

For many reasons impairment is an enduring, ubiquitous phenomenon of professional life. First, instead of responsibly discharging the responsibility toward self-regulation, professions and professionals sometimes abuse their power or office (Gellhorn, 1976). Second, professionals tend to protect inept colleagues (Goode, 1967). Third, professional impairment does not receive much attention in the education and training of those who are entering a profession. While medical students may be quick to identify and chastise a patient who has a serious emotional or drinking problem, they are less likely to learn how to recognize or respond constructively to self-impairment or to impairment in a colleague. Fourth, some professions foster impairment. The idealized image of the competitive, self-reliant practitioner drives professionals to succeed and to work in isolation, patterns of behavior that are conducive to impairment.

Even if a medical professional knows about professional impairment, he or she may not see it (Talbott and Benson, 1980). Medical professionals are autonomous practitioners, which means that they tend to be self-supervising. Where contact is occasional they may not have the opportunity to discern that a colleague is impaired, or feel responsible for doing something if they suspect it. Where contact is frequent, they may cover for their impaired colleague. To the extent that medical professionals practice as independent contractors without supervision or sustained periods of collaboration and regular contact, the ability to see that a professional is impaired is impeded. To the extent that medical professionals work together, collegiality may supplant professional concern.

Initial signs of impairment are frequently quite subtle and are not likely to be obvious to someone who is not looking for them. Moreover, just as few individuals are looking for impairment, few wish to discover that someone is impaired. The ability to recognize impairment is affected by the willingness to see it. Missed appointments, tardiness, sloppiness in one's work might be attributed to a passing stress and not taken as signs of something that is seriously wrong. A friendly inquiry met with a plausible response may be enough to assuage concern about a colleague.

Professionals may sympathize or identify with a troubled colleague. Given how much time, money, and effort professionals invest to establish their careers, the potential consequences of finding impairment can be enough to cause any particular professional to accommodate rather than to report a colleague who is in trouble. The tendency of professionals to protect an inept colleague limits society's ability to respond to the impaired professional (Goode, 1967).

Fear of possible recrimination from the individual and from peers also affects the professional's response to the suspicion or recognition that a colleague is impaired. The professional may think that reporting or taking action on impairment in another may expose him or her to civil liability. Even if reporting a colleague poses no genuine threat of legal action, peers may punish an individual for initiating the process of exposing a colleague to shame and to institutional or legal action. These and other pressures may suffice to make even conscientious professionals reluctant to report an apparently impaired colleague.

The legal, professional, and institutional response to professional impairment remains harsh. The impaired professional who has been reported is likely to encounter problems at his or her place of employment and to experience difficulties in licensure and insurance. Depending on the nature and severity of the impairment, rehabilitation and recovery may not restore his or her former status.

Confronting or reporting an impaired professional may be more difficult because that person is unable or unwilling to recognize that he or she is impaired. Admitting to impairment may damage others' image of the impaired person and his or her reputation in the community. It may be fatal to a career, bringing to an end all that the individual has worked for and hopes to accomplish.

Unfortunately, the risk an impaired professional poses—to himself or herself and to others—does not disappear or diminish if the impairment is ignored or unaddressed. On the contrary, it is likely to worsen. To ignore or dismiss the signs of impairment creates and sustains a potentially tragic situation. When the professional's impairment manifests itself, it is likely to be severe. At that point, those around the impaired professional are likely to be asked why no one intervened sooner, when the harm done could have been avoided or minimized.

What to do

Professional impairment requires a variety of responses. Professional schools need to integrate this topic into the education and training of students. Professionals themselves, as well as employers and health-care institutions, need to improve their ability to recognize impairment, and to respond constructively to the plight of the impaired professional. Increased supervision and enhanced scrutiny of applications for initial and continued employment can help, especially if programs of support and assistance are available on a confidential basis. To the extent that it is made easier for professionals to help themselves, the number of impaired practitioners will be reduced. Unfortunately, not everyone who needs help will volunteer for it.

U.S. law requires professionals to report impaired colleagues, and grants immunity from liability when they do, largely in response to the Health Care Quality Improvement Act and increasing concern about impaired as well as incompetent practitioners. In addition to making reporting of impairment mandatory, some states make failure to report it grounds for disciplinary action, although the actual enforcement of such statutes remains lax. Because the purpose of the law is prophylactic and arises out of the state's interest in protecting the public against harm, actual harm to a patient need not occur in order for a physician to be considered impaired. Because professional regulation is governed by state, not federal, law and because this is an area of the law that is in constant flux, the specific requirements, immunities, and programs vary considerably (Walzer, 1990).

Can anything be done to prevent professional impairment? Professional schools can help by ensuring that their students are prepared for the rigors of professional life. This requires alerting students to what those rigors will be and assessing how well students deal with the pressure of their professional education and training. If professional schools can teach students to cope with the demands of their field, and to identify and address personal and professional problems before they become severe, they can reduce the incidence of impairment.

To the extent that the expectations of what it means to be a professional create and sustain conditions that are conducive to impairment, society may reduce the incidence of impairment by creating different expectations. Nothing suggests that individuals must compete in isolation in order to succeed professionally. Whatever can be done to reduce the incidence of impairment without compromising the commitment to professionalism and quality of care should be done (Gorovitz, 1984). It makes no more sense to place the burden of this problem on the individual professional than it does to make it someone else's problem. If we sincerely wish to address impairment and prevent harm, we must define it, examine its causes, identify those who are at risk, and intervene effectively and productively.

Increasing awareness of the extent to which prejudice against persons with disabilities permeates society should also lead to some changes in how professional impairment is addressed. Most statutes defining professional impairment refer to the existence of a physical or mental disability as a condition that can be regarded as impairing, reflecting global perceptions about persons with disabilities that have come to be regarded as anachronistic and unwarranted. The Americans with Disabilities Act (1993) prohibits discrimination against persons with disabilities in such areas as employment and public services. It is intended to reduce or, ideally, eliminate actions and decisions made concerning persons with disabilities that reflect prejudicial attitudes about physical and mental disability. It is too early to tell how much and what sort of impact legislation such as the Americans with Disabilities Act will have on how impairment is defined and addressed. Given the fact that this legislation already has had an impact on the licensure of professionals, it is fair to expect that it will alter how states, employers, and institutions address some aspects of professional impairment to the extent that the law already has moved from a punitive toward a rehabilitative approach to impairment. The Americans with Disabilities Act may not only help professionals receive the services they need but also ensure that the rehabilitated professional will be able to return to work (Piltch et al., 1993).

Unfortunately, given the history of professions and the power that professionalization confers, we should not expect the situation to improve markedly. Unless professionals are willing to share or yield the power that they have worked so hard to secure, we can expect that professionals will address impairment only to the extent that they must in order to preserve their professional sovereignty. Until society redefines the professions in ways that reduce the insolence of office that professionalism fosters (Walzer, 1983), power, not ethics, will determine what society's response to the impaired professional will be.

GILES R. SCOFIELD

For a further discussion of topics mentioned in this entry, see the entries DISABILITY, *articles on* ATTITUDES AND SOCIOLOGICAL PERSPECTIVES, *and* LEGAL ISSUES; LICENSING, DISCIPLINE, AND REGULATION IN THE HEALTH PROFESSIONS; MEDICAL EDUCATION; MENTAL ILLNESS; MENTALLY DISABLED AND MENTALLY ILL PERSONS; PROFESSIONAL–PATIENT RELATIONSHIP; PROFESSION AND PROFESSIONAL ETHICS; *and* SUBSTANCE ABUSE. *For a discussion of related ideas, see the entries* COMPETENCE; RESPONSIBILITY; *and* TRUST. *Other relevant material may be found under the entries* MEDICINE AS A PROFESSION; *and* NURSING AS A PROFESSION.

Bibliography

ABBOTT, ANDREW D. 1988. *The System of Professions: An Essay on the Division of Expert Labor.* Chicago: University of Chicago Press.

ANNAS, GEORGE J. 1978. "Who to Call When the Doctor Is Sick." *Hastings Center Report* 8, no. 6:18–20.

CURRAN, RICHARD F. 1984. "Hospital, Heal Thyself: Coping with Impaired Providers and Other Hospital Employees." *QRB: Quality Review Bulletin* 10, no. 11:335–339.

FREIDSON, ELIOT. 1970. *Profession of Medicine: A Study of the Sociology of Applied Knowledge.* New York: Dodd, Mead.

GELLHORN, WALTER. 1976. "The Abuse of Occupational Licensing." *University of Chicago Law Review* 44:6–27.

GOODE, WILLIAM J. 1967. "The Protection of the Inept." *American Sociological Review* 32, no. 1:5–19.

GOROVITZ, SAMUEL. 1984. "Preparing for the Perils of Practice." *Hastings Center Report* 14, no.6:38–41.

LA PUMA, JOHN, and SCHIEDERMAYER, DAVID. 1994. *Ethics Consultation: A Practical Guide.* Boston: Jones and Bartlett.

MORREIM, E. HAAVI. 1993. "Am I My Brother's Warden? Responding to the Unethical or Incompetent Colleague." *Hastings Center Report* 23, no. 3:19–27.

MORROW, CAROL K. 1984. "Doctors Helping Doctors." *Hastings Center Report* 14, no. 6:32–38.

NELSON, JAMES LINDEMANN, and JENNINGS, BRUCE. 1992. "Properly Diagnosing Impairment." *QRB: Quality Review Bulletin* 18, no. 3:24–25.

PILTCH, DEBORAH L.; KATZ, JAMIE W.; and VALLES, JANINE. 1993. "The Americans with Disabilities Act and Professional Licensing." *Mental and Physical Disability Law Reporter* 17, no. 5:556–562.

RUESCHEMEYER, DIETRICH. 1986. *Power and the Division of Labour.* Stanford, Calif.: Stanford University Press.

TALBOTT, GEORGE D., and BENSON, EDWARD B. 1980. "Impaired Physicians: The Dilemma of Identification." *Postgraduate Medicine* 68, no. 6:56–64.

WALZER, MICHAEL. 1983. *Spheres of Justice: A Defense of Pluralism and Equality.* New York: Basic Books.

WALZER, ROBERT S. 1990. "Impaired Physicians: An Overview and Update of the Legal Issues." *Journal of Legal Medicine* 11, no. 2:131–198.

INCOMPETENCE

See COMPETENCE.

INDIA

See MEDICAL ETHICS, HISTORY OF, *section on* SOUTH AND EAST ASIA, *article on* INDIA. *See also* EUGENICS AND RELIGIOUS LAW, *article on* HINDUISM AND BUDDHISM; HINDUISM; *and* POPULATION ETHICS, *section on* RELIGIOUS TRADITIONS, *article on* HINDU PERSPECTIVES.

INDONESIA

See MEDICAL ETHICS, HISTORY OF, *section on* SOUTH AND EAST ASIA, *article on* SOUTHEAST ASIAN COUNTRIES.

INDUSTRIAL HEALTH

See OCCUPATIONAL SAFETY AND HEALTH. *See also* HAZARDOUS WASTES AND TOXIC SUBSTANCES.

INFANTICIDE

See INFANTS, *articles on* HISTORY OF INFANTICIDE, *and* ETHICAL ISSUES. *See also* CHILDREN, *article on* HISTORY OF CHILDHOOD.

INFANTS

I. MEDICAL ASPECTS AND ISSUES IN THE CARE OF INFANTS

The most widely discussed ethical dilemmas involving infants pertain to decisions to withhold or withdraw life-sustaining medical treatment. Such discussions tend to focus on the microethical world of the acute-care hospital or neonatal intensive-care unit (NICU) and are framed in terms of the morality of a particular decision for a particular patient at a particular time. Such decisions are controversial because, in the United States and some other countries with liberal political traditions, the prevailing legal and moral standard for decisions to withhold life-sustaining treatment is reliance on the expressed preferences of patients. Infants cannot express preferences or participate in such decisions, so the decisions must be made by others. Traditionally, parents were empowered to make such decisions, but recent legal developments provide children with independent rights. Parents are not permitted to make decisions that would directly endanger the life, or seriously imperil the health, of their child. In other words, they are required to make decisions that are in the child's interest. However, determining what is in the child's interests may not be straightforward, and different people may judge it differently in different situations.

Because of this emphasis on individual patient decisions, not as much attention is given to macroethical issues that also influence child health, such as the just allocation of resources, or the limits of societal responsibilities to improve the health of all infants. Infants may live or die as the result of decisions made by doctors and parents in NICUs, but their survival is also affected by the decisions made by legislators and policymakers. In the United States, for example, the overall infant mortality rate is nine per 1000, yet African-American infants die at nearly twice that rate. Portions of several U.S. urban areas have infant mortality rates similar to those of underdeveloped countries. The disproportion between infant mortality rates for the most and least fortunate Americans is partly a consequence of a health-care system in which preventive care and prenatal care are relatively inaccessible, while access to neonatal intensive care is guaranteed by law.

Discussions of macroethical issues generally involve terms that are hard to apply to the individual case, while discussions of individual cases often ignore larger issues of resource allocation and social justice. Thus, the value of a program to provide universal access to prenatal care or to supplemental food for pregnant women can be conceptualized only in terms of the average number of lives that will be saved. The saving of any particular life cannot be attributed to such programs. To focus on individual lives while ignoring statistical trends distorts values in a way that is both insidious and hard to avoid. This discussion will examine both macroethical allocation issues and microethical clinical care issues.

Macroethical issues

Infant mortality is defined as death before one year of age. In some ways, the infant mortality rate defines the achievable goals of neonatal medicine. At the lower limits, infant mortality rates give an indication of what is "natural," that is, how many infant deaths are unavoidable in spite of medical or social interventions. Short of this limit, the infant mortality rate suggests something about how many infant deaths a society is willing to tolerate.

The infant mortality rate is a curious statistic, because it measures an effect that is associated with various causes. Thus, it may be used as an indicator of the success or failure of many different types of programs. It is often used as a measure of social welfare, with comparisons of infant mortality rates between countries or ethnic groups allowing comparisons of the adequacy of social services. It can also be used to evaluate the cost effectiveness of particular medical interventions. High infant mortality rates have been used in the United States to argue for a wide variety of interventions, including universal access to prenatal care, widespread use of neonatal intensive care, increased funding for Head Start programs, national programs to provide nutritional supplements to women, infants, and children, family planning programs, legalized abortions, and decreased military expenditures.

Infant mortality is divided into two components, neonatal mortality and postneonatal mortality. Neonatal mortality is death before twenty-eight days of age, and postneonatal mortality is death between twenty-eight days of age and a baby's first birthday. Factors lowering neonatal mortality rates can be divided into those that increase birth weight and those that decrease mortality for babies at a given birth weight. Postneonatal mortality is related less to birth weight than to immunization rates and the prevalence of infectious disease.

Higher birth weight is strongly associated with decreased infant mortality because babies of low birth weight (LBW) are generally either premature or ill. Prematurity is associated with mortality because crucial body functions or body organ systems may be underdeveloped and not function properly at birth. One of the most important influences on birth weight is maternal health status. Mothers with poor nutritional status have infants of lower birth weight. Programs that improve maternal nutrition have been shown to increase birth weight (Rush et al., 1988). The nutritional improvements that resulted from participation in the Women, Infants and Children (WIC) supplemental food program in the early 1980s, for example, led to a 1 to 2 percent increase in birth weight and a 16 to 20 percent decrease in the proportion of LBW babies (U.S. General Accounting Office, 1984).

In most studies, race is associated with birth weight. African-Americans have, on average, babies of significantly lower birth weight than people of other racial backgrounds. It is difficult to disentangle the contributions of race, socioeconomic status, cultural influences (such as diet and family structure), and access to medical care. Access to prenatal and other health care can lead to improvements in birth weight, even in high-risk populations (Geronimus, 1986). But it is hard to define precisely how or how much prenatal care actually helps, because access to prenatal care is associated with many other factors that also have a beneficial effect on birth weight, such as a higher socioeconomic status and better parental education. In studies that carefully control for socioeconomic status and access to medical care, access to prenatal care does not eradicate the racial difference in LBW (Schoendorf et al., 1992).

Availability of family-planning services (i.e., programs that provide contraception and abortion) has been shown to be associated with decreases in infant mortality (Starfield, 1985). According to one study, the estimated impact of a reduction of the number of abortions in the United States to the 1969 rate of four per 1,000 pregnancies would be to increase neonatal mortality rates by 25 percent for whites and by 6 percent for blacks (Hadley, 1992). Family-planning programs allow women to decide when to become pregnant and have children, leading to improved maternal health, babies of higher birth weight, and lower infant mortality.

Macroallocation decisions, or laws, programs, or judgments made by the government, policymakers, or society as a whole, affect trends in birth weight. Such decisions become the major underlying influence on the extent of the need for neonatal intensive care. In the United States, systematic neglect of preventive medicine and family planning has led to an exceptionally high need for neonatal intensive care. As a result, physicians in the United States have pioneered developments that lower birth-weight-specific mortality. The interventions that collectively comprise neonatal intensive care are the only known mechanisms for lowering birth-weight-specific mortality rates.

Postneonatal infant mortality is largely accounted for by a few diseases. The most prevalent causes are the Sudden Infant Death Syndrome (SIDS) and congenital anomalies. Deaths due to congenital anomalies are generally not preventable. Deaths due to SIDS and other diseases are considered preventable. Like neonatal mortality, postneonatal mortality is a phenomenon affected by macroallocative political decisions.

Postneonatal mortality rates have been steadily falling throughout the twentieth century. The U.S. postneonatal mortality rate has declined from over sixty postneonatal deaths per 1,000 live births in 1900 to fewer than four deaths in 1987. However, the international standing of the United States in postneonatal mortality deteriorated from third in 1950 to sixteenth in 1986. Studies show a slowdown in the decline in postneonatal mortality between 1970 to 1981 and 1981 to 1986 in Canada, England and Wales, the Netherlands, and the United States, where continual advances in health care have been accompanied by skyrocketing costs and a growing segment of the population without access to affordable health care. Norway actually experienced increases during this period. Only France, which implemented programs to increase access to prenatal and pediatric care, showed an acceleration in the rate's decline during the 1980s. Canada, which adopted a government-sponsored health-care system, maintained the most rapid rate of decline between 1950 and 1986 (Kleinman and Kiely, 1990). While it is difficult to determine the causal factors that precisely account for such associations (Kleinman et al., 1991), the relatively striking changes in different countries suggest that the underlying causes of the differences are political rather than biological and relate to the structure and organization of health-care services for high-risk populations.

Different responses to allocation issues cannot make the microethical issues go away. There will always be sick newborns, even in countries with comprehensive social programs and universal access to family planning and prenatal care. Allocation choices cannot eliminate microethical dilemmas, but they can affect the frequency with which such dilemmas arise, and the context within which they must be resolved.

Microethical issues

In developed countries, LBW is the most important factor associated with infant mortality. Low birth weight is defined as weight at birth of less than 2,500 grams (or about five pounds and eight ounces). Very low birth weight (VLBW) is birth weight below 1,500 grams (or about three pounds). Infant mortality rates increase as birth weight decreases. Fifty percent of babies whose birth weight is less than 800 grams die in the first month of life, compared to 0.5 percent of babies whose birth weight is over 2,500 grams. In spite of the grim statistics, survival is possible for newborns who weigh as little as 500 grams.

Major advances in the treatment of LBW infants occurred during the 1970s, 1980s, and 1990s. Two medical interventions in particular have made the survival of VLBW babies possible: mechanical ventilation and total parenteral nutrition. Mechanical ventilation allows treatment of respiratory distress syndrome, a common problem in premature babies, by pumping oxygen-enriched air into the infant's lungs through a tube inserted into the infant's trachea. Parenteral nutrition allows infants who are too immature to feed to obtain adequate nutrition through intravenous lines and to survive and thrive.

Most babies who die in NICUs do so in the first seventy-two hours of life, even if all available treatment is provided. It is difficult to predict which babies will survive. In the early 1990s, researchers tried to refine prognostic assessment tools in order to define a subpopulation for whom continued treatment might be considered futile (Tyson et al., 1991). This tactic did not prove very successful. Almost any group of infants with a high likelihood of dying will include babies who survive in spite of a dismal prognosis. As a result, many caregivers opt to provide intensive care to all viable babies and allow the babies to "declare themselves," either by stabilizing or by deteriorating. Once a baby deteriorates to the point where survival is considered unlikely, or where the baby will survive only with serious neurologic damage, many neonatologists are willing to withhold or withdraw therapy (Lantos et al., 1992). Treatment issues for babies with two common neonatal conditions—respiratory distress syndrome and intraventricular hemorrhage—illustrate the ethical factors involved in the care of infants.

Respiratory distress syndrome/bronchopulmonary dysplasia. Respiratory distress syndrome (RDS), also known as hyaline membrane disease, is the most common condition affecting premature babies. Treatment of RDS requires high-pressure mechanical ventilators using high concentrations of oxygen. The high concentration of oxygen and high pressures required to deliver that oxygen can damage the infant's delicate lung tissue, leading to a chronic lung disease called bronchopulmonary dysplasia (BPD). Although the exact cause of BPD is unclear, it is associated with premature birth, RDS, oxygen supplementation, and mechanical ventilation (Northway, 1992) and is characterized by dependence on oxygen beyond twenty-eight days of age. In some cases, an infant's lung disease may be so severe that he or she remains permanently dependent on mechanical ventilation. Of infants treated with oxygen and mechanical ventilation, nearly one-third develop BPD. The percentage is even higher among infants at lower birth weights.

BPD illustrates an ethical paradigm for decision making in neonatal intensive care. It can lead to early death, prolonged disease with eventual death, survival with chronic lung disease, or unimpaired survival. Prognosis for any individual newborn is uncertain at birth. Although prognostication becomes more accurate as children get older, significant uncertainty remains. Thus, decision makers must consider not only the severity of illness and its impact on quality of life; they must also consider that any prediction about survival or quality of life will be probabilistic. Furthermore, in evaluating quality of life, the availability of home care using life-sustaining technology such as mechanical ventilation offers some new hope for these children, although the hope comes at an enormous economic and emotional cost (Lantos and Kohrman, 1992).

Intraventricular hemorrhage (IVH). Like RDS, intraventricular hemorrhage (IVH) is not so much a disease as it is a condition that arises because of the immaturity of the circulatory system in the fetal brain. The outcome for infants with IVH depends on the degree of brain injury associated with the hemorrhage (Guzzeta et al., 1992). The more immature the infant, the more likely it is that a hemorrhage will occur. Twenty percent of infants smaller than 1,500-gram birth weight have an IVH (Hanigan et al., 1991). The hemorrhages are graded from I to IV depending on severity, with the prognosis for normal development decreasing with increasing severity of bleeding. An infant with a grade I or II hemorrhage has no greater risk of developmental handicaps than one with no hemorrhage. Grade IV hemorrhages involve bleeding into the substance of the brain. Infants with grade IV hemorrhages are seven times more likely to have major handicaps than infants with no hemorrhage (Faranoff and Martin, 1992). However, even for infants with grade IV hemorrhage, a normal outcome is possible, though unlikely.

Ethical issues in neonates with RDS and IVH. Neonatal RDS and IVH both present ethical dilemmas at two points. First, when premature infants develop RDS or IVH, questions arise about whether life-sustaining treatment should be withdrawn. Studies show that doctors may decide not to initiate mechanical ventilation for babies weighing less than 800 grams (Hack et al., 1991). The circumstances and procedures for arriving at these decisions are complex (Rostain, 1986). Decisions might be based on concerns about the prognosis for survival, about the quality of life for survivors with chronic lung disease, about the just allocation of scarce intensive-care resources, or about the economic and emotional cost to families of long-term neonatal intensive care. Often, neonatologists respond to prognostic uncertainty with a wait-and-see attitude, continuing treatment along with further observation until it is possible to make a precise prognostication. This leads to the second ethical dilemma.

If decisions to withhold treatment are put off early in the course of treatment because the prognosis is uncertain, doctors must define some clinical outcome that would be considered unacceptable at some defined point in the course of an illness. For infants who develop BPD, a number of long-term consequences might be considered. Such infants have compromised pulmonary func-

tion and an increased incidence of pulmonary infections and asthma. Some remain ventilator-dependent. Children with BPD grow poorly. BPD may be associated with developmental delay. Overall mortality for children with BPD is around 25 percent, but is presumably worse for children with severe or progressive disease (Boynton, 1988). Any one of these factors might justify a conclusion that prolongation of life is not in the child's best interests. For infants with IVH, decisions reflect the degree of neurodevelopmental impairment, which may range from persistent vegetative state to mild cerebral palsy or learning disabilities, and the presence of associated neurologic problems, such as seizures or apnea.

These two diseases are paradigmatic of the type of clinical dilemmas that arise in the neonatal intensive care unit. A number of other diseases or conditions present different clinical issues. In each of them, the clinical questions point to two issues: (1) How unlikely is survival, even with continued treatment? and (2) How bad will the child's quality of life be if he or she does survive? Much of the literature of neonatal bioethics has focused on infants with particular congenital anomalies, such as trisomy 21 (Down syndrome) or myelomeningocele (spina bifida). These are conditions for which treatment will generally lead to survival, but in which survival is associated with mental retardation or physical disabilities. The types of considerations relevant to infants with these conditions are similar to those associated with intraventricular hemorrhage, in that they are based on qualitative predictions of neurologic outcomes and quantitative estimates of how likely each possible outcome might be. While each disease has unique elements that must be considered, the ethical considerations remain the same.

Conclusion

Any discussion of the ethical dilemmas in the care of infants must consider both macro- and microethical issues. The macroethical issues are more difficult to frame in the traditional nosology of bioethics, since they involve implicit societal choices concerning the value of infant lives. Nevertheless, the macro issues can be fruitfully examined by comparing events and policies in different countries or societies as if those were willful decisions made by ethically accountable individuals. Although this approach is somewhat metaphoric, it has been used by others (Calabresi and Bobbitt, 1978).

In evaluating microethical issues, it is easy to miss the forest for the trees. The facts of any medical case will necessarily be probabilistic. Ethicists who engage these questions need to base arguments not only on moral principles but also on statistical realities. Individual circumstances differ widely, and the highly particularistic knowledge necessary to evaluate prognosis for any individual baby can be daunting. Nevertheless, most ethical analyses turn on epidemiologic data regarding likelihood of survival and anticipated quality of life.

JOHN D. LANTOS
KATHRYN L. MOSELEY

Directly related to this article are the other articles in this entry: HISTORY OF INFANTICIDE, ETHICAL ISSUES, *and* PUBLIC-POLICY AND LEGAL ISSUES. *For a further discussion of topics mentioned in this article, see the entries* DEATH AND DYING: EUTHANASIA AND SUSTAINING LIFE; ETHICS, *article on* TASK OF ETHICS; HEALTH-CARE RESOURCES, ALLOCATION OF, *article on* MACROALLOCATION; IATROGENIC ILLNESS AND INJURY; *and* PUBLIC HEALTH, *article on* PUBLIC-HEALTH METHODS: EPIDEMIOLOGY AND BIOSTATISTICS. *For a further discussion of surrogate decision making, see the entry* DEATH AND DYING: EUTHANASIA AND SUSTAINING LIFE, *article on* ETHICAL ISSUES. *For a discussion of related ideas, see the entries* JUSTICE; LIFE, QUALITY OF; *and* VALUE AND VALUATION.

Bibliography

BOYNTON, BRUCE R. 1988. "The Epidemiology of Bronchopulmonary Dysplasia." In *Bronchopulmonary Dysplasia: Contemporary Issues in Fetal and Neonatal Medicine,* pp. 19–32. Edited by T. Allen Merritt, William H. Northway, and Bruce R. Boynton. Boston: Blackwell Scientific.

CALABRESI, GUIDO, and BOBBITT, PHILIP. 1978. *Tragic Choices.* New York: W. W. Norton.

FARANOFF, AVROY A., and MARTIN, RICHARD J. 1992. *Neonatal-Perinatal Medicine: Diseases of the Fetus and Infant.* 5th ed. St. Louis: Mosby Year Book.

GERONIMUS, ARLINE T. 1986. "The Effects of Race, Residence, and Prenatal Care on the Relationship of Maternal Age to Neonatal Mortality." *American Journal of Public Health* 76, no. 12:1416–1421.

GUZZETTA, FRANCO; SHAKLEFORD, GARY D.; VOLPE, SARA; PERLMAN, JEFFREY; and VOLPE, JOSEPH J. 1986. "Periventricular Intraparenchymal Echodensities in the Premature Newborn: Critical Determinant of Neurologic Outcome." *Pediatrics* 78, no. 6:995–1006.

HACK, MAUREEN; HORBAR, JEFFREY D.; MALLOY, MICHAEL H.; TYSON, JOHN E.; WRIGHT, ELIZABETH; and WRIGHT, LINDA. 1991. "Very Low Birth Weight Outcomes of the National Institute of Child Health and Human Development Network." *Pediatrics* 87, no. 5:587–597.

HADLEY, JACK. 1992. *More Medical Care, Better Health? An Economic Analysis of Mortality Rates.* Washington, D.C.: Urban Institute Press.

HANIGAN, WILLIAM C.; MORGAN, ANDREW M.; ANDERSON, ROBERT J.; BRADLE, PATRICIA; COHEN, HOWARD S.;

CUSACK, THOMAS J.; THOMAS-MCCAULEY, TINA; and MILLER, TIM. 1991. "Incidence and Neurodevelopmental Outcome of Periventricular Hemorrhage and Hydrocephalus in a Regional Population of Very Low Birth Weight Infants." *Neurosurgery* 29, no. 5:701–806.

KLEINMAN, JOEL C.; FINGERHUT, LOIS A.; and PRAGER, KATE. 1991. "Differences in Infant Mortality by Race, Nativity Status, and Other Maternal Characteristics." *American Journal of Diseases of Children* 145, no. 2:194–199.

KLEINMAN, JOEL C., and KIELY, JOHN L. 1990. "Postneonatal Mortality in the United States: An International Perspective." *Pediatrics* 86 (suppl. no. 6, pt. 2):1091–1097.

LANTOS, JOHN D., and KOHRMAN, ARTHUR F. 1992. "Ethical Aspects of Pediatric Home Care." *Pediatrics* 89, no. 5, pt. 1:920–924.

LANTOS, JOHN D.; MEADOW, WILLIAM; MILES, STEVEN H.; EKWO, EDEM; PATON, JOHN; HAGEMAN, JOSEPH R.; and SIEGLER, MARK. 1992. "Providing and Forgoing Resuscitative Therapies for Babies of Very Low Birth Weight." *Journal of Clinical Ethics* 3, no. 4:283–287.

NORTHWAY, WILLIAM H. 1992. "Bronchopulmonary Dysplasia: Twenty-Five Years Later." *Pediatrics* 89, no. 5, pt. 1: 969–973.

NORTHWAY, WILLIAM H.; ROSAN, ROBERT D.; and PORTER, DAVID Y. 1967. "Pulmonary Disease Following Respiratory Therapy of Hyaline-Membrane Disease: Bronchopulmonary Dysplasia." *New England Journal of Medicine* 276, no. 7:357–368.

ROSTAIN, ANTHONY. 1986. "Deciding to Forego Life-Sustaining Treatment in the Intensive Care Nursery: A Sociologic Account." *Perspectives in Biological Medicine* 30, no. 1:117–134.

RUSH, DAVID; SLOAN, NANCY L.; LEIGHTON, JESSICA; ALVIR, JOSE M.; HORVITZ, DANIEL G.; SEAVER, W. BURLEIGH; GARBOWSKI, GAIL C.; JOHNSON, SALLY S.; KULKA, RICHARD A.; HOLT, MIMI; DEVORE, JAMES W.; LYNCH, JUDITH T.; WOODSIDE, M. BEEBE; and SHANKLIN, DAVID S. 1988. "V. Longitudinal Study of Pregnant Women." *American Journal of Clinical Nutrition* 48 (suppl. 2): 439–483.

SCHOENDORF, KENNETH C.; HOGUE, CAROL J. R.; KLEINMAN, JOEL C.; and ROWLEY, DIANE. 1992. "Mortality Among Infants of Black as Compared with White College-Educated Parents." *New England Journal of Medicine* 326, no. 23:1522–1526.

STARFIELD, BARBARA. 1985. *The Effectiveness of Medical Care: Validating Clinical Wisdom.* Baltimore: Johns Hopkins University Press.

TYSON, JON; WRIGHT, ELIZABETH; MALLOY, MIKE; and WRIGHT, LINDA. 1991. "How Predictable Is the Outcome and Care of Ventilated Extreme Low Birth Weight Infants?" NICDH Neonatal Research Network, Bethesda, Md. Abstracted in *Pediatric Research* 29, no. 4, pt. 2: 237A, 1991.

U.S. GENERAL ACCOUNTING OFFICE. 1984. *WIC Evaluations Provide Some Favorable but No Conclusive Evidence on the Effects Expected for the Special Supplemental Program for Women, Infants, and Children.* GAO/PEMD–84–4. Washington, D.C.: Author.

II. HISTORY OF INFANTICIDE

In many societies infanticide, the deliberate killing of infants, was not only tolerated but also sometimes promoted as a solution to the problem of unwanted infants, whether deformed or healthy. This article provides a historical account of infanticide in Western societies, beginning with its practice in Graeco-Roman antiquity and concluding with modern evidence for infanticide.

Infanticide in antiquity

In Greek society, an infant's worth was measured by its potential to fulfill a useful function in society. Thus, Plato maintained that society was better served if deformed newborns were "hidden away, in some appropriate manner that must be kept secret," a practice that likely included infanticide (Plato, *Republic*, 460). Similarly, Aristotle wrote in *Politics*: "As to the exposure and rearing of children, let there be a law that no deformed child shall live." Aristotle also condoned abandonment as a method of population control, although he recommended early abortion in regions where the "regular customs hinder any of those born being exposed" (Aristotle, *Politics*, 1335b). In Sparta, where military strength was highly valued, infanticide may have reached its zenith. Plutarch gives an account of the Spartan custom: "But if it was ill born and deformed they sent it to . . . a chasm-like place at the foot of Mount Taygetus, in the conviction that the life of that which nature had not well-equipped at the very beginning for health and strength, was of no advantage, either to itself or to the state" (Plutarch, *Life of Lycurgus*, 16).

It is difficult to distinguish between infanticide, with the intent to kill the infant, and abandonment, which may or may not have involved this intention. Failure to distinguish between the two has made accurate assessment of each difficult (Boswell, 1988). Historians have generally interpreted the Greek word for abandonment, translated as "exposure, putting out, or hiding away," as equivalent to infanticide. However, the Greek terms for abandonment do not convey the sense of injury or harm associated with infanticide. Historical evidence is not clear as to whether abandoned infants usually died or if those who abandoned them intended their death. Often abandonment was viewed as an alternative to infanticide. Nevertheless, it is reasonable to infer that some deformed and healthy infants, particularly females, were exposed with the intent that they would not survive. Further, it is likely that direct infanticide was practiced for both eugenic purposes and population control. Laws neither prohibited the killing of defective infants nor protected healthy infants from death by exposure.

Evidence from classical sources suggests that infanticide was practiced widely and with impunity in Roman society. While Romans continued the practice of disposing of defective infants for eugenic and economic reasons, an additional motivation stemmed from the Roman belief in the phenomenon of unnatural events, or *prodigia* (Amundsen, 1987). The Greeks saw deformities in newborns as natural occurrences. In contrast, the Romans viewed *portentosi*, meaning "unnatural" or "monstrous" births, as ominous or numinous signs that needed to be destroyed in order to rid the community of guilt and fear. The historian Livy of the first century B.C.E. wrote about the birth of an infant who was both unusually large and of indeterminate gender:

> [M]en were troubled again by the report that at Frusino there had been born a child as large as a four year old, and not so much a wonder for size as because . . . it was uncertain whether male or female. In fact the soothsayers summoned from Etruria said it was a terrible and loathsome portent; it must be removed from Roman territory, far away from contact with earth, and drowned in the sea. They put it alive into a chest, carried it out to sea and threw it overboard. (Livy, *Histories*, 37.27)

Roman literature is rife with testimony to such killings. According to the Laws of the Twelve Tables (5th century B.C.E., considered to be the basis of Roman law), deformed children, *puer ad deformitatem*, were to be killed quickly. Historians disagree whether the law required that these infants be killed or whether it merely allowed infanticide. In any case, Roman society appears to have accepted infanticide as a reasonable solution to the problem of deformed infants both for eugenic and superstitious motives. In a gynecological treatise entitled "How to Recognize a Newborn Worth Rearing," the Graeco-Roman physician Soranus (1st–2nd century C.E.) specifies that such an infant "immediately cries with proper vigor, is perfect in all its parts, members and senses [and] has been born at the due time, best at the end of nine months. And by conditions contrary to those mentioned, the infant not worth rearing is recognized" (Soranus, *Gynecology*, pp. 79–80).

Seneca argued that the practice of infanticide is rationally motivated: "Mad dogs we knock on the head; the fierce and savage ox we slay; sickly sheep we put to the knife to keep them from infecting the flock; unnatural progeny we destroy; we drown even children who at birth are weakly and abnormal. Yet it is not anger, but reason that separates the harmful from the sound" (Seneca, *Moral Essays*, 1.15). Even if it were not legally mandated, it is unlikely infanticide was penalized in Roman society given the tradition of *patria potestas*, which granted fathers absolute authority over other members of the family. Roman fathers had power of life and death over their children and were allowed to execute even a grown son (Boswell, 1988). The most likely victims, however, were infants, especially deformed ones, or female children who—even when healthy—were considered of little social value.

Some Roman philosophers objected to abandonment and infanticide. Musonius Rufus, writing in the first century C.E., opposed infanticide because it reduced the population. Epictetus, a Stoic philosopher and a contemporary of Musonius, condemned abandonment as a violation of the natural affection that parents should have for their offspring. Such apparent concern for the infant was not based on a belief in the child's intrinsic right to life, but was motivated by the desires to follow natural law and to increase the population. Thus, although evidence for the practice of infanticide under the Roman empire is somewhat inconclusive, Roman law and custom apparently did not prohibit parents from killing their children.

Early Jewish and Christian traditions

Jewish scholars were among the first to clearly condemn the killing of infants. Jews believed that humans were created in the image of their creator, Yahweh. Hence, all human life was sacred from the moment of birth. The Torah speaks of defective individuals as Yahweh's creations and it mandates protection to the blind, the deaf, the weak, and others who are needy (Lev. 19:14). Human life had intrinsic value by virtue of divine endowment, not merely instrumental value by virtue of social utility, as in classical Greek and Roman society.

The first-century Jewish philosopher Philo denounced infanticide and emphasized adults' duties toward children. His account equated abandonment with infanticide:

> Some [parents] do the deed with their own hands; with monstrous cruelty and barbarity they stifle and throttle the first breath which the infants draw or throw them into a river or into the depths of the sea, after attaching some heavy substance to make them sink more quickly under its weight. Others take them to be exposed in some desert place, hoping, they themselves say, that they may be saved, but leaving them in actual truth to suffer the most distressing fate. For all the beasts that feed in human flesh visit the spot and feast unhindered on the infants, a fine banquet provided by their sole guardians, those who above all others should keep them safe, their fathers and mothers.

Philo further condemned the practice by claiming, "Infanticide undoubtedly is murder, since the displeasure of the law is not concerned with ages but with a breach to the human race" (Philo, *Works*, vol. 7).

However, it was the advent of Christianity, rooted in Judaism, that significantly altered public attitudes toward the practice of infanticide. Christians inherited the Jewish doctrine that humans were divinely created, including the emphasis on the sanctity of all human life.

Believers were urged to emulate Christ's self-sacrificing love through benevolence and charity, providing a new rationale for philanthropy (Ferngren, 1987a). The consequences of this philanthropy were seen in Christian charities and endeavors for the poor, the sick, and the needy. Rescue and care of exposed infants was viewed as a special Christian duty. During the medieval period through the nineteenth century, Christians established foundling hospitals, institutions for abandoned and unwanted children.

Two other Christian concepts important for their effect on the practice of infanticide were original sin and its correlative ritual of infant baptism, thought to have become common during the third century. Christians believed that infants who died without baptism were condemned to eternal hell. Because baptisms were performed only on holy days, not necessarily soon after birth, many parents already were committed to raising the child by the time of the ritual. Thus, baptism served as an important deterrent to both abandonment and infanticide.

Although Jews and Christians vigorously opposed infanticide, their opposition had little impact until Christianity became widespread and officially recognized in the fourth century. A church council in Spain issued the first canon against infanticide in 305 C.E., and soon after, both local and ecumenical councils throughout Europe took similar actions. The penalty prescribed by the church for infanticide was either penance or excommunication.

The first secular law concerning the killing of children was issued in 318 C.E. by Constantine, the first Christian emperor. However, the law mentions children killing parents as well as parents killing children and thus was not directed specifically against infanticide. In 374 C.E., Valentinian enacted legislation declaring infanticide to be murder and punishable by law. Soon after, a statute was issued that appears to have prohibited exposure of infants. Although Christian emperors promulgated many laws reflecting Christian morality, fear of losing salvation made the penitential system of the churches far more effective in influencing moral behavior than did state legislation. Church leaders continued to put pressure on the state, bringing about a series of legal codes aimed at protecting newborn children.

Although the laws did not distinguish between healthy and defective infants, one may assume that Christian condemnation of infanticide extended to all infants. Early Christian apologists reflect this position. Saint Augustine argued that differences between healthy and deformed people should be seen in the same light as racial and ethnic diversity:

> If whole peoples have been monsters, we must explain the phenomenon as we explain the individual monsters

who are born among us. God is the Creator of all; He knows best where and when and what is, or was, best for Him to create, since He deliberately fashioned the beauty of the whole out of both the similarity and dissimilarity of its parts. . . . It would be impossible to list all the human offspring who have been very different from the parents from whom they were certainly born. Still all these monsters undeniably owe their origin to Adam. (Augustine, *City of God*, 16.8)

Augustine's writings show a concern for children unusual in his time, placing the infant and the child under the protection of the Lord.

Despite decisive changes in attitudes and laws, infanticide persisted even after the official triumph of Christianity as the imperial religion. While the practice may have diminished, episodic killing of infants continued throughout Western history. What changed in subsequent periods were the motivations, methods, and penalties associated with infanticide as well as the options available to parents of unwanted children.

Medieval period

Christianity's beliefs mixed with pagan myth, superstition, and folklore during Europe's medieval period. This commingling had significant implications for deformed infants and the practice of infanticide. Some thought, for example, that parental sexual behavior or "ill-timed passions" generated abnormal births or that sexual relations during menstruation, pregnancy, or lactation resulted in dire consequences for the unborn. In addition, the birth of an anomalous infant was sometimes attributed to demonic intervention: Such births were seen as the product of either a sexual liaison between the mother/witch and the devil or a changeling left by the devil as punishment for parental sins. Parents, particularly mothers, were held morally responsible for their infants' abnormalities.

The changeling myth, derived from pagan sources, maintained that fairies, motivated by jealousy, substituted an elf child for the real child (Haffter, 1968). This version did not impute guilt to the parents; instead, blame was placed on demon fairies of the underworld and their envy of humans. Once the myth was Christianized, however, it became the devil who stole the real child and left a demon-child in its place. Thus, God allowed parents to be punished for impiety or for bearing children outside matrimony. This change transformed the rationalization for the birth of defective infants from external forces to parental responsibility. Brutal and frequently lethal methods were employed either to exorcise the devil from the child or to compel the devil to return the normal child. Few infants survived the ordeal. However, violent infanticide of this sort was probably the

exception rather than the rule, even during the Middle Ages.

There was some secular legislation against infanticide, particularly in the later medieval period, and the crime was usually considered to be homicide. But overlaying (suffocation in the parental bed), the most frequent cause of infanticide, was easy to conceal and intent was nearly impossible to establish, thus making prosecution extremely difficult. When cases of infanticide did reach secular courts, the accused were readily acquitted on pleas of insanity or poverty. Secular authorities displayed remarkable ambivalence toward the killing of infants. By law it was considered a serious crime, yet in practice it was generally excused (Damme, 1978).

Throughout most of the medieval period, infanticide was regulated largely by church courts rather than civil courts. Ecclesiastical penalties for married women convicted of infanticide were also remarkably light, considering the Church's position. Punishment involved penance and was comparable to that imposed for sexual offenses such as adultery and fornication. Once the penance had been performed, the guilty person was not prosecuted in civil courts. The relatively light penance and the failure of secular authorities to prosecute cases of infanticide suggests that the crime was considered something less than homicide (Helmholz, 1974). Cases involving unwed mothers, however, were treated differently. Unmarried mothers who killed their infants were often accused of being witches. In fact, infanticide was the most common charge brought against "witches" during the Middle Ages. Unlike their married counterparts, alleged witches were punished severely, usually by drowning, burial alive, or impalement.

The only reference to the status of infants under medieval secular laws was a civil law definition of a freeman, which appears to have excluded both illegitimate and seriously deformed infants from what little protection the law offered: "Among freemen there may not be reckoned those who are born of unlawful intercourse . . . nor those who are created pervertedly, against the way of human kind, as for example, if a woman bring forth a monster or a prodigy" (Fleta 1.5, "Of Different Kinds of Children"). As legal historian Catherine Damme comments, "Clearly, these pitiful non-persons were vulnerable to the murderous attacks of their progenitors" (Damme, 1978, p. 7).

Although direct infanticide was practiced to some extent, the more common and insidious cause of infant death during the Middle Ages was abandonment. The distinction between infanticide and abandonment became increasingly important because abandonment was generally regarded as a venial offense, punishable only if the child died. In the early Middle Ages, abandonment was widespread, motivated primarily by poverty and illegitimacy. Although a few churchmen believed it was equivalent to infanticide, two forms of abandonment were virtually institutionalized: oblation (or donating infants to the Church) and leaving infants at foundling hospitals. From a Christian point of view, both were improvements over the morally objectionable practices of exposure and infanticide. A canonical decree of the tenth century urged women to leave their illegitimate infants at the church rather than kill them (Boswell, 1988). Although oblates were tied irrevocably to the Church for life, the Church provided food, clothing, and a secure monastic life.

Foundling homes were established to diminish the practice of exposure and to provide a humane solution to infanticide. In reality, however, the foundling home often was equivalent to consigning the child to death through neglect, disease, and sometimes more direct action. Once infants arrived at a foundling home, they frequently were sent to the country with a wet nurse who was likely to be negligent and more interested in a steady flow of babies than in nurturing. Death rates were high, especially for female infants (Trexler, 1973). Markedly high demographic ratios of males to females throughout Europe during this period suggest that selective female infanticide may have been widely practiced. The disparity between male and female deaths was probably due to greater social value for males and a greater likelihood that, when put into foundling homes, they would be reclaimed by their parents. Thus, such institutions did little to secure the lives of unwanted infants. They were successful only in transferring the problem of unwanted infants from a public arena to an institutional one, shielding society from the realities of abandoned children and possibly encouraging the very practice they were intended to alleviate.

Renaissance and Reformation

During the sixteenth and seventeenth centuries there was a concerted effort to stem the practice of infanticide throughout Europe. Despite a dramatic surge in reported cases, it is not clear whether or not the increase meant more frequent practice; urbanization undoubtedly made it more difficult to destroy infants secretly. Authorities were more successful at promulgating harsh legislation aimed at ending the practice and were also increasingly vigilant in prosecuting murdering mothers. An intense focus on the problems of poverty and sexual promiscuity and their purported ties to infanticide led to laws that were strongly moral in tone and selective against unmarried mothers.

The first attempt to strengthen and unify infanticide laws under the Holy Roman Empire was a statute known as the Carolina, issued in 1532 by Emperor Charles V. The law decreed that those found guilty were to be buried alive, or impaled, or drowned. The law also made concealment of pregnancy a crime, as it was presumed that such secrecy indicated infanticidal intentions. Many judges, under the pretext of the Carolina, "engaged in a policy of terror," the most notorious being the Saxon jurist Benedict Carpozof, who claimed that he assisted in the executions of 20,000 women (Piers, 1978, p. 69). The Carolina was only the first in a series of laws over the next few centuries that dealt severely with alleged infanticidal mothers.

In England, Henry VIII's split from the Roman Catholic church resulted in increased secular control. Growing concern about sexual immorality and criminality among the swelling numbers of urban poor led to the enactment of several social control laws. The Poor Law of 1576 (18 Eliz. I, c.3) made bearing bastard children a crime. The fact that punishment was severe and involved substantial social disgrace for the mother increased the incentive for these women to commit infanticide. It is not surprising, therefore, that English criminal court records show that the number of indictments and guilty verdicts for infanticide rose dramatically after 1576. Most cases involved bastard children, and concealment of pregnancy was mentioned frequently (Hoffer and Hull, 1981).

The reasons for the increased zeal in punishing illegitimacy are somewhat obscure, but Puritan interests seem to have played a role. The 1623 Jacobean infanticide statute (21 Jac. I, c.27), influenced by the Puritan element in parliament, allowed courts to convict on the basis of circumstantial evidence of concealment and prior sexual misconduct. The law presumed that the child was born alive and then killed unless the mother could prove otherwise. Prosecutions of infanticide showed a fourfold increase immediately following its enactment (Hoffer and Hull, 1981).

Ideas about the role of witches in the death of infants, even the deaths of children in foundling hospitals, persisted. Infanticide and witchcraft were so strongly interrelated during this period that their rates of indictments rose and fell in parallel. Witchcraft continued to play a major part in the drama of infanticide until the early 1800s.

Foundling hospitals continued to remove unwanted and abandoned children from public view throughout the sixteenth and seventeenth centuries. As in earlier centuries, the fate of these children was precarious. Overcrowded conditions, disease, lack of enough wet nurses, and general neglect continued to claim the lives of many of the institutions' charges.

The overwhelming majority of the victims of infanticide during this period were children born out of wedlock. Demographic information does not show the strong gender bias seen in the medieval years, nor is there evidence that defective newborns were consistently selected out. Apparently the shame associated with immoral sexual behavior was the primary selective force associated with the killing of infants.

Eighteenth and nineteenth centuries

In the eighteenth century, a steep decline occurred in indictments for infanticide; the courts showed greater leniency toward those accused of killing their children. In addition, illegitimacy was more common; as a result the stigma associated with it lessened and its strong correlation to infanticide began to diminish. Attitudes toward parenting changed as well, with a new emphasis on the emotional nurturing of children. Wet-nursing lost popularity, and it became more common for children to spend their early months with their mothers. The greater value placed on children resulted in increased beneficence in child rearing, and so parents were probably less likely to kill their offspring. In any case, juries were less willing to convict parents of infanticide solely on the basis of concealment.

New defenses for the suspected infanticidal mother were developed and more readily accepted by juries. One of the first of these defenses, known as "benefit of linen," was based on evidence that the mother had made linen for the baby before its birth and therefore had no intention to kill it. This line of argument became very popular after 1700 and virtually guaranteed acquittal. Another major defense commonly used was the "want of help" plea. Various accidents and calamities, such as failure to tie the umbilical cord, falls of either the mother or baby, illness of the mother, and unheeded cries for help, all effectively helped to sway jurors.

Efforts to reform the English infanticide statute of 1624 began in 1773 but were not successful until 1803. In the ambivalence of eighteenth-century English society, infanticide was considered homicide yet somehow not quite the equivalent of killing an adult. Despite the failure of reform resolutions until the nineteenth century, juries tended to ignore the severe infanticide law aimed selectively at unwed mothers.

A similar trend occurred in Prussia during the reign of Frederick the Great. In his *Dissertation sur les raisons d'établir ou d'abroger les lois* (1756), Frederick argued that the prevalence of infanticide was due to the harsh penalties for illegitimacy. He therefore abolished laws penalizing pregnancies out of wedlock and eventually provided legal protection for unwed mothers. Scholars throughout Europe, including Cesare Beccaria, Voltaire, Johann Heinrich Pestalozzi, and Johann Wolfgang von Goethe, also called for legal reform and urged authorities to prevent the circumstances leading to infanticide.

Despite moderately successful reform efforts, however, infanticide did not disappear. During the nineteenth century high rates of illegitimate births continued; so, consequently, did infant killing. Corpses of infants found in privies, parks, rivers, and other public places fueled the perception that infanticide was reaching intolerable proportions. This perception may or may not have represented an actual increase in the incidence of the crime, but it did serve to stimulate an unprecedented public outcry. By the mid-nineteenth century, the concern over the "slaughter of innocents" appeared in the press (Behlmer, 1979). The British newspaper *Morning Star* (June 23, 1863) declared, "This crime is positively becoming a national institution"; and the *Pall Mall Gazette* (April 30, 1866) protested, "It is exceedingly unpleasant to find ourselves stigmatized in foreign newspapers . . . as a nation of infanticides. . . . 13,000 children are yearly murdered by their mothers in heretical England." The *Saturday Review* (1865, pp. 161–162) asserted that infanticide "is the characteristic at once of the rudest barbarism and of that more terrible epoch of national life when the wheel has gone its full circle, and society falls to pieces by the vices of civilization."

Physicians were among those who led reform efforts. In his essay on infanticide in 1862, William Burke Ryan wrote passionately against the horrors of infant murder; he and several colleagues formed the Infant Life Protection Society. By 1870 the group had achieved many of its goals, including mandatory registration of all births. In 1872, Parliament passed the first Infant Life Protection Act requiring registration of all "baby farms," houses with more than one child under the age of one.

Legal prosecution of infanticide also underwent significant changes. Ellenborough's Act of 1803, which replaced the Infanticide Act of 1623, reinstated the common-law presumption of stillbirth, shifting the burden of proof from the defendant (mother) back to the prosecutor. In 1828 the law was expanded to include legitimate as well as illegitimate births, removing the obvious selection against unwed mothers. The fact that courts consistently acquitted the accused or mitigated penalties on the basis of insanity is testimony to the court's continued hesitancy to consider infanticide the moral equivalent of murder. There was a "visceral feeling that such a crime simply could not be a rational act. . . . the minds of the jury and jurist could not accept that such a heinous act could be committed by a rational person—the accused's mind had to be deranged, if only temporarily" (Damme, 1978, p. 14).

Twentieth century

The most notorious instances of infanticide in the twentieth century were committed secretly in Nazi Germany, under the auspices of the Committee for the Scientific

Treatment of Severe, Genetically Determined Illness. Doctors, nurses, and teachers were required to register all children with congenital abnormalities or mental retardation. Failure to comply meant civil penalties or imprisonment. Defective children were removed from their homes and routinely euthanized at hospitals by morphine injection, gas, lethal poisons, or sometimes starvation. To ensure secrecy, the bodies were cremated immediately. Parents who protected their children were sent to labor camps and their children were taken from them. Documents reveal substantial public support for the euthanasia of defective children, even from parents with abnormal children (Proctor, 1988).

Calls for legalized euthanasia also arose from the United States, where it was justified primarily as a way of limiting the social costs associated with defective infants. W. A. Gould, writing in the *Journal of the American Institute of Homeopathy,* cited the "elimination of the unfit" in ancient Sparta as a defense of the economic arguments for euthanasia in the twentieth century (Gould, 1933). In 1938, W. G. Lennox advocated the "privilege of death for the congenitally mindless and for the incurable sick who wish to die" because saving these lives "adds a load to the back of society" (Lennox, 1938, p. 454). But as the realities of the Nazi extermination programs began to surface in the United States in the 1940s, promotion of euthanasia in general began to decline.

Yet in 1942, Foster Kennedy, professor of neurology at Cornell Medical College, wrote an article entitled "The Problem of Social Control of the Congenital Defective" advocating "euthanasia for those hopeless ones who should never have been born—Nature's mistakes." Kennedy believed "we have too many feebleminded people among us," and it was most humane to relieve defective individuals of their tortured and useless existence. Furthermore, he maintained that in diagnosis and prognosis there could be no mistakes in this "category" of children. A Gallup poll conducted twelve years earlier indicated that Kennedy's position probably was not without support within the American community. According to the poll, 45 percent of Americans in 1930 favored euthanasia of anomalous infants (Proctor, 1988, p. 180).

Conclusion

Authors who have explored the ethical dimensions of infanticide have frequently prefaced their discussions with surveys of its practice throughout history. The ostensible purpose of these discussions generally has been to provide a broader, less culturally bound perspective. However, Stephen Post argues that many writers selectively present "a one-sided and reductionist view of the history of infanticide to support their position . . . that

active killing of neonates is morally acceptable" (Post, 1988, p. 14). He contends that the extent of infanticide has been misrepresented and overstated. The argument is that commentators on the history of infanticide have drawn, at least to some extent, from historical surveys plagued by interpretations that tend to view history in a positivist or linear fashion. The French historian Phillipe Ariès maintains that the idea of a separate childhood was unknown until the later Middle Ages (Ariès, 1962). Similarly, Lloyd DeMause contends: "The further back in history one goes, the lower the level of child care, and the more likely children are to be killed, abandoned, beaten, terrorized, and sexually abused" (DeMause, 1974, p. 1).

Revisionist historians, focusing on social, economic, and cultural forces, offer a significantly altered perspective on infanticide. While infanticide has been practiced continuously throughout Western history, it is not obvious that filicidal tendencies are widespread among parents. On the contrary, parents have usually resorted to infanticide only in exceptional circumstances. Although accurate estimates of the frequency of infanticide are almost nonexistent (largely due to inadequate and inconsistent recordkeeping), the prevalence of infanticide throughout Western history seems to have been episodic. Rates of infant killing have shown a tendency to rise and fall depending on prevailing economic and social forces. There have been striking discrepancies between the official position of the law, the frequency of the crime, the rate of prosecutions, the severity of punishment, and public sentiment concerning infanticide. Although the law has been relatively consistent in prohibiting its practice, the law has not always been an accurate gauge of societal values. Finally, the availability of alternatives to infanticide—including abandonment, foundling hospitals, oblation, contraception, and abortion—appears to have had more impact on its practice than have official prohibitions.

CINDY BOUILLON-JENSEN

Directly related to this article are the other articles in this entry: MEDICAL ASPECTS AND ISSUES IN THE CARE OF INFANTS, ETHICAL ISSUES. *and* PUBLIC-POLICY AND LEGAL ISSUES. *Also directly related are the entries* HOMICIDE; *and* PERSON. *For a further discussion of topics mentioned in this article, see the entries* DISABILITY, *articles on* ATTITUDES AND SOCIOLOGICAL PERSPECTIVES, *and* PHILOSOPHICAL AND THEOLOGICAL PERSPECTIVES; EUGENICS; MEDICAL ETHICS, HISTORY OF, *section on* EUROPE, *subsection on* ANCIENT AND MEDIEVAL; NATIONAL SOCIALISM; *and* WOMEN, *article on* HISTORICAL AND CROSS-CULTURAL PERSPECTIVES. *For a discussion of related ideas, see the entries* ABORTION, *section on* RELIGIOUS TRADITIONS;

DEATH, *article on* WESTERN RELIGIOUS THOUGHT; DEATH AND DYING: EUTHANASIA AND SUSTAINING LIFE, *articles on* HISTORICAL ASPECTS, *and* ETHICAL ISSUES; EUGENICS AND RELIGIOUS LAW; FAMILY; LIFE; *and* REPRODUCTIVE TECHNOLOGIES, *article on* SEX SELECTION.

Bibliography

AMUNDSEN, DARREL W. 1987. "Medicine and the Birth of Defective Children: Approaches of the Ancient World." In *Euthanasia and the Newborn: Conflicts Regarding Saving Lives*, pp. 3–22. Edited by Richard C. McMillan, H. Tristram Engelhardt, Jr., and Stuart F. Spicker. Boston: D. Reidel.

ARIÈS, PHILLIPE. 1962. *Centuries of Childhood: A Social History of Family Life.* Translated by Robert Baldick. New York: Vintage Books.

BEHLMER, GEORGE K. 1979. "Deadly Motherhood: Infanticide and Medical Opinion in Mid-Victorian England." *Journal of the History of Medicine and Allied Sciences* 34, no. 4: 403–427.

BOSWELL, JOHN. 1988. *The Kindness of Strangers: The Abandonment of Children in Western Europe from Late Antiquity to the Renaissance.* New York: Pantheon.

DAMME, CATHERINE. 1978. "Infanticide: The Worth of an Infant Under Law." *Medical History* 22, no. 1:1–24.

DEMAUSE, LLOYD, ed. 1974. *The History of Childhood: The Untold Story of Child Abuse.* New York: Psychohistory Press.

FERNGREN, GARY B. 1987a. "The *Imago Dei* and the Sanctity of Life: The Origins of an Idea." In *Euthanasia and the Newborn: Conflicts Regarding Saving Lives*, pp. 23–45. Edited by Richard C. McMillan, H. Tristram Engelhardt, Jr., and Stuart F. Spicker. Boston: D. Reidel.

———. 1987b. "The Status of Defective Newborns from Late Antiquity to the Reformation." In *Euthanasia and the Newborn: Conflicts Regarding Saving Lives*, pp. 46–64. Edited by Richard C. McMillan, H. Tristram Engelhardt, Jr., and Stuart F. Spicker. Boston: D. Reidel.

GOULD, W. A. 1993. "Euthanasia." *Journal of the Institute of Homeopathy* 27:82.

HAFFTER, CARL. 1968. "The Changeling: History and Psychodynamics of Attitudes to Handicapped Children in European Folklore." *Journal of the History of the Behavioral Sciences* 4, no. 1:55–61.

HANAWALT, BARBARA. 1977. "Childrearing Among Lower Classes of Late Medieval England." *Journal of Interdisciplinary History* 8, no. 1:1–22.

HELMHOLZ, R. H. 1974. "Infanticide in the Province of Canterbury During the Fifteenth Century." *History of Childhood Quarterly* 2, no. 3:379–390.

HOFFER, PETER C., and HULL, N. E. H. 1981. *Murdering Mothers: Infanticide in England and New England*, pp. 1558–1803. New York: New York University Press.

KELLUM, BARBARA A. 1974. "Infanticide in England in the Later Middle Ages." *History of Childhood Quarterly* 1, no. 3:367–388.

LANGER, WILLIAM L. 1974. "Infanticide: A Historical Survey." *History of Childhood Quarterly* 1, no. 3:353–365.

LENNOX, W. G. 1938. "Should They Live? Certain Economic Aspects of Medicine." *American Scholar* 7:454–466.

PIERS, MARIA W. 1978. *Infanticide.* New York: W. W. Norton.

POST, STEPHEN. 1988. "History, Infanticide, and Imperiled Newborns." *Hastings Center Report* 18:14–17.

PROCTOR, RICHARD. 1988. *Racial Hygiene: Medicine Under the Nazis.* Cambridge, Mass.: Harvard University Press.

TREXLER, RICHARD C. 1973. "Infanticide in Florence: New Sources and First Results." *History of Childhood Quarterly* 1, no. 1:98–116.

WRIGHTSON, KEITH. 1975. "Infanticide in Earlier Seventeenth-Century England." *Local Population Studies* no. 15 (Autumn):10–22.

III. ETHICAL ISSUES

The birth of a baby can be one of the most satisfying, fulfilling experiences of a parent's life or a couple's marriage. After months of "infanticipating," the experiences connected with the first few hours and days of the baby's life can be intensely rewarding for the parents, providing them with joy, gratitude, and perhaps humility as they contemplate the new life that is now entrusted to them for care and support. If they are religious believers, they may be inclined to think of the baby's life as a divine gift and to regard their parental role as involving responsible stewardship over that gift. At the very least, they will probably be thankful that the baby has a normal brain, the correct number of fingers and toes, and the rest of a physical endowment that would suggest normal human development.

Unfortunately, in a small minority of cases the months of parental dreams and plans for a normal baby turn out to be false hope. In some instances, even when prenatal diagnosis has already indicated that the baby will not be normal, there may still be parental surprise and disappointment at the range of medical problems and the degree of neurologic impairment the child has. In other instances, when prenatal diagnosis was not done and the potential parents had no opportunity for anticipatory grief over the loss of a normal baby, the birth of a premature and/or congenitally disabled infant can have an enormous emotional impact on the parents that severely tests their most deeply held beliefs, values, and hopes for the future.

The birth of such a baby can also reflect the diversity of ethical perspectives that exist among parents, physicians, and other persons regarding the value of infants with life-threatening medical conditions, especially when the projected future lives of these children are filled with a mixture of neurologic impairments, mental and physical disabilities, and, sometimes, considerable medical uncertainty regarding the degree of those disabilities. For many persons, such cases raise important substantive questions: What is the moral status of infants with mental and physical disabilities? Should all of these infants receive life-sustaining medical interventions regardless of the severity of their medical conditions? What should be the ethical standard according to which a few infants would not receive life-sustaining efforts? Is there any moral difference between withholding and withdrawing life-sustaining treatments? Are there important moral differences between decisions about life-sustaining treatment in cases of severely disabled infants compared with cases of adults who have never been autonomous because of severe mental retardation? Would it be justifiable, in rare cases, intentionally to kill any of these infants?

Cases of premature and disabled infants also raise important procedural questions: Who should have the authority to make these life-and-death decisions? Should physicians, and in particular neonatologists, make these decisions because of their greater technical knowledge and experience with similar cases? Should the infant's parents decide because of their roles in conceiving and caring for the child, and because of their greater emotional and financial stake in the child's death or disabled life? Should a collective body (e.g., a pediatric ethics committee) make the borderline decisions?

In addition, important questions are sometimes raised about contextual and methodological matters related to decisions about the care of infants: What lessons can we learn about caring and nurturing from parents who have learned to cope with and transcend one of life's personal tragedies? Is a philosophical approach that focuses on principles, rights, interests, and obligations the correct model for ethical analysis? Do theological claims about the sanctity of life, the meaning of suffering, and the importance of stewardship over life have a significant place in decisions about the appropriate level of care for infants, whether normal or abnormal in some way? To what extent should the realities of medical economics influence the decision about whether a premature and severely disabled infant lives or dies? How much should decision makers in individual cases consider the implications of their decisions in terms of public policy?

This article has five parts: (1) a brief historical overview; (2) international perspectives among pediatricians; (3) alternative perspectives on the moral status of infants; (4) perspectives on abating life-sustaining treatment; and (5) the emerging mainstream ethical perspective. Additional information on some of these points is found in the other articles in this entry.

Historical overview

Throughout history, as at the present time, the birth of a baby has often been the occasion for joy, celebration, and thanksgiving. In earlier centuries, the birth of a healthy, normal baby was frequently the occasion for celebration because the baby, especially if the infant was male, offered future promise for the family: another hunter for food supplies, another worker for the field or factory, another opportunity for continuing the family lineage. The birth of a baby was often an occasion for celebration for another reason: the mother had survived the dangers inherent in pregnancy and childbirth, dangers that posed a significant risk to maternal health and life in every pregnancy before the advent of modern medicine.

However, not all births were celebratory occasions. In many societies and in virtually all historical periods, very young infants, female infants, bastards, and infants and older children believed to be "defective" in some way were frequently killed. The intentional destruction of infants and children through starvation, drowning, strangulation, burning, smothering, poisoning, exposure, and a variety of lethal weapons was a tragically common practice. Such practices were widely accepted ways of dealing with unwanted children, with the responses of governments varying from required infanticidal practices (e.g., in Sparta), to acceptance of or at least indifference to the killing of female infants (e.g., in China and India), to considerable uncertainty as to how to punish parents who may have committed an illegal act by killing one of their children under questionable circumstances.

Mothers and fathers have historically had several possible reasons for killing one or more of their children. Some of them have killed for economic reasons: A dead child would mean one less mouth to feed. Others have killed their infants because of social customs and pressures: An illegitimate child, an "extra" child beyond a certain number, or another female child was especially vulnerable. Still other parents have killed their children because the infants were physically or mentally abnormal, with their congenital abnormalities being interpreted as works of the devil, signs of fate, punishment for the sins of the parents, or tricks played by witches (Weir, 1984).

Some of these older explanations of congenital disabilities seem strange now, but two features of traditional infanticidal practices remain a part of the modern world. First, infants are still sometimes killed by their parents or, perhaps more commonly, abandoned without food, shelter, or parental protection. No society is exempt from such events, with media reports of dead or abandoned babies coming from China, India, Brazil, the United States, Romania, and other countries. Second, even for parents who cannot imagine killing their own children, the birth of an extremely premature and/or severely disabled infant is a mixed blessing. For that reason, parental decisions about medical efforts to prolong a child's life frequently involve concerns about the future of the family as well as considerations about the welfare of the child.

In many parts of the world, such decisions, whether made by a child's parents or physicians, are strikingly similar to decisions made about sick and disabled children in earlier historical periods because many countries still lack the medicines, the medical and nursing personnel, and the medical technology that are common to the rest of the world. In technologically developed countries, by contrast, the development of neonatal intensive-care units (NICUs), neonatologists and other pediatric subspecialists, sophisticated medical technology, new medicines, and new surgical techniques has brought unprecedented opportunities and challenges to physicians, parents, nurses, and all other persons interested in prolonging the lives and improving the health of critically ill children. Likewise, changes in neonatal medicine since the 1970s have meant that physicians, parents, or some combination of health-care professionals in a hospital can sometimes decide that the appropriate course of moral action in a case is not to initiate or continue life-sustaining treatments, given the child's severe neurologic impairments and likelihood of continued suffering.

Such decisions—not to use medical technology to sustain an extremely premature or severely disabled infant's life—are usually difficult and sometimes controversial. In the United States, public and professional responses to publicized pediatric cases in the 1980s generated two efforts at regulating selective nontreatment decisions. The two attempts at regulation, while not always in conflict, reflected two quite different ethical perspectives regarding how and by whom selective nontreatment decisions should be made.

One effort at regulation took the form of two sets of published federal regulations during the administration of President Ronald Reagan. The "Baby Doe" regulations, first proposed in 1983, and the subsequent child-abuse regulations, established in 1985, differed in legal philosophy, implementation, and influence. Yet both agreed on the ethical perspective that should govern life-and-death decisions made in NICUs and pediatric intensive-care units (PICUs): Every infant, unless permanently unconscious, irretrievably dying, or salvageable only with treatment that would be "virtually futile and inhumane," should be given life-sustaining treatment, no matter how small, young, or disabled the infant might be.

The other effort at regulation was made by the U.S. President's Commission for the Study of Ethical Problems in Medicine (1983), the American Academy of Pediatrics, and numerous writers on ethics in pediatric medicine. Given the complexity of some pediatric cases and the life-and-death nature of selective nontreatment decisions, the common recommendation was to have an ethics committee consult on the cases and give advice to the physicians in the cases. The ethical perspective at the heart of this recommendation was straightforward: In truly difficult cases, the most prudent procedure for decision making is the achievement of consensus by a multidisciplinary committee that is knowledgeable, impartial, emotionally stable, and consistent from case to case.

Similar efforts at regulating selective nontreatment decisions in NICUs and PICUs have not occurred in other countries having technological medicine. In Britain and Australia, for example, governments interested in regulating assisted reproduction technologies to protect pre-embryos have not had a similar interest in regulating selective nontreatment decisions to protect young infants, either from premature deaths or from profoundly impaired lives. Likewise, neither the governments nor the medical societies in these countries have chosen to establish pediatric ethics committees, preferring instead to leave decisions to abate life-sustaining treatment for young infants to the discretion of the physicians and parents of the children.

Nevertheless, some themes and problems are common as decision makers in technologically advanced countries confront the difficult choices presented by premature and disabled infants. First, the ongoing technological development of pediatrics (e.g., the use of exogenous surfactants and high-frequency oscillatory ventilation for treating pulmonary problems) has resulted in improved mortality and morbidity rates for numerous infants and young children. Second, unprecedented surgical techniques (e.g., surgery for short-bowel syndrome and for hypoplastic left ventricle) have resulted in the prolongation of life for many infants who would have died without surgery only a few years ago. Third, these technological and surgical achievements have created a trend in some pediatric subspecialties toward overtreatment of premature and disabled infants, a trend that seems to be contrary to the best interests of some of these children (Caplan et al., 1992). Fourth, even with the technological progress in pediatrics, neonatologists and the parents with whom they work in individual cases are still frequently confronted with an inescapable problem: medical uncertainty regarding the degree and range of disability a neurologically impaired child will have, if the child survives with medical treatment (Hastings Center, 1987).

Compared with earlier historical periods, the period of technological medicine has produced unprecedented changes and challenges for parents, physicians, and other persons concerned about the care of infants. The rapidity and extent of the change is noticeable in the types of cases that now present the greatest ethical challenges for parents and physicians in NICUs. In the 1970s and 1980s, considerable debate centered on whether infants with Down syndrome plus complications and infants with myelomeningocele should receive surgical correction of their physical abnormalities. In the 1990s these types of cases have largely been replaced as ethical challenges by other kinds: (1) cases of extremely premature neonates with birth weights below 600 grams, gestational ages of approximately twenty-four weeks, and severe cardiac, pulmonary, and neurologic impairments; (2) cases of very small and disabled neonates whose low birth weights and disabilities are the result of factors during pregnancy, such as maternal malnutrition, infection (e.g., HIV and AIDS), smoking, consumption of alcohol, or use of cocaine and other drugs; and (3) cases of neonates with anencephaly whose organs could be transplanted into other infants, if the parents of the anencephalic infants were to consent and the law were to permit the transplantation (Walters, 1991).

International perspectives among pediatricians

The roles of physicians, parents, and nurses in the care of premature and disabled infants vary significantly from country to country. In general, pediatricians in countries that in recent decades have been characterized by authoritarian or totalitarian political regimes tend to take a similar approach to decisions made in NICUs: The decisions to treat or not to treat are made by physicians with only minimal participation by parents, nurses, or other health professionals. By contrast, pediatricians in democratic societies tend to have a more democratic attitude toward decisions made in NICUs: With some variation from physician to physician, the decisions to treat or not to treat are often made in consultation with the parents of the imperiled infants, with some physicians also finding merit in having pediatric ethics committees consult on some of the truly difficult decisions.

For example, one study indicated significant differences between pediatricians in Poland and pediatricians in Australia. The majority of both groups of physicians indicated that they had been confronted with the necessity of making decisions regarding the withholding or withdrawing of life-sustaining treatment from severely disabled infants. However, their views regarding the substantive and procedural features of such decisions were quite different. Whereas virtually all the pediatricians surveyed in Australia (98.2 percent) indicated that they did not believe that "every possible effort" should be made to sustain life in every case, half of the pediatricians surveyed in Poland (50 percent) stated that they thought that all possible efforts at sustaining life should be made in every case. Regarding specific diagnostic cases, significant numbers of Australian pediatricians thought that life-sustaining treatment could be withheld or withdrawn in cases of anencephaly and microcephaly

(29.7 percent of the responding physicians), spina bifida and myelomeningocele (25.2 percent), extreme prematurity (9.0 percent), Down syndrome with complications (16.2 percent), and brain damage with projected mental retardation (26.1 percent). By contrast, the pediatricians in Poland, while agreeing with the Australian physicians regarding cases of extreme prematurity and brain damage, were much more reluctant to abate life-sustaining treatment for infants having microcephaly, spina bifida, or Down syndrome (Szawarski and Tulczynski, 1988).

The differences between the Australian and Polish pediatricians were even more significant when they were asked about the procedural aspects of decisions that would probably result in an infant's death. The majority of responding Australian pediatricians indicated that they discussed such decisions with other physicians (90.9 percent), the parents of the infant (90.1 percent), and nurses (84.7 percent). The Polish pediatricians, by contrast, almost always consulted with other physicians (99.0 percent) but rarely discussed the decisions with the parents (8.1 percent) or nurses (4.3 percent).

Another study suggested that there are differences among pediatricians in the United States, Sweden, Britain, and Australia on both substantive and procedural aspects of selective nontreatment decisions. According to this interpretive study, the dominant practice among American pediatricians, especially neonatologists, is to initiate aggressive life-sustaining treatments early, continue those medical interventions while diagnostic tests are being done and various pediatric specialists are consulted, and talk with parents about the alternative of abating treatment only when the parents bring up the subject or when a grim prognosis becomes increasingly clear. This perspective is described as a "wait until certainty" approach, an approach involving a clear ethical choice: Saving an infant who will have severe-to-profound disabilities is preferable to permitting the death of an infant who could have lived a tolerable life. This strategy ensures that all errors are in one direction: the promotion of the infant's life, even a severely disabled life. Treatment that sustains the infant's life can therefore be terminated only when death or profoundly impaired life is inevitable (Rhoden, 1986).

This study suggests that pediatricians in Sweden have a different perspective, one that is described as a "statistical prognostic" strategy. This approach seeks to minimize the number of infants whose deaths would come slowly as well as those whose lives would be characterized by profound disabilities. At the risk of sacrificing some potentially normal infants to avoid prolonging the lives of severely impaired infants, this approach uses statistical data, like birth weight, gestational age, and early diagnostic tests, to make selective nontreatment decisions. This strategy also ensures that all errors are in one direction: the promotion of healthy life, even at the cost of allowing some infants to die who could have lived with disabling conditions.

Pediatricians in Britain and Australia are described in the study as having medical and ethical perspectives that frequently differ from those of their American and Swedish counterparts. In contrast to many pediatricians in the United States, pediatricians in Britain and Australia are willing to withhold or withdraw treatment with much less prognostic certainty. Yet in contrast to many pediatricians in Sweden, British and Australian pediatricians are willing to engage in time-limited trials to give various treatments a chance to work, even when the child being treated is likely to have ongoing disabilities. Called an "individualized prognostic" strategy, this approach reflects an ethical perspective that realizes the inherent uncertainty in medicine, permits some role for parental discretion, and affirms the appropriateness of selective nontreatment decisions once a child's prognosis appears poor (Rhoden, 1986).

In much of the world, the ethical perspectives among physicians are quite different from the approaches described above because the provision of care to infants takes place outside the confines of technological medicine. In the People's Republic of China, India, the countries of the former Soviet Union, and many of the other countries in the world, the differences in medical management that have just been described have no significance. The shortages of medicine, the obsolescence of medical equipment, the inadequacies of prenatal care, the limited number of pediatricians, and the ongoing problems of malnutrition and infectious disease contribute to a social context in which the lives of infants are frequently short and often characterized by disease and disability.

Alternative perspectives on the moral status of infants

Ethical perspectives on the care of infants are significantly influenced by views that are held regarding the ontological status and moral standing of infants, whether premature, disabled, or normal. What kind of entity is it whose life, health status, or death is at stake in the decisions made by physicians and/or parents? Is a neonate, in terms of ontological status, the same as an older child and an adult? Does an infant count as a person, in the same way that you and I count as persons? Or are questions about personhood irrelevant in terms of the moral standing that adults choose to grant infants? In terms of moral standing, what kinds of moral rights do infants possess? Do human infants possess full moral standing, making them morally equal to adult persons? Is the moral standing of neonates to be understood as

somehow less than that of human adults but more than of human fetuses, or are fetuses, neonates, and adults to be understood as morally the same?

For many philosophers in recent years, questions related to the moral standing of infants have been addressed in the broader context of a discussion about ontological status and, more specifically, the meaning of personhood. One approach is to define "person" as meaning "a living being with full moral standing." According to this definition, all persons have such standing, leaving open the question of just which characteristics give that standing.

Given this general philosophical perspective on personhood, at least three positions can be identified that link the ontological status of neonates with the moral standard granted to infants. The first position holds that all neonates, whether normal or neurologically impaired, count as actual persons in the same way that you and I count as persons. According to this view, the personhood of neonates is merely an extension of the personhood possessed earlier by fetuses. With this ontological status, neonates, like all other actual persons, have the moral right not to be killed or prematurely allowed to die, since the possession of personhood entails full moral standing, regardless of the age of the person. Personhood, according to this view, is based on genetic code or some other characteristic possessed at conception, not on possession of consciousness, self-awareness, rationality, or any other neurological characteristic.

The second position holds that in order to count as persons, infants (and other beings, whether human or nonhuman) must possess the intrinsic qualities or traits often defined by philosophers as being the threefold combination of consciousness, self-awareness, and at least minimum rationality (Feinberg, 1986). If infants lack these core properties, they have an ontological status that is more similar to the status of human fetuses than to the status of older children or adults. Holders of this view claim that all neonates, including normal babies, fail to pass the neurologic tests for personhood and are thus to be classified as nonpersons. In this view, all neonates lack the cognitive qualities that make a human into a person. In addition, the notion of potential personhood is discarded as flawed, largely because the advocates of this second position argue that personhood cannot be possessed in varying degrees. Holders of this second view also claim that only those who have the neurological characteristics of persons possess the rights of persons, including the right not to be killed or prematurely allowed to die. The result, in terms of the moral standing of neonates, is straightforward: Neonates do not possess the moral rights of persons, leaving them at risk of being killed or prematurely allowed to die unless their parents and physicians are motivated by psychological or legal considerations to sustain their lives (Tooley, 1983).

The third position stands between the other positions. It identifies the same neurological characteristics of personhood, but according to this view, most neonates (those lacking severe neurologic impairment) are to be regarded as potential persons, not yet possessing the ontological status of actual persons but on the way to the possession of the core properties of personhood through the normal course of human development. Agreeing with advocates of the first two positions on the linkage between ontological status and moral standing, philosophers holding the third position maintain that when infants develop and subsequently become persons, they will acquire full moral standing. Until that time, including during the neonatal period, they are regarded as having a prima facie claim not to be killed, prematurely allowed to die, or significantly harmed in some other way, precisely because they will subsequently and naturally become actual persons.

The differences in these philosophical views have practical consequences in terms of the ways that adults value the lives of infants, including infants who may be extremely premature or severely disabled. Advocates of the first position tend to call for life-sustaining treatment to be administered to all infants in NICUs regardless of birth weight, gestational age, or neurological status, because all infants are actual persons in possession of the full panoply of moral rights common to persons. By contrast, any parents or physicians in NICUs who regard neonates as nonpersons (and who believe that only persons bear the rights borne by persons) are likely to be ready to withhold or withdraw treatment much more quickly, if the law permits them to do so, because the infant lives that are lost do not yet count for much morally. For advocates of the third position, the concept of potential personhood provides an intellectual framework in which difficult prognostic judgments make some sense. In this view, at least part of the difficulty in making decisions to provide life-sustaining treatment or to abate treatment, especially in cases of severe neurologic impairment, has to do with judgments about whether a particular baby has the potential even to become a person in the normal course of his or her development.

Other perspectives on the moral status of infants, some of which are grounded in theological ethics, suggest that the philosophical debate about the personhood of infants is intellectually restrictive and of little practical significance. For example, one fairly common view is that the moral standing of infants cannot depend on whether they meet a philosophically strict definition of personhood, because all infants fail to meet that standard. Rather, what is important is a social understanding of "person" according to which infants are regarded by their parents, physicians, and others "as if" they were persons. This social sense of personhood involves the imputing of personlike rights to infants because of their special roles in families and in society. The practical consequence of this view is that infants, who are given the imputed status of "person" in a social sense, have the same kind of moral standing as older human beings who are persons in a more formal sense (Engelhardt, 1978).

Another widely held view is that the personhood question simply does not apply to infants, either in a strict sense or in a social sense. Rather, what is important is that infants are understood to have moral standing as "fellow human beings." Advocates of this view may regard fetuses and infants as having equal moral standing as human beings, or they may have a developmental view in which viable fetuses and infants, but not nonviable fetuses, have equal moral standing as human beings. Either way, infants are regarded as having the same kinds of moral rights that older human beings have, including the right not to be killed or allowed to die prematurely unless, in unusual cases, the burdens of continued life are regarded as outweighing the benefits of that life to the child (Fletcher, 1975). Holders of this view give the same moral standing to infants and fetuses as do holders of the first position above, but deny that these beings have to be called persons.

The personhood approach to the moral status of infants, according to another theological view, is unrelated to the possession of the neurological characteristics identified with personhood discussed above for another reason. The limiting of an infant's value to the question of whether that infant possesses the intrinsic properties of personhood entirely omits another approach to the understanding of the value that infants have: namely, a relational view of value that results from interpersonal bonding, affection, and care by parents and other adults. Even when an infant has a future that will, because of neurologic impairments, be characterized by developmental delay and mental retardation, the parents of the child still usually go through a process of bonding with the child. That process of bonding, which involves the replacement of a hoped-for child with a healthy attachment to the child one has been given, results in a valuing of the child by parents that is surely equal to the valuing of normal children by their parents (May, 1984).

A related view is that philosophical arguments about the moral status of infants need to be supplemented, if not replaced, by an experiential ethic of care. This view emphasizes the importance of the various perspectives that parents, physicians, nurses, and other persons bring to pediatric cases. Rather than focusing on the ontological and moral status of infants, most commonly with questions related to the possession of personhood and moral rights, this approach concentrates on the various values and virtues present, or possible, in the context of decision making about an infant's impending death or projected life with disabilities. The practical result is that questions in difficult cases are raised not only about what should be done for the patient but also about what kinds of moral agents the parents, physicians, and nurses should be as they provide care for an imperiled infant (Reich, 1987).

Ethical perspectives on abating life-sustaining treatment

The ethical perspective that became enacted into the "Baby Doe" regulations and child abuse regulations was only one of the ethical perspectives on the medical care of infants that received considerable attention in the United States in the 1970s–1990s. Other ethical perspectives have also been widely held, both before and after the federal regulations became policy.

For example, for some persons the important ethical question is not whether a given infant can be salvaged through medical treatment. Rather, the important question is what quality of life the child will probably have later, especially if the child's future is predicted to be dominated by severe-to-profound neurologic impairments, multiple surgeries, and numerous other medical problems. The question is sometimes posed in terms of the future relational potential possessed by a child with severe neurologic impairments, with the moral judgment being that an infant who lacks relational capacity will never have the quality of life that would justify the continuation of the child's life (McCormick, 1974).

A closely related ethical perspective focuses on a child's best interests. For persons holding this position, the important question is whether the life-sustaining treatment that could be given to imperiled newborns will, on balance, provide the infants with more benefits than burdens. Since quality-of-life projections can sometimes extend to include persons other than the patient, this position's strength is in framing the ethical debate primarily in terms of the patient's best interests, not the interests of the family or society (U.S. President's Commission, 1983).

Another ethical perspective emphasizes procedural issues. According to this view, the most important aspect of decisions not to sustain some infants' lives is the question of who should make these difficult decisions. Advocates of this position maintain that in most cases, the parents of a premature or disabled infant are the appropriate decision makers.

A very different ethical perspective on selective treatment decisions also has some advocates. As described in the previous section, some philosophers hold that life-sustaining treatment can morally be withheld or withdrawn from any infant, regardless of birth weight or disability, because the only deaths that matter are the deaths of persons, and no infants meet the requirements of personhood.

Three of these ethical perspectives continue to play major roles in selective nontreatment decisions, with the dominant perspective in individual cases varying from hospital to hospital, physician to physician, parent to parent, case to case. The perspective that calls for life-sustaining treatment to be administered to all infants who are conscious, not dying, and for whom treatment is not "virtually futile and inhumane" remains influential, even if the federal regulations that reflect this perspective have been largely unenforced throughout the country. The reasons for its continuing influence are twofold. First, this perspective is consistent with the reasons that motivate neonatologists to do the work they do: to prolong and enhance the lives of the youngest, smallest, most disabled, and most vulnerable human beings among us. Second, this perspective offers the simplest way of dealing with the multiple problems that constitute the "ethics lab" known as the NICU: It minimizes the factor of medical and moral uncertainty in cases, the role of parents as decision makers, and any considerations of the harm that may be done through prolonged, aggressive efforts to salvage imperiled young lives.

The second perspective that remains influential is the position that emphasizes the role of parents as decision makers. Advocates of this view rarely suggest that parents alone should make the selective nontreatment decisions that could result in the deaths of their children, or that parents should be given unlimited discretion in making such decisions. Rather, the claim that is often made is that parents should, in response to appropriate medical information and advice, have reasonable discretion in making a life-and-death decision regarding their child in the NICU, subject to certain ethical and legal constraints. They are the ones, after all, who may be saddled with the enormous financial costs of neonatal intensive care. They are the ones, in addition to the child, who will have to deal with the child's ongoing medical problems, repeated hospitalizations and surgeries, neurologic abnormalities, and developmental delays. They are the ones who will have to struggle to sustain their marriage, their family life, their careers, and their own physical and mental health.

The third perspective that remains influential is the patient's-best-interests position. Advocates of this position acknowledge the medical and moral uncertainty inherent in many cases, affirm an important role for parents as decision makers, and recognize that the same medical and surgical interventions that produce great benefit for some patients can produce undue harm for others. In contrast to the parental perspective, proponents of this view emphasize that the focal point of decision making in neonatal and pediatric cases should be the best interests of the patient, even when the patient's interests conflict with the interests of the parents. In this manner, the patient's-best-interests position emphasizes the linkage between life-sustaining medical treatment and patient-centered considerations regarding the quality of life—without broadening quality-of-life judgments to include the family, the society, or arbitrary standards for normalcy and acceptability, as quality-of-life projections sometimes do.

The emerging mainstream perspective

If any of these positions can be correctly designated as the mainstream ethical position, at least in the United States, it is the patient's-best-interests position. Advocates of this position are concerned about the treatment-related harms that sometimes occur when neonatologists and other pediatric subspecialists persist, perhaps under the influence of the federal regulations, in overtreating infants who have extremely low birth weights and severe disabling conditions but who are neither unconscious nor dying. At the same time, proponents of the best-interests view are reluctant to grant the parents of premature and disabled infants as much discretion in deciding to abate life-sustaining treatment as some parents would like to have.

In clinical cases, the best-interests position relies on eight variables that help to determine whether to initiate, continue, or abate life-sustaining treatment: (1) the severity of the patient's medical condition, as determined by diagnostic evaluation and comparison with (a) all infants and (b) infants having the same medical condition; (2) the achievability of curative or corrective treatment, in an effort to determine what is meant by "beneficial" treatment in a given case; (3) the important medical goals in the case, such as the prolongation of life, the effective relief of pain and other suffering, and the amelioration of disabling conditions; (4) the presence of serious neurologic impairments, such as permanent unconsciousness or severe mental retardation; (5) the extent of the infant's suffering, as determined by the signs of suffering that infants send by means of elevated blood pressure, elevated heart rate, degree of agitation, and crying; (6) the multiplicity of other serious medical problems, with the most serious cases usually involving a combination of neurologic, cardiac, pulmonary, renal, and other medical complications; (7) the life expectancy of the infant, because some of the severe congenital anomalies involve a life expectancy of only a few weeks or months; and (8) the proportionality of treatment-related benefits and burdens to the infant, a medical and ethical "bottom line" for determining whether life-sustaining treatment or the abatement of such treatment is in a particular infant's best interests (Weir and Bale, 1989).

Even with these variables, the ethical analysis of cases involving neonates or other young pediatric patients is anything but easy. Although there are numerous cases about which almost everyone agrees, there continue to be many cases that combine unprecedented medical and moral territory, advances in medical management and technology, medical uncertainty, and ethical conflicts between physicians and parents in such a way as to present serious ethical challenges to all the parties involved in the cases. In such instances, the discernment of the infant's best interests can be a challenging and humbling experience.

ROBERT F. WEIR

Directly related to this article are the other articles in this entry: MEDICAL ASPECTS AND ISSUES IN THE CARE OF INFANTS, HISTORY OF INFANTICIDE, *and* PUBLIC-POLICY AND LEGAL ISSUES. *For a further discussion of topics mentioned in this article, see the entries* ABUSE, INTERPERSONAL, *article on* CHILD ABUSE; AIDS; CARE, *article on* CONTEMPORARY ETHICS OF CARE; CHILDREN; CLINICAL ETHICS, *article on* INSTITUTIONAL ETHICS COMMITTEES; DEATH AND DYING: EUTHANASIA AND SUSTAINING LIFE; FAMILY; GENETIC TESTING AND SCREENING; HUMAN NATURE; LIFE, QUALITY OF, *article on* QUALITY OF LIFE IN CLINICAL DECISIONS; MEDICAL ETHICS, HISTORY OF, *section on* EUROPE, *subsection on* ANCIENT AND MEDIEVAL, *article on* GREECE AND ROME, *and subsection on* CONTEMPORARY PERIOD; *and section on* SOUTH AND EAST ASIA, *subsection on* CHINA, *and article on* INDIA; MENTALLY DISABLED AND MENTALLY ILL PERSONS; OBLIGATION AND SUPEREROGATION; PERSON; RIGHTS; SURGERY; TEAMS, HEALTH-CARE; *and* TECHNOLOGY. *For a discussion of related ideas, see the entries* COMPASSION; CONFLICT OF INTEREST; DISABILITY; HARM; HEALTH-CARE FINANCING; INFORMATION DISCLOSURE; LIFE; *and* PAIN AND SUFFERING.

Bibliography

CAPLAN, ARTHUR L.; BLANK, ROBERT H.; and MERRICK, JANNA C., eds. 1992. *Compelled Compassion: Government Intervention in the Treatment of Critically Ill Newborns.* Totowa, N.J.: Humana.

ENGELHARDT, H. TRISTRAM, JR. 1978. "Medicine and the Concept of Person." In *Ethical Issues in Death and Dying,* pp. 271–284. Edited by Tom Beauchamp and Seymour Perlin. Englewood Cliffs, N.J.: Prentice-Hall.

FEINBERG, JOEL. 1986. "Abortion." In *Matters of Life and Death: New Introductory Essays in Moral Philosophy.* 2d ed., pp. 256–293. Edited by Tom L. Beauchamp and Tom Regan. New York: Random House.

FLETCHER, JOHN C. 1975. "Abortion, Euthanasia, and Care of Defective Newborns." *New England Journal of Medicine* 292, no. 2:75–78.

FRADER, JOEL. 1986. "Forgoing Life-Sustaining Food and Water: Newborns." In *By No Extraordinary Means: The Choice to Forgo Life-Sustaining Food and Water*, pp. 180–185. Edited by Joanne Lynn. Bloomington: Indiana University Press.

HASTINGS CENTER. 1987. "Imperiled Newborns." *Hastings Center Report* 17, no. 6:5–32.

HORAN, DENNIS J., and DELAHOYDE, MELINDA, eds. 1982. *Infanticide and the Handicapped Newborn*. Provo, Utah: Brigham Young University Press.

KOPELMAN, LORETTA M.; IRONS, THOMAS G.; and KOPELMAN, ARTHUR E. 1988. "Neonatologists Judge the 'Baby Doe' Regulations." *New England Journal of Medicine* 318, no. 11:677–683.

KUHSE, HELGA, and SINGER, PETER. 1985. *Should the Baby Live?: The Problem of Handicapped Infants*. Oxford: Oxford University Press.

MAGNET, JOSEPH E., and KLUGE, EIKE-HENNER W. 1985. *Withholding Treatment from Defective Newborn Children*. Cowansville, Quebec: Brown Legal Publications.

MAY, WILLIAM F. 1984. "Parenting, Bonding, and Valuing the Retarded." In *Ethics and Mental Retardation*, pp. 141–160. Edited by Loretta M. Kopelman and John C. Moskop. Dordrecht, Netherlands: D. Reidel.

MCCORMICK, RICHARD A. 1974. "To Save or Let Die: The Dilemma of Modern Medicine." *Journal of the American Medical Association* 229, no. 2:172–176.

MURRAY, THOMAS H., and CAPLAN, ARTHUR L., eds. 1985. *Which Babies Shall Live? Humanistic Dimensions of the Care of Imperiled Newborns*. Clifton, N.J.: Humana.

PARIS, JOHN J.; CRONE, ROBERT K.; and REARDON, FRANK. 1990. "Physicians' Refusal of Requested Treatment: The Case of Baby L." *New England Journal of Medicine* 322, no. 14:1012–1015.

REICH, WARREN THOMAS. 1987. "Caring for Life in the First of It: Moral Paradigms for Perinatal and Neonatal Ethics." *Seminars in Perinatology* 11, no. 3:279–287.

RHODEN, NANCY K. 1986. "Treating Baby Doe: The Ethics of Uncertainty." *Hastings Center Report* 16, no. 4:34–42.

RHODEN, NANCY K., and ARRAS, JOHN D. 1985. "Withholding Treatment from Baby Doe: From Discrimination to Child Abuse." *Milbank Memorial Fund Quarterly* 63, no. 1:18–51.

SHELP, EARL E. 1986. *Born to Die? Deciding the Fate of Critically Ill Newborns*. New York: Free Press.

SHINNAR, SHLOMO, and ARRAS, JOHN D. 1989. "Ethical Issues in the Use of Anencephalic Infants as Organ Donors." *Neurologic Clinics* 7, no. 4:729–743.

STRONG, CARSON. 1984. "The Neonatologist's Duty to Patient and Parents." *Hastings Center Report* 14, no. 4:10–16.

SZAWARSKI, ZBIGNIEW, and TULCZYNSKI, ALEKSANDER. 1988. "Treatment of Defective Newborns—A Survey of Paediatricians in Poland." *Journal of Medical Ethics* 14, no. 1: 11–17.

TODRES, I. DAVID; GUILLEMIN, JEANNE; GRODIN, MICHAEL A.; and BATTEN, DICK. 1988. "Life-Saving Therapy for Newborns: A Questionnaire Survey in the State of Massachusetts." *Pediatrics* 81, no. 5:643–649.

TOOLEY, MICHAEL. 1983. *Abortion and Infanticide*. Oxford: At the Clarendon Press.

U.S. PRESIDENT'S COMMISSION FOR THE STUDY OF ETHICAL PROBLEMS IN MEDICINE AND BIOMEDICAL AND BEHAVIORAL RESEARCH. 1983. "Seriously Ill Newborns." In *Deciding to Forego Life-Sustaining Treatment: A Report on the Ethical, Medical, and Legal Issues in Treatment Decisions*, pp. 197–229. Washington, D.C.: U.S. Government Printing Office.

WALTERS, JAMES W. 1991. "Report from North America: Anencephalic Infants as Organ Sources." *Bioethics* 5, no. 4:326–341.

WEIR, ROBERT F. 1984. *Selective Nontreatment of Handicapped Newborns: Moral Dilemmas in Neonatal Medicine*. New York: Oxford University Press.

WEIR, ROBERT F., and BALE, JAMES F., JR. 1989. "Selective Nontreatment of Neurologically Impaired Neonates." *Neurologic Clinics* 7, no. 4:807–822.

IV. PUBLIC-POLICY AND LEGAL ISSUES

Medical decisions regarding infants vary in the seriousness of their consequences for infants, families, health providers, and society. They range from decisions about home birth and male circumcision—debatable but generally agreed to be matters of private choice—to vaccination, genetic screening, female genital mutilation, and artificial life support for a critically ill newborn. In the United States, parents' legal right to select even the most invasive treatment—or to refuse lifesaving measures—was nearly unquestioned until recently; it has become the subject of litigation, extensive scholarly comment, and public concern. Because much of the legal and public-policy debate has focused on infants who require life support, decision making will be discussed here in that context.

The infant's interests

The increasing complexity of decisions about the treatment and nontreatment of infants has exacerbated the struggle over who may decide these issues. Advances in medical technology, surgical procedures, and pharmaceuticals allow severely compromised infants to survive, often for prolonged periods of time. These new technologies also usually entail painful, invasive procedures for the infant and the possibility of adverse effects that further attenuate the infant's already fragile hold on life. For example, medical expertise allows the resuscitation of many more premature infants than would have survived in the past; but these infants frequently need prolonged ventilatory assistance and frequent invasive tests.

They are also at increased risk both for cerebral hemorrhages, which create severe neurological and mental deficits, and for serious adverse effects of treatment, such as blindness and deafness.

Decisions on treatment have traditionally rested with parents, health-care providers, or some combination of the two. Since the 1980s, the decision-making powers of these parties have been challenged. In the United States, the older body of law has been partially eroded by legislative enactments and court decisions that focus instead on the rights of the infant (Cooper, 1992). Indeed, recognition of the infant's individual rights arising from the celebrated 1982 Baby Doe case became the basis for substantial federal intervention in medical practice and family life.

Baby Doe was afflicted with Down syndrome, a chromosomal abnormality resulting in mental retardation and a propensity for cardiac and other congenital malformations. The infant had such a congenital defect, a tracheo-esophageal fistula (an abnormal passage connecting the trachea and esophagus), which if not surgically corrected results in death. The parents, after consultation and with the concurrence of their attending physician, refused to consent to the surgery, primarily on the ground that a child with Down syndrome could not attain a "minimally acceptable quality of life." That conclusion was, and continues to be, strongly disputed. A trial court, however, ruled that the parents had the right to refuse surgery for their child (*In re Infant Doe*, 1982).

Immediately after the infant's death, President Ronald Reagan directed the U.S. Department of Health and Human Services (DHHS) to issue regulations protecting handicapped infants from treatment discrimination by parents, health-care providers, or both. Through the regulations, issued in March of 1983, DHHS claimed authority under the Rehabilitation Act of 1973 to order health-care facilities receiving federal assistance to provide sustenance and aggressive medical treatment to handicapped infants. The regulations required posting signs announcing the new federal protection in treatment areas of hospitals; established teams, soon nicknamed "Baby Doe Squads," to investigate alleged instances of treatment discrimination; and provided for a toll-free hotline to facilitate the reporting of discrimination (Lawton et al., 1985). Most health-care providers, as well as many members of the public and of Congress, reacted negatively. A prestigious national group studying health-care decisions—the U.S. President's Commission for the Study of Ethical Problems in Medicine and Biomedical and Behavioral Research—and the American Academy of Pediatrics (AAP) strongly criticized the regulations. The AAP, along with several other parties, sought help from the federal courts, which invalidated the regulations only a few weeks after they became final (*American Academy of Pediatrics* v. *Heckler*, 1983).

DHHS next produced the "Baby Doe II" regulations, modifying the requirements for signs and providing for an infant-care review committee in each hospital in place of the outside investigative team. These regulations too were rejected—ultimately by the U.S. Supreme Court—on the ground that the Rehabilitation Act did not give DHHS any authority to regulate parental decisions about infant treatment (*Bowen* v. *American Hospital Association*, 1986).

In a final effort to influence the care of newborns, even if indirectly, Congress enacted the Child Abuse Amendments of 1984, which directed DHHS to develop regulations governing infant care and guidelines for hospital infant-care review committees. As of 1985, federal funding for state child-abuse prevention and treatment efforts was conditioned on compliance; only a few states had declined the funding. Under the amendments, the Child Protection Service of a state is the only party that may initiate an action of neglect. Still, the fact that the act broadened the definition of child abuse to include "withholding of medically indicated treatment" affects physician practice standards. The amendments require that a disabled infant receive appropriate nutrition, hydration, medication, and the "most effective" treatment according to the reasonable judgment of the treating physician. In only three situations may treatment be withheld: (1) when the child is chronically and irreversibly comatose; (2) when treatment could not save the child's life for any substantial length of time; or (3) when the treatment would be inhumane and "virtually futile" with respect to survival. The distinction between inability to save the life (situation 2) and "virtually futile" (situation 3) lies in the "degree of probability or uncertainty in determining the futility of treatment" (Boyd and Thompson, 1990). This distinction has become increasingly difficult to draw, in the context of both withdrawal and continuation of treatment. With respect to the latter, for example, in the case of Baby "K," a mother fought successfully to continue extraordinary medical intervention to preserve the life of her irreversibly comatose anencephalic child, despite the fact that such treatment is virtually futile in terms of ultimate survival (Baby "K," 1994).

The U.S. President's Commission disagreed with the Reagan administration on its Baby Doe regulations and proposed that the standard for infant treatment or nontreatment be based on the "best interests" of the infant. This standard was a variation of the substituted judgment standard that is often applied to incapacitated but once competent patients. In such cases, a proxy attempts to make treatment decisions as she or he believes the patient would, if able. For newborns, the commission recommended that decision makers attempt to assess the best interests of the infant "by reference to more objective, societally shared criteria." In sum, the commission recommended that decision makers "choose a course that will promote the patient's well-being as it would be conceived by a reasonable person in the patient's circumstances" (U.S. President's Commission, 1983, pp. 135–136). Numerous courts have since adopted the "best interests" standard in making infant treatment decisions.

Ascertaining the infant's best interests generally falls to the primary caregivers—in most cases, the parents, who, although assisted by numerous directors, nurses, and social workers, frequently must make and bear the brunt of these difficult decisions. Unfortunately, the guidelines available to decision makers from the commission and subsequent case law are far from concrete. In describing the "best interests" standard, the commission stressed that normal adults must not impose their values or external concerns upon the beleaguered infant. In its guidelines, the commission stated that futile treatment for severely compromised infants with a life span of hours or days, such as anencephalics, need not be provided; at the other end of the spectrum, the commission condemned the withholding of treatment for a correctable problem when the infant was afflicted with an unrelated, non-life-threatening disorder, such as Down syndrome (U.S. President's Commission, 1983). However, for the vast territory in between, there is little guidance.

Determining the best interests of a compromised infant using the commission's guidelines presents considerable problems of interpretation (Rhoden, 1985). Some, including C. Everett Koop, former U.S. Surgeon General, believe that the best interests of the infant require providing maximum treatment in virtually all cases (Smith, 1992; Wells, 1988; Wells et al., 1990). In this view, infants express their interest in surviving by responding positively to treatment (Cooper, 1992). Others believe that nontreatment may be justified when the infant's life can be viewed as an injury rather than a gift to the infant; an "injury" is inferred when there is no prospect of meaningful life, which might occur because life expectancy is very short, there are severe mental deficits, and no curative or corrective treatments are available (Weir, 1994).

Some argue that the rational interests of the infant in treatment or nontreatment should not be limited to avoiding suffering (including the pain of treatment) and to minimizing physical and mental deficits, but should also include factors such as the burden of treatment on family and society (Wells et al., 1990; Smith, 1992). Such a view holds that when an infant's condition lacks any "'truly human' qualities" or "relational potential,"

the best decision is not to treat (Smith, 1992, p. 56). Certainly, one can presume that an infant has an interest in his or her "standing and memory within the family" (Mitchell, 1989, p. 341). If so, the infant's best interests cannot be determined in isolation from the feelings and concerns of others. Although such "quality of life" considerations are given short shrift under the current federal law and under the President's Commission's best-interests standard, they may well be inevitable (Rhoden, 1985). Heretofore the courts have both embraced and enhanced quality-of-life concerns in deciding controversial issues. No consensus has yet emerged.

Parents' interests

U.S. jurisprudence still strongly favors parents as decision makers for children's medical care, although it does not accord the preference constitutional status (*Cruzan v. Director, Missouri Department of Health,* 1990). Though some dispute the basis for a parental preference—asking whether it is for the parents' sake, the children's, or society's (Schneider, 1988)—the law is willing to assume that parents, with physicians' help, can best judge the child's interest and will best protect it. Moreover, it seems fair to defer to those who will live intimately with the results of the decisions. As explained below, however, the wisdom of this presumption is challenged on many fronts, both from within and outside the legal establishment. In any case, parental authority is conditional. It is settled law that the state may intervene if necessary, superseding parents' authority by proving them unable or unwilling to guard the child's welfare. In extreme cases, parents may be criminally liable for failing to fulfill the responsibility to provide ordinary care.

Critics of leaving decisions about the treatment for dangerously ill newborns solely or primarily to parents question how well parents are able to judge an infant's needs. Certainly the task is daunting, since the medical specialists on whom parents depend often cannot predict a child's chances of survival or normality with any certainty at the point when decisions must be made, nor adequately warn of the suffering that treatment may eventually entail (Bouregy, 1988). In addition, parents come to the task exhausted by childbirth and the child's medical crisis, grief-stricken and in near shock (Jellinek et al., 1992). There is evidence that physicians do not always share essential information with parents and that parents often absorb poorly the limited information they receive (Perlman et al., 1991). Even observers who find parents the best possible decision makers speak of their vulnerability during the crisis, especially to manipulation by others (Rushton and Glover, 1990). On the other hand, parents may wholly reject medical guidance. Several have protested the removal of a dead infant from life support; and in one notorious incident, a father,

Rudy Linares, disconnected his infant son's respirator and held off nurses at gunpoint until the boy died. (For an excellent analysis of the issues discussed in this article, see Gostin, 1989.)

A second criticism of giving parents authority is that they may deliberately elect not to satisfy an infant's dire needs. In this view, it is naive to posit an identity of interest between infant and parent. Parents guard their own interests, those of the family as a unit, and those of current and future siblings—all of which may be gravely threatened by the newborn. Some observers of such behavior describe it neutrally. To a sociobiologist, "individual infants may attempt to extract greater investment from their parents than the parents have been selected to give," causing parents to reduce their investment in the child (Hrdy, 1992, p. 410). A philosopher writing on the subject actively encourages parents to weigh the child's interests, including life itself, against others' needs: "The neonate is not born into the family circle so much as outside it, awaiting inclusion or exclusion. The moral problem the parents must confront is whether the child should become a part of the family unit" (Blustein, 1989, p. 166). But other commentators condemn any deviation on the part of parents from pursuit of the child's interest. Among these were the proponents of the Baby Doe regulations and, later, a majority of the U.S. Supreme Court, which noted that family members "may have a strong feeling—a feeling not at all ignoble or unworthy, but not entirely disinterested either—that they do not wish to witness the continuation of the life of a loved one which they regard as hopeless, meaningless, and even degrading" (*Cruzan v. Director, Missouri Department of Health*, 1990, p. 286).

Practitioners—doctors, lawyers, and social workers—also observe parents acting from mixed motives in accepting or rejecting medical care. By forgoing treatment, they may hope to spare the infant suffering and lessen their own, avoid financial and other burdens on the family, and prevent the child's eventual institutionalization (Newman, 1989). They may instinctively—and with good reason—fear the damage to parent–child relations created by medicine's lifesaving technology (Boyce, 1992; Kratochvil et al., 1991). Not infrequently, the parents' religious beliefs discourage medical intervention. On the other hand, a parent may insist on extraordinary measures in an attempt to be faithful to their understanding of their religion's tenets, as well as to assuage perceived guilt; or to please the other parent, friends, and family; or from selfless devotion to the child that the parent cannot reconcile with consenting to death (Nelson and Nelson, 1992).

By whatever means and for whatever reasons, parents usually prove effective advocates for their treatment preference. (An exception is where parents cannot agree on treatment. When this occurs, neither is likely to re-main the primary decision maker [*Jane Doe*, 1992].) Deference to parents was especially prevalent before Baby Doe. Surveys of physicians in the 1970s suggest either their deference to parents or a marked congruence between parents' and physicians' choices for infants. Three studies are particularly revealing because they ask the very question later placed in issue by Baby Doe: whether lifesaving treatment that would be given to other newborns may be withheld from a child with Down syndrome. In each survey, most physicians either would not recommend treatment or would acquiesce in a parental decision to reject it (U.S. President's Commission, 1983). According to Angela Holder, when courts review parents' decisions, parents usually lose if they stand alone against physicians; but bolstered by respectable medical advice, they generally prevail against legal challenges from other physicians, health-facility administrators, lawyers, or government agencies (Holder, 1985).

However, the differing views of the intrinsic value of the infant's life described above are not mirrored in the law. The law is relatively clear in its expectation of parents, though the mandate may be excruciatingly difficult to follow. Firmly rejecting any intermediate status for newborns, federal and state constitutions, as well as statutory and decisional law, accord equal status to all living human beings. Parents must act in their child's interest, weighing the immediate physical and long-term emotional suffering for the infant to be expected from aggressive treatment against the consequences of no or lesser treatment. Thus, while some object to consideration of the infant's quality of life in these decisions, such factoring is central to the parents' legal duty.

Health-care providers' interests

Historically, treatment decisions rested with the midwife or physician caring for the newborn and its mother. Although parents ostensibly "owned" their children, they routinely ceded control to the health-care provider. During the twentieth century, the decision-making model shifted to one in which the parent and the provider jointly decided on medical intervention for the infant. In recent decades, the parents' role has markedly increased as a result of a greater number of treatment options and increased parental knowledge and awareness (Cooper, 1992).

Organized medicine has not opposed this development. A 1975 AAP survey indicated broad support among pediatricians for the proposition that infant treatment decisions should be made jointly by the parents and physician, with the parents taking the pivotal role. The Society of Critical Care Medicine's Task Force on Ethics recommends that parents set priorities for treatment of critically ill pediatric patients (Task Force on Ethics, 1990). The American Medical Association also defers to parents but would require them to decide on the basis of the best-interests standard proposed by the President's Commission.

Physicians readily acknowledge the frequent conflicts between their dual commitment to save lives and to alleviate suffering. In reality, these factors are rarely the only ones that affect the physician treating a critically ill infant. Health-care providers may have varying philosophies with respect to treatment of infants afflicted with certain disabilities; they may also be influenced by their research agendas, possess insufficient knowledge to assess accurately the infant's disability and prognosis, or be influenced by real or perceived risk of legal liability (Rushton and Glover, 1990). In addition, physicians focus on the diagnosis, rather than on the prognosis and long-term care of their infant patients (Perlman et al., 1991). As a result of all these factors, physicians may not be optimally effective partners for the parents in the decision-making process. For example, an obstetrician may act in a paternalistic fashion toward his or her patient, the mother, seeking to protect her from the tragedy of dealing with the fate of an impaired infant. Alternatively, a neonatalogist may be overly optimistic in judging and discussing with the parents the infant's potential for meaningful life (Cooper, 1992).

Frequently, nurses serve as the primary information conduit between doctors and parents, and naturally there are biases inherent in their perspective, too. Because they are the health-care providers who care for patients most intimately, they may personalize severely disabled infants beyond reality in order to deal with the burden of nursing them on a day-to-day basis. As a result, nurses may be incapable of advocating against treatment when it is futile and thus be unable to serve as effective advocates for either the infant or the family. In addition, they are limited by the practical realities of their role in the employment hierarchy of the hospital (Mitchell, 1989).

In some cases, health-care facilities and providers may overtreat a severely compromised infant to avoid legal liability. The Linares case, while an extreme example, arose from tensions that are often present. There, despite their acknowledged sympathy and agreement with the father's desire for his son's death, the health-care providers insisted for many months on treating the infant. They did so, they said later, because they believed that state law required continued life support. Critics alleged that individual health-care providers and the facility (through its lawyer) had abandoned the best interests of both the child and the family to protect themselves. Indeed, some see an "overwhelming fear of possible, indeed theoretical, adverse legal repercussions" among health-care providers (Nelson and Cranford, 1989, p. 3210). The Baby "K" case, which casts doubt

on the physician's freedom to refuse to provide treatment he or she considers futile, suggests that fear of legal reprisal is not unfounded.

Providers are also strongly motivated by sympathy. Some physicians assert that when patients' lives are extended beyond hope of recovery, it is usually because the patient's family is unwilling to accept the inevitability of death (Emanuel, 1994). When this occurs, although it may be ethically justifiable and legally defensible for a physician to withhold or withdraw treatment, physicians frequently accede to parental demand (Nelson and Nelson, 1992).

Society's interests

A society such as that of the United States has numerous, sometimes contradictory, interests in the health care of infants. These include preservation of the life and health of the next generation; the guarantee of rights to individuals; the support of families; the conservation and wise expenditure of economic resources; the maintenance of a just and predictable legal system; and the compromise—or at least the orderly expression—of clashing values of groups within society. Two of these issues, cost and the social effect of litigating treatment decisions, are discussed below.

Concern for the cost of neonatal intensive care—the most expensive element in the care of infants—preceded the currently intense focus on health costs in general. This treatment is the exception to the rule that the United States directs resources disproportionately to adults, especially the elderly. Technological advances in the treatment of newborns halved the neonatal death rate between 1970 and 1980 (U.S. President's Commission, 1983). Since then, the extraordinary cost of the technology has helped to focus attention on how many and which infants should be treated.

Many families cannot cover the cost, and there is debate over whether the resources available for a particular infant should be taken into account by decision makers. Most commentators share the view expressed in a seminal article on the subject: "Just as a parent is not obligated to attempt to save a drowning child if the parent cannot swim, neither is he obligated to incur enormous expense in providing treatment with a slight chance of success" (Robertson, 1975, p. 236; see also Newman, 1989). No judicial decision, however, accepts the proposition that personal resources should dictate life or death. Usually, the issue is avoided in litigation. When it is specifically cited, a typical court reply is that the "cost of care in human or financial terms is irrelevant" (*Beth, Care and Protection of,* 1992, p. 1383).

Whether or not cost should affect decisions on treatment, there is evidence that it does. Although providers may not abandon a patient without incurring liability, a study comparing medical need to the services sick newborns receive indicates that health-care providers do not allocate services solely according to need, but are instead influenced by the newborn's insurance coverage—private, governmental, or none (Braveman et al., 1991). Governmental insurance is less attractive to providers than private insurance because government does not reimburse the full cost of care. Thus, at times it appears that while society insists on extending the life of premature and seriously ill infants, it simultaneously refuses to absorb the cost of their immediate and long-term care—a result described as "political hypocrisy in its cruelest form" (Holder, 1985, p. 113).

A second salient issue for society is whether it has erred by assigning this category of treatment decisions increasingly to the courts. Criticism of the failure to treat Baby Doe was widespread and severe, but the legal processes that ensued were also criticized. Numerous objections are raised to the removal of medical decisions from the private sphere. The judicial system may be too cumbersome and costly and may further traumatize family members and invade their privacy. The publicity surrounding infant-care cases may prevent other parents from exercising their right to forgo treatment. In addition, the practice of medicine is negatively affected. Explicit direction from some courts to extend life whenever possible and the implicit threat of litigation reinforce U.S. medicine's alleged tendency to overtreat (Newman, 1989). For example, one in three neonatologists state that the Baby Doe regulations require treatment not in an infant's best interest (Fost, 1989). Finally, in investigating and deciding these cases, judges and other officials must choose among competing moral and religious philosophies, a problematic choice in a society that values diversity (Newman, 1989).

Obviously, the law is disadvantaged in attempting to supervise medical care for particular infants. In most jurisdictions, understanding of the legal requirements for forgoing treatment is imperfect, even among lawyers (see Gostin, 1989). The scarcity of prosecutions and precedents suggests a high degree of social ambivalence on this subject—"a troubling disjunction between the law on the books, which seems to make neonatal euthanasia criminal, and the law in action, which does not punish it" (Schneider, 1988, p. 152). According to Carl Schneider, there is no social consensus on the central questions: What is human life? When is death preferable to life? What do parents owe their children? What does society owe the suffering? As a result, he and others see a tendency to abandon the search for substantive principles in the law and instead adopt procedures for reviewing individual cases (Schneider, 1988).

One such procedure is the assignment of a role in decision making to institutional ethics committees. Virtually unknown before 1983 (fewer than 1 percent of

U.S. hospitals had committees), they came to prominence through two avenues. First, the influential U.S. President's Commission report in 1983 recommended their use; second, the establishment of committees became a major point of compromise in negotiations between the government and health-care providers over the Baby Doe regulations (Lawton et al., 1985). By 1986 the American Academy of Pediatrics, which had strongly endorsed the committees, found them in 60 percent of hospitals.

In some instances, the committees have functioned as it was hoped they would. For example, in the case of Baby "L," a physician applied to the hospital's ethics committee for permission to cease extraordinary treatment of an infant who was capable only of pain perception and to transfer the infant to another facility and provider. The parent opposed this action and sought an opinion from the courts. The court upheld the hospital and physician's decision and allowed transfer of the child to a facility willing to continue treatment (Paris et al., 1990). In the case of Baby "K," however, a hospital's ethics committee failed to persuade either the parent or the trial court that treatment was futile.

Concerns are expressed about the committees' role, makeup, criteria for decision making, influence, results, and effectiveness. Are they intended to advise or to bind? If the latter, do they deprive parents or infants of constitutional rights? Are they instruments of the medical establishment rather than havens for patients? How reflective of the entire community is their membership? Do they diffuse moral responsibility? Do they—and should they—help to reduce liability? (Newman, 1989; U.S. President's Commission, 1983). Despite such questions, ethics committees appear entrenched as a visible representative of society in controversies over care for infants.

Conclusion

Long-standing respect for parent and health-care provider discretion in making infant treatment decisions has been partially replaced by a greater emphasis on the rights of the infant. As a result, the roles of the infant, parents, health-care providers, and, in the larger context, society, in making these difficult decisions are undergoing reexamination. Although institutional infant-care review committees occasionally serve as forums for such decision making, a number of these cases continue to be referred to the courts, where little, if any, consensus has emerged.

ANNE M. DELLINGER
PATRICIA C. KUSZLER

Directly related to this article are the other articles in this entry: MEDICAL ASPECTS AND ISSUES IN THE CARE OF IN-

FANTS, HISTORY OF INFANTICIDE, *and* ETHICAL ISSUES. *For a further discussion of topics mentioned in this article, see the entries* ABUSE, INTERPERSONAL, *article on* CHILD ABUSE; ARTIFICIAL ORGANS AND LIFE-SUPPORT SYSTEMS; CIRCUMCISION, *article on* MALE CIRCUMCISION; CLINICAL ETHICS, *article on* INSTITUTIONAL ETHICS COMMITTEES; DEATH AND DYING: EUTHANASIA AND SUSTAINING LIFE; FAMILY; FIDELITY AND LOYALTY; FUTURE GENERATIONS, OBLIGATIONS TO; HARM; LAW AND BIOETHICS; LIFE, QUALITY OF, *article on* QUALITY OF LIFE IN CLINICAL DECISIONS; PATERNALISM; *and* RIGHTS. *For a discussion of related ideas, see the entries* AIDS; AUTONOMY; BENEFICENCE; CONFLICT OF INTEREST; FETUS; HEALTH-CARE FINANCING; INFORMATION DISCLOSURE; MENTALLY ILL AND MENTALLY DISABLED PERSONS; *and* PAIN AND SUFFERING.

Bibliography

American Academy of Pediatrics v. Heckler. 1983. 561 F.Supp. 395 (D.D.C.).

Baby "K," In re. 1993. No. 93–1899, No. 93–1923, No. 93–1924.

Beth, Care and Protection of, In re. 1992. 587 N.E.2d 1377 (Mass.).

BLUSTEIN, JEFFREY. 1989. "The Rights Approach and the Intimacy Approach: Family Suffering and Care of Defective Newborns." *Mount Sinai Journal of Medicine* 56, no. 3: 164–167.

BOUREGY, WILLIAM L. 1988. "Parental Refusal of Consent for Treatment of Handicapped Newborns: Comparing Case Results in England and the United States." *New York Law School Journal of International and Comparative Law* 9: 379–433.

Bowen v. American Hospital Association. 1986. 476 U.S. 610.

BOYCE, W. THOMAS. 1992. "The Vulnerable Child: New Evidence, New Approaches." *Advances in Pediatrics* 39:1–33.

BOYD, DIANE E., and THOMPSON, PETER J. 1990. "United States Commission on Civil Rights—Medical Discrimination Against Children with Disabilities: An Abstract." *Journal of Contemporary Health Law and Policy* 6:379–410.

BRAVEMAN, PAULA A.; EGERTER, SUSAN; BENNETT, TRUDE; and SHOWSTACK, JONATHAN. 1991. "Differences in Hospital Resource Allocation Among Sick Newborns According to Insurance Coverage." *Journal of the American Medical Association* 255, no. 23:3300–3308.

COOPER, REBECCA. 1992. "Delivery Room Resuscitation of the High Risk Infant: A Conflict of Rights." *Catholic Lawyer* 33, no. 4:325–360.

Cruzan v. Director, Missouri Department of Health. 1990. 497 U.S. 261.

EMANUEL, EZEKIEL J. 1994. "A Look at . . . Health Care Quandaries: Who Won't Pull the Plug?" *Washington Post,* January 2, p. C3.

FOST, NORMAN. 1989. "Do the Right Thing: Samuel Linares and Defensive Law." *Law, Medicine and Health Care* 17, no. 4:330–334.

GOLDMAN, GILBERT M.; STRATTON, KAREN M.; and BROWN,

MAX DOUGLAS. 1989. "What Actually Happened: An Informed Review of the Linares Incident." *Law, Medicine and Health Care* 17, no. 4:298–307.

GOSTIN, LARRY O., ed. 1989. "Family Privacy and Persistent Vegetative State." *Law, Medicine and Health Care* 17, no. 4:295–346. Special section.

HOLDER, ANGELA. 1985. "The Child and Death." In her *Legal Issues in Pediatrics and Adolescent Medicine,* pp. 82–122. New Haven, Conn.: Yale University Press.

HRDY, SARAH BLAFFER. 1992. "Fitness Tradeoffs in the History and Evolution of Delegated Mothering with Special Reference to Wet-Nursing, Abandonment, and Infanticide." *Ethnology and Sociobiology* 13 (September–November): 409–442.

Infant Doe, In re. 1982. No. GU 8204–004A (Cir. Ct. Monroe County, Ind., Apr. 12); *writ of mandamus* dismissed *subnom. state ex. rel. Infant Doe v. Baker* no. 482 140 (Sup. Ct. Ind. May 27, 1982); cert. denied 104 S. Ct. 394 (1983).

Jane Doe, In re. 1992. 418 S.E.2d 3 (Ga.).

JELLINEK, MICHAEL S.; CATLIN, ELIZABETH A.; TODRES, I. DAVID; and CASSEM, EDWIN H. 1992. "Facing Tragic Decisions with Parents in the Neonatal Intensive Care Unit: Clinical Perspectives." *Pediatrics* 89, no. 1:119–122.

KRATOCHVIL, MARIANNE; ROBERTSON, CHARLENE; and KYLE, JANIS. 1991. "Parents' View of Parent–Child Relationship Eight Years After Neonatal Intensive Care." *Social Work in Health Care* 16, no. 1:95–118.

LAWTON, STEPHAN E.; CARDER, ELIZABETH B.; and WEISMAN, ANNE W. 1985. "Recent Governmental Action Regarding the Treatment of Seriously Ill Newborns." *Journal of College and University Law* 11, no. 4:405–416.

MITCHELL, CHRISTINE. 1989. "On Heroes and Villains in the Linares Drama." *Law, Medicine and Health Care* 17, no. 4:339–346.

NELSON, LAWRENCE J., and CRANFORD, ROBERT. 1989. "Legal Advice, Moral Paralysis, and the Death of Samuel Linares." *Law, Medicine and Health Care* 17, no. 4:316–324.

NELSON, LAWRENCE J., and NELSON, ROBERT M. 1992. "Ethics and the Provision of Futile, Harmful, or Burdensome Treatment to Children." *Critical Care Medicine* 20, no. 3:427–433.

NEWMAN, STEPHAN A. 1989. "Baby Doe, Congress, and the States: Challenging the Federal Treatment Standard for Impaired Infants." *American Journal of Law and Medicine* 15, no. 1:1–60.

PARIS, JOHN J.; CRONE, ROBERT K.; and REARDON, FRANK. 1990. "Physicians' Refusal of Requested Treatment: The Case of Baby L." *New England Journal of Medicine* 322, no. 14:1012–1015.

PERLMAN, NITZA B.; FREEDMAN, JONATHAN L.; ABRAMOVITCH, RENA; WHITE, HILARY; KIRPALANI, HARESH; and PERLMAN, MAX. 1991. "Informational Needs of Parents of Sick Neonates." *Pediatrics* 88, no. 3:512–518.

RHODEN, NANCY K. 1985. "Treatment Dilemmas for Imperiled Newborns: Why Quality of Life Counts." *Southern California Law Review* 58, no. 5:1283–1347.

ROBERTSON, J. A. 1975. "Involuntary Euthanasia of Defective Newborns: A Legal Analysis." *Stanford Law Review* 27:213–269.

RUSHTON, CINDY HYLTON, and GLOVER, JACQUELINE J. 1990. "Involving Parents in Decisions to Forgo Life-Sustaining Treatment for Critically Ill Infants and Children." *Clinical Issues in Critical Care Nursing* 1, no. 1:206–214.

SCHNEIDER, CARL E. 1988. "Rights Discourse and Neonatal Euthanasia." *California Law Review* 76, no. 1:151–176.

SMITH, GEORGE. 1988. "Murder, She Wrote or Was It Merely Selective Nontreatment?" *Journal of Contemporary Health Law and Policy* 8:49–71.

TASK FORCE ON ETHICS OF THE SOCIETY OF CRITICAL CARE MEDICINE. 1990. "Consensus Report on the Ethics of Forgoing Life-Sustaining Treatments in the Critically Ill." *Critical Care Medicine* 18, no. 12:1435–1439.

U.S. PRESIDENT'S COMMISSION FOR THE STUDY OF ETHICAL PROBLEMS IN MEDICINE AND BIOMEDICAL AND BEHAVIORAL RESEARCH. 1983. *Deciding to Forgo Life-Sustaining Treatment: A Report of the Ethical, Medical, and Legal Issues in Treatment Decisions.* Washington, D.C.: Author.

WEIR, ROBERT F. 1994. *Selective Nontreatment of Handicapped Newborns: Moral Dilemmas in Neonatal Care.* Oxford: Oxford University Press.

WELLS, CELIA. 1988. "Whose Baby Is It?" *Journal of Law and Society* 15, no. 4:323–341.

WELLS, CELIA; ALLDRIDGE, PETER; and MORGAN, DEREK. 1990. "An Unsuitable Case for Treatment." *New Law Journal* 140 (November 2), no. 6478:1544–1545.

INFORMATION DISCLOSURE

I. Attitudes Toward Truth-Telling
   Kate H. Brown
II. Ethical Issues
   Andrew Jameton

I. ATTITUDES TOWARD TRUTH-TELLING

Ethicists, health professionals, and social scientists have paid considerable attention to the issue of information disclosure in clinical settings worldwide. Attitudinal research involving innumerable samples of clinicians, patients, families, and the public has examined the questions of whether "truth" should be told to patients, and if so, what truths, how much, by whom, when, and how. Opinions about how these questions should be answered have been assessed and analyzed in regard to an array of circumstances, illnesses, and conditions, each presenting special considerations. For instance, patients and practitioners have been asked about the wisdom and desirability of disclosing the risks of experimentation, terminal prognoses, or specific diagnoses—including but not limited to cancer, mental illness, HIV, and genetic predispositions. Whether revealing such information is a benefit or a burden to patients may be a question as old as the healer–patient relationship. Even as this ancient question remains unsettled, however, new puzzles about disclosure are created by new diseases, health-care technologies, roles, and organizational structures. This article reviews recent attitudinal trends regarding information disclosure in a number of areas of clinical concern.

To tell or not to tell?

Many of the attitudinal surveys about information disclosure in clinical settings have focused on whether physicians should reveal diagnoses to patients, particularly when the diagnosis implies a terminal prognosis. These studies have documented a marked difference in physicians' attitudes over time. Until the 1970s, surveys of U.S. physicians indicated their clear preference for protecting patients from the news of impending death from cancer. Then, beginning in the 1970s, there was evidence of a shift. Dennis Novack and his colleagues (1979), replicating a 1961 study by Donald Oken, found a complete reversal of the earlier findings. Ninety-seven percent of these physicians, compared with 10 percent in the first sample, reported that it was their general policy to provide patients with the full details of their condition.

Other countries have witnessed similar, although not as dramatic, trends indicating an increasing willingness of physicians to talk with patients about their impending death. A study of family practice physicians in the United States, Canada, and Britain provides a useful comparison of current practice in these three countries. Responding to hypothetical vignettes, physicians indicated their relative willingness to divulge information about the possibility of multiple sclerosis and cancer to patients. In general, the U.S. sample was most likely to tell patients about the suspected diseases (55 and 79 percent), Canadian physicians were moderately likely to tell patients (49 and 67 percent), and British physicians least likely to do so (45 and 44 percent). Even in Japan, where the majority of physicians remain hesitant to reveal diagnoses of malignancy (especially cancers) to patients, there is increasing public and professional debate about this traditional practice (Hattori et al., 1991).

Of course, what survey respondents say they do is not always a measure of actual behavior. This methodological shortcoming is well illustrated by Kathryn Taylor's (1988) study of Canadian oncologists who reported they routinely discuss the results of breast biopsies with patients. A comparison between observational and interview data revealed that despite their perceptions of their behavior, very few of the physicians actually communicated positive biopsy results to patients in a clear and direct manner.

Since the 1960s legal requirements for informed consent have undoubtedly influenced the change in physicians' attitudes toward disclosure of information to patients. These laws generally require that patients be given explicit information about the risks and benefits of procedures, drugs, and clinical trials. However, even where the practice of informed consent is law, physicians vary in terms of what information is revealed and how it is disclosed. An international study (Taylor and Kelner, 1987) polling oncologists in Canada, Australia, France, Sweden, the United States, England, and Italy about their attitudes toward informed consent for breast cancer treatment trials found that these physicians used a wide range of discretion in the amount of detail they gave to patients; their disclosures depended more on their assessments of patients' needs than on regard for legal regulations pertaining to disclosure. Other studies document a similar pattern of clinicians' preference for discretionary use of partial disclosure of drug side effects (Keown et al., 1984) or the possible complications associated with a medical procedure (Kessler, 1977).

Why tell a lie?

A number of studies have investigated different reasons why physicians equivocate to patients with lies, half-truths, vague accounts, or avoidance, especially when it comes to the disclosure of bad news. A common explanation for such behavior derives from the belief that disclosure can set off a destructive interplay of psychological and physical processes that result in worsening of patients' conditions (Meador, 1992). In the case of informed consent for a painful procedure or risky clinical trial, some authors warn that the power of suggestion can exacerbate pain and side effects unnecessarily or that the truth will lead subjects to decline to participate in randomized treatment (Simes et al., 1986). Other studies contradict this reasoning with evidence that patients' coping skills are enhanced, cooperation with treatment is increased, and levels of anxiety are reduced when they are provided with adequate information about their condition (Ell et al., 1989).

Several authors focus on the importance of the context of disclosure to explain clinicians' decisions about what to tell patients and others. For instance, Dennis Novack et al. (1989) found that most in their sample of U.S. internists would willingly engage in deception if, in their judgment, circumstances called for it. Responding to hypothetical cases, these physicians said they would misrepresent facts if to do so would benefit a patient or circumvent a stupid regulation; one-third of the sample answered that they would evade or mislead in order to protect themselves if they had mistakenly contributed to a patient's death. Another study reported

that opinions regarding when it is best to tell patients about genetic predispositions or anomalies will vary if the information is relevant to imminent reproductive decisions (Wertz and Fletcher, 1987). Haavi Morreim raises important questions about whether and how new practice arrangements and reimbursement procedures in the United States will affect "physicians' obligations to discuss these economic changes openly with patients and to help them find their way through an increasingly complex maze of resource rules and restrictions" (1991, p. 276).

Physicians often express confidence in their "gut reactions" to assess their patients' ability and desire to hear bad news (Still and Todd, 1986). Consequently, they are apt to recommend flexibility and individualized consideration of patients' needs. Given the psychological, clinical, and linguistic complexity of communication about illness, it is important to honor this sentiment.

However, a number of researchers have shown that physicians' decisions regarding information disclosure may well be influenced by their culturally constructed role expectations and rules for communication (Todd and Still, 1984; Takahaski, 1990). In pluralistic societies, physicians and patients may not share assumptions about appropriate disclosure. Moreover, role expectations are subject to change over time, creating confusion about what is to be revealed and by whom. Research has shown that the introduction of new clinical roles (e.g., radiologists; Vallely and Mills, 1990) and the expansion of old ones (e.g., nurses; Davis and Jameton, 1987) can complicate role expectations and raise questions about who on the clinical team is or should be responsible for giving information to patients.

Furthermore, the asymmetry of power and knowledge inherent in the physician–patient relationship can confound communication efforts (Waitzkin, 1985), especially when it is exaggerated by social class differences (Mathews, 1983). In addition, physicians' own discomfort with death (Eggerman and Dustin, 1985) and their lack of explicit training in communication skills can limit their effectiveness in breaking bad news and handling patients' reactions to it. To the extent that these factors cloud clinical judgment about disclosure, physicians may not be serving their patients' interests when solely relying on their intuition and medical expertise.

The patient's perspective

In contrast with the variable nature of physicians' attitudes about disclosing terminal diagnoses, many surveys of patients over time and across cultures indicate they would prefer to have knowledge of their diagnosis, treatment course, and prognosis. As early as 1950, William Kelly and Stanley Friesen found that 89 percent of their respondents in the United States wanted to know their diagnosis of cancer. Subsequent studies in the United States (Blanchard et al., 1988), Australia (Reynolds et al., 1981), Scotland (Reid et al., 1988), and Canada (Sutherland et al., 1989) report that similarly high proportions of patients with cancer would like to hear from their physicians about the nature of their malignancies.

Many patients seem to want information about other diagnoses besides cancer. For instance, a 1988 study of ambulatory patients in the United States reported that over 90 percent would want to know if they were found to have Alzheimer's disease (Erde et al., 1988). Cross-national studies report that parents want to know information about the diagnoses and prognoses of their children's diseases, including leukemia (Greenberg et al., 1984), spina bifida and Down syndrome (Murdoch, 1983), and severe mental handicaps (Quine and Pahl, 1986). Highlighting the difference between patients and physicians, Ruth Faden and her colleagues found that patients' parents in the United States wanted "far more detailed disclosures than physicians routinely offer[ed]" about epilepsy medication (1981, p. 718). This patient–parent sample wanted detailed information even if it would make them feel anxious, and they were willing to take and pay for the extra time required during an office visit for this depth of information.

However, not everyone desires complete disclosure of diagnoses, prognoses, or risks inherent in their medical choices. Circumstances and cultural interpretations influence what patients and families desire to know and how they want to be told. For example, the context of disclosure was significant to a sample in the United States who reported that they would prefer that the news of the unexpected death of a relative be couched in a temporary lie if they received it from a physician by telephone; in person, they would prefer immediate and full notification (Viswanathan et al., 1986). A study about informed-consent practice associated with elective circumcisions on male newborns in the United States showed that parents' commitment to traditional, religious, and social values superseded their interest in hearing about medical risks of this surgery (Christensen-Szalanski et al., 1987).

In companion articles, Antonella Surbone and Edmund Pellegrino reason that variation in our expectations for disclosure of information is based on different cultural understandings of patient autonomy as it relates to truth-telling. Surbone observes, "In Italian culture autonomy (*autonomia*) is often synonymous for isolation (*isolamento*) . . . [so] protecting the ill family member from painful information is seen as essential for keeping the family together and not allowing the ill member to suffer alone" (1992, p. 1662). Given such an interpretation, Pellegrino advises that "to thrust the truth or the decision on a patient who expects to be buffered

against news of impending death is a gratuitous and harmful misinterpretation of the moral foundations for respect for autonomy" (1992, p. 1735).

Similar reasoning informs Nicholas Christakis's recommendation that researchers be sensitive to cultural definitions of personhood and ethical norms governing informed consent for AIDS vaccine trials in Africa (1988). On the other hand, Carel IJsselmuiden and Ruth Faden (1992) caution against the use of cultural arguments supporting the wholesale disregard of informed consent, especially in the context of contemporary African society, where radical changes have restructured traditional communal beliefs and social organization. They argue that the appeal to cultural sensitivity may well mask other, less benign motives related to expediency of experimentation and development of pharmaceutical markets among African populations.

HIV/AIDS and information disclosure

The AIDS epidemic has brought additional challenges to the issue of truth-telling in clinical settings. Until effective pharmaceutical therapies are developed, HIV will remain a fatal condition and thus will bear the psychological and social weight of this prognosis. Furthermore, in the United States and elsewhere, the virus carries a stigma due to its association with socially marginalized populations: homosexuals, illegal intravenous drug users, and prostitutes. The very real threat of discrimination and abuse of persons who are HIV-positive has brought renewed seriousness to the need for safeguarding patient confidentiality and has necessitated careful examination of decisions to disclose patients' HIV status to patients and others. At the same time, however, clinicians often must balance this concern for patient confidentiality with their duty to warn others who may be at risk of unprotected exposure to the virus.

A number of studies have explored the question of who should know someone's HIV status. The patient? Not all patients who are tested for HIV want to know their test results (Lyter et al., 1987). Nor is it clear whether children with HIV will benefit from learning about their diagnosis, and if so, at what age.

Attention has also been paid to the question of who, besides the person with HIV, needs to be informed about that person's infection. Samuel Perry and his colleagues (1990) surveyed forty gay men in New York about whom they voluntarily told when they learned of their positive test results. Most of the sample had told their personal physicians and current sexual partners; however, most had not tried to contact their former sexual partners. A Los Angeles study of men with HIV reported that half of those who had been sexually active since learning of their condition had kept their infection secret from one or more partners (Marks et al., 1991). If patients with HIV are reluctant to talk about their infection, who should disclose this information to those at risk? A South Carolina study of sexual partners showed that a contact-tracing program through the health department was acceptable to that research sample (Jones et al., 1990).

Health providers do not agree on the issue of who should know someone's HIV status. According to a study of mainland United States and Puerto Rican health providers' opinions, the range of people who should know about a mother's or infant's HIV is subjective and seemingly without limit, potentially including many clinical and administrative hospital personnel, as well as patients' formal and informal support systems (Dougherty et al., 1990). The issue of whether health providers with HIV should disclose this information to their patients raises special concern among health providers, their patients, and the public (Gramelspacher et al., 1990).

Conclusion

This review of research about attitudes toward information disclosure reveals a diversity of opinion on the subject. Numerous factors enter into considerations of whether and what to tell patients and research subjects about their conditions, treatments, or risks of experimentation. Variation in cultural expectations for patients and their caregivers influences what information will be told, to whom, and in what manner. Personal and social characteristics of providers and patients, such as their age, social class, and orientation to death, also shape the content and process of communication in clinical encounters. The specific clinical, environmental, and economic circumstances of such encounters can further define preferences for what is told and how it is told. Given this contextual complexity, ethical concerns regarding information disclosure are likely to continue to demand sensitivity, thoughtfulness, and skillful communication from clinicians, patients, and ethicists in the future.

KATE H. BROWN

Directly related to this article is the companion article in this entry: ETHICAL ISSUES. *For a further discussion of topics mentioned in this article, see the entries* AIDS; CONFIDENTIALITY; DEATH; DEATH, ATTITUDES TOWARD; HARM; INFORMED CONSENT; LAW AND BIOETHICS; *and* PROFESSIONAL–PATIENT RELATIONSHIP. *This article will find application in the entries* AUTONOMY; *and* PATERNALISM. *For a discussion of related ideas, see the entries* CONFLICT OF INTEREST; FAMILY; FIDELITY AND LOYALTY; HOMOSEXUALITY; MEDICAL INFORMATION SYSTEMS; PAIN AND SUFFERING; PRIVILEGED COMMUNICATIONS; PROSTITUTION; SUICIDE; *and* TRUST.

Bibliography

BLANCHARD, CHRISTINA G.; LABRECQUE, MARK S.; RUCK-DESCHEL, JOHN C.; and BLANCHARD, EDWARD B. 1988. "Information and Decision-Making Preferences of Hospitalized Adult Cancer Patients." *Social Science and Medicine* 27, no. 11:1139–1145.

CHRISTAKIS, NICHOLAS A. 1988. "The Ethical Design of an AIDS Vaccine Trial in Africa." *Hastings Center Report* 18, no. 3:31–37.

CHRISTENSEN-SZALANSKI, JAY J.; BOYCE, W. THOMAS; HARREL, HARRIET; and GARDNER, MARY M. 1987. "Circumcision and Informed Consent: Is More Information Always Better?" *Medical Care* 25, no. 9:856–867.

DAVIS, ANNE J., and JAMETON, ANDREW L. 1987. "Nursing and Medical Student Attitudes Toward Nursing Disclosure of Information to Patients: A Pilot Study." *Journal of Advanced Nursing* 12, no. 6:691–698.

DOUGHERTY, CHARLES; BROWN, KATE; PINCH, WINIFRED; ALLEGRETTI, JOSEPH; EDWARDS, BARBA; and MCCARTHY, VIRGINIA. 1990. "Ethical Challenges of Pediatric AIDS." *Medical Ethics* 5, no. 4:1–2, 10.

EGGERMAN, SINDA, and DUSTIN, DICK. 1985. "Death Orientation and Communication with the Terminally Ill." *Omega* 16, no. 3:255–265.

ELL, KATHLEEN; NISHIMOTO, ROBERT; MORVAY, TZIPORA; MANTELL, JOANNE; and HAMOVITCH, MAURICE A. 1989. "A Longitudinal Analysis of Psychological Adaptation Among Survivors of Cancer." *Cancer* 63, no. 2: 406–413.

ERDE, EDMUND L.; NADAL, EVAN C.; and SCHOLL, THERESA O. 1988. "On Truth Telling and the Diagnosis of Alzheimer's Disease." *Journal of Family Practice* 26, no. 4:401–406.

FADEN, RUTH R.; BECKER, CATHERINE; LEWIS, CAROL; FREEMAN, JOHN; and FADEN, ALAN I. 1981. "Disclosure of Information to Patients in Medical Care." *Medical Care* 19, no. 7:718–733.

GRAMELSPACHER, GREGORY P.; MILES, STEPHEN H.; and CASSEL, CHRISTINE K. 1990. "When the Doctor Has AIDS." *Journal of Infectious Diseases* 162, no. 2:534–537.

GREENBERG, LARRIE W.; JEWETT, LESLIE S.; GLUCK, RITA S.; CHAMPION, LORRAINE A.; LEIKIN, SANFORD L.; ALTIERI, MICHAEL F.; and LIPNICK, ROBERT N. 1984. "Giving Information for a Life-Threatening Diagnosis: Parents' and Oncologists' Perceptions." *American Journal of Diseases of Children* 138, no. 7:649–653.

HATTORI, HIROYUKI; SALZBURG, STEPHAN M.; KIANG, WINSTON P.; FUJIMIYA, TATSUYA; TEJIMA, YUTAKA; and FURUNO, JUNJI. 1991. "The Patient's Right to Information in Japan—Legal Rules and Doctor's Opinions." *Social Science and Medicine* 32, no. 9:1007–1016.

HOFFMASTER, C. BARRY; STEWART, MOIRA A.; and CHRISTIE, RONALD J. 1991. "Ethical Decision Making by Family Doctors in Canada, Britain, and the United States." *Social Science and Medicine* 33, no. 6:647–653.

IJSSELMUIDEN, CAREL B., and FADEN, RUTH R. 1992. "Research and Informed Consent in Africa—Another Look." *New England Journal of Medicine* 326, no. 12:830–833.

JONES, JEFFREY L.; WYKOFF, RANDOLPH F.; HOLLIS, SHIRLEY

L.; LONGSHORE, SHARON T.; GAMBLE, WILLIAM B.; and GUNN, ROBERT A. 1990. "Partner Acceptance of Health Department Notification of HIV Exposure, South Carolina." *Journal of the American Medical Association* 264, no. 10:1284–1286.

KELLY, WILLIAM D., and FRIESEN, STANLEY R. 1950. "Do Cancer Patients Want to Be Told?" *Surgery* 27, no. 6: 822–826.

KEOWN, CHARLES; SLOVIC, PAUL; and LICHTENSTEIN, SARAH. 1984. "Attitudes of Physicians, Pharmacists, and Laypersons Toward Seriousness and Need for Disclosure of Prescription Drug Side Effects." *Health Psychology* 3, no. 1: 1–11.

KESSLER, HOWARD W. 1977. "Preoperative Education and the Informed Patient." *Legal Aspects of Medical Practice* 5, no. 10:46–49.

LYTER, DAVID W.; VALDISERRI, RONALD O.; KINGSLEY, LAWRENCE A.; AMOROSO, WILLIAM P.; and RINALDO, CHARLES R., JR. 1987. "The HIV Antibody Test: Why Gay and Bisexual Men Want or Do Not Want to Know Their Results." *Public Health Reports* 102, no. 5:468–474.

MARKS, GARY; RICHARDSON, JEAN L.; and MALDONADO, NORMA. 1991. "Self-Disclosure of HIV Infection to Sexual Partners." *American Journal of Public Health* 81, no. 10:1321–1322.

MATHEWS, JOAN J. 1983. "The Communication Process in Clinical Settings." *Social Science and Medicine* 17, no. 18:1371–1378.

MEADOR, CLIFTON K. 1992. "Hex Death: Voodoo Magic or Persuasion?" *Southern Medical Journal* 85, no. 3:244–247.

MORREIM, E. HAAVI. 1991. "Economic Disclosure and Economic Advocacy: New Duties in the Medical Standard of Care." *Journal of Legal Medicine* 12, no. 3:275–329.

MURDOCH, J. C. 1983. "Communication of the Diagnosis of Down's Syndrome and Spina Bifida in Scotland." *Journal of Mental Deficiency Research* 27, pt. 4:247–253.

NOVACK, DENNIS H.; DETERING, BARBARA J.; ARNOLD, ROBERT; FORROW, LACHLAN; LADINSKY, MORISSA; and PEZZULLO, JOHN C. 1989. "Physicians' Attitudes Toward Using Deception to Resolve Difficult Ethical Problems." *Journal of the American Medical Association* 261, no. 20:2980–2985.

NOVACK, DENNIS H.; PLUMER, ROBIN; SMITH, RAYMOND L.; OCHITILL, HERBERT; MORROW, GARY R.; and BENNETT, JOHN M. 1979. "Changes in Physicians' Attitudes Toward Telling the Cancer Patient." *Journal of the American Medical Association* 241, no. 9:897–900.

PELLEGRINO, EDMUND D. 1992. "Is Truth Telling to the Patient a Cultural Artifact?" *Journal of the American Medical Association* 268, no. 13:1734–1735.

PERRY, SAMUEL; RYAN, JOANNE; FOGEL, KAREN; FISHMAN, BARUCH; and JACOBSBERG, LAWRENCE. 1990. "Voluntarily Informing Others of Positive HIV Test Results: Patterns of Notification by Infected Gay Men." *Hospital and Community Psychiatry* 41, no. 5:549–551.

QUINE, LYN, and PAHL, JAN. 1986. "First Diagnosis of Severe Mental Handicap: Characteristics of Unsatisfactory Encounters Between Doctors and Parents." *Social Science and Medicine* 22, no. 1:53–62.

REID, A.; BENNETT-EMSLIE, G.; ADAMS, L.; and KAYE, S. B. 1988. "What Should We Tell Patients with Cancer?" *Scottish Medical Journal* 33, no. 3:260.

REYNOLDS, PATRICIA M.; SANSON-FISHER, R. W.; POOLE, A. DESMOND; HARKER, JENNIFER; and BYRNE, MICHAEL J. 1981. "Cancer and Communication: Information-giving in an Oncology Clinic." *British Medical Journal* 282, no. 6274:1449–1451.

SIMES, R. J.; TATTERSALL, M. H. N.; COATES, A. S.; RAGHAVEN, D.; SOLOMON, H. J.; and SMARTT, H. 1986. "Randomized Comparison of Procedures for Obtaining Consent in Clinical Trials of Treatment for Cancer." *British Medical Journal* 293, no. 6554:1065–1068.

STILL, ARTHUR W., and TODD, CHRIS J. 1986. "Role Ambiguity in General Practice: The Care of Patients Dying at Home." *Social Science and Medicine* 23, no. 5:519–525.

SURBONE, ANTONELLA. 1992. "Truth Telling to the Patient." *Journal of the American Medical Association* 268, no. 13:1661–1662.

SUTHERLAND, H. J.; LLEWELLYN-THOMAS, H. A.; LOCKWOOD, G. A.; TRITCHLER, D. L.; and TILL, J. E. 1989. "Cancer Patients: Their Desire for Information and Participation in Treatment Decisions." *Journal of the Royal Society of Medicine* 82, no. 5:261–263.

TAKAHASHI, YOSHITOMO. 1990. "Informing a Patient of Malignant Illness: Commentary from a Cross-Cultural Viewpoint." *Death Studies* 14, no. 1:83–91.

TAYLOR, KATHRYN M. 1988. "Physicians and the Disclosure of Undesirable Information." In *Biomedicine Examined,* pp. 441–463. Edited by Margaret M. Lock and Deborah R. Gordon. Dordrecht, Netherlands: Kluwer.

TAYLOR, KATHRYN M., and KELNER, MERRIJOY. 1987. "Informed Consent: The Physician's Perspective." *Social Science and Medicine* 24, no. 2:135–143.

TODD, CHRIS J., and STILL, ARTHUR W. 1984. "Communication Between General Practitioners and Patients Dying at Home." *Social Science and Medicine* 18, no. 8:667–672.

VALLELY, STEPHEN R., and MILLS, J. O. MANTON. 1990. "Should Radiologists Talk to Patients?" *British Medical Journal* 300, no. 6724:305–306.

VISWANATHAN, RAMASWAMY; CLARK, JULIAN J.; and VISWANATHAN, KUSUM. 1986. "Physicians' and the Public's Attitudes on Communication About Death." *Archives of Internal Medicine* 146, no. 10:2029–2033.

WAITZKIN, HOWARD. 1985. "Information Giving in Medical Care." *Journal of Health and Social Behavior* 26, no. 2: 81–101.

WERTZ, DOROTHY C.; and FLETCHER, JOHN C. 1987. "Communicating Genetic Risks." *Science, Technology, and Human Values* 12, nos. 3–4:60–66.

II. ETHICAL ISSUES

Since 1970, ethically recommended health-care practice in the United States has increasingly supported a high level of information disclosure to patients. This article reviews the change, notes some reasons for it, and explores several concerns about disclosure and its implications for particular information types.

Philosophical background of current opinion

Generally, philosophical discussion has supported veracity as a moral principle, obligation, or virtue. Veracity draws its strength from the complex support it provides to diverse values—respecting others, avoiding coercion and manipulation, supporting community, maintaining reciprocity in relationships, supporting the value of communication generally, eliminating the costs and complexities of deception, refraining from unduly assuming responsibility, and maintaining trust.

Philosophers have generally treated veracity as an obligation flowing from more fundamental theoretical principles, such as utility, religious duty, respect for persons, or some combination of beneficence, fidelity, and autonomy. John Stuart Mill, for instance, regarded truth-telling as justified by utilitarian considerations, and W. D. Ross included honesty among the duties of fidelity. A few have given it more basic status. Some theologians, such as Dietrich Bonhoeffer, have set truth telling in the context of greater religious truths and treated false doctrines as forms of deception. Aristotle described falsehood as "in itself mean and culpable" (Bok, 1978, p. 24); G. J. Warnock listed veracity as a major virtue with the same status as beneficence and justice. Immanuel Kant and Augustine are notable for having defended truth-telling most strongly. In a brief article, Kant argued that it would be wrong to lie even to a murderer seeking the hiding place of an intended victim.

However, not all theorists have defended veracity; Henry Sidgwick denied that it could stand as a "definite moral axiom" because of its variable applications and numerous exceptions (Bok, 1978, p. 293). David Nyberg argued that trusting relationships among people normally require "the adroit management of deception" (Nyberg, 1993, p. 24). Moreover, most philosophers have defended deception in at least some cases. Plato defended lying to the public for the sake of society as a whole, and many philosophers have warranted deception when truthfulness might result in serious harm (Bok, 1978).

Application to health care

Until the late twentieth century, philosophers often regarded a physician's withholding a fatal diagnosis from a patient as a stock exception to general precepts of veracity. Philosophers and physicians regarded the distress expected from such news as sufficiently harmful to outweigh the presumption favoring disclosure. Withholding a fatal diagnosis functioned as a paradigm for sharing other medical information with patients. The ethical tradition concerning the doctor–patient relationship thus tended, with some notable exceptions such as Worthington Hooker and Richard Cabot, to emphasize the obligations of confidentiality and to ignore and even deprecate disclosure (Radovsky, 1985). Oaths and codes omitted truth telling, and precepts and discussions of talking with patients tended to recommend caution in revealing information. Ethicists perceived the doctor–patient relationship as oriented to therapy, reassurance, and avoiding harm; physicians were to provide lies and truth instrumentally only insofar as they aided therapy.

Since the 1960s, opinion on the role of disclosure in health care has changed rapidly in the United States. The patients' rights movement and the rise of bioethics have created a climate of opinion supporting honest disclosure of medical information. The affirmation in 1972 of "A Patient's Bill of Rights" by the Board of Trustees of the American Hospital Association notably marked this shift in opinion. The bill stated, "The patient has the right to obtain from his physician complete current information concerning his diagnosis, treatment, and prognosis in terms the patient can be reasonably expected to understand" (Lee and Jacobs, 1973, p. 41).

These changes in opinion developed in concert with the spread of informed consent as standard practice in research and therapy. Informed consent derived from a view of respect for persons that emphasized an individual's power to make decisions adequately. This view required honest disclosure. Thus, most ethicists in the 1970s and 1980s supported fuller disclosure as a means of respecting patient autonomy (Katz, 1984).

The patients' rights movement favored empowering patients and increasing their control over medical care. As Howard Waitzkin argued in his observations of physicians' communications with patients, the traditional pattern of withholding information reflected a habit of dominating patients and keeping the course of therapy firmly under professional control (Waitzkin, 1991). Reformers saw a wider patient understanding of care as supporting a less paternalistic and more contractual relationship, as well as empowering particular classes of patients, such as women and people of color. Susan Sherwin, for example, identified one of the main tasks of feminist health-care ethics as being to increase equity "by distributing the specialized knowledge on health matters in ways that allow persons maximum control over their own health" (Sherwin, 1992, p. 93).

The codes of ethics of the health professions began to reflect this important shift in opinion. The American Nurses' Association's Code for Nurses linked disclosure with truth-telling and self-determination: "Clients have the moral right . . . to be given accurate information, and all the information necessary for making informed judgments." The code counseled nurses to avoid "claims that are false, fraudulent, misleading, deceptive, or unfair" in their relations with the public (American Nurses' Association, 1985, p. 2). The 1980 revision of the American Medical Association's "Principles of Medical

Ethics" included the principle, "A physician shall deal honestly with patients and colleagues, and strive to expose those physicians deficient in character or competence, or who engage in fraud or deception" (Council on Ethical and Judicial Affairs, 1989, p. ix). The American College of Physicians' (ACP) Ethics Manual recommended that patients be "well informed to make health care decisions and work intelligently in partnership with the physician." The manual advised that communication can "dispel uncertainty and fear and enhance healing and patient satisfaction." In general, the ACP held, "disclosure to patients is a fundamental ethical requirement" (1992, p. 950). Subspecialty ethics codes—such as those of the American Academy of Orthopaedic Surgeons, the World Psychiatric Association, and the American College of Obstetricians and Gynecologists—also began to include recommendations supporting veracity.

Changing contexts for veracity in health care

While a high level of disclosure became the recommended practice, cross-currents of thought emerged regarding the motivations for informing patients. First, observers discussed the psychological benefits and risks of giving patients bad news. Second, the increasingly institutional setting of health-care practice influenced patterns of disclosure. Third, discussion distinguished the obligation to disclose information from the obligation to refrain from lying. Fourth, the uncertainty of medicine modulated the obligation to disclose. Finally, an increasing philosophical emphasis on relational aspects of practitioner–patient ethics broadened the foundations for veracity beyond the single element of respect for autonomy.

Healthy disclosure.   Medical works prior to the 1970s tended to assume that revealing a fatal diagnosis would cause patients to experience painful emotions, commit suicide, refuse needed care, or give up hope and die more swiftly. In her important work *Lying: Moral Choice in Public and Private Life*, Sissela Bok argued that traditionalists exaggerated such problems. Patients generally want to be informed, and the benefits to a well-informed and cooperating patient outweigh the risks of disclosure (Bok, 1978). Others supplied case histories illustrating the emotional perils of withholding a terminal diagnosis from vulnerable and trusting patients (Dunbar, 1990; Sherwin, 1992).

Elisabeth Kübler-Ross provided crucial support for the psychological benefits of disclosure by her research on the emotional processes of coming to terms with expected death. In extensive interviews with dying cancer patients, she observed that patients' initial negativity was normally followed by a staged sequence of feelings resolving in acceptance with hope. She regarded disclo-

sure as part of the healthy process of maintaining ongoing communication with dying patients, and her stage theory permitted clinicians to engage in a therapeutic process around disclosure of a fatal diagnosis. The hospice movement accepted this perspective as key to humane care of the dying. Kübler-Ross nevertheless strongly opposed disclosing detailed predictions of life expectancy (Kübler-Ross, 1969).

Patients' powerful emotional reactions and personal transformations during grave illnesses involve caregivers in intimate, significant connections with patients. The belief that knowledge of death is healthy has changed the image of the clinician from that of maintaining a cool distance to one of performing emotional work with patients (Hochschild, 1983). Ethicists often suggested that health professionals who withheld information from patients reflected several concerns: denial of their own and the patient's fear of dying, unconscious wishes to foster dependency in their clients, concern that discussing death constituted admitting failure, and manipulation of hope to encourage more extensive treatment choices.

Some commentators have challenged the positive emotional benefits of discussing death. Ernest Becker argued that the fear of death is too powerfully terrifying to permit most people to accept it (Becker, 1973). Some studies have found at least a few patients showing regret over being informed (Temmerman, 1992). Others have criticized the cold delivery of information, the image of the physician "bearing down" on the patient with bad news (Byrne, 1990). But in most of the literature, the question has become not whether to tell but how to tell; sharing bad news involves timing and a commitment to continuing empathy, compassion, reassurance, and conversation (Buckman, 1992; Kessel, 1979; Kübler-Ross, 1969; Radovsky, 1985).

The institutional context.   Expanding health-care delivery organizations and complex technologies have multiplied the number of personnel providing patient care. These changes have magnified the obstacles to easily orchestrated and effective deception; a physician must not only deceive the patient and family but also involve dozens of other staff in the process. Institutional growth has also increased the need for accurate recordkeeping to cope with the expanding quantity of information.

Although information flow to patients has traditionally been the responsibility of physicians, other health-care team members spend more time with patients, have the knowledge and opportunity to disclose information to patients and their families, and belong to professions assuming responsibility for educating patients. Coordinating communication has become an organizational challenge as hospital staffing has become more efficient, patient acuity greater, and lengths of stay shorter (Zussman, 1993). Who should talk with the patient when the physician is absent poses ethical questions for staff members, who may feel reluctant to provide information without explicit delegation even though disclosure may be timely for the patient. Nurses experience ethical conflicts when physicians order them to withhold information to which patients are entitled (Chadwick and Tadd, 1992). Staff members may make promises to patients and their families about disclosure, promises that other staff members cannot keep.

Legally, the information in the hospital record belongs to the patient (Annas, 1992), but patients are not employees, and so patients' rights are hard to define procedurally. Patients' responsibility to provide honest disclosure to health-care staff similarly lacks explicit definition. Thus, although large health-care institutions have fostered a need for improved communication with patients and made systematic deception difficult, smoothing the flow of appropriate information to patients presents a daunting institutional task.

Disclosure and deception. The principle of veracity suffers ambiguity; it may simply prohibit lying and deception, or it may express a broader obligation to disclose information. Ethicists have tended to deploy arguments against lying and deception to support a high level of disclosure in health care, because lying and deception have often accompanied withholding information in maintaining illusory hopes. But, one can avoid lies and deception and yet disclose scant information. Since the obligation of full disclosure is role-dependent, supporting it involves considerations beyond criticizing deception. Arguments for full disclosure require normative arguments concerning appropriate relationships of health-care professionals and institutions to patients in their service.

In health care, the principle of full disclosure stands in a reciprocal relationship to the obligation to keep confidentiality. Clinicians often have an obligation to disclose information to the patient, and at the same time, keep the same information from others. Moral judgment requires appreciating the range of application of both principles, that is, knowing which information should be disclosed or withheld in what circumstances (Jonsen and Toulmin, 1988). The more formal arguments justifying disclosure parallel the arguments for informed consent by appealing to autonomy, but broader notions of serving patient psychological good and building relationships provide less clear guidance as to the full extent of disclosure. Although favoring disclosure of a fatal diagnosis, as the worst possible news, has tended to encourage wide disclosure of less frightening information, it is still unclear what patients should or should not be told about hospital procedures, student participation in procedures, financial information, names of manufacturers, opinions on the skills of clinicians, personal information about practitioners, mistakes, and so on.

Doubts and uncertainties. The phrase "information disclosure" connotes a level of certainty absent from many diagnoses, prognoses, and therapeutic options. Do guesses and projections "belong" to the patient as much as the contents of the case record? Kathryn Taylor observed that physicians diagnosing cancer often exaggerate their uncertainty in order to soften the blow of a diagnosis or suppress it in order to hide feelings of doubt (Taylor, 1988). Physicians diagnosing symptoms often consider unlikely possibilities, which would frighten patients if shared unnecessarily with them. Nurses may discover or obtain information about which they are uncertain or lack authority to know and wonder whether or not to share it with patients.

Prevailing uncertainty has motivated some physicians to argue that the truth is so uncertain and variable that veracity is irrelevant to patient care. They argue that prospects and options can be framed in so many ways that clinicians inevitably control patient decisions. Even in the relatively well-studied area of informed consent, what to tell about unlikely dangers remains a contested area. Although some physicians have chosen to limit disclosure on the grounds of uncertainty, David Hilfiker characterized giving false reassurances and concealing uncertainty as forms of dishonest misrepresentation (Hilfiker, 1985).

Building relationships. Although bioethics in the 1970s and 1980s rooted disclosure in autonomous decision making, the practice of disclosure has become so widespread in the United States that it has received support on broader grounds. Feminist ethics began to shift the basis of philosophical discussion from the language of autonomy to the language of caring and community. This trend, by diminishing the use of rights language, might have relaxed the new emphasis on disclosure; however, the trend expanded grounds for it, and a conception of the practitioner–patient relationship developed that sees disclosure as a key element in a good professional–patient relationship, apart from its role in decision making.

Lorraine Code, for instance, noted that there is "no stark dichotomy between interdependence and autonomy" (Code, 1991, p. 74). Howard Brody recommended that as part of the ongoing "conversation" between physicians and patients, physicians should "think out loud" (Brody, 1992, p. 116) in order to share medical reasoning more fully with patients. Charles Lidz and his colleagues found that patients generally wanted procedures explained to them, not to participate in decision making, but as a sign of respect and to assist in therapy (Lidz et al., 1983). Annette Baier advocated the necessity of going beyond the contract model and of appreciating disclosure in a context in which power relationships are unequal (Baier, 1986). Baier emphasized trust in relationships as a priority over decision making. Trust thrives most readily in relationships free of deception and where good mutual communication maintains connections between people.

Specific concerns in disclosure

Although terminal diagnoses have served as the paradigm for exploring disclosure, they cover only a portion of the possible concerns involving communication with patients. This section briefly describes a few of the other concerns. Many can arise, such as using placebos; therapeutic privilege; giving patients information about the costs of care; disclosing brain death to the family; lying to an insurance company to obtain coverage for a treatment or diagnostic test; falsifying records to help patients escape war service or school busing; reporting an accidentally discovered serious condition to the patient when the doctor–patient relationship is undefined; offering information to patients concerning futile therapeutic options; deceptively introducing medical students to patients as "doctor"; concealing the histocompatibility (mutual tolerance of tissues or organs to be grafted) of an unwilling potential organ donor; revealing to patients that a caregiver has tested positive for the human immunodeficiency virus (HIV); revealing HIV diagnoses to patients; encouraging patients to disclose HIV diagnoses to sexual partners; communicating psychiatric interpretations to patients; expecting disclosure by patients to health professionals; and disclosing genetic information to patients.

Diseases lacking effective treatment. When a diagnostic test can predict a dread and incurable disease—such as Huntington or Alzheimer's disease—some physicians consider the possibility of withholding the diagnosis. An instrumental view of communication tends to support the view that the burden to the patient of knowing outweighs the value of disclosure. This concern arose with regard to Huntington disease when a levodopa test became available in the early 1970s; the concern was renewed when genetic marker tests became available in 1983. Although some critics continued to express reservations, genetic counselors tended to find that disclosure helped both patient and family to make long-range plans. Gwen Terrenoire emphasized that a consensus favoring testing and disclosure resulted from counselors working with organized patient groups involved with Huntington disease (Terrenoire, 1992). In 1989, the Huntington Disease Society of America published guidelines for testing for the condition. They recommended counseling patients prior to the screening

decision and before disclosing results. They also recommended against screening patients who have conditions that diminish judgment, while thoroughly evaluating them for suicide risk (DeGrazia, 1991).

Disclosing diagnostic tests. Hospitals and clinics often screen patients upon admission for a wide range of conditions without informing them of the reasons for testing. Services may standardly screen for HIV, sexually transmitted diseases, or pregnancy without informing the patient. They may also wish to make surreptitious tests when they believe a patient is claiming false symptoms. One case study described a patient as suffering from mysterious bruising, which could most probably be explained by drug abuse; she denied taking drugs and refused to permit a blood test. Physicians considered whether to administer the diagnostic test without informing her of its purpose. The discussants of the case argued that a contractual model of the doctor–patient relationship is inadequate because patients frequently lie to physicians and are poor historians. They suggested also that such tests need not be disclosed since they yield such diverse results; they are often based on guesses; and their interpretation depends on patient histories (Vanderpool and Weiss, 1984).

Revealing mistakes to patients. Surely, practitioners should tell patients of mistakes pertinent to their welfare or requiring changes in treatment plans. However, the possibility of lawsuits, the fear of losing patient confidence, painful feelings of incompetence, and solidarity between health-care team members often outweigh patient benefits in frankness regarding errors. Charles Bosk observed that discussion of medical errors tends to be highly ritualized, confined to well-defined hospital subgroups, and used to reaffirm a strong collective sense of competence (Bosk, 1980). Hilfiker, however, in a remarkably frank discussion of his own errors, recommended that patients can be accepting of physician limitations, that maintenance of illusions about competence tends ultimately to undermine trust in physicians, and that hiding mistakes tends to alienate caregivers from the healing process of confessing and handling mistakes (Hilfiker, 1985). The ACP Ethics Manual also recommends disclosing significant "procedural or judgment errors" (ACP, 1992, p. 950).

Patient refusal of information. The bioethics literature has debated the proper handling of patient refusals of information (Ost, 1984; Strasser, 1986). On the one hand, the literature usually has regarded refusing information as an autonomous choice and therefore has supported it: A caregiver may ethically choose to respect a patient's wish to rely more heavily on the caregiver. Raanan Gillon argued that "forcing" information on a patient is both harmful and disrespectful of autonomy (Gillon, 1990). The issue can also be regarded as a feature of relational style; Edmund Pellegrino noted that "some patients need a more authoritative approach than others" (Pellegrino, 1992, p. 1735).

On the other hand, autonomy is not the only basis for disclosure; caregivers have some role-dependent duties to disclose information to the reluctant; and patients have responsibilities as well as rights to use information on their own behalf. Some information may be so surprising and crucial for patients or so necessary for a working partnership that caregivers have an obligation to disclose despite patient protests. Caregivers may feel that a patient's denial is slowing recovery, or that patients may have a duty to act on information, such as that they are HIV-positive, in order to protect others. It is thus doubtful that the question of refusals can be answered generally.

Disclosure to family members. Kübler-Ross suggested entrusting some information to family members rather than the patient (Kübler-Ross, 1969); this has also been the pattern reported in several countries, such as Hungary, Italy, Japan, and China. This approach may result from seeing the patient as "an extension of the family" (Christakis and Fox, 1992, p. 1101), respecting the family as a strongly interdependent unit, or wishing others to carry the burden of knowledge. Yoshitomo Takahashi reported that some Japanese practitioners consider talking about death as threatening family relationships and separating the patient from others (Takahashi, 1990), and Eric Feldman noted that many Japanese practitioners perceive disclosing terminal diagnoses as "a callous practice" (Feldman, 1985, p. 21). However, supporters of patient autonomy have expressed concern that leaving the patient uninformed is more likely to isolate the patient psychologically (Quill and Townsend, 1991). From both perspectives, the main concern appears to be to include the dying patient in the community, but it is difficult to make reliable cross-cultural generalizations because recommended practices, actual practices, and patient attitudes often vary widely within each culture.

Difficult questions balancing disclosure and confidentiality arise in keeping family members appropriately informed along with the patient. The family may be the recipient of disclosure when an unconscious patient is admitted to the hospital; when the patient recovers competency, the pattern of leaving the family in charge may continue or the family may become excluded from communication. Or family members may give clinicians important information about the patient and ask that the patient not be told; however, the ACP Ethics Manual holds that practitioners are "not obliged" to keep such secrets and should "use sensitivity and judgment" in disclosing such information (ACP, 1992, p. 949).

Disclosure in the social arena. Although bioethical discussion has focused primarily on disclosure and honesty at the bedside, similar issues arise in the larger health-care arena. For instance, a study of advertising in medical journals showed that a high proportion of pharmaceutical advertisements failed to meet U.S. Food and Drug Administration standards for honesty (Wilkes et al., 1992). Many physicians rely on advertisements and pharmaceutical representatives for their information. Consequently, deceiving physicians leads to misinformed patients.

Occupational and public-health physicians face conflicts affecting disclosure. For instance, some clinicians and medical researchers cooperated for many years in industry suppression of information on the carcinogenicity of asbestos (Lilienfeld, 1991); other health professionals have been active in political struggles over posting health warnings on cigarette and alcohol labels. In recent years, the U.S. Occupational Safety and Health Administration has expanded workers' rights to know about their exposure to toxic materials in the workplace, although the complexity of state and federal regulations makes application difficult. Pressures arising from fear of litigation, protection of trade secrets, and concern for individual confidentiality create tensions in pursuing public-health goals of improving public health by keeping workers and the public better informed of their exposure (Ashford and Caldart, 1985).

Conclusion

Beneath this sketch of disclosure lie a number of ethical concerns of great subtlety and depth. Brief reflection on honesty links veracity primarily to telling others what one believes. But, the complex interactions between clinicians and patients require clinicians to consider carefully how patients interpret their words; skill in listening to patients has often been identified as the key element in effective patient teaching. Moreover, health professionals bear serious duties to service and science that require them to examine honestly the limits of their knowledge, the help they can promise, and their insights into the meanings of illness and death. Thus, accepting honest disclosure calls upon professionals to reflect deeply on the relationship of medical science to health, the consequences of individual service to public health, and the impact of health-care institutions and practices on the public's understanding of health, illness, and death.

ANDREW JAMETON

Directly related to this article is the companion article in this entry: ATTITUDES TOWARD TRUTH-TELLING. *Also directly related are the entries* INFORMED CONSENT, *articles on* MEANING AND ELEMENTS OF INFORMED CONSENT, *and* CLINICAL ASPECTS OF CONSENT IN HEALTH CARE; FIDELITY AND LOYALTY; PROFESSIONAL–PATIENT RELATION-

SHIP, *article on* ETHICAL ISSUES; *and* PATIENTS' RIGHTS, *article on* ORIGIN AND NATURE OF PATIENTS' RIGHTS. *This article will find application in the entries* ALTERNATIVE THERAPIES, *article on* ETHICAL AND LEGAL ISSUES; DEATH AND DYING: EUTHANASIA AND SUSTAINING LIFE; GENETIC COUNSELING; IATROGENIC ILLNESS AND INJURY; *and* RESEARCH POLICY, *article on* GENERAL GUIDELINES. *For a discussion of related ideas, see the entries* AUTONOMY; BENEFICENCE; FREEDOM AND COERCION; HARM; PATERNALISM; RISK; *and* TRUST. *Other relevant material may be found under the entries* COMMUNICATION, BIOMEDICAL; DEATH, ATTITUDES TOWARD; EXPERT TESTIMONY; FRAUD, THEFT, AND PLAGIARISM; MEDICAL CODES AND OATHS; MEDICINE AS A PROFESSION; RESEARCH, UNETHICAL; *and* WHISTLEBLOWING. *See also the* APPENDIX (CODES, OATHS, AND DIRECTIVES RELATED TO BIOETHICS), SECTION II: ETHICAL DIRECTIVES FOR THE PRACTICE OF MEDICINE, SECTION III: ETHICAL DIRECTIVES FOR OTHER HEALTH-CARE PROFESSIONS, *and* SECTION IV: ETHICAL DIRECTIVES FOR HUMAN RESEARCH.

Bibliography

AMERICAN COLLEGE OF PHYSICIANS (ACP). 1992. "American College of Physicians Ethics Manual: Third Edition." *Annals of Internal Medicine* 117, no. 11:947–960.

AMERICAN NURSES' ASSOCIATION. 1985. *Code for Nurses: With Interpretive Statements.* Washington, D.C.: Author.

ANNAS, GEORGE J. 1992. *The Rights of Patients: The Basic ACLU Guide to Patient Rights.* 2d ed., rev. Totowa, N.J.: Humana.

ASHFORD, NICHOLAS A., and CALDART, CHARLES C. 1985. "The 'Right to Know': Toxics Information Transfer in the Workplace." *Annual Review of Public Health* 6:383–401.

BAIER, ANNETTE. 1986. "Trust and Antitrust." *Ethics* 96, no. 2:231–260.

BECKER, ERNEST. 1973. *The Denial of Death.* New York: Free Press.

BOK, SISSELA. 1978. *Lying: Moral Choice in Public and Private Life.* New York: Vintage.

BOSK, CHARLES L. 1980. "Occupational Rituals in Patient Management." *New England Journal of Medicine* 303, no. 2:71–76.

BRODY, HOWARD. 1992. *The Healer's Power.* New Haven, Conn.: Yale University Press.

BUCKMAN, ROBERT, and KASON, YVONNE. 1992. *How to Break Bad News: A Guide for Health Professionals.* Baltimore: Johns Hopkins University Press.

BYRNE, PETER. 1990. "Comments on an Obstructed Death— A Case Conference Revisited." *Journal of Medical Ethics* 16, no. 2:88–89.

CHADWICK, RUTH F., and TADD, WIN. 1992. *Ethics & Nursing Practice: A Case Study Approach.* Hampshire, U.K.: Macmillan.

CHRISTAKIS, NICHOLAS A., and FOX, RENÉE C. 1992. "Informed Consent in Africa." *New England Journal of Medicine* 327, no. 15:1101–1102.

CODE, LORRAINE. 1991. *What Can She Know? Feminist Theory and the Construction of Knowledge.* Ithaca, N.Y.: Cornell University Press.

COUNCIL ON ETHICAL AND JUDICIAL AFFAIRS. AMERICAN MEDICAL ASSOCIATION. 1989. "Principles of Medical Ethics." In *Current Opinions,* p. ix. Chicago: American Medical Association.

DEGRAZIA, DAVID. 1991. "The Ethical Justification for Minimal Paternalism in the Use of the Predictive Test for Huntington's Disease." *Journal of Clinical Ethics* 2, no. 4:219–228.

DUNBAR, SCOTT. 1990. "An Obstructed Death and Medical Ethics." *Journal of Medical Ethics* 16, no. 2:83–87.

FELDMAN, ERIC. 1985. "Medical Ethics the Japanese Way." *Hastings Center Report* 15, no. 5:21–24.

GILLON, RAANAN. 1990. "Deceit, Principles and Philosophical Medical Ethics." *Journal of Medical Ethics* 16, no. 2: 59–60.

HILFIKER, DAVID. 1985. *Healing the Wounds: A Physician Looks at His Work.* New York: Pantheon.

HOCHSCHILD, ARLIE R. 1983. *The Managed Heart: Commercialization of Human Feeling.* Berkeley: University of California Press.

JONSEN, ALBERT R., and TOULMIN, STEPHEN E. 1988. *The Abuse of Casuistry: A History of Moral Reasoning.* Berkeley: University of California Press.

KATZ, JAY. 1984. *The Silent World of Doctor and Patient.* New York: Free Press.

KESSEL, NEIL. 1979. "Reassurance." *Lancet* 1, no. 8126: 1128–1133.

KÜBLER-ROSS, ELISABETH. 1969. *On Death and Dying.* New York: Macmillan.

LEE, ANDRE L., and JACOBS, GODFREY. 1973. "Workshop Airs Patients' Rights." *Hospitals* 47, no. 4:39–43.

LIDZ, CHARLES W.; MEISEL, ALAN; OSTERWEIS, MARIAN; HOLDEN, JANICE L.; MARX, JOHN H.; and MUNETZ, MARK R. 1983. "Barriers to Informed Consent." *Annals of Internal Medicine* 99, no. 4:539–543.

LILIENFELD, DAVID E. 1991. "The Silence: The Asbestos Industry and Early Occupational Cancer Research—A Case Study." *American Journal of Public Health* 81, no. 16: 791–800.

NYBERG, DAVID. 1993. *The Varnished Truth: Truth Telling and Deceiving in Ordinary Life.* Chicago: University of Chicago Press.

OST, DAVID E. 1984. "The 'Right' Not to Know." *Journal of Medicine and Philosophy* 9, no. 3:301–312.

PELLEGRINO, EDMUND D. 1992. "Is Truth Telling to the Patient a Cultural Artifact?" *Journal of the American Medical Association* 268, no. 13:1734–1735.

QUILL, TIMOTHY E., and TOWNSEND, PENELOPE. 1991. "Bad News: Delivery, Dialogue, and Dilemmas." *Archives of Internal Medicine* 151, no. 3:463–468.

RADOVSKY, SAUL S. 1985. "Bearing the News." *New England Journal of Medicine* 313, no. 9:586–588.

SHERWIN, SUSAN. 1992. *No Longer Patient: Feminist Ethics and Health Care.* Philadelphia: Temple University Press.

STRASSER, MARK. 1986. "Mill and the Right to Remain Uninformed." *Journal of Medicine and Philosophy* 11, no. 3: 265–278.

TAKAHASHI, YOSHITOMO. 1990. "Informing a Patient of a Malignant Illness: Commentary from a Cross-Cultural Viewpoint." *Death Studies* 14, no. 1:83–91.

TAYLOR, KATHRYN M. 1988. "Physicians and the Disclosure of Undesirable Information." In *Biomedicine Examined*, pp. 441–463. Edited by Margaret M. Lock and Deborah R. Gordon. Dordrecht, Netherlands: Kluwer.

TEMMERMAN, MARLEEN. 1992. "Informed Consent in Africa." *New England Journal of Medicine* 327, no. 15:1102–1103.

TERRENOIRE, GWEN. 1992. "Huntington's Disease and the Ethics of Genetic Prediction." *Journal of Medical Ethics* 18, no. 2:79–85.

VANDERPOOL, HAROLD Y., and WEISS, GARY B. 1984. "Patient Truthfulness: A Test of Models of the Physician-Patient Relationship." *Journal of Medicine and Philosophy* 9, no. 4:353–372.

WAITZKIN, HOWARD. 1991. *The Politics of Medical Encounters: How Patients and Doctors Deal with Social Problems.* New Haven, Conn.: Yale University Press.

WILKES, MICHAEL S.; DOBLIN, BRUCE H.; and SHAPIRO, MARTIN F. 1992. "Pharmaceutical Advertisements in Leading Medical Journals: Experts' Assessments." *Annals of Internal Medicine* 116, no. 11:912–919.

ZUSSMAN, ROBERT. 1993. "Life in the Hospital: A Review." *Milbank Quarterly* 71, no. 1:167–185.

INFORMATION SYSTEMS, MEDICAL

See MEDICAL INFORMATION SYSTEMS.

INFORMED CONSENT

I. HISTORY OF INFORMED CONSENT

Informed consent is not an ancient concept with a rich medical tradition. The term "informed consent" first appeared in 1957, and serious discussion of the concept began only around 1972. As the idea of informed consent evolved, discussion of appropriate guidelines moved increasingly from a narrow focus on the physician's or researcher's obligation to disclose information to the quality of a patient's or subject's understanding of information and right to authorize or refuse a biomedical intervention.

Early history of associated ideas

Prior to the late 1950s, there was no firm ground in which a commitment to informed consent could take root. This is not to say, however, that there is no relevant history of the physician's or researcher's management of information in the encounter with patients and subjects. The major writings of prominent figures in ancient, medieval, and modern medicine contain a storehouse of information about commitments to disclosure and discussion in medical practice. But it is a disappointing history from the perspective of informed consent. Beginning with the classic text of ancient medicine, the Hippocratic Corpus, the primary focus of medical ethics became the obligation of physicians to provide medical benefits to patients and to protect them from harm. Thepurpose of medicine as expressed in the Hippocratic oath was to benefit the sick and keep them from harm and injustice. Managing information in interactions with patients was portrayed as a matter of prudence and discretion. The Hippocratic writings did not hint even at obligations of veracity.

Throughout the ancient, medieval, and early modern periods, medical ethics developed predominantly within the profession of medicine. With few exceptions, no serious consideration was given to issues of either consent or self-determination by patients and research subjects. The proper principles, practices, and virtues of truthfulness in disclosure were occasionally discussed, but the perspective was largely one of maximizing medical benefits through the careful management of medical information. The central concern was how to make disclosures without harming patients by revealing their condition too abruptly and starkly. Withholding information and even outright deception were regularly justified as morally appropriate means of avoiding such harm. The emphasis on the principle "First, do no harm" even promoted the idea that a health-care professional is obligated not to make disclosures because to do so would be to risk a harmful outcome.

Eighteenth and nineteenth centuries

Benjamin Rush and John Gregory are sometimes cited for their enlightened views about disclosure and public education in the eighteenth century. However, neither was advocating informed consent; they wanted patients to be sufficiently educated so that they could understand physicians' recommendations and therefore be motivated to comply. They were not even optimistic that patients would form their own opinions and make appropriate medical choices. For example, Rush advised physicians to "yield to [patients] in matters of little consequence, but maintain an inflexible authority over them in matters that are essential to life" (Rush, 1786, p. 323). Gregory (1772) was quick to underscore that the physician must be keenly aware of the harm that untimely revelations might cause. There is no assertion of the importance of respecting rights of self-determination for patients or of obtaining consent for any purpose other than a medically good outcome. Gregory and Rush appreciated the value of information and dialogue from the patient's point of view, but the idea of informed consent was not foreshadowed in their writings.

Thomas Percival's historic *Medical Ethics* (1803) continues in this same tradition. It makes no more mention of consent solicitation and respect for decision making by patients than had previous codes and treatises. Percival did, however, struggle with the issue of truth-telling. He held that the patient's right to the truth must yield to the obligation to benefit the patient in cases of conflict, thereby recommending benevolent deception. Percival maintained that

> [T]o a patient . . . who makes inquiries which, if faithfully answered, might prove fatal to him, it would be a gross and unfeeling wrong to reveal the truth. His right to it is suspended, and even annihilated; because, its beneficial nature being reversed, it would be deeply injurious to himself, to his family, and to the public. And he has the strongest claim, from the trust reposed in his physician, as well as from the common principles of humanity, to be guarded against whatever would be detrimental to him. . . . The only point at issue is, whether the practitioner shall sacrifice that delicate sense of veracity, which is so ornamental to, and indeed forms a characteristic excellence of the virtuous man, to this claim of professional justice and social duty. (Percival, 1803, pp. 165–166)

Percival was struggling against the arguments of his friend, the Rev. Thomas Gisborne, who opposed practices of giving false assertions intended to raise patients' hopes and lying for the patient's benefit: "The physician . . . is invariably bound never to represent the uncertainty or danger as less than he actually believes it to be" (Gisborne, 1794, p. 401). From Percival's perspective, the physician does not lie or act improperly in beneficent acts of deception and falsehood, as long as the objective is to give hope to the dejected or sick patient.

The American Medical Association (AMA) accepted virtually without modification the Percival paradigm in its 1847 "Code of Medical Ethics." Many of the above passages appear almost verbatim in this code as the AMA position on the obligations of physicians in regard to truth-telling (AMA, 1847). This code and most codes of medical ethics before and since do not include rules of veracity although many codes today do contain rules for obtaining an informed consent. For more than a century thereafter, American and British medical ethics developed under Percival's vision.

There was, however, a notable nineteenth-century exception to the consensus that surrounded Percival's recommendations. Connecticut physician Worthington Hooker was the first champion of the rights of patients to information, in opposition to the model of benevolent deception that had reigned from Hippocrates to the AMA (Hooker, 1849). He and Harvard professor of medicine Richard Clarke Cabot were the best known among physicians who championed this model prior to the second half of the twentieth century. Moreover, there may never have been a figure who, in regard to truth-telling, swam so much against the stream of indigenous medical tradition as Hooker.

Hooker's arguments are novel and ingenious but do not amount to a recommendation of informed consent. Hooker was concerned with "the general effect of deception" on society and on medical institutions. He thought the effect disastrous. But in Hooker no more than in the AMA Code is there a recommendation to obtain the permission of patients or to respect autonomy for the sake of autonomy. Hooker's concerns were with expediency in disclosure and truth-telling rather than with the promotion of autonomous decision making or informed consent. The idea that patients should be enabled to understand their situation so that they are able to participate with physicians in decisions about medical treatment was an idea whose time was yet to come.

Although the nineteenth century saw no hint of a rule or practice of informed consent in clinical medicine, consent practices were not entirely absent. Evidence exists in surgery records of consent-seeking practices and rudimentary rules for obtaining consent since at least the middle of the nineteenth century (Pernick, 1982). However, the consents thus obtained do not appear to have been meaningful informed consents, because they had little to do with the patient's right to decide after being appropriately informed. Practices of obtaining consent in surgery prior to the 1950s were pragmatic responses to a combination of concerns about medical reputation, malpractice suits, and practicality in medical institutions. It is at best physically difficult and interpersonally awkward to perform surgery on a patient without obtaining the patient's permission. Such practices of obtaining permission, however, do not constitute practices of obtaining informed consent, although they did provide a modest nineteenth-century grounding for this twentieth-century concept.

The situation is similar in research involving human subjects. Little evidence exists that, until recently, requirements of informed consent had a significant hold on the practice of investigators. In the nineteenth century, for example, it was common for research to be conducted on slaves and servants without acquiescence or consent on the part of the subject. By contrast, at the turn of the century, American army surgeon Walter Reed's yellow-fever experiments involved formal procedures for obtaining the consent of potential subjects. Although deficient by contemporary standards of disclosure and consent, these procedures recognized the right of the individual to refuse or authorize participation in the research. The extent to which this principle became ingrained in the ethics of research by the mid-twentieth century is a matter of historical controversy. Although it has often been reported that the obtaining of informed and voluntary consent was essential to the ethics of research and was commonplace in biomedical investigation, it is unclear that consent seeking on the part of investigators was standard practice. Anecdotal evidence suggests that biomedical research often proceeded without adequate consent at least into the 1960s.

Early twentieth-century legal history

The legal history of disclosure obligations and rights of self-determination for patients evolved gradually. It is the nature of legal precedent that each decision, relying on earlier court opinions, joins a chain of authority that incorporates the relevant language and reasoning from the cited cases. In this way, a few early consent cases built on each other to eventuate in a legal doctrine. The best known and ultimately the most influential of these early cases is *Schloendorff* v. *New York Hospital* (1914). *Schloendorff* used rights of "self-determination" to justify imposing an obligation to obtain a patient's consent. Subsequent cases that followed and relied upon *Schloendorff* implicitly adopted its justifactory rationale. In this way, self-determination came to be the primary rationale or justification for legal requirements that consent be obtained from patients.

In the early twentieth century, the behavior of physicians was often egregious, and courts did not shrink from using ringing language and sweeping principles to denounce it. The same language was then applied as precedent in later cases in which physicians' behavior was less outrageous. As the informed-consent doctrine developed and problems grew more subtle, the law could have turned away from the language of self-determination but instead increasingly relied on this rationale as its fundamental premise. The language in the early cases suggests that rights of freedom from bodily invasion contain rights of medical decision making by patients.

The 1950s and 1960s: Law and medicine

The emerging legal doctrine of informed consent first brought the concept of informed consent to the attention of the medical community. "The doctrine of in-

formed consent" is a legal doctrine; and informed consent has often been treated as synonymous with this legal doctrine. A remarkable series of cases in the second half of the twentieth century brought informed consent to the attention of lawyers and physicians alike.

During the 1950s and 1960s, the traditional duty to obtain consent evolved into a new, explicit duty to disclose certain types of information and then to obtain consent. This development needed a new term; and so "informed" was added onto "consent," creating the expression "informed consent," in the landmark decision in *Salgo* v. *Leland Stanford, Jr. University Board of Trustees* (1957). The *Salgo* court suggested, without accompanying analysis, that the duty to disclose the risks and alternatives of treatment was not a new duty but a logical extension of the already established duty to disclose the treatment's nature and consequences. Nonetheless, *Salgo* clearly introduced new elements into the law. The *Salgo* court was not interested merely in whether a recognizable consent had been given to the proposed procedures. Instead, *Salgo* focused strongly on the problem of whether the consent had been adequately informed. The court thus created not only the language but the substance of informed consent by invoking the same right of self-determination that had heretofore applied only to a less robust consent requirement.

Shortly thereafter, two opinions by the Kansas Supreme Court in the case of *Natanson* v. *Kline* (1960) pioneered the use of the legal charge of negligence in informed-consent cases, rather than that of battery. The court established the duty of disclosure as the obligation "to disclose and explain to the patient in language as simple as necessary the nature of the ailment, the nature of the proposed treatment, the probability of success or of alternatives, and perhaps the risks of unfortunate results and unforeseen conditions within the body" (*Natanson* v. *Kline*, 1960). Thus, the *Natanson* court required essentially the same extensive disclosure—of the nature, consequences, risks, and alternatives of a proposed procedure—as had *Salgo*. After *Natanson*, battery and negligence appeared virtually identical in their disclosure requirements for informed consent.

Not surprisingly, the number of articles in the medical literature on issues of consent increased substantially following these and other legal cases. Typically written by lawyers, these reports functioned to alert physicians both to informed consent as a new legal development and to potential malpractice risk. How physicians reacted to these legal developments in the 1950s and 1960s is not well documented, but a handful of empirical studies of informed consent in clinical medicine provides some insights. A study done in the early to mid-1960s indicates that a preoperative consent form was not yet a ubiquitous feature of the practice of surgery. Surgeons at several hospitals refused to participate in this study precisely because they were not using a consent form for surgery.

This indifference to consent procedures seems to have changed by the late 1960s, when most physicians appear to have come to recognize both a moral and a legal duty to obtain consent for certain procedures and to provide some kind of disclosure. There is also evidence, however, that physicians' views about proper consent practices even in the late 1960s differed markedly from the consensus of opinion and convention today. For example, in one study, half of the physicians surveyed thought it medically proper, and 30 percent ethically proper, for a physician to perform a mastectomy with no authorization from the patient other than her signature on the blanket consent form required for hospital admission; more than half the physicians thought that it was ethically appropriate for a physician not to tell a cancer patient that she had been enrolled in a double-blind clinical trial of an experimental anticancer drug.

On the basis of the volume of commentary in the medical literature, many physicians before the 1970s were at least dimly aware of informed consent. Empirical studies conducted at the time suggest that there was at least enough documentable consent seeking in such areas as surgery, organ donation, and angiography to warrant empirical investigation. Also during this period, the procedure-specific consent form was gaining acceptance, although it was not yet universally in use. Whether in the 1960s physicians generally regarded informed consent as a legal nuisance or as an important moral problem is unclear, but an explosion of commentary on informed consent emerged in the medical literature in the early 1970s. Much of this commentary was negative: Physicians saw the demands of informed consent as impossible to fulfill and—at least in some cases—inconsistent with good patient care. In tone the articles ranged from serious critique to caustic parody. Predictions were voiced that fearful patients would refuse needed surgery after disclosure. In much of this literature, only the legal, not the moral dimensions of informed-consent requirements were recognized. This began to change in the 1970s, with the ascendancy of an interdisciplinary approach to medical ethics. Gradually, informed consent became a moral as well as a legal issue.

The 1950s and 1960s: Biomedical research

The histories of informed consent in research and in clinical medicine have developed largely as separate pieces in a larger mosaic of biomedical ethics, and these pieces have never been well integrated even when they developed side by side. Research ethics prior to World War II was no more influential on research practices than the parallel history of clinical-medicine ethics was on clinical practices. But one event that unquestionably influenced thought about informed consent was the Nuremberg trials. The Nuremberg military tribunals unambiguously condemned the sinister political motivation of Nazi experiments in their review of "crimes against humanity." A list of ten principles constituted the Nuremberg Code. Principle One of the code states, without qualification, that the primary consideration in research is the subject's voluntary consent, which is "absolutely essential" (Germany [Territory Under Allied Occupation], 1947).

The Nuremberg Code served as a model for many professional and governmental codes formulated in the 1950s and 1960s, but several other incidents involving consent violations subsequently moved the discussion of post-Nuremberg problems into the public arena. Thus began a rich and complex interplay of influences on research ethics: scholarly publications, journalism, public outrage, legislation, and case law. In the United States, one of the first incidents to achieve notoriety in research ethics involved a study conducted at the Jewish Chronic Disease Hospital (JCDH) in Brooklyn, New York. In July 1963, Dr. Chester Southam of the Sloan-Kettering Institute for Cancer Research persuaded the hospital's medical director, Emmanuel E. Mandel, to permit research involving injection of a suspension of foreign, live cancer cells into twenty-two patients at the JCDH. The objective was to discover whether a decline in the body's capacity to reject cancer transplants was caused by the cancer or by debilitation. Patients without cancer were needed to supply the answer. Southam had convinced Mandel that although the research was nontherapeutic, such research was routinely done without consent. Some patients were informed orally that they were involved in an experiment, but it was not disclosed that they were being given injections of cancer cells. No written consent was attempted, and some subjects were incompetent to give informed consent. The Board of Regents of the State University of New York later censured Southam and Mandel for their role in the research. They were found guilty of fraud, deceit, and unprofessional conduct (*Hyman* v. *Jewish Chronic Disease Hospital*, 1964).

Another major controversy about the ethics of research in the United States developed at Willowbrook State School, an institution for "mentally defective" children in Staten Island, New York. Beginning in 1956, Saul Krugman and his associates began a series of experiments to develop an effective prophylactic agent for infectious hepatitis. They deliberately infected newly admitted patients with isolated strains of the virus based on parental consents obtained under controversial circumstances that may have been manipulative. The issues in the Willowbrook case are more complex than those in the Jewish Chronic Disease Hospital case, and today there are those who still defend, at least in part, the ethics of these experiments. Krugman's research unit was eventually closed, but closure on the debate about the ethics of the studies conducted in the unit was never achieved (New York University, 1972).

The most notorious case of prolonged and knowing violation of subjects' rights in the United States was a Public Health Service (PHS) study initiated in the early 1930s. Originally designed as one of the first syphilis-control demonstrations in the United States, the stated purpose of the Tuskegee syphilis study, as it is now called, was to compare the health and longevity of an untreated syphilitic population with a nonsyphilitic but otherwise similar population. These subjects, all African-American males, knew neither the name nor the nature of their disease. That they were participants in a nontherapeutic experiment also went undisclosed. They were informed only that they were receiving free treatment for "bad blood," a term local African-Americans associated with a host of unrelated ailments, but which the white physicians allegedly assumed was a local euphemism for syphilis (Jones, 1981).

Perhaps the most remarkable thing about Tuskegee was that, although the study was reviewed several times between 1932 and 1970 by PHS officials and medical societies as well as reported in thirteen articles in prestigious medical and public-health journals, it continued uninterrupted and without serious challenge. It was not until 1972 that the U.S. Department of Health, Education and Welfare (DHEW) appointed an ad hoc advisory panel to review the study and the department's policies and procedures for the protection of human subjects. The panel found that neither DHEW nor any other government agency had a uniform or adequate policy for reviewing experimental procedures or securing subjects' consents.

The 1970s and 1980s

Although the Jewish Chronic Disease Hospital case, the Willowbrook study, and the Tuskegee study had a profound effect on public consciousness with respect to the ethics of research and medicine, these events are insufficient to explain why informed consent became the focus of so much attention in both case law and biomedical ethics between the late 1960s and the late 1980s. Many hypotheses can be invoked to explain this phenomenon. Perhaps the most accurate explanation is that law and ethics, as well as medicine itself, were all affected by issues and concerns in the wider society about individual liberties and social equality, made dramatic by an increasingly technological, powerful, and impersonal medical-care system. It seems likely that in-

creased legal interest in the right of self-determination and increased philosophical interest in the principle of respect for autonomy and individualism were instances of the new rights orientation that various social movements had introduced. The issues raised by civil rights, women's rights, the consumer movement, and the rights of prisoners and the mentally ill often included health-care components and helped reinforce public acceptance of rights applied to health care. Informed consent was swept along with this body of social concerns, which propelled the new bioethics throughout the 1970s.

Three 1972 court decisions are widely recognized as informed consent landmarks: *Canterbury v. Spence, Cobbs v. Grant,* and *Wilkinson v. Vesey. Canterbury* had a massive influence. In its most significant and dramatic finding, the *Canterbury* court moved in the direction of a more patient-oriented standard of disclosure:

> The patient's right of self-decision can be effectively exercised only if the patient possesses enough information to enable an intelligent choice. The patient should make his own determination on treatment. Informed consent is a basic social policy for which exceptions are permitted (1) where the patient is unconscious or otherwise incapable of consenting, and harm from failure to treat is imminent; or (2) when risk-disclosure poses such a serious psychological threat of detriment to the patient as to be medically contraindicated. Social policy does not accept the paternalistic view that the physician may remain silent because divulgence might prompt the patient to forego needed therapy. Rational, informed patients should not be expected to act uniformly, even under similar circumstances, in agreeing to or refusing treatment. (*Canterbury v. Spence,* 1972)

As the impact of *Canterbury* filtered down to medical practice, the U.S. National Commission for the Protection of Human Subjects of Biomedical and Behavioral Research began in 1974 what would be a four-year struggle with a variety of concerns about informed consent in research involving human subjects. The commission developed an abstract schema of basic ethical principles for research ethics that gave informed consent a major role (U.S. National Commission, 1978):

Principle of	applies to	Guidelines for
Respect for Persons		Informed Consent
Beneficence		Risk/Benefit Assessment
Justice		Selection of Subjects

Under this schema, the purpose of consent provisions is not protection from risk, as some earlier federal policies had implied, but rather the protection of autonomy and personal dignity, including the personal dignity of incompetent persons incapable of acting autonomously (for whose involvement a third party must consent). This conclusion develops an explicit philosophical position on informed consent for the first time in a government-sponsored document.

Among the most important publications in the medical literature to appear during this period was a statement by the Judicial Council of the American Medical Association in 1981. For the first time, the AMA recognized informed consent as "a basic social policy" necessary to enable patients to make their own choices even if the physician disagrees. The AMA's statement is a testament to the impact of the law of informed consent on medical ethics: The AMA's position closely followed the language of *Canterbury* v. *Spence* (Judicial Council, 1981).

The U.S. President's Commission for the Study of Ethical Problems in Medicine and Biomedical and Behavioral Research provides further evidence regarding the status informed consent had achieved by the 1980s. The commission was first convened in January 1980, with informed consent as a main item on its agenda. In 1982 it produced a three-volume report that dealt directly with informed consent: *Making Health Care Decisions: The Ethical and Legal Implications of Informed Consent in the Patient–Practitioner Relationship.* The commission argued that although informed consent has emerged primarily from a history in law, its requirements are essentially moral and policy-oriented. It held that informed consent is ultimately based on the principle that competent persons are entitled to make their own decisions from their own values and goals, but that the context of informed consent and any claim of "valid consent" must derive from active, shared decision making. The principle of self-determination was described as the "bedrock" of the commission's viewpoint.

In addition to the efforts of the U.S. President's Commission and the statement of the AMA, the 1980s saw the publication of several books devoted to the subject of informed consent, as well as hundreds of journal articles, and the passage of procedure-specific informed-consent laws and regulations. These events provide powerful testimony of the importance of informed consent in moral and legal thinking about medicine in the United States. By themselves, however, they tell us little about physicians' or researchers' actual consent practices or opinions or about how informed consent was viewed or experienced by patients and subjects.

As might be expected, the empirical evidence on this subject is mixed, although it is clear that procedures of informed consent have taken a firm hold in some parts of medical practice. For example, routine practice encourages the obtaining of signatures on consent forms and the disclosing of information about alternative treatments, risks, and benefits. The best data on this

subject are the findings of a national survey conducted for the U.S. President's Commission by Louis Harris and Associates in 1982. Almost all of the physicians surveyed indicated that they obtained written consent from their patients before in-patient surgery or the administration of general anesthesia. At least 85 percent said they usually obtained some kind of consent—written or oral—for minor office surgery, setting of fractures, local anesthesia, invasive diagnostic procedures, and radiation therapy. Only blood tests and prescriptions appear to have proceeded frequently without patient consent, although about half of the physicians reported obtaining oral consent (Harris, 1982).

The overall impression conveyed by this survey is that the explosion of interest in informed consent in the 1970s had a powerful impact on medical practice. However, evidence from the Harris survey and other sources questions the meaningfulness of the increase in consent-related activity. The overwhelming impression from the empirical literature and from reported clinical experience is that the actual process of soliciting informed consent often falls short of a serious show of respect for the decisional authority of patients. As the authors of one empirical study of physician–patient interactions put it, "despite the doctrine of informed consent, it is the physician, and not the patient, who, in effect, makes the treatment decision" (Siminoff and Fetting, 1991, p. 817).

The history of informed consent, then, indicates that medicine has undergone widespread changes under the influence of legal and moral requirements of informed consent, but it also reminds us that informed consent is an evolving process, not a set of events whose history has passed.

TOM L. BEAUCHAMP
RUTH R. FADEN

Directly related to this article are the other articles in this entry: MEANING AND ELEMENTS OF INFORMED CONSENT, CONSENT ISSUES IN HUMAN RESEARCH, CLINICAL ASPECTS OF CONSENT IN HEALTH CARE, LEGAL AND ETHICAL ISSUES OF CONSENT IN HEALTH CARE (*with its* POSTSCRIPT), *and* ISSUES OF CONSENT IN MENTAL-HEALTH CARE. *For a further discussion of topics mentioned in this article, see the entries* AUTONOMY; INFORMATION DISCLOSURE; PATERNALISM; PATIENTS' RIGHTS, *especially the article on* ORIGIN AND NATURE OF PATIENTS' RIGHTS; *and* PROFESSIONAL–PATIENT RELATIONSHIP. *This article will find application in the entries* RESEARCH, HUMAN: HISTORICAL ASPECTS; *and* RESEARCH POLICY. *For a discussion of related ideas, see the entries* HARM; LAW AND BIOETHICS; MEDICAL ETHICS, HISTORY OF, *section on* THE AMERICAS, *article on* UNITED STATES IN THE TWENTIETH CENTURY; PATIENTS' RESPONSIBILITIES;

RESEARCH, UNETHICAL; RESEARCH ETHICS COMMIT-
TEES; RIGHTS; *and* RISK. *Other relevant material may be
found in the entry* MEDICAL CODES AND OATHS, *article
on* HISTORY. *See also the* APPENDIX (CODES, OATHS,
AND DIRECTIVES RELATED TO BIOETHICS), SECTION II:
ETHICAL DIRECTIVES FOR THE PRACTICE OF MEDICINE,
especially OATH OF HIPPOCRATES, *and* CODE OF ETHICS
[1847] *of the* AMERICAN MEDICAL ASSOCIATION; *and* SEC-
TION IV: ETHICAL DIRECTIVES FOR HUMAN RESEARCH,
especially the NUREMBERG CODE, *and the* DECLARATION
OF HELSINKI *of the* WORLD MEDICAL ASSOCIATION.

Bibliography

AMERICAN MEDICAL ASSOCIATION. 1847. "Code of Medical
Ethics." In *Proceedings of the National Medical Conventions,
Held in New York, May 1846, and in Philadelphia, May
1847.* Adopted May 6 and submitted for publication in
Philadelphia. Philadelphia: Author.
———. JUDICIAL COUNCIL. 1981. *Current Opinions of the Ju-
dicial Council of the American Medical Association.* Chi-
cago: American Medical Association.
Canterbury v. Spence. 1972. 464 F.2d 772 (D.C. Cir.), *cert.
denied* 409 U.S. 1064.
Cobbs v. Grant. 1972. 104 Cal. Rptr. 505, 502 P.2d 1.
FADEN, RUTH R.; BEAUCHAMP, TOM L.; and KING, NANCY M.
P. 1986. *A History and Theory of Informed Consent.* New
York: Oxford University Press.
GERMANY (TERRITORY UNDER ALLIED OCCUPATION, 1945–
1955: U.S. ZONE) MILITARY TRIBUNALS. 1947. "Permis-
sible Military Experiments." In vol. 2 of *Trials of War
Criminals Before Nuremberg Tribunals Under Control Law
No. 10,* pp. 181–184. Washington, D.C.: U.S. Govern-
ment Printing Office.
GISBORNE, THOMAS. 1794. *An Enquiry into the Duties of Men
in the Higher and Middle Classes of Society in Great Britain,
Resulting from Their Respective Stations, Professions, and
Employments.* London: B. and J. White.
GREGORY, JOHN. 1772. *Lectures on the Duties and Qualifications
of a Physician.* New ed. London: Strahan & Cadell.
HARRIS, LOUIS, and ASSOCIATES. 1982. "Views of Informed
Consent and Decisionmaking: Parallel Surveys of Physi-
cians and the Public." In vol. 2 of *Making Health Care
Decisions,* pp. 17–316. Washington, D.C.: U.S. Presi-
dent's Commission for the Study of Ethical Problems in
Medicine and Biomedical and Behavioral Research.
HOOKER, WORTHINGTON. 1849. *Physician and Patient; or, A
Practical View of the Mutual Duties, Relations and Interests
of the Medical Professions and the Community.* New York:
Baker and Scribner.
Hyman v. Jewish Chronic Disease Hospital. 1964. 251 N.Y. 2d
818 (App. Div.); 206 N.E. 2d 338 (1965).
JONES, JAMES H. 1981. *Bad Blood: The Tuskegee Syphilis Exper-
iment.* New York: Free Press.
KATZ, JAY. 1984. *The Silent World of Doctor and Patient.* New
York: Free Press.

Natanson v. Kline. 1960. 186 Kan. 393, 350 P.2d 1093, opin-
ion on denial of motion for rehearing, 187 Kan. 186, 354
P.2d 670.
NEW YORK UNIVERSITY. POST-GRADUATE SCHOOL. 1972. *Pro-
ceedings of the Symposium on Ethical Issues in Human Ex-
perimentation: The Case of Willowbrook State Hospital
Research, May 4.* New York: New York University Medical
Center.
PERCIVAL, THOMAS. 1803. *Medical Ethics; or, A Code of Insti-
tutes and Precepts, Adapted to the Professional Conduct of
Physicians and Surgeons.* Manchester, England: S. Russell.
PERNICK, MARTIN S. 1982. "The Patient's Role in Medical
Decisionmaking: A Social History of Informed Consent
in Medical Therapy." In vol. 2 of *Making Health Care De-
cisions.* Washington, D.C.: U.S. President's Commission
for the Study of Ethical Problems in Medicine and
Biomedical and Behavioral Research.
RUSH, BENJAMIN. 1786. *An Oration . . . Containing an Enquiry
into the Influence of Physical Causes upon the Moral Faculty.*
Philadelphia: Charles Cist.
Salgo v. Leland Stanford, Jr. University Board of Trustees. 1957.
317 P.2d 170 (Cal.).
Schloendorff v. Society of New York Hospital. 1914. 211 N.Y.
125, 129, 105 N.E. 92.
SIMINOFF, L. A., and FETTING, J. H. 1991. "Factors Affecting
Treatment Decisions for a Life-Threatening Illness: The
Case of Medical Treatment of Breast Cancer." *Social Sci-
ence and Medicine* 32, no. 7:813–818.
U.S. PRESIDENT'S COMMISSION FOR THE STUDY OF ETHICAL
PROBLEMS IN MEDICINE AND BIOMEDICAL AND BEHAV-
IORAL RESEARCH. 1982. *Making Health Care Decisions: A
Report on the Ethical and Legal Implications of Informed Con-
sent in the Patient–Practitioner Relationship.* 3 vols. Wash-
ington, D.C.: Author.
Wilkinson v. Vesey. 1972. 295 A.2d 676 (R.I.).

II. MEANING AND ELEMENTS OF INFORMED CONSENT

Appropriate criteria must be identified to define and
classify an act of informed consent properly. If overde-
manding criteria such as "full disclosure and complete
understanding" are adopted, an informed consent becomes impossible to obtain. Conversely, if underdemanding criteria such as "the patient signed the form"
are used, an informed consent becomes too easy to obtain and the term loses all moral significance. Many interactions between a physician and a patient or an
investigator and a subject that have been called informed consents have been so labeled only because they
rest on underdemanding criteria; they are inappropriately referred to as informed consents. For example,
a physician's truthful disclosure to a patient has often
been declared the essence of informed consent, as if a
patient's silence following disclosure could constitute an
informed consent. The existence of such inadequate un-

derstandings of informed consent can be explained in part by empirical information about physicians' beliefs about informed consent.

Contemporary assumptions in medicine

Data about the relevant beliefs of physicians in the United States were gathered in a 1982 survey of physicians conducted by Louis Harris and Associates. One question of this survey asked physicians, "What does the term informed consent mean to you?" In their answers, only 26 percent of physicians indicated that informed consent has something to do with a patient's giving permission, consenting, or agreeing to treatment. In a related question, only 9 percent indicated that it involves the patient's making a choice or stating a preference about his or her treatment (Harris and Associates, 1982; U.S. President's Commission, 1982). Similar results were found in a survey of Japanese physicians (Hattori et al., 1991).

The majority of these physicians appear to regard disclosure as the primary (and perhaps sole) element of informed consent. That is, they conceive of informed consent as explaining to patients the nature of their medical conditions together with a recommended treatment plan. But if physicians regard informed consent as nothing more than an event of conveying information to patients, rather than a process of discussion with and obtaining permission from the patient, then claims that they regularly "obtain consents" from their patients before initiating medical procedures are both vague and unreliable.

Other polls conducted in the United States indicate that the majority of physicians understand an informed consent to be either a signed consent form or a disclosure. Some also conclude that no evidence exists that informed-consent practices are widespread in clinical medicine and that many agreements by patients that are called informed consents in some clinical settings fall far short of being meaningful informed consents (Lidz and Meisel, 1982).

The elements of informed consent

Literature of bioethics often analyzes informed consent in terms of the following elements: (1) disclosure; (2) comprehension; (3) voluntariness; (4) competence; and (5) consent (see U.S. National Commission, 1978, U.S. President's Commission, 1982; Meisel and Roth, 1981). This analysis is sometimes joined with a corresponding thesis that these elements collectively define informed consent. The postulate is that a person gives an informed consent to an intervention if and only if the person receives a thorough disclosure about the procedure, comprehends the disclosed information, acts voluntarily, is competent to act, and consents.

This definition is attractive because of its consistency with standard usage of informed consent in medicine and law. However, medical convention and malpractice law have special orientations that tend to distort the meaning of informed consent in ways that need correction. Analyses that use the five elements listed above, as well as conventional usage in law and medicine, are best suited for cataloguing the analytical parts of informed consent and for delineating moral and legal requirements of informed consent, not for conceptually analyzing the meaning of informed consent. Neither requirements nor parts amounts to a definition.

The U.S. Supreme Court addressed the definition of informed consent in *Planned Parenthood of Central Missouri v. Danforth* as follows: "One might well wonder . . . what 'informed consent' of a patient is. . . . We are content to accept, as the meaning, the giving of information to the patient as to just what would be done and as to its consequences . . ." (*Planned Parenthood of Central Missouri v. Danforth*, 1976, p. 67). The essential element or part of informed consent, as described here, is disclosure, an analysis that recalls the assumptions made by physicians in the Harris poll (Harris and Associates, 1982). However, as we will see, nothing about an informed consent requires disclosure as part of its meaning, and this element does not amount to a definition. Moreover, to make disclosure the sole or even the major condition of informed consent incorporates questionable assumptions about medical authority, physician responsibility, and legal liability. These norms delineate an obligation to make disclosures so that a consent can be informed, rather than a meaning of informed consent. Even all five of the above elements merged as a set do not satisfactorily capture the meaning of informed consent.

Both the elements and the meaning of informed consent, then, need a more comprehensive treatment. The following seven categories express the analytical components of informed consent more adequately than the above five categories—although this sevenfold list does not adequately express the meaning of informed consent either (Beauchamp and Childress, 1994):

I. Threshold elements (preconditions)
   1. Competence (to understand and decide)
   2. Voluntariness (in deciding)
II. Information elements
   3. Disclosure (of material information)
   4. Recommendation (of a plan)
   5. Understanding (of terms 3 and 4)
III. Consent elements
   6. Decision (in favor of a plan)
   7. Authorization (of the chosen plan)

The language of material information in (3) is pivotal for an adequate analysis of the elements of disclosure (3) and understanding (5). Critics of legal requirements of informed consent have often held that procedures sometimes have so many risks and benefits that they cannot be disclosed and explained in a reasonable period of time or in an understandable framework. The demands in this misreading of the nature and requirements of informed consent must be pruned, as many courts have pointed out. Material risks are the risks a reasonable patient needs to understand in order to decide among the alternatives; only these risks and benefits need to be disclosed and understood.

Corresponding to each of the above elements, one could construct informed-consent requirements. That is, there could be disclosure requirements, comprehension requirements, noninfluence requirements, competence requirements, authorization requirements, and so forth. These requirements would specify the conditions that must be satisfied for a consent to be valid.

Two meanings of informed consent

Translating the above seven elements directly into a definition or meaning of informed consent invites confusion, because the term "informed consent" has subtleties not captured by these elements. A subtlety that has generated considerable misunderstanding is that two very different meanings of informed consent operate in current literature and social practices.

In the first meaning, an informed consent is an autonomous authorization of a medical intervention or of involvement in research by individual patients or subjects. An autonomous authorization requires more than merely acquiescing in, yielding to, or complying with an arrangement or a proposal made by a physician or investigator. A person gives an informed consent in this first sense if and only if the person, with substantial understanding and in substantial absence of control by others, intentionally authorizes a health professional to do something. A person who intentionally refuses to authorize an intervention but otherwise satisfies these conditions gives an informed refusal. This first sense derives from the philosophical premises that informed consent is fundamentally a matter of protecting and enabling autonomous or self-determining choice by patients and subjects and that final authority for making decisions about medical treatment or research participation properly rests with patients and subjects, not physicians or research scientists.

In the second meaning, informed consent is analyzed in terms of institutional and policy rules of consent. This sense expresses the mainstream conception in the regulatory rules of federal agencies and in health-care institutions. Here "informed consent" refers only to a legally or institutionally effective approval by a patient or subject. An approval is therefore effective or valid if it conforms to the rules that govern specific institutions, whatever the operative rules may be. In this sense, unlike the first, conditions and requirements of informed consent are relative to a social and institutional context and need not be autonomous authorizations. This meaning is driven by demands in the legal and health-care systems for a generally applicable and efficient consent mechanism by which responsibilities and violations can be readily and fairly assessed (Faden et al. 1986).

Under these two contrasting understandings of informed consent, a patient or subject can give an informed consent in the first sense, but not in the second sense, and vice versa. For example, if the person consenting is a minor and therefore not of legal age, he or she cannot give an effective or valid consent under the prevailing institutional rules; a consent is invalid even if the minor gives the consent autonomously and responsibly. ("Mature minor" laws do sometimes make an exception and give minors the right to authorize medical treatments in a limited range of circumstances.)

The relationship between the two meanings

Rules governing effective authorization have often not been premised on a carefully delineated conception of autonomous decision making, but current literature in bioethics suggests that any justifiable analysis of informed consent must be rooted in autonomous choice by patients and subjects. An act is increasingly recognized in this literature as an informed consent only if (1) a patient or subject agrees to an intervention based on an understanding of material information; (2) the agreement is not controlled by influences that engineer the outcome; and (3) an authorization for an intervention is given by the patient or subject with the understanding that it is an authorization.

In principle, although less clearly in practice, these conditions of informed consent (in the sense of an individual's autonomous authorization) can function as model standards for fashioning the institutional and policy requirements for effective consent. The model of autonomous choice would then serve as the benchmark against which the moral adequacy of prevailing rules and practices should be evaluated. The postulate that policies governing informed consent in the second sense should be formulated to conform to the standards of informed consent in the first sense is grounded in the premise that the primary goal of informed consent in medical care and in research is to enable potential subjects and patients to make autonomous decisions about whether to grant or refuse authorization for medical and research interventions (Katz, 1984).

It does not follow that institutional policies regarding informed consent are justifiable only if they rank the protection of decision making above all other values.

Consent requirements imposed by institutions should be formulated and evaluated against a range of social and institutional considerations. The preservation of autonomous choice is the first but not the only consideration. For example, a patient's need for education and counseling in order to achieve a substantial understanding of a medical situation must be balanced against the interests of other patients and of society in maintaining a productive and efficient health-care system. Accordingly, institutional policies must consider what is fair and reasonable to require of health-care professionals and researchers and what the effect would be of alternative consent requirements on efficiency and effectiveness in the delivery of health care and the advancement of science.

TOM L. BEAUCHAMP
RUTH R. FADEN

Directly related to this article are the other articles in this entry: HISTORY OF INFORMED CONSENT, CONSENT ISSUES IN HUMAN RESEARCH, CLINICAL ASPECTS OF CONSENT IN HEALTH CARE, LEGAL AND ETHICAL ISSUES OF CONSENT IN HEALTH CARE (*with its* POSTSCRIPT), *and* ISSUES OF CONSENT IN MENTAL-HEALTH CARE. *For a further discussion of topics mentioned in this article, see the entries* AUTONOMY; COMPETENCE; INFORMATION DISCLOSURE; *and* PROFESSIONAL–PATIENT RELATIONSHIP. *Other relevant material may be found in the entries* FREEDOM AND COERCION; *and* RISK.

Bibliography

APPELBAUM, PAUL S.; LIDZ, CHARLES W.; and MEISEL, ALAN. 1987. *Informed Consent: Legal Theory and Clinical Practice.* New York: Oxford University Press.

BEAUCHAMP, TOM L., and CHILDRESS, JAMES F. 1994. *Principles of Biomedical Ethics.* 4th ed. New York: Oxford University Press.

FADEN, RUTH R., and BEAUCHAMP, TOM L.; and KING, NANCY M. P. 1986. *A History and Theory of Informed Consent.* New York: Oxford University Press.

HARRIS, LOUIS, and ASSOCIATES. 1982. "Views of Informed Consent and Decisionmaking: Parallel Surveys of Physicians and the Public." In vol. 2 of *Making Health Care Decisions,* pp. 17–316. Washington, D.C.: U.S. President's Commission for the Study of Ethical Problems in Medicine and Biomedical and Behavioral Research.

HATTORI, HIROYUKI; SALZBURG, STEPHAN M.; KIANG, WINSTON P.; FUJIMIYA, TATSUGA; TEJIMA, YUTAKA; and FURUNO, JUNJI. 1991. "The Patient's Right to Information in Japan—Legal Rules and Doctor's Opinions." *Social Science and Medicine* 32, no. 9:1007–1016.

KATZ, JAY. 1984. *The Silent World of Doctor and Patient.* New York: Free Press.

LEVINE, ROBERT J. 1988. *Ethics and Regulation of Clinical Research.* 2d ed. New Haven, Conn.: Yale University Press.

LIDZ, CHARLES W., and MEISEL, ALAN. 1982. "Informed Consent and the Structure of Medical Care." In vol. 2 of *Making Health Care Decisions,* pp. 317–410. Washington, D.C.: U.S. President's Commission for the Study of Ethical Problems in Medicine and Biomedical and Behavioral Research.

MEISEL, ALAN, and ROTH, LOREN H. 1981. "What We Do and Do Not Know About Informed Consent." *Journal of the American Medical Association* 246, no. 21:2473–2477.

MERZ, JON F., and FISCHOFF, BARUCH. 1990. "Informed Consent Does Not Mean Rational Consent: Cognitive Limitations on Decision–Making." *Journal of Legal Medicine* 11, no. 3:321–350.

Planned Parenthood of Central Missouri v. Danforth. 1976. 423 U.S. 52.

U.S. NATIONAL COMMISSION FOR THE PROTECTION OF HUMAN SUBJECTS OF BIOMEDICAL AND BEHAVIORAL RESEARCH. 1978. The *Belmont Report: Ethical Principles and Guidelines for the Protection of Human Subjects of Biomedical and Behavioral Research.* DHEW Publication (OS) 78-0012. Washington, D.C.: Department of Health, Education, and Welfare.

U.S. PRESIDENT'S COMMISSION FOR THE STUDY OF ETHICAL PROBLEMS IN MEDICINE AND BIOMEDICAL AND BEHAVIORAL RESEARCH. 1982. *Making Health Care Decisions: A Report on the Ethical and Legal Implications of Informed Consent in the Patient-Practitioner Relationship.* 3 vols. Washington, D.C.: Author.

III. CONSENT ISSUES IN HUMAN RESEARCH

"The voluntary consent of the human subject is absolutely essential." This, the first sentence of the Nuremberg Code, signals the centrality of the consent requirement in research involving human subjects (Germany [Territory Under Allied Occupation], 1947, p. 181). Before the Nuremberg Code was written in 1947 as a response to the atrocities committed in the name of science by Nazi physician-researchers, statements of medical and other professional organizations apparently made no mention of the necessity of consent. Ironically, the only nations known to have promulgated regulations that established a requirement for consent to research were Prussia and Germany (Perley et al., 1992). Subsequently, the tendency to focus on informed consent has been reinforced by public outcry over the inadequacy of consent in certain U.S. judicial landmark cases, such as *Willowbrook, Jewish Chronic Disease Hospital, Tea Room Trade,* and *Tuskegee* (Katz et al., 1972; Levine, 1986). Indeed, the issue of informed consent has so dominated recent discussion of the ethics of research that one might be led to think erroneously that other ethical issues (e.g., research design, selection of subjects) are either less important or more satisfactorily resolved.

Grounding of informed consent

Philosophical basis. The philosophical foundations of the requirement for informed consent may be found in several lines of reasoning (Veatch, 1981; Faden et al., 1986; Brock, 1987). Based upon the Hippocratic admonition "to help, or at least, to do no harm," one can justify seeking consent for the benefit of the patient; to do so provides a mechanism for ascertaining what the patient would consider a benefit. Allowing the individual to decide what he or she considers beneficial is consistent with the perspective affirmed in U.S. public policy that competent persons are generally the best protectors of their own well-being (Brock, 1987). However, a focus solely on patient benefit would allow physicians and scientists not to seek consent when they judge that doing so might harm patients or subjects. Thus this justification alone does not suffice to establish a requirement to seek consent.

The requirement can also be justified on grounds of social benefit: The practice of seeking consent may contribute to producing the "greatest good for the greatest number" by forestalling suspicion about research, thus ensuring a subject population and increasing the efficiency of the research enterprise. Again, however, the justification fails to stand alone, since it can also be used to justify not seeking consent; the social good might be better served by avoiding the inefficient and frequently time-consuming consent process. Some commentators express concern that, carried to its extreme, the social-benefit argument might support the use of unwilling subjects, as in Nazi Germany (Caplan, 1992); such a position would necessarily rest on a very limited vision of the relevant social consequences.

The firmest grounding for the requirement to seek consent is the ethical principle "respect for persons," which according to the U.S. National Commission for the Protection of Human Subjects of Biomedical and Behavioral Research (hereafter, U.S. National Commission) "incorporates at least two basic ethical convictions: first, that individuals should be treated as autonomous agents, and second, that persons with diminished autonomy and thus in need of protection are entitled to such protection" (U.S. National Commission, 1978, p. 4). Although this term suggests a Kantian or deontological grounding of the principle, this was not the intent of the commission; a substantially similar principle, self-determination, may be grounded in rule utilitarianism (Brock, 1987). In a legal context, Justice Benjamin Cardozo in 1914 stated that "every human being of adult years and sound mind has a right to determine what shall be done with his own body" (Katz, 1984, p. 51). To return to the Kantian terms that will be used often in this article, this principle ensures that the research subject will be treated as an end and not merely as a means to another's end (Beauchamp and Childress, 1989). Thus the purpose of the consent requirement is not to minimize risk but to give persons the right to choose.

Religious basis. Several fundamental tenets of the Judaeo-Christian tradition also provide grounding for the requirement to seek consent. This tradition affirms that each human life is a gift from God and is of infinite and immeasurable worth (the "sanctity of life"). The infinite worth of the individual requires that persons treat each other with respect and not interfere in each other's lives without consent. The consent requirement can also be grounded explicitly in the notion of covenant. Seeking consent is an affirmation of the basic faithfulness or care required by the fundamental covenantal nature of human existence (Ramsey, 1970).

Legal basis. The legal grounding for the requirement for consent to research (Annas et al., 1977; Fried, 1974) is based on the outcome of litigation of disputes arising almost exclusively in the context of medical practice. There is virtually no case law on the basis of which legal standards for consent to research, as distinguished from practice, might be defined (there is one Canadian case, *Halushka* v. *University of Saskatchewan*). The law defines, in general, the circumstances under which a patient, or by extension, a subject, may recover damages for having been wronged or harmed as a consequence of failure to negotiate adequate consent.

The legal bases for the consent requirement—which also shed light on the ethical dimensions of consent—are twofold (Annas et al., 1977). First, failure to obtain proper consent was traditionally treated as a battery action. Closely related to the principles of respect for persons and self-determination, the law of battery makes it wrong a priori to touch, treat, or do research upon a person without the person's consent. Whether or not harm befalls the patient/subject is irrelevant: It is the unconsented-to touching that is wrong.

The modern trend in malpractice litigation is to treat cases based upon failure to obtain proper consent as negligence rather than battery actions. The negligence doctrine combines elements of patient benefit and self-determination. To bring a negligence action, a patient/subject must prove that the physician had a duty toward the patient; that the duty was breached; that damage occurred to the patient; and that the damage was caused by the breach. In contrast to battery actions, negligence actions remove as a basis for the requirement for consent the simple notion that unconsented-to touching is a wrong. Rather, such touching is wrong (actionable) only if it is negligent and results in harm; otherwise, the patient/subject cannot recover damages. Under both battery and negligence doctrines, consent is invalid if any information is withheld that might be considered material to the decision to give consent.

Functions of informed consent

Jay Katz and Alexander Capron identified the following functions of informed consent: to promote individual autonomy; encourage rational decision making; avoid fraud and duress; involve the public; encourage self-scrutiny by the physician-investigator; and reduce the civil and/or criminal liability of the investigator and his or her institution (Katz and Capron, 1975).

In general, the negotiations for informed consent are designed to safeguard the rights and welfare of the subject, while documentation that the negotiations have been conducted properly safeguards the investigator and institution (Levine, 1986). The net effect of the documentation may, in fact, be harmful to the interests of the subject. Retaining a signed consent form tends to give the advantage to the investigator in any adversary proceeding. Moreover, the availability of such documents in institutional records may lead to violations of privacy and confidentiality. Consequently, federal regulations permit waivers of the requirement for consent forms when the principal threat to the subject would be a breach of confidentiality and "the only record linking the subject and the research would be the consent document" ("Documentation of Informed Consent," 1993, 46.117c).

Those who are interested in making operational the requirement for consent have a tendency to focus nearly all of their attention on the consent form. Federal regulations prescribe what information must be included in and excluded from these forms. Members of institutional review boards and researchers collaborate in a struggle to create reproachless forms. This seems to reflect an assumption that the consent form is an appropriate instrumentality through which researchers might fulfill their obligation not to treat persons merely as means. Most commentators on informed consent disagree, however, seeing consent as a continuing process rather than an event symbolized by the signing of a form; for example, Robert Levine (1986) characterizes informed consent as a discussion or negotiation, while Katz (1984) envisions consent as a searching conversation.

Whether or not negotiations for informed consent to research should be conducted according to different standards than consent to practice is controversial. Alvan Feinstein observes that it is the custom to adhere to a double standard: "An act that receives no special concern when performed as part of clinical practice may become a major ethical or legal issue if done as part of a formally designed investigation" (Feinstein, 1974, p. 331). In his view there is less need for formality in the negotiations for informed consent to a relationship where the interests of research and practice are conjoined—for example, as in research conducted by a physician-investigator who has the aim of demonstrating

the safety and/or efficacy of a nonvalidated therapeutic maneuver—than when the only purpose of the investigator–subject relationship is to perform research. Capron, on the other hand, asserts: "Higher requirements for informed consent should be imposed in therapy than in investigation, particularly when an element of honest experimentation is joined with therapy" (Capron, 1972, p. 574). Levine (1986) concludes that patients are entitled to the same degree of thoroughness of negotiations for informed consent as are subjects of research. However, patients may be offered the opportunity to delegate some (but not all) decision-making authority to a physician, while subjects should rarely be offered this option. The most important distinction is that the prospective subject should be informed that in research, in contrast with practice, the subject will be at least in part a means and perhaps primarily a means to an end identified by someone else.

Two interpretations of the consent requirement

Interpretations of the meaning and application of informed consent reflect a tension between respecting the autonomy of persons and protecting them from harm. Hans Jonas (1970) and Paul Ramsey (1970) have developed a covenantal model in which subjects are respected and protected by ensuring that they give truly informed consent. Benjamin Freedman (1975) stresses the individual's freedom of choice, whether or not the choice is informed.

For Jonas and Ramsey, the consent requirement is derived from the duty to treat persons as ends, not merely as means. In research, subjects are "used" as means to the end of acquiring knowledge. (In Jonas's terms, they are "sacrificed" for the collective good.) Such "use" of persons is justified only if the subjects so identify with the purposes of the research that they will those purposes as their own ends. Only then are they not being "used," but instead they have become, in Ramsey's term, "co-adventurers." The consent requirement thus affirms a basic covenantal bond between the researcher and the subject and ensures respect for the subject as an end, not merely a means.

To establish a true covenant, the subject's consent must be informed. Only subjects who genuinely know the purposes and appreciate the risks of research can assume those risks and adopt those purposes as their own ends. Ideal subjects, therefore, would be researchers themselves (Jonas, 1970). The less one understands the risks and identifies with the purposes of research, the less valid is one's consent. Jonas therefore established a "descending order of permissibility" for the recruitment ("conscription") of volunteers. Both Ramsey and Jonas restrict the use of subjects unable to consent or to understand what is involved, permitting the use of such subjects only in research directly related to their own condition (Jonas) or their own survival and well-being (Ramsey).

This interpretation reflects certain assumptions that can be challenged. First, while neither Jonas nor Ramsey focuses exclusively on patients as subjects, their approach appears to be influenced largely by the medical practice model. That approach may not be adequate to deal with research not based on the medical practice model—for example, social-science research.

Second, while Ramsey argues that it is wrong to use a person in research without consent irrespective of risk (because one can be "wronged" without being "harmed"), he nonetheless appears to share with Jonas the assumption that most research is risky and involves "sacrifice" on the part of the subject. In fact, most research does not present risk of physical or psychological harm; rather, it presents inconvenience (e.g., of urine collection) and discomforts (e.g., of needle sticks) (Levine, 1986). Even Phase I drug testing, involving the first administration of new drugs to humans and usually assumed to be highly risky, has been estimated to present subjects with "risks" slightly greater than those involved in secretarial work and substantially less than those assumed by window washers and miners (Levine, 1986).

But the most important challenge is Freedman's (1975) alternative interpretation and use of the basic principles. Like Jonas and Ramsey, Freedman derives the consent requirement from the duty to have respect for persons. Unlike Jonas and Ramsey, however, he interprets the requirement of respect for persons to allow the possibility of a "valid but ignorant" consent.

Freedman proposes that striving for "fully informed consent" is generally undesirable, and that what is required is "valid consent," not necessarily "informed consent." To be valid, consent must be responsible and voluntary. Thus valid consent "entails only the imparting of that information which the patient/subject requires in order to make a responsible decision" (Freedman, 1975, p. 34). A choice based upon less or other information than another responsible person might consider essential is not necessarily a sign of irresponsibility. Overprotection is a form of dehumanization and lack of respect; for example, to classify persons as incompetent in order to protect them from their own judgment is the worst form of abuse.

This approach also has several weaknesses. Much hinges on what is taken to be a responsible choice. Freedman suggests that responsibility is a dispositional characteristic and is to be judged in terms of the person, not in terms of a particular choice. However, there is still an element of paternalism introduced in judging another to be a responsible person. Moreover, this approach may not provide sufficient protection for those subjects who tend too readily to abdicate responsibility for choice.

It is clear that debates over the interpretation of informed consent depend on interpretations of the basic ethical principle of respect for persons and the extent to which that principle requires protection from harm or respect for autonomy.

Informed consent: Conditions and exceptions

According to the Nuremberg Code, to consent to participate in research one must (1) be "so situated as to be able to exercise free power of choice"; (2) have the "legal capacity" to give consent; (3) have "sufficient . . . comprehension" to make an "enlightened" decision; and (4) have "sufficient knowledge" on which to decide (Germany [Territory Under Allied Occupation], 1947, p. 181). Recent discussion emphasizes the knowledge or information component of consent—hence the term "informed consent" (Katz, 1984). Nuremberg's focus on freedom of choice rather than on the quantity or quality of information transmitted is represented by its use of the term "voluntary consent," not "informed consent." It is worth recalling that a demand for informed consent at the expense of other styles of self-determination such as Freedman's responsible choice is not necessarily respectful of persons. Most commentators agree that compromise of any one of the four conditions specified by the Nuremberg Code jeopardizes the ethical acceptability of the consent.

"Free power of choice." The Nuremberg Code proscribes "any element of force, fraud, deceit, duress, overreaching, or other ulterior forms of constraint or coercion" (Germany [Territory Under Allied Occupation], 1947, p. 181) in obtaining consent. Any flagrant coercion—for instance, when competent, comprehending persons are forced to submit to research against their expressed will—clearly renders consent invalid. There may be more subtle or indirect "constraints" or "coercions" when prospective subjects are highly dependent, impoverished, or "junior or subordinate members of a hierarchical group" (Council for International Organizations of Medical Sciences [CIOMS], 1993, p. 30). Some argue that consent obtained from such persons violates the intent of the Nuremberg Code. This argument has been posed most sharply with respect to prisoners and other institutionalized populations, since institutionalization often involves both dependency and impoverishment. (Biomedical research involving prisoners as subjects has become quite rare since 1976 when the U.S. National Commission recommended very stringent standards for its justification [Dubler and Sidel, 1989].) Some argue that consent to participate in research is not valid when it is given (1) to procure financial reward in situations offering few alternatives for remuneration; (2) to seek release from an institution either by evidencing "good behavior" or by ameliorating the condition for which one was confined; or (3) to please physicians or authorities on whom one's continued welfare depends (Branson 1977).

Cornel West (1976) argues, however, that such indirect forms of constraint do not constitute coercion in a strict sense and thus do not render consent involuntary. "Coercion," says West, consists in a threat to render one's circumstances worse if one does not do something. Hence, a threat to withdraw basic necessities of existence, or in some other way to render a prison inmate's situation worse if he or she declines to participate in research, would constitute coercion and render consent invalid. Similarly, to condition release from prison upon participation would constitute coercion, since it would make the inmate's situation worse by removing normal alternatives for seeking release. But the provision of better living conditions in exchange for participation in research does not constitute a threat to make conditions worse; rather, it is an enticement to make conditions better. While enticement and bribery can invalidate consent by undermining the rational grounds for choice, they do not undermine the voluntariness of the choice (Cohen, 1978). Similarly, a desire to "get well" or to favorably influence institutional authorities is not an "ulterior" constraint in the strict sense of the Nuremberg Code, though it may be a very real psychological constraint.

Other commentators, however, are less concerned with a sharp distinction between coercion and other forms of constraint or undue influence (Levine, 1986; CIOMS, 1993). Even outside such total institutions as prisons there are many situations in which junior or subordinate members of hierarchical groups may be exploited or manipulated. Such persons may assume that their willingness to consent to research may be rewarded by preferential treatment or that their refusals could provoke retaliation by those in positions of authority in the system. Whether or not such assumptions are justified, it is the assumptions themselves that make such persons susceptible to manipulation. Examples of such persons are medical or nursing students, subordinate hospital and laboratory personnel, employees of pharmaceutical firms, and members of the military services. Other persons whose dependency status can be exploited include residents of nursing homes, people receiving welfare benefits, patients in emergency rooms, and those with incurable diseases.

Apart from those populations identified by regulations and ethical codes as requiring "special protection"—fetuses, children, prisoners, and those who are incompetent by reason of mental incapacity—there is no clear consensus about how to respond to the problems presented by those whose capacity to consent may be limited by virtue of their dependency status. For example, while some medical schools have policies that forbid the involvement of medical students as research subjects, others have required investigators to invite them to participate in certain complex projects, reasoning that their highly sophisticated understanding of the risks, benefits, and purposes of such projects ensures a high quality of consent (Levine, 1986). Involvement of medical students, it is further argued, is consistent with Jonas's "descending order of permissibility" and contributes to their socialization into the medical profession.

While most regulations and ethical codes proscribe undue material inducements, there is no consensus on what this means. Some commentators argue that in most cases in which competent adults are recruited to serve as subjects in research that presents only slight increases above minimal risk, the role of the research subject is similar to that of an employee (Levine, 1986). Consequently, the amounts of cash payments or other material inducements can be determined by ordinary market factors. Others protest that because participation in research entails "selling one's body" as opposed to "selling one's labor" the role of the research subject might be considered more akin to prostitution than to any other type of employment (Wartofsky, 1976). According to this view, research subjects should not be paid at all; rather they should be motivated by altruism.

Attempts to regulate the amounts of permissible material inducements are inevitably problematic (Levine, 1986). Setting the rates at a low level results in inequitable distribution of the burdens of participation among those who have no opportunities to earn more money for each unit of their time. Higher rates may overwhelm the capacity of the impoverished to decline participation.

Competence and comprehension. The Nuremberg Code requires both "legal capacity" to consent (often called "competence") and "sufficient understanding" to reach an "enlightened" decision. Definitions of competence often include elements of comprehension, for example, to evaluate relevant information, to understand the consequences of action, and to reach a decision for rational reasons (Stanley and Stanley, 1982).

Joseph Goldstein charges that linking determinations of competence to assessments of comprehension is "pernicious," since refusal to participate in research might be judged "irrational" by the investigator and then used as grounds for declaring the person incompetent. Because the purpose of the informed consent requirement is to guarantee the exercise of free choice, not to judge its rationality, Goldstein argues, competence should be presumed; only a "showing that the patient is comatose" should ordinarily be accepted as proof of incompetence (Goldstein, 1978).

Assessments of incompetence. The various standards employed for assessing competence are variations of four basic themes (Stanley and Stanley, 1982).

1. *Reasonable outcome of choice.* This is a highly paternalistic standard in that the individual's right to self-determination is respected only if he or she makes the "right" choice—that is, one that accords with what the competency reviewer either considers reasonable or presumes a reasonable person might make.
2. *Factual comprehension.* The individual is required to understand, or at least be able to understand, the information divulged during the consent negotiation.
3. *Choice based on rational reasons.* Individuals must demonstrate a capacity for rational manipulation of information. They may, for example, be required to show that they not only understand the risks and benefits but also have weighed them in relation to their personal situations.
4. *Appreciation of the nature of the situation.* Individuals must demonstrate not only comprehension of the consent information but also the ability to use the information in a rational manner. Furthermore, they must appreciate the fact that they are being invited to become research subjects and what that implies.

While there is disagreement as to the grounds for assessing incompetence, most commentators agree that such assessments are limited in several ways (Faden et al., 1986). First, a judgment of incompetence may apply only to certain areas of decision making, for example, to one's legal but not to one's personal affairs. Second, confinement to a mental institution is not in itself equivalent to a determination of incompetence. Third, some who are legally competent are functionally incompetent, while some who are legally incompetent are functionally competent.

The Nuremberg Code does not permit the use of subjects lacking legal capacity or comprehension. Most subsequent codes and discussions allow their use with certain restrictions: for example, that mentally competent adults are not suitable subjects, that the veto of a legally incompetent but minimally comprehending subject is binding, and that consent or permission of the legal guardian must be obtained (Levine, 1986).

According to the U.S. President's Commission for the Study of Ethical Problems in Medicine and Biomedical and Behavioral Research (hereafter, U.S. President's Commission), "decisionmaking capacity requires, to a greater or lesser degree: (1) possession of a set of values and goals; (2) the ability to communicate and understand information; and (3) the ability to reason and deliberate about one's choices" (U.S. President's

Commission, 1982, p. 57). Moreover, individuals may have sufficient capacity to make some decisions but not others (Brock, 1987; Kopelman, 1990). In the words of the U.S. President's Commission:

> Since the assessment [of capacity] must balance possibly competing considerations of well-being and self-determination, [one should] take into account the potential consequences of the patient's decision. When the consequences for well-being are substantial, there is a greater need to be certain that the patient possesses the necessary level of capacity. . . . Thus a particular patient may be capable of deciding about a relatively inconsequential medication, but not about the amputation of a gangrenous limb. (U.S. President's Commission, 1982, p. 60)

Proxy consent. The debate between Paul Ramsey and Richard McCormick over the legitimacy of proxy consent to authorize the participation of an incompetent person in research is one of the classics in the brief history of bioethics. Adopting the battery argument, Ramsey claimed that the use of a nonconsenting subject is wrong whether or not there is risk, simply because it involves an unconsented touching. Unconsented touching is not wrongful, however, when it is for the good of the individual. Hence, proxy consent may be given for the use of nonconsenting subjects in research only when it includes therapeutic interventions related to the subject's own recovery (Ramsey, 1970).

However, Ramsey acknowledged that benefit does not always justify unconsented touching; such touching of a competent adult is wrong even if it benefits that person. Why, then, can benefit be presumed to justify such touching for a child (or other subject unable to give consent)? McCormick proposed that the validity of such interventions rests on the presumption that the child, if capable, would consent to therapy. This presumption in turn derives from a child's obligation to seek therapy, an obligation that the child possesses simply as a human being (McCormick, 1974). Because children have an obligation to seek their own well-being, we presume they would consent if they could, and thus presume also that proxy consent on their behalf would not violate respect for them as persons.

By analogy, McCormick suggested that, as members of a moral community, children have other obligations to which one would presume their consent and give proxy consent on their behalf. One such obligation is to contribute to the general welfare when such contribution requires little or no sacrifice. Hence, nonconsenting subjects may be used in research not directly related to their own benefit so long as the research fulfills an important social need and involves no discernible risk. Ramsey countered this argument with respect to children, claiming that McCormick's position fails to recognize that children are not adults with a full range of duties and obligations. Instead, they have rights that must be protected by adults (Ramsey, 1976).

Adopting this premise about the nature of the child as a moral being, Freedman drew different conclusions. Since a child is not a moral being in the same sense as an adult, he argued, the concept of wrongful touching does not apply. The child has no right to be left alone but only a right to be protected. Hence, Freedman concludes that the only relevant moral issue is the risk involved in the research, and, like McCormick, that children could be used in research unrelated to their therapy, provided it presents them no discernible risk (Freedman, 1975). Thus, the debate centers on the status of the child (a paradigmatic incompetent) as a moral being and on interpretations of the requirements of respect for persons.

Although disagreements persist over both standards of competence and the use of incompetent subjects, one issue seems to have been settled by the U.S. National Commission in several of its reports (Levine, 1986). Parents, guardians, and, in some cases, other "responsible relatives" may give "permission" (a term that replaces "proxy consent") to involve an incompetent in research if there is no more than minimal risk, if incompetents who are capable of giving their "assents" (knowledgeable agreements that do not meet the legal standards for informed consent) do so, and if certain other criteria are satisfied. If there is more than minimal risk, the standards for ethical justification of the involvement of incompetents are more stringent.

Disclosure of information. The Nuremberg Code requires that the subject be told "the nature, duration, and purpose of the experiment; the method and means by which it is to be conducted; all inconveniences and hazards reasonably to be expected; and the effects upon his health or person which may possibly come (Germany, [Territory Under Allied Occupation], 1947, p. 182)." These requirements have been modified by subsequent codes and regulations. U.S. federal regulations require (1) a statement of the purpose of the research and a description of its procedures; (2) a description of foreseeable risks and discomforts; (3) a description of benefits; (4) disclosure of appropriate alternatives, if any; (5) a statement of the extent of confidentiality; (6) an explanation of the availability of medical treatment for injury and compensation for disability; (7) an explanation of whom to contact for answers to questions; and (8) a statement that participation is voluntary and that neither refusal to participate nor withdrawal at any time will result in a loss of benefits to which the subject is otherwise entitled ("General Requirements," 1993). The regulations further specify six additional elements of information to be provided when appropriate: (1) additional risks to the subject or to the

fetus if the subject becomes pregnant; (2) circumstances in which a subject's participation may be terminated without his or her consent; (3) additional costs to the subject that may result from participation; (4) the consequences of a subject's decision to withdraw and procedures for orderly termination of participation; (5) a commitment to divulge significant new findings developed during the research that may relate to the subject's continued willingness to participate; and (6) the approximate number of subjects in the study. Finally, the regulations forbid requirements that subjects waive any of their legal rights as well as releases of the investigator, sponsor, or institution from liability for negligence.

While these requirements have the force of law, they are by no means exhaustive of possible standards for disclosure. To them one might add the following: a clear invitation to participate in research, distinguishing maneuvers required for research purposes from those necessary for therapy; an explanation of why that particular person is invited (selected); a suggestion that the prospective subject might wish to discuss the research with another person; and an identification of the source of funding for the research. Robert Veatch would add the names of members of any review boards that had approved the research and an explanation of the right, if any, to continue receiving treatments found useful (Veatch, 1978). In short, there is no universal agreement on standards for disclosure of information or on what it takes for a person to have "sufficient knowledge" to give "informed" consent.

Those who agree on the need for disclosure of information in a particular category—the risks, for example—often disagree on the nature of the information that must be made known. The Nuremberg Code requires explication of hazards "reasonably" to be expected. Does this include a very slight chance of a substantial harm, or a substantial chance of a very slight harm? Neither the quality nor the probability of the risks to be divulged has been clearly determined legally.

Disagreements over particulars arise in part from disagreements about underlying standards: Is disclosure to be determined by (1) general medical practice or opinion; (2) the requirements of a "reasonable person"; or (3) the idiosyncratic judgment of the individual? While the legal trend may be shifting from the first to the second, it may be argued that only the third, the "subjective standard," is truly compatible with the requirement of respect for the autonomy of the individual person (Faden and Beauchamp, 1986; Veatch, 1978).

Yet even those who adopt the subjective standard disagree as to its implications. As noted earlier, Freedman (1975) holds that the idiosyncratic judgment of the individual is overriding, to the point that the prospective subject can choose to have less information than a "reasonable" person might require. Veatch, however, argues that anyone refusing to accept as much information as would be expected of a "reasonable person" should not be accepted as a subject (Veatch, 1978).

In the context of medical practice, two exceptions to the requirement for informed consent are recognized—"emergency exception" and "therapeutic privilege." The former, which permits the doctor to proceed without delay to administer urgently required therapy in emergencies, is included in a limited form in the regulations of the U.S. Food and Drug Administration; in some "life-threatening" emergencies in which informed consent is "infeasible," physician-investigators are authorized to employ investigational drugs and devices (Levine, 1986). There is continuing controversy over whether the emergency exception can be invoked to justify "deferred consent," that is, postponement of soliciting the consent of the subject or permission of the next-of-kin for up to several days after the subject has been enrolled in a research protocol in an emergency (Levine, 1991; Prentice et al., 1994). The therapeutic-privilege exception to the informed-consent rule permits the doctor to withhold information when, in his or her judgment, disclosure would be detrimental to the patient's interests or well-being (Levine, 1986). Most commentators agree that invoking the doctrine of therapeutic privilege to assure a subject's cooperation in a research project is almost never appropriate; it gives the investigator entirely too much license to serve vested interests by withholding information that might be material to a prospective subject's decision. U.S. federal regulations do not explicitly endorse the use of the therapeutic-privilege exception in research, although some authors have suggested that they could be interpreted as an implicit endorsement (Levine, 1986).

The success of some research activities is contingent upon withholding from the subjects information about their purposes or procedures or, in some cases, by deliberate deception (providing false information). U.S. federal regulations permit "waivers and alterations" of consent requirements if there is no more than minimal risk; if the waiver or alteration will not adversely affect subjects' rights or welfare; if without the waiver or alteration the research "could not practicably be carried out"; and if the subjects will be debriefed (given a full and accurate explanation afterward) when appropriate ("General Requirements," 1993, 46.116d). Diana Baumrind opposes deceptive practices, arguing not only that they violate the principle of respect for persons but also that in the long run they will invalidate research on scientific grounds (Baumrind, 1979). Various proposals have been made to minimize the need for and harmful effects of deceptive practices: Subjects might be invited to consent to incomplete disclosure with a promise of full disclosure at the termination of the research; sub-jects might be told as much as possible and asked to consent for specified limits of time and risk; or approval of the plans to withhold information from or to deceive subjects might be sought from "surrogate" populations that resemble the actual intended subject populations in relevant respects (Levine, 1986).

Conclusions

The use of a person as a research subject can be justified only if that person, or one authorized to speak on his or her behalf, consents to such use. The legal and ethical requirement for consent is grounded in fundamental tenets of the Judaeo-Christian religious tradition as well as in basic ethical principles that create the universal obligation to treat persons as ends and not merely as means to another's end. The consent requirement also reflects the perspective that competent persons are generally the best protectors of their own well-being. Most major disagreements over the form and substance of the consent requirement derive from conflicting interpretations of one or more of the basic principles.

A widespread tendency among researchers to focus on consent forms seems to reflect an assumption that the consent form is an appropriate instrumentality through which they might fulfill their obligation not to treat persons merely as means. Most commentators on informed consent disagree, however, seeing consent as a continuing process rather than a single event consummated by the signing of a form. Moreover, while the primary purposes of informed consent are to foster self-determination and to empower prospective subjects to protect their own well-being and other interests, the primary purpose of its written documentation is to protect the investigator, the institution, and the research sponsor from legal liability.

ROBERT J. LEVINE

Directly related to this article are the other articles in this entry: HISTORY OF INFORMED CONSENT, MEANING AND ELEMENTS OF INFORMED CONSENT, CLINICAL ASPECTS OF CONSENT IN HEALTH CARE, LEGAL AND ETHICAL ISSUES OF CONSENT IN HEALTH CARE (*with its* POSTSCRIPT), *and* ISSUES OF CONSENT IN MENTAL-HEALTH CARE. *For a further discussion of topics mentioned in this article, see the entries* COMPETENCE; FREEDOM AND COERCION; INFORMATION DISCLOSURE; RESEARCH POLICY, *article on* RISK AND VULNERABLE GROUPS; *and* RIGHTS, *especially article on* SYSTEMATIC ANALYSIS. *This article will find application in the entries* AUTOEXPERIMENTATION; MEDICAL ETHICS, HISTORY OF, *section on* THE AMERICAS, *article on* UNITED STATES IN THE TWENTIETH CENTURY; *and section on* EUROPE, *subsection on* CONTEMPORARY PERIOD, *article on* GERMAN-SPEAKING COUNTRIES AND SWITZERLAND; MILITARY PERSONNEL AS RESEARCH SUBJECTS; PRISoners, *article on* RESEARCH ISSUES; RESEARCH, HUMAN: HISTORICAL ASPECTS; RESEARCH, UNETHICAL; *and* STUDENTS AS RESEARCH SUBJECTS. *For a discussion of related ideas, see the entries* AUTONOMY; BENEFICENCE; MINORITIES AS RESEARCH SUBJECTS; MULTINATIONAL RESEARCH; PRIVACY AND CONFIDENTIALITY IN RESEARCH; *and* RESEARCH ETHICS COMMITTEES. *Other relevant material may be found in the entries* HARM; NATIONAL SOCIALISM; PATIENTS' RESPONSIBILITIES; *and* RISK. *See also the* APPENDIX (CODES, OATHS, AND DIRECTIVES RELATED TO BIOETHICS), SECTION IV: ETHICAL DIRECTIVES FOR HUMAN RESEARCH, *especially the* NUREMBERG CODE.

Bibliography

ANNAS, GEORGE J.; GLANTZ, LEONARD H.; and KATZ, BARBARA F. 1977. *Informed Consent to Human Experimentation: The Subject's Dilemma.* Cambridge, Mass.: Ballinger.

BAUMRIND, DIANA. 1979. "IRBs and Social Science Research: The Costs of Deception." *IRB* 1, no. 6:1–4.

BEAUCHAMP, TOM L., and CHILDRESS, JAMES F. 1989. *Principles of Biomedical Ethics.* 3d ed. New York: Oxford University Press.

BRANSON, ROY. 1977. "Prison Research: National Commission Says 'No, Unless . . .'" *Hastings Center Report* 7, no. 1:15–21.

BROCK, DAN W. 1987. "Informed Consent." In *Health Care Ethics: An Introduction,* pp. 98–126. Edited by Donald VanDeVeer and Tom Regan. Philadelphia: Temple University Press.

CAPRON, ALEXANDER MORGAN. 1972. "The Law of Genetic Therapy." In *Experimentation with Human Beings: The Authority of the Investigator, Subject, Professions, and State in the Human Experimentation Process,* pp. 574–575. Edited by Jay Katz, Alexander Morgan Capron, and Eleanor Glass Swift. New York: Russell Sage Foundation.

COHEN, CARL. 1978. "Medical Experimentation on Prisoners." *Perspectives in Biology and Medicine* 21, no. 3: 357–372.

COUNCIL FOR INTERNATIONAL ORGANIZATIONS OF MEDICAL SCIENCES (CIOMS). 1993. *International Ethical Guidelines for Biomedical Research Involving Human Subjects.* Geneva: Author.

"Documentation of Informed Consent." 1993. 45 *Code of Federal Regulations* 46.117.

DUBLER, NANCY N., and SIDEL, VICTOR W. 1989. "On Research on HIV Infection and AIDS in Correctional Institutions." *Milbank Memorial Quarterly* 67, no. 2:171–207.

FADEN, RUTH R.; BEAUCHAMP, TOM L. and KING, NANCY M. P. 1986. *A History and Theory of Informed Consent.* New York: Oxford University Press.

FEINSTEIN, ALVAN R. 1974. "Clinical Biostatistics. XXVI: Medical Ethics and the Architecture of Clinical Research." *Clinical Pharmacology and Therapeutics* 15, no. 3:316–334.

FREEDMAN, BENJAMIN. 1975. "A Moral Theory of Informed Consent." *Hastings Center Report* 5, no. 4:32–39.

FRIED, CHARLES. 1974. *Medical Experimentation: Personal Integrity and Social Policy.* Amsterdam: North-Holland.

"General Requirements for Informed Consent." 1993. 45 *Code of Federal Regulations* 46.116.

GERMANY (TERRITORY UNDER ALLIED OCCUPATION, 1945–1955: U.S. ZONE) MILITARY TRIBUNALS. 1947. "Permissible Medical Experiments." In *Trials of War Criminals Before the Nuremberg Tribunals Under Control Law No. 10,* pp. 181–184. Washington, D.C.: U.S. Government Printing Office.

GOLDSTEIN, JOSEPH. 1978. "On the Right of the 'Institutionalized Mentally Infirm' to Consent to or Refuse to Participate as Subjects in Biomedical and Behavioral Research." *Appendix to Report and Recommendations: Research Involving Those Institutionalized as Mentally Infirm:* DHEW publication no. (OS) 78-0007. Bethesda, Md.: U.S. National Commission for the Protection of Human Subjects of Biomedical and Behavioral Research.

Halushka v. *University of Saskatchewan.* 1965. 52 W.W.R. 608 (Sask. C.A.).

INGELFINGER, FRANZ J. 1972. "Informed (But Uneducated) Consent." *New England Journal of Medicine* 287, no. 9: 465–466.

JONAS, HANS. 1970. "Philosophical Reflections on Experimenting with Human Subjects." In *Experimentation with Human Subjects,* pp. 1–31. Edited by Paul A. Freund. New York: George Braziller.

KATZ, JAY. 1984. *The Silent World of Doctor and Patient.* New York: Free Press.

KATZ, JAY, and CAPRON, ALEXANDER MORGAN. 1975. *Catastrophic Diseases: Who Decides What? A Psychosocial and Legal Analysis of the Problems Posed by Hemodialysis and Organ Transplantation.* New York: Russell Sage Foundation.

KATZ, JAY; CAPRON, ALEXANDER MORGAN; and SWIFT, ELEANOR GLASS, eds. 1972. *Experimentation with Human Beings: The Authority of the Investigator, Subject, Professions, and State in the Human Experimentation Process.* New York: Russell Sage Foundation.

KOPELMAN, LORETTA M. 1990. "On the Evaluative Nature of Competency and Capacity Judgments." *International Journal of Law and Psychiatry* 13, no. 4:309–329.

LEVINE, ROBERT J. 1986. *Ethics and Regulation of Clinical Research.* 2d ed. Baltimore: Urban & Schwarzenberg.

———. 1991. "Deferred Consent." *Controlled Clinical Trials* 12, no. 4:546–550.

McCORMICK, RICHARD A. 1974. "Proxy Consent in the Experimentation Situation." *Perspectives in Biology and Medicine* 18, no. 1:2–20.

———. 1976. "A Reply to Paul Ramsey: Experimentation in Children: Sharing in Sociality." *Hastings Center Report* 6, no. 6:41–46.

PERLEY, SHARON; FLUSS, SEV S.; BANKOWSKI, ZBIGNIEW; and SIMON, FRANÇOISE. 1992. "The Nuremberg Code: An International Overview." In *The Nazi Doctors and the Nuremberg Code: Human Rights in Human Experimentation,* pp. 149–173. Edited by George J. Annas and Michael A. Grodin. New York: Oxford University Press.

PRENTICE, ERNEST D.; ANTONSON, DEAN L.; LEIBROCK, LYAL G.; PRABHU, VIKRAM C.; KELSO, TIMOTHY K.; and

Sears, Thomas D. 1994. "An Update on the PEG-SOD Study Involving Incompetent Subjects: FDA Permits an Exception from Informed Consent Requirements." *IRB* 16, nos. 1–2:16–18.

Ramsey, Paul. 1970. *The Patient as Person: Explorations in Medical Ethics.* New Haven, Conn.: Yale University Press.

———. 1976. "A Reply to Richard McCormick: The Enforcement of Morals: Nontherapeutic Research on Children." *Hastings Center Report* 6, no. 4:21–30.

Stanley, Barbara H., and Stanley, Michael. 1982. "Testing Competency in Psychiatric Patients." *IRB* 4, no. 8:1–6.

U.S. National Commission for the Protection of Human Subjects of Biomedical and Behavioral Research. 1978. *The Belmont Report: Ethical Principles and Guidelines for the Protection of Human Subjects of Research.* DHEW publication nos. (OS) 78-0012 to (OS) 78-0014. Bethesda, Md.: Author.

U.S. President's Commission for the Study of Ethical Problems in Medicine and Biomedical and Behavioral Research. 1982. *Making Health Care Decisions: A Report on the Ethical and Legal Implications of Informed Consent in the Patient-Practitioner Relationship.* Stock no. 040-000-00459-9. Washington, D.C.: Author.

Veatch, Robert M. 1978. "Three Theories of Informed Consent: Philosophical Foundations and Policy Implications." In *The Belmont Report: Ethical Principles and Guidelines for the Protection of Human Subjects of Research: Appendix II,* pp. 26-1–26-66. DHEW publication no. (OS) 78-0014. Bethesda, Md.: U.S. National Commission for the Protection of Human Subjects of Biomedical and Behavioral Research.

———. 1981. *A Theory of Medical Ethics.* New York: Basic Books.

Wartofsky, Marx W. 1976. "On Doing It for Money." In *Appendix to Report and Recommendations: Research Involving Prisoners,* pp. 3-1–3-24. DHEW publication no. (OS) 76-132. Bethesda, Md.: U.S. National Commission for the Protection of Human Subjects of Biomedical and Behavioral Research.

West, Cornel R. 1976. "Philosophical Perspective on the Participation of Prisoners in Experimental Research." In *Appendix to Report and Recommendations: Research Involving Prisoners,* pp. 2-1–2-22. DHEW publication no. (OS) 76-132. Bethesda, Md.: U.S. National Commission for the Protection of Human Subjects of Biomedical and Behavioral Research.

IV. CLINICAL ASPECTS OF CONSENT IN HEALTH CARE

Health-care decision making is an everyday event, not only for doctors and patients but also for nurses, psychologists, social workers, emergency medical technicians, dentists, and other health professionals. Since the 1960s, however, the cultural ideal of how those decisions should be made has changed considerably. The concept that medical decision making should rely exclu-sively on the physician's expertise has been replaced by a model in which health-care professionals share information and discuss alternatives with patients who then make the ultimate decisions about treatment. This article reviews the origins in the United States of this ideal in the doctrine of informed consent, discusses various arguments against its use in clinical decision making, and describes a model for effectively incorporating it into clinical practice with competent patients.

The concept of informed consent gained its initial support as part of the general societal trend toward broadening access to decision making during the 1960s. Thus, the initial support for informed consent came from legal and philosophic circles rather than from health-care professionals. In the legal arena, informed consent has been used to develop minimal standards for doctor-patient interactions and clinical decision making (Appelbaum et al., 1987). Although there are some differences by jurisdiction, widely accepted legal standards require that health-care professionals inform patients of the risks, benefits, and alternatives of all proposed treatments and then allow the patient to choose among acceptable therapeutic alternatives. In academia, informed consent has served as a cornerstone for the development of the discipline of bioethics. Based on the importance of autonomy in moral discourse, philosophers have argued that health-care professionals are obligated to engage patients in discussions regarding the goals of therapy and the alternatives for reaching those goals and that patients are the final decision makers regarding all therapeutic decisions.

There also has been some support for informed consent within academic medicine, but there seems to be little enthusiasm for it in routine medical practice (Lidz et al., 1984). Physicians typically think of informed consent as a legal requirement for a signed piece of paper that is at best a waste of time and at worst a bureaucratic, legalistic interference with their care for patients. Rather than seeing informed consent as a process that promotes good communication and patient autonomy, many health-care professionals view informed consent as a complex, legally prescribed recitation of risks and benefits that only frightens or confuses patients. There are various objections to informed consent that clinicians often make, and it will be useful to review those objections here.

Objections to informed consent

Consent cannot be truly "informed." Many practicing clinicians report that their patients are unable to understand the complex medical information necessary for a fully rational weighing of alternative treatments. There is considerable research support for this view. A variety of studies document that patients recall only a small percentage of the information that professionals present to them (Meisel and Roth, 1981); that they are not as good decision makers when they are sick as at other times (Sherlock, 1986); and that they often make decisions based on medically trivial factors. Informed consent thus appears either to promote uninformed, and thus suboptimal, decisions or to encourage patients to blindly accept health-care professionals' recommendations. In either case informed consent appears to be a charade, and a dangerous one at that.

That patients often do have difficulty understanding important aspects of medical decisions does not mean that health-care professionals are the best decision makers about the patient's treatment. Knowledge about medical facts is not enough. Wise house buyers will have a structural engineer check over an old house, but few would be willing to allow the engineer to choose their house for them. Just as structural engineers cannot decide which house a family should buy because they lack knowledge about the family's pattern of living, personal tastes, and potential family growth, health-care professionals cannot scientifically deduce the best treatment for a specific patient simply from the medical facts. Because what matters to individuals about their health depends on their lifestyles, past experiences, and values, choosing the "optimal therapy" is not a purely "objective" matter (U.S. President's Commission, 1982). Thus, patients and health-care professionals both contribute essential knowledge to the decision-making process—patients bring their knowledge of their personal situation, goals, and values, and health-care professionals bring their expertise on the nature of the problem and the technology that may be used to meet the patient's goals (see Brock, 1991).

Informed-consent disclosures, even if they are well done, may not lead to what clinicians might consider optimal decisions. Most people make major life decisions, such as whom to marry and which occupation to take up, based on faulty or incomplete information. Patients' lack of understanding of medical information in choosing treatment is probably no worse than their lack of information in choosing a spouse, nor are medical decisions more important than spousal choice. Respecting patient autonomy means allowing individuals to make their own decisions even if the health-care professional disagrees with them. Informed-consent disclosures can improve patient decisions, but they cannot be expected to lead to perfect decisions.

Moreover, although sick persons have some defects in their rational abilities, so do health-care professionals. There are no data that demonstrate that health-care professionals' reasoning abilities are better than patients. In fact, some of the most famous research on the diffi-

culties individuals have with the rational use of probabilistic data involves physicians (Dawson and Ackes, 1987). Health professionals must be careful not to be too pessimistic about patients' ability to become informed decision makers. Patients may not be able to become as technically well-informed as professionals, but they clearly can understand and make decisions based on relevant information. A recent study, for example, showed that patients' decisions regarding life-sustaining treatment changed when they were given accurate information about the therapy's chance of success (Murphy et al., 1994).

Most important, the difficulty of educating sick persons does not justify unilateral decision making. Rather, it places a special obligation on health-care professionals to communicate clearly with patients. Using technical jargon, trying to give all of the available information in one visit, and not asking what the patient wants to know is a recipe for confusing even the most intelligent patient. A growing literature, for example, discusses the problems patients have understanding uncertainty about treatment outcomes and suggests ways to help patients deal with such uncertainty (Katz, 1984). Health-care professionals also need to become more familiar with different cultural patterns of communication in order to talk with patients from different cultural backgrounds. For example, although a simple, factual discussion of depression and its treatment may be acceptable to most middle-class Americans, it would be seen as inappropriate by a first-generation Vietnamese male (Hahn, 1982), whose culture discourages viewing depression as a disease. There is no reason, in principle, why a person who daily makes decisions at home and work cannot, with help, understand the medical data sufficiently to become involved in medical decisions. Health-care professionals must learn how best to present that help.

Patients do not wish to be involved in decision making. Many health-care professionals believe that it is unfair to force patients to make decisions regarding their medical care. After all, they argue, patients pay their health-care professionals to make medical decisions. The empirical literature partially supports the view that patients want professionals to make treatment decisions for them (Steele et al., 1987). For example, in a study of male patients' preferences about medical decision making regarding hypertension, only 53 percent wanted to participate at all in the decision-making process (Strull et al., 1984).

There is no reason to force patients to be involved in decisions if they do not want to be. However, unless the health professional asks, he or she cannot know how involved a patient wants to be. Indeed, patients may not always want to be involved in decision making, since many have been socialized into believing that "the doctor knows best." This is particularly true for poorer patients. Studies have shown that physicians wrongly assume that because patients with fewer socioeconomic resources ask fewer questions, they do not want as much information. These patients may in fact want just as much information, but they have been socialized into a different way of interacting with health-care professionals (Waitzkin, 1984).

Patients may choose to allow someone else to make the decision for them. However, when a patient asks, "What would you do if you were me?" the underlying question may be, "As an expert in biomedicine, what alternative do you think will best maximize my values or interest?" If this is the case, the health-care professional should respond by making a recommendation and justifying it in terms of the patient's values or interests. More frequently, the patient is asking, "If you had this disease, what therapy would you choose?" This question presumes that the professional and patient have the same values, needs, and problems, something that is often not true. Health-care professionals should respond by pointing this out and by emphasizing the importance of the patients' values in the decision-making process.

Although many patients do not want to be actively involved in decision making, they almost always want more information concerning their illness than the health-care professional gives them. Health-care professionals should not assume that just because patients do not wish to choose their therapy, they do not want information. Patients may desire information so as to increase compliance or make modifications in other areas of their lives, as well as to make medical decisions.

There are harmful effects of informing patients. Health-care professionals often justify withholding information from patients because of their belief that informing patients would be psychologically damaging and therefore contrary to the principle of nonmaleficence. Many health-care professionals, however, overestimate potential psychological harm and neglect the positive effects of full disclosure (Faden et al., 1986). Moreover, bad news can often be communicated in a way that ameliorates the psychological effects of the disclosure (Quill and Townsend, 1991). Truth-telling must be distinguished from "truth dumping." Explanation of the care that can be provided, and empathic attention to the patient's fears and uncertainties can often prevent or mitigate otherwise more painful news.

Informed consent takes too much time. Respecting autonomy and promoting patient well-being, the values served through informed consent, are fundamental to good medicine. However, adhering to the ideals of medical practice takes time, time to help patients understand their illness and work through their emotional reactions to stressful information; to discuss each party's preconceptions and to clarify the therapeutic goals; to decide on a treatment plan; and to elicit questions about diagnosis and treatment.

In U.S. health care, time is money. As many commentators have noted, physicians are less well reimbursed for talking to patients than for performing invasive tests. This may discourage doctors from spending enough time discussing treatment options with patients. Changes in physician reimbursement, such as the Relative-Value Based Scale, which are designed to increase reimbursement for cognitive skills, including the time it takes to discuss diagnosis and treatment with patients, will encourage physicians to discuss patients' preferences with them. The ultimate justification for spending time to facilitate patient decisions, however, is the same as that for spending any time in medical care: that patients will be better cared for.

Clinical approaches to informed consent

Many of the problems in implementing informed consent result at least in part from the way informed consent has been implemented in clinical practice. Informed consent has become synonymous with the "consent form," a legal invention with a legitimate role in documenting that informed consent has taken place, but hardly a substitute for the discussion process leading to informed consent (Andrews, 1984).

A pro forma approach: An event model of informed consent. In many clinical settings, consent begins when "it is time to get consent," typically just prior to the administration of treatment. The process of getting the patients' consent consists of the recitation by a physician or nurse of the list of material risks and benefits and a request that the patient sign for the proposed treatment. This "conversation" is a very limited one that emphasizes the transfer of information from the physician or nurse to the patient. This procedure does meet the minimal legal requirements for informed consent efficiently. However, it does not meet the higher ethical goal of informed consent, which is to empower patients by educating and involving them in their treatment plans. Instead, it imposes an almost empty ritual on an unchanged relationship between health-care provider and patient (Katz, 1984).

The procedure just described assumes that care involves a series of discrete, circumscribed decisions. In fact, much of clinical medicine consists of a series of frequent, interwoven decisions that must be repeatedly reconsidered as more information becomes available. When "it is time to get consent," there may be nothing left to decide. Consider the operative consent form obtained the evening prior to an operation. After patients have discussed with their families whether to be admitted to the hospital, rearranged their work and child-care schedules for admission, and undergone a long and painful diagnostic workup, the decision to have surgery seems preordained. The evening before the operation, patients do not seriously evaluate the operation's risks and benefits; consent is pro forma. No wonder some health-care professionals feel that "consent" is a waste of time and energy.

The event model for gathering informed consent falls far short of meeting the ethical goal of ensuring patient participation in the decision-making process. Rather than engaging the patient as an active participant in the decision-making process, the patient's role is to agree to or veto the health-care professionals' recommendations. Little attempt is made to elicit patient preferences and to consider how treatment might address them.

A dialogical approach: The process model of informed consent. Fortunately, it is possible to fulfill legal requirements for informed consent while maximizing active patient participation in the clinical setting. An alternative to the event model described above, which sees informed consent as an aberration from clinical practice, the process model attempts to integrate informed consent into all aspects of clinical care (Appelbaum et al., 1987). The process model of informed consent assumes that each party has something to contribute to the decision-making process. The physician brings technical knowledge and experience in treating patients with similar problems. Patients bring knowledge about their life circumstances and the ability to assess the effect that treatment may have on them. Open discussion makes it possible for the patient and the physician to examine critically their views and to determine what might be optimal treatment.

The process model also recognizes that medical care rarely involves only one decision, made at a single point in time. Decisions about care frequently begin with the suspicion that something is wrong and that treatment may be necessary, and end only when the patient leaves follow-up care. Decisions involve diagnostic as well as therapeutic interventions. Some decisions are made in one visit, while others occur over a prolonged period of time. Although some interactions between health-care professional and patient involve explicit decisions, decisions are made at each interaction, even if the decision is only to continue treatment. The process model also recognizes that various health-care professionals may play a role in making sure that the patients' consent is informed. For example, a woman deciding on various breast cancer treatments may talk with an oncologist and a surgeon about the risks of various treatments, with a nurse about the side effects of medication, with a social worker about financial issues in treatment, and with a

patient-support group about her husband's reaction to a possible mastectomy.

Ideally, then, informed consent involves shared decision making over a period of time, that is, a dialogue throughout the course of the patient's relationship with various health-care professionals. Such a dialogue aims to facilitate patient participation and to strengthen the therapeutic alliance.

Tasks involved in informed consent

Consent is a series of interrelated tasks. First, the patient and professional must agree on the problem that will be the focus of their work together (Eisenthal and Lazare, 1976). Most nonemergency consultations involve complex negotiations between health-care professional and patient regarding the definition of the patient's problem. The patient may see the problem as a routine physical examination for a work release, the need for advice, or the investigation of a physical symptom. If professionals are to respond effectively to the patients' goals, they must find out the reason for the visit. Whereas physicians typically focus on biomedical information and its implications, patients typically view the problem in the context of their social situation (Fisher and Todd, 1983). The differences between the patient's perceptions of the problem and the professional's must be explicitly worked through since agreement regarding the focus of the interactions lead to increased patient satisfaction and compliance with further treatment plans (Meichenbaum and Turk, 1987).

Even when the professional and patient have agreed on what the problem is, substantial misunderstanding may arise regarding the treatment goals. The patient may expect the medically impossible, or may expect outcomes based on knowledge of life circumstances about which the physician is unaware. Since assessing the risks and benefits of any treatment option depends on therapeutic goals, the professional and patient must agree on the goals the therapy aims to accomplish.

Finding out what the patient wants is more complicated than merely inquiring, "What do you want?" A patient typically does not come to the professional with well-developed preferences regarding medical therapy except "to get better," with little understanding of what this may involve. As a patient's knowledge and perspective change over the course of an illness, so too may the patient's views regarding the therapeutic goals.

Because clinicians provide much of the medical information needed to ensure that the patient's preferences are grounded in medical possibility, health-care professionals play a significant role in how a patient's preferences evolve. It is important that they understand that patients may reasonably hold different goals from those their practitioners hold. This is particularly true when they come from different economic strata. For example, a physician's emphasis on the most medically sophisticated care may pale in the light of the patient's financial problems. Therapeutic goals, like the definition of the problem, require ongoing clarification and negotiation.

After agreeing upon the problem and the therapeutic goals, the health-care professional and the patient must choose the best way to achieve them. If patients have been involved in the prior two steps, the decision about a treatment plan will more likely reflect their values than if they are merely asked to assent to the clinician's strategy.

Health-care professionals often ask how much information they must supply to ensure that the patient is an informed participant in the decision-making process (Mazur, 1986). There is a more important question: Has the information been provided in a manner that the patient can understand? While the law only requires that health-care professionals inform patients, morally valid consent requires that patients understand the information conveyed. Ensuring patient understanding requires attention to the quality as well as the quantity of information presented (Faden, 1977).

A great deal of empirical data has been collected concerning problems with consent forms. These forms have been criticized, for example, as being unintelligible because of their length and use of technical language (Appelbaum et al., 1987). Health-care professionals thus need to be aware of, and facile in using, a variety of methods to increase patients' comprehension of information; these include verbal techniques, written information, or interactive videodiscs (Stanley et al., 1984).

Still, the question of how much information to present remains. The legal standards regarding information disclosure—what a reasonable patient would find essential to making a decision or what a reasonably prudent physician would disclose—are not particularly helpful. Howard Brody has suggested two important features: (1) The physician must disclose the basis on which the proposed treatment or the alternative possible treatments have been chosen; and (2) the patient must be encouraged to ask questions, suggested by the disclosure about the physician's reasoning, and the questions need to be answered to the patient's satisfaction (Brody, 1989). Health-care professionals must also inform patients when controversy exists about the various therapeutic options. Similarly, patients should also be told the degree to which the recommendation is based on established scientific evidence versus personal experience or educated guesses.

Two other factors will influence the amount of information that should be given: the importance of the decision, given the patient's situation and goals, and the amount of consensus within the health-care professions regarding the agreed-upon therapy. For example, a low-risk intervention, such as giving influenza vaccines to elderly patients, offers a clear-cut benefit with minimal risk. In this case, the professional should describe the intervention and recommend it because of its benefits. A detailed description of the infrequent risks is not needed unless the patient asks or is known to be skeptical of medical interventions. Interventions that present greater risks or a less clear-cut risk–benefit ratio require a longer description—for example, the decision to administer AZT to an HIV (human immunodeficiency virus)-positive, asymptomatic woman with a CD4 count of 400. In neither case is a discussion of pathophysiology or biochemistry necessary. It must be emphasized that there is no formula for deciding how much a patient needs to be told. The amount of information necessary will depend on the patient's individual situation, values, and goals.

Finally, an adequate decision-making process requires continual updating of information, monitoring of expectations, and evaluation of the patient's progress in reaching the chosen or revised goals. Thus the final step in informed consent is follow-up. This step is particularly important for patients with chronic diseases in which modifications of the treatment plan are often necessary.

The process model of informed consent just described has many advantages. Because it assumes many short conversations over time rather than one long interaction, it can be more easily integrated into the professional's ambulatory practice than the event model; it allows patients to be much more involved in decision making and ensures that treatment is more consistent with their values. Furthermore, the continual monitoring of patients' understanding of their disease, the treatment, and its progress is likely to reduce misunderstandings and increase their investment in, and adherence to, the treatment plan. Thus, the process model of informed consent is likely to promote both patient autonomy and well-being.

There are situations in which this approach is not very helpful. Some health-care professionals, anesthesiologists or emergency medical technicians, for example, are not likely to have ongoing relationships with patients. In emergencies, there is not time for a decision to develop through a series of short conversations. In these cases, informed consent may more closely approximate the event model. However, since most medical care is delivered by primary-care practitioners in an ambulatory setting, the process model of informed consent is more helpful.

ROBERT M. ARNOLD
CHARLES W. LIDZ

Directly related to this article are the other articles in this entry, especially the articles on HISTORY OF INFORMED CONSENT, MEANING AND ELEMENTS OF INFORMED CONSENT, *and* LEGAL AND ETHICAL ISSUES OF CONSENT IN HEALTH CARE (*with its* POSTSCRIPT). *Also directly related are the entries* AUTONOMY; COMPETENCY; CLINICAL ETHICS, *article on* ELEMENTS AND METHODOLOGIES; *and* INFORMATION DISCLOSURE. *This article will find application in the entries* DEATH AND DYING: EUTHANASIA AND SUSTAINING LIFE; GENETIC COUNSELING, *article on* ETHICAL ISSUES; PROFESSIONAL–PATIENT RELATIONSHIP, *article on* ETHICAL ISSUES; *and* SURGERY. *Other relevant material may be found under the entries* BENEFICENCE; FREEDOM AND COERCION; HOSPITAL, *article on* CONTEMPORARY ETHICAL PROBLEMS; LAW AND BIOETHICS; LIFE, QUALITY OF, *article on* QUALITY OF LIFE IN CLINICAL DECISIONS; MEDICAL CODES AND OATHS, *article on* ETHICAL ANALYSIS; PATERNALISM; PATIENTS' RIGHTS, *article on* ORIGIN AND NATURE OF PATIENTS' RIGHTS; *and* RIGHTS, *article on* RIGHTS IN BIOETHICS.

Bibliography

ANDREWS, LORI B. 1984. "Informed Consent Status and the Decision-making Process." *Journal of Legal Medicine* 5, no. 2:163–217. The author criticizes current laws for their emphasis on how much information a physician provides rather than whether the patient understands the information provided.

APPELBAUM, PAUL S.; LIDZ, CHARLES W.; and MEISEL, ALAN. 1987. *Informed Consent: Legal Theory and Clinical Practice.* New York: Oxford University Press. A clinically based review of the theory and practice of informed consent.

BROCK, DAN W. 1991. "The Ideal of Shared Decision Making Between Physicians and Patients." *Kennedy Institute of Ethics Journal* 1, no. 1:28–47. A philosophically interesting description of what shared decision making might mean.

BRODY, HOWARD. 1989. "Transparency: Informed Consent in Primary Care." *Hastings Center Report* 19, no. 5:5–9. The author proposes a new standard for determining how much information a physician must provide a patient in order to obtain informed consent.

DAWSON, NEAL V., and ARKES, HAL R. 1987. "Systematic Errors in Medical Decision Making: Judgment Limitations." *Journal of General Internal Medicine* 2, no. 3:183–187.

EISENTHAL, SHERMAN, and LAZARE, AARON. 1976. "Evaluation of the Initial Interview in a Walk-in Clinic." *Journal of Nervous and Mental Disease* 162, no. 3:169–176.

FADEN, RUTH R. 1977. "Disclosure and Informed Consent: Does It Matter How We Tell It?" *Health Education Monographs* 5, no. 3:198–214.

FADEN, RUTH R.; BEAUCHAMP, TOM L.; and KING, NANCY M. P. 1986. *A History and Theory of Informed Consent.* New York: Oxford University Press. A comprehensive look at the history and philosophical theory of informed consent. An excellent reference.

FISHER, SUE, and TODD, ALEXANDRA D., eds. 1983. *The Social Organization of Doctor-Patient Communication.* Washington, D.C.: Center for Applied Linguistics. A series of papers that analyze the empirical relationships between social class, gender, and medical interactions.

GADOW, SALLY. 1980. "Existential Advocacy: Philosophic Foundation of Nursing." In *Nursing: Images and Ideals: Opening Dialogue with the Humanities,* pp. 79–101. Edited by Stuart F. Spicker and Sally Gadow. New York: Springer. An attempt to define the role of nurse to make informed consent central to what it is to be a nurse.

HAHN, ROBERT A. 1982. "Culture and Informed Consent: An Anthropological Perspective." In vol. 2 of *Making Health Care Decisions: The Ethical and Legal Implications of Informed Consent in the Patient-Practitioner Relationship.* Washington, D.C.: U.S. President's Commission for the Study of Ethical Problems in Medicine and Biomedical and Behavioral Research.

KATZ, JAY. 1984. *The Silent World of Doctor and Patient.* New York: Free Press. A psychoanalytically based view of doctor–patient communication problems. The author offers important suggestions for rethinking the doctor–patient relationship to increase shared decision making.

LIDZ, CHARLES W.; MEISEL, ALAN; ZERUBAVEL, EVIATAR; CARTER, MARY; SESTAK, REGINA M.; and ROTH, LOREN H., eds. 1984. *Informed Consent: A Study of Decision-Making in Psychiatry.* New York: Guilford. An in-depth study of how physicians, psychologists, nurses, and social workers do and do not obtain informed consent in a psychiatric hospital.

MAZUR, DENNIS J. 1986. "What Should Patients Be Told Prior to a Medical Procedure? Ethical and Legal Perspectives on Medical Informed Consent." *American Journal of Medicine* 81, no. 6:1051–1054.

MEICHENBAUM, DONALD, and TURK, DENNIS. 1987. *Facilitating Treatment Adherence: A Practitioner's Guidebook.* New York: Plenum Press.

MEISEL, ALAN, and ROTH, LOREN H. 1981. "What We Do and Do Not Know About Informed Consent." *Journal of the American Medical Association* 246, no. 21:2473–2477.

MURPHY, DONALD J.; BURROWS, DAVID; SANTILLI, SARA; KEMP, ANNE W.; TENNER, SCOTT; KRELING, BARBARA; and TENO, JOAN. 1994. "The Influence of the Probability of Survival on Patients' Preferences Regarding Cardiopulmonary Resuscitation." *New England Journal of Medicine* 330, no. 8:545–549.

QUILL, TIMOTHY E., and TOWNSEND, PENELOPE. 1991. "Bad News: Delivery, Dialogue, and Dilemmas." *Archives of Internal Medicine* 151:463–468. A practical article on giving bad news to patients.

SHERLOCK, RICHARD. 1986. "Reasonable Men and Sick Human Beings." *American Journal of Medicine* 80, no. 1:2–4.

STANLEY, BARBARA; GUIDO, JEANNINE; STANLEY, MICHAEL; and SHORTELL, DIANN. 1984. "The Elderly Patient and Informed Consent: Empirical Findings." *Journal of the American Medical Association* 252, no. 10:1302–1306.

STEEL, DAVID J.; BLACKWELL, BARRY; GUTMANN, MARY C.; and JACKSON, THOMAS C. 1987. "The Activated Patient: Dogma, Dream or Desideratum." *Patient Education and Counseling* 10, no. 1:3–23. An excellent review of articles studying the degree to which patients want to be involved in decision making.

STRULL, WILLIAM M.; LO, BERNARD; and CHARLES, GERARD. 1984. "Do Patients Want to Participate in Medical Decision-making?" *Journal of the American Medical Association* 252, no. 21:2990–2994.

U.S. PRESIDENT'S COMMISSION FOR THE STUDY OF ETHICAL PROBLEMS IN MEDICINE AND BIOMEDICAL AND BEHAVIORAL RESEARCH. 1982. *Making Health Care Decisions: A Report on the Ethical and Legal Implications of Informed Consent in the Patient-Practitioner Relationship.* Washington, D.C.: Author. A landmark analysis of informed consent. Volume 1 summarizes what has become the consensus of opinion about informed consent. Volumes 2 and 3 contain philosophical, sociological, and anthropological studies of informed consent.

WAITZKIN, HOWARD. 1984. "Doctor-Patient Communication: Clinical Implications of Social Scientific Research." *Journal of the American Medical Association* 252, no. 17:2441–2446.

———. 1991. *The Politics of Medical Encounters: How Patients and Doctors Deal with Social Problems.* New Haven, Conn.: Yale University Press.

WEST, CANDACE. 1984. *Routine Complications: Troubles with Talk Between Doctors and Patients.* Bloomington: Indiana University Press.

V. LEGAL AND ETHICAL ISSUES OF CONSENT IN HEALTH CARE

This article, by Jay Katz, is reprinted from the first edition, where it carried the title "Informed Consent in the Therapeutic Relationship: II. Legal and Ethical Aspects." It is followed immediately by a "Postscript," prepared by Angela R. Holder for purposes of updating the original article.

The doctrine of informed consent, introduced into U.S. case law in 1957, represents judges' groping efforts to delineate physicians' duties to inform patients of the benefits and risks of diagnostic and treatment alternatives, including the consequences of no treatment, as well as to obtain patients' consent (*Salgo v. Stanford University,* 1957). The doctrine's avowed purpose was to protect patients' right to "thoroughgoing self-determination" (*Natanson v. Kline,* 1960). The legal implications of informed consent, however, remain unclear. The doctrine is in fact more of a slogan, which judges have been too timid or too wise to translate into law, at least as yet. It has been employed with little care but great passion to voice a dream of personal freedom and individual dignity. Though its legal impact in protecting patients' right to self–decision making has been scant, the threat of informed consent has opened profound issues for the traditional practice of medicine.

The medical framework

It has been insufficiently recognized, particularly by judges, that disclosure and consent, except in the most rudimentary fashion, are obligations alien to medical practice. Hippocrates' admonitions to physicians are still followed today: "Perform [these duties] calmly and adroitly, concealing most things from the patient while you are attending to him. Give necessary orders with cheerfulness and serenity, turning his attention away from what is being done to him; sometimes reprove sharply and emphatically, and sometimes comfort with solicitude and attention, revealing nothing of the patient's future or present condition" (Hippocrates, 1923). Thus it is not surprising that the Hippocratic oath is silent on the duty of physicians to inform, or even converse with, patients. Similarly Dr. Thomas Percival, whose 1803 book *Medical Ethics* influenced profoundly the subsequent codifications of medical ethics in England and the United States, commented only once on the discourse between physicians and patients, restricting his remarks to "gloomy prognostications." Even in that context he advised that "friends of the patient" be primarily informed, though he added that the patient may be told "if absolutely necessary" (Percival, 1927, p. 91). The Code of Ethics of the American Medical Association, adopted in 1847, and the Principles of Medical Ethics of the American Medical Association, adopted in 1903 and 1912, repeat, in almost the same words, Percival's statement. The AMA Principles of Medical Ethics, endorsed in 1957, delete Percival's wording entirely and substitute the vague admonition that "physicians . . . should make available to their patients . ,. . the benefits of their professional attainments." The pertinent sections of the *Opinions of the Judicial Council of the AMA,* interpreting the principles, note only the surgeon's obligation to disclose "all facts relevant to the need and performance of the operation" and the experimenter's obligation, when using new drugs and procedures, to obtain "the voluntary consent of the person" (American Medical Association Judicial Council, 1969). Nine years later, the AMA House of Delegates in endorsing, with modifications, the Declaration of Helsinki, asked that investigators, when engaged "in clinical [research] primarily for treatment," make relevant disclosures to and obtain the voluntary consent of patients or their legally authorized representative.

Thus in the context of therapy no authoritative statement encouraging disclosure and consent has ever been promulgated by the medical profession. The AMA's tersely worded surgical exception was compelled by the law of malpractice. Its experimental exception represented primarily an acquiescence to the U.S. Public Health Service and the U.S. Department of Health, Education, and Welfare requirements, which in turn were formulated in response to congressional concerns about research practices. When disclosure and consent prior to the conduct of therapeutic research were endorsed by the AMA, it did not extend those requirements to *all* patient care but limited the exception to "clinical [research] primarily for treatment."

Two significant conclusions can be drawn: (1) "Informed consent" is a creature of law and not a medical prescription. A duty to inform patients has never been promulgated by the medical profession, though individual physicians have made interesting, but as a rule unsystematic, comments on this topic. Judges have been insufficiently aware of the deeply ingrained Hippocratic tradition against disclosure and, instead, seem to have assumed that individual physicians lack of disclosure was aberrant with respect to standard medical practice, and hence "negligent," in the sense of "forgetful" or "inadvertent," conduct. (2) When judges were confronted with claims of lack of informed consent, no medical precedent, no medical position papers, and no analytic medical thinking existed on this subject. Thus physicians were ill prepared to shape judges' notions on informed consent with thoughtful and systematic positions of their own.

The legal framework

With the historical movement from feudalism to individualism, consent, respect for the dignity of human beings, and the right of individuals to shape their own lives became important principles of English common law and, in turn, of American common law. Yet, as these principles gained greater acceptance, questions arose in many areas of law about the capacity of human beings to make their own decisions and about the need to protect them from their own "folly." The tug of war between advocates of thoroughgoing self-determination and those of paternalism has continued unabated. The informed-consent doctrine manifests this struggle. While in physician–patient interactions the legal trend during the past two decades has been to increase somewhat the right of patients to greater freedom of choice, the informed-consent doctrine has not had as far-reaching an impact on patients' self-determination as many commentators have assumed. This fact has been insufficiently appreciated and has led to confusion, further compounded by the courts' rhetoric that seemed to promise more than it delivered.

Consent to medical and surgical interventions is an ancient legal requirement. Historically an intentional touching without consent was adjudicated in battery. The law has not changed at all in this regard, and a surgeon who operates on a patient without permission is legally liable, even if the operation is successful. In such instances any inquiry into medical need or negligent conduct becomes irrelevant, for what is at issue is the disregard of the person's right to exercise control over his body. The jurisprudential basis of these claims is personal freedom:

> . . . under a free government at least, the free citizen's first and greatest right, which underlies all others—the right to himself—is the subject of universal acquiescence, and this right necessarily forbids a physician or surgeon, however skillful or eminent . . . to violate without permission the bodily integrity of his patient by . . . operating on him without his consent. . . . (*Pratt v. Davis*, 1906)

But what does consent mean? In battery cases it means only that the physician must inform the patient what he proposes to do and that the patient must agree. Medical emergencies and patients' incompetence are the only exceptions to this requirement.

In mid-twentieth century, judges gradually confronted the question whether patients are entitled not only to know what a doctor proposes to do but also to decide whether the intervention is advisable in the light of its risks and benefits and the available alternatives, including no treatment. Such awareness of patients' informational needs is a modern phenomenon, influenced by the simultaneous growth of product liability and consumer law.

The law of fraud and deceit has always protected patients from doctors' flagrant misrepresentations, and in theory patients have always been entitled to ask whatever questions they pleased. What the doctrine of informed consent sought to add is the proposition that physicians are now under an affirmative duty to offer to acquaint patients with the important risks and plausible alternatives to the proposed procedure. The underlying rationale for that duty was stated in *Natanson v. Kline*:

> Anglo-American law starts with the premise of thorough-going self-determination. It follows that each man is considered to be master of his own body, and he may, if he be of sound mind, expressly prohibit the performance of life-saving surgery, or other medical treatment. A doctor might well believe that an operation or form of treatment is desirable or necessary but the law does not permit him to substitute his own judgment for that of the patient by any form of artifice or deception. (*Natanson v. Kline*, 1960)

The language employed by the *Natanson* court in support of an affirmative duty to disclose derives from the language of the law of battery, which clearly makes the patient the ultimate decision maker with respect to his body. Thus the courts reasoned, with battery principles very much in mind, that significant protection of patients' right to decide their medical fate required not merely perfunctory assent but a truly "informed consent," based on an adequate understanding of the medical and surgical options available to them.

Yet in the same breath judges also attempted to intrude as little as possible on traditional medical practices. In doing so their impulse to protect the right of individual self-determination collided with their equally strong desire to maintain the authority and practices of the professions. Law has always respected the arcane expertise of physicians and has never held them liable if they practiced "good medicine." The law of consent in battery represented no aberration from this principle since most physicians agree that patients at least deserve to know the nature of the proposed procedure. However, the new duty of disclosure that the law, in the name of self-determination, threatened to impose upon physicians was something quite different. For the vast majority of physicians significant disclosure is not at all part of standard medical practice. Most doctors believe that patients are neither emotionally nor intellectually equipped to be medical decision makers, that they must be guided past childish fears into "rational" therapy, and that disclosures of uncertainty, gloomy prognosis and dire risks often seriously undermine cure. Physicians began to wonder whether law was now asking them to practice "bad" medicine.

In the early informed-consent cases, judges simply did not resolve the conflict between self-determination and professional practices and authority. The result was distressing confusion. In obeisance to the venerable ideal of self-determination, courts purported to establish, as a matter of law, the physician's

> . . . obligation . . . to disclose and explain to the patient in language as simple as necessary the nature of the ailment, the nature of the proposed treatment, the probability of success or of alternatives, and perhaps the risks of unfortunate results and unforeseen conditions within the body. (*Natanson v. Kline*)

The threat of such an obligation greatly disturbed the medical profession. It recognized that serious implementation of such a standard would significantly alter medical practice. Physicians argued that in order fully to serve patients' best interests, they must have the authority to exercise medical judgment in managing patients. Courts likewise bowed to this judgment. In the very sentence that introduced the ambiguous but exuberant new phrase "informed consent," the court showed its deference to medical judgment and its hesitancy to disturb traditional practice:

> . . . in discussing the element of risk a certain amount of discretion must be employed consistent with the full disclosure of facts necessary to an informed consent. (*Salgo v. Stanford University*)

Thus the extent to which evolving case law, under the banner of individualism, was challenging traditional medical practice—which for millennia has treated patients paternally as children—remained confusing. In those earlier cases (*Salgo v. Stanford University*, *Natanson v. Kline*) judges were profoundly allegiant to both points of view, but the balance was soon tipped decisively in favor of protecting medical practices.

Battery or negligence. The striking ambivalence of judges toward the doctrine of informed consent manifested itself in the competition between battery and negligence doctrines as a means of analyzing and deciding the claims of lack of informed consent. Battery offered a more rigorous protection of patients' right to self-determination. The inquiry into disclosure and consent would not be governed by professional practices but instead would rest on the question: Has the physician met his expanded informational responsibility so that the patient is able to exercise a choice among treatment options? A negative answer to this question would show that the physician's actions constitute trespass, rendering him liable for an unauthorized and "offensive" contact (*Dow v. Kaiser Foundation*).

However, in virtually every jurisdiction judges resolved the competition in favor of negligence law. In doing so, judges were able to defer to medical judgment by evaluating the adequacy of disclosure against the medical professional standard of care, asserting that this standard will govern those duties as it does other medical obligations. As a consequence, physicians remain free to exercise the wisdom of their profession and are liable only for failure to disclose what a reasonable doctor would have revealed. Furthermore, negligence theory does not redress mere dignitary injuries, irrespective of physical injuries, and requires proof that the patient, fully informed, would have refused the proposed treatment. Interferences with self-determination, standing alone, are not compensated.

In rejecting battery, judges made much of the fact that such an action required "intent," while negligence involved "inadvertence"; it was the latter, they believed, that accounted for the lack of disclosure. They overlooked that the withholding of information on the part of physicians is generally quite intentional, dictated by the very exercise of medical judgment that the law of negligence seeks to respect. In stating that the nondisclosures were "collateral" to the central information about the nature of the proposed procedure and hence not required for a valid consent, judges discarded the very idea of informed consent—namely, that absence of expanded disclosure vitiates consent. They refused to extend the inquiry to the total informational needs of patients, without which patients' capacity for self–decision making remains incomplete. At bottom, the rejection of an expanded battery theory and of its proposed requirement of informed consent followed from the threat they posed to the authority of doctors and traditional medical practice.

Thus informed consent, based on patients thoroughgoing self-determination, was a misnomer from the time the phrase was born. To be sure, a new cause of action has emerged for failure to inform of the risks of, and in most jurisdictions alternatives to, treatment. Some duty to disclose risks and alternatives, the courts were willing to say, exists; the extent of that duty is defined by the disclosure practice of a reasonable physician in the circumstances of the case. The new claim is firmly rooted in the law of negligent malpractice, in that plaintiffs are still required to prove the professional standard of care by means of medical expert witnesses. In these, the majority of jurisdictions, traditional medical practice—which generally opposes disclosure—has scarcely been threatened at all in legal reality. The legal life of informed consent, except for dicta about self-determination and the hybrid negligence law promulgated in a handful of jurisdictions, was almost over as soon as it began. Judges had briefly toyed with the idea of patients' self-determination and then largely cast it aside. Good medicine, as defined by doctors, remains good law almost everywhere.

Modifications in professional standard of care. In a few jurisdictions, beginning in 1972 in the District of Columbia with the decision in *Canterbury* v. *Spence,* the new cause of action for failure to inform combined elements of battery with negligence, creating a legal hybrid. The court purported to abandon the professional standard of care with respect to disclosure, asserting that

> . . . respect for the patient's right of self-determination on particular therapy demands a standard set by law for physicians rather than one which physicians may or may not impose upon themselves. (*Canterbury* v. *Spence*)

Thus the court laid down a judge-made rule of disclosure of risks and alternatives, which for all practical purposes resembled an expanded battery standard of disclosure.

The preoccupation with risk disclosure, however, continued unabated. From the very beginning, despite all the talk about "informed consent," judges did not lay down any rules for a careful inquiry into the nature and quality of consent, which on its face any meaningful implementation of the doctrine required. Instead major emphasis was placed on risk disclosures. Since in the cases before courts plaintiff-patients only complained of the injurious results of treatment, this emphasis is understandable. Yet to focus solely on risks is to bypass the principal issue of self-determination—namely, whether the physician kept the patient from arriving at his own decision. The *Canterbury* court, too, restricted its con-

cerns largely to risk disclosures and added the requirement that

> an unrevealed risk that should have been made known must materialize for otherwise the omission, however, unpardonable, is legally without consequence. (*Canterbury* v. *Spence*)

Thus the court foreclosed legal redress for the patient who, fully informed of the potential effects of, for example, a maiming operation, would have chosen an alternative medical course, even though some of the risks did not materialize.

But to the extent these jurisdictions have abandoned the professional standard of disclosure, traditional medical practice has been challenged; "good medicine," in the eyes of the profession, may no longer be a sufficient defense. Seemingly, in these jurisdictions self-determination has begun to encroach upon the province of medical paternalism. That encroachment, however, may be substantially an illusion, for the touted abandonment of the professional standard of disclosure in *Canterbury* was far from complete. Medical judgment to truncate full disclosure must be "given its due," the court said, when "it enters the picture." The court left ambiguous when the plaintiff must establish the appropriate standard of disclosure by an expert witness, or when he must produce such a witness in order to rebut a defendant-physician's claim that good medical judgment was exercised.

What is clear is that the physician has a "therapeutic privilege" not to disclose information where such disclosure would pose a threat to the "well-being" of the patient. But the ambit of this privilege as well as the relationship of its invocation to a directed verdict is not clear, and this for "good" reasons: Even in these most liberal jurisdictions with respect to patients' rights, courts still cannot face squarely the question of how much they are willing to challenge the traditional medical wisdom of nondisclosure. The law remains ambiguous with respect to this, the core issue of informed consent.

Tensions between self-determination and paternalism. Beyond its allegiance to medical paternalism, noted above, the *Canterbury* court showed its preference for paternalism in another way. Under negligence law, the courts have stated that lack of disclosure cannot be said to have caused the patient's injury unless the patient, if adequately informed, would have declined the procedure; this is the crucial problem of causation in informed-consent cases. Such an approach to causation is quite appropriate where law seeks not to compensate interference with self-determination, but only physical injuries resulting from inadequate disclosure. Yet the *Canterbury* court, and every court that has considered the matter subsequently, held that the decision whether or not to undertake therapy must be examined not from the point of view of the patient-plaintiff but from that of a "prudent person in the patient's position," limiting the inquiry to whether a "reasonable patient" would have agreed to the procedure. This substitution of a community standard of a "reasonable" person cuts the heart out of the courts purported respect for individual self-determination. Questions of the influence of hindsight and bitterness are familiar to juries, as is the problem of self-serving testimony generally. While those are delicate problems, they do not justify abrogating the very right at issue in cases of informed consent: the right of individual choice, which may be precisely the right to be an "unreasonable" person.

Epilogue on law. Thus law has proceeded feebly toward the objective of patients' self-determination. While a new cause of action, occasionally hybridized with battery, has emerged for the negligent failure to disclose risks and alternative treatments, it remains a far cry from the avowed purpose of the informed-consent doctrine, namely, to secure patients' autonomy and right to self-determination. In not tampering significantly with the medical wisdom of nondisclosure, yet creating a new cause of action based on traditional disclosure requirements, courts may have accomplished a different result, very much in line with other purposes of tort law—namely, to provide physically injured patients with greater opportunities for seeking compensation whenever it can be argued that disclosure might have avoided such injuries. In doing so judges may have hoped, through the anticipatory tremors of dicta, to urge doctors to consider modifying their traditional disclosure practices. But judges have been unwilling, at least as yet, to implement earnestly patients' right to self-determination.

Whither informed consent?

The disquiet that the doctrine of informed consent has created among physicians cannot be fully explained by the small incremental step courts have taken to assure greater patient participation in medical decision making. More likely it was aroused by the uncertainty over the scope of the doctrine and by an appreciation that medical practice, indeed all professional practice, would be radically changed if fidelity to thoroughgoing self-determination were to prevail. In what follows, some of the issues raised by the idea of an informed-consent doctrine, based on a premise of self-determination, will be discussed.

Patients. Traditionally patients have been viewed as ignorant about medical matters, fearful about being sick, childlike by virtual of their illness, ill-equipped to sort out what is in their best medical inter-

est, and prone to make decisions detrimental to their welfare (Parsons). Thus physicians have asserted that it makes little sense to consult patients on treatment options: far better to interact with them as beloved children and decide for them. In the light of such deeply held convictions, many physicians are genuinely puzzled by any informed-consent requirement. Moreover, its possible detrimental impact on compassion, reassurance, and hope—ancient prescriptions for patient care—has raised grave ethical questions for the medical profession.

Those concerns should not be dismissed lightly. What may be at issue, however, is not an intrinsic incapacity of patients to participate in medical decision making. For not all patients, and probably not even most, are too uneducated, too frightened, or too regressed to understand the benefits and risks of treatment options available to them. Moreover, their capacities for decision making are affected to varying degrees, for example, by the nature of the disease process, its prognosis, acuteness, painfulness, etc., as well as by the personality of patients. The medical literature is largely silent on the question of who—under what circumstances and with what conditions—should or should not be allowed to participate fully in medical decision making.

But why has not the sorting-out process, distinguishing between those patients who do and those who do not have the capacity for decision making, been undertaken long ago? One answer suggests itself: Once those patients have been identified who, in principle, can make decisions on their own behalf, physicians would be compelled to confront the questions of whether to interact with them on a level of greater equality; whether to share with them the uncertainties and unknowns of medical diagnosis, treatment, and prognosis; and whether to communicate to them their professional limitations as well as the lack of expert consensus about treatment alternatives. Such an open dialogue would expose the uncertainties inherent in most medical interventions; and to the extent medicine's helpful and curative power depends on the faith and confidence which the physician projects, patients may be harmed by disclosure and consent.

Physicians' objections to informed consent, therefore, may have less to do with the incompetence of patients as such than with an unrecognized concern of the doctrine's impact on the dynamics of cure. Put another way, the all too sweeping traditional view of patients has misled doctors into believing that medicine's opposition to informed consent is largely based on patients' incompetence, rather than on an apprehension, however dimly perceived, that disclosure would bring into view much about the practice of medicine that physicians seek to hide from themselves and their patients; for example, the uncertainties and disagreements about the treatments employed; the curative impact of physicians' and patients' beliefs in the unquestioned effectiveness of their prescriptions rather than the prescriptions themselves; the difficulty in sorting out the contributions that *vis medicatrix naturae* ("the healing power of nature") makes to the healing process; the impact of patients' suggestibility to cure, etc. Thus the question: When does informed consent interfere with physicians' effectiveness and with the dynamics of cure?

Little attention has been paid to the fact that the practice of Hippocratic medicine makes patients more incompetent than they need be. Indeed patients' incompetence can become a self-fulfilling prophecy as a consequence of medical practices. That the stress of illness leads to psychological regression, to chronologically earlier modes of functioning, has been recognized for a long time. Precious little, however, is known about the contributions that physicians' attitudes toward and interactions with their patients make to the regressive pull. Also, little is known about the extent to which regression can be avoided by not keeping patients in the dark, by inviting them to participate in decision making, and by addressing and nurturing the intact, mature parts of their functioning. This uncharted territory requires exploration in order to determine what strains will be imposed on physicians and patients alike, if Anna Freud's admonition to students of the Western Reserve Medical School is heeded:

> . . . you must not be tempted to treat [the patient] as a child. You must be tolerant toward him as you would be toward a child and as respectful as you would be towards a fellow adult because he has only gone back to childhood as far as he's ill. He also has another part of his personality which has remained intact and that part of him will resent it deeply, if you make too much use of your authority. (quoted in Katz, 1972, p. 637)

Physicians.   Traditionally physicians have asserted that their integrity, training, professional dedication to patients' best medical interests, and commitment to "doing no harm" are sufficient safeguards for patients. The complexities inherent in medical decision making, physicians maintain, require that trust be patients' guiding principle. The idea of informed consent does not question the integrity, training, or dedication of doctors. Without them, informed consent would be of little value. What the idea of informed consent does question is the necessity and appropriateness of physicians' making all decisions for their patients; it calls for a careful scrutiny of which decisions belong to the doctor and which to the patient.

Physicians have preferences about treatment options that may not necessarily be shared by patients. For example, no professional consensus exists about the treatment of breast cancer. The advantages and disadvantages of lumpectomy, simple mastectomy, radical mastectomy, radiation therapy, chemotherapy, and various combinations among these are subject to much controversy. Dr. Bernard Fisher, chairman of the National Surgical Adjuvant Breast Cancer Project, has said that we simply do not know which method is best (Fisher, 1970). Thus the question must be answered: How extensive an opportunity must patients be given to select which alternative? Informed consent challenges the stereotypical notion that physicians should assume the entire burden of deciding what treatment *all* patients, *whatever* their condition, should undergo. Indeed, can the assumption of this burden be defined purely on medical grounds in the first place? Is not the decision in favor of one treatment for breast cancer over another, like many other treatment decisions, a combination of medical, emotional, aesthetic, religious, philosophical, social, interpersonal, and personal judgments? Which of these component judgments belong to the physician and which to the patient?

Much needs to be investigated in order to learn the practical human limits of any new obligations to disclose and to obtain consent:

1. Informing patients for purposes of decision making requires learning new ways of interacting and communicating with patients. Such questions as the following will have to be answered: What background information must patients receive in order to help them formulate their questions? How should physicians respond to "precipitous" consents or refusals? How deeply should doctors probe for understanding? What constitutes irrelevant information that only tends to confuse? What words and explanations facilitate comprehension? Physicians have not been in the habit of posing such questions.

2. Underlying informed consent is the assumption that physicians have considerable knowledge about their particular specialties, keep abreast of new developments, and are aware of what is happening in other fields of medicine that impinge on their area of professional interest. This is not so; indeed, it may be asking too much. Moreover, since physicians have their preferences for particular modes of treatment, can they be expected to present an unbiased picture of alternative treatments?

3. Physicians have consistently asserted that informed consent interferes with compassion (Silk, 1976). Doctors believe that, in order to maintain hope or to avoid the imposition of unnecessary suffering, patients in the throes of a terminal illness, and other patients as well, should not be dealt with honestly. But the evidence for such allegations is lacking. When physicians are asked to support them with clinical data, they are largely unable to do so (Oken, 1961). Indeed, the few studies that have been con-

ducted suggest that most patients do not seem to yearn for hope based on deception, but for hope based on a reassurance that they will not be abandoned, that everything possible will be done for them, and that physicians will deal truthfully with them. Moreover, evidence is accumulating that informed patients become more cooperative, more capable of dealing with discomfort and pain, and more responsible. Whether the often alleged conflict between "compassionate" silence and "cruel" disclosure is myth or reality remains to be seen. Disclosure may turn out to be a greater burden to those who have to interact with patients than to the patients themselves.

4. Informed consent confronts the role of faith in the cure of disease and the complex problems created by the uncertainties inherent in medical practice. To some extent the two issues are intertwined. The effectiveness of a therapeutic program, it has often been said, depends on three variables: the "feeling of trust or faith the patient has in his doctor and therefore in his therapy . . . the faith or confidence the physician has in himself and in the line of therapy he proposes to use . . . and the therapy [itself]" (Hoffer, 1967, p. 124). Informed consent could interfere with the first two variables and thus undermine the effectiveness of treatment. Precisely because of the uncertainties in medical decision making, the physician, to begin with, defends himself against those uncertainties by being more certain about what he is doing than he realistically can be. There is perhaps some unconscious wisdom in what he has been doing since Hippocrates' days, for the unquestioned faith the doctor has in his own therapy is also therapeutic in its own right. Thus, to be a more effective healer, a physician may need to defend himself against his uncertainties by believing himself to be more powerful than he is. That defense will be threatened by informed consent, for it would now require him to be more aware of what he does not know, and therapeutic effectiveness in turn might suffer. Finally, patients' response to treatment also depends on faith in the physician and his medicines. Knowing of the "ifs" and "buts" may shake patients' faith and undermine the therapeutic impact of suggestibility, which contributes so much to recovery from illness.

Physicians' traditional counterphobic reaction to uncertainty, adopting a sense of conviction that what seems right to them is the only correct thing to do, has other consequences as well. Defensive reactions against uncertainty have led to overenthusiasm for particular treatments that have been applied much more widely than an unbiased evaluation would dictate. The ubiquitous tonsillectomies performed to the psychological detriment of untold children is a classical example. Moreover, by not acknowledging uncertainty to themselves, doctors cannot acknowledge it to their patients. Thus consciously and unconsciously physicians avoid the terrifying confrontation of uncertainty, particularly when associated with poor prognosis. As a result, communications with patients take the form of an evasive monologue. The dialogue that might reveal these uncertainties is discouraged (Davis, 1960).

While disclosure of information would reduce patients' ignorance, it would also diminish doctors' power within the physician–patient relationship. As Waitzkin and Stoeckle (1972) have observed, the "physician enhances his power to the extent that he can maintain the patient's uncertainty about the course of illness, efficacy of therapy, or specific future actions of the physician himself" (p. 187). Thus new questions arise: What consequences would a diminution of authority have on physicians effectiveness as healers? How would patients react to less powerful doctors? Would they accept them or turn to new faith healers?

Limits of self-determination.   Patients' capacity for self-determination has been challenged on the grounds that neither total understanding nor total freedom of choice is possible (Ingelfinger, 1972). This of course is true. Any informed-consent doctrine, to be realistic, must take into account the biological, psychological, intellectual, and social constraints imposed upon thought and action. But those inherent constraints, which affect all human beings, do not necessarily justify treating patients as incompetents. Competence does not imply total understanding or total freedom of choice.

What needs to be explored is the extent to which medicine, like law, should presume competence rather than incompetence, in interactions with patients. Neither presumption comports fully with the psychobiology of human beings; both of them express value judgments on how best to interact with human beings. Once the value judgment is made, one can decide on the additional safeguards needed to avoid the harm that any fiction about human behavior introduces.

The idea of informed consent asks for a presumption in favor of competence. If that is accepted, it may also follow that human beings should be allowed to strike their own bargains, however improvident. The then Circuit Judge Warren E. Burger, in commenting on a judicial decision to order a blood transfusion for a Jehovah's Witness, had this to say: "Nothing in [Justice Brandeis's 'right to be let alone' philosophy, suggests that he] thought an individual possessed these rights only as to *sensible* beliefs, *valid* thought, *reasonable* emotions or *well-founded* sensations. I suggest he intended to include a great many foolish, unreasonable and even absurd ideas which do not conform such as refusing medical treatment even at great risk" (*Application of President of Georgetown College,* 1964). A physician may wish, and even should try, to presuade his patients to agree to what he believes would serve their medical interests best; but timately he may have to bow to his patients' decision, however "senseless" or "unreasonable," or withdraw from further participation. The alternatives, deception or coercion, may be worse, for either would victimize not only patients but physicians as well.

Conclusion

The narrow scope that courts have given to the informed-consent doctrine may reflect a deeply held belief that the exercise of self-determination by patients is often against the best interests of otherwise responsible adults and that those interests deserve greater protection than personal freedom. It may also reflect a judicial recognition of law's limited capacity to regulate effectively the physician–patient relationship. Therefore, once having suggested that patients deserve at least a little openness in communication, courts may have concluded that they had gone as far as they could. Judges, at least for the time being, have largely left it up to the medical profession to confront the question of patients' greater participation in medical decision making.

Despite their snail's pace, the courts' approach may have merit. Implementing a right of self-determination has tremendous consequences for medical practice. Many difficult problems, each with vast ethical implications, need to be considered by the medical profession. Thus introspection and education, responsive to the legal and professional problems that new patterns of physician–patient interaction will create, may ultimately provide firmer foundations for new patterns of physician–patient interactions than forced change through outside regulation. The latter, however, may increase if the profession does not rise to the challenge of addressing these long-neglected problems.

JAY KATZ

POSTSCRIPT

General developments

Although case law has not materially changed since 1978, when the *Encyclopedia of Bioethics* was first published, courts have expanded the concept of informed consent to cover more situations and more categories of patients. The duty of disclosure is now seen in new contexts, such as the duty of a physician to inform a patient of the consequences of refusing treatment (e.g., *Truman* v. *Thomas*, 1980; *Battenfield* v. *Gregory*, 1991). The doctrine is no longer centered on the concept of "unwanted touching," so in most (but not all) states, physicians can be liable for failure to explain the possible side effects of drugs they prescribe. On the other hand, some state legislatures have enacted statutes substantially restricting a patient's right to sue a physician for damages for failure to obtain informed consent.

The most profound change in the legal concept of informed consent has come with the expansion of its principles to persons other than the clearly competent, literate adults involved in the pre-1980 cases. Much of the litigation in the 1980s and 1990s involves the rights of minors, psychiatric patients, pregnant women, the elderly, and the incompetent. Issues of the patient's right to information and decision making may now arise at the end of life, including situations in which the patient or family insists on treatment that physicians believe to be futile, and situations in which families wish life-sustaining therapy terminated while physicians want to continue it.

Special situations

Pregnant patients.   During the 1980s, there was a series of cases in which pregnant women were subjected to court-ordered treatments, such as cesarean sections, that they had wished to refuse. These court orders were granted on the theory that the fetus was "medically neglected" under state child-abuse laws. After Angela Carder, a terminally ill pregnant woman whose husband and mother refused to consent to a cesarean, died along with her very premature infant following court-ordered surgery (A.C., 1990), professional organizations began to issue statements urging that such refusals of treatment be respected.

Minors.   With increasing frequency, young people over the age of fourteen or so are gaining greater autonomy in decision making about health-care matters. This includes decisions about "Do Not Resuscitate" orders when young patients are terminally ill (*Belcher* v. *Charleston*, 1992; *Swan*, 1990) as well as in less serious situations (*Cardwell* v. *Bechtol*, 1987). There is also an increased awareness among physicians of the need to provide confidential care to adolescents. Of course, if such care is provided, the young person alone must consent, since the parents will not be informed (Council on Scientific Affairs, 1993).

Psychiatric patients.   Admission, even involuntary commitment, to a mental hospital does not preclude a patient's ability and right to consent to many aspects of his or her care, including agreeing to or refusing medication. In order to lose such a right to consent, the patient must be found by a court to be incompetent as well as mentally ill. Moreover, a psychiatric patient is presumed as capable of giving informed consent to participate in research as he or she is of making decisions about treatment.

Limits on self-determination

Informed consent does not mean that a patient is always entitled to have whatever care he or she wishes. A physician who deems a therapy "nonbeneficial" does not have to provide it. An institution in which a patient is hospitalized, however, may not have the right to discontinue life-prolonging therapy over the patient's or the family's objection even if the physicians see no hope of recovery. Of course, a physician is never obligated to provide treatment he or she believes is worthless (e.g., laetrile for a cancer patient) when other qualified practitioners would agree with that assessment, or treatment he or she believes unnecessary, such as prescription of an antibiotic for a cold. If the treatment is one in which the physician does not believe or is not willing to provide, but one accepted by even a small minority of "mainstream" physicians, the physician may have an obligation to refer the patient to someone who will use the alternative therapy the patient wants.

Economic constraints on self-determination

Could physicians be found liable if they fail to inform a patient about a very expensive therapy they are quite sure the patient cannot afford, even if the physicians cannot offer an alternative? For example, many states do not pay for transplant surgery for adult Medicaid patients. If a Medicaid patient with breast cancer has had a recurrence after conventional chemotherapy, is the physician obligated to tell her about bone marrow transplants with high-dose chemotherapy, which can cost $100,000 or more, if the state will not pay for it? It would seem that the physician would have such an obligation. No court has ever suggested that a patient has the right only to information about the treatment alternatives that the patient's third-party payer is willing to fund.

As an increasing number of patients find their way into health-maintenance organizations or other managed-care programs, where their physicians may be salaried employees of the organization, this problem is likely to become more acute. Presumably the organization, wishing to control costs, will not want patients to know about expensive therapies they are unwilling to provide, and thus will pressure their employee-physicians not to inform patients about those treatments. It is likely that the economic factors in health care will be the leading issue in informed-consent litigation for some time to come.

ANGELA RODDEY HOLDER

Directly related to this article are the other articles in this entry: HISTORY OF INFORMED CONSENT, MEANING AND ELEMENTS OF INFORMED CONSENT, CONSENT ISSUES IN HUMAN RESEARCH, CLINICAL ASPECTS OF CONSENT IN HEALTH CARE, *and* ISSUES OF CONSENT IN MENTAL-HEALTH CARE. *For a further discussion of topics mentioned in this article, see the entries* ADOLESCENTS; ALTERNATIVE THERAPIES; CHILDREN, *articles on* RIGHTS OF CHILDREN,

and HEALTH-CARE AND RESEARCH ISSUES; COMPASSION; HEALTH-CARE FINANCING; INFORMATION DISCLOSURE; PATERNALISM; *and* PROFESSIONAL–PATIENT RELATIONSHIP. *For a discussion of related ideas, see the entries* COMPETENCE; PATIENTS' RIGHTS, *article on* ORIGIN AND NATURE OF PATIENTS' RIGHTS; RISK; *and* VALUE AND VALUATION. *See also the* APPENDIX (CODES, OATHS, AND DIRECTIVES RELATED TO BIOETHICS), SECTION I: DIRECTIVES ON HEALTH-RELATED RIGHTS AND PATIENT RESPONSIBILITIES, A PATIENT'S BILL OF RIGHTS *of the* AMERICAN HOSPITAL ASSOCIATION, *and* SECTION II: ETHICAL DIRECTIVES FOR THE PRACTICE OF MEDICINE, PRINCIPLES OF MEDICAL ETHICS *and* CURRENT OPINIONS *of the* AMERICAN MEDICAL ASSOCIATION, *and* FUNDAMENTAL ELEMENTS OF THE PATIENT–PHYSICIAN RELATIONSHIP *of the* AMERICAN MEDICAL ASSOCIATION.

Bibliography (article)

AMERICAN MEDICAL ASSOCIATION. JUDICIAL COUNCIL. 1969. "Principles of Medical Ethics." In *Opinions and Reports of the Judicial Council*, pp. vi–vii. Chicago: Author.

Application of President of Georgetown College. 1964. 331 F. 2d 1010 (D.C. Cir.). *Certiorari denied.* 377 U.S. 978. 12 L. Ed. 2d 746. 84 S. Ct. 1883.

BURGER, WARREN E. 1968. "Reflections on Law and Experimental Medicine." *UCLA Law Review* 15:436–442.

Canterbury v. Spence. 1972. 464 F.2d 772 (D.C.C.A.).

Cobbs v. Grant. 1972. 104 Cal. Rptr. 505. 502 P.2d 1.

DAVIS, FRED. 1960. "Uncertainty in Medical Prognosis: Clinical and Functional." *American Journal of Sociology* 66: 41–47.

Dow v. Kaiser Foundation. 1970. 12 Cal. App.3d 488. 90 Cal. Rptr. 747 (Ct. App.).

Estate of Brooks, in re., 1965. 32 Ill. 2d 361. 205 N.E.2d 435.

FISHER, BERNARD. 1970. "The Surgical Dilemma in the Primary Therapy of Invasive Breast Cancer: A Critical Appraisal." *Current Problems in Surgery*, October, pp. 1–53.

GLASS, ELEANOR S. 1970. "Restructuring Informed Consent: Legal Therapy for the Doctor–Patient Relationship." *Yale Law Journal* 79:1533–1576.

HENDERSON, L. J. 1935. "Physician and Patient as a Social System." *New England Journal of Medicine* 212:819–823.

HIPPOCRATES. 1923. "Decorum." In *Hippocrates.* Translated by W. H. S. Jones. Loeb Classical Library. London: William Heinemann.

HOFFER, A. 1967. "A Theoretical Examination of Double-Blind Design." *Canadian Medical Association Journal* 97:123–127.

INGELFINGER, F. J. 1972. "Informed (but Uneducated) Consent." *New England Journal of Medicine* 287:465–466.

KATZ, JAY, ed. 1972. *Experimentation with Human Beings: The Authority of the Investigator, Subject, Professions, and State in the Human Experimentation Process.* New York: Russell Sage Foundation.

KATZ, JAY, and CAPRON, ALEXANDER MORGAN. 1975. *Catastrophic Diseases: Who Decides What? A Psychosocial and Legal Analysis of the Problems Posed by Hemodialysis and*

Organ Transplantation. New York: Russell Sage Foundation.

McCoid, Allan H. 1957. "A Reappraisal of Liability for Unauthorized Medical Treatment." *Minnesota Law Review* 41:381–434.

Mohr v. Williams. 1905. 104 N.W. 12 (Minn.).

Natanson v. Kline. 1960. 186 Kan. 393. 350 P.2d 1093. 187 Kan. 186. 354 P.2d 670.

Oken, Donald. 1961. "What to Tell Cancer Patients: A Study of Medical Attitudes." *Journal of the American Medical Association* 175:1120–1128.

Parsons, Talcott. 1951. *The Social System.* Glencoe, Ill.: Free Press.

Percival, Thomas. 1927. *Medical Ethics.* Edited by Chauncey D. Leake. Baltimore: Williams & Wilkins.

Plante, Marcus L. 1968. "An Analysis of 'Informed Consent.'" *Fordham Law Review* 36:639–672.

Pratt v. Davis. 1906. 118 Ill. App. 161 (1905). Aff. 224 Ill. 300. 79 N.E. 562.

Salgo v. Stanford University. 1957. 317 P.2d 170 (Cal. 1st Dist. Ct. App.).

Schloendorff v. New York Hospital. 1914. 105 N.E. 92 (N.Y.).

Silk, Arthur D. 1976. "A Physician's Plea: Recognize Limitations of Informed Consent." *American Medical News,* 12 April, p. 19.

Waitzkin, H., and Stoeckle, J. D. 1972. "The Communication of Information About Illness: Clinical, Sociological, and Methodological Considerations." *Advances in Psychosomatic Medicine* 8:180–215.

Wilkinson v. Vesey. 1972. 295 A.2d 676 (R.I.).

Bibliography (postscript)

A. C., In Re. 1990. 573 A.2d 1235 (D.C. App.).

Angell, Marcia. 1991. "The Case of Helga Wanglie: A New Kind of 'Right to Die' Case." *New England Journal of Medicine* 325:511–512.

Appelbaum, Paul S.; Lidz, Charles W.; and Meisel, Alan. 1987. *Informed Consent: Legal Theory and Clinical Practice.* New York: Oxford University Press.

Battenfield v. Gregory. 1991. 247 N.J. Super. 538, 589 A.2d 1059.

Belcher v. Charleston Area Medical Center. 1992. 188 W. Va. 105, 422 S.E.2d 827.

Board of Trustees. American Medical Association. 1990. "Legal Interventions During Pregnancy: Court-Ordered Medical Treatments and Legal Penalties for Potentially Harmful Behavior by Pregnant Women." *Journal of the American Medical Association* 264:2663–2670.

Cardwell v. Bechtol. 1987. 724 S.W.2d 739, Tenn.

Council on Scientific Affairs. American Medical Association. 1993. "Confidential Health Services for Adolescents." *Journal of the American Medical Association* 269, no. 11:1420–1424.

Holder, Angela R. 1987. "Minors' Rights to Consent to Medical Care." *Journal of the American Medical Association* 357:3400–3402.

Katz, Jay. 1984. *The Silent World of Doctor and Patient.* New York: Free Press.

Lidz, Charles W.; Meisel, Alan; Zerubavel, Eviatar; Carter, Mary; Sestak, Regina M.; and Roth, Loren H., eds. 1984. *Informed Consent: A Study of Decision-Making in Psychiatry.* New York: Guilford.

Rozovsky, Fay A. 1990. *Consent to Treatment: A Practical Guide.* 2d ed. Boston: Little, Brown.

Swan, In re. 1990. 569 A.2d 1202 (Me.).

Teno, Joan M.; Lynn, Joanne; Phillips, Russell S.; Murphy, Donald; Youngner, Stuart J.; Bellamy, Paul; Connors, Alfred F., Jr.; Desbiens, Norman A.; Fulkerson, William; and Kraus, William A. 1994. "Do Formal Advance Directives Affect Resuscitation Decisions and Use of Resources for Seriously Ill Patients?" *Journal of Clinical Ethics* 5:23.

Truman v. Thomas. 1980. 165 Cal. Rptr. 308, 611 P.2d 902.

VI. ISSUES OF CONSENT IN MENTAL-HEALTH CARE

Informed consent in medicine involves at least three overlapping doctrines. First, it describes an ethical doctrine addressing the sometimes conflicting obligations of physicians to respect patients' autonomy in decision making and to provide the best treatment. Second, it refers to a legal doctrine guaranteeing certain rights and privileges of patients in determining their treatment. And third, informed consent describes aspects of an evolving ideal for the doctor–patient relationship, particularly with regard to the sharing of information, decision making, and power. All three concerns—the ethical obligations of physicians, the legal protection of patients, and the evolution of the doctor–patient relationship—are relevant to mental-health care as well as to the general practice of medicine.

Informed consent in the mental-health field, however, merits distinct attention because of the historically differential treatment of involuntarily hospitalized mental patients, the recent development of a distinct body of case law and legislation regarding consent procedures for the hospitalized mentally ill, and the centrality of competency concerns in the doctor–patient relationship. Justice Benjamin Cardozo of the U.S. Supreme Court declared in 1914 that "every human being of adult years and sound mind has a right to determine what shall be done with his body" (*Schloendorff v. New York Hospital,* 1914, p. 126). The question of the rights of those with "unsound" minds regarding treatment decisions has been the focus of a more recent debate.

The doctrine of informed consent summarizes one of the critical ethical issues in health care—the extent to which patient rights should be overridden by physicians' paternalistic effort to treat sickness. While Cardozo considered treatment without consent a battery (a violation of bodily integrity as opposed to negligence or civil-rights violation) early in the twentieth century, patient-centered practice has emerged only since the 1960s, as the physician's therapeutic privilege only slowly gave way to the liberal state's valuation of individual rights. Even today, the doctor–patient relationship can hardly be called a paradigm of liberalism: Sick people and their families are dependent in many ways on caregivers.

While the consumer metaphor receives wide treatment, the inequality of information and power will not permit typical market-driven, contractual relationships between health professionals and patients (Brennan, 1991). Medical ethics supports a value structure on the part of professionals that emphasizes altruistic commitment to the patient. The physicians' obligations are not restricted to those obligations borne by citizens of the liberal state. Rather they are defined by the patient's needs.

Along with this commitment, however, there was long expected a quid pro quo in which the patient was to follow the physician's advice. The physician was to act selflessly but was also expected to retain paternalistic prerogatives unlike those found elsewhere in liberalism. In effect, the patient's autonomy was diminished by the state of sickness and the agreement to seek therapy.

The contrast between the therapeutic relationship and typical relationships in the liberal state is heightened in the case of mental health. In mental health, the presumption often is that the patient is incapable to some extent of making decisions for himself or herself. The need for the professional's paternalism is therefore much greater. Indeed, the dependence of the patient on the physician, and the mutuality that develops in the face of disease, is arguably greater in the mental-health context (Burt, 1982).

As a result, the move to establishment of patients' rights generally, and informed consent in particular, has been slower in mental health. In addition, given the prominence of the police power of the state in mental-health decisions, the role of the courts in defining a more liberal relationship between doctor and patient has been much greater. Since the 1960s, judicial intervention has combined with the recognized failures of state hospitals, resulting in widespread deinstitutionalization, and the availability of psychiatric pharmaceuticals has led to a complete reformation of psychiatric practices.

Prior to the 1960s in the United States, involuntary commitment to psychiatric facilities was presumptively therapeutic, and commitment on the basis of a mental disorder was equivalent to a determination of mental incompetence for a wide variety of decisions the patient faced, including treatment. The basic orientation toward patients was paternalistic, and the fundamental ethical obligation of the physician was to do what he or she perceived was best for the patient.

Since then, changes in commitment laws and practices have delineated more explicitly, and perhaps more accurately, society's interests in confining persons to psychiatric facilities. Involuntary hospitalization has been scrutinized by the courts, which have decided that institutionalization is not always in the service of treatment, and that it is certainly not tantamount to a determination of patients' incompetence to make significant decisions.

This historical development has in turn led to significant changes in the decision-making process for persons severely compromised by their mental disorders. Using informed consent as a legitimate norm for the doctor–patient relationship, judges have addressed a variety of situations in which meaningful patient participation is in doubt because of disturbances in the patient's mental processes. The five components of informed consent have been summarized as disclosure, comprehension, voluntariness, competence, and consent (Appelbaum et al., 1987). It is not clear whether these conditions can be met when psychiatric disturbances alter patients' ability to comprehend information, to think reasonably on the basis of that information, and to act (decide) voluntarily in a manner consistent with their comprehension and reasoning. Other significant questions arise: For example, what is the standard for patient participation; how is patient competence determined; and how are decisions to be made when a patient is determined incapable of providing informed consent? The potentially coercive nature of institutional settings raises additional concerns about the voluntariness of patient participation in the consent process.

The judicial answers to such questions have emphasized process. Increasingly, judge-imposed procedural conditions have been integrated in the determination of incompetence, treatment decisions, and approval of arrangements that substitute outside parties for patients in decision making. Such procedures have in turn led to a "second generation" of concerns, as the legal doctrine of informed consent has been used to reiterate the rights of patients, particularly those involuntarily hospitalized. These concerns have included practical considerations, given the cost, time, and at times questionable efficacy of these judicial or quasi-judicial proceedings; clinical considerations, given the impact of a legal process on an ongoing treatment relationship; and moral considerations, given the plight of many mentally ill persons who do not receive treatment because they cannot or will not consent to it.

Finally, as specific case law and legislation have moved toward defining a patient's right to informed consent or, if that is not possible because of incompetence, to certain procedural guarantees, there has been more elaborate discussion of what constitutes valid informed consent. Questions have been raised about the degree of patient comprehension and rationality necessary for meaningful consent, the degree to which the risks and benefits of the decision affect competency standards, and the degree to which the patient's decision itself should be involved in assessing competency. While these considerations are relevant to all medical decision making and while irrationality can also be found in nonpsychiatric patients and doctors, the nature of both mental disorders and institutional practice make these issues particularly relevant to mental-health care and often lead to legal intervention between psychiatrists and their patients.

The law of informed consent in mental health

Much of what occurs in the practice of psychiatry is ethically uncontroversial. For instance, competent outpatients are allowed to refuse therapy as are other medical patients. An involuntary hospitalization of a competent patient is often a matter of the police power of the state. But two distinct scenarios continue to provoke lively debate and notable case law. The first, and the one with the longest tradition, is the refusal by the involuntarily hospitalized patient to take medications. In the mid-1970s, rights advocates initiated a number of suits that argued for the right of involuntarily committed patients to make decisions about drug therapy. They followed closely on the heels of the *Kaimowitz* decision, which questioned the ability of prisoners to consent freely to experimental medical care (Burt, 1982). These suits were resolved only after nearly a decade of litigation, first in federal courts, later in state courts. Arguably the most prominent was the *Rogers* litigation in Massachusetts, which began in 1979 with a federal class action that alleged that forced medication and isolation policies were unconstitutional violations of the right to privacy. Judge Joseph Tauro agreed with plaintiffs and also alluded to violations of the First Amendment free-speech protections (*Rogers v. Okin*, 1979). Relying on state law, he also ruled that commitment determinations were distinct from those of competence; hence, involuntarily hospitalized patients could be considered competent. The *Rogers* opinion was condemned by the leadership of psychiatry, but hailed by civil libertarians (Roth, 1986).

On appeal, the First Circuit Court noted that language in the U.S. Constitution supporting patients' rights was unclear and ruled that the police power of the state could override those rights at times, but generally upheld the district court (*Rogers v. Okin*, 1979). The U.S. Supreme Court, however, vacated the circuit court decision, sending it back to state court on the ground that state law might be more protective of the involuntarily hospitalized than federal law would be. Meanwhile, decisions by the Supreme Court concerning involuntarily committed mentally retarded patients (*Youngberg v. Romeo*, 1982) and mentally retarded individuals housed in inadequate state facilities (*Pennhurst*

State School and Hospital v. Halderman, 1984) significantly decreased the ability of federal courts to enforce state law against officials of that state.

The result was to force the litigation back into the state court. In 1983, the Massachusetts Supreme Judicial Court reinforced the original federal district court ruling, setting forth a procedural format, including judicial determination of competence (*Rogers v. Commissioner of the Department of Mental Health*, 1983). The prerogatives available to psychiatrists under the guise of the police power of the state were restricted, and specific criteria were set forth as the basis for a competency determination. Many other state courts have since adopted this kind of protection for the involuntarily hospitalized mentally ill (*Rivers v. Katz*, 1986).

Most courts, however, have stopped short of judicial involvement in the competency determinations (*Rennie v. Klein*, 1981) while still restricting the use of the police power. In the decision of *Washington v. Harper* (1990), the U.S. Supreme Court ruled acceptable a process for review of forced medication that relied upon an in-house panel consisting of a psychiatrist, a psychologist, and a corrections official, and rejected the need for a formal judicially supervised hearing.

Jurisdictions that demand formal judicial oversight of treatment decisions have now had sufficient experience to allow some empirical analysis. In Massachusetts, for instance, only 3.4 percent of cases requiring a so-called *Rogers* determination have resulted in court backing for the patient's preference (Schouten and Gutheil, 1990). Years of litigation, and now experience with a variety of procedural formats for determining competence, have done little, however, to resolve the disagreements between civil rights advocates and those advocating some form of restraint (Brakel and David, 1991). Meanwhile, academic debates about the meaning and definition of competence continue to thrive.

The second scenario in which informed-consent issues figure prominently in treatment decisions is the result of a 1990 U.S. Supreme Court decision that raises questions about the constitutional protection for patients' voluntary decisions to be committed. Just as before the *Rogers* litigation, there was an implicit assumption that involuntarily committed individuals were incompetent to make treatment decisions, so, too, was it assumed that a mentally ill individual who sought hospitalization was competent to do so. The decision of *Zinermon v. Burch* (1990) upset this assumption.

While in a psychotic state, Darrell Burch signed himself into a community mental-health center and then into a state hospital. After discharge, he claimed that his consent to admission had not been informed as is guaranteed by Florida state law, a fact acknowledged by Florida officials. More important, Burch alleged that his constitutional rights had been violated by Florida officials because there was no process to guarantee that consent was informed, specifically because there was no determination of competence. The U.S. Supreme Court agreed and required Florida to develop procedures to determine competence and to steer incompetent patients away from the voluntary commitment process.

The holding in the case is quite narrow and applies only to those jurisdictions that mandate patient informed consent before voluntary hospitalization. However, the Court did suggest that patients might have a liberty interest in "avoiding confinement in a mental hospital," and therefore that a competency determination might be necessary before any voluntary confinement. This hint of a new protected interest has been decried by psychiatrists who point out the costs of enforcing these new rights (Appelbaum, 1990).

It seems unlikely that the U.S. Supreme Court will require formal hearings for voluntary hospitalizations, a move that would essentially make all hospitalization procedures, voluntary and involuntary, equivalent. In the leading case of *Parham* v. *J.R.* (1979), as well as the case of *Washington* v. *Harper* (1990), the Court highlighted concerns about the administrative costs in its decisions to reject the use of specific hearings. Nonetheless, from a completely different perspective, *Zinermon* v. *Burch* (1990) highlights the same set of tensions found in *Rogers*. The question remains: To what extent should individual rights, whether or not constitutionally protected, justify extensive judicial oversight procedures before psychiatric care can proceed?

Beyond competency

The foregoing legal analysis suggests the centrality of competence to discussions of informed consent in mental health. The debate over competence often features dramatically different legal and medical understandings of the mentally ill patient who refuses therapy. Laurence Tancredi has insightfully noted that psychiatrists, like most physicians, believe that the existence of disease calls for therapy, and that refusal to accept therapy raises questions about the patient's competence (Tancredi, 1980). Lawyers do not assume this and demand attention to the individual and his or her rights. This demand has increasingly led to the use of situation-specific criteria to judge competence and to ever more subtle methods of conceptualizing the judgment (Saks, 1991).

But competence is a term that is never easily defined, and a mental state that can be very difficult to recognize. Indeed, there are a multitude of standards of competence (Macklin, 1982). In the early 1980s, Paul Appelbaum and Loren Roth listed criteria to determine competence, such as evidencing a choice, rational manipulation of information, appreciation of the nature of the situation, and factual understanding of the issues (Appelbaum and Roth, 1982). Yet most of these are vague enough to be controversial in any one case.

Actual competency judgments often involve concerns other than patient' capacities, particularly whether the patient is assenting to or refusing treatment. For example, in situations where a patient is agreeing to highly beneficial treatment with low risk, a low standard of competency may be more appropriate than in situations where a patient is asked to consider risky treatment.

This analysis has been extended to suggest that the law should take other values into account when establishing procedures to determine a patient's competency to participate in consent decisions (Winick, 1991). These procedures, it is argued, should acknowledge that the patient's capacities to express choice, to reason about alternatives, or to understand decisions may be more critical in certain circumstances than in others. Specifically, when patients assent to, rather than refuse, proposed treatments, lower standards for patient competency may be beneficial. This doctrine of "therapeutic jurisprudence" attempts to accept the patient's decision as informed consent more readily when the decision coincides with the recommendations of physicians. This is arguably a more reasonable integration of the conflicting autonomy and beneficence values at the center of the informed consent debate and may be preferable to extensive judicial procedures in cases when patients already agree with their physicians' proposed standard treatments.

A related approach to the determination of competency also rests on the nature of the patient's decision as well as the nature of his or her mental capacities. Charles Culver and Bernard Gert have argued that courts and clinicians should more explicitly examine the rationality of decisions and in certain circumstances override "competent" patients' highly irrational choices (Culver and Gert, 1990). This, they suggest, would clarify the underlying conflict of beneficence and autonomy values at stake, which is observed by current practices of incorporating rationality concerns in competency determinations. Such an approach also incorporates broader concerns about procedures ostensibly directed at support of mental patients' self-determination rights.

In addition to these considerations regarding the rights of patients and the ethical dilemmas of physicians, the informed-consent process addresses the nature and quality of the doctor–patient relationship. In this sense, Jay Katz, among others, has advocated a more profound discussion of choices between patients and doctors, in which doctors actively try to foster patient reflection and more extended conversation about possible treatments (Katz, 1984). Both legal reform and professional debate of informed consent in mental health have focused primarily on exceptions to a hypothetical standard of acceptable informed consent. Thus, the matter of patient competence has received considerable attention, and indeed, considerable changes have been effected for those severely ill patients deemed not competent to participate in an informed-consent process. However, legal exceptions based on incompetence and ethical concerns about competing beneficence values do not preclude pursuit of the goal of fostering expanded dialogue between all patients and doctors.

The impact upon the rest of psychiatric practice of legal efforts to curb paternalistic and potentially coercive behavior toward incompetent hospitalized patients is not clear. In general, formal informed-consent considerations related to disclosure and discussion in psychiatric treatment and research seem to be regarded as standard practice. Whether there has been a more profound shift in attitude and practice, consistent with goals of fostering patient reflection and involvement, remains unclear.

Several psychiatrists have raised the concern that the societal emphasis on patients' rights regarding consent has resulted in morally unacceptable deprivation and misery for many persons who are unable or unwilling to consent to treatment. Focusing on the plight of the homeless mentally ill, H. Richard Lamb has advocated for an increased willingness on the part of clinicians to initiate involuntary treatment and hospitalization (Lamb, 1990). Lamb asserts that a too passive approach in engaging many homeless mentally ill persons is ethically questionable; he asks, "Does society have the right to deny involuntary treatment to this population? . . . Are we physicians who care for the sick or are we not? . . . Are we a caring society or are we not?" (Lamb, 1990, p. 5). Along these lines, a few communities have established assertive outreach programs which are willing to engage mentally ill persons on a voluntary basis but are far less reluctant to pursue involuntary treatment if the person is unable or unwilling to consent to treatment. Others have emphasized that the refusal of hospitalization by many mentally ill persons may reflect legitimate and more broadly held antipathy for state institutions and advocate that psychiatrists should more readily accept the role of the judiciary, the legitimacy of patient's wishes, and the nonpsychiatric social causes of homelessness (Mossman and Perlin, 1992).

In practice, many mental-health services have responded to the demands for greater liberty for patients and for more assertive treatment of severely ill persons through the development of voluntary and involuntary alternatives to prolonged commitment to state hospitals. These alternatives include court-ordered outpatient treatment and medication usage, alternative community-based treatment sites, and mandated external control over patients' funds and resources. Through these

interventions, patients' liberty demands can be partially met, albeit on a paternalistic basis. The argument here is that this is a reasonable and ethical compromise; patients are forced to give up part of their freedom in return for treatment in a less restrictive setting. While these alternatives offer new compromises between the rights of the patient and the paternalistic concerns of society, their acceptance by the courts and their acceptance by society have not been fully evaluated. The development of these alternatives does perhaps reflect a broadening of the dialogue between patients and doctors, in part due to the more general acceptance of the doctrine of informed consent in the mental-health field.

Conclusion

Numerous changes in psychiatric decision making have occurred because of the judiciary's acceptance of informed consent as a standard in patient care. In the mental-health field, those most affected by these changes have been patients hospitalized with more severe disorders. Previously, involuntary commitment was assumed to afford physicians broad paternalistic authority over many decisions in patients' lives. The courts have carefully and specifically defined incompetent patients and have instituted a variety of judicial procedures that share substitute decision making among reviewing physicians, the court, guardians, and other third parties.

The central issues, however, remain: first, balancing these concerns for patients' autonomy with concerns for their welfare, and second, promoting a more meaningful discussion between patients and mental-health clinicians. Changes spurred by the legal doctrine of informed consent have moved the fulcrum toward support for patients' self-determination.

ALAN P. BROWN
TROYEN A. BRENNAN

Directly related to this article are the other articles in this entry, especially the articles on MEANING AND ELEMENTS OF INFORMED CONSENT, *and* CONSENT ISSUES IN HUMAN RESEARCH. *For a further discussion of topics mentioned in this article, see the entries* AUTONOMY; COMPETENCE; PATIENTS' RIGHTS, *article on* MENTAL PATIENTS' RIGHTS; *and* PROFESSIONAL–PATIENT RELATIONSHIP. *This article will find application in the entries* MENTAL-HEALTH SERVICES; MENTAL-HEALTH THERAPIES; *and* MENTALLY DISABLED AND MENTALLY ILL PERSONS. *For a discussion of related ideas, see the entries* BENEFICENCE; DIVIDED LOYALTIES IN MENTAL-HEALTH CARE; INSTITUTIONALIZATION AND DEINSTITUTIONALIZATION; PATERNALISM; PRIVACY IN HEALTH CARE; *and* RIGHTS. *See also the* APPENDIX (CODES, OATHS, AND DIRECTIVES RELATED TO BIOETHICS), SECTION I: DIRECTIVES ON HEALTH-RELATED RIGHTS AND PATIENT RESPONSIBILI-

TIES, RIGHTS OF MENTALLY RETARDED PERSONS *of the* UNITED NATIONS, *and* A PATIENT'S BILL OF RIGHTS *of the* AMERICAN HOSPITAL ASSOCIATION; *and* SECTION III: ETHICAL DIRECTIVES FOR OTHER HEALTH-CARE PROFESSIONS, ETHICAL PRINCIPLES OF PSYCHOLOGISTS *of the* AMERICAN PSYCHOLOGICAL ASSOCIATION.

Bibliography

ANNAS, GEORGE J. 1991. "The Health Care Proxy and the Living Will." *New England Journal of Medicine* 324, no. 17:1210–1213.

APPELBAUM, PAUL S. 1990. "Voluntary Hospitalization and Due Process: The Dilemma of *Zinermon v. Burch.*" *Hospital and Community Psychiatry* 41, no. 10:1059–1062.

APPELBAUM, PAUL S.; LIDZ, CHARLES W.; and MEISEL, ALAN. 1987. *Informed Consent: Legal Theory and Clinical Practice.* New York: Oxford University Press.

APPELBAUM, PAUL S., and ROTH, LOREN H. 1982. "Competency to Consent to Research: A Psychiatric Overview." *Archives of General Psychiatry* 39, no. 8:951–958.

BRAKEL, SAMUEL JAN, and DAVIS, JOHN M. 1991. "Taking Harms Seriously: Involuntary Patients and the Right to Refuse Treatment." *Indiana Law Review* 25, no. 1: 429–473.

BRENNAN, TROYEN A. 1991. *Just Doctoring: Medical Ethics in the Liberal State.* Berkeley: University of California Press.

BURT, ROBERT. 1982. *Taking Care of Strangers: The Rule of Law in Doctor-Patient Relations.* New York: Free Press.

CULVER, CHARLES M., and GERT, BERNARD. 1990. "The Inadequacy of Incompetence." *Milbank Quarterly* 68, no. 4:619–643.

DRESSER, REBECCA. 1984. "Bound to Treatment: The Ulysses Contract." *Hastings Center Report* 14, no. 3:13–16.

KATZ, JAY. 1984. *The Silent World of Doctor and Patient.* New York: Free Press.

LAMB, H. RICHARD. 1990. "Will We Save the Homeless Mentally Ill?" *American Journal of Psychiatry* 147, no. 5: 649–651.

MACKLIN, RUTH. 1982. "Some Problems in Gaining Informed Consent from Psychiatric Patients." *Emory Law Journal* 31:345.

Mills v. Rogers, 1982. 457 U.S. 291.

MOSSMAN, DOUGLAS, and PERLIN, MICHAEL L. 1992. "Psychiatry and the Homeless Mentally Ill: A Reply to Dr. Lamb." *American Journal of Psychiatry* 149, no. 7: 951–957.

Opinion of Justices. 1983. 123 N.H. 554, 465 A. 2d 484.

Parham v. J. R. 1979. 442 U.S. 584.

Pennhurst State School and Hospital v. Halderman. 1984. 104 S.Ct. 900.

Rennie v. Klein. 1981. 653 F. 2d 836 (3rd Cir.); *vacated* 458 U.S. 1119 (1982).

Rivers v. Katz. 1986. 67 N.Y. 2d 485, 495 N.E. 2d 337, 504 N.Y.S. 2d 74.

ROGERS, JOSEPH A., and CENTIFANTI, J. BENEDICT. 1991. "Beyond 'Self-Paternalism': Response to Rosenson and Kasten." *Schizophrenia Bulletin* 17, no. 1:9–14.

Rogers v. Commissioner of Mental Health. 1983. 390 Mass. 489, 458 N.E. 2d 308.

Rogers v. Okin. 1979. 478 F. Supp. 1342 (D. Mass); *aff'd in part, rev'd in part,* 634 F.2d 650 (1st Cir. 1980); *vacated sub nom. Mills v. Rogers,* 457 U.S. 291 (1982).

ROTH, LOREN. 1986. "The Right to Refuse Psychiatric Treatment: Law and Medicine at the Interface." *Emory Law Journal* 35, no. 1:139–161.

SAKS, ELYN R. 1991. "Competency to Refuse Treatment." *North Carolina Law Review* 69, no. 4:945–999.

Schloendorff v. New York Hospital. 1914. 211 N.Y. 125, 129; 105 N.E. 92.

SCHOUTEN, RONALD, and GUTHEIL, THOMAS G. 1990. "Aftermath of the Rogers Decision: Assessing the Costs." *American Journal of Psychiatry* 147, no. 10:1348–1352.

SCHWARTZ, H. I., and ROTH, LOREN H. 1989. "Informed Consent and Competency in Psychiatric Practice." *Psychiatric Update: American Psychiatric Association Annual Review of Psychiatry* 8:409–431.

TANCREDI, LAURENCE R. 1980. "The Rights of Mental Patients: Weighing the Interests." *Journal of Health Policy, Politics and the Law* 5, no. 2:199–204.

Washington v. Harper. 1990. 494 U.S. 210.

WINICK, BRUCE J. 1991. "Competency to Consent to Treatment: The Distinction Between Assent and Objection." In *Essays in Therapeutic Jurisprudence,* pp. 41–81. Edited by David B. Wexler and Bruce J. Winick. Durham, N.C.: Carolina Academic Press.

Youngberg v. Romeo. 1982. 457 U.S. 307.

Zinermon v. Burch. 1990. 494 U.S. 113.

INJURY AND INJURY CONTROL

The factual assertions used to demonstrate the importance of injuries as a public-health problem are well known: Injuries are the leading cause of death for the majority of the human life span; injuries deprive people of more potential years of life than any single disease; and the cost of injuries, whether measured in dollars or in human suffering, is staggering (Rice et al., 1989). Injuries are generally defined by those working in the field of injury prevention as human damage due to the acute transfer of energy or the lack of essentials such as oxygen (as in asphyxiation) or heat (as in hypothermic injuries) (National Committee for Injury Prevention and Control, 1989).

Actions taken to control injury provide prototypical clashes between the personal liberty of the individual and the goals of public health. These conflicts—referred to in ethical terminology as conflicts between paternalistic beneficence and individual autonomy—are experienced in such public interventions as those that mandate helmet use by motorcyclists or that require the wearing of seat belts by drivers and passengers in automobiles. However, injury control also illuminates how public health makes progress by redefining the nature of the problem—in this case, by shifting from the term "accident" (which points to the individual who is injured or an "act of God" as the responsible agent) to "injury" (which suggests that equipment, environment, and those responsible for equipment and environment share responsibility).

Historical development

Although injuries have plagued the human race since its earliest times, it is only in the twentieth century that science has been applied to this public-health problem. For most of history, and to some extent up to the present, injuries have been misperceived as the equivalent of accidents; that is, chance occurrences that are basically unpredictable, and therefore unpreventable. The notions that some people are accident-prone, and therefore we should expect them to be injured, and that people are injured as punishment for a prior moral offense, have substantially retarded the ability to approach injuries and injury prevention scientifically.

A turning point in the historical development of injury control occurred in the early 1960s, when scientists first recognized that injuries, like diseases, had agents that interacted with hosts in specific environments to produce human damage (Gibson, 1961; Haddon, 1963). By modifying the agent (which was recognized as transferred energy), the human host, or the environment, one could substantially reduce the likelihood and/or the severity of an injury. William Haddon is generally recognized as the individual who most clearly "moved injury prevention into the mainstream of public health research and policy" (Baker, 1989). He developed the conceptual tools for the analyses of injury etiology and prevention that form the foundation of modern injury control.

In the decades that followed, scientists applied epidemiologic methods to the investigation of injuries and developed a new body of knowledge on how, when, where, and to whom injuries occur. Data are now available to dispel definitively the notion that injuries occur at random. The clear patterns of injury, which include identified high-risk groups (e.g., elderly persons at risk for hip fractures), geographic patterns (e.g., the distribution of firearm fatalities in the United States), and temporal trends (e.g., the increasing rate of adolescent suicide), make injuries both predictable and, more important, preventable (Baker et al., 1992). Interventions can be focused on high-risk persons and sites, and the effects of the interventions can be scientifically evaluated by comparisons of injury rates.

Shifting conceptions: Environmental and product modification

Notwithstanding these significant advances in the science of injury control, the field remains troubled by popular misconceptions that impede effective prevention programs. The reduction of injuries is still considered a matter of common sense by many. Unlike disease prevention, which is generally recognized to depend upon expert knowledge, injury prevention is commonly misperceived as a matter of an individual's responsibility rather than of public policy, and the importance of expert advice in preventing injuries is often not acknowledged. Thus the false orientation that the only way to prevent injuries is to teach people to be careful remains a popular bias, even among key decision makers who are in a position to protect millions from injury.

The exclusive focus on the behavior of individuals for the prevention of injuries characterizes what was once known as accident prevention. Accidents were understood as the result of imprudent behavior; the remedy was to teach people to be constantly careful and vigilant. An example of this is the early approach to reducing highway fatalities. The method relied upon was improvement of drivers' skills through education and frequent reminders to be careful delivered in public service announcements. By the mid-1960s, however, there was a growing awareness that lives could be saved by shifting the focus of attention from the driver to the highway and the automobile. Crashes were recognized as foreseeable events. By altering the construction of vehicles and highways, the human cargo of the vehicles would not have to suffer serious injuries if and when a crash occurred.

The U.S. Congress took notice of the increasing number of highway fatalities and the opportunity to reduce this toll by mandating "crashworthy" vehicles. In 1966, Congress passed the National Traffic and Motor Vehicle Safety Act, which provided for the creation of motor vehicle safety standards. These standards, which anticipated driver error and provided a more forgiving environment within the vehicle, have saved tens of thousands of lives (Robertson, 1981).

The idea of paying attention to products as well as behaviors has not been restricted to highway safety. Efforts to prevent childhood scald injuries from hot tap water provide an example of this trend toward product alteration. Hot water coming out of faucets in homes is often at a temperature that can cause a severe burn injury to a child's skin in a matter of a few seconds. Rather than relying on parents to keep young children away from faucets, efforts have been made to direct the parents to turn down the setting on their water heaters so that water will not be discharged at temperatures greater than 125°F (Katcher et al., 1989). This prevention strategy, however, still relies upon motivating parents to reset the water heater. An even more effective strategy has been to influence appliance manufacturers to set the heaters at the proper level before they leave the factory, thus eliminating the need to modify parental behavior.

A general principle of injury control, illustrated by the prevention of scald injuries, is to shift the focus of prevention from the individual to the community (Beauchamp, 1989; Barry, 1975). Legislation and regulation that require safer products and environments are more effective in preventing injuries than are efforts to have individuals control their own behaviors. When safety legislation or regulation has been difficult to accomplish because of strongly resistant political influences, litigation has been used. An example of this is product liability litigation, which transfers the cost of injuries from a dangerous product back to the manufacturer, thus giving the manufacturer a strong incentive to improve the safety aspects of its product (Teret, 1986).

Altering behaviors: Paternalism and prevention

Sometimes product modification is not available to achieve a desired prevention strategy, and reliance upon altering behaviors is necessary. Such is the case with motorcycle helmet use. The effectiveness of helmet use in preventing or reducing the severity of head injuries is well established, but helmet use is not universally accepted by motorcyclists. Legislation requiring helmet use is effective both in increasing the use rates and in decreasing motorcyclist death rates. These laws, however, have been bitterly fought by some motorcyclists, and most states have passed and then repealed mandatory helmet use laws.

The debate over motorcycle helmet laws has raised many issues that apply to other areas of mandating safe behaviors. The propriety of governmental paternalism, the relevance of who pays the costs of injuries, and the constitutionality of laws that interfere with personal decisions are all included in the helmet issue. Assuming a definition of paternalism as institutional interference with individual action for the sake of some greater good, motorcyclists question whether their enforced safety is a good substantial enough to deny them their freedom of choice to ride without a helmet.

Opponents of helmet laws categorize such laws as "hard" legal paternalism, in that the laws regulate voluntary behavior that can harm only the motorcyclist (see Feinberg, 1986, p. 12, for distinction between "hard" and "soft" legal paternalism). Proponents of the laws point out that the increased harm inflicted on a helmetless motorcyclist eventually affects the public as a whole. The public pays about 85 percent of the costs of motorcyclists' injuries; helmet laws would reduce the human capital costs by about $400 million per year in the United States (Rice et al., 1989).

Arguments have been raised that the solution to the cost-of-injury problem is to require adequate medical insurance of those who choose to assume risks, but the flaws of this argument are apparent. Some motorcyclists will not purchase insurance, through lack of money or indifference; and it would be unacceptable to have the

injuries of these motorcyclists go without medical attention (Dworkin, 1983).

The motorcycle helmet issue illustrates a problem that permeates the field of injury prevention. As a society, Americans will still permit the manufacture and marketing of some inherently dangerous products, and then rely upon limited efforts to control the behavior of the individuals to whom these products are distributed. Guns provide a striking example. There are about 38,000 firearm fatalities each year in the United States, and most of the policy to reduce this toll focuses on modifying the behavior of the individual who possesses a gun. There are few effective regulations governing the number and types of guns that can be manufactured in the United States (Webster et al., 1991).

The future success of injury prevention appears to be highly dependent upon the willingness of government to regulate business. The products people use and the built environments in which they place themselves are highly determinative of the risk of injury. Since people do not always act in a prudent fashion, and since government is unwilling and unable to mandate such behavior, the greatest opportunity to reduce the incidence and severity of injury rests in the regulation of products and environments.

STEPHEN P. TERET
MICHAEL D. TERET

Directly related to this entry are the entries PUBLIC HEALTH, *article on* HISTORY OF PUBLIC HEALTH; PATERNALISM; AUTONOMY; *and* RISK. *For a further discussion of topics mentioned in this entry, see the entry* PUBLIC HEALTH, *article on* PUBLIC-HEALTH METHODS: EPIDEMIOLOGY AND BIOSTATISTICS. *For a discussion of related ideas, see the entry* PUBLIC HEALTH AND THE LAW. *Other relevant material may be found in the entry* TECHNOLOGY, *article on* PHILOSOPHY OF TECHNOLOGY.

Bibliography

BAKER, SUSAN P. 1989. "Injury Science Comes of Age." *Journal of the American Medical Association* 262, no. 16:2284–2285.

BAKER, SUSAN P.; O'NEILL, BRIAN; GINSBERG, MARVIN J.; and LI, GUOHUA. 1991. *The Injury Fact Book.* 2d ed. New York: Oxford University Press.

BARRY, PATRICIA Z. 1975. "Individual Versus Community Orientation in the Prevention of Injuries." *Preventive Medicine* 4, no. 1:47–56.

BEAUCHAMP, DAN E. 1989. "Injury, Community and the Republic." *Law, Medicine and Health Care* 17, no. 1:42–49.

DWORKIN, GERALD. 1983. "Paternalism." In *Paternalism*, pp. 19–34. Edited by Rolf E. Sartorius. Minneapolis: University of Minnesota Press.

FEINBERG, JOEL. 1986. *Harm to Self: The Moral Limits of the Criminal Law.* New York: Oxford University Press.

GIBSON, JAMES J. 1961. "The Contribution of Experimental Psychology to the Formulation of the Problem of Safety—A Brief for Basic Research." In *Behavioral Approaches to Accident Research*, pp. 77–89. By the Conference on Research in Accident Prevention. New York: Association for the Aid of Crippled Children.

HADDON, WILLIAM, JR. 1963. "A Note Concerning Accident Theory and Research with Special Reference to Motor Vehicle Accidents." *Annals of the New York Academy of Sciences* 107:635–646.

KATCHER, MURRAY L.; LANDRY, GREGORY L.; and SHAPIRO, MARY MELVIN. 1989. "Liquid-Crystal Thermometer Use in Pediatric Office Counseling About Tap Water Burn Prevention." *Pediatrics* 83, no. 5:766–771.

NATIONAL COMMITTEE FOR INJURY PREVENTION AND CONTROL. 1989. *Injury Prevention: Meeting the Challenge*. New York: Oxford University Press.

RICE, DOROTHY P.; MacKENZIE, ELLEN J.; JONES, ALISON S.; KAUFMAN, SHARON R.; deLISSOVOY, GREGORY V.; MAX, WENDY; McLOUGHLIN, ELIZABETH; MILLER, TED R.; ROBERTSON, LEON S.; SALKEVER, DAVID S.; and SMITH, GORDON S. 1989. *Cost of Injury in the United States: A Report to Congress*. Edited by Ida V. S. W. Red. San Francisco: Institute for Health and Aging, University of California, and Injury Prevention Center, Johns Hopkins University.

ROBERTSON, LEON S. 1981. "Automobile Safety Regulations and Death Reductions in the United States." *American Journal of Public Health* 71, no. 8:818–822.

TERET, STEPHEN P. 1986. "Litigating for the Public's Health." *American Journal of Public Health* 76, no. 8:1027–1029.

WEBSTER, DANIEL W.; CHAULK, C. PATRICK; TERET, STEPHEN P.; and WINTEMUTE, GAREN J. 1991. "Reducing Firearm Injuries." *Issues in Science and Technology* 7, no. 3:73–79.

INSEMINATION, ARTIFICIAL

See REPRODUCTIVE TECHNOLOGIES, *articles on* ARTIFICIAL INSEMINATION, ETHICAL ISSUES, *and* LEGAL AND REGULATORY ISSUES.

INSTITUTIONAL ETHICS COMMITTEES

See CLINICAL ETHICS, *article on* INSTITUTIONAL ETHICS COMMITTEES.

INSTITUTIONALIZATION AND DEINSTITUTIONALIZATION

Deinstitutionalization, the mass exodus of mentally ill persons from state hospitals into the community, was accomplished in the United States during the seventh and eighth decades of the twentieth century. We have taken away from the chronically and severely mentally ill the almost total asylum from the pressures of the world and the care, however imperfect, that they received in these institutions. The central ethical question is: Does society not have an obligation to provide the care and treatment that they need in the community? The fact that a significant proportion of this population is now living in the streets, in jails, and in other squalid conditions is evidence that adequate community care has not been provided. Moreover, it may be that some mentally ill persons who cannot be effectively treated in the community have been deinstitutionalized. Does society not have an obligation to correct this situation as well?

Before the current era of deinstitutionalization, chronically and severely mentally ill persons were usually institutionalized for life in large state mental hospitals. This institutionalization often began after a first acute mental breakdown in adolescence or early adulthood. Sometimes these patients went into remission in the hospital and were discharged, but at the point of their next psychotic episode were rehospitalized, often never to return to the community.

In the 1960s, British social psychiatrist John Wing and others observed that persons who spent long periods in mental hospitals developed what has come to be known as "institutionalism," a syndrome characterized by lack of initiative, apathy, withdrawal, submissiveness to authority, and excessive dependence on the institution (Wing and Brown, 1970). Sociologist Erving Goffman argued that in what he called "total institutions," such as state mental hospitals, impersonal treatment can strip away a patient's dignity and individuality and foster regression (Goffman, 1961). The deviant person is locked into a degraded, stigmatized, deviant role. Goffman and others believed that the social environment in institutions could strongly influence the emergence of psychotic symptoms and behavior.

Other investigators, however, observed that institutionalism may not be entirely the outcome of living in dehumanizing institutions; at least in part, it may be characteristic of the schizophrenic process itself. With deinstitutionalization, these researchers observed that many chronically and severely mentally ill persons who were liable to institutionalism seemed to develop dependence on any other way of life that provided minimal social stimulation and allowed them to be socially inactive. They gravitated toward a lifestyle that allowed them to remain free from symptoms and painful and depressive feelings.

Is this dependent, inactive lifestyle bad? For many deinstitutionalized persons, it may lead to unnecessary regression and impede their social and vocational functioning; thus, for these patients deinstitutionalization should be discouraged. However, this restricted lifestyle may meet the needs of many deinstitutionalized individuals and help them stay in the community. Mental-health professionals and society at large need to recognize the crippling limitations of mental illness that do not yield to current treatment methods. They also need to be clear about the importance of providing adequate care for this vulnerable group of severely mentally ill persons so that the end result is not like the fate of the mentally ill in the back wards of state hospitals—neglect, abysmal conditions, extreme regression, and marked deterioration of their mental states. For those persons who can be restored to social and vocational functioning only to a degree, many mental-health professionals advocate lowered expectations and the provision of reasonable comfort and a dignified, undemanding life.

The origins of deinstitutionalization

In 1955, the number of persons in state hospitals in the United States reached its highest point: 559,000 persons were institutionalized in state mental hospitals out of a total national population of 165 million. In 1992, there were approximately 101,000 institutionalized persons out of a population of 248 million. In about 35 years, the United States reduced its number of occupied state hospital beds from 339 per 100,000 population to 41 per 100,000. Some individual states have gone even further. In California, for example, there are now 14 state hospital beds per 100,000 population, including forensic patients (committed through the legal system); nonforensic beds number only 8.3 per 100,000. State mental hospitals had fulfilled the function for society of keeping the mentally ill out of sight and thus out of mind. At the same time, before the advent of modern psychoactive medications, the controls and structure provided by the state hospitals, as well as the granting of asylum, may have been necessary for many of the long-term mentally ill. Unfortunately, the ways in which structure and asylum were achieved, and the everyday abuses of state hospital life, such as neglect, abysmal living conditions, and deterioration of the patients' mental states, left scars on the mental-health professions and on the reputation of state hospitals, as well as on the patients. Periodic public outcries about these deplorable conditions, documented by journalists such as Albert Deutsch in his influential book *The Shame of the States* (1948), set the stage for deinstitutionalization. These concerns, shared by mental-health professionals, led to the formation by Congress of the Joint Commission on Mental Illness and Health (1961), which issued recommendations for community alternatives to state hospitals. When psychoactive medications appeared in the 1950s, along with a new philosophy of social treatment, the majority of the chronic psychotic population seemed to have been left in an environment that was no longer necessary or even appropriate.

Other factors also came into play. First, the conviction that mental patients receive better and more humanitarian treatment in the community than in state hospitals far away from home was a philosophical keystone of the community mental-health movement. Another motivating force was concern that the system of indefinite commitment and institutionalization of psychiatric patients deprived them of their civil rights. Finally, many financially strapped state governments wished to shift some of the fiscal burden for these patients to federal and local governments, that is, to federal Supplemental Security Income (SSI) and Medicaid, and to local law-enforcement and emergency-health and mental-health services.

The process of deinstitutionalization was accelerated in 1963 by two developments at the federal level. Under the provisions of categorical Aid to the Disabled (ATD), the mentally ill became eligible (by administrative order of the Secretary of Health, Education and Welfare) for federal financial support in the community. Moreover, Congress passed legislation to facilitate the establishment of community mental-health centers. With ATD, psychiatric patients and mental-health professionals acting on their behalf now had access to federal grants-in-aid, in many places supplemented by the state. This enabled patients to support themselves or be supported either at home or in such facilities as board-and-care homes (boarding homes) or old hotels, at little cost to the state. ATD is now the Supplemental Security Income referred to above, and is administered by the Social Security Administration. Instead of maintaining patients in a state hospital, the states, even those that provided generous ATD supplements, found the cost of maintaining these patients in the community to be far less than the cost of maintaining them in state hospitals. Although the amount of money available to patients under ATD was not a princely sum, it was sufficient to pay for a board-and-care home or to maintain a low standard of living elsewhere in the community.

Many individuals in the community discovered that they could earn substantial additional income by taking former mental patients into their homes, even at the rates allowed by the ATD grants. Some entrepreneurs set up board-and-care homes holding as many as one hundred persons or more in large, old houses and converted apartment buildings and rooming houses. Although these board-and-care-home operators were not skilled in the management of psychiatric patients, they were able to accommodate tens of thousands of persons who had formerly been in state hospitals and who did not now have major behavior problems (primarily because they were being treated with the antipsychotic drugs).

In 1963, too, Congress passed the Mental Retardation Facilities and Community Mental Health Centers Construction Act, amended in 1965 to provide grants for the initial costs of staffing newly constructed centers. This legislation was a strong incentive to the development of community programs with the potential to treat people whose main recourse previously had been the state hospital. However, although rehabilitative services and precare and aftercare services were among the ten services eligible for funding, an agency did not have to offer them in order to qualify for funding as a comprehensive community mental-health center. Many community mental-health centers chose to focus on persons with neuroses and problems of living—the healthy but unhappy. The chronically and severely mentally ill were often just as neglected in the community as they had been in the hospitals.

Sweeping changes in the commitment laws of the various states also contributed to deinstitutionalization. In California, for instance, the Lanterman-Petris-Short Act of 1968 provided further impetus for the movement of patients out of hospitals. Underlying this legislation was a concern for the civil rights of the psychiatric patient. (Much of this concern came from civil-rights groups and individuals outside the mental-health professions.) The act made the involuntary commitment of psychiatric patients a much more complex process. Holding psychiatric patients indefinitely against their will in mental hospitals became much more difficult. Thus, the initial stage of what had formerly been the career of the long-term hospitalized patient—namely, an involuntary, indefinite commitment—became a thing of the past.

Deinstitutionalization in practice

One of the most important lessons to be drawn from the experience with deinstitutionalization was almost totally unforeseen by its advocates. The most difficult problem is not the fate of those patients discharged into the community after many years of hospitalization. Rather, the problem that has proved most vexing, and that has presented the most difficult ethical dilemmas, has been the treatment of the generation that has grown up since deinstitutionalization. It is largely from this generation that the homeless mentally ill are drawn. The large homeless population with major mental illness—that is, schizophrenia, schizoaffective disorder, bipolar illness, and major depression with psychotic features—tends to be young.

Why is this so? In the older generation of long-stay, hospitalized patients, chances are that most of those who are least appropriate for discharge—because of their propensity to physical violence, very poor coping skills, or marked degree of manifest pathology—will not be discharged, or if they are discharged and fail, will not be sent into the community again.

Those who have been hospitalized for long periods have been institutionalized to passivity. For the most part, they have come to do what they are told. This is not presented as a beneficial effect of long-term hospi-

talization, but simply as a clinical observation. When those for whom discharge from the hospital is feasible and appropriate are placed in a community living situation with sufficient support and structure, most (though by no means all) tend to stay where they are placed and to accept treatment.

The chronically and severely mentally ill persons of the new generation, however, have not been institutionalized to passivity. Not only have they not spent long years in hospitals, they have probably had difficulty just getting admitted to an acute hospital, whether or not they wanted to be admitted, and even greater difficulty staying there for more than a short period on any one admission. Acute psychiatric inpatient care is extremely expensive, and there is a great reluctance to use scarce mental-health funds to provide it.

Existential problems in the community

A young person just beginning to deal with life's demands struggles to achieve some measure of independence, to choose and succeed at a vocation, to establish satisfying interpersonal relationships and attain some degree of intimacy, and to acquire some sense of identity. Lacking the abilities to withstand stress and to form meaningful interpersonal relationships, the mentally ill person's efforts often lead only to failure. The result may be a still more determined, often frantic effort with a greatly increased level of anxiety and desperation. Ultimately, this may lead to another failure accompanied by feelings of despair. For a person predisposed to retreats into acute mental breakdowns the result is predictably stormy, with acute psychotic breaks, and repeated—and usually brief—hospitalizations often related to these desperate attempts to achieve. The situation becomes even worse when such persons are in an environment where unrealistic expectations emanate not just from within themselves, but also from families and mental-health professionals.

Before deinstitutionalization, these "new chronic patients" would have been institutionalized, often from the time of their first mental breakdown in adolescence or early adulthood. After their initial failures in trying to cope with the vicissitudes of life and of living in the community, such patients would have been exposed no longer to these stresses, but given a permanent place of asylum from the demands of the world.

Such an approach now tends to be the exception, not the rule; since large-scale deinstitutionalization began, hospital stays tend to be brief. In this sense, the majority of "new" long-term patients are the products of deinstitutionalization. To observe this is not to imply that we should turn the clock back and return to a system of total institutionalization for all chronically and severely mentally ill patients. In the community, most of these patients can have something very precious—

their liberty, to the extent they can handle it. Furthermore, if the resources are provided, they can realize their potential to pass some of life's milestones successfully. Nevertheless, it is this new generation of chronically and severely mentally ill persons that poses the greatest ethical challenge to deinstitutionalizataion and the most difficult clinical problems in community treatment and that has swelled the ranks of the homeless and the incarcerated mentally ill.

Problems in treatment

As recently as 1950, there were no psychoactive drugs to bring chronically and severely mentally ill persons out of their world of autistic fantasy and help them return to the community. Even today, many patients fail to take psychoactive medications because of disturbing side effects, denial of illness, or, in some cases, the desire to avoid the depression and anxiety that result when they see their reality too clearly; grandiosity and a blurring of reality may make their lives more bearable than a relative drug-induced normality.

A large proportion of the new chronic patients tends to deny the need for mental-health treatment and to eschew the identity of the chronic mental patient. Admitting mental illness seems to many of these persons to be admitting failure. Becoming part of the mental-health system seems to them like joining an army of misfits. Many of these persons also have substance-abuse disorders and/or medicate themselves with street drugs. Another contributing factor is the natural rebelliousness of youth.

The problem becomes worse for those whose illnesses are more severe. These persons' problems are again illustrated by the problems of the homeless mentally ill. Evidence is beginning to emerge that the homeless mentally ill are more severely ill than the mentally ill in general. At Bellevue Hospital in New York City, for example, approximately 50 percent of inpatients who were homeless are transferred to state hospitals for long-term care as a result of the severity of their illnesses, as opposed to 8 percent of other Bellevue psychiatric inpatients.

Functions of the state hospital

Valid concerns about the shortcomings and antitherapeutic aspects of state hospitals in the United States often overshadowed the fact that the state hospitals fulfilled some crucial functions for the chronically and severely mentally ill. The term "asylum" was in many ways appropriate; these imperfect institutions did provide asylum and sanctuary from the pressures of the world with which, in varying degrees, most of these patients were unable to cope. They also provided medical care, patient monitoring, respite for the patient's family, and a social network for the patient, as well as food, shelter, and needed support and structure.

Furthermore, in the state hospitals, the treatment and services that did exist were in one place and under one administration. In the community the situation is very different. Services and treatment are under various administrative jurisdictions and in various locations. Even the mentally healthy have difficulty dealing with a number of bureaucracies, both governmental and private, and having their needs met. Patients can easily get lost in the community. In a hospital, they may have been neglected, but at least their whereabouts were known.

These problems have led to the recognition of the importance of case management. Many of America's homeless mentally ill would not be on the streets if they were on the caseload of a professional or paraprofessional trained to deal with the problems of the chronically mentally ill, monitor these patients (with considerable persistence when necessary), and facilitate their receiving services.

The fact that the chronically mentally ill have been deinstitutionalized does not mean they no longer need social support, protection, and relief, either periodic or continuous, from external stimuli and the pressures of life. In short, they need asylum and sanctuary in the community. Unfortunately, because the old state hospitals were called asylums, the word "asylum" took on an almost sinister connotation. Only in recent years has the word again become respectable, signifying the function of providing asylum, rather than asylum as a place.

The concept of asylum and sanctuary in the community becomes important in postdischarge planning because, while some chronically mentally ill patients eventually attain high levels of social and vocational functioning, others have difficulty meeting simple demands of living on their own, even with long-term rehabilitative help. Whatever degree of rehabilitation is possible for each patient cannot take place unless support and protection in the community—from family, treatment program, therapist, family-care home, or board-and-care home—are provided at the same time. Moreover, if we do not take into account the need for asylum and sanctuary in the community from many of the stresses of life, living in the community may not be possible for many chronically and severely mentally ill persons.

Ingredients of a system of community care

Has community care in the United States been better for the chronically and severely mentally ill than institutionalized care? The answer appears to be both yes and no. With deinstitutionalization, for instance, some chronically dysfunctional and mentally disordered individuals gradually, over a period of years, succeed in their strivings for independence, a vocation, intimacy, and a sense of identity. For them, deinstitutionalization has indeed been a success. We have also learned much about what good community care should be: a comprehensive and integrated system of care, with designated responsibility, accountability, and adequate fiscal resources.

More specifically, such care requires an adequate number and ample range of graded, stepwise, supervised community-housing settings; adequate, comprehensive, and accessible psychiatric and rehabilitative services provided assertively and through outreach services when necessary; and available and accessible crisis services. A system of responsibility for the chronically and severely mentally ill living in the community should ensure that each patient has one case manager, a mental-health professional or paraprofessional who is responsible for seeing that the appropriate psychiatric and medical assessments are carried out; who formulates, in collaboration with the patient, an individualized treatment and rehabilitation plan, including the proper pharmacotherapy; and who monitors the patient, and assists him or her in receiving services. Respite care, a period when families can be relieved of the responsibilities of caring for their mentally ill relatives, is needed for the more than 50 percent of the chronically and severely mentally ill population in the United States who live with their families, so that the family is better able to provide a support system. The entire burden of deinstitutionalization should not be allowed to fall on families, as it sometimes has.

Setting up such a comprehensive and integrated system of care for the chronically and severely mentally ill in the United States has proven far more difficult to accomplish than was envisioned. A large proportion of the many hundreds of thousands of chronically and severely mentally ill persons has not been well served in the community. In addition, some patients who cannot be effectively treated in the community have been deinstitutionalized. Probably only a relatively small minority of long-term mentally ill persons requires a highly structured, locked, twenty-four-hour setting for adequate intermediate or long-term management. But for members of this small minority, much institutional management may be critical—for their sake and for the sake of the community. Attempts to treat persons characterized by such problems as assaultive behavior; severe, overt major psychopathology; grossly inappropriate social behavior; reluctance to take psychoactive medications; inability to adjust to open settings; problems with drugs and alcohol; and self-destructive behavior in the community have required an inordinate amount of time and effort from mental-health professionals, various social agencies, and the criminal-justice system. Many patients have been lost to the mental-health system because their treatment needs have not been met, and these people are on the streets or in jail.

The result has often been seen as a series of failures on the part of both mentally ill persons and mental-health professionals. As a consequence, a number of long-term mentally ill persons have become alienated from the system that has not met their needs, and some mental-health professionals have become disenchanted with the treatment of these persons. The heat of the debate in the United States over the issue of whether or not to provide intermediate and long-term hospitalization has tended to obscure the benefits of community treatment for the great majority of the long-term mentally ill, who do not require such highly structured, twenty-four-hour care.

Where to treat—hospital versus community—should not be an ideological issue; it is a decision best based on the clinical needs of each person. Unfortunately, efforts to deinstitutionalize have, in practice, too often confused locus of care and quality of care. Where mentally ill persons are treated has been seen as more important than how they are treated. Care in the community has often been assumed by definition to be better than hospital care. In actuality, poor care can be found in both hospital and community settings.

Independence

For many long-term mentally ill persons, nothing is more difficult to attain and sustain than independence. The issue of supervised versus unsupervised housing provides an example. Professionals would like to see their patients living in their own apartments and managing on their own, perhaps with some outpatient support. But, as described in the 1992 American Psychiatric Association Task Force's report on the homeless mentally ill (American Psychiatric Association, 1992), the experience of deinstitutionalization has shown that most long-term, severely mentally ill persons living in unsupervised mainstream housing in the community find the ordinary stresses of managing on their own more than they can handle. After a while they tend to not take their medications and to neglect their nutrition. Their lives unravel; eventually they find their way back to the hospital or to the streets.

Mentally ill persons value independence highly, but they often underestimate their dependency needs and their needs for structure—in this instance to have a living situation where their medication is dispensed to them and their meals are provided. Professionals need to be realistic about their patients' potential for independence, even if the patients are not.

Freedom

What about the issue of freedom? The chronically mentally ill enjoy much more liberty than when they were institutionalized; in most cases, as was discussed earlier, this is appropriate. But that freedom may well be damaging to some patients if they are given more than they can handle. Many of those on the streets and in the jails suffer from the lack of structure and organization in their lives; they need, because of their illnesses, to have these elements imposed upon them.

However, involuntary treatment presents an extremely difficult ethical dilemma. Our beliefs in civil liberties come into conflict with our concern for the welfare of chronically and severely mentally ill persons. A basis for facing this dilemma is provided by the belief that the mentally ill have a fundamental right to treatment, even if at times the treatment must be involuntary when, because of severe mental illness, they present a serious threat to their own welfare or that of others and are not able to make a rational decision about accepting treatment. Reaching out to patients and working with them to accept help on a voluntary basis is certainly a mandatory first step. But if this fails and the patient is at serious risk, professionals with direct responsibility for patients usually see that ethically they cannot simply stop there.

In such cases, humane commitment laws facilitate a prompt return to acute inpatient treatment when such treatment is needed. Ongoing measures, such as conservatorship or guardianship, court-mandated outpatient treatment, and appointing a payee for the person's disability check are components of a treatment philosophy and practice that recognizes that external controls such as these are a positive therapeutic approach for mentally ill persons who lack the internal controls to deal with their impulses and to cope with life's demands. Such external controls may help interrupt a self-destructive, chaotic life on the streets and in and out of jails and hospitals.

Conclusion

Deinstitutionalization must be preceded by careful planning and the establishment of community services. In fact, community services set up in the United States have in most cases been swamped by the number of patients coming out of the hospitals or who are already in the community and in need of care. Clearly, deinstitutionalization should be implemented only to the extent that each chronically and severely mentally ill person in the community can be properly and adequately housed and treated. Those who implement a policy of deinstitutionalization must take into account not only those already in hospitals but those mentally ill persons who are reaching an age where their mental illness is becoming manifest and who will never be long-term hospitalized mental patients.

For this latter group, it is essential that there be a system of case management with staff who understand their problems and their needs, as well as a range of su-

pervised housing in the community that is sufficiently structured to accommodate those who require it. Although adequate case management, appropriate housing, and treatment should greatly decrease the need for involuntary treatment, there should still be a willingness to use it when it becomes necessary. It also needs to be recognized that there is a significant subpopulation of the chronically and severely mentally ill who should not be deinstitutionalized.

Having dismantled such a large proportion of the institutions for the mentally ill, we continue to face the grave ethical and clinical question of whether we still have an obligation to provide care and treatment in the community for the mentally ill who used to inhabit these institutions. It is a matter of priorities among the various social needs of our society. Mental-health professionals, at least those in public service, are coming around to giving this population the highest priority. With regard to legislators and the general public, there is much more ambivalence, and the chronically and severely mentally ill often fare poorly in the struggle over setting priorities and allocating funds.

H. RICHARD LAMB

Directly related to this entry are the entries MENTAL-HEALTH SERVICES; MENTAL-HEALTH THERAPIES; MENTALLY DISABLED AND MENTALLY ILL PERSONS, *article on* HEALTH-CARE ISSUES; *and* PATIENTS' RIGHTS, *article on* MENTAL PATIENTS' RIGHTS. *For a further discussion of topics mentioned in this entry, see the entries* AUTONOMY; BEHAVIOR CONTROL; CHRONIC CARE; FREEDOM AND COERCION; HEALTH-CARE RESOURCES, ALLOCATION OF; JUSTICE; LONG-TERM CARE, *article on* CONCEPT AND POLICIES; *and* RIGHTS. *For a discussion of related ideas, see the entries* MENTAL HEALTH, *article on* MEANING OF MENTAL HEALTH; *and* MENTAL ILLNESS, *articles on* CONCEPTIONS OF MENTAL ILLNESS, *and* ISSUES IN DIAGNOSIS. *Other relevant material may be found under the entries* DISABILITY, *article on* ATTITUDES AND SOCIOLOGICAL PERSPECTIVES; INFORMED CONSENT, *article on* ISSUES OF CONSENT IN MENTAL-HEALTH CARE; PSYCHIATRY, ABUSES OF; PSYCHOPHARMACOLOGY; PSYCHOSURGERY; *and* SUBSTANCE ABUSE, *article on* ADDICTION AND DEPENDENCE.

Bibliography

AMERICAN PSYCHIATRIC ASSOCIATION. 1992. *Treating the Homeless Mentally Ill: A Task Force Report of the American Psychiatric Association.* Edited by H. Richard Lamb, Leona L. Bachrach, and Frederic I. Kass. Washington, D.C.: Author.

BACHRACH, LEONA L. 1976. *Deinstitutionalization: An Analytical Review and Sociological Perspective.* Washington, D.C.: U.S. Government Printing Office.

———. 1984. "Asylum and Chronically Ill Psychiatric Patients." *American Journal of Psychiatry* 141, no. 8: 975–978.

BAUM, ALICE S., and BURNES, DONALD W. 1993. *A Nation in Denial: The Truth About Homelessness.* Boulder, Colo.: Westview.

CURSON, DAVID A.; PANTELIS, CHRISTOS; WARD, JAN; and BARNES, THOMAS R. E. 1992. "Institutionalism and Schizophrenia 30 Years On: Clinical Poverty and the Social Environment in Three British Mental Hospitals in 1960 Compared with a Fourth in 1990." *British Journal of Psychiatry* 160 (February):230–241.

DEUTSCH, ALBERT. 1948. *The Shame of the States.* New York: Harcourt, Brace.

GOFFMAN, ERVING. 1961. *Asylums: Essays on the Social Situation of Mental Patients and Other Inmates.* New York: Doubleday.

ISAAC, RAEL JEAN, and ARMAT, VIRGINIA C. 1990. *Madness in the Streets: How Psychiatry and the Law Abandoned the Mentally Ill.* New York: Free Press.

JOINT COMMISSION ON MENTAL ILLNESS AND HEALTH. 1961. *Action for Mental Health: Final Report.* New York: Basic Books.

LAMB, H. RICHARD. 1982. *Treating the Long-Term Mentally Ill.* San Francisco: Jossey-Bass.

———. 1988. "Deinstitutionalization at the Crossroads." *Hospital and Community Psychiatry* 39, no. 9:941–945.

———, ed. 1984. *The Homeless Mentally Ill: A Task Force Report of the American Psychiatric Association.* Washington, D.C.: American Psychiatric Association.

MANDERSCHEID, RONALD W., and SONNENSCHEIN, MARY ANNE, eds. 1992. *Mental Health, United States 1992.* Washington, D.C.: U.S. Government Printing Office. Gives the number of persons in state hospitals in 1992.

MARCUS, LUIS R.; COHEN, NEAL L.; NARDACCI, DAVID; and BRITTAIN, JOAN. 1990. "Psychiatry Takes to the Streets: The New York City Initiative for the Homeless Mentally Ill." *American Journal of Psychiatry* 147, no. 11:1557–1561. Describes the program at Bellevue Hospital.

MINKOFF, KENNETH. 1987. "Beyond Deinstitutionalization: A New Ideology for the Postinstitutional Era." *Hospital and Community Psychiatry* 39, no. 9:945–950.

THORNICROFT, GRAHAM, and BEBBINGTON, PAUL. 1989. "Deinstitutionalization—From Hospital Closure to Service Development." *British Journal of Psychiatry* 155 (December):739–753.

TORREY, E. FULLER. 1988. *Nowhere to Go: The Tragic Odyssey of the Homeless Mentally Ill.* New York: Harper & Row.

WING, JOHN K. 1990. "The Functions of Asylum." *British Journal of Psychiatry* 157 (December):822–827.

WING, JOHN K., and BROWN, GEORGE W. 1970. *Institutionalism and Schizophrenia: A Comparative Study of Three Mental Hospitals 1960–1968.* Cambridge: At the University Press.

INSTITUTIONAL REVIEW BOARDS

See RESEARCH ETHICS COMMITTEES.

INSURANCE, HEALTH

See HEALTH-CARE FINANCING, *article on* HEALTH-CARE INSURANCE.

INTEGRITY

See CONSCIENCE.

INTERNATIONAL CODES OF MEDICAL ETHICS

See MEDICAL CODES AND OATHS. *See also the* APPENDIX (CODES, OATHS, AND DIRECTIVES RELATED TO BIOETHICS), SECTION I: DIRECTIVES ON HEALTH-RELATED RIGHTS AND PATIENT RESPONSIBILITIES; SECTION II: ETHICAL DIRECTIVES FOR THE PRACTICE OF MEDICINE; *and* SECTION III: ETHICAL DIRECTIVES FOR OTHER HEALTH-CARE PROFESSIONS.

INTERNATIONAL HEALTH

International health has two meanings. The first is the systematic comparison of the factors that affect the health of human populations. The second, more familiar meaning refers to the organized activity by donor countries or international agencies to improve the health of developing societies and regions. This essay deals mostly with ethical issues arising from organized efforts to improve health in poor countries, although ethical conflicts arising from research activity in poor countries will not be ignored.

Organization of international health activities

Among intergovernmental organizations, the World Health Organization (WHO) is the preeminent integrating body, acting through six regional headquarters and representatives in many countries. Other members of the United Nations (U.N.) family, such as the U.N. Development Program, the U.N. High Commission for Refugees, the U.N. Fund for Population Activities, and the U.N. Children's Fund (UNICEF), also undertake international health activities. The World Bank and regional (Asian, African, and Interamerican) development banks play a significant role, primarily in limited local projects. Official development agencies such as the U.S. Agency for International Development (USAID) and analogous groups in most other industrialized countries form an important interface between their own governments, those of other countries, and multilateral agencies. Many charitable foundations and thousands of professional, religious, and secular private voluntary organizations (PVOs) work internationally in disaster relief, the welfare of children, the provision of general medical care, and the alleviation of specific health conditions such as tuberculosis, malnutrition, and blindness. Many PVOs function primarily to relieve suffering rather than to promote health, which is the general goal of intergovernmental organizations.

The international health arena necessarily includes national health departments and ministries, which are obligated to undertake certain activities, including the collection of vital statistics and data on the occurrence of officially reportable diseases. In practice, few reliable data exist for the least developed nations and regions.

Moral obligations of wealthy countries toward poorer ones

Especially since the end of World War II, there has been a conventionally accepted view that wealthier governments have a moral responsibility to provide aid to poor countries. Three issues are involved: the needs of extremely poor people in extremely poor countries; the large and growing inequalities between those with excess resources and those with insufficient resources; and historical relationships considered unjust and requiring restitution and/or compensation (Singer, 1986). The force of the moral argument is diminished to the extent that foreign aid is viewed as a politically motivated transfer of funds to encourage favorable behaviors or to reward friendly governments for their support. During the 1980s, the growth of external debt in many developing nations, and consequent structural adjustment policies mandated by the International Monetary Fund, have led to austerity budgets and the decay of social welfare services, including health care.

Commercial transactions and military assistance aside, cash flows from developed to developing countries take many forms. Charitable donations, freely given by individuals or groups motivated by beneficence, equity, and distributive justice, are channeled through private voluntary organizations, religious or secular, including major foundations.

Ethical issues arise from the asymmetries of power and influence among the donor and recipient nations. Contentious issues in the interaction of industrialized and developing countries include charges of unfairness concerning coercion to adopt, or to relinquish, certain values and behaviors; the transfer of inappropriate advanced medical technologies; inequitable regulations respecting patents and marketing policies for pharmaceuticals, including inducements to physicians; the trade in infant formulas and alleged discouragement of breast-feeding; the growing international commerce in tobacco products; the migration of health professionals from poor to wealthy countries; and the shipment of noxious wastes from wealthy to poor countries.

The growth of modern biomedical science has led to increasing pressure to obtain sites for clinical trials of new pharmaceutical products and vaccines, including those intended for diseases found primarily in developing countries. The ethical standards applied to research conducted by investigators of one country on subjects of another should be no less exacting than they would be for research carried out within the initiating country (CIOMS, 1982).

A second group of ethical issues arises from sharp cultural and religious differences in societal goals, moral teachings, the meaning of justice, and the perceptions of individual autonomy. Attitudes vary among national societies and cultural groups about the treatment of children, women, the elderly, or the handicapped; those with mental illness, Hansen's Disease (leprosy), or AIDS; or members of societal subgroups such as homosexuals or certain ethnic minorities. The activities of foreign donor agencies may conflict with local traditions regarding abortion, family planning, child labor, or a host of other concerns. The terms of reference of any bilateral agreement for health-related activities must be spelled out in detail, with care to maintain respect for the ethical precepts of the host country. In some countries, official policy or habitual practice results in systematic abuse of groups of people. Foreign workers to whom this is ethically unacceptable must face the dilemma of either terminating their programs or remaining to try to effect change.

The Western principle of informed consent is predicated on the notion of respect for persons as individuals and as autonomous agents. Some societies, especially in Africa, put greater stress on the connectedness of the individual with the community and define a person by his or her relations to others (Christakis, 1988). Where the notion of persons as autonomous individuals is not dominant, the consent process may shift from the individual to the family or to the community (LaVertu and Linares, 1990). However, consent through a community leader "proxy" could be susceptible to inducement, bribe, or fraud, and individuals could be reluctant to disagree with the declaration of the selected community leader, even if they have grave reservations about participation in the trial. Where several different codes of informed consent may be applicable, investigators as a rule should adhere to the most stringent.

Varying concepts of the causality of disease and the significance of health, illness, and death used by well-intentioned outside researchers may generate great conflict. For example, mothers in many societies are reluctant to speak about deceased children, particularly with strangers, while researchers consider such information essential to design programs to save the lives of other children. It must be carefully considered whether the data obtained compensate for their cost in psychological trauma to the mothers. International ethical guidelines for epidemiological studies have been issued (Bankowski et al., 1991).

A third group of ethical issues stems from the mixed motives of foreign assistance. Assistance comes from donor countries through multilateral organizations such as development banks, or directly from the donor government. Often there are strings attached; donor country motivations and politics vary widely. These mixed motives may sometimes be only irritants; at other times they may raise profound internal conflicts concerning host country policies. Other, more altruistic assistance is furnished directly from the donor government to the recipient government, as grants or low-interest loans, which account for a very large proportion of the net capital inflow of many very poor nations.

Donor country motivations and policies regarding assistance vary widely. In many instances assistance is "tied," or restricted to donor country origin and sources for procurement of commodities, for the vessels in which to ship them, or for recruitment of expert technical assistance in project design or implementation. In some instances bilateral assistance is tied to certain sectors, or even to specific programs or projects that would not have been the first priority of the recipient country's government. Programs such as family planning are particularly sensitive among certain groups in both recipient and donor countries, the former fearing unwarranted interference or even genocidal intentions; the latter, as in the case of official U.S. policy in the 1980s, refusing to fund some kinds of activities, such as abortion services. Conflicts in goals and values become more apparent when the donor nations insist on furthering their own policy objectives with little priority given to the recipient's needs. Some authorities from both donor and recipient countries worry that long-continued assistance will create economic and political dependency.

The pursuit of pragmatic foreign policies may be in conflict with enunciated donor country ethical principles or economic development goals, but may be necessary to obtain popular and legislative support for assistance programs at home. Similarly, some developing-country authorities may feel obligated in international forums to support public-health programs that, once adopted, compete for scarce funds with other health activities considered of higher priority.

Of all categories of assistance, food aid is often criticized because the transferred products may disrupt normal markets for local producers, create a preference for imported foods, or cause a shift in agricultural production away from local foods and toward export products. Moreover, the foods shipped may represent those in surplus in the donor country, reflecting subsidies to support home country producers, and may not be those requested or desired by the recipients.

Primary health care

One aspect of international health in recent years has been the attempt by the WHO to make "health for all" a centerpiece of an international struggle for justice. In 1977 the WHO announced as a target "the attainment by all citizens of the world of a level of health that will permit them to lead a socially and economically productive life" by the year 2000. The following year a WHO/UNICEF international conference, held at Alma Ata in Kazakhstan, determined that primary health care was the best means to achieve health for all. The *Declaration of Alma Ata* defined primary health care as

> essential health care based on practical, scientifically sound and socially acceptable methods and technology made universally accessible to individuals and families in the community through their full participation and at a cost that the community and country can afford to maintain at every stage of their development in a spirit of self-reliance and self-determination. It forms an integral part both of the country's health system, of which it is the central function and focus, and of the overall social and economic development of the community.

Proponents of such "comprehensive primary health care" believe that health is indivisible and inseparable from other aspects of daily life, that community participation is essential in planning and implementation, and that control should rest on empowering local people, not outside experts, to make decisions about their own health needs and the means to achieve them. The associated concepts of autonomy, equity, social justice, and right to health constitute the core of this perspective. A contrasting viewpoint is held by those who advocate the practical concept of "selective primary health care," which determines priorities selected by health professionals in relation to their prevalence, morbidity, mortality, cost, negative impact on the community, and feasibility of control.

Child survival programs in developing countries

Efforts to reduce infant and child mortality, largely under the banners of the WHO, UNICEF, USAID, and other organizations, have centered on universal immunization, the control of diarrheal and acute respiratory diseases, maternal and child health, and similar themes. Such programs are justified on both humanitarian and utilitarian grounds. One common moral consideration engendered by these activities is whether the lives of infants should be saved, only to have them die at an age when they will comprehend their own death (Woolley,

1990). There has been little formal discussion in the international health literature of the grim prospect that reducing infant mortality may only postpone early death a few years, and may actually increase total suffering.

A second, more Malthusian argument cites unrelenting environmental pressure from increasing population growth, with resultant degradation of fragile tropical ecosystems. Maurice King has argued for a more ecologically sound international public health, one that takes into account the impact of saving lives on ecosystems such as tropical rain forests. It would be more acceptable, King argues, for a large international agency to have a more ecological and long-term orientation in its decisions than it would for an individual physician or even a mission society (King, 1990a). He discusses the need to strike a moral balance between the sanctity of individual human life and the need to sustain the collective environment, between the present and the future, and between the utilitarian "greatest good" and the deontological "absolute duty." He suggests that in the absence of complementary ecologically sustained measures, especially family planning and ecological support, it may be better that lifesaving measures such as the use of oral rehydration solutions for infant diarrheal disease not be introduced on a public-health scale (King, 1990b).

A frequently heard justification for child survival activities is that a reduction in child mortality will lead eventually to a decline in the birthrate, because parents who are confident that their children will not die will have fewer children. The argument cites the historical demographic transition in countries now more developed, in which reductions in child mortality have preceded sustained declines in fertility. Cynthia Lloyd and Serguey Ivanov (1987, p. 26) point out that this observation does not permit us to conclude that reducing infant mortality and improving the health of children will automatically and immediately be followed by a decline in the birthrate. For both practical and ethical reasons, it is of paramount importance to learn whether shifts in mortality and fertility are causally related, and the degree to which both coincide with advances in the standard of living.

Conclusion

Each nation has the primary responsibility for its own development, including policies to assure adequacy, equity, and justice regarding the health care of its citizens. Governments should encourage individuals and communities to become informed and participate actively in protecting their own health. On the other hand, all nations are interdependent in many ways, including commerce and scientific knowledge, the need for global information about health conditions, and the obligation to work cooperatively for control of cosmopolitan threats and global diseases such as AIDS and tuberculosis. Interdependence carries significant moral responsibility to promote international health activities that are beneficial to all involved. The wealthier countries must not apply their superior resources to exploit poor governments or peoples for commercial advantage, or to build scientific knowledge in cultural or unethical ways, or to deal with poorer countries paternalistically or moralistically, offending deeply held religious beliefs.

PAUL F. BASCH

Directly related to this entry are the entries PUBLIC HEALTH; JUSTICE; BENEFICIENCE; *and* FOOD POLICY. *For a further discussion of topics mentioned in this entry, see the entries* INFORMED CONSENT, *article on* MEANING AND ELEMENTS OF INFORMED CONSENT; *and* MULTINATIONAL RESEARCH. *For a discussion of related ideas, see the entry* AIDS, *article on* PUBLIC-HEALTH ISSUES. *Other relevant material may be found under* POPULATION POLICIES.

Bibliography

BANKOWSKI, Z.; BRYANT, JOHN H.; and LAST, JOHN M. 1991. *Ethics and Epidemiology: International Guidelines.* Geneva: Council for International Organization of Medical Sciences.

BASCH, PAUL F. 1990. *Textbook of International Health.* New York: Oxford University Press.

CHRISTAKIS, NICHOLAS A. 1988. "The Ethical Design of an AIDS Vaccine Trial in Africa." *Hastings Center Report* 18:31–37.

COUNCIL FOR INTERNATIONAL ORGANIZATIONS OF MEDICAL SCIENCES (CIOMS). 1982. *Proposed International Guidelines for Biomedical Research Involving Human Subjects.* Geneva: Author.

KING, MAURICE. 1990a. "Public Health and the Ethics of Sustainability." *Tropical and Geographical Medicine* 42, no. 3:197–206.

———. 1990b. "Health Is a Sustainable State." *Lancet* 36, no. 8716:664–667.

LAVERTU, DIANA SERRANO, and LINARES, ANA MARÍA. 1990. "Ethical Principles of Biomedical Research on Human Subjects: Their Application and Limitations in Latin America and the Caribbean." *Bulletin of the Pan American Health Organization* 24, no. 4:469–479.

LLOYD, CYNTHIA B., and IVANOV, SERGUEY. 1987. "The Effects of Improved Child Survival on Family Planning Practice and Fertility." Vol. 7 of *Technical Background Papers Prepared for the International Conference on Better Health for Women and Children Through Family Planning.* New York: The Population Council.

SINGER, HANS. 1986. "The Ethics of Foreign Aid." In *Rights and Obligations in North-South Relations: Ethical Dimensions of Global Problems.* Edited by Moorhead Wright. London: Macmillan.

WOOLLEY, F. ROSS. 1990. "Medical Ethics, Technology and Public Health." *Asia-Pacific Journal of Public Health* 4:228–233.

INTERPRETATION

When we fall ill, we start trying to say what it is like compared with how it was and in relation to how we thought it was going to be and may still turn out to be. Thus do we locate ourselves in our story as we understand it and seek the counsel of others to help us make sense of an unexpected turn of events, an illness or injury that resists being written off, and therefore must be written into the script of our lives.

Interpreting illness

What the caregiver is expected to do in such encounters is not to solve a problem but to follow a story—about pain and discomfort, to be sure, but also about love, loss, loyalty, and the like. Interpretive medical ethics begins with patients and doctors (or nurses or family) talking with each other about what the hurt is like and why it hurts like that just now. There is no logical movement from premises to conclusion. One looks to the acceptability of events, their appropriateness rather than their necessity. The emphasis is on contingency, and the interpretive task is to relate the current episode to what has transpired in the story thus far and to what is anticipated by introducing a medical explanation or procedure. Following, then, is not merely a matter of trailing along or keeping track but of becoming aware and getting the gist of the development of the story. Nor is the caregiver the reader and the patient the text. Rather, the two of them together are interpreters of the illness and joint authors of the illness narrative. Interpretation is a time-honored means of making sense of human events.

Hermeneutics and the varieties of interpretation

Classical beginnings. Not until the nineteenth century was it possible plausibly to claim, as Friedrich Nietzsche did, that "everything is interpretation." Nonetheless, the interpretive arts are ancient. The origin of the term "hermeneutics" is Greek—*hermeneia,* or interpretation—probably after Hermes, who made human sense of the sometimes obscure utterances of the gods. Aristotle wrote a treatise on interpretation. Philo of Alexandria interpreted the Mosaic law allegorically. Writing in the third century C.E., Origen was the first

Christian theologian to articulate a theory of interpretation according to which Scripture was understood to yield multiple—literal, moral, and mystical—meanings. In the fourth century, Augustine adopted and refined a later version of this theory, and in the Middle Ages the Scholastics applied it in countless practical manuals of biblical exegesis. With the rise of modernity and, in particular, with the translation of the Bible into the vernacular, the long-held view that Holy Writ was accessible only to ecclesiastical experts gradually gave way to the idea that the sense of sacred texts is available to any devout reader who has mastered the requisite techniques of textual analysis.

Well into the eighteenth century textual analysis aimed at deciphering and then making contemporary sense of the self-evident word of God—exegesis followed by exposition. The rise of historical self-consciousness and of modern historical criticism unsettled this view, so that by the time of Friedrich Schleiermacher (1768–1834), hermeneutics was being secularized. The question was not, What are the right rules for getting at the hidden meaning of a text? but, How is understanding of human meaning possible at all in light of the seminal influence of cultural context on sacred text? Now that "original meaning" had become problematic, perhaps inaccessible, was any meaning available at all? Thus did Schleiermacher, generally regarded as the founder of modern hermeneutics, bring discussions of textual analysis to bear on the process of understanding itself, not with the aim of uncovering universals but with a view to explicating the texts of lived experience.

We make sense of our lives, Schleiermacher observed, by means of a kind of practical divination.

> Hermeneutics is not to be limited to written texts. I often make use of hermeneutics in personal conversation when, discontented with the ordinary level of understanding, I wish to explore how my friend has moved from one thought to another or to try to trace out the views, judgements and aspirations which led him to speak about a given subject in just this way and no other. Who does not try in meaningful conversation to lift out its main points, to try to grasp its internal coherence, to pursue all its subtle intimations further? (Schleiermacher, 1986, p. 66)

The conversation metaphor at the center of Schleiermacher's theory of understanding is the touchstone of modern hermeneutics.

Interpretation begins in efforts at understanding of an ordinary sort. We size up situations in which we find ourselves. We move through these situations guided by readings taken in transit. As circumstances change, or cues become unclear, we make midcourse corrections. When messages are mixed or obstacles to understanding arise, the fluid motion of our lives is interrupted and we pause long enough to step back and figure out why.

In practice, the art of interpretation consists of an oscillating movement—conjecturing (Schleiermacher says "divining," a kind of educated guess), then comparing this conjecture with similar previous experiences, conjecturing, comparing, and so on—talking with the text of experience until an understanding is reached. "The hermeneutical principle . . . is that just as the whole is understood from the parts, so the parts can be understood only from the whole" (Schleiermacher, 1986, p. 75). This oscillating movement occurs within a circle of meaning. "Just as hermeneutics would be unable to begin its work if what is to be understood were completely foreign, so there would be no reason for hermeneutics to begin if nothing were strange between speaker and hearer" (Schleiermacher, 1986, p. 65). It is a strangeness that engages the interpreter's attention, but if that strangeness is thoroughgoing, the hermeneutic work cannot proceed. The possibility of dialogue presupposes at least some similarity of language or experience or disposition.

Wilhelm Dilthey (1833–1911) appropriated and broadened the scope of Schleiermacher's hermeneutical ideas beyond the realm of written texts and spoken word to human expression generally. To Dilthey's mind, the human world in all its manifestations resembles a text that requires reading. Dilthey drew a distinction between elementary and higher forms of understanding that serves much the same purpose as Schleiermacher's metaphor of conversation. It holds intact the vital connections between hermeneutics as a formal method and ordinary interpretation. In the world of the everyday, we make countless "judgements about the character and capacities of individuals. We constantly take account of interpretations of individual gestures, facial expressions, actions or combinations of these . . . to gain insight into the people surrounding us so that we can make sure how far we can count on them" (Dilthey, 1988, p. 157).

Understanding emerges from the interaction of such life experience with self-understanding, an idea reminiscent of Schleiermacher's dialogical approach. By means of an act of sympathetic imagination, the interpreter projects himself or herself into the experience of another. Piecing together the outward and visible signs of another's expressions, the interpreter envisages an inward and invisible narrative of lived experience. According to Dilthey, higher understanding "is only possible if the context which exists in one's own experience . . . is always . . . present and ready" (Dilthey, 1988, p. 159)—an alertness to possibility and a receptive disposition in the absence of which much that is significant will go unnoticed or unrecognized, with the result that interpretation will be either sidetracked or stymied.

The early Dilthey believed that self-understanding was a sufficient basis for understanding others. In his mature work, however, he incorporated into his conception of understanding both an intuitive grasping and a reliving and reconstructing of the experience of another. Understanding is now not an immediate but a reflective process mediated by the imagination (Dilthey says "filtered through the consciousness") of the interpreter. Although Dilthey successfully preserved Schleiermacher's insight into the conversational character of interpretation and brought it to bear on lived experience and its representations generally, his notion that the interpreter can enter another's experience left his formulation vulnerable to the charge of Romanticist tendencies.

Phenomenological influences.   The work of twentieth-century continental theorists in the tradition of phenomenological inquiry, such as Hans Georg Gadamer (1900–) and Paul Ricoeur (1913–), may be viewed as an extension of Dilthey's insights. Gadamer reevaluates the Romantic idea of tradition, arguing that Romanticism provided a useful corrective to the Enlightenment dream of Reason in that it acknowledged the influence of tradition and the need to critically evaluate and renew it. This appreciation for the historical and cultural embeddedness of all knowledge and understanding is common to hermeneutical and phenomenological modes of reflection and reasoning. Both are characterized by a critical attentiveness to the relation of language and experience. Like Schleiermacher and Dilthey, Gadamer appeals to the kind of provisional, customary understanding aimed at an ordinary conversation, but he eschews the notion that an interpreter can enter the mind or grasp the intention of an interlocutor or of the author of a text requiring interpretation. "To understand what a person says is . . . to agree about the object, not to get inside another person and relive his experience" (Gadamer, 1975, p. 345).

Phenomenologists argue that what is given to the interpreter is the previously interpreted world and an invitation to speak and be spoken to: "It is the function of the dialogue that in saying or stating something a challenging relation with the other evolves, a response is provoked, and the response provides the interpretation of the other's interpretation." The purpose of the conversation is not to prove anything but to understand someone or something—intelligibility and appropriation rather than validation. The aim is not to get "back" to some foundational principle or "up" to some higher principle but to strive toward some common ground, shared at least long enough to keep the conversation going. Participation is the phenomenologist's alternative to the search for foundations: "By sharing, by our participating in the things in which we are participating, we enrich them. . . . The whole life of tradition consists exactly in this enrichment so that life is our culture and our past:

the whole inner store of our lives is always extending by participating" (Gadamer, 1984, p. 64). Critics such as Jürgen Habermas (1980) and Karl-Otto Apel see in Gadamer's view a linguistic idealism that succumbs to contextual relativism. A hermeneutic that lacks external reference points is vulnerable to ideological social and economic distortions of tradition emanating from beyond the self-contained, internally driven interpretive dialogue.

As does Gadamer, Ricoeur links the phenomenological approach to hermeneutics, but he has a more literary orientation. For him, the goal of hermeneutics is understanding by means of discernment and appropriation. This was as true for Schleiermacher and Dilthey as it is for Ricoeur, but though the aim is identical and the means are similar, the starting point is significantly different. Schleiermacher and Dilthey began, as we have seen, with dialogue, and developed their interpretive approach by analogy to ordinary conversation. For Ricoeur the Romantic tradition in hermeneutics did not sufficiently appreciate that dialogue is itself interpretive. Just as one does not begin a conversation without presupposition, so the activity of discernment does not set out *ab ovo* but always begins *in via*, with its own stock of inherited maxims, metaphors, and meanings.

Ricoeur contends that hermeneutics consists in a dialectic of comprehending and explaining, which is not a linear extension of the speaking and hearing that constitute dialogue. He stipulates the task of hermeneutics as understanding the experience of self and other taken together as text. The text that requires interpretation is a web of relations connecting self to other. Meaning is constructed by persons-in-relation reading the texts of relationships—texts that "speak of possible worlds and of possible ways of orienting oneself in these worlds" (Ricoeur, 1981, p. 177). Reading is not a deciphering of signs or a search for something hidden behind the text, but a search for something disclosed by the text. (Ricoeur uses the phrase "in front of it," implying that it is between text and reader.) Such meaning is not there literally to be discovered, nor is the stuff of experience merely the material out of which meaning is to be constructed. Such meaning as experience has is located contextually and articulated metaphorically, in the mutual give-and-take of dialogical discernment and appropriation. "To understand is not to project oneself into the text but to expose oneself to it; it is to receive a self enlarged by the appropriation of the proposed worlds which interpretation unfolds" (Ricoeur, 1981, p. 94).

Interpretive bioethics

The meaning of malady emerges in a dialogue with the text of affliction. The analogy between cultural or textual analysis and ordinary conversations between pa-

tients and those who care for them, though not exact in every detail, is suggestive. The interpreter of the text of a life event or of a novel, poem, or play imaginatively places the text in illuminating contexts (a cultural milieu, a literary genre) and then closely reads its lines and between its lines. So, too, in the therapeutic encounter the caregiver turns a trained ear to a particular patient's account of misfortune or malaise, places it in the company of similar accounts he or she has heard before, and then attends not only to what is said but also to what is unspoken and to what is unspeakable, all the while conversing with the patient to test the fit of the patient's experience with similar experiences. This requires a capacity to imagine illness or injury from the patient's perspective and an awareness of the impossibility of identifying with the patient's experience: a kind of listening with the third ear—an awareness of setting and significance and an alertness to narrative possibility.

Interpretation of the birth of a retarded child. William F. May makes use of an interpretive approach in his reflections on the birth of a retarded child. As an alternative to what he calls a possessional view of the self, May advances a relational view. The operant terms here are not qualities, capacities, and properties possessed by the self, or diminished, compromised, or altogether lacking in the self. Rather, May uses the familiar theological concept of covenant to inquire into the ways in which parents and their children are bound to each other. Instead of setting out from the classificatory scheme family: human; genus: child; species: retarded, May probes the meaning of human parenting and its bearing on the relationship between parent and child. "Bonding describes the way in which two people settle into one another's bone marrow and kidneys, imagination and bowels. Bonding does not demand a mystical merger of identity between two partners, but it establishes a tie so powerful that neither can undertake much without reckoning with the consequences for the being and well-being of the other" (May, 1991, p. 36).

Moral analysis of parenting begins in the observation that the newborn is a stranger and one who is to remain in the parents' midst. Beyond getting used to that odd fact, the presence of a child means a partial loss of freedom on the parents' part. Time, attention, and affection heretofore directed elsewhere will now be required by the child. Furthermore, while giving birth is an affirmation and expresses hope, it also provokes anxiety about the future. These are potential obstacles to the bonding of parent and newborn. They must be successfully negotiated if the bond is to "take."

Against this background, May undertakes to interpret bonding between parents and a retarded child. "Bearing a retarded child imposes upon the parents an experience that corresponds structurally to those great turning points (and associated rites of passage) in traditional societies that transported people from one stage of life to another—birth, puberty, marriage, and death" (May, 1991, p. 43). These turning points include three moments: a break with the past, a turbulent transition, and entry into a new life.

The first moment is dominated for the parents by the necessity of burying the dream of the child they had expected and of getting used to the alienation engendered by the retarded child's irremediable dependency. "In a variety of ways, the retarded child disconnects its family from the culture at large. . . . [The parents] become estranged in their own culture. Loyalty to this child requires a reconsidered relation to much else" (May, 1991, p. 45). This first moment is a moment of irreversible loss.

In the period of transition, family members try to claim the child that they have and to reconstruct their lives in relation to this child. This is the time of the dark night of the soul, when the experience of bereftness deepens and widens into ordeal. Now others are needed to help navigate the transition—skilled professionals and other parents who have lived through similar ordeals.

The final moment is that of embarkation on the difficult journey to a new life. May likens it to induction into the sacred in traditional societies: "Bonding takes hold in the parents when the event they originally perceived as blank and intractable fate now seizes them as destiny in which they imperfectly but humanly find their identity and calling" (May, 1991, p. 52). This covenant is not sustained by the parents alone. The child also nourishes the parents. By asking the question of how we should value retarded children in relational terms, we (parents and professionals) are reminded that we, too, are needy in our own ways—if not just now, that we once were and will be again. In recognizing this reciprocity of need, we gain humility. In acknowledging our solidarity with the afflicted, we reaffirm the ties that bind us and, to recall Ricoeur's formulation, we receive a self enlarged.

May demonstrates how an interpretive approach can operate in medical ethics, in an effort to make sense of malady. Retelling the story of the birth of a retarded child in the theological language of covenant may yield understanding and care.

Interpreting injury.   James Dickey's poem "The Scarred Girl" (Dickey, 1963) presents a different kind of interpretive challenge, one prompted by injury. The scarred girl lies heavily bandaged because an accident threw her face-first into the windshield of the car in which she was riding. Just prior to the accident "the windshield held"—it was intact, it shielded her in the vehicle, and it framed a pastoral scene. In a flash, at the moment of impact, this peaceful scene, this peaceful life, and the girl's beauty were painfully, uselessly broken.

For our mind's eye, the poet conflates the girl's face and the car's windshield. They splinter simultaneously. We know from experience that a shattered windshield cannot be repaired. We infer from the poem's title that the girl's face cannot be completely restored. But for all the brute facticity of brokenness here, this poem is about "the process and hurt of . . . healing."

The poet imagines what the scarred girl is thinking: "All glass may yet be whole"—and her fractured face "restored and undamaged." These are more than mere thoughts, they are a yearning and a dawning. It comes to the girl that the country field and the animals framed by the windshield and shattered on impact can be restored. The restoration will depend on her. The fate of the fragmented meadow and the broken cattle rests in her hands, or rather in her way of seeing. The meadow and the cattle "know that her visage contains/The process and hurt of their healing." Her point of view, her life, her attitude can restore "the glass of the world."

But there is another field here, the one the girl does not think of. It is a battlefield on which a war for her beauty is already lost. Her face is not only buried under bandages but is dead and gone. The girl's "visage" contains the clue to the restoration of the glass of the world. Blinded by the bandages, she thinks of the world as she last saw it, flashing and fractured. But when the wrappings come off, she will see through the looking glass as through a window to "pastures of earth and of heaven/Restored and undamaged, the cattle/Risen out of their jagged graves." She will remember them as they were before the deadly crash. And her memory will be the means of their resurrection.

All this "she thinks." And all the while the shattered field anxiously awaits the girl's reaction to what she will see in the mirror when first she views her own "unimagined face." We who hold the mirror dread what may come, but that is because we do not see beyond the scars to what the girl recognizes—herself, in the mirror. She looks squarely at her face and does not flinch. Her face is red, raw, odd, and calm. It is a new face and "entire." Her old face is gone, but this one is whole in its own way. She will never forget her former beauty (it will "hover near for the rest of her life"), but her new face, a semblance of the old ("plainly in sight"), will be the one that she will live with. This is the "newborn countenance put upon everything," the scarred girl's outlook that accompanies her new face. In place of resurrection and restoration there is reconciliation. The scarred girl is reconciled. It is "the only way."

Interpretation in medical practice

The poet moves imaginatively from perception to construction as the doctor moves from hunch to generalization—that is, from this particular case to cases of this sort—with the aim of making sense of an experience that resists meaning. The caregiver's interpretive advantage, like that of the poet, is owed to his or her access to a repertoire of cases into which this patient's case is likely to fit. The fit will not be exact, of course. The interpretation of morally vexing cases does not admit of precision because circumstances cannot be fixed, steadied, or held fast—and circumstances alter cases. Nonetheless, an interpretation may be close enough to shed light. Familiarity with a range of cases of a kind, artfully combined with a particular patient's distinctive experience, illuminates the case at hand (Jonsen, 1986).

Interpretation is at the heart of medical practice because an experience of illness does not occur in general. It is always someone's experience. Fitting a particular case to a general run of cases requires an act of imagination. Interrupted by an episode of illness or injury, the patient's story requires retelling, now with a new chapter to accommodate the unanticipated turn of events. The story's very intelligibility to the girl herself and to those who care for her is dependent on, may in fact be tantamount to, what Ricoeur calls its followability.

The automobile accident in Dickey's poem has disrupted the girl's life story, making it temporarily unintelligible, unfollowable. To follow a story is to proceed forward in the midst of contingencies, but always with an expectation that finds its fulfillment in the provisional conclusion of the story. This conclusion is not the logical implication of premises (this is a conversation, not an argument) but an end, or better, the *sense* of an ending deemed suitable in that it provides a vantage point from which the story may be seen as whole, at least for the time being (Kermode, 1967).

Perplexed at an instance of human suffering, we offer a conjecture about its meaning. Once we have a tentative grasp on that meaning, we compare the particularities of this concrete situation with other similar situations in order to test our intuitive grasp of the current perplexity. The next movement is a return to the case at hand with a view to testing the fit of the general interpretation of cases of this type to our reading of this case, and so on, back and forth, conjecturing, comparing, until a plausible fresh interpretation is discerned. The oscillating movement of interpretation takes place within a circle of meaning, beyond which there is no recourse to definitive meaning.

The lived experience of illness may be approached in this way, as a text requiring reading—ideally, by a patient and a caregiver comparing notes. Thus construed, the patient–caregiver relationship is collaborative, and the work of healing commences not when the caregiver makes the diagnosis but when text and readers converge in a common narrative. Narrative evolves by projecting a limited set of possibilities, each with moral implications. It proceeds by creating expectations and by plausibly situating them and unfolding them in the direction of future expectations. In just this way, most medical practice is a storied practice. Contrary to the impression created by the stainless-steel apparatus and vital-sign monitors of rescue medicine, what is required of the caregiver in patient encounters is less often swift judgment and deft action than a discerning reading of the situation at hand. What does the ailment in question mean? Is the suffering to be relieved or endured, and in what measure? What can one reasonably expect to be the result of this or that intervention? Are there fates worse than death? Answers to such questions must be thought through and talked about person by person, case by case. In this process of reflection and conversation, defensible courses of action evolve.

Thinking about morality and medicine interpretively prompts a shift away from an exclusive concentration on abstract, normative ethics toward reflections on the narrative, symbolic, and rhetorical dimensions of relations between patients and caregivers. After more than a decade of dominance by formal analytical approaches, medical ethics is increasingly being shaped by cultural, historical, literary, and theological approaches. Bioethics continues to concern itself with morally troubling aspects of medical care, but the approach is less that of principles and applications than of cases and interpretations. Whereas the former method is deductive and didactic, the latter is conversational, mutual, and constructive, phenomenological and pragmatic.

RONALD A. CARSON

Directly related to this entry is the entry NARRATIVE. *For a further discussion of topics mentioned in this entry, see the entries* CASUISTRY; HEALING; HEALTH AND DISEASE, *article on* THE EXPERIENCE OF HEALTH AND ILLNESS; LIFE; LITERATURE; PAIN AND SUFFERING; PROFESSIONAL–PATIENT RELATIONSHIP; *and* VALUE AND VALUATION. *This entry will find application in the entries* BIOETHICS; *and* CLINICAL ETHICS. *For a discussion of related ideas, see the entries* CARE; ETHICS, *especially the article on* NORMATIVE ETHICAL THEORIES; FAMILY; *and* VIRTUE AND CHARACTER. *Other relevant material may be found under the entry* ADVERTISING.

Bibliography

BAIER, ANNETTE. 1985. "Theory and Reflective Practices." In her *Postures of the Mind: Essays on Mind and Morals*, pp. 207–227. Minneapolis: University of Minnesota Press.

BAKHTIN, MIKHAEL M. 1981. *The Dialogic Imagination: Four Essays.* Translated by Michael Holquist. Austin: University of Texas Press.

BRODY, HOWARD. 1987. *Stories of Sickness.* New Haven, Conn.: Yale University Press.

CARSON, RONALD A. 1990. "Interpretive Bioethics: The Way of Discernment." *Theoretical Medicine* 11, no. 1:51–59.

CASSELL, ERIC J. 1991. *The Nature of Suffering and the Goals of Medicine.* New York: Oxford University Press.

CROSMAN, ROBERT. 1980. "Do Readers Make Meaning?" In *The Reader in the Text: Essays on Audience and Interpretation.* Edited by Susan R. Suleiman and Inge Crosman Wimmers. Princeton, N.J.: Princeton University Press.

DICKEY, JAMES. 1992. [1963]. *The Scarred Girl.* In his *The Whole Motion: Collected Poems, 1945–1992,* pp. 153–154. Hanover, N.H.: University Press of New England. Originally published in the *New Yorker,* June 1, 1963.

DILTHEY, WILHELM. 1988. "The Understanding of Other Persons and Their Life-Expressions." In *The Hermeneutics Reader: Texts of the German Tradition from the Enlightenment to the Present,* pp. 152–164. Edited by Kurt Mueller-Vollmer. New York: Continuum.

GADAMER, HANS GEORG. 1975. *Truth and Method.* New York: Seabury.

———. 1981. *Reason in the Age of Science.* Cambridge, Mass.: MIT Press.

———. 1987. "The Problem of Historical Consciousness." In *Interpretive Social Science: A Second Look,* pp. 82–140. Edited by Paul Rabinow and William M. Sullivan. Berkeley: University of California Press.

GEERTZ, CLIFFORD. 1973. "Thick Description: Toward an Interpretive Theory of Culture." In his *The Interpretation of Cultures: Selected Essays.* New York: Basic Books.

GUSTAFSON, JAMES M. 1990. "Moral Discourse About Medicine: A Variety of Forms." *Journal of Medicine and Philosophy* 15, no. 2:125–142.

HABERMAS, JÜRGEN. 1980. "The Hermeneutic Claim to Universality." In *Contemporary Hermeneutics.* Edited by Josef Bleicher. London: Routledge & Kegan Paul.

HAUERWAS, STANLEY. 1974. "The Self as Story: A Reconsideration of the Relation of Religion and Morality from the Agent's Perspective." In his *Vision and Virtue: Essays in Christian Ethical Reflection,* pp. 68–89. Notre Dame, Ind.: University of Notre Dame Press.

HOLMES, HELEN BEQUAERT, and PURDY, LAURA M., eds. 1992. *Feminist Perspectives in Medical Ethics.* Bloomington: Indiana University Press.

HUNTER, KATHRYN MONTGOMERY. 1991. *Doctors' Stories: The Narrative Structure of Medical Knowledge.* Princeton, N.J.: Princeton University Press.

ISER, WOLFGANG. 1974. "The Reading Process: A Phenomenological Approach." In *New Directions in Literary History,* pp. 125–145. Edited by Ralph Cohen. Baltimore: Johns Hopkins University Press.

JONSEN, ALBERT R. 1986. "Casuistry and Clinical Ethics." *Theoretical Medicine* 7, no. 1:65–74.

KERMODE, FRANK. 1967. *The Sense of an Ending: Studies in the Theory of Fiction.* New York: Oxford University Press.

KLEINMAN, ARTHUR. 1988. *The Illness Narratives: Suffering, Healing, and the Human Condition.* New York: Basic Books.

LEDER, DREW. 1990. "Clinical Interpretation: The Hermeneutics of Medicine." *Theoretical Medicine* 11, no. 1:9–24.

MAY, WILLIAM F. 1991. *The Patient's Ordeal.* Bloomington: Indiana University Press.

MINK, LOUIS O. 1987. *Historical Understanding.* Edited by Brian Fay, Eugene O. Golob, and Richard T. Vann. Ithaca, N.Y.: Cornell University Press.

NUSSBAUM, MARTHA C. 1992. *Love's Knowledge: Essays on Philosophy and Literature.* New York: Oxford University Press.

RICOEUR, PAUL. 1981. *Hermeneutics and the Human Sciences: Essays on Language, Action and Interpretation.* Edited by John B. Thompson. Cambridge: At the University Press.

SCHAFER, ROY. 1992. *Retelling a Life: Narration and Dialogue in Psychoanalysis.* New York: Basic Books.

SCHLEIERMACHER, FRIEDRICH. 1986. "The Academy Addresses of 1829: On the Concept of Hermeneutics with Reference to F. A. Wolf's Instruction and Ast's Textbook." In *The Interpretation of Texts,* p. 66. Vol. 1 of *Hermeneutical Inquiry.* Edited by David E. Klemm. Atlanta, Ga.: Scholars Press.

STOUT, JEFFREY. 1988. *Ethics After Babel: The Languages of Morals and Their Discourses.* Boston: Beacon Press.

TAYLOR, CHARLES. 1987. "Overcoming Epistemology." In *After Philosophy: End or Transformation?* pp. 464–488. Edited by Kenneth Baynes, James Bohman, and Thomas McCarthy. Cambridge, Mass.: MIT Press.

TOOMBS, S. KAY. 1992. *The Meaning of Illness: A Phenomenological Account of the Different Perspectives of Physician and Patient.* Dordrecht, Netherlands: Kluwer.

TRACY, DAVID. 1987. *Plurality and Ambiguity: Hermeneutics, Religion, Hope.* San Francisco: Harper & Row.

WALZER, MICHAEL. 1987. *Interpretation and Social Criticism.* Cambridge, Mass.: Harvard University Press.

ZANER, RICHARD M. 1988. *Ethics and the Clinical Encounter.* Englewood Cliffs, N.J.: Prentice-Hall.

IN VITRO FERTILIZATION

See REPRODUCTIVE TECHNOLOGIES, *articles on* IN VITRO FERTILIZATION AND EMBRYO TRANSFER, ETHICAL ISSUES, *and* LEGAL AND REGULATORY ISSUES.

INVOLUNTARY COMMITMENT

See COMMITMENT TO MENTAL INSTITUTIONS. *See also* INFORMED CONSENT, *article on* ISSUES OF CONSENT IN MENTAL-HEALTH CARE; INSTITUTIONALIZATION AND DEINSTITUTIONALIZATION; *and* PATIENTS' RIGHTS, *article on* MENTAL PATIENTS' RIGHTS.

IRAN

See MEDICAL ETHICS, HISTORY OF, *section on* NEAR AND MIDDLE EAST, *article on* IRAN.

IRAQ

See MEDICAL ETHICS, HISTORY OF, *section on* NEAR AND MIDDLE EAST, *article on* CONTEMPORARY ARAB WORLD.

IRELAND, NORTHERN

See MEDICAL ETHICS, HISTORY OF, *section on* EUROPE, *subsection on* CONTEMPORARY PERIOD, *article on* UNITED KINGDOM.

IRELAND, REPUBLIC OF

See MEDICAL ETHICS, HISTORY OF, *section on* EUROPE, *subsection on* CONTEMPORARY PERIOD, *article on* REPUBLIC OF IRELAND.

IRREVERSIBLE COMA

See DEATH, DEFINITION AND DETERMINATION OF. *See also* DEATH AND DYING: EUTHANASIA AND SUSTAINING LIFE.

ISLAM

Islam, the last of the Abrahamic religions (literally meaning "submission [to God's will]"), was proclaimed by Muhammad (born ca. 570 C.E.), the prophet of Islam and the founder of Islamic public order in the seventh century C.E. in Arabia. This article will focus on the historical development of Islam, its fundamental teachings, Islamic legal thought, the Islamic theological and ethical tradition, Islamic mysticism, and Islam and modernity. Throughout the article an attempt will be made to relate religious-moral belief to practice, thereby indicating implications of the tradition in molding attitudes toward maintenance and preservation of life, including ways of dealing with suffering, pain, illness, death, and connected issues.

Historical development

Seventh-century Arabia was socially and politically ripe for the emergence of new leadership. When Muhammad was growing up in Mecca, a city that had become an important center of a flourishing trade between Byzantium and nations on the Indian Ocean, he was aware of the social inequities and injustices that existed in the tribal society dominated by a political oligarchy made up of a few powerful chiefs. Monotheistic traditions like Judaism and Christianity were known to the Arabs; but they had persisted in worshiping their pagan deities, who dwelt in sanctuaries in and around Mecca. The most important shrine in Mecca was the Kaaba, a rectangular building, to which tribes made annual pilgrimage, using the occasion to trade with people who came from all over Arabia.

Religious practices and attitudes before Islam, then, were determined by the tribal aristocracy who also upheld tribal values: "bravery in battle, patience in misfortune, persistence in revenge, protection of the weak, defiance of the strong," generosity, and hospitality as part of their moral code (Watt, 1953, p. 20). The growth of Mecca as a commercial center where individuals acted more freely in their own private interest than in the interest of the tribe, had weakened this tribal ethic to the extent that weaker members of a tribe and those who had been marginalized were left without security. Islam emerged in the midst of a serious socioeconomic imbalance between the rich and the poor, between extreme forms of individualism and tribal solidarity.

Muhammad was born into the Hashimite clan of the powerful Quraysh tribe in Mecca. His father died before he was born, and his mother died when he was six years old. In accordance with Arab tribal norms, he was brought up first by his grandfather, then, following the grandfather's death, by his uncle, with whom he traveled on trade missions to Syria. As a young man he was employed by a wealthy Meccan woman, Khadija, as her trade agent. He was twenty-five when he accepted a marriage offer from Khadija, who was fifteen years his senior. When Muhammad received his prophetic call at the age of forty, Khadija was the first person to become "muslim" ("believer in Islam").

This was the beginning of Islam as a struggle to establish a monotheistic faith and create an ethical public order embodying divine justice and mercy. Meccan leadership resisted Muhammad and persecuted him and his followers, who were drawn mainly from among the poor and disenfranchised. Under unbearable conditions, Muhammad decided to emigrate to Medina, an oasis town in the north, where two warring Arab tribes had invited him to arbitrate their affairs. This emigration in 622 C.E. marks the beginning of the Muslim calendar and the genesis of the first Islamic polity: Muhammad as a statesman instituted a series of reforms to create his community, *umma,* on the basis of religious affiliation. It also established a distinctive feature of Islamic faith, which does not admit the separation between the religious and temporal spheres of human activity, and has insisted on the ideal unity of civil and moral authority under the divinely ordained legal system, the *shari'a.*

Muhammad died in 632 C.E., having brought the whole of Arabia under the Medina government. However, he had left no explicit instructions regarding succession to his religious-political authority. The early Muslim leaders who succeeded him as caliphs exercised

Muhammad's political authority, making political and military decisions that led to the expansion of Muslim domains beyond Arabia. The community leaders were convinced that the Islamic domain, and not necessarily Islamic faith, was to prevail over all other nations. This conviction, in addition to the political need to consolidate the Muslim polity threatened by internal tribal strife, became the driving force behind the early territorial expansion. Within a century Muslim armies had conquered the region from the Nile in North Africa to the Oxus in Central Asia and as far as India. This vast empire required an Islamic legal system for the administration of the highly developed political systems of the conquered Persian and Byzantine regions. Muslim jurists formulated a comprehensive legal code, using the ethical and legal principles set forth in the Qur'an, the collected revelations of Muhammad, and the precedents set by the Prophet and the early community, in addition to the customary law in the conquered regions.

Differences of opinion on certain critical issues emerged as soon as Muhammad died. The question of succession to Muhammad was one of the major issues that divided the community into the Sunni and the Shia. Those supporting the candidacy of Abu Bakr (d. 634), an elderly associate of the Prophet, as caliph (political successor) formed the majority of the community, who gradually came to be known as the Sunnis; those who acclaimed 'Ali (d. ca. 660), Muhammad's cousin and son-in-law, as the imam (religious and political leader) designated by the Prophet, formed the minority group, known as the Shia ("partisans").

The dispute had profound implications beyond the political. The ideal nature of prophetic prestige in the community, established both in the Qur'an through persistent admonition to obey the prophet and through the prophet's personal exercise of discretionary power in shaping the public order, meant acknowledgment of an authority whose decisions in all spheres affecting Muslim life would be binding on posterity.

The early years of military victories over the Persians and the Byzantines were followed by the civil wars that broke out in 656 c.e. under Muhammad's third successor, 'Uthman. The tension occasioned by the existence of political and social injustices in the Muslim polity gave rise to two distinct, and in some ways contradictory, attitudes among Muslims: quietist and activist. The supporters of a quietist posture supported authoritarian politics, which feigned unquestioning and immediate obedience to almost any de facto Muslim authority who publicly promised to uphold Islamic norms. The exponents of an activist posture supported radical politics and taught that under certain circumstances, it was imperative to remove an unjust authority from power. Gradually the quietist and authoritarian stance became associated with the majority of the Sunnite

Muslims. The activist and radical stance came to be associated with Shiite Islam.

By the end of the third Islamic century (ninth–tenth c.e.), these two distinct responses to the question of political-religious authority were expounded by the Sunni and Shia schools of thought. Despite the disintegration of the caliphal authority in the thirteenth century c.e., the Muslim community has continued to live in the shadow of the idealized history of early Islam, when the religious and secular authority was united under the divinely guided caliph.

Fundamental teachings

The two authoritative sources of Islamic teachings are the Qur'an, regarded by Muslims as the book of God, and the *sunna*, the exemplary conduct of the Prophet. The Qur'an consists of the revelations Muhammad received intermittently from the time of his call as prophet in 610 c.e. until his death in 632. Muslims believe that the Qur'an was directly communicated to the Prophet by God through the archangel Gabriel; accordingly, it is regarded as inerrant and immutably preserved. It has served as the source for ethical and theological doctrines and principles for the public organization. The *sunna* (meaning "trodden path") has functioned as the elaboration of the Qur'anic revelation, providing details about each and every precept and deed purportedly traced back to the Prophet's own precedent. The narratives that carried such information were designated as *hadith*. In the ninth century, Muslim scholars developed an elaborate system for the theological and legal classification of these *hadith* to deduce certain beliefs and practices.

The *hadith* literature describes the Muslim creed and practice as "the Five Pillars of Islam." The First Pillar is the *shahada*, the profession of faith: "There is no deity but God, and Muhammad is the messenger of God." Belief in God constitutes the integrity of human existence, individually and as a member of society. The Qur'an speaks about God as the being whose presence is felt in everything that exists; everything that happens is an indicator of the divine. God is the "knower of the Unseen and the Visible; . . . the All-Merciful, the All-compassionate, . . . the Sovereign Lord, the All-holy, the Giver of peace, the Keeper of faith, the All-preserver, the All-mighty, the All-powerful, the Most High" (Qur'an, 59:23). Faith in God results in being safe, well integrated, sound, and at peace.

Life is the gift of God, and the body is the divine trust given to humankind to enable it to serve God as completely and fully as the wonderful creation of God has made that serving possible. The humble origin of humans is established by the Qur'anic reference to their creation from "dry clay of black mud formed into shape"

(15:26). Through the well-proportioned creation of the human body and the perpetual guidance provided to perfect it both spiritually and morally, human beings have been given the trusteeship of their body. On the Day of Resurrection, all parts of the human body will have to account for the actions of the person whose bodily organs they formed. God has set limits on what human beings may do with their own bodies. Suicide, homicide, and torturing one's body in any form are regarded as transgressions.

The Qur'anic affirmation of bodily resurrection has determined many religious-moral decisions regarding cadavers. Dead bodies should be buried reverently, as soon as possible. Islamic law prohibits mutilation of the cadaver and, thus, cremation. Under certain circumstances, in order to determine the cause of death, autopsy is permitted. Postmortem dissection is permitted, for instance, to retrieve a valuable object belonging to another person that might have been swallowed by a deceased person. There was doubt about the use of human cadavers for medical research until fairly recently.

The rulings are now well established in regard to the cadavers of non-Muslims, which do not require any monetary compensation for their mutilation (as required by the *shari'a* for the cadaver of a Muslim). However, if the research for a cure of a disease is dependent on the dissection of a Muslim cadaver, then most Sunni and Shi'ite jurists rule it permissible and, as a precautionary measure, require the payment of compensation to the family of the deceased (*Fiqh al-tabib* [Islamic Laws for Physicians], 1993, pp. 159–180). Some recent rulings from Shi'ite jurists make no distinction between a Muslim and a non-Muslim cadaver, thereby permitting research and use of organs for transplantation (*Fiqh al-tabib* [Islamic Laws for Physicians], 1993).

The Qur'an affirms reverence for human life in reference to a similar commandment given to other monotheists: "We decreed for the Children of Israel that whosoever killeth a human being for other than manslaughter or corruption in the earth, it shall be as if he had killed all humankind, and whoso saveth the life of one, it shall be as if he saved the life of all humankind" (5:32). This passage has provided modern Muslim jurists with religious documentation to legitimize medical advances in saving human lives. It has also served as an incentive to protect humanity against peril by choosing to save oneself and others from perdition and to serve humanity as service to God.

The corollary of the belief in God's guidance is human accountability to further divine purposes on earth. The purpose of creation is to allow human beings, created with cognition and volition, freely to accept the responsibility of perfecting their existence by working with the laws of nature grasped by the divinely endowed innate disposition (*fitra*) and by understanding princi-

ples of causality that regulate their well-being. The Qur'an emphasizes God's benevolence, all-forgivingness, and mercy. But it also accentuates God's justice, and stresses that humanity should develop moral and spiritual awareness (*taqwa*) in fulfilling everyday requirements of life.

Human existence is not free of tension and inner stresses caused by rejection of truth (*kufr*) and impairment of moral consciousness. To help humanity, God sends prophets "to remind" humanity of its covenant with God (Qur'an, 7:172). There have been 124,000 prophets from the beginning of history, of whom five (Noah, Abraham, Moses, Jesus, and Muhammad) are regarded as "messengers" sent to organize their people on the basis of the guidance revealed by God.

The Second Pillar is daily worship (*salat*), required five times a day: at dawn, midday, afternoon, evening, and night. These very short prayers entail bowing and prostrations. A Muslim may worship anywhere, preferably in a congregation, facing Mecca. Muslims are required to worship as a community on Fridays at midday and on two major religious holidays, celebrating the end of Ramadan and the completion of the pilgrimage in Mecca. The congregational prayer gives expression to the believer's religious commitment within the community. Women are exempt from the obligation of congregational participation, and the tradition recommends that they worship in the privacy of their homes. However, they have always worshiped at designated areas in the mosque, apart from men. The Qur'an prescribes physical purity for the worshiper through the performance of ablutions, and a full washing after sexual intercourse or a long illness, prior to undertaking worship. Women are required to perform a full washing after the menstrual cycle and childbirth, because blood is regarded as ritually unclean. Islamic law prescribes regular cleansing and physical hygiene as expressions of one's faith.

Prayer in Islam is regarded as therapeutic. Besides seeking medical treatment, Muslims are encouraged to seek healing, especially of psychological illnesses, by praying to God. Many illnesses, according to the teachings of the Prophet, are caused by psychological conditions like anxiety, sorrow, fear, loneliness, and so on. Hence, prayer restores the serenity and tranquillity of the soul.

The Third Pillar is the mandatory "alms levy" (*zakat*). The obligation to share what one possesses with those less fortunate is stressed throughout the Qur'an. The Muslim definition of the virtuous life includes charitable support of widows, wayfarers, orphans, and the needy. Islamic law includes technical regulations about how much *zakat* is due and upon what property it is to be levied. These legal rulings, which originated before the disintegration of the Islamic public order, do not necessarily prevail in contemporary Muslim nations. Although *zakat* has for the most part been left to the conscience of Muslims, the obligation to be charitable and contribute to the general welfare of the community continues to be emphasized. In a number of poor Muslim countries this benevolence, provided by wealthy individuals, has underwritten badly needed health care for those who cannot afford the rising cost of medical treatment. It has also led to the creation of private charitable foundations that compete with the cumbersome and poorly administered government welfare institutions.

The Fourth Pillar is the fast during the month of Ramadan. Since the Muslim calendar, which has been in use since the seventh century, is lunar, the month of fasting moves throughout the year over a period of time, because the lunar year is shorter than the solar. Ramadan is regarded as the holy month during which the Qur'an was revealed to Muhammad. During the fast, which lasts from dawn to dusk, Muslims are required to refrain not only from eating, smoking, and drinking but also from sexual intercourse and acts leading to sensual behavior. The fasting is meant to alter the pattern of life for a month, and Muslims are required to make necessary adjustments in their normal schedules of work and study. The end of the month is marked by a festival, 'Id al-fitr, after which life returns to normal.

Instituted to cultivate individual spiritual and moral self-control, Ramadan also provides a community experience in which families and friends share both fasting and evening meals in the spirit of thanksgiving. Like prayer, fasting possesses therapeutic value. Prophetic medical tradition prescribes fasting for various kinds of ailments, including psychological problems caused by fear and anxiety. It was regarded as a remedy for excessive sexual drive.

The Fifth Pillar is the pilgrimage, the *hajj*, which all Muslims are required to undertake once in their lives, provided they have the financial means. The rituals of the pilgrimage at Mecca are a collective commemoration of the sacrifice story of Abraham and of lessons to be derived from it. Its spiritual objective is to inculcate a form of asceticism accompanied by renunciation of worldly desires (sexual intercourse, use of perfumes, and so on) and concern with the hereafter. The experience brings together Muslims of diverse cultures and nationalities to achieve a purity of existence and a communion with God that will exalt the pilgrim for the rest of his or her life.

Islamic legal thought

Islamic jurisprudence (*fiqh*) was developed to determine normative Islamic conduct as detailed in the *shari'a*, the sacred law. The *shari'a*, the divinely ordained blueprint for human conduct, is inherently and essentially religious. The juridical inquiry that led to the *shari'a* code was comprehensive because it necessarily dealt with every case of conscience covering God-human relations, as well as the ethical content of interpersonal relations in every possible sphere of human activity. Most of the legal activity, however, went into settling more formal interpersonal activities that affected the morals of the community. These activities dealt with the obligation of doing good to Muslims and guarding the interests of the community.

Islamic legal theory recognized four sources for judicial decisions: the Qur'an, the *sunna*, consensus (*ijma*') of the early community of the Muslims, and analogy (*qiyas*), a method of reasoning from data furnished by the Qur'an and the *sunna* in an attempt to estimate the unknown from the known ruling. Al-Shafi'i (d. 820), a rigorous legal thinker, systematically and comprehensively linked the four sources in order to derive the *shari'a* to cover all possible contingencies. The legal precedents and principles provided by the Qur'an and *sunna* were used to develop an elaborate system of rules of jurisprudence. Human conduct was to be determined in terms of how much legal weight was borne by a particular rule that rendered a given practice obligatory or merely recommended.

For instance, if it is deemed that by risking one's life, one may be able to save another person from impending death, then the law permits not only donation but also sale of a needed body part or an organ after a careful risk-benefit analysis. Vital organs like eyes are excepted in this ruling. Likewise, it had to be decided whether an obligatory act, because of its social relevance and the degree of applicability of a given rule or precedent, was to be enforced by penalties in the courts or left to God's judgment in the hereafter.

In family law, the rights of women, children, and other dependents were protected against the male head of the family, who, on the average, was stronger than a woman and more independent, being free of pregnancy and having to care for children. Islamic marital rules encouraged individual responsibility by strengthening the nuclear family. *Shari'a* protected the prerogative of the male because he was required to support the household; the woman was protected primarily by her family. Muslim jurists gave the husband one-sided divorce privileges because for a woman to divorce a man would mean to unsettle her husband's economic investment. Under these rules a husband could divorce a wife almost at will; a wife who wished to leave her husband had to show good reason.

The main legal check upon the man in divorce was essentially financial and a matter of contract between equal parties that included a provision about the bridal gift. Part of the gift, which might be substantial, was paid at the time of marriage; if a husband divorced his wife without special reason, he had to pay her the rest. The equality of women in the *shari'a* carried with it an important financial independence. The Muslim woman could own property that could not be touched by any male relative, including her husband, who was required to support her from his own funds. Moreover, she had a personal status that might allow her to go into business on her own. However, this potential female independence was curbed primarily by cultural means, keeping marriages within the extended family, so that property would not leave the family through women marrying out.

Muslim jurists, although tending to give the male an extensive prerogative, presupposed a considerable social role for women. The Qur'anic injunction to propriety was stretched by means of the *sunna* to impose seclusion. The veil was presented simply in terms of personal modesty; the female apartments, in terms of family privacy. It was not intended to become a form of social distinction, as it did with upper-class women living in rigorous segregation. Among the latter it became a mark of a woman of a quality that she was secluded from all men but those in her own family.

Segregation of the sexes as required by the *shari'a* has led to untold problems in the teaching and practice of medicine today. The problems cover such areas as closely examining and touching the reproductive organs (male-female, female-male, male-male, and female-female); looking at photographs of naked persons for studying physiology and anatomy; taking the pulse and other vital signs of patients of opposite sex. While the classical decisions were prohibitive in all these cases, the majority of the modern Muslim jurists have casuistically accommodated the need to carry out necessary medical training, research, and treatment.

In the patriarchal family structure, and not necessarily in the *shari'a*, women were assigned a subordinate role in the household and community. Through certain cultural practices women's reproductive capacity was controlled. In some parts of the Muslim world women are subjected to traditional practices that are often harmful to their well-being and that of their children. One of the controversial and persistent practices is female circumcision (*khafd* or *khifad*), without which it is believed that girls cannot attain the status of womanhood. Islamic views on female circumcision are ambiguous. While Islam does not condone the practice, neither does it forbid it. The operation was performed long before the rise of Islam. It is not a practice in many Muslim countries, including Saudi Arabia, Tunisia, Iran, and Turkey. There is nothing in the Qur'an that justifies female circumcision, especially its most severe

form, infibulation. The Prophet opposed the custom as found among pre-Islamic Arabs, since he considered it harmful to women's sexual well-being. Yet the official juridical position among the majority of Sunni jurists is that female circumcision is sanctioned by the *sunna*. However, the *shari'a* does not regard it as obligatory. It is merely a recommended act.

As Islamic jurisprudence became highly technical, disputes about method and judicial opinions crystallized into legal schools designated by the names of prominent jurists. The legal school that followed the Iraqi tradition was called Hanafi, after Abu Hanifa (d. 767), the great imam (teacher) in Iraq. Those who adhered to the rulings of Malik ibn Anas (d. 795), in Arabia and elsewhere, were known as Malikis. Al-Shafi'i founded a legal school in Egypt whose influence spread widely to other regions of the Muslim world. Another school was associated with Ahmad ibn Hanbal (d. 855), who compiled a work on *hadith* reports that became the source for juridical decisions of those who followed him. Shiites developed their own legal school, whose leading authority was the imam Ja'far al-Sadiq (d. 765).

Normally, Muslims accepted one of the legal schools prevalent in their region. Most Sunnites follow Hanafi or Shafi'i; the Shiites follow the Ja'fari school. In the absence of an organized "church" and ordained "clergy" in Islam, determination of valid religious praxis was left to the qualified scholar of religious law. Hence, there emerged a living tradition, with different interpretations of the Qur'anic laws and prophetic traditions, giving rise to different schools of the *shari'a*.

The scope of *shari'a*, understood as the norm of the Muslim community as a community, was defined by two essential areas of human life: acts of worship, both public and private, connected with the pillars of faith; and acts of public order that ensure individual justice. The *shari'a* reflected Muslim endeavors to ensure that Islam pervaded the whole of life. However, many areas of human existence, including the ethical problems connected with the medical treatment of ailments, received little systematic attention in the classical formulations of the legal thought.

Islamic theological and ethical tradition

In the first half of the eighth century, the debates about qualified leadership, the existence of injustices in the community, and the appropriate response to redress the situation, formed the rudiments of the earliest systematic theology of the group called Mu'tazilites. Before them, some Muslim thinkers had developed theological arguments, including a doctrine of God and human responsibility, in defense of the Islamic revelation and the prophethood of Muhammad when these were challenged by other monotheists. The Mu'tazilites undertook to show that there was nothing repugnant to reason in the Islamic revelation. Their theological system was worked out under five headings: (1) belief in God's unity, which rejected anything that smacked of anthropomorphism; (2) the justice of God, which denied any ascriptions of injustice to God's judgment of human beings, with the consequence that humans alone were responsible for all their acts, and thus punishable for their evil ones; (3) the impending judgment, which underscored the importance of daily righteousness and rejected laxity in matters of faith; (4) the middle position of the Muslim sinner, who, because of disobeying God's commandments was neither condemned to Hell nor rewarded with Paradise but was regarded as reformable; and (5) the duty to command the good and forbid the evil in order to ensure an ethical social order.

In defining God's creation and governance of the world, these early Muslim theologians sought to demonstrate the primacy of revelation. At the same time, their theology reflected Hellenic influences. From the ninth century on, translations of the full Greek philosophic and scientific heritage became available in Arabic. The result was the development of a technical vocabulary and a pattern of syntax that enriched theological terminology.

The Ash'arites, reacting to Mu'tazilite rationalism, limited speculative theology to a defense of the doctrines given in the *hadith* reports, which were regarded as more reliable than abstract reason in deducing individual doctrines. The Ash'arites emphasized the absolute will and power of God, and denied nature and humankind any decisive role. What humans perceive as causation, they believed, is actually God's habitual behavior. In their response to the Mu'tazilite view on the objective nature of good and evil, and in their effort to maintain the effectiveness of a God, at once omnipotent and omnibenevolent, who could and did intervene in human affairs, they maintained that good and evil are what God decrees them to be. Accordingly, they cannot be known from nature but must be discovered in the sources of revelation, like the Qur'an and the Prophet's example. There are no inherently unchanging essences and natural laws that self-subsistent reason can discern. God transcends the order of nature. Hence, the notion of free will is incompatible with the divine transcendence, which determines all actions directly.

Ash'arite theological views remained dominant well into modern times, and had a profound effect upon scientific (and particularly medical) theory and practice among the Sunnites. The attitude of resignation, a byproduct of belief in predestination, is summed up in the Sunni creedal confession: "What reaches you could not possibly have missed you; and what misses you could not possibly have reached you" (*Fiqh akbar*, art. 3, in Wensinck, 1965, p. 103). This belief in overpowering destiny was bound to have negative implications for some Sunni Muslims encountering adversities caused by illness and other forms of suffering. The Shiite theological and ethical doctrines were based on the Mu'tazilite thesis about the justice of God and the objective nature of moral values.

Positive sciences, especially medicine and astronomy, emerged from the rationalism of Muslim theologians influenced by translations of the works on these subjects from Greek into Arabic. Nature studies in Islamic civilization were pursued by intellectuals who contributed to the Mu'tazilite and Shiite rational theology. Human nature was studied in order to deduce rational principles that could help direct human life to create an ideal society. Ethics and politics were regarded as rational knowledge necessary to harmonize human existence in the universe.

At the practical level, medicine involved the training necessary to apply techniques that demonstrated tact and insight in the treatment of patients. Medical practice was based on a tradition of clinical observation, which became the source for encyclopedic works like the *Canon* (*al-Qanun*) of Avicenna (d. 1037). Since dissection of human cadavers was impossible because of the prohibition in Islamic law against mutilation of the dead and the requirement of immediate burial, physicians treated their patients partly on the basis of their knowledge of anatomy and partly by relying on their understanding of the rationality and harmony of the cosmos. Diagnosis and prognosis were also based on their insights about psychological and environmental factors. Despite the disapproval of some orthodox Muslims, who rejected Greek medicine as not provided for in the Prophetic medical tradition, many of these Greek-influenced philosopher-physicians came to be known as the *hakim* (wise). Prophetic medicine (*al-tibb al-nabawi*) was believed to have arisen to counter the authority of Greek-based medical tradition by positing the notion that certainty in knowledge, including medicine, depended upon revealed sources. However, although seemingly based on the Qur'an and statements attributed to the Prophet, Prophetic medicine actually was the remnant of the medicine customarily practiced among the Arabs in the pre-Islamic age.

Islamic mysticism

In the early days of the Islamic empire under the Umayyads (eighth century), the mysticism that began as an ascetic reaction to growing worldliness in the Muslim community became institutionalized. Sufism, as Islamic mysticism came to be known, aimed to interiorize the formally undertaken ritual acts, and emphasized rigorous self-assessment and self-discipline for the achievement of spiritual and moral perfection. In its early form Sufism was mainly a form of ascetic piety that involved ridding oneself of any dependence on satisfying one's desires, in order to devote oneself entirely to God. Mystical practices developed by the Sufi masters comprised a moral process to gain the relative personal clarity that comes at moments of retreat and reflection. A further dimension of this reflection was to cultivate an ability to face reality about oneself and to love any being capable of needing love. The mystic experienced more intense levels of awareness, which could take ecstatic forms, including ecstatic love of God.

This aspect of Sufism brought the mystics into direct conflict with orthodox Muslims. Sufi teaching that a symbolic and spiritual fulfillment of religious duties was as good as the actual rites was seen by orthodox Muslims as a kind of antinomian behavior within the community that considered literal adherence to the requirements of law as the valid form of religiosity. In general, Sufis increasingly tended to minimize religious differences among various faiths and cultivated humanism based on universalistic spiritual and moral qualities.

By the eleventh century the Sufi masters had developed a new form of religious orientation that brought about the acceptance of Sufism in many parts of the Islamic world. Near the end of the twelfth century, several formal Sufi brotherhoods or orders (*tariqa*), in which women also participated, were organized. Each order taught a pattern of invocation and meditation that used devotional practices to organize a group of novices under a master. Special controls of breath and bodily posture accompanied invocative words or syllables to make possible more intense concentration. The orthodox, who had been suspicious of early elitist Sufism, were now persuaded to accept the Sufism of the masses and to try to discipline it. The ultimate approval of Sufism as a genuine form of Islamic piety was facilitated by Abu Hamid al-Ghazali (d. 1111), who taught Islamic law and theology in Baghdad. His writings in connection with his personal spiritual crisis at the height of his professional success demonstrated that Sufism could be a powerful discipline for curing doubt and experiencing truth.

A number of Sufi masters served as analysts for younger Sufis, helping them to understand their psychic states and making sense of their place in the universe. In the premodern Islamic world, where medical treatment was not generally available to an average person, some prominent Sufis practiced traditional medicine based on the theory of the four humors that kept the body functioning. Herb remedies were used to treat ailments caused by imbalance in the four qualities of the body (hot and cold, moist and dry), which led to an imbalance of the humors. Other Sufis treated physical and psychic disorders through the writing of talismans and amulets. Talismans, some using sections of the Qur'an, and exorcism are used in treating mental disorders even today in rural areas of the Islamic world.

Islam and modernity

The modern age brought Islam and Muslims face to face with intellectual as well as political challenges both from within and from without. From within, Muslims faced the deterioration of Islamic religious life caused by centuries of stagnation and petrification of doctrines and beliefs. From without, the hegemony of the West since the mid-nineteenth century resulted in alien domination of Muslim societies. Since that time, Muslims have endeavored to strike a balance between the divine promise of earthly success to Muslims and their tenuous contemporary situation by introducing internal reforms to prevent further degeneration of Islamic life, and by resisting any form of domination of Muslim societies by the Western powers.

Islamic fundamentalism in modern times stems from the acute awareness among Muslims of a conflict between the religion that promises worldly as well as eternal prosperity to its followers, on the one hand, and the historical development of the Muslim world, which points to the breach of a divine promise, on the other. Muslim leaders call for a return to the original teachings of Islam in the Qur'an and the Prophet's exemplary life. To regain the power and prestige of early Islam, they propose fashioning the modern nation-state on ideals derived from the practices of the original Muslim community. Muslim brotherhoods throughout the Islamic world have joined forces to implement strictly religious reform in a modern society, requiring adherence to the restrictive traditional social-cultural norms.

Resistance to modern secular ideologies and their implications has posed a greater challenge to the Muslim leadership. It has meant providing an Islamic alternative to intentionally imported or externally imposed sociopolitical systems. Such an alternative entails creative interpretation of religious ideas and symbols. Thus far, the traditional Muslim leadership has not succeeded in providing such an alternative as the only viable solution to the multifarious problems faced by the Muslim societies.

A case in point is provided by enormous problems that have arisen with the technological advancement in medicine. Muslim jurists are faced with a crisis because, by its own standards, Islamic jurisprudence has ceased to progress toward some further stage of development. The methods of inquiry and the forms of argument have disclosed inadequacies to furnish solutions to concrete problems faced by the community. Hence, important questions connected with the role of female physicians and patients in a male-dominated profession; conflict between rigorous religious observance and medical education; state policy toward family planning; and social and cultural factors that affect women's health adversely are among numerous pressing issues that remain to be authoritatively resolved.

The judicial decisions issued so far in various Muslim countries, where conferences on bioethics have been held in the last three decades, are mostly in the form of supposition or opinion, and lack the intellectual rigor to become part of state-sponsored health policy.

The greatest challenge to Muslim leadership, both religious and political, remains that of correcting the social and political injustices endured by the common people, who encounter a modern, materialist world over which they have minimal control.

Muslims living as a minority outside the geographical sphere of Islam face the challenge of integration and assimilation in the non-Muslim social universe. Muslim communities belonging to various ethnocultural groups in the West, including North America, are engaged in working out socially interactive strategies that will enable them to establish their identity as Western Muslims. African-American Muslims in North America have reminded the immigrant Muslims of the difficult process of integrating ethnic-cultural and religious identities in modern secular society. African-American Muslims, having been part of American society for a long time, have emerged with a rare ability to combine the most relevant and applicable facets of the modern American social universe and their adopted religion, Islam.

ABDULAZIZ SACHEDINA

Directly related to this entry is the entry MEDICAL ETHICS, HISTORY OF, *section on* NEAR AND MIDDLE EAST, *articles on* IRAN, *and* CONTEMPORARY ARAB WORLD; *and section on* AFRICA, *article on* SUB-SAHARAN COUNTRIES. *Also directly related are the entries* EUGENICS AND RELIGIOUS LAW, *article on* ISLAM; POPULATION ETHICS, *section on* RELIGIOUS TRADITIONS, *article on* ISLAMIC PERSPECTIVES; *and* ABORTION, *section on* RELIGIOUS TRADITIONS, *article on* ISLAMIC PERSPECTIVES. *For a further discussion of topics mentioned in this entry, see the entries* BODY, *article on* CULTURAL AND RELIGIOUS PERSPECTIVES; CIRCUMCISION, *article on* FEMALE CIRCUMCISION; *and* SUICIDE. *For a discussion of related ideas, see the entries* ETHICS, *article on* RELIGION AND MORALITY; FAMILY; HUMAN NATURE; LAW AND BIOETHICS; SEXUAL ETHICS; *and* VALUES AND VALUATION. *See also the entries* ENVIRONMENT AND RE-LIGION; *and* WOMEN, *article on* HISTORICAL AND CROSS-CULTURAL PERSPECTIVES.

Bibliography

ASSAAD, MARIE BASSILI. 1979. *Female Circumcision in Egypt: Current Research and Social Implications.* Cairo: American University, Social Research Centre.

BAKAR, OSMAN. 1986. "Islam and Bioethics." *Greek Orthodox Theological Review* 31, nos. 1-2:157–179.

BURGEL, J. CHRISTOPH. 1973. "Psychosomatic Methods of Cures in the Islamic Middle Ages." *Humaniora Islamica* 1:157–172.

———. 1976. "Secular and Religious Features of Medieval Arabic Medicine." In *Asian Medical Systems: A Comparative Study,* pp. 44–62. Edited by Charles M. Leslie. Berkeley: University of California Press.

CAMPBELL, DONALD EDWARD H. 1926. *Arabian Medicine and Its Influence on the Middle Ages.* 2 vols. Trubner's Oriental Series. London: K. Paul, Trench, Trubner.

EBRAHIM, ABUL FADL MOHSIN. 1991. *Abortion, Birth Control and Surrogate Parenting: An Islamic Perspective.* Indianapolis: American Trust.

ELGOOD, CYRIL. 1951. *A Medical History of Persia and the Eastern Caliphate from the Earliest Times Until the Year A.D. 1932.* Cambridge: At the University Press.

———. 1962. "Tibb-ul-Nabbi or Medicine of the Prophet: Being a Translation of Two Works of the Same Name. I. The Tibb-ul-Nabbi of al-Suyuti. II. The Tibb-ul-Nabbi of Mahmud bin Mohamed al-Chaghhayni, Together with Introduction, Notes and a Glossary." *Osiris* 14:33–192.

Fiqh al-tabib [Islamic Laws for Physicians]. 1993. Compiled by Mustafa Najafi, Mas'ud Salihi, and Mas'ud Firdawsi. International Congress on Medical Ethics. Tehran, July 14–16.

GIORGIS, BELKIS WOLDE. 1981. *Female Circumcision in Africa.* Addis Ababa: U.N. Economic Commission for Africa.

HODGSON, MARSHALL G. S. 1974. *The Venture of Islam: Conscience and History in a World Civilization,* vol. 1. Chicago: University of Chicago Press.

Islam and Family Planning. 1974. International Islamic Conference (Rabat, Morocco, 1971). 2 vols. Beirut: International Planned Parenthood Federation, Middle East and North Africa Region.

Islamic Medical Wisdom: The Tibb al-A'imma. 1991. Translated by Batool Ispahany. Edited by Andrew J. Newman. London: Muhammadi Trust.

MASOOM, SEYED HOSSEIN FATTAHY. 1992. *Collection of Articles from the Seminar on Islam's Views in Medicine.* Mashhad: Ferdowsi University Press. In Persian.

MUSALLAM, BASIM F. 1983. *Sex and Society in Islam: Birth Control Before the Nineteenth Century.* Cambridge: At the University Press.

PLESSNER, MARTIN. 1974. "The Natural Sciences and Medicine." In *The Legacy of Islam.* 2d ed. Edited by Joseph Schacht with C. E. Bosworth. Oxford: Clarendon Press.

Rahman, Fazlur. 1980. *Major Themes of the Qur'an*. Minneapolis: Bibliotheca Islamica.

———. 1989. *Health and Medicine in the Islamic Tradition: Change and Identity*. New York: Crossroad.

Rispler-Chaim, Vardan. 1993. *Islamic Medical Ethics in the Twentieth Century*. Leiden, Netherlands: E. J. Brill.

Rosenthal, Franz. 1969. "The Defence of Medicine in the Medieval Muslim World." *Bulletin of the History of Medicine* 43, no. 6:519–532.

Sachedina, Abdulaziz A. 1988. "Islamic Views on Organ Transplantation." *Transplantation Proceedings* 20, no. 1 (Supp. 1):1084–1088.

Watt, W. Montgomery. 1968. *Muhammad at Mecca*. Oxford: Clarendon Press.

Wensinck, A. J. 1965. [1932]. *The Muslim Creed: Its Genesis and Historical Development*. London: Frank Cass.

ISRAEL

See Medical Ethics, History of, *section on* near and middle east, *articles on* ancient near east, *and* israel. *See also* Abortion, *section on* religious traditions, *article on* jewish perspectives; Eugenics and Religious Law, *article on* judaism; Judaism; *and* Population Ethics, *section on* religious traditions, *article on* jewish perspectives.

ITALY

See Medical Ethics, History of, *section on* europe, *subsection on* contemporary period, *article on* southern europe.

J

JAINISM

The Jaina religious tradition originated in India. Its adherents currently number approximately seven million, most of them living in India. According to tradition, the founders of the faith were not emissaries or embodiments of a supreme being, but were human beings who through their own efforts reached an elevated spiritual state called Kevala, characterized as blissful, omniscient solitude free from all karmic suffering and hence liberated from rebirth. According to Jaina lore, twenty-four persons known as Tīrthaṅkaras crossed over the river of rebirth and conquered the influences of negative karma. They then established and promulgated the Jaina religion. Their stories extend back into the prehistory of India. Historical records exist for the two most recent Tīrthaṅkaras: Parśvanatha, who lived around 850 B.C.E., and Vardhamāna Mahāvīra, the Jina or Conqueror, whose approximate dates are 599–527 B.C.E. The term "Jaina" means "follower or disciple of the Jina."

The belief structure and lifestyle of the Jainas are closely linked. In Jainism, there is no creator God. Rather, the Jaina religion is rooted in a unique respect for all life forms that serves as the basis for a sophisticated system of ethics based on the observance of nonviolence (ahiṃsā).

According to the Jainas, there are two categories of reality: one possesses life (jīva); the other is lifeless (ajīva). However, unlike Western definitions of life, which require "metabolism, growth, response to stimulation, and reproduction," the Jainas regard even seemingly inanimate objects as possessing life. The universe is said to be suffused with countless life forces grouped in five categories: earth, water, fire, and air bodies; microorganisms (nigoda); plants; animals; and humans. These jīva take the shape of their particular life form, whether it be large as a whale or small as a pebble. Each of these life forces is involved in a process of transmigration, moving after death into a new form.

According to Jaina tradition, sticky particles of nonliving matter called karmas adhere to jīvas when acts of desire, passion, or violence are committed. Though not visible to the naked eye, six subtle color distinguish this karma. Black, blue, and gray are associated with sinful or brutish karma, and yellow with less serious offenses. Pink and white indicate that one's karmic burden is being lessened. Through unethical passionate or violent behavior, one increases the inhibiting influence of darker, heavier karma. Through adherence to the Jaina code of ethics, one can expel the negative karma and cultivate the purer forms. Eventually, the goal of Jainism entails breaking free from all karmic influence. In this state, referred to as Kevala, one gains omniscience and freedom from rebirth, dwelling eternally in energy, consciousness, and bliss.

Jaina ethics consists of taking vows (vrata) designed to eliminate karma. Both lay Jainas and members of monastic orders are expected to observe these vows, though the rules for nuns and monks are much more stringent. Earliest Jaina tradition lists four vows: nonviolence (ahiṃsā), truthfulness (satya), not stealing (as-

teya), and nonpossession (*aparigraha*). Vardhamāna Mahavīra is credited with adding a fifth vow, chastity (*brahmacarya*). Scriptures such as the *Acārāṅga Sūtra* serve as authoritative sources for religious life.

From ancient times to the present, Jaina monks and nuns have served as preceptors and living symbols of this tradition. Though there are many "lineages" within the Jaina tradition, all modern Jainas can be classified as belonging to either the Śvetāmbara (White Clad) or the Digambara (Sky Clad) group. In the former group, all monks and nuns wear white robes. In the latter group, the highest order of monks renounces all possessions, including clothing. Both sects allow women to take advanced religious vows, though only the Śvetāmbara allow women to take final vows.

Jaina monks and nuns wander throughout India, teaching the lay community about the lives of earlier saints, advocating the practice of nonviolence, and discussing such topics as the all-pervasiveness of life forms and the karmic effects of behavior. Depending upon the rules of their particular subsect, they may cover their mouths with cloth to avoid injuring insects and microorganisms, or gently sweep the path in front of them to remove insects. In 1949, Acārya Tulsi, head of the Terāpanthi Śvetāmbara monastic order, began teaching a twelvefold system of vows, including modern adaptations such as "not to resort to unethical practices in elections" and "to avoid contributing to pollution."

Although these vows are most intently observed by members of monastic communities, the Jaina lay community has developed a culture anchored in the practice of nonviolence. Lay Jainas generally enter professions in which they can avoid violent action that would increase the depth and darkness of one's karma. Many Jainas engage in trade and commerce, provided that animal products and weaponry are not involved. All Jainas, both laypersons and members of religious orders, are lacto-vegetarians.

Although the Jaina system was originally conceived as outlining a path of personal liberation and spiritual enlightenment, many of the practices inspired by a desire to avoid the accumulation of karma have found new relevance in the modern ethical context, especially vegetarianism, animal protection, attitudes toward death, and the Jaina ideal of tolerance.

Jainas regard vegetarianism as a way to ensure that one does not accumulate the negative karmas associated with animal slaughter. In modern medical terms, it also purifies one's body, minimizing the violence done to the body that is often associated with the consumption of meat. Jaina eating habits, rooted in the ancient doctrine of nonviolence, are compatible with modern, scientific concerns about enhancing personal health through a low-fat, low-cholesterol diet.

Respect for animals has long been a mainstay of Jaina tradition. Throughout Indian history Jainas have lobbied for animal protection, building shelters and providing food for lost or wounded animals, and successfully campaigning to ban animal sacrifice in most parts of India. The Mogul emperor Akbar (1556–1605), influenced by Jaina monks, proclaimed days of restraint from hunting and renounced the consumption of several types of meat. Jaina laypersons periodically visit slaughterhouses and purchase animals for release and protection. In India, pharmaceutical companies owned by Jainas, though required to test medicines on animals, rehabilitate their test animals and then release them.

Jaina tradition regards the death of an older person to be both natural and an opportunity for spiritual advancement. For many centuries, Jainas of advanced age or infirmity have engaged in a practice known as *sallekhanā*, referred to by modern Therāpanthi Śvetāmbara Jainas as *santhārā*. Rather than prolonging death when the process of decline becomes irreversible, some Jainas obtain permission from their religious preceptor to engage in a fast unto death. This final ritual is deemed in Samantabhadra's *Ratnakaranḍaśrāvakācāra*, a Jaina text of the second century, as acceptable only in "calamity, severe famine, old age, or illness from which there is no escape." One first renounces food, then milk, then water, and is encouraged to "depart from the body repeating the *nammokkāra mantra* [prayer] until the last." The Jainas assert that such a fast is neither suicide, which is done out of despair or hopelessness, nor euthanasia, which requires the assistance of a second party and a violent act. This practice, associated with a quest for spiritual freedom, embodies the Jaina ideal of encountering and embracing death without fear.

In a more philosophical vein, the Jainas have developed an ethic of debate, according to which each position or opinion is given provisional status. Any statement or perspective is said to be perhaps true or partially true, including the religious views held by non-Jainas. This ethic both reflects and fosters an attitude of tolerance for which the Jainas have become well known. Mahatma Gandhi, Albert Schweitzer, and Leo Tolstoy were all influenced by Jaina principles.

Technology and modernity present new challenges to the Jaina tradition in that they have spawned new forms of violence not discussed in the original Jaina texts. At Jaina Viśva Bhārati, a university dedicated to the teaching of Jainism located in western India, a curriculum has been developed to help apply Jaina principles to contemporary life, to minimize conflict among groups of people, and to encourage sensitivity to ecological issues.

The Jaina worldview sees the world as a biocosmology, a reality suffused with life. From the perspective of bioethics, this religion is unique in its advocacy of vegetarianism, animal protection, tolerance of multiple perspectives, and philosophical approach to the inevitability of death.

CHRISTOPHER KEY CHAPPLE

Directly related to this entry is the entry MEDICAL ETHICS, HISTORY OF, *section on* SOUTH AND EAST ASIA, *article on* INDIA. *For a further discussion of topics mentioned in this entry, see the entries* ANIMAL WELFARE AND RIGHTS, *articles on* VEGETARIANISM, *and* ETHICAL PERSPECTIVES ON THE TREATMENT AND STATUS OF ANIMALS; DEATH, *article on* EASTERN THOUGHT; DEATH, ATTITUDES TOWARD; *and* ENVIRONMENT AND RELIGION. *See also the entry* ETHICS, *article on* RELIGION AND MORALITY.

Bibliography

CHAPPLE, CHRISTOPHER KEY. 1993. *Nonviolence to Animals, Earth, and Self in Asian Traditions.* Albany: State University of New York Press.

JACOBI, HERMANN, trans. 1884–1895. *Jaina Sutras.* 2 vols. Oxford: Oxford University Press.

JAINI, JAGOMANDERLAL. 1916. *Outlines of Jainism.* Cambridge: At the University Press.

JAINI, PADMANABH S. 1979. *The Jaina Path of Purification.* Berkeley: University of California Press.

———. 1991. *Gender and Salvation: Jaina Debates on the Spiritual Liberation of Women.* Berkeley: University of California Press.

TATIA, NATHMAL. 1951. *Studies in Jaina Philosophy.* Banaras: Jain Cultural Research Society.

TOBIAS, MICHAEL. 1991. *Life Force: The World of Jainism.* Berkeley, Calif.: Asian Humanities Press.

JAPAN

See MEDICAL ETHICS, HISTORY OF, *section on* SOUTH AND EAST ASIA, *article on* GENERAL SURVEY; *and subsection on* JAPAN, *articles on* JAPAN THROUGH THE NINETEENTH CENTURY, *and* CONTEMPORARY JAPAN. *See also* BUDDHISM; CONFUCIANISM; EUGENICS AND RELIGIOUS LAW, *article on* HINDUISM AND BUDDHISM; POPULATION ETHICS, *section on* RELIGIOUS TRADITIONS, *article on* BUDDHIST PERSPECTIVES; *and* TAOISM.

JEHOVAH'S WITNESSES

See ALTERNATIVE THERAPIES; *and* PROTESTANTISM. *See also* BLOOD TRANSFUSION; DEATH AND DYING: EUTHANASIA AND SUSTAINING LIFE, *articles on* ETHICAL ISSUES, *and* PROFESSIONAL AND PUBLIC POLICIES; *and* PATIENTS' RIGHTS.

JOURNALISM AND BIOMEDICINE

See COMMUNICATION, BIOMEDICAL, *article on* MEDIA AND MEDICINE.

JUDAISM

As a specific discipline, bioethics is as new to Judaism as it is to human culture in general. To be sure, every cultural tradition throughout history has developed various ethical norms or rules to govern the different areas of human action. But it is only with the great innovations in biomedical science and technology during the second half of the twentieth century that there has been a need for a distinct schematization of traditional rules, and even the formulation of new ones, for this increasingly complex area of human action.

Judaism is no exception to this general cultural phenomenon. Indeed, Jewish ethicists have been particularly eager to make a Jewish contribution to bioethics, not least of all because of the great interest Jews have always taken in medical practice throughout history, and because many Jewish scholars maintain that there is no area of human action, however unprecedented, to which the rules formulated in the Jewish tradition do not somehow apply. Furthermore, the increasingly cross-cultural context of bioethics gives Jewish ethicists a much larger audience of interested parties than they have had heretofore.

Origins and development of Jewish bioethics

Historically, Judaism has seen the normative authority of Jewish life, both communal and individual, as stemming from a twofold teaching (Torah): Scripture and Tradition, or the Written Torah and the Oral Torah. The Written Torah consists of the divinely mandated precepts of the first five books of the Hebrew Bible. The Oral Torah consists largely of the legislation of the rabbis of the Talmudic period (first century B.C.E. to the sixth century C.E.) along with a few ancient traditions (*halakhot*) accepted as having been revealed to Moses at Mount Sinai. Regarding many ethical (as opposed to ritual) norms, moreover, especially those dealing with basic human questions of life and death, Judaism has seen the Torah's commandments as binding on all humankind, at least in theory. This area of the law has been designated as "Noahide Law," the descendants of Noah being the name for humankind. Since it has long been accepted that there cannot be a double standard differentiating between Jews and non-Jews in questions of life and death (*Sanhedrin* 59a; *Tosafot* s. v. "leika"), and since virtually all medical treatment and so much contemporary Jewish discussion of bioethical issues is conducted in the context of a pluralistic society, this universal aspect of Jewish law has become the most prevalent standard for the formulation of most Jewish views on the subject.

Scriptural law is subject to human interpretation, but it cannot be amended or repealed (Num. 15:23; Deut. 4:2; *Kiddushin* 29a; cf. *Sotah* 9.9) because it is taken to be the direct word of God. Because rabbinic law is considered human-made law only, although legislated by authority sanctioned by Scripture (*Shabbat* 23a), it has been much easier to change and adapt than scriptural law. Rabbinic legislation, at least in theory, admits of amendment and repeal (*Eduyot* 1.5), but since the demise of the Sanhedrin as the central Jewish legislative authority, reinterpretation of already existing norms has been the method of changing rabbinic law. Since the actual practical rules of any area of Jewish law—certainly those pertaining to bioethics—are much more rabbinic than scriptural, the authorized range for the exercise of human reason is the widest.

Within the immediate confines of the traditional Jewish community, the method of judgment employed in Jewish bioethics is not different from the method employed in any other area of Jewish law. The basic scriptural norm is located, its rabbinic elaborations are traced through the Talmud and related literature, its authoritative structure is determined, relevant precedents (if there are any) are culled from the vast literature of legal responsa by individual rabbinical authorities, and finally the person accepted by a community of Jews as their legal authority frequently seeks the counsel of learned colleagues. This process involves the ordering and application of rules to apply adequately to a case at hand, and occasionally the recognition of more basic principles behind the rules as well as procedures that direct their application. More and more frequently, in the cases posed by the new medical technology we see a greater role for principles. It is often much more difficult to find appropriate rules for the novel situations at hand, and principles must more directly guide the formulation of rather tenuous analogies from existing rules. Also, in the context of cross-cultural discussion of bioethical issues, the general guidance suggested by principles is sought much more than the governance of the rules of a singular tradition.

Theological and moral principles in Jewish bioethics

A number of theological-moral principles operate in Jewish discussions of bioethics. The most prominent of these principles are God as creator, God as covenanter, the sanctity of human life, human benevolence, the authority of medical expertise, and the personal prerogatives of the patient.

God as creator. All the great Jewish theologians throughout history have emphasized that the first principle of Judaism is that God is the creator and Lord of the entire universe, who maintains its perpetual order (*ma'aseh beresheet*), its "nature." Accordingly, God is considered to be the only possessor of absolute property rights. All creatures are the subjects of varying privileges granted by their divine creator. In accordance with its exalted status as the image of God, the human creature is given duties (*mitsvot*; Gen. 2:16) as well as the highest privileges (Gen. 1:26). However, whatever powers humans have are legitimate only when they are seen as from God for the sake of God, and not as the possessions of the individual or the community in any way. "Indeed, all lives are Mine" (Ezek. 18:4).

This principle is at the very heart of the differences between Jewish law and the secular norms based on the primacy of human autonomy or utility. This is especially apparent in the current intense debates concerning the beginning of human life in relation to abortion, and concerning the end of human life in relation to euthanasia. Arguments insisting upon a "right" to abortion or a "right" to euthanasia, be that "right" the individual's or the community's, essentially deny divine creatorship and lordship as the fundamental norm, which is contrary to what Judaism teaches. Therefore, one can see that the most intense debates in bioethics are quite often more about theological principles than ethical precepts as such.

God as covenanter. God is not only the creator of the universe and its perpetual Lord but is also in intimate historical relationship with the people of Israel. This relationship is called the "covenant" (*berit*). According to Moses Maimonides (1135–1204) and other Jewish theologians, Christians and Muslims, who also see themselves as related to this covenantal God, share in some of this covenantal intimacy (*Mishneh Torah: Melakhim*, chap. 11, uncensored ed.). This theological principle impinges upon the main issues of bioethics because it largely determines the status of human personhood as the "image of God" (*tselem Elohim*), a term that seems to designate the essential human capacity for a direct personal relationship with God. Accordingly, human persons are not seen as being primarily defined by innate capacities such as intelligence or freedom of choice, because these qualities vary too much from person to person and are not possessed by everyone born into the human race. Thus, according to the first-century sage Ben Azzai, the most all-encompassing principle of the entire Torah is expressed in the verse "This is the book of the human generations" (Gen. 5:1; quoted in *Palestinian Talmud: Nedarim* 9.3/41c). This means that full personhood is gained solely by one's birth to human parents, and not by less comprehensive criteria based on such capacities as rationality or freedom of choice.

The principle of God as covenanter is also at the heart of the issue of care for the sick. If the sick have the privilege of making special claims upon those able to care for them, claims that translate into the duties of caretakers, then these privileges and duties are rooted in God's care for his creation, care that is epitomized by God's covenantal involvement with Israel. This is clearly seen in the role of prayer in the treatment of illness, both the special privilege of the prayers of the sick themselves (*Shabbat* 12b) and the duty of those who care for them to pray for them as well (*Nedarim* 40a). In fact, the Talmud interprets the scriptural command that the sufferer from the disease *tsara'at* (mistranslated as "leprosy"—but actually a skin disease with symptoms close to those of eczema or psoriasis) publicly declare himself "unclean! unclean!" (Lev. 13:45)—to be a cry to those hearing these words of anguish to pray for the sufferer (*Mo'ed Qatan* 5a). In another Talmudic text this requirement is extended to include prayer for the plight of anyone suffering from any other illness of calamity (*Sotah* 32b). Those with whom God has covenanted must show genuine sympathy to one another. The extension of this sympathy is, finally, seen as reaching even to nonmembers of the covenant in the interest of peace and general goodwill (*Gittin* 61a).

The sanctity of human life. The term "sanctity of human life" does not appear in the classical Jewish sources but is an accurate expression of the principle that "one human life is not pushed aside for another" (*Ohalot* 7.6; see also *Tosefta: Terumot* 7.20), that is, that one human life has no more inherent value than another, that the blood of one person "is not redder than someone else's" (*Pesahim* 25b; cf. *Sefer Hasidim*, ed. Parma, no. 252; Luria, *Yam shel Shlomoh: Baba Kama*, 8.59). The underlying assumption of the basic sanctity of each individual human life is expressed by the *Mishnah*: "Whoever saves even one human life, it is as if he saved an entire world" (*Sanhedrin* 4.5; *Palestinian Talmud: Sanhedrin* 4.5/22a).

However, this does not mean that the value of any human life is infinite. In certain cases Judaism demands martyrdom, especially when continued life requires that the God of Israel be denied (*Sanhedrin* 74a). Moreover, at times, priorities are assigned when only one life in a particular situation can be saved as opposed to all lives in that same situation being lost (*Horayot* 3.7–8; *Tosefta: Terumot* 7.20; *Baba Metsia* 62a; *Sanhedrin* 72b). It is in the realm of ritual practice that the sanctity of human life and the duty to rescue are paramount (*Yoma* 85b). Any doubt is to be resolved in favor of human life; thus the practice of any ritual act that endangers human life

is proscribed (*Shabbat* 129a). The classic example of this is the rule that rescue efforts are to be conducted on the Sabbath or on the Day of Atonement, irrespective of whatever labors are involved, as long as there is any chance that human life might be saved (*Yoma* 85a). But once the death of the person endangered is ascertained, all ritual restraints are in effect once more (*Tosefta Shabbat* 17.19; *Shabbat* 30b, 151b).

The principle of the sanctity of human life can be seen most clearly operating in cases of nonviability, that is, when there is no reasonable expectation of survival. Thus a child born so defective as to be considered nonviable is still to be nursed by its mother (*Yevamot* 80b, *Rashi* and *Bach* thereto; also, *Tosefta: Ketubot* 5.5; *Tosefta: Niddah* 2.5), that is, not abandoned to die, as was the case in many ancient cultures. And a human life in the very last stages of its existence, in its death throes, is not to be extinguished on the assumption that death is inevitable (*Shabbat* 151b).

There is debate among later authorities as to what measures may or may not be taken to extend the death throes called *goses* (Isserles's note on *Shulhan Arukh: Yoreh De'ah* 339.1; cf. *Bach* on *Tur: Yoreh De'ah* 339). This debate anticipates current ones as to whether one can distinguish between active and passive euthanasia. Those authorities who argued that not extending the death agony automatically shortens the life of the patient would seem to support the view that no cogent distinction can be made in euthanasia: either one must permit it per se (as Judaism clearly does not) or one must prohibit it per se (as Judaism seemingly does). This is based on a rejection in the Talmud of any "double effect" rationale (*Shabbat* 75a).

However, the treatment of pain is something that may be done as an end in itself as long as it is not simultaneous with the actual death of the patient (*Avodah Zarah* 18a). Moreover, one is allowed to pray for the death of the patient in cases where agony is extreme and there is no real hope for recovery (*Ran* on *Nedarim* 40a re *Ketubot* 104a). Yet this is always an appeal for divine action and not an endorsement of humans acting in place of God. Even in cases of extreme suffering, the taking of human life is never to be the purpose of any intervention (*Avodah Zarah* 18a). Whereas a cure cannot always be effected, care is always mandated until the very end of human life. That is why, for example, a dying person is not to be left alone even when there is very little time left (*Shulhan Arukh: Yoreh De'ah* 339.4).

Human benevolence. The duty to care for the sick, and to heal them whenever possible (*biqur holim*, literally, "visitation of the sick"), is derived from two different sets of biblical and rabbinic sources. The difference in the selection of the sources indicates two distinct approaches to the issue of medical treatment in general.

Maimonides, who was the prototypical rabbi-physician for later generations, categorized the specific duty to care for the sick as a rabbinically mandated act stemming from the general duty of benevolence commanded in Scripture: "You shall love your neighbor as yourself" (Lev. 19:18), which, undoubtedly basing himself on earlier rabbinic sources (*Shabbat* 31a; *Targum Jonathan* on Lev. 19:18), he paraphrased as "Everything you want others to do for you, you do" (*Mishneh Torah: Evel* 14.1). As for the duty actually to save a human life, Maimonides based this directly on the scripturally mandated act: "Do not stand idly by your neighbor's blood" (Lev. 19:16), that is, whoever can save a life and does not do so has violated a negative commandment (*Mishneh Torah: Rotseah* 1.13).

Finally, he located the specific duty to heal the sick by those competent to do so in the scriptural command concerning the duty to return lost property to its owner (Deut. 22:2). He reasoned, as the Talmud had earlier (*Sanhedrin* 73a), that if one is to return someone else's lost property, then certainly one is to return someone else's "lost body" to him or her—namely, the bodily function lost through illness or injury (*Mishnah Commentary: Nedarim* 4.4). All of this is quite consistent with Maimonides's high regard for the regularity of the natural order and the role of medicine as part of the general human attitude of respect for that order and cooperation with its inherent teleology (*Guide of the Perplexed*, 2.40). Any special role for medicine, by separating it from the commandment of general benevolence, might very well lead to its being considered a magical function. This would contradict the essentially scientific role of medicine insisted on by Maimonides (*Mishnah Commentary: Pesahim* 4.10).

Many commentators wondered why Maimonides never quoted the most direct Talmudic source for the duty to heal the sick: "It was taught in the School of Rabbi Ishmael that from the words of Scripture 'he shall surely provide for his healing' (Exod. 21:19) we derive permission for a physician to heal" (*Baba Kama* 85a). Perhaps he did not think that the verse itself supported this inference, since the text refers directly to the duty of an assailant to pay the medical bills of his or her victim, not the duty of the physician to heal. Also, the use of the word "permission" (*reshut*) might have seemed to him too weak to ground a duty, since it seems only to allow an option.

Nevertheless, Moses Nahmanides (1194–1270) does use this Talmudic text, reflecting his entirely different approach to the practice of medicine. He sees this use of the word "permission" as being an answer to those who might say that medicine is an unwarranted interference with divine healing. Just as a judge is not inter-

fering with God's dispensing justice, he argued, so is a physician not interfering with God's dispensing healing. Both judge and physician have the exalted role of participating directly in acts that are seen as essentially divine (*Torat Ha'Adam*, ed. Chavel, 41–43). Both roles are forms of *imitatio dei*. This follows from Nahmanides's emphasis that medicine is needed by those in less than a full state of grace, who are within the confines of nature alone, and that the truly righteous will not need any such human intervention, being assured of direct divine attention (*Torah Commentary:* Lev. 26:11).

Nahmanides's connection of medical treatment with what the rabbis called "following after God's attributes" (*middotav*) has a precedent in the rabbinic location of the duty to attend to the sick in God's visitation of Abraham immediately after his circumcision (*Sotah* 14a re Gen. 18:1; also *Baba Metsia* 30b re Exod. 18:20; 86b). Indeed, attending to the needs of the sick has been seen in Jewish tradition as being more than general benevolence; it is an act having even mystical connotations. This appears in the many biblical texts that see illness and healing as specifically supernatural interventions (e.g., Gen. 18:14, 25:21–22; Exod. 15:26; Lev. 26:16; Num. 5:21; Deut. 28:20–22, 32:39; 2 Kings 5:7–8, 20:1–5; Jer. 17:14; Ps. 103:1–3; 2 Chron. 16:12). The rabbis, too, saw any affliction as being God's special visitation that calls for a special human response (*Berakhot* 5a re Isa. 53:10; cf. *Shabbat* 55a–b).

Protection of the human condition. The human condition is always to be the subject of care, and its infirmities are to be cured if possible. The question of the relation between care and cure is especially acute today, when the new means to extend life provided by advances in medical technology are seen by many as simultaneously compromising care by extending the agony of the terminally ill. Contemporary Jewish bioethicists certainly struggle with this problem as much as any other group. One can find no sufficient body of rules on this subject in the tradition, because the death agony in the past was seen as being quite brief (*Mordecai: Mo'ed Qatan* no. 864). There do not seem to be any rules at hand for dealing with persons in irreversible comas lasting weeks, months, or even years.

Some precedent for this dilemma, however, can be found in an eighteenth-century responsum by Rabbi Jacob Reischer. He asked whether one may risk one's life by undergoing surgery that has a chance to prolong it, but also a chance to terminate it sooner than would be the case if nothing were done and nature were left to run its course. Reischer permitted such surgery if there was reasonable consensus of medical opinion that there was a good chance for success (*Shevut Ya'agov: Yoreh De'ah* no. 75). But without this consensus, it seems that the patient might have the right to refuse what is in effect an unwarranted invasion of his or her body.

The most immediate phenomenon that medicine treats is pain. Whereas the patient knows he or she is alive by inference from consciousness, one is immediately conscious of the presence of pain. Pain is a primary datum for all sentient beings (Maimonides, *Guide of the Perplexed*, 3.48). Jewish tradition mandates the treatment of unbearable pain in much the same way it mandates the treatment of mortal danger to human life. This can be seen by looking at the laws pertaining to the Sabbath, which is the most important religious observance in Judaism (*Palestinian Talmud: Nedarim* 3.9/38b). Just as the Sabbath is to be violated in case of a threat to human life (*sakkanat nefesh*), so may medical procedures normally prohibited on the Sabbath be performed when they can alleviate bodily pain. Such procedures as lancing a painful boil (*Shabbat* 107a; *Tosafot* s.v. "u-memai") and a woman removing by hand milk from her engorged breasts (*Shabbat* 135a; *Tosafot* s.v. "mipnei") are mentioned in the Talmud.

The great public-health problem of AIDS entails another challenge to Jewish tradition and its ability to rule in the interest of protecting the human condition of all sufferers from any disease whatsoever. That challenge arises when it must be determined what is to be done with those who have contracted AIDS through acts that the normative tradition regards as sinful. Most AIDS sufferers have contracted the disease through male homosexual acts and intravenous drug use. These acts are proscribed by Scripture and Jewish tradition (Lev. 18:22; Maimonides, *Mishneh Torah: Ishut*, 1.4; *De'ot* 4.1). Furthermore, one Talmudic text minimally prescribes neglect for those who are seen to be "habitual sinners" (*Avodah Zarah* 26b). Nevertheless, the important twentieth-century authority Rabbi Abraham Isaiah Karelitz contended that this harsh law no longer applies because its intention is to dissuade sinners, and in this day and age such harshness would be counterproductive (*Hazon Ish: Yoreh De'ah* sec. 2). His opinion has rarely been contested, for it is not unprecedented (*Teshuvot Ha-Rosh* 17.1). This legal opinion is important because it removes the one main impediment in the tradition for treating AIDS patients with the same concern as those suffering from any illness not contracted through acts the tradition considers illicit.

Medical expertise. Jewish tradition has long recognized that a trained medical profession is a requirement of a humanly sufficient society. This can be seen in the Talmud's ruling (*Sanhedrin* 17b; cf. *Baba Batra* 21a; *Bach* on *Tur: Hoshen Mishpat* 156) that no educated Jew should live in a locality where there is no physician (*rofe*). Because of this, members of the medical profession have special duties and special privileges connected with these duties.

The first duty of medical professionals is to attend to whoever requires their attention. The centrality of this duty is seen in the interpretation by Rashi, the great eleventh-century commentator on the Bible and the Talmud, of the rather bizarre statement in the *Mishnah* that "the best of the physicians are destined for hell" (*Kiddushin* 4.14). Rashi takes this to be an indictment of persons who are physicians rather than of the institution of medicine as such (Nahmanides, *Torat Ha'Adam*, ed. Chavel, 43). He emphasizes the frequent carelessness and arrogance of physicians, and that they often refuse to treat the poor. This final indictment presupposes that lack of funds should not be an impediment to a person's right to medical treatment (*Tur: Yoreh De'ah* 336; see also *Ketubot* 67b re Deut. 15:8).

Medical practitioners are considered to be "experts" (*beqi'im*), and thus have a professional status (*Yoma* 8.5). Hence they are to be publicly licensed (*Avodah Zarah* 26b–27a). Publicly licensed medical professionals are exempt from paying damages to their patients unless it can be proven that they were grossly negligent or actually malicious in performing their medical duties (*Tosefta: Baba Kama* 9.11, 6.17; *Gittin* 3.8). Based on the analogy between physicians and judges, Nahmanides (*Torat Ha'Adam*, ed. Chavel, 41) sees the basis of this unusual dispensation from civil and even criminal liability in the Talmud's acceptance of the inherent subjectivity of judgment in even the most precise human activities: "The judge only has what his eyes see" (*Sanhedrin* 6b). However, this dispensation applies only to licensed personnel and does not extend to unlicensed personnel, even if they are otherwise "expert" (*Sanhedrin* 44).

Because medical professionals are engaged in an activity commanded by the Torah (*mitsvah*), they are not to be paid directly for their services because no one is to receive direct monetary benefit for the performance of a commandment (*Sanhedrin* 44 re *Bekhorot* 29a; see also *Rosh Hashanah* 28a). In this respect they are like Torah scholars, who are to study and teach the Torah for its own sake and not for the sake of any monetary benefit (*Avot* 4.5; *Nedarim* 37a). Nevertheless, based on this analogy, one cannot be expected regularly to deplete his or her own income when benefiting someone else. If this were the case, only those of independent wealth could possibly function either as scholars or as physicians, or in any other necessary communal function. For this reason, then, both scholars and medical personnel, being deemed necessary for a well-functioning Jewish community, are to be paid, not for what they actually do but for what they do not do—in other words, what they would be paid if they were making a living doing something else. This legal fiction is called "payment for idleness" (*sekhar betalah*).

Medical personnel are exposed to the danger of contagion in treating persons suffering from diseases. The question arises of how much danger they are required to expose themselves to in the course of their work, and how much danger is considered to be above and beyond the call of duty. This question has become especially acute today with the proliferation of a number of highly contagious diseases, such as hepatitis B.

In cases of clear and direct danger to one's own life, Jewish tradition mandates the priority of one's own life (*Baba Metsia* 62a re Lev. 25:36) irrespective of whether one is a layperson or a professional. Acts above and beyond the call of duty are considered forms of supererogatory piety. Such acts cannot be seen as being derived from a universal rule applicable to everyone and anyone, however meritorious they might be to the person performing them (*Palestinian Talmud: Terumot* 8.4/46b). However, the real moral problem arises in cases where there is possible danger (*safeq sakkanah*) to those involved in treating the sick. There is a passage in the Talmud that states, "When there is a plague in the city, gather up your legs" (*Baba Kama* 60b re Isa. 26:20; Deut. 32:25), which implies that one should save oneself in the face of possible danger.

Nevertheless, the sixteenth-century commentator Rabbi Solomon Luria argued that in the absence of clear and direct danger to oneself, one ought to remain in the city if one is able to save other lives there. He also indicates that those who had already suffered from "the plague" (he probably meant smallpox) were in no danger of further recurrence and so should remain in the city to help others in distress (*Yam shel Shlomoh: Baba Kama* 6.26). Earlier, Rabbi Joseph Karo (1488–1575) had ruled that one was to expose oneself to possible danger if this enabled one to save other human lives (*Kesef Mishneh* on Maimonides, *Mishneh Torah: Rotseah* 1.14; *Bet Yosef* on *Tur: Hoshen Mishpat* 426; cf. Rabbi David ibn Zimra, *Teshuvot Ha-Radbaz* 3, no. 627). Of course, the difference between certain possible danger can be decided only on an ad hoc basis. Nevertheless, the distinction must always be kept in mind, that is, one can rule neither that health-care personnel must treat every patient nor that they may absolve themselves from treating any patient whom they consider at all dangerous to their well-being.

Medical professionals are to keep abreast of scientific developments that affect their ability to treat patients. Along these lines, the tenth-century authority Sherira Gaon argued that the medical opinions of the rabbis of the Talmud, unlike their legal opinions, had no inherent value and should be accepted or rejected solely on the basis of whether they are actually effective (Jakobovits, 1975). Maimonides made the same point two centuries later (*Mishnah Commentary: Yoma* 8.4). In cases where human viability is to be determined, Maimonides ruled that current medical opinion is the criterion to rely on (*Mishneh Torah: Rotseah* 2.8; cf. *Shehitah* 10.13). As in all scientific questions, it is irrelevant whether those offering the accepted opinion are Jews (*Pesahim* 94b; Maimonides, *Shemonah Peraqim,* intro.).

However, other authorities were more conservative in their treatment of the medical counsels of the rabbis of the Talmud. Some of them held that the cures prescribed by the Talmud are ineffective in later times because human nature has changed significantly (*Mo'ed Qatan* 11a; *Tosafot* s.v. "kavra"; Isserles's note on *Shulhan Arukh: Even Ha'Ezer* 156.4). This view denies that earlier sages were deficient in any knowledge whatsoever, a point in keeping with the general rabbinic tendency to consider past sages always to have been wiser than present sages (*Shabbat* 112b). Thus, present sages are taken to be incapable of making some of the fine scientific distinctions that were made by past sages in medical issues pertaining to the law (Isserles's note on *Shulhan Arukh: Orah Hayyim* 330.5).

Nevertheless, whether one accepts changed medical practice on the more radical grounds suggested by Sherira Gaon and Maimonides, or on the more conservative grounds suggested by the tosafists (medieval Franco-German glossators on the Talmud) the Isserles, the fact is that no Jewish authority sees the medical remedies from the Talmud or any other classical source as being valid in the present. This has enabled the most religiously traditional Jewish medical professionals to take advantage of all the current and future advances in medical technology.

Personal prerogatives of the patient.   Current bioethics has stressed the personal prerogatives of those who are ill so that they can take a more active and responsible role in their own treatment and not simply be the passive "patients" of medical professionals. Most advocates of patient activism in medical treatment have looked to the modern principle of autonomy for grounding—namely, that human individuals are essentially their own masters. Clearly, the theocentric Jewish tradition does not underwrite autonomy in this strong sense of the term. However, it does supply the basis for allowing patients to take an active role for other reasons.

Pain, for example, is to be treated immediately, and the patient is considered the final authority in determining just how much pain he or she can stand, even if that personal determination contradicts expert opinion. It is assumed that the person is the best judge of his or her own condition at this most elementary level of experience (*Yoma* 83a re Prov. 14:10; see also *Baba Kama* 8.1). This judgment by the suffering person can exempt that person from the same ritual obligations (such as fasting) as an expert's judgment concerning a life-threatening condition can. Unbearable pain is considered worse than death, and to escape it, anything short of direct killing is exonerated (*Ketubot* 33a; *Shir Ha-Shirim Rabbah* 2.18; Rabbi Tsvi Hirsch Chajes, *Tiferet Yisrael,* beg.).

A second personal prerogative of the patient is the right to be told the exact nature of his or her illness and the opinion of the experts about whether death is imminent. Thus the Talmud rules that when it is determined that one's death is imminent, one is to be told so that there may still be time for the patient to offer the deathbed confession known as *vidui* (*Shabbat* 32a). This is considered extremely important because whether one dies in a state of repentance could very well affect whether one merits the life of the world to come (*Sanhedrin* 6.2). If the life in this world is considered a preparation for the unending life of the world to come (*Avot* 4.16), and if no one but the person himself or herself can make the proper preparation, then it follows that one may not be kept in ignorance about the gravity of one's condition. Only persons considered too emotionally unstable to be able to make proper use of this information are to be spared (Nahmanides, *Torat Ha'Adam,* ed. Chavel, 46).

The stages of human life

Judaism is concerned with the human condition from conception to death. Especially at the edges of life, where there is much public dispute, Jewish teachings have been very much in the forefront of current debate.

Abortion.   The abortion debate has usually centered on the question of when human personhood begins. Those on the "pro-life" side of the issue argue that human personhood begins at conception, and abortion is therefore murder. Those on the "pro-choice" side of the issue argue that human personhood begins at birth, and abortion is therefore not murder and ought to be the option of the individual pregnant woman.

In Jewish tradition there seem to be two differing views as to when human personhood begins. One view (*Sanhedrin* 57b re Gen. 9:6; see also *Sanhedrin* 91b re Job 10:12) is that it begins at conception; another view (*Ohalot* 7.6; *Sanhedrin* 72b; *Rashi* s.v. "yatsa rosho") is that it begins at birth. Nevertheless, these views are more statements of principle than actual rules. Rules are not directly derived from principles in Jewish law (*Baba Batra* 130b). Instead, principles are formulated to explain rules, coordinate them with other rules, and guide their application. Therefore, one should not automatically deduce from principles defining human personhood just what the rule concerning abortion is to be.

The rule proscribes abortion unless there is a threat to the life or health of the mother. Those who hold that personhood begins at conception thus see abortion as being akin to murder (although, on technical legal grounds, not literally murder that is liable for capital punishment; see *Niddah* 5.3; *Niddah* 44b re Lev. 24:17). They would tend to be more conservative in judging what constitutes a threat to the life or health of the mother. Yet even they would judge some abortions (however few) to be mandated. Those who hold that personhood begins at birth, and who are thus likely to be more liberal in judging just what constitutes a threat to the mother's life or health, still hold that abortion is usually proscribed because even fetal life has enough rights of its own (*Yoma* 82a; *Rashi* s.v. "ubar"). It may not be destroyed unless it is a threat (*rodef*) to the mother's life or health. Even assuming that the fetus is still considered part of the mother's body in utero (*Sanhedrin* 80b) does not lead to permission for elective abortion because self-mutilation is proscribed (*Baba Kama* 91b).

Hence traditionalist authorities, however they might view the actual beginnings of human personhood in principle, all regard abortion as generally proscribed, and permitted only under specific conditions. Their practical debates all center on the interpretation of the exceptions to the general proscription of abortion. In that sense, the more conservative authorities are no more absolutely "pro-life" than the more liberal authorities are absolutely "pro-choice." In fact, abortion is not an option at all. Either it is proscribed in most cases, or it is prescribed in some exceptional cases. Nonetheless, less traditionalist Jewish feminists have argued that the whole issue of abortion must be reconsidered inasmuch as it most directly affects women, and women's voices have been absent from the legal debates about it in the Jewish community heretofore (see Davis, 1991).

Definition of death.   The question of precisely when human life ends is an issue of much current debate among contemporary Jewish bioethicists. Some of the more conservatively inclined have insisted that the traditional criteria for determining death be literally interpreted: the cessation of spontaneous reflexes, heartbeat, and breath (*Yoma* 85a; *Teshuvot Hatam Sofer: Yoreh De'ah* no. 338). Yet other Jewish bioethicists, more liberally inclined, or more influenced by current scientific trends, have argued that "brain death" can constitute a ground for taking a patient off a respirator, inasmuch as breathing in this case is not being done by the patient, but by a machine (Task Force on Death and Dying, 1972). In fact, not doing this might constitute a violation of Jewish law, the prohibition against leaving the dead unburied (*Sanhedrin* 46b re Deut. 21:23). However, the motive behind this innovation, whether stated or not, is that the interpreters of Jewish law must accept growing medical consensus on any major issue if their rulings are to be taken seriously in the general society, where even the most pious Jews receive their medical treatment.

DAVID NOVAK

Directly related to this entry is the entry MEDICAL ETHICS, HISTORY OF, *section on* NEAR AND MIDDLE EAST, *article*

on ISRAEL. *Also directly related are the entries* ABOR-
TION, *section on* RELIGIOUS TRADITIONS, *article on* JEW-
ISH PERSPECTIVES; EUGENICS AND RELIGIOUS LAW,
article on JUDAISM; *and* POPULATION ETHICS, *section on*
RELIGIOUS TRADITIONS, *article on* JEWISH PERSPEC-
TIVES. *For a further discussion of topics mentioned in this
entry, see the entries* BENEFICENCE; DEATH, DEFINI-
TION AND DETERMINATION OF, *article on* CRITERIA FOR
DEATH; DEATH AND DYING: EUTHANASIA AND SUS-
TAINING LIFE, *article on* ETHICAL ISSUES; HOSPICE AND
END-OF-LIFE CARE; INFANTS, *article on* MEDICAL AS-
PECTS AND ISSUES IN THE CARE OF INFANTS; IN-
FORMATION DISCLOSURE; MEDICAL MALPRACTICE;
OBLIGATION AND SUPEREROGATION; *and* PERSON. *For
discussion of related ideas, see the entries* DEATH, *article
on* WESTERN RELIGIOUS THOUGHT; *and* DOUBLE EF-
FECT. *See also the entry* ETHICS, *article on* RELIGION AND
MORALITY.

Bibliography

Biblical, rabbinic, and medieval sources are cited in the text.

Modern Responsa

FEINSTEIN, MOSES. 1959–1973. *Igrot Mosheh.* 7 vols. New
York: M. Feinstein.

WALDENBERG, ELIEZER. 1945–1992. *Sefer Sheelot u-teshuvot:
Tsits Eliezer.* 19 vols. Jerusalem: E. Waldenberg.

WEINBERG, YECHIEL. 1961–1969. *Seride Esh: Sheelot u-te shu-
vot, hidushim u-veurim.* 4 vols. Jerusalem: Mosad ha-Rav
Kuk.

YOSEF, OVADIA. 1986. *Yabia omer: . . . sheelot u-teshuvat.* 2nd
ed. 6 vols. Jerusalem: Mosad ha-Rav Kuk.

General Works

DAVIS, DENA S. 1991. "Beyond Rabbi Hiyya's Wife: Women's
Voices in Jewish Bioethics." *Second Opinion* 16 (March):
10–30.

FELDMAN, DAVID M. 1968. *Birth Control in Jewish Law: Marital
Relations, Contraception, and Abortion as Set Forth in the
Classic Texts of Jewish Law.* New York: New York Univer-
sity Press.

———. 1986. *Health and Medicine in the Jewish Tradition.* New
York: Crossroad.

FRIEDENWALD, HARRY. 1944. *The Jews and Medicine.* 2 vols.
Baltimore: Johns Hopkins University Press.

JAKOBOVITS, IMMANUEL. 1975. *Jewish Medical Ethics: A Comparative and Historical Study of the Jewish Religious Attitude
to Medicine and Its Practice.* New York: Bloch.

KLEIN, ISSAC. 1979. *A Guide to Jewish Religious Practice.* New
York: Jewish Theological Seminary of America.

NOVAK, DAVID. 1974–1976. *Law and Theology in Judaism.* 2
vols. New York: KTAV.

———. 1985. *Halakah in a Theological Dimension.* Chico,
Calif.: Scholars Press.

ROSNER, FRED, and BLEICH, J. DAVID, eds. 1978. *Jewish Bioethics.* New York: Hebrew Publishing.

TASK FORCE ON DEATH AND DYING OF THE INSTITUTE OF SO-
CIETY, ETHICS, AND LIFE SCIENCES. 1972. "Refinements
in Criteria for the Determination of Death: An Appraisal." *Journal of the American Medical Association* 221,
no. 1:48–53.

ZIMMELS, HIRSCH JACOB. 1952. *Magicians, Theologians, and
Doctors: Studies of Folk-Medicine and Folklore as Reflected
in the Rabbinical Responsa, 12th–19th Centuries.* London:
E. Goldston.

JUSTICE

At some time or another, virtually all of us become involved in disputes about justice. Sometimes our involvement in such disputes is rooted in the fact that we
believe ourselves to be victims of some form of injustice;
sometimes our involvement is rooted in the fact that
others believe us to be the perpetrators or at least the
beneficiaries of some form of injustice affecting them.
Sometimes the injustice at issue seems to require for its
elimination a drastic reform, or even a revolutionary
change in the political system. Sometimes it seems to
require only some electoral pressure or administrative
decision, as may be required in ending a war. Whatever
the origin and whatever the practical effect, such disputes about justice are difficult to avoid, especially when
one is dealing with issues, like the distribution of income
or health-care resources, that have widespread social effects.

Reasonable resolutions of such disputes require a
critical evaluation of the alternative conceptions of justice available to us. In philosophical debate at the end
of the twentieth century, five major conceptions of justice are defended: (1) a libertarian conception, which
takes liberty to be the ultimate political ideal; (2) a socialist conception, which takes equality to be the ultimate political ideal; (3) a welfare liberal conception,
which takes contractual fairness or maximal utility to be
the ultimate political ideal; (4) a communitarian conception, which takes the common good to be the ultimate political ideal; and (5) a feminist conception,
which takes a gender-free society to be the ultimate political ideal.

All these conceptions of justice have certain features in common. Each regards its requirements as belonging to the domain of obligation rather than to the
domain of charity; they simply disagree about where to
draw the line between these two domains. Each is also
concerned with giving people what they deserve or
should rightfully possess; they simply disagree about
what it is that people deserve or rightfully possess. These
common features constitute a generally accepted core
definition of justice. What we need to do, however, is
examine the aspects of each of these conceptions of justice over which there is serious disagreement in order to
determine which conception, if any, is most defensible.

Libertarian justice

Libertarians frequently cite the work of Friedrich A. Hayek, particularly *The Constitution of Liberty* (1960), as an intellectual source of their view. Hayek argues that the libertarian ideal of liberty requires "equality before the law" and "reward according to market value" but not "substantial equality" or "reward according to merit." Hayek further argues that the inequalities due to up-bringing, inheritance, and education that are permitted by an ideal of liberty actually tend to benefit society as a whole.

In basic accord with Hayek, contemporary libertarians define "liberty" as "the state of being unconstrained by other persons from doing what one wants." Libertarians go on to characterize their moral and political ideal as requiring that each person have the greatest amount of liberty commensurate with the same liberty for all. From this ideal, libertarians claim that a number of more specific requirements—in particular a right to life; a right to freedom of speech, press, and assembly; and a right to property—can be derived.

The libertarians' right to life is not a right to receive from others the goods and resources necessary for pre-serving one's life; it is simply a right not to be killed. So understood, the right to life is not a right to receive wel-fare. In fact, there are no welfare rights in the libertarian view. Accordingly, the libertarian's understanding of the right to property is not a right to receive from others the goods and resources necessary for one's welfare but, rather, a right to acquire goods and resources either by initial acquisition or by voluntary agreement.

By defending rights such as these, libertarians can support only a limited role for government. That role is simply to prevent and punish initial acts of coercion—the only wrongful acts for libertarians.

Libertarians do not deny that it is a good thing for people to have sufficient goods and resources to meet their basic nutritional needs and basic health-care needs, but they do deny that government has a duty to provide for such needs. Some good things, such as the provision of welfare and health care to the needy, are requirements of charity rather than justice, libertarians claim. Accordingly, failure to make such provisions is neither blameworthy nor punishable.

A basic difficulty with the libertarian's conception of justice is the claim that rights to life and property, as the libertarian understands these rights, derive from an ideal of liberty. Why should we think that an ideal of liberty requires a right to life and a right to property that excludes a right to welfare? Surely it would seem that a right to property, as the libertarian understands it, might well justify a rich person's depriving a poor person of the liberty to acquire the goods and resources necessary for meeting basic nutritional needs. How, then, could we appeal to an ideal of liberty to justify such a deprivation

of liberty? Surely we couldn't claim that such a depri-vation is justified for the sake of preserving a rich per-son's freedom to use the goods and resources he or she possesses to meet luxury needs. By any neutral assess-ment, it would seem that the liberty of the deserving poor not to be interfered with when taking from the sur-plus possessions of the rich what they require to meet their basic needs would have priority over the liberty of the rich not to be interfered with when using their sur-plus possessions to meet their luxury needs. But if this is the case, a right to welfare—and possibly a right to equal opportunity as well—would be grounded in the libertar-ian's own ideal of liberty.

Socialist justice

In contrast with libertarians, socialists take equality to be the ultimate political ideal. In the *Communist Mani-festo* (1848), Karl Marx and Friedrich Engels maintained that the abolition of bourgeois property and bourgeois family structure is a necessary first requirement for build-ing a society that accords with the political ideal of equality. In the *Critique of the Gotha Programme* (1891), Marx provided a much more positive account of what is required to build a society based on the political ideal of equality. In such a society, Marx claimed, the distribu-tion of social goods must conform, at least initially, to the principle "from each according to his ability to each according to his contribution." But when the highest stage of communist society has been reached, Marx added, distribution will conform to the principle "from each according to his ability to each according to his need."

At first hearing, this conception might sound ridic-ulous to someone brought up in a capitalist society. The obvious objection is, how can you get people to contrib-ute according to their ability if income is distributed on the basis of their needs and not on the basis of their contributions?

The answer, according to a socialist conception of justice, is to make the work that must be done in a so-ciety as enjoyable, in itself, as possible. As a result, peo-ple will want to do the work they are capable of doing because they find it intrinsically rewarding. For a start, socialists might try to get people to accept currently ex-isting intrinsically rewarding jobs at lower salaries—top executives, for example, to work for $300,000 rather than $900,000, a year. Yet ultimately, socialists hope to make all jobs as rewarding as possible, so that after peo-ple are no longer working primarily for external rewards while making their best contributions to society, distri-bution can proceed on the basis of need.

Socialists propose to implement their ideal of equal-ity by giving workers democratic control over the work-place. They believe that if workers have more to say about how they do their work, they will find their work intrinsically more rewarding. As a consequence, they will be more motivated to work, because their work itself will be meeting their needs. Socialists believe that extending democracy to the workplace will necessarily lead to socialization of the means of production and the end of private property. Socialists, of course, do not deny that civil disobedience or even revolutionary action may be needed to overcome opposition to extending democracy to the workplace.

However, even with democratic control of the workplace, some jobs, such as collecting garbage or changing bedpans, probably cannot be made intrinsically rewarding. Socialists propose to divide such jobs up in some equitable manner. Some people might, for example, collect garbage one day a week and then work at a more rewarding job for the rest of the week. Others would change bedpans or do some other menial work for one day a week and then work at a more rewarding job the other days of the week. Socialists believe that by making jobs intrinsically as rewarding as possible, in part through democratic control of the workplace and an equitable assignment of unrewarding tasks, people will contribute according to their ability even when distribution proceeds according to need.

Another difficulty raised concerning the socialist conception of justice is in the proclaimed necessity of abolishing private property and socializing the means of production. It seems perfectly possible to give workers more control over their workplace while the means of production remain privately owned. Of course, private ownership would have a somewhat different character in a society with democratic control of the workplace, but it need not cease to be private ownership. After all, private ownership would also have a somewhat different character in a society where private holdings, and hence bargaining power, were distributed more equally than they are in most capitalist societies, yet it would not cease to be private ownership. Accordingly, we could imagine a society where the means of production are privately owned but where—because ownership is so widely dispersed throughout the society and because of the degree of democratic control of the workplace—many of the criticisms socialists make of existing capitalist societies would no longer apply.

Welfare liberal justice: The contractarian perspective

Finding merit in both the libertarian's ideal of liberty and the socialist's ideal of equality, welfare liberals attempt to combine both liberty and equality into one political ideal that can be characterized as contractual fairness or maximal utility.

A classic example of the contractual approach to welfare liberal justice is found in the political works of Immanuel Kant, who claimed that a civil state ought to be founded on an original contract satisfying the requirements of freedom (the freedom to seek happiness in whatever way one sees fit as long as one does not infringe upon the freedom of others to pursue a similar end), equality (the equal right of each person to restrict others from using his or her freedom in ways that deny equal freedom to all), and independence (which is necessarily presupposed for each person by the free agreement of the original contract).

According to Kant (*Theory and Practice*, Part II, 1792), the original contract, which ought to be the foundation of every civil state, does not have to "actually exist as a fact." It suffices that the laws of a civil state are such that people would agree to them under conditions in which the requirements of freedom, equality, and independence obtain. Laws that accord with this original contract would then, Kant claimed, give all members of society the right to reach any degree of rank that they could earn through their labor, industry, and good fortune. Thus, the equality demanded by the original contract would not, in Kant's view, exclude a considerable amount of economic liberty.

The Kantian ideal of a hypothetical contract as the moral foundation for a welfare liberal conception of justice has been further developed by John Rawls in A *Theory of Justice* (1971). Rawls, like Kant, argues that principles of justice are those that free and rational persons who are concerned to advance their own interests would accept in an initial position of equality. Yet Rawls goes beyond Kant by interpreting the conditions of his "original position" to explicitly require a "veil of ignorance." This veil of ignorance, Rawls claims, has the effect of depriving persons in the original position of the knowledge they would need to advance their own interests in ways that are morally arbitrary.

According to Rawls, the principles of justice that would be derived in the original position are the following:

1. Special conception of justice
   a. A principle of equal political liberty
   b. A principle of equal opportunity
   c. A principle requiring that the distribution of economic goods work to the greatest advantage of the least advantaged.
2. General conception of justice
   A principle requiring that the distribution of all social goods work to the greatest advantage of the least advantaged.

The general conception of justice differs from the special conception of justice by allowing trade-offs between political liberty and other social goods. According to Rawls, persons in the original position would want the special conception of justice to be applied in place of the general conception of justice whenever social conditions allow all representative persons to benefit from the exercise of their political liberties.

Rawls holds that these principles of justice would be chosen in the original position because persons so situated would find it reasonable to follow the conservative dictates of the "maximin strategy" and *maximize the minimum*, thereby securing for themselves the highest minimum payoff.

Rawls's defense of a welfare liberal conception of justice has been challenged in a variety of ways. Some critics have endorsed Rawls's contractual approach while disagreeing with him over what principles of justice would be derived from it. These critics usually attempt to undermine the use of a maximin strategy in the original position. Other critics, however, have found fault with the contractual approach itself. Libertarians, for example, have challenged the moral adequcy of the very ideal of contractual fairness because they claim that it conflicts with their ideal of liberty.

This second challenge to the ideal of contractual fairness is potentially the more damaging because, if valid, it would force its supporters to embrace some other political ideal. This challenge, however, would fail if it were shown that the libertarian's own ideal of liberty, when correctly interpreted, leads to much the same practical requirements as are usually associated with the welfare liberal ideal of contractual fairness.

Welfare liberal justice:
The utilitarian perspective

One way to avoid the challenges that have been directed at a contractarian defense of welfare liberal justice is to find some alternative way of defending it. Historically, utilitarianism has been thought to provide such an alternative defense. It has been claimed that the requirements of a welfare liberal conception of justice can be derived from considerations of utility in such a way that following these requirements will result in the maximization of total happiness or satisfaction in society. The best-known classical defense of this utilitarian approach is certainly that presented by John Stuart Mill in *Utilitarianism* (1861).

In Chapter 5 of this work, Mill surveyed various types of actions and situations that are ordinarily described as just or unjust and concluded that justice simply denotes a certain class of fundamental rules, the adherence to which is essential for maximizing social utility. Thus Mill rejected the idea that justice and social utility are ultimately distinct ideals, maintaining instead that justice is in fact derivable from the ideal of social utility.

Nevertheless, a serious problem remains for the utilitarian defense of welfare liberal justice. There would appear to be ways of maximizing overall social utility that do injustice to particular individuals. Think of the Roman practice of throwing Christians to the lions for the enjoyment of all those in the Colosseum. Did this unjust practice not maximize overall social utility?

John Rawls (1971) makes the same point somewhat differently. He criticizes utilitarianism for regarding society as a whole as if it were just one person, and thereby treating the desires and satisfactions of separate persons as if they were the desires and satisfactions of just one person. In this way, Rawls claims, utilitarianism fails to preserve the distinction between persons. But is Rawls right? It may well be that a proper assessment of the relative merits of the contractual and utilitarian approaches to welfare liberal justice will turn on this very issue.

Communitarian justice

Another prominent political ideal defended by contemporary philosophers is the communitarian ideal of the common good. Many contemporary defenders of a communitarian conception of justice regard their conception as rooted in Aristotelian moral theory. In the *Nicomachean Ethics* (1962), Aristotle distinguished between different varieties of justice. He first distinguished between justice as the whole of virtue and justice as a particular part of virtue. In the former sense, justice is understood as what is lawful, and the just person is equivalent to the moral person. In the latter sense, justice is understood as what is fair or equal, and the just person is the one who takes only a proper share. Aristotle focused his discussion on justice in the latter sense, which further divides into distributive justice, corrective justice, and justice in exchange. Each of these varieties of justice can be understood to be concerned with achieving equality. For distributive justice, it is equality between equals; for corrective justice, it is equality between punishment and the crime; and for justice in exchange, it is equality between whatever goods are exchanged. Aristotle also claimed that justice has both its natural and conventional aspects: this twofold character of justice seems to be behind his discussion of equity, in which equity, a natural standard, is described as a corrective to legal justice, a conventional standard.

Few of the distinctions Aristotle made seem tied to the acceptance of any particular conception of justice. One could, for example, accept the view that justice requires formal equality, but then specify the equality that is required in different ways. Even the ideal of justice as giving people what they deserve, which has its roots in Aristotle's account of distributive justice, is also subject to various interpretations. An analysis of the concept of desert would show that there is no conceptual difficulty with claiming, for example, that everyone deserves to have his or her needs satisfied or that everyone deserves an equal share of the goods distributed by society. Consequently, Aristotle's account is helpful primarily for clarifying the distinctions belonging to the concept of justice that can be made without committing oneself to any particular conception of justice.

Yet rather than draw out the particular requirements of their own conception of justice, contemporary communitarians have frequently chosen to defend their conception by attacking other conceptions of justice; by and large, they have focused their attacks on the welfare liberal conception of justice. Alasdair MacIntyre, for example, argues in "The Privatization of the Good" (1990a) that virtually all forms of liberalism attempt to separate rules defining right action from conceptions of the human good. MacIntyre contends that these forms of liberalism not only fail but must fail because the rules defining right action cannot be adequately grounded apart from a conception of the good. For this reason, MacIntyre claims, only a version of a communitarian theory of justice that grounds rules supporting right action in a complete conception of the good can ever hope to be adequate.

But why cannot we view most forms of liberalism as attempting to ground moral rules on part of a conception of the good—specifically, that part of a conception of the good that is more easily recognized, and needs to be publicly recognized, as good? For Rawls, this partial conception of the good is a conception of contractual fairness, according to which no one deserves his or her native abilities or initial starting place in society. If this way of interpreting liberalism is correct, in order to evaluate welfare liberal and communitarian conceptions of justice properly, we would need to do a comparative analysis of their conceptions of the good and their practical requirements. Moreover, there is reason to think that once the practical requirements of both liberal and communitarian conceptions of justice are compared, they will be quite similar.

Feminist justice

Defenders of a feminist conception of justice present a distinctive challenging critique to defenders of other conceptions of justice. In *The Subjection of Women* (1869), John Stuart Mill, one of the earliest male defenders of women's liberation, argued that the subjection of women was never justified but was imposed on women because they were physically weaker than men; later this subjection was confirmed by law. Mill argued that society must remove the legal restrictions that deny women the same opportunities enjoyed by men. However, Mill did not consider whether, because of past discrimination against women, it may be necessary to do more than

simply removing legal restrictions: he did not consider whether positive assistance may also be required.

Usually it is not enough simply to remove unequal restrictions to make a competition fair among those who have been participating. Positive assistance to those who have been disadvantaged in the past may also be required, as would be the case in a race where some were unfairly impeded by having to carry ten-pound weights for part of the race. To render the outcome of such a race fair, we might want to transfer the ten-pound weights to the other runners in the race for an equal period of time. Similarly, positive assistance, such as affirmative-action programs, may be necessary if women who have been disadvantaged in the past are going to be able to compete fairly with men.

In *Justice, Gender and the Family* (1989), Susan Okin argues for the feminist ideal of a gender-free society, that is, one in which basic rights and duties are not assigned on the basis of a person's sex. Being male or female is not the grounds for determining what basic rights and duties a person has in a gender-free society. Since a conception of justice is usually thought to provide the ultimate grounds for the assignment of rights and duties, we can refer to this ideal of a gender-free society as "feminist justice."

Okin goes on to consider whether John Rawls's welfare liberal conception of justice can support the ideal of a gender-free society. Noting Rawls's failure to apply his original position-type thinking to family structures, Okin is skeptical about the possibility of using a welfare liberal ideal to support feminist justice. She contends that in a gender-structured society like that of the United States, male philosophers cannot achieve the sympathetic imagination required to see things from the standpoint of women. In a gender-structured society, Okin claims, male philosophers cannot do the original position-type thinking required by the welfare liberal ideal because they lack the ability to put themselves in the position of women. According to Okin, original position-type thinking can really be achieved only in a gender-free society.

Yet, at the same time that Okin despairs of doing original position-type thinking in a gender-structured society, she purportedly does a considerable amount of just that type of thinking. For example, she claims that Rawls's principles of justice "would seem to require a radical rethinking not only of the division of labor within families but also of all the nonfamily institutions that assume it" (Okin, 1989, p. 104). She also claims that "the abolition of gender seems essential for the fulfillment of Rawls's criterion of political justice" (Okin, 1989, p. 104). So Okin's own work would seem to indicate that we can do such thinking and that her reasons for thinking we cannot are not persuasive. To do original position-type thinking, it is not necessary that everyone be able to put themselves imaginatively in the position of everyone else. All that is necessary is that some people be able to do so. Some people may not be able to do original position-type thinking because they have been deprived of a proper moral education. Others may be able to do original position-type thinking only after they have been forced to mend their ways and live morally for a time.

Of course, even among men and women in a gender-structured society who are in a broad sense capable of a sense of justice, some may not be able to do such original position-type thinking with respect to the proper relationships between men and women; these men and women may be able to do so only after the laws and social practices in our society have significantly shifted toward a more gender-free society. But this inability of some to do original position-type thinking does not render it impossible for others who have effectively used the opportunities for moral development available to them to achieve the sympathetic imagination necessary for original position-type thinking with respect to the proper relationships between men and women.

What conclusion should we draw from this discussion of libertarian, socialist, welfare liberal, communitarian, and feminist conceptions of justice? Should we draw the conclusion defended by Alasdair MacIntyre in *After Virtue* (1981) that such conceptions of justice are incommensurable and, hence, there is no rational way of deciding between them? Many philosophers have challenged this view, and even MacIntyre, in *Three Rival Versions of Moral Enquiry* (1990b), has significantly qualified it, now claiming that it is possible to argue across conceptions of justice.

Another conclusion that we might draw from this discussion of conceptions of justice is that if the ideal of liberty of libertarian justice can be shown to require the same rights to welfare and equal opportunity that are required by the welfare liberal conception of justice, and if the communication critique of welfare liberalism can be rebutted, it may be possible to reconcile, at a practical level, the differences between welfare liberal justice, socialist justice, and feminist justice. If this can be done, all that would be necessary to reasonably resolve disputes about justice would be to clarify what the shared practical requirements of these conceptions of justice are and simply to act on them.

The provision of just health care

Assuming that it is possible to show that libertarian, welfare liberal, socialist, communitarian, and feminist conceptions of justice have the same practical requirements as a right to welfare and a right to equal op-

portunity, then in order to determine the morally appropriate level of health care, it would be necessary to determine what provision of health care would be required by these rights. Since a right to welfare and a right to equal opportunity are usually associated with a welfare liberal conception of justice, it would seem reasonable to use John Rawls's original position decision procedure—a procedure favored by welfare liberals—to determine what level of health care would be required by a right to welfare and a right to equal opportunity.

In *Just Health Care* (1985) and *Am I My Parents' Keeper?* (1988), Norman Daniels develops just such an account of health care. Daniels imagines people behind a veil of ignorance trying to determine how they should allocate health-care services over their lifetimes. Behind this veil of ignorance, people are to imagine themselves ignorant of their actual age so that they could be young or old. Daniels claims that people using this Rawlsian decision procedure would reserve certain life-extending technologies for their younger years and thus maximize their chances of living a normal life span, even if that meant reducing the medical resources that would be available in their old age.

The consequences of using a Rawlsian decision procedure to determine the morally appropriate level of health care required by a right to welfare and a right to equal opportunity are (1) a focus on death-preventing level of health care for the young, (2) a focus on a life-enhancing health care for both young and old, and (3) a willingness to cut back on death-preventing health care for the old to some extent when it conflicts with (1) and possibly when it conflicts with (2) as well.

Yet these consequences remain indeterminate until we can specify the amount of resources that are to be devoted to health care rather than to meeting the various other needs and wants that people have. It will not do simply to have each person choose the level of health care that he or she prefers because we cannot assume that everyone will have sufficient income to purchase whatever level of health care he or she wants or needs. Rather, there seem to be two options.

One option is to specify an optimal and affordable level of health care and then guarantee this level of health care to all legitimate claimants. The other option is to specify a decent minimal level of health care and guarantee that level of health care to all legitimate claimants, but then allow higher levels of health care to be purchased by whoever has the income and desire to do so. Of course, both these options will leave some people dissatisfied. The equal-health-care option will leave dissatisfied people who would have preferred and could have afforded a higher level of health care that would have been available under the multitiered health-care option. The multitiered health-care option will leave dissatisfied people who would receive only the decent minimum level of health care under that option but who want or need more health care than they will be receiving. Is there any just resolution of this conflict?

Assuming again that we are trying to determine the morally appropriate level of health care required by a right to welfare and a right to equal opportunity, it is surely the case that nothing less than a guaranteed decent minimum level of health care to all legitimate claimants would be morally acceptable. But is a multi-tiered option for health care morally permissible, or is the option of an equal level of health care morally required?

To answer this question, we must take into account all the morally legitimate claimants to our available resources. They include not only the members of the particular society to which we happen to belong but also distant peoples and future generations as well. Once we recognize how numerous are the morally legitimate claimants on the available resources, it becomes clear that all that we can hope to do is provide a decent minimal level of health care to all claimants. Given the morally legitimate claims that distant peoples and future generations make on our available resources, it is unlikely that we will have sufficient resources to allow people to purchase higher levels of health care (the multi-tiered option). Morally, we would seem to have no other choice than to favor the same level of health care for everybody (the equal-health-care option).

In preferring the equal-health-care option, we appealed not to the ideal of equality itself but, rather, to the goal of providing all legitimate claimants with a decent minimum level of health care. Given that available resources are limited, to meet the goal of providing a decent minimum of health care to all legitimate claimants, equality of health care for all legitimate claimants is required. In this context, no one can have more than equality if everyone is to have enough. This choice would clearly be favored by people behind a Rawlsian veil of ignorance, assuming that the hypothetical choosers are understood to represent all morally legitimate claimants.

Nor could one reasonably object to the ideal of including distant peoples and future generations within the class of morally legitimate claimants, because each of the five conceptions assumes that each human being has the same basic rights. So if these basic rights that each human being has include a right to welfare and a right to equal opportunity, the requirements to provide each human being with a decent minimum of health care would clearly follow.

Nevertheless, there remains the question of how to specify this minimum level of health care that all legitimate claimants are to receive. The problem here is how to specify how much of the available resources should go to providing everyone with a decent minimum of health care rather than providing for the satisfaction of people's other needs and wants. Yet here, too, the question seems resolvable with the aid of a Rawlsian hypothetical choice procedure. We simply need to introduce behind the veil of ignorance the knowledge of the relevant technology for meeting people's basic needs and the knowledge of available resources to decide how much of the resources should be devoted to providing a decent minimum level of health care and how much should be devoted to meeting the other needs and wants that people have.

In this way, we should be able to determine what specific requirements of just health care are grounded in a right to welfare and a right to equal opportunity. Moreover, these specific requirements of just health care would be further supported if it can be shown that the rights from which these health-care requirements are derived are themselves the shared practical requirements of libertarian, welfare liberal, socialist, communitarian, and feminist conceptions of justice.

JAMES P. STERBA

Directly related to this entry are the entries FEMINISM; HEALTH-CARE RESOURCES, ALLOCATION OF; SOCIAL MEDICINE; *and* UTILITY. *For a further discussion of topics mentioned in this entry, see the entries* CARE; ECONOMIC CONCEPTS IN HEALTH CARE; ETHICS, *article on* SOCIAL AND POLITICAL THEORIES; HEALTH POLICY, *article on* POLITICS AND HEALTH CARE; NATIONAL SOCIALISM; PATIENTS' RIGHTS; *and* RIGHTS. *Other relevant material may be found under the entries* BIOETHICS; FUTURE GENERATIONS, OBLIGATIONS TO; HEALTH-CARE FINANCING; *and* OBLIGATION AND SUPEREROGATION. *This entry will find application in the entries* ABORTION, *section on* CONTEMPORARY ETHICAL AND LEGAL ASPECTS, *article on* CONTEMPORARY ETHICAL PERSPECTIVES; AGING AND THE AGED, *article on* HEALTH-CARE AND RESEARCH ISSUES; AIDS; ALTERNATIVE THERAPIES, *article on* ETHICAL AND LEGAL ISSUES; BIOTECHNOLOGY; CHILDREN, *article on* RIGHTS OF CHILDREN; CIVIL DISOBEDIENCE AND HEALTH CARE; DEATH AND DYING: EUTHANASIA AND SUSTAINING LIFE, *article on* ETHICAL ISSUES; DEATH PENALTY; DISABILITY, *article on* HEALTH CARE AND PHYSICAL DISABILITY; EUGENICS, *article on* ETHICAL ISSUES; FAMILY; FERTILITY CONTROL, *article on* ETHICAL ISSUES; FOOD POLICY; GENETIC TESTING AND SCREENING, *article on* ETHICAL ISSUES; HARM; HEALTH-CARE DELIVERY, *article on* HEALTH-CARE SYSTEMS; HEALTH SCREENING AND TESTING IN THE PUBLIC-HEALTH CONTEXT; HOSPICE AND END-OF-LIFE CARE; INFANTS, *article on* ETHICAL ISSUES; KIDNEY DIALYSIS; MENTAL-HEALTH SERVICES; OCCUPATIONAL SAFETY AND

HEALTH, *article on* ETHICAL ISSUES; ORGAN AND TISSUE TRANSPLANTS, *article on* ETHICAL AND LEGAL ISSUES; PUBLIC HEALTH, *article on* PHILOSOPHY OF PUBLIC HEALTH; PUBLIC POLICY AND BIOETHICS; REPRODUCTIVE TECHNOLOGIES, *article on* ETHICAL ISSUES; TRIAGE; *and* WOMEN, *article on* HEALTH-CARE ISSUES.

Bibliography

ARISTOTLE. 1962. *Nicomachean Ethics,* bk. 5. Translated by Martin Ostwald. Indianapolis, Ind.: Bobbs-Merrill.

BRODY, BARUCH A. 1981. "Health Care for the Haves and Have Nots: Toward a Just Basis of Distribution." In *Justice and Health Care,* pp. 151–159. Edited by Earl E. Shelp. Dordrecht, Netherlands: D. Reidel.

BUCHANAN, ALAN E. 1984. "The Right to a Decent Minimum of Health Care." *Philosophy and Public Affairs* 13, no. 1: 55–78.

DANIELS, NORMAN. 1985. *Just Health Care.* Cambridge: At the University Press.

———. 1988. *Am I My Parents' Keeper? An Essay on Justice Between the Young and the Old.* New York: Oxford University Press.

GIBBARD, ALAN. 1982. "The Prospective Pareto Principle and Equity of Access to Health Care." *Milbank Memorial Fund Quarterly/Health and Society* 60, no. 3:399–428.

GUTMANN, AMY. 1981. "For and Against Equal Access to Health Care." *Milbank Memorial Fund Quarterly/Health and Society* 59, no. 4:542–560.

HAYEK, FRIEDRICH A. 1960. *The Constitution of Liberty.* Chicago: University of Chicago Press.

JAGGAR, ALISON M. 1983. *Feminist Politics and Human Nature.* Totowa, N.J.: Rowman & Allanheld.

MACINTYRE, ALASDAIR C. 1981. *After Virtue: A Study in Moral Theory.* Notre Dame, Ind.: University of Notre Dame Press.

———. 1990a. "The Privatization of the Good: An Inaugural Lecture." *Review of Politics* 52, no. 3:344–361.

———. 1990b. *Three Rival Versions of Moral Enquiry: Encyclopaedia, Genealogy, and Tradition.* Notre Dame, Ind.: University of Notre Dame Press.

MARX, KARL. 1977. [1891]. *Critique of the Gotha Programme.* Edited by C. P. Dutt. New York: International Publishers.

MARX, KARL, and ENGELS, FRIEDRICH. 1992. [1848]. *The Communist Manifesto.* Edited by David McLellan. Oxford: Oxford University Press.

MILL, JOHN STUART. 1979. [1861]. *Utilitarianism,* ch. 5. Indianapolis, Ind.: Hackett.

———. 1988. [1869]. *The Subjection of Women.* Indianapolis, Ind.: Hackett.

NIELSON, KAI. 1985. *Liberty and Equality: A Defense of Radical Egalitarianism.* Totowa, N.J.: Rowman & Allanheld.

NOZICK, ROBERT. 1974. *Anarchy, State, and Utopia.* New York: Basic Books.

OKIN, SUSAN M. 1989. *Justice, Gender and the Family.* New York: Basic Books.

RAWLS, JOHN. 1971. *A Theory of Justice.* Cambridge, Mass.: Harvard University Press.

SOMMERS, CHRISTINA. 1989. "Philosophers Against the Family." In *Person to Person,* pp. 182–195. Edited by George Graham and Hugh LaFollette. Philadelphia: Temple University Press.

STERBA, JAMES P. 1988. *How to Make People Just.* Totowa, N.J.: Rowman & Littlefield.

U.S. PRESIDENT'S COMMISSION FOR THE STUDY OF ETHICAL PROBLEMS IN MEDICINE AND BIOMEDICAL AND BEHAVIOR RESEARCH. 1983. Vol. 1 of *Securing Access to Health Care: A Report on the Ethical Implications of Differences in the Availability of Health Services.* Washington, D.C.: U.S. Government Printing Office.

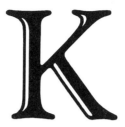

K

KIDNEY DIALYSIS

Two principal therapies exist for patients who develop irreversible kidney failure and require renal replacement therapy to survive: kidney dialysis and kidney transplantation. The topic of kidney transplantation is addressed elsewhere in the Encyclopedia. This entry discusses kidney dialysis.

The two main techniques for kidney dialysis are hemodialysis and peritoneal dialysis. In hemodialysis, blood is pumped from a patient's body by a dialysis machine to a dialyzer—a filter composed of thousands of thin plastic membranes that uses diffusion to remove waste products—and then returned to the body. The time a hemodialysis treatment takes varies with the patient's size and remaining kidney function; most patients are treated for three to four hours three times a week in a dialysis unit staffed by nurses and technicians. In peritoneal dialysis, a fluid containing dextrose and electrolytes is infused into the abdominal cavity; this fluid, working by osmosis, draws waste products from the blood into the abdominal cavity and then is drained from the abdominal cavity and discarded. Most patients on peritoneal dialysis perform four procedures daily about six hours apart to drain out the fluid with the accumulated wastes and instill two liters of fresh fluid. This technique is called continuous ambulatory peritoneal dialysis (CAPD). An automated form of peritoneal dialysis, called continuous cycling peritoneal dialysis (CCPD), is also available.

Both hemodialysis and peritoneal dialysis require a means to enter the body, called an access. In hemodialysis, access to the blood is obtained by removing blood through plastic catheters inserted directly into blood vessels or through needles inserted into surgically created conduits, called fistulas, from arteries to veins. In peritoneal dialysis, access to the abdominal cavity is obtained with a plastic catheter, which is surgically implanted into the abdominal wall with the tip of the catheter positioned in the abdominal cavity.

Dialysis is a benefit to patients with severe kidney failure because it removes metabolic waste products and excess fluid, electrolytes, and minerals that build up in the blood when the kidneys are not functioning normally. Without the removal of these substances, patients become very weak, short of breath, and lethargic and eventually die. While dialysis is lifesaving for these patients and some can return to their prior level of functioning, most do not, because they do not feel well. Despite dialysis and medications, patients may experience anemia, bone pain and weakness, hypertension, heart disease, strokes, infections or clotting of the dialysis access, and bleeding. In addition to these medical problems, dialysis may impose other burdens on dialysis patients and their families, including extra costs for medications and for transportation to the dialysis center, loss of time spent in the treatments and travel to the dialysis center, and loss of control over the patient and family schedule to accommodate dialysis treatments. For these reasons, renal transplantation is considered to be the preferable form of treatment for severe kidney-failure patients who are able to undergo this major surgical procedure.

Kidney dialysis predates other life-sustaining therapies. In 1945 in the Netherlands, Willem Kolff first used hemodialysis to save the life of a woman with acute renal failure. In subsequent years, Kolff and others improved hemodialysis, but it could not be provided to patients with chronic, irreversible renal failure, or what has been called end-stage renal disease (ESRD), until 1960, when Belding Scribner of Seattle, Washington, used plastic tubes in a shunt that could be left in an artery and vein for repeated dialysis access.

By most standards, kidney dialysis can be considered a successful life-sustaining treatment. In the United States alone, since the inception of the Medicare-funded ESRD program in 1973, several hundred thousand patients have had their lives sustained by dialysis, and at least some of them have survived for longer than twenty-five years. This program has been costly, however; in 1989, for example, the cost per year of keeping these patients alive in the United States exceeded six billion dollars. Because dialysis preceded many other modern life-sustaining medical technologies, and because initially there was a scarcity of resources to pay for it, many of the ethical concerns subsequently discussed for other modern medical technologies were initially debated regarding dialysis: patient selection criteria, access to treatment, the just allocation of scarce resources, the right to die (by having dialysis withheld or withdrawn), and conflicts of interest (in dialysis unit ownership). This entry examines a number of these concerns in the United States ESRD program and compares them with those in other countries.

Patient-selection criteria

The first ethical concern to arise for physicians was how to select patients for dialysis. In the early 1960s in the United States, 10,000 people were estimated to be dying of renal failure every year, but there were not enough dialysis machines or trained physicians and nurses to treat these patients. Furthermore, the cost of treatment for one patient for one year, $15,000, was prohibitively expensive for most patients. Dialysis centers like the Seattle Artificial Kidney Center, founded in 1962, were able to treat only a small number of patients. It was therefore necessary to restrict the number of patients selected for dialysis.

The problem of selecting patients had major ramifications because the patients denied access would die. The solution of the physicians of the Seattle dialysis center was to ask the county medical society to appoint a committee of seven laypersons to make the selection decisions for them from among persons they had identified as being medically appropriate. The doctors recognized that the selection decision went beyond medicine and would entail value judgments about who should have access to dialysis and be granted the privilege of continued life. Historian David Rothman says that their decision to have laypersons engaged in life-and-death decision making was the historic event that signaled the entrance of bioethics into medicine (Rothman, 1991). Bioethics scholar Albert Jonsen believes that the field of bioethics emerged in response to these events in Seattle because they caused a nationwide controversy that stimulated the reflection of scholars regarding a radically new problem at the time, the allocation of scarce lifesaving resources (Jonsen, 1990).

The doctors regarded children and patients over the age of forty-five as medically unsuitable, but they gave the committee members no other guidelines with which to work. At first the committee members considered choosing patients by lottery, but they rejected this idea because they believed that difficult ethical decisions *could* be made about who should live and who should die. In the first few meetings, the committee members agreed on factors they would weigh in making their decisions: age and sex of the patient, marital status and number of dependents, income, net worth, emotional stability, educational background, occupation, and future potential. They also decided to limit potential candidates to residents of the state of Washington.

As the selection process evolved, a pattern emerged of the values the committee was using to reach its decisions. They weighed very heavily a person's character and contribution to society (Alexander, 1962).

Once public, the Seattle dialysis patient-selection process was subjected to harsh criticism. The committee was castigated for using middle-class American values and social-worth criteria to make decisions (Fox and Swazey, 1978). The selection process was felt to have been unfair and to have undermined American society's view of equality and the value of human life.

In 1972, lobbying efforts by nephrologists, patients, their families, and friends culminated in the passage by the U.S. Congress of Public Law 92-603 with Section 2991. This legislation classified patients with a diagnosis of chronic renal failure as disabled, authorized Medicare entitlement for them, and provided the financial resources to pay for their dialysis. The only requirement for this entitlement was that the patients or their spouses or (if dependent children) parents were insured or entitled to monthly benefits under Social Security.

When Congress passed this legislation, its members believed that money should not be an obstacle to providing lifesaving therapy (Rettig, 1976, 1991). Although the legislation stated that patients should be screened for "appropriateness" for dialysis and transplantation, the primary concern was to make dialysis available to those who needed it. Neither Congress nor physicians thought it necessary for the government to determine patient-selection criteria.

By 1978, many U.S. physicians believed that it was morally unjustified to deny dialysis treatment to any patient with ESRD (Fox and Swazey, 1978). As a consequence, patients who would not previously have been accepted as dialysis candidates were started on treatment. A decade later, the first report of the U.S. Renal Data System documented the progressively greater acceptance rate of patients onto dialysis (U.S. Renal Data System, 1989), and subsequent reports have shown that the rise in the number of dialysis patients could be explained in part by the inclusion of patients who had poor prognoses, especially the elderly and those with diabetic nephropathy (Hull and Parker, 1990). As more of these people were started on dialysis, the patient mortality per year rose steadily.

Observers have raised concerns about the appropriateness of treating patients with a limited life expectancy and limited quality of life because of numerous simultaneous medical conditions (Fox, 1981; Levinsky and Rettig, 1991). Specifically, questions have been raised about the appropriateness of providing dialysis to two groups of patients: those with a limited life expectancy despite the use of dialysis and those with severe neurological disease. The first group includes patients with kidney failure and other life-threatening illnesses, such as atherosclerotic cardiovascular disease, cancer, chronic pulmonary disease, and AIDS. The second group includes patients whose neurological disease renders them unable to relate to others, such as those in a persistent vegetative state or with severe dementia or cerebrovascular disease (Rettig and Levinsky, 1991).

The Institute of Medicine Committee for the Study of the Medicare End-Stage Renal Disease Program, which issued its report in 1991, acknowledged that the existence of the public entitlement for treatment of ESRD does not obligate physicians to treat all patients who have kidney failure with dialysis or transplantation (Levinsky and Rettig, 1991). For some kidney-failure patients, the burdens of dialysis may substantially outweigh the benefits; the provision of dialysis to these patients would violate the medical maxim "Be of benefit and do no harm." This committee recommended that guidelines be developed for identifying such patients and that the guidelines allow physicians discretion in assessing individual patients. Subsequent studies have demonstrated that nephrologists differ on how they make decisions to start or stop dialysis for patients (Moss et al., 1993; Singer, 1992). The guidelines might help nephrologists make such decisions more uniformly, with

greater ease, and in a way that promotes patient benefit and the appropriate use of dialysis resources.

Access to dialysis and the just allocation of scarce resources

In the late 1980s, as the cost of the ESRD program increased and as the United States experienced record-breaking budget deficits, questions began to be raised about continued federal funding for the ESRD program. Observers wondered if the money was well spent or if more good could be done with the same resources for other patients (Moskop, 1987).

One response to the increasing cost of the ESRD program was to call for increased efficiency. Some urged that measures be taken to maximize the use of resources in the program by treating patients, if possible, with less costly home dialysis and transplantation (Dottes, 1991; Roberts et al., 1980).

Even as the ESRD program became more efficient, its cost continued to rise as the number of patients in the program increased each year. It was apparent that if the cost was to be contained, patient-selection criteria would have to be reintroduced. In one study, medical directors of dialysis units were asked what criteria they used to select patients for dialysis and how those criteria would change if resources were further limited and access to dialysis was restricted. About half used prognosis and medical benefit in their patient-selection decisions, but more than 95 percent said they would use these criteria in situations of significant scarcity (Kilner, 1988).

In the early 1990s, the ESRD program satisfied neither of the first principles of distributive justice: equality and utility. On neither a macro- nor a microallocation level did the ESRD program provide equality of access. On the macroallocation level, observers asked, as a matter of fairness and equality, why the federal government should provide almost total support for one group of patients with end-stage disease—those with ESRD—and deny such support to those whose failing organs happened to be hearts, lungs, or livers (Moskop, 1987; Rettig, 1991). On a microallocation level, only 93 percent of patients with ESRD have been eligible for Medicare ESRD benefits. The poor and ethnic minorities are thought to constitute most of the ineligible, and their numbers doubled between 1980 and 1990. The Institute of Medicine Committee for the Study of the Medicare End-Stage Renal Disease Program recommended that the U.S. Congress extend Medicare entitlement to all citizens and resident aliens with ESRD (Rettig and Levinsky, 1991).

From a utilitarian perspective, the ESRD program could not be argued to be maximizing the good for the greatest number. While in 1990 more than 30 million

Americans were without basic health insurance, the cost to treat one ESRD patient—of whom there were about 200,000—was nearly $40,000 per year. Despite the high cost, ESRD patient one-year mortality approached 25 percent; for many, as Anita Dottes noted, life on dialysis was synonymous with physical incapacitation, dependency, chronic depression, and disrupted family functioning (Dottes, 1991).

Withholding and withdrawing dialysis

Withdrawal from dialysis is the third most common cause of dialysis-patient death. In one large study, dialysis withdrawal accounted for 22 percent of deaths (Neu and Kjellstrand, 1986). Older patients and those with diabetes were found to be most likely to stop dialysis. By the late 1980s, as the percentage of diabetic and older patients (those sixty-five or over) on dialysis increased, withdrawal from dialysis had become more common. According to a survey done in 1990, most dialysis units had withdrawn one or more patients from dialysis in the preceding year (Moss et al., 1993).

Because of the increased frequency of decisions to withhold and withdraw dialysis in the 1980s and early 1990s, the clinical practices of nephrologists in reaching these decisions with patients and families generated heightened interest. Discussions of the ethics and process of withholding or withdrawing dialysis became more frequent (Hastings Center, 1987; U.S. President's Commission, 1983). Two ethical justifications were given for withholding or withdrawing dialysis: the patient's right to refuse dialysis, which was based on the right of self-determination, and an unfavorable balance of benefits to burdens to the patient that continued life with dialysis would entail. Nephrologists and ethicists recommended that decisions to start or stop dialysis be made on a case-by-case basis, because individual patients evaluate benefits and burdens differently. They noted that such decisions should result from a process of shared decision making between the nephrologist and the patient with decision-making capacity. If the patient lacked decision-making capacity, the decisions should be made on the basis of the patient's expressed wishes (given either verbally or in a written advance directive) or, if these were unknown, the patient's best interests. They also advised that in such cases a surrogate be selected to participate with the physician in making decisions for the patient.

Questions were identified to help nephrologists evaluate a patient's request to stop dialysis. For example, why does the patient want to stop? Does the patient mean what he or she says and say what he or she means? Does the patient have decision-making capacity, or is his or her capacity altered by depression, encephalopathy, or another disorder? Are there any changes that can be made that might improve life on dialysis for the patient? How do the patient's family and close friends view his or her request? Would the patient be willing to continue on dialysis while factors responsible for the patient's request to stop are addressed?

If, after patient evaluation based on these questions, the patient still requested discontinuation of dialysis, nephrologists were counseled to honor the competent patient's request. In several studies, nine out of ten nephrologists indicated that they would stop dialysis at the request of a patient with decision-making capacity (Moss et al., 1993; Singer, 1992).

In half or more of the cases in which decisions have been made to withdraw dialysis, patients have lacked decision-making capacity. Nephrologists have expressed a willingness to stop dialysis of "irreversibly incompetent" patients who had clearly said they would not want dialysis in such a condition, but they have disagreed about stopping dialysis in patients without clear advance directives (Singer, 1992). In general, there has been a presumption in favor of continued dialysis for patients who cannot or have not expressed their wishes. The patient's right to forgo dialysis in certain situations has therefore usually been difficult to exercise.

The Patient Self-Determination Act, which applied to institutions participating in Medicare and Medicaid and which became effective December 1, 1991, was intended to educate health-care professionals and patients about advance directives and to encourage patients to complete them. Although the ESRD program is almost entirely funded by Medicare, dialysis units were inadvertently left out of the act. Nonetheless, the completion of advance directives by dialysis patients has been specifically recommended for two reasons: (1) the elderly, who constitute roughly half of the dialysis population, are those who are most likely to withdraw or be withdrawn from dialysis; (2) unless an advance directive to withhold cardiopulmonary resuscitation (CPR) is given, it will automatically be provided, and CPR rarely leads to extended survival in dialysis patients (Moss et al., 1992).

When patients lack decision-making capacity and have not completed advance directives, ethically complex issues may arise in the decision whether to start or stop dialysis. Many nephrologists have indicated that they would consult an ethics committee, if available, for assistance in making decisions in different cases (Moss et al., 1993). Ethics consultations are most frequently requested for decisions regarding the withholding or withdrawing of life-sustaining therapy such as dialysis.

The effect of reimbursement

Reimbursement has affected both dialysis techniques and quality of care provided to dialysis patients. Since the ESRD program began in 1973, payments for dialysis treatments have decreased while patient mortality, adjusted for age and for other medical conditions, has remained stable. With experience and improvements in dialysis techniques, a decrease in mortality might have been expected.

When the U.S. Congress established the Medicare ESRD program, the highest estimate for cost of the program by 1977 was $250 million; the actual cost was approximately $1 billion (Fox and Swazey, 1978). At least two major reasons were held to be responsible for the higher cost: the increasing number of patients being started on dialysis, some of whom would have been "unthinkable" dialysis candidates ten years earlier, and the growth of in-center dialysis while the use of less costly home dialysis declined.

In the United States between 1972 and 1980, the proportion of patients on home dialysis decreased from 43 percent to 11 percent. Home hemodialysis was estimated to cost $7,000 per year less than in-center hemodialysis, but patients were discouraged from dialyzing at home because the Medicare regulations imposed a financial and administrative burden on home dialysis patients. While these disincentives to home dialysis were recognized almost immediately, it took the U.S. Congress five years to pass legislation providing incentives for home dialysis and transplantation (Roberts et al., 1980).

By 1981, cost was federal policymakers' primary concern about the ESRD program. More than 5 percent of the total Medicare budget was being spent on dialysis and transplant patients, who represented less than 0.2 percent of the active Medicare patient population. In 1983 and again in 1986, federal reimbursement rates for dialysis were reduced. By 1989, the average reimbursement rate—adjusted for inflation—for freestanding dialysis units was 61 percent lower than it had been when the program began (Rettig and Levinsky, 1991).

By the end of the 1980s, six key changes had occurred as a result, at least in part, of the decreasing reimbursement: (1) more patients were dialyzed in freestanding than in hospital-based dialysis units; (2) CAPD and CCPD had replaced home hemodialysis as the primary methods of home dialysis; (3) most dialysis units were reusing dialyzers; (4) the average duration of a dialysis treatment had been shortened; (5) the staffing in almost all dialysis units had decreased; and (6) physicians made rounds on patients in dialysis units less often than they had done.

Changes in the regulations for reimbursement during the mid-1980s made it financially advantageous for hospital-based dialysis units to move out of hospitals and for new units to be started as freestanding operations. Though many of the emergency services available in a hospital were not present in freestanding dialysis units,

dialysis in freestanding units was actually associated with a lower risk of death (Held et al., 1987).

Despite more than a doubling of the dialysis population, the absolute number of patients on home hemodialysis continued to decrease, and by 1989 there were more than five times as many patients on CAPD/CCPD at home as there were on home hemodialysis. CAPD replaced home hemodialysis as the preferred home-dialysis method for several reasons, including that it was conceptually simpler and that it did not require a machine, a trained partner, or modifications to the plumbing system in the patient's home. Most studies indicated that there was no difference in the death rates for patients treated with in-center hemodialysis and those treated with CAPD.

Dialyzer reuse was one response of dialysis units to the decreasing reimbursement. Expensive dialyzers could be reused ten to twenty times or more, rather than be discarded after one use, with considerable savings. Only 16 percent of dialysis units were reusing hemodialyzers in the 1970s; by 1988, 67 percent of units were. Initial opposition by patient groups to dialyzer reuse, because of concerns about the safety and efficacy of used dialyzers, abated as studies showed that dialysis with used dialyzers resulted in fewer patient symptoms because the inflammatory response to dialysis with used dialyzers was less than it was with new ones. By the mid-1980s, researchers reported that the relative risk of death for dialysis patients who were treated in a dialysis unit that had been reusing dialyzers for several years was significantly less than that for units that were not reusing dialyzers (Held et al., 1987).

Another way dialysis units saved money was to shorten the dialysis treatment time. Shortened dialysis times reduced the labor costs per treatment. However, the effect of this on the quality of care was a major concern; the length of dialysis had been regarded as a key determinant of its effectiveness. Researchers have subsequently shown that short dialysis treatment times were associated with increased patient mortality. The observation that quality of care suffered as an indirect result of decreased Medicare reimbursement indicated the clinical consequences of financial decisions to cut reimbursement.

In response to reductions in reimbursement and increases in labor costs, quality and number of staff in dialysis units were also reduced. Dialysis units were reported to have fewer registered and licensed nurses and more nursing assistants and technicians providing patient care. Furthermore, even though dialysis patients were on average older and sicker at the end of the 1980s than they had been in the early 1970s, the patient-to-staff ratio increased from 3:1 to more than 4:1. While there was no direct evidence that these changes in dialysis staffing patterns hurt the quality of patient care, those in the dialysis community held this opinion (Rettig and Levinsky, 1991).

Conflicts of interest

A conflict of interest occurs when there is a clash between a physician's personal financial gain and the welfare of his or her patients. While a conflict of interest generally exists for all physicians who practice fee-for-service medicine, there is a potentially greater conflict of interest for physicians who share in the ownership of for-profit dialysis units in which they treat patients. Physicians who receive a share of the profits are financially rewarded for reducing costs. Although measures to reduce costs may simply lead to greater efficiency, they may also compromise patient welfare if they entail decreasing dialysis time; purchasing cheaper, possibly less effective dialyzers and dialysis machines; and hiring fewer registered nurses, social workers, and dietitians. In the past, for-profit dialysis companies were quite open about their policy of giving physicians a financial stake in their companies. Such companies flourished under the ESRD program (Kolata, 1980).

Since the early 1980s, over half the patients in the ESRD program have been dialyzed in for-profit units. Physicians and dialysis units are paid on a per-patient and per-treatment basis, respectively, under the ESRD program, and the 1987 acceptance rate of patients to dialysis in the United States was higher than anywhere else in the world (Hull and Parker, 1990). This higher rate has been at least partly attributed to the acceptance on dialysis in the United States of a much greater number of patients with poor prognoses. While some might argue that this high acceptance rate was a sign that nephrologists and dialysis units were seeking to increase their incomes, others have commented that many physicians believed they were obligated to dialyze all patients with end-stage renal disease, since the federal government was bearing the costs (Fox, 1981).

In the early 1990s, the concerns about conflicts of interest heightened. Short dialysis times were found disproportionately in for-profit units and associated with increased mortality. The nephrologist who owned all or a share of a for-profit unit was confronted with a clear conflict of interest, and he or she was believed to be treading a very fine line between maintaining adequate profit to keep the dialysis unit open and compromising patient care.

A decade earlier, nephrologist and *New England Journal of Medicine* editor Arnold Relman had anticipated the predicament nephrologist owners of dialysis units would face. He had warned that the private enterprise system—the so-called new medical-industrial complex—had a particularly striking effect on the practice of dialysis, and he urged physicians to separate themselves totally from any financial participation so as to maintain their integrity as professionals (Relman, 1980). Education of nephrologists about these issues, both in training and in continuing education courses, may help them to identify present and potential conflicts of interest and resolve them in a way that places patients' interests first.

International perspective

In 1988 there were more than 300,000 patients worldwide whose lives were maintained with dialysis. Whereas the United States had the highest acceptance rate per million population, Japan had the highest prevalence rate. It is possible to compare the dialysis programs in countries that have a national renal disease registry—Canada, the United States, Japan, and Australia—or have dialysis facilities that report to the European Dialysis and Transplant Association. In 1987, the approximate numbers of dialysis patients (and the prevalence rate per million population) for countries with some of the largest programs were as follows: the United States, 150,000 dialysis patients (403); Japan, 80,000 (671); West Germany, 18,000 (320); France, 13,000 (254); Canada, 11,000 (186); and Australia, 6,000 (152) (Hull and Parker, 1990). The number of patients per million population treated with dialysis and transplantation correlates highly with the gross national product per capita. Countries with a per capita gross national product of less than $3,000 per year treat a negligible number of patients with dialysis and transplantation. Approximately three-quarters of the world's population live in these poorer countries.

Economics have affected how dialysis programs in most countries have developed. Two contrasting examples are Japan and the United Kingdom. Japan is the richest country in the world and has been a leader in the development of plastic materials used in dialyzers. Japan's reimbursement rate per dialysis treatment is estimated to be more than twice the rate in the United States, and 95 percent of the health care there is covered by national health insurance. Acceptance of elderly patients and those with diabetes approaches that of the United States, and 97 percent of patients are treated with in-center hemodialysis and 3 percent with CAPD. In 1988, Japan had the highest prevalence rate for dialysis in the world: 778 per million population. The high Japanese prevalence rate is due in large part to the low number of Japanese ESRD patients who undergo transplantation, only 3 percent, compared to more than 20 percent in the United States. The low Japanese transplantation rate has been attributed to Japanese cultural values that find the practices of organ procurement from brain-dead donors and transplantation unacceptable.

In the United Kingdom, the National Health Service (NHS) is responsible for financing essentially all dialysis. It spends less than half the amount spent per person for health care in the United States, and in 1987 the prevalence rate for dialysis and transplantation was 271 per million population. To provide ESRD replacement therapy most cost-effectively, the NHS has emphasized transplantation and home dialysis. In-center hemodialysis comprises less than 25 percent of ESRD treatment. Also, patient selection in the United Kingdom has differed from that in Japan, the United States, and other Western European countries. Patients who were incapable of performing independent dialysis, who were unlikely to receive kidney transplants, or who were over the age of fifty-five were more likely to be excluded from dialysis in the United Kingdom. Patient access to dialysis in the United Kingdom has been restricted in two other ways. First, patients may not refer themselves to consultant nephrologists who have been shown to be more likely to accept patients for dialysis than general practitioners. Second, the number of dialysis units per million population is a third to a quarter the number in other European countries, such as France, Spain, and Italy. The revelation of age discrimination in the late 1970s drew widespread criticism. Since then dialysis treatment programs in the United Kingdom have expanded to accommodate older patients.

In other parts of the world, where dialysis technology and money for health care are limited, two sets of criteria have been used to select patients for dialysis. In India, China, Egypt, Libya, Tunisia, Algeria, Morocco, Kenya, and South Africa, money and political influence play an important role in deciding which patients will have access to dialysis and transplantation. In Eastern Europe, ESRD patients with primary renal disease who have a lower mortality and who are more likely to be rehabilitated tend to be selected (Kjellstrand and Dossetor, 1992).

Conclusion

Since the capability to treat patients with chronic renal failure was first developed in 1960, economic limits have generated the two foremost ethical dilemmas in the field of dialysis: how resources should be allocated to scarce life-sustaining therapies like dialysis and how patients should be selected to receive these resources. In the United States, an entitlement to dialysis was created to eliminate the ethical dilemma of patient selection. The existence of this entitlement led to widening patient-selection criteria and a more expensive dialysis program. In the early 1990s, dialysis in the United States was in a midlife crisis of sorts—successful in that it was growing in numbers of patients treated but causing concern about the cost, value, and quality of care it was providing.

Everyone was displeased with the federally funded program: the providers, who felt they were being strangled by inflationary pressures; the patients, who were concerned about deteriorating quality; federal policymakers, who were upset about rising costs; and the public, who did not want to pay for it in increased taxes.

Some in the United States argued that dialysis is precisely the kind of life-sustaining technology that should not be developed, because of its limited benefit to many and its high cost (Callahan, 1987). The dialysis community countered that dialysis has been successful in saving thousands of lives; however, they identified three areas requiring reform: (1) dialysis reimbursement levels, so they would be adequate to support the costs of excellent patient care; (2) the quality of patient care, so patient morbidity and mortality would be reduced; and (3) guidelines for dialysis initiation and withdrawal, so only patients who have a reasonable expectation of benefit from it would receive it.

Since its inception, dialysis has raised many ethical concerns to be analyzed and resolved that have subsequently been issues for other expensive modern medical technologies. Because of the unsettled state of dialysis in the early 1990s, it may continue to do so in the future.

ALVIN H. MOSS

For a further discussion of topics mentioned in this entry, see the entries AGING AND THE AGED, *article on* HEALTH-CARE AND RESEARCH ISSUES; AIDS, *article on* HEALTH-CARE AND RESEARCH ISSUES; ARTIFICIAL ORGANS AND LIFE-SUPPORT SYSTEMS; AUTONOMY; BIOTECHNOLOGY; CHRONIC CARE; CLINICAL ETHICS, *article on* CLINICAL ETHICS CONSULTATION; COMPETENCE; CONFLICT OF INTEREST; DEATH AND DYING: EUTHANASIA AND SUSTAINING LIFE, *article on* ADVANCE DIRECTIVES; ECONOMIC CONCEPTS IN HEALTH CARE; HEALTH-CARE FINANCING, *article on* MEDICARE; HEALTH-CARE RESOURCES, ALLOCATION OF; LIFE, QUALITY OF; *and* UTILITY. *Other relevant material may be found under the entries* BENEFICENCE; HARM; JUSTICE; ORGAN AND TISSUE TRANSPLANTS, *article on* ETHICAL AND LEGAL ISSUES; PATIENTS' RIGHTS, *article on* ORIGIN AND NATURE OF PATIENTS' RIGHTS; RIGHTS, *article on* RIGHTS IN BIOETHICS; *and* TECHNOLOGY.

Bibliography

ALEXANDER, SHANA. 1962. "They Decide Who Lives, Who Dies." *Life,* November 9, p. 4.

CALLAHAN, DANIEL. 1987. *Setting Limits: Medical Goals in an Aging Society.* New York: Simon and Schuster.

DOTTES, ANITA L. 1991. "Should All Individuals with End-Stage Renal Disease Be Dialyzed?" *Contemporary Dialysis and Nephrology* 12:19–30.

Fox, Renée C. 1981. "Exclusion from Dialysis: A Sociologic and Legal Perspective." *Kidney International* 19, no. 5: 739–751.

Fox, Renée C., and Swazey, Judith P. 1978. *The Courage to Fail: A Social View of Organ Transplants and Dialysis.* 2d ed., rev. Chicago: University of Chicago Press.

Hastings Center. 1987. *Guidelines on the Termination of Life-Sustaining Treatment and the Care of the Dying.* Bloomington: Indiana University Press.

Held, Philip J.; Levin, Nathan W.; Bovbjerg, Randall R.; Pauly, Mark V.; and Diamond, Louis H. 1991. "Mortality and Duration of Hemodialysis Treatment." *Journal of the American Medical Association* 265, no. 7:871–875.

Held, Philip J.; Pauly, Mark V.; and Diamond, Louis. 1987. "Survival Analysis of Patients Undergoing Dialysis." *Journal of the American Medical Association* 257, no. 5:645–650.

Hull, Alan R., and Parker, Tom F., III. 1990. "Proceedings from the Morbidity, Mortality and Prescription of Dialysis Symposium, Dallas TX, September 15 to 17, 1989." *American Journal of Kidney Diseases* 15, no. 5:375–383.

Jonsen, Albert R. 1990. *The New Medicine and the Old Ethics.* Cambridge, Mass.: Harvard University Press.

Kilner, John F. 1988. "Selecting Patients When Resources Are Limited: A Study of U.S. Medical Directors of Kidney Dialysis and Transplantation Facilities." *American Journal of Public Health* 78, no. 2:144–147.

Kjellstrand, Carl M., and Dossetor, John B., eds. 1992. *Ethical Problems in Dialysis and Transplantation.* Dordrecht, Netherlands: Kluwer.

Kolata, Gina Bari. 1980. "NMC Thrives Selling Dialysis." *Science* 208, no. 4442:379–382.

Levinsky, Norman G., and Rettig, Richard A. 1991. "The Medicare End-Stage Renal Disease Program: A Report from the Institute of Medicine." *New England Journal of Medicine* 324, no. 16:1143–1148.

Moskop, John C. 1987. "The Moral Limits to Federal Funding for Kidney Disease." *Hastings Center Report* 17, no. 2:11–15.

Moss, Alvin H.; Holley, Jean L.; and Upton, Matthew B. 1992. "Outcomes of Cardiopulmonary Resuscitation in Dialysis Patients." *Journal of the American Society of Nephrology* 3, no. 6:1238–1243.

Moss, Alvin H.; Stocking, Carol B.; Sachs, Greg A.; and Siegler, Mark. 1993. "Variation in the Attitudes of Dialysis Unit Medical Directors toward Reported Decisions to Withhold and Withdraw Dialysis." *Journal of the American Society of Nephrology* 4, no. 2:229–234.

Neu, Steven, and Kjellstrand, Carl M. 1986. "Stopping Long-Term Dialysis: An Empirical Study of Withdrawal of Life-Supporting Treatment." *New England Journal of Medicine* 314, no. 1:14–20.

Relman, Arnold S. 1980. "The New Medical-Industrial Complex." *New England Journal of Medicine* 303, no. 17:963–970.

Rettig, Richard A. 1976. "The Policy Debate on Patient Care Financing for Victims of End-Stage Renal Disease." *Law and Contemporary Problems* 40, no. 4:196–230.

———. 1991. "Origins of the Medicare Kidney Disease Entitlement: The Social Security Amendments of 1972." In *Biomedical Politics,* pp. 176–208. Edited by Kathi E. Hanna. Washington, D.C.: National Academy Press.

Rettig, Richard A., and Levinsky, Norman G. 1991. *Kidney Failure and the Federal Government.* Washington, D.C.: National Academy Press.

Roberts, Stephen D.; Maxwell, Douglas R.; and Gross, Thomas L. 1980. "Cost Effective Care of End-Stage Renal Disease: A Billion Dollar Question." *Annals of Internal Medicine* 92, no. 2, pt. 1:243–248.

Rothman, David J. 1991. *Strangers at the Bedside: A History of How Law and Bioethics Transformed Medical Decision Making.* New York: Basic Books.

Singer, Peter A. 1992. "Nephrologists' Experience with and Attitudes Towards Decisions to Forego Dialysis: The End-Stage Renal Disease Network of New England." *Journal of the American Society of Nephrology* 2, no. 7:1235–1240.

U.S. President's Commission for the Study of Ethical Problems in Medicine and Biomedical and Behavioral Research. 1983. *Deciding to Forego Life-Sustaining Treatment: A Report on the Ethical, Medical, and Legal Issues in Treatment Decisions.* Washington, D.C.: U.S. Government Printing Office.

U.S. Renal Data System. 1989. *Annual Data Report, 1989.* Bethesda, Md.: National Institutes of Health, National Institute of Diabetes and Digestive and Kidney Diseases, Division of Kidney, Urologic, and Hematologic Diseases.

KIDNEY TRANSPLANTATION

See Organ and Tissue Procurement; *and* Organ and Tissue Transplants. *See also* Artificial Organs and Life-Support Systems.

KILLING AND LETTING DIE

See Action; Death and Dying: Euthanasia and Sustaining Life, *articles on* ethical issues, *and* professional and public policies. *See also* Double Effect.

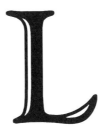

LABORATORY TESTING

Laboratory testing is an essential part of contemporary health care in developed countries and a major contributor to the high costs of that care. Consider, for example, the case of Mrs. K., hospitalized in the intensive-care unit of a New York City hospital for twenty-five days in 1983 until her death after multiple organ failure. Charges for her hospital stay (not including doctor bills) totaled $47,311. Of this total, the second highest category of charges (after $12,000 in intensive-care room charges) was for laboratory services: $11,201 (Hellerstein, 1984). Despite the high volume and costs of laboratory testing, the moral dimensions of this activity did not attract much attention or commentary for many years. Beginning in 1985, however, the development and use of a diagnostic test for human immunodeficiency virus (HIV) focused widespread attention on a number of moral issues in testing, including informed consent, confidentiality, accuracy, access, and safety (Bayer et al., 1986). In the 1990s the U.S. Human Genome Project directed renewed attention to all of these moral issues as they bear on myriad new tests for various genetic conditions (Fost, 1993).

The term "laboratory testing" does not denote a single specific practice but rather a set of similar practices performed in several different settings, by different kinds of professionals, for a number of reasons. Primary-care physicians perform routine tests in small office labs; highly specialized pathologists and technicians carry out more complicated tests in large hospital or independent commercial labs. Tests are performed for medical reasons (to diagnose a patient's disease), legal reasons (to identify the source of blood or tissue samples in a criminal investigation), financial reasons (to qualify for life insurance), and social reasons (to identify drug abuse by airline pilots). Not surprisingly, these different settings, actors, and purposes raise different ethical issues. This review will begin with the moral interests of the patient and then broaden its focus to include other relevant interests and perspectives.

Because laboratory testing is an integral part of health care, patients' expectations regarding testing can be understood as applications of their more general health-care interests. Patients have general interests in securing access to effective and affordable health care, avoiding unnecessary care, controlling what is done to or for them, knowing about their condition and its treatment, and limiting others' access to sensitive personal information about themselves. Applying these general patient interests to laboratory testing, we can construct a scenario that approaches the ideal from the patient's point of view. In this scenario, all patients have ready access to accurate and affordable laboratory tests. Patients are not subjected to unnecessary tests, and over-reliance on testing does not result in neglect of other diagnostic tools, such as history taking and physician examination (see Eichna, 1980; Griner and Glaser, 1982). All material information about proposed tests and test results is shared with patients, and patients give their implicit or explicit consent, as appropriate, for all tests. Test results are kept strictly confidential and given only to those directly involved in the care of the particular patient.

Others, including health-care professionals, third parties, and society at large, have interests that sometimes conflict with patient interests. Let us now consider how these other interests can conflict with specific patient interests in the context of laboratory testing.

Access to testing

Because laboratory tests can provide information essential for the diagnosis and treatment of disease, they offer obvious benefits for patients. Modern clinical laboratories equipped to perform technologically sophisticated tests are costly enterprises, however, and lack of resources precludes access to most laboratory testing for most of the world's people. Even in affluent nations like the United States, where testing is widely available, its costs contribute to the rapidly escalating overall cost of health care. In one clinical chemistry laboratory in a large university medical center over a ten-year period (1980–1990), the number of billable tests performed increased an average 12.1 percent annually, from some 300,000 tests in 1980 to 650,000 tests in 1990, and gross billings increased a striking 25.8 percent annually, from $5.6 million in 1980 to $19 million in 1990 (Benge et al., 1993). Hospitals like this one may have raised laboratory testing prices artificially high in order to shift the cost of caring for Medicare and uninsured patients on to patients with retrospective, fee-for-service private health insurance (Conn, 1993). Despite such cost shifting by some providers, indigent patients still encounter obstacles to receiving needed health care; broader access to care in the United States awaits basic reforms in the overall distribution and financing of health care (see, e.g., Callahan, 1990; *Clinton Administration*, 1993).

Access to testing can also be limited for nonfinancial reasons. HIV screening of all prospective blood donors, for example, was proposed early in 1985 in order to protect the nation's blood supply. Because gay men and members of other groups at higher risk for AIDS (acquired immunodeficiency syndrome) had been asked, since 1983, to refrain from donating blood, it appeared that these persons would not have access to the newly developing screening tests. To resolve this problem, the federal government eventually agreed to fund alternative testing sites where persons at risk for infection could receive testing (Silverman and Silverman, 1985).

Access to testing is not a benefit unless the tests performed provide generally accurate information about a patient's condition. Quality control is, therefore, an essential part of laboratory testing. Concerns about quality control in laboratory testing led to the passage of the Clinical Laboratory Improvement Act of 1967 (CLIA '67) and the Clinical Laboratory Improvement Amendments of 1988 (CLIA '88) by the U.S. Congress (Centers for Disease Control, 1992). CLIA '88 was designed to extend quality-assurance regulations to all clinical laboratories, including small physician office labs. New quality-control and personnel standards in this area bring with them additional costs, however, and so illustrate a tension between ensuring quality, on the one hand, and promoting easy access to testing and controlling its costs, on the other. In written comments on the first CLIA '88 implementation regulations proposed by the Health Care Financing Administration (HCFA) in 1990, some 60,000 physicians argued that the regulations were unduly burdensome and would force them to close their office labs. In response to those criticisms, HCFA relaxed its requirements significantly in the revised final clinical laboratory regulations issued in February 1992 (Anderson, 1992).

Unnecessary testing

In contrast to the lack of access to testing for some patients, other patients are subjected to unnecessary testing, that is, tests that do not make a useful contribution to these patients' care. Patients' interests in avoiding the financial and physical burdens of unnecessary testing may conflict with a variety interests of their caregivers. An informal list of reasons physicians order laboratory tests compiled by Lundberg (1983) includes peer pressure, public relations, legal requirements, medicolegal need, CYA, personal profit, hospital profit, research, curiosity, insecurity, frustration at nothing else to do, to buy time, "fishing expeditions," personal education, to report to an attending physician, and habit.

Defensive medicine is perhaps the most commonly cited reason for ordering medically unnecessary tests. Physicians may order a laboratory test, despite their belief that it will not make a significant contribution to the care of the patient, in order to protect themselves from the threat of malpractice liability. There are, however, reasons for questioning whether this threat is genuine or serious enough to justify self-interested action by physicians at some financial, and often physical, cost to patients. The standard of care required of physicians is based on what is "reasonable and necessary." Unnecessary medical tests should, therefore, not be part of the standard of care. Paradoxically, if all physicians rush to do unnecessary tests for defensive purposes, such tests may become "standard" in the sense that everyone does them. Increasing emphasis on outcomes research and practice guidelines may help to eliminate such inappropriate standards.

Performing medically unnecessary laboratory tests in order to profit financially from the revenues they generate is a clear violation of the physician's professional responsibility to act in the patient's best interests. Concerns about tests ordered for financial gain are especially pronounced when physicians refer patients to independent clinical laboratories in which they have an ownership interest (called self-referrals). U.S. federal legislation enacted in 1989 prohibits most physician referrals of Medicare patients to clinical laboratories in which they hold an interest (Iglehart, 1990).

Knowledge and control

Patients want to be treated, to be sure, but they also want to be informed about their condition and its treatment and to have an active role in decisions about their health care. These latter two interests are expressed in the legal doctrine of informed consent to treatment, which requires that competent patients be given the opportunity to consent to or refuse proposed treatment on the basis of information about treatment benefits, risks, and alternatives (U.S. President's Commission, 1982). The amount of information to be communicated and the nature of the consent process vary with the treatment in question. In the case of routine lab tests on blood and urine, for example, where the purpose of the test is simple and obvious and the risks of testing are minimal, little or no additional information about the tests may be required, and consent may be implicit in the act of seeking care. Other kinds of lab tests, however, where the purposes of testing are complicated and the physical or psychosocial risks of testing are significant (e.g., HIV testing, tumor biopsies, genetic testing), may require a much more formal information and consent procedure. Informed consent for genetic testing of a couple for cystic fibrosis carrier status, for example, may require extensive counseling regarding the nature of cystic fibrosis, the limitations of current tests, treatment options, procreative options including abortion, and possible psychosocial consequences, such as discrimination in insurance and employment (Fost, 1993). In view of the significant consequences of a diagnosis of HIV infection, many states have specially mandated written informed consent for HIV testing (Gostin, 1989).

Lawmakers have seen fit to limit individual control over testing decisions in the interests of specific third parties and of society at large. In the United States, for example, HIV screening is mandatory for blood donors, military recruits, active-duty military personnel, prospective immigrants, and federal and some state prison inmates. Commentators have praised mandatory HIV screening of blood donors for its success in protecting the blood supply but have criticized other mandatory screening programs for their high cost, limited contribution to public health, and compromise of individual rights (Field, 1990; Gostin, 1989). For example, two U.S. states, Illinois and Louisiana, adopted mandatory premarital HIV screening programs in the 1980s, but both repealed their programs within two years. In its first year of operation (1988), the Illinois program identified only twenty-three HIV-positive persons among 159,000 tested, at a total cost of $5.6 million (Field, 1990).

Some health professionals and hospitals have proposed policies of routine HIV testing of all hospital patients or all patients undergoing elective surgery (see Hagen et al., 1988). Routine HIV screening would clearly benefit those patients who learn from the screening that they are HIV-infected and begin therapy to prevent or postpone its complications (Jewett and Hecht, 1993). Such benefits do not, however, seem great enough to justify the abandonment of informed consent for HIV testing, nor are they usually the primary reason proponents defend these policies. Rather, proponents point out that routine screening would enable caregivers to take appropriate precautions to protect their own safety in caring for HIV-infected patients. Opponents of such policies argue that the universal blood and body fluid precautions for health-care settings first recommended by the Centers for Disease Control in 1985 and mandated by the Occupational Safety and Health Administration in 1991 are the most effective means of protection against disease transmission, and therefore routine hospital screening for HIV infection is neither necessary nor desirable (Moskop, 1990).

Confidentiality

Access to the information generated by laboratory testing is necessary for managing patient care and for informing patients about their condition and its treatment. Much, if not most, of the information produced by lab tests is quite technical and is meaningful only to trained professionals, but some information, such as diagnosis of HIV infection, a sexually transmitted or genetic disease, cancer, or pregnancy, is potentially very sensitive. Patients often have an interest in keeping this information confidential and in limiting disclosure of test results to those who have a need to know in order to provide effective care for them.

Despite the obvious moral significance of these confidentiality interests, social policy limits confidentiality in a variety of ways in order to address the needs and interests of others (Dickens, 1988). For example, physicians report information about infectious diseases to state and federal agencies for epidemiological and public-health purposes, such as identifying and notifying the contacts of sexually transmitted disease and HIV patients regarding their risks. Contact tracing of HIV-infected patients, once strenuously resisted by AIDS advocacy organizations in the name of confidentiality, has gained wider acceptance and endorsement by professional organizations for its public-health value and for enabling infected persons to secure early treatment

(Bayer, 1991). Similarly, physicians and genetic counselors may feel a duty to disclose information about a patient's serious genetic condition to relatives who are at significant risk of developing the same condition or passing it on to their children, even if the patient is unwilling to permit such disclosure (Fost, 1993). The proper balance between the duty to respect confidentiality and the duty to warn in these cases remains deeply controversial.

This entry has reviewed some of the major issues in laboratory testing but by no means exhausted the field. For example, the increasing use of sophisticated DNA typing in criminal investigations and trials (Annas, 1992) and the use of laboratory testing by employers and insurance companies (U.S. Congress, 1991; Murray, 1993) raise complex moral and legal questions. Laboratory testing has become, and will remain, a topic of lively moral concern.

JOHN C. MOSKOP

Directly related to this entry is the entry HEALTH SCREENING AND TESTING IN THE PUBLIC-HEALTH CONTEXT. *For a further discussion of topics mentioned in this entry, see the entries* AIDS; ALLIED HEALTH PROFESSIONS; CONFIDENTIALITY; HEALTH-CARE FINANCING, *especially the article on* PROFIT AND COMMERCIALISM; INFORMATION DISCLOSURE; INFORMED CONSENT; *and* MEDICAL MALPRACTICE. *This entry will find application in the entry* GENETIC TESTING AND SCREENING.

Bibliography

ANDERSON, JANE M. 1992. "CLIA's Final Rules Arrive." *Medical World News* 33, no. 3:19–25.

ANNAS, GEORGE J. 1992. "Setting Standards for the Use of DNA Typing Results in the Courtroom—The State of the Art." *New England Journal of Medicine* 326, no. 24: 1641–1644.

BAYER, RONALD. 1991. "Public Health Policy and the AIDS Epidemic: An End to HIV Exceptionalism?" *New England Journal of Medicine* 324, no. 21:1500–1504.

BAYER, RONALD; LEVINE, CAROL; and WOLF, SUSAN M. 1986. "HIV Antibody Screening: An Ethical Framework for Evaluating Proposed Programs." *Journal of the American Medical Association* 256, no. 13:1768–1774.

BENGE, HERMAN; CSAKO, GYORGY; and PARL, FRITZ F. 1993. "A 10-Year Analysis of 'Revenues,' Costs, Staffing, and Workload in an Academic Medical Center Clinical Chemistry Laboratory." *Clinical Chemistry* 39, no. 9: 1780–1787.

CALLAHAN, DANIEL. 1990. *What Kind of Life: The Limits of Medical Progress.* New York: Simon and Schuster.

CENTERS FOR DISEASE CONTROL. 1992. "Regulations for Implementing Clinical Laboratory Improvement Amendments of 1988: A Summary." *Journal of the American Medical Association* 267, no. 13:1725–1727, 1731–1734.

Clinton Administration Description of President's Health Care Reform Plan, "American Health Security Act of 1993." 1993. Washington, D.C.: Bureau of National Affairs.

CONN, REX B. 1993. "Health Care Reform and the Clinical Laboratory." *Clinical Chemistry* 39, no. 9:1759–1760.

DICKENS, BERNARD M. 1988. "Legal Limits of AIDS Confidentiality." *Journal of the American Medical Association* 259, no. 23:3449–3451.

EICHNA, LUDWIG W. 1980. "Medical-School Education, 1975–1979: A Student's Perspective." *New England Journal of Medicine* 303, no. 13:727–734.

FIELD, MARTHA A. 1990. "Testing for AIDS: Uses and Abuses." *American Journal of Law and Medicine* 16, nos. 1–2:33–106.

FOST, NORMAN. 1993. "Genetic Diagnosis and Treatment: Ethical Considerations." *American Journal of Diseases of Children* 147, no. 11:1190–1195.

GOSTIN, LARRY O. 1989. "Public Health Strategies for Confronting AIDS: Legislative and Regulatory Policy in the United States." *Journal of the American Medical Association* 261, no. 11:1621–1629.

GRINER, PAUL F., and GLASER, ROBERT J. 1982. "Misuse of Laboratory Tests and Diagnostic Procedures." *New England Journal of Medicine* 307, no. 21:1336–1339.

HAGEN, MICHAEL D.; MEYER, KLEMENS B.; and PAUKER, STEPHEN G. 1988. "Routine Preoperative Screening for HIV: Does the Risk to the Surgeon Outweigh the Risk to the Patient?" *Journal of the American Medical Association* 259, no. 9:1357–1359.

HELLERSTEIN, DAVID. 1984. "The Slow, Costly Death of Mrs. K——." *Harper's*, March, pp. 84–89.

IGLEHART, JOHN K. 1990. "Congress Moves to Regulate Self-Referral and Physicians' Ownership of Clinical Laboratories." *New England Journal of Medicine* 322, no. 23: 1682–1687.

JEWETT, JOHN F., and HECHT, FREDERICK M. 1993. "Preventive Health Care for Adults with HIV Infection." *Journal of the American Medical Association* 269, no. 9:1144–1153.

LUNDBERG, GEORGE D. 1983. "Perseveration of Laboratory Test Ordering: A Syndrome Affecting Clinicians." *Journal of the American Medical Association* 249, no. 5:639.

MOSKOP, JOHN C. 1990. "AIDS and Hospitals: The Policy Options." *Hospitals and Health Services Administration* 35, no. 2:159–171.

MURRAY, THOMAS H. 1993. "Genetics and Just Health Care: A Genome Task Force Report." *Kennedy Institute of Ethics Journal* 3, no. 3:327–331.

SILVERMAN, MERVYN F., and SILVERMAN, DEBORAH B. 1985. "AIDS and the Threat to Public Health." *Hastings Center Report* 15, no. 4 (suppl.):19–22.

U.S. CONGRESS. OFFICE OF TECHNOLOGY ASSESSMENT. 1991. *Medical Monitoring and Screening in the Workplace: Results of a Survey—Background Paper.* OTA-BP-BA-67. Washington, D.C.: Author.

U.S. PRESIDENT'S COMMISSION FOR THE STUDY OF ETHICAL PROBLEMS IN MEDICINE AND BIOMEDICAL AND BEHAVIORAL RESEARCH. 1982. *Making Health Care Decisions: A Report on the Ethical and Legal Implications of Informed Consent in the Patient-Practitioner Relationship.* Washington, D.C.: Author.

LAND ETHIC

See ENVIRONMENTAL ETHICS, *article on* LAND ETHIC.

LATIN AMERICA

See MEDICAL ETHICS, HISTORY OF, *section on* THE AMERICAS, *article on* LATIN AMERICA.

LAW AND BIOETHICS

Bioethics began as, and remains, an interdisciplinary field. If developments in biology and medicine have fueled the bioethics train and philosophy has laid down the tracks on which it has run, then law has been the engineer at the controls of the locomotive and statutes and court decisions have thrown the switches that guided the train through the rail yards. Law's influence on bioethics has been so pronounced as to be unmistakable, yet so pervasive as sometimes to be unnoticed.

It might be argued that law's role was pronounced for purely historical reasons: Bioethics began as an American phenomenon and hence was shaped by certain aspects of American culture. Lacking an established church or a single heritage of values, though committed to the rule of law and to the equality of all persons, Americans have a habit of turning to courts to resolve moral conflicts. Moreover, other features of the terrain also indicated a major role for the law. Bioethics frequently presents central civic issues, among them these: When does a human entity first become (or cease being) a legal person? What conduct of health-care professionals treating incurably ill patients would constitute murder? May parents be paid for transferring to other persons the rights of custody and control over their children? Does the prospect of gaining knowledge of potential benefit to the community ever justify using people without their consent or even their knowledge?

Dependence on the legal system to settle many ethical and social issues generated by medicine and the life sciences does more than merely provide a means for resolving disputes. Reliance on the legal system denotes that an issue should be understood as having two opposing sides that will do battle for their respective rights to act in a particular fashion or to restrain the other side from acting in a contrary fashion. Moreover, as a means of discovering and articulating principles, the law favors certain implicit and explicit values.

The relationship of law and bioethics has not, however, been unidirectional: Bioethics has also affected the law. While much of law is concerned with commerce and institutions, both public and private, bioethics is essentially about people and about the fundamental choices that determine and even define their lives. If the law has brought to bioethical cases an attention to rights and procedure, bioethics has enriched legal analysis with life-and-death dramas. It would strain the point to say that medicine saved the law, as Stephen Toulmin observed medicine did for philosophy (Toulmin, 1982). But the ethical dilemmas arising from medicine and its associated scientific disciplines have helped to humanize the law, providing a setting in which the central struggles of our times—of individual rights and the collective good, of liberty as against equity and equality, of justice and fairness, of personal wishes versus expert judgment or the will of the majority—are played out with unparalleled urgency and vitality. When the question is whether a life is worth living, for example, the answer is consequential. And when legal institutions falter in answering such questions, then lawyers and others are reminded that perfect legal solutions may not exist for all bioethical dilemmas. Bioethics raises fundamental challenges for theorists as well as practitioners of the law about the harm that society may impose upon a minority in order to uphold values believed to be of fundamental importance to the majority, or the limits of the law as a guide to human conduct. Yet the focus of this essay is not the theoretical connection between morality and law, but rather the law as a practical force in shaping and defining bioethics.

What is the law?

Sources of law. The term "law" carries a number of meanings. In ordinary speech, it usually refers to specific criminal or regulatory provisions ("It's against the law to . . ."). This usage also reflects the common equation of law with statutes, denoting not just criminal statutes but also those governing civil or procedural matters, such as the ownership of property or how one is called for jury duty. A fuller understanding of the law would emphasize other important sources. Of particular prominence today are the detailed and voluminous regulations issued by governmental departments and administrative agencies to implement the powers and carry out the duties conferred on them by statutes. Although statutes are sometimes quite detailed, many areas of human activity (especially of an industrial or commercial nature) are so complex that the legislature must almost of necessity confine itself to framing the basic legal structure, while delegating the task of supplying all the details to those with greater time and expertise at the administrative level, subject to various degrees of public, executive, legislative, and judicial oversight.

Especially in countries, including the United States, whose legal systems are derived from the English model, judicial decisions are a source of law at least as important as statutes. In some decisions, judges interpret statutes and hence give meaning and shape to them; while in others, judges decide issues not directly addressed by statutes and effectively make new law. At one time, when statutory rules covered only a small portion of human affairs, most of English law consisted of judicial resolution of individual disputes, collectively known as "the common law." To this day, many areas of law have a strong common-law flavor, which is constantly reinforced and renewed by judges' decisions about novel issues. Even in countries with civil-law systems based on Roman law or the Napoleonic Code, judges participate in the crafting of the law by their interpretation of code provisions.

Finally, in legal systems that follow the model of the United States, in which all activities of the government—including making and interpreting the law—are subject to limits specified in a constitution, no statement of the law would be complete without reference to the text of that supreme law, as well as the authoritative interpretations of its provisions by the courts.

Even these sources—statutes, regulations, judicial decisions, and the constitutions—do not exhaust the meaning of "the law," which also connotes the legal system, the institutions, and the processes through which the law is applied. In this sense, the law encompasses the processes and rules of courts and administrative bodies (for example, on admission of evidence), as well as the more informal standards or practices that are reflected in the action of those law-applying people and institutions (such as public prosecutors or bureaucrats) who have wide discretion in administering statutes and regulations. Within their sphere of authority, the law is what they say it is. Indeed, to the extent they are not expressly forbidden, the customs and practices of people in any field may properly be described as part of the law, though those customs and practices may formally be denominated "law" only when explicitly incorporated into a judicial opinion, statute, or regulation.

Seen in this way, the law is a basic framework for society; it is a system not only for promulgating official policies and procedures and for administrating prosecutorial, judicial, and regulatory affairs but also for providing explicit or implicit sanction for the private arrangements through which activities and relationships are ordered. Of course, many people would not identify the law as the source for the way they conduct their affairs. Instead, they would point to the influence of family and community customs or values, as well as to explicit moral or religious teachings. But as members of society, they must still operate within the law; this means that if their private arrangements run afoul of the expectations of society as embodied in the law, these arrangements may be limited or nullified. For example, in a number of U.S. jurisdictions, legislatures or judges

have declared contracts for women to bear children for couples (so-called surrogate motherhood) to be null and void, as against public policy, even though a purported contract is freely and knowingly agreed to by all parties.

The existence of such private ordering as an important but often overlooked source of lawmaking also serves as a reminder that even in a society, such as the United States, with a high proportion of lawyers, lawmaking is not restricted to lawyers. From the local to the national level, many members of the legislative and executive branches of government are not lawyers; indeed, the federal constitution does not even require that judges be legally trained. Law is one of the three traditional learned professions (along with medicine and the clergy). Its members are licensed by the state and admitted "as officers of the court" to practice "at the bar of justice." Accordingly, like physicians, they are governed by ethical standards articulated by their profession through its associations as well as through the decisions of judges passing on cases of alleged transgression of professional obligations.

Around the world, most legal education occurs in schools affiliated with universities. Characterizing legal education in the early twentieth century as akin to a trade school, Thorstein Veblen opined that "the law school belongs in the modern university no more than a school of fencing or dancing" (Veblen, 1965 [1918], p. 211); but this complaint is no longer justified, if indeed it ever was. Today, schools provide much more than mere vocational training, and scholarship is not limited to exegesis of doctrine; it encompasses empirical, normative, and theoretical work. Nonetheless, the law is a practical field, not simply one of the liberal arts and sciences.

Divisions of the law.   Traditionally, for purposes of basic study and classification, law has been divided along such doctrinal lines as tort law, criminal law, contract law, constitutional law, equitable remedies, property law, wills and trusts, and civil and criminal procedure. Each of these areas is characterized by prototypical relationships among parties and a set of analytic and practical devices for structuring those relationships and determining the outcomes of disputes. In recent years, legal scholarship has taken on several additional layers.

One is an enrichment of the tools brought to the law's tasks by combining with another discipline: legal anthropology, law and economics, legal history, law and literature, law and philosophy, law and psychology or psychoanalysis, sociology of law, and law and religion, to mention prominent examples. Each of these combined subdisciplines has not only a methodology but also its own theories and assumptions. Furthermore, additional schools of thought have arisen—such as legal realism, critical legal studies, feminism, and critical race studies—that provide perspectives on the law by combining the tools of several disciplines and a set of attitudes toward legal, social, economic, and personal relationships. Plainly, a person working in an interdisciplinary field may bring one of the analytic perspectives to bear—for instance, a feminist approach to legal history or a legal-realist perspective on law and economics.

A third way of dividing the domain of law is by focusing on its application to specialized types of personal, commercial, institutional, and sociopolitical activities. (The range of specialized areas of the law seems virtually limitless; attorneys now practice antitrust law, art law, bankruptcy law, civil-rights law, commercial law, education law, employment and labor law, entertainment law, family law, insurance law, intellectual-property law, juvenile and dependency law, media and broadcast law, mental-health law, probate law, public and private international law, regulated industries law, sports law, securities law, and even space law, to name a few.) Whether from an academic or a practice vantage point, specialized fields of law usually link traditional doctrinal categories with information and methods derived from the disciplinary and analytic approaches just described. For example, people working in family law will draw not only on legal doctrines from remedies, from property law, from wills and trusts, and from criminal and civil law and procedure, but also on psychological, sociological, or feminist analyses and perspectives; while those pursuing antitrust law will draw not only on various aspects of business law and criminal and civil law but also on law and economics studies and perhaps historical and sociological analysis as well.

Health law. Traditionally, medicine and law intersected in civil or criminal cases in which proof of medical facts was at issue. From the medical side, those involved were usually pathologists, who became specialists in "forensic medicine," as the field was known to prosecutors and criminal-defense attorneys; on the legal side, torts specialists who handled a large proportion of malpractice cases (and some of whom held degrees in both law and medicine) described their expertise as encompassing "medical law." With the tremendous growth in health care and research beginning in the mid-1960s, health-care law—or more simply health law—emerged as a new field that includes these areas and more. It is one of the fastest-growing, most diverse, and most exciting legal specialties.

Health law draws on practically the entire corpus of traditional doctrinal fields—civil, criminal, constitutional, property, and procedural—as well as many other specialized areas, such as labor, insurance, antitrust, and government regulation. Practitioners represent hospitals and other health-care providers; academic research centers; physicians, nurses, and other health-care professionals and nonprofessional employees; insurance carriers and employers that provide health insurance as an employee benefit; manufacturers and distributors of drugs and medical devices; patients and their families; and governmental departments and agencies that finance and regulate the individuals and institutions providing health care. Although cases involving ethical dilemmas are the ones that draw public attention, they are the exception for most health lawyers, who are more likely to spend their time drafting contracts for the purchase of goods and services; bargaining about insurance reimbursement; preparing staff bylaws, checking professional peer activities, or handling other issues that arise in accreditation, credentialing, or certification of practitioners or institutions; negotiating with government agents about licensing, taxation, and environmental controls; or litigating a case of professional malpractice (Macdonald et al., 1991).

The impact of law on bioethics

The relationship of law and bioethics is complex and multifaceted. One need not share the view of a leading legal commentator—"American law, not philosophy or medicine, is primarily responsible for the agenda, development, and current state of American bioethics" (Annas, 1993, p. 3)—to conclude that the law has strongly influenced the methodology of bioethics, the central focus of bioethics, and the values of bioethics. "And—to the considerable extent that bioethics is an American invention and export—the influence of American law has been felt even in societies in which legal institutions play a less pronounced role than they do in the United States" (Capron, 1994, p. 43). Law's role in shaping bioethics has at least five facets.

Famous legal cases. Notable cases have played a major role not merely in the development of bioethics but also in making it, by the 1990s, a prominent part of private reflection and public discourse. Difficult ethical issues are nothing new to the health professions. Yet until recently, issues were examined largely behind closed doors by physicians and nurses and an occasional theologian. In democratic societies, legal proceedings are usually open (though sometimes parties are permitted to use fictitious names, to help preserve their privacy). Consequently, the media are able not merely to report about a difficult decision that must be taken but also to put a human face on it by recounting the drama as it unfolds in the hearing room.

And bioethics cases are often very dramatic. A familiar example: As Karen Quinlan's parents argued during 1975–1976 in the New Jersey courts for authority to order her ventilator turned off, her photograph appeared so often in the media that it was probably more familiar to most Americans than the faces of their local members of Congress. Likewise, bioethical breaches—particularly scandalous ones, such as the Nazi physicians' experiments on concentration camp prisoners and the Tuskeegee syphilis study—not only generate landmark judicial rulings but also provoke adoption of new statutory or administrative law.

Methodology.   Related to the addressing of bioethical cases through the law is a second facet, the law's largely inductive methodology. This method is especially associated with the common law, the process through which judges render decisions specific to the facts of the individual cases before them that are grounded in, or justified by, the decisions in prior cases whose facts are sufficiently analogous. Not only do judges often apply the same methodology when interpreting statutes, but legislatures, in drafting statutes, usually operate concretely and incrementally, building on court decisions and existing legislation (or borrowing from other jurisdictions) rather than attempting to operationalize grand principles. The law's fact-based, inductive method provides a counterpoint to the "principlism" that characterizes much philosophically oriented analysis in bioethics. Of course, this approach is not unique to the law, but it reinforces other case-based traditions in ethics, such as casuistry and Jewish ethics.

Procedural emphasis.   Third, recognizing that midlevel ethical principles such as autonomy, beneficence, justice, and nonmaleficence cannot solve most bioethical dilemmas (which arise precisely when conflict occurs among these unranked principles), and that pluralistic societies do not necessarily hold enough moral views in common to agree upon the correct resolution of most controversies, many bioethicists have welcomed "a procedural ethic, based on respect of the freedom of the moral agents involved, even without establishing the correctness of any particular moral sense" (Engelhardt, 1986, p. 45). This emphasis on procedure is familiar to lawyers, though the suggestion that bioethics should concentrate on acceptable decision-making processes rather than substantive rules draws objections from some legal scholars who see in proceduralism the risk of a slide into "the arbitrary exercise of power" (Annas, 1988, p. xiii).

Even when they have mandated that procedures be followed, the courts have not insisted that bioethical disagreements outside court employ all the procedural niceties that attach to judicial proceedings. Indeed, judges, legislators, and administrators alike have not always been very clear about the mandate and membership, much less the process, of institutional committees to make judgments about medical treatment and research. For example, in its landmark *Quinlan* decision, the New Jersey Supreme Court held that the guardians of unconscious patients could order life-sustaining treatment forgone with the agreement of the treating physician, provided a multiprofessional committee at the

hospital concurred; yet it said nothing about how that committee should gather, hear, or evaluate evidence or otherwise reach conclusions (*In re Quinlan*, 1976).

Rights orientation.   The issues in bioethics are some of the most sensitive and most divisive confronted by our society, not least because of the rapid development of the life sciences. In both the laboratory and the clinic, novel problems are constantly generated by new capabilities for organ transplantation and mechanical replacement, for genetic diagnosis and therapy, for assisting reproduction, for sustaining life, for modifying human behavior, and for myriad other means of altering nature; such problems also arise out of major changes in the way health services are organized and financed. These developments and changes challenge existing social and professional norms; where those challenges are substantial and intractable, the people involved not infrequently turn to courts, legislatures, or executive agencies to protect their rights. "The concept of rights . . . has its most natural use when a political society is divided, and appeals to cooperation or a common goal are pointless" (Dworkin, 1977, p. 184).

Concern over abuses of patients and research subjects has been a major theme in bioethics, reinforced repeatedly by instances in which health-care professionals and institutions have acted—sometimes from good motives and occasionally not—to the detriment of people in their care. The law has offered bioethics not just a procedural response but also a long tradition of protecting people from harm by assertion of their rights; indeed, a rights orientation seems inherent in the law's perspective on the relationship of the health-care system to patients and research subjects.

Certain risks to patients arise from the imbalance inherent in this relationship—the vulnerability and dependence that illness creates, physicians' superior knowledge and technical mastery, and the way the organization of health care enhances professionals' power and prestige. From ancient times, medical ethics proclaimed the duties of beneficence and fidelity to patients' interests in order to guard against harm to patients. Yet, as bioethicists have pointed out from the first, this traditional view of medical ethics is problematic because physicians not only promised to serve their patients' interests but often took it upon themselves to define those interests. Lawyers aided this assault on medical paternalism with concepts borrowed from civil-rights law, such as political liberty and equality of treatment. From the 1960s onward, bioethicists adopting this stance "had much in common with the new roster of rights agitators" for consumers, racial and sexual minorities, and women (Rothman, 1991, p. 245).

The increase in the rights orientation coincided with the increasing effectiveness of medical interventions. Armed with wonder drugs, high-tech surgery, and new methods of resuscitation and intensive care, physicians saw their power to influence their patients' futures increase dramatically from the middle of the twentieth century; and that power became the subject of disputes concerning how it was to be distributed in the physician–patient relationship. Legal commentators suggested—and most bioethicists embraced—a reformulation of that relationship in terms of patients' rights (Annas and Healy, 1974). The dominance of the rights orientation dismays many health-care professionals, who lament the adversarial tone they feel law has introduced into the practice of medicine. There may be a legitimate complaint here, but physicians have historically denied that they are making anything but medical decisions for patients. It has taken bioethicists to point out that once alternatives become available, the choice between them is usually based on value judgments, not medical judgments, and doctors have no special expertise that justifies their values taking precedence over patients' values. Rights are crucial to dealing with power inequality, even where one might prefer to conceive of relationships in terms of caring and connection. This tension remains a recurring theme in law and bioethics.

Although the incorporation of such central legal doctrines as informed consent into the core of bioethics can hardly be doubted, the transformative effects of law on medical practice are less clear. Commentators such as George Annas, who take a patients' rights approach, find many instances where those rights are still abused (Annas, 1988); whereas scholars such as Jay Katz, who look at physicians' behavior, emphasize that powerful factors in physicians' training and psychology have prevented them from adopting a stance of open discussion and shared decision making (Katz, 1984). At the same time, other critics argue that the authority the law took from physicians is often transferred to lawyers and judges, not to patients; and that moreover, by replacing professional discretion with legal rules, the law has given physicians the unintended message that they need not exercise ethical judgment (Hyman, 1990). Even if physicians do not react in this fashion, the law's inclination to view relationships in terms of rights changes the way bioethical issues are analyzed and potentially displaces other forms of moral discourse traditionally associated with medicine. For example, by emphasizing what one has the right to do without helping to define what is the right thing to do, the law may have undermined the specifically moral aspects of bioethics (Schneider, 1994). "[N]othing but confusion of thought can result," as Justice Oliver Wendell Holmes observed, "from assuming that the rights of man in a moral sense are equally rights in the sense of the Constitution and the law" (Holmes, 1920, p. 172).

Specific values. Besides leading toward a rights orientation, the reliance upon the legal system imports specific values. These values are not unique to the legal system, though they tend to be associated with it, nor are they controversial, though they are not without consequence. That is, when one of these values is given preference in the resolution of a problem, other values, such as those that may be favored by medicine or by other philosophical systems, are likely to be overridden. The values usually associated with the law include justice, as opposed to progress or efficiency; equality, as opposed to inherent differences or measures of quality; due process, as opposed to scientific proof; and individual self-determination over one's life and body, as opposed to beneficence, psychological interdependence, or communal welfare. The law's values are generally those of liberal society: personal autonomy within a setting of ordered liberty in which individuals have wide but not unlimited freedom. Especially in pluralistic democracies, the law sets boundaries on the enforcement of majoritarian morality, thereby protecting many individual choices from interference.

Not all liberal societies treat the values involved in the same way. For example, although revolutions in France and the United States in the late eighteenth century drew on the same sources in articulating basic rights, the Declaration of the Rights of Man and the Citizen in France in 1789—unlike the Declaration of Independence in the United States in 1776—emphasized that individuals have duties as well as rights (Glendon, 1991). This difference between the American and European views of rights, which persists to this day, has important implications as bioethicists attempt to address such issues as self-risking behavior and limits on the allocation of scarce community resources to health care.

Law and bioethics as a field

As a field of study, law and bioethics can be viewed from several perspectives. First, from the vantage point of a nonlawyer doing bioethics—whether at a policy level or in individual clinical situations—one needs at least some understanding of the law and legal institutions. Moreover, institutional ethics committees usually include at least one lawyer, who can provide analytic abilities as well as expertise on statutory, regulatory, and case law.

Second, "law and bioethics" is a subject of increasing interest to students, scholars, and practitioners of law. In one view, law and bioethics can be seen as a subset of health law that deals with medical decision making, genetic and reproductive technology, human subjects research, and the like. In fact, health-law casebooks today typically include chapters or sections on bioethics. But this view does not fully capture the way in which bioethics is generally conceived. By the early 1960s, long before health law emerged as a separate field, courses dealing with bioethics were being taught at American law schools, although the first casebook with the title *Cases, Materials, and Problems in Bioethics and Law* was not published until 1981 (Shapiro and Spece, 1981). That volume, like other legal books dealing with bioethical issues, not only describes "the new biology" and recounts the dilemmas engendered by modern medicine and biotechnology; it also discusses ethical theories and concepts, such as proportionality and personhood, that have crept from ethics into legal opinions. Nonetheless, law and bioethics is not just a subset of law and philosophy (or law and religion), since attention is usually focused on philosophical concepts not for their own sake but as they relate to understanding society's appropriate responses to technical developments that deeply affect people's lives and relationships. Most of the text of such books is drawn from reports of medical and scientific developments and from the rich array of relevant cases, statutes, and regulations, as well as commentaries about them (Capron and Michel, 1993).

In addition to academic attention, law and bioethics has been examined through commissions established by national and state governments through statutes and executive orders. These bodies have advanced bioethical analysis and promulgated legislative and administrative proposals (U.S. Congress, 1993).

Although people looking at the topic "law and bioethics" from the perspective of the latter field are likely to view it as a legitimate area of scholarship and practice, it is largely unrecognized among lawyers at large, who treat it neither as one of the distinctive "law and . . ." interdisciplinary fields nor as a distinct special application of law ("bioethics law") akin to employment law, sports law, and the like. The Association of American Law Schools does not categorize courses or teachers under such a heading, nor does the *Index to Legal Periodicals*, despite the existence in law journals of bioethics symposia as far back as the late 1960s (Capron and Michel, 1993). The literature of law and bioethics is not found only in law reviews or, for that matter, in scholarly journals of other disciplines such as philosophy. It also appears in medical and health-policy journals and in bioethics publications, such as the *Hastings Center Report*, the *Kennedy Institute of Ethics Journal*, and the *Journal of Law, Medicine, and Ethics*.

One important aspect of legal scholarship that can legitimately be said to be part of the "law and bioethics" literature is abortion. Recent treatments of this subject have been enriched by feminist legal analysis, which itself is greatly influenced by theorists such as Carol Gilligan and Nel Noddings, whose work concerns moral development and the different ways in which women and men may resolve moral dilemmas. This influence is perceptible not only in subjects dealing directly with women, such as abortion, maternal–fetal issues, and reproductive technology, but also in less obvious places such as analyses of ethics committees. Since feminist analysis emphasizes relationships and nurturance, it is not surprising to see that as the literature of law and bioethics moves beyond the rights orientation, feminist insights become important in developing a better legal understanding of the relationship between patients and health caregivers (Capron and Michel, 1993).

Conclusion

Scholars differ on the precise influence the law has had in shaping the content, methods, and focus of the interdisciplinary field of bioethics, but all would agree that the influence has been significant. Both those who applaud and those who bemoan the law's influence seem to agree that the law has done more than merely allow the enforcement of, or provide redress for breach of, existing moral rights possessed by participants in the health-care system. Rather, the law has—through its orientation toward rights and through the values implicit in the processes it has fostered—established new rights and preferred certain values over others. On the positive side, this has helped promote the autonomy of patients and subjects, the openness of the processes by which decisions are reached, and equality of respect and concern for all participants. On the negative side, it has diminished the sense of community and of duties that attach to rights, while increasing many providers' sense of adversariness in their relationship to patients.

In a society in which ethical standards were sufficiently complete to address even novel technical problems, widely enough shared to be accepted without question by all or nearly all persons, and consistent and coherent enough never to lead to uncertain or contradictory results, bioethics might operate with little reference to the law. As Grant Gilmore observed, "A reasonably just society will reflect its values in a reasonably just law. The better the society, the less law there will be. In Heaven there will be no law and the lion will lie down with the lamb" (Gilmore, 1975, p. 1044). Until that time, the law will continue to play a large role in bioethics—not only providing a relatively neutral means through which troubling issues can be addressed and contended points resolved in a manner that is socially sanctioned, but also shaping bioethics through its concerns for justice and fair procedures, equality, and personal self-determination.

ALEXANDER MORGAN CAPRON

Directly related to this entry are the entries BIOETHICS; LAW AND MORALITY; *and* MEDICAL ETHICS, HISTORY OF, *section on* THE AMERICAS, *article on* UNITED STATES IN THE

TWENTIETH CENTURY. *For a further discussion of topics mentioned in this entry, see the entries* AUTONOMY; CASUISTRY; FEMINISM; PATIENTS' RIGHTS; PROFESSIONAL–PATIENT RELATIONSHIP; *and* RIGHTS. *This entry will find application in the entries* BIOTECHNOLOGY; GENOME MAPPING AND SEQUENCING; HOMICIDE; INFORMED CONSENT; PERSON; *and* PUBLIC HEALTH AND THE LAW. *For a discussion of related ideas, see the entries* CARE; JUSTICE; PATIENTS' RESPONSIBILITIES; *and* RESEARCH, UNETHICAL.

Bibliography

ANNAS, GEORGE J. 1988. *Judging Medicine.* Clifton, N.J.: Humana Press. A lively collection of essays on law and the life sciences; most are focused on a noteworthy case, statute, or similar provocation.

———. 1993. *Standard of Care: The Law of American Bioethics.* New York: Oxford University Press. More of the same.

ANNAS, GEORGE J., and HEALY, JOSEPH M., JR. 1974. "The Patient Rights Advocate: Redefining the Doctor–Patient Relationship in the Hospital Context." *Vanderbilt Law Review* 27:243–269.

CAPRON, ALEXANDER MORGAN. 1994. "Why Law and the Life Sciences?" *Hastings Center Report* 24, no. 3:42–44.

CAPRON, ALEXANDER MORGAN, and MICHEL, VICKI. 1993. "Law and Bioethics." *Loyola of Los Angeles Law Review* 27 (November):25–40. Compares and contrasts law and bioethics with other interdisciplinary legal fields and traces the history of the field in teaching and scholarship.

DWORKIN, RONALD. 1977. *Taking Rights Seriously.* London: Gerald Duckworth.

ENGELHARDT, H. TRISTRAM, JR. 1986. *The Foundations of Bioethics.* New York: Oxford University Press.

GILMORE, GRANT. 1975. "The Storrs Lectures: The Age of Anxiety." *Yale Law Journal* 84, no. 5:1022–1044.

GLENDON, MARY ANN. 1991. *Rights Talk: The Impoverishment of Political Discourse.* New York: Free Press.

HOLMES, OLIVER WENDELL. 1920. "The Path of the Law." In his *Collected Legal Papers.* New York: Harcourt, Brace.

HYMAN, D. A. 1990. "How Law Killed Ethics." *Perspectives in Biology and Medicine* 34:134–151.

KATZ, JAY. 1984. *The Silent World of Doctor and Patient.* New York: Free Press. The classic account of the prospects for, and barriers to, truly informed and voluntary patient choice.

MACDONALD, MICHAEL G.; KAUFMAN, ROBERT M.; CAPRON, ALEXANDER MORGAN; and BIRNBAUM, IRWIN M., eds. 1991. *Treatise on Health Care Law.* New York: Matthew Bender. Standard treatise, updated semiannually, that includes fifteen chapters covering business issues in health care (from financing and organization to medical malpractice and insurance) and eight chapters on ethics-related issues (from confidentiality and consent to mental health, reproduction, and human subjects research).

Quinlan, In re. 1976. 70 N.J. 10, 355 A.2d 747, cert. denied sub nom. *Ginger v. New Jersey,* 429 U.S. 922.

ROTHMAN, DAVID J. 1991. *Strangers at the Bedside: A History of How Law and Bioethics Transformed Medical Decision-making.* New York: Basic Books. A historian's account of twenty-five years of change in health-care practices in light of cases on informed consent and forgoing treatment, ethics committees, government commissions, and pressure from academics and bioethics think tanks.

SCHNEIDER, CARL E. 1994. "Bioethics in the Language of the Law." *Hastings Center Report* 24, no. 4:16–22.

SHAPIRO, MICHAEL H., and SPECE, ROY G., JR. 1981. *Cases, Materials, and Problems in Bioethics and Law.* St. Paul, Minn.: West. A pioneering casebook for law school courses.

TOULMIN, STEVEN. 1982. "How Medicine Saved the Life of Ethics." *Perspectives in Life and Medicine* 25:736–750.

U.S. CONGRESS. OFFICE OF TECHNOLOGY ASSESSMENT. 1993. *Biomedical Ethics in U.S. Public Policy.* Washington, D.C.: Author. Describes and assesses government efforts to study and make recommendations about ethical issues in medicine and research; includes an appendix on activities outside the United States.

VEBLEN, THORSTEIN. 1965. [1918]. *The Higher Learning in America: A Memorandum on the Conduct of Universities by Business Men.* New York: B. W. Huebsch.

LAW AND ENVIRONMENTAL POLICY

See ENVIRONMENTAL POLICY AND LAW.

LAW AND GENETICS

See GENETICS AND THE LAW.

LAW AND MORALITY

Bioethical problems are often discussed in legal as well as in moral contexts. Lawyers as well as ethicists are involved with such questions as abortion, euthanasia, and experimentation upon human beings. This is not surprising; the law is seriously concerned with protecting such basic rights as life, bodily integrity, and privacy— the rights involved in these ethical questions.

The overlap between law and morality has been a source of the substantial debate about the relation between law and morality, a debate not confined to the bioethical context. It is best divided into two main issues, although the discussion of these issues often overlaps: (1) What, if any, bearing does the moral status of a rule have on its status as a law? (2) To what extent, if any, should the legal system be used to enforce moral perspectives?

Moral status and legal status

Western legal thought has been dominated by a natural-law tradition. There are many variants of this tradition, and the differences among them will be discussed below; what they have in common is a belief in a body of laws governing all people at all times, and in a source for those laws other than the customs and institutions of a given society. Such beliefs are frequently accompanied by the additional beliefs that no society is authorized to create laws that conflict directly with natural laws, and that any such conflicting laws may therefore be invalid. In short, the natural-law tradition asserts the existence of a set of laws whose status as laws is based upon their moral status.

The beginning of this tradition lies in the ancient world. Aristotle (384–322 B.C.E.) drew a distinction between the part of justice that is natural and should have the same force everywhere, and the part that is legal and has its force only in those places where it has been adopted by the people who live there. That distinction was developed extensively by the Stoics, who emphasized two further points about natural justice: that it is based upon right reason and that it is in agreement with nature. Cicero (106–43 B.C.E.), whose legal writings are based upon the Stoic tradition, emphasized the claim that no legislation can alter the validity of natural laws, which remain binding on all people. Some of these ideas were incorporated into Roman law, and the later Roman lawyers probably identified *jus naturale* (the philosophical notion of natural law) with *jus gentium* (a system of laws that had developed in the Roman world and governed the relations among free men independently of their nationality). This identification strengthened the idea of natural law as universal law.

These classical ideas gave rise to a number of different natural-law traditions, the two most important of which are the religious tradition culminating in the writings of Saint Thomas Aquinas (1224–1274) and the secular tradition, exemplified by Hugo Grotius (1583–1645) and John Locke (1632–1704).

Saint Thomas Aquinas defined a law as an ordinance of reason for the common good, promulgated by the individual who has the care of the community. He then distinguished four types of laws: eternal laws, natural laws, human laws, and divine laws. The eternal laws are laws promulgated by God on the basis of divine reason. The natural laws are the eternal laws implanted by God in human beings, in that human beings are naturally inclined toward their proper acts and ends. In short, Saint Thomas postulated an eternal, unchanging set of laws implanted by God in human beings and knowable by reason. Human laws are valid only insofar as they do not conflict with divinely promulgated, unchanging laws. Valid human laws either are conclusions drawn from the basic natural laws or are determinations of details left undetermined by the natural laws.

The natural-law theories of Grotius and Locke also contain theological references, and Saint Thomas does emphasize the rational basis of natural law. Nevertheless, Grotius and Locke represent a different tradition of natural law, one that puts more emphasis on natural law as rationally derivable than on natural law as divinely ordained. In addition, their tradition, especially in the writings of Locke, puts great emphasis on the natural law's protection of natural rights, rights that all human beings have independently of the state and its laws. Locke explicitly drew the conclusion that a state loses its legitimacy insofar as its laws are in violation of natural rights, such as the right to life or liberty.

These natural-law traditions continue to influence discussions about the relation between the law and bioethics. Writers influenced by the theological version of the natural-law tradition continue to argue that any valid law must be in conformity with the divinely ordained natural law. Thus, many Roman Catholic writers (e.g., Grisez and Boyle, 1979) argue that there must be civil laws prohibiting abortion and euthanasia because those procedures are in conflict with the natural law. To those who would object that this is an illegitimate use of the law to enforce morality, these writers reply that it is the very nature of legitimate law to prohibit such activities. The most important recent reiteration of this view is found in the 1987 statement from the Congregation for the Doctrine of the Faith entitled *Instruction on Respect for Human Life in its Origin and on the Dignity of Procreation*. Having argued that abortion from the moment of conception and various forms of assisted reproduction are immoral, the Congregation goes on to claim that there must be laws prohibiting both because "The task of the civil law is to ensure the common good of people through the recognition of and the defence of fundamental rights and through the promotion of peace and of public morality" (1987, p. 35).

Writers influenced by the ideas of natural-rights thinkers like Locke continue to argue that no purported law is legitimate if it allows the violation of the basic rights of human beings. This type of argumentation is particularly prevalent in countries such as the United States, where the courts possess the ability to declare laws unconstitutional when they infringe upon basic human rights. U.S. Supreme Court decisions from *Griswold v. Connecticut* (1965), in which the Supreme Court ruled that a Connecticut law prohibiting the use of contraceptives is unconstitutional, to *Roe v. Wade* (1973), in which the Supreme Court ruled that women have a constitutional right to abortions at least in the first two trimesters, have indicated that jurists are prepared to extend those rights to include ones not explicitly mentioned in the Constitution, suggesting to many—but by no means all—commentators that they are implicitly invoking some natural-law theory of rights.

The natural-law tradition has not been universally accepted. There has also been a long tradition of thinkers, dating back to antiquity, who have insisted that the only laws that exist are those adopted by a given society, and that there is no necessary connection between the legal status of a law and its moral status. Defenders of this position, the position of legal positivism, are not opposed to the moral criticism of individual laws and of whole legal institutions; positivists often advocate changes in the law on the basis of moral considerations. But the positivists insist that an immoral law, however much it should be changed, remains valid as a law until it is repealed by the society's appropriate social mechanisms.

Jeremy Bentham (1748–1832) and John Austin (1790–1859) were the two most influential proponents of this view, although earlier figures like Jean Bodin (1530–1596) and Thomas Hobbes (1588–1679) should also be mentioned. The basic thesis of positivism has often been conflated with another of Austin's theories, the imperative theory of law, which held that law is the command of the sovereign. Since this latter theory has not survived critical examination, it is crucial to distinguish it from the basic theme of positivism: that what the law is, is a separate question from what the law ought to be. H. L. A. Hart, the most influential contemporary positivist, placed particular emphasis on drawing this distinction.

Some legal positivists have taken their view to mean that laws must be obeyed no matter how immoral they are. But the most important positivists, Bentham and Austin, clearly argued that there are circumstances in which an immoral law should be violated despite its status as a law; this of course weakens the force of the claim that a law retains its status as a law despite its immorality.

In any case, legal positivists insist that questions about the relation between law and morality must be settled independently of questions about what the law is. The legal status of a rule is independent of its moral status. This leads us, therefore, to the second of our questions: When ought the law to be used to enforce certain moral positions?

Use of the legal system to enforce morality

The law is clearly used on some occasions to enforce moral viewpoints. We believe that murder is wrong and that the coercive mechanism of the law should be used to prevent murders. However, even if we believe that euthanasia is wrong or that one should come to the aid of others in distress, should the law be used to enforce these beliefs?

John Stuart Mill (1806–1873), in his classic *On Liberty* (1859), advocated the liberal answer to that question—that society should use the coercive mechanisms of the law only to prevent actions that harm someone other than the performer or another who has consented to the performance of the action. In other words, Mill argued that the social enforcement of morality was inappropriate when only the agent or others who had consented would be harmed. In his elaboration of this position in *The Moral Limits of the Criminal Law* (1984–1988), the most important elaboration of the liberal position in the twentieth century, Joel Feinberg has argued that actions might be criminalized if they were profoundly offensive, even if not harmful, to others.

Mill's followers have therefore opposed the existence of laws creating "victimless crimes," among which they have included laws against suicide and voluntary euthanasia, unless such laws are required to protect against mistake and abuse. They have also approved of court decisions that allow rational adults to refuse medical treatment on religious or on other grounds, even though the refusal would result in their dying.

A number of points must be kept in mind about the liberal position. First, it does not require legislation prohibiting all actions that harm others. Whether there should be legislation will depend upon such factors as the existence of harmful consequences and the possibility of enforcement. All that the liberal position entails is that such actions, because they harm others, are candidates for appropriate legal prohibition.

Second, actions that harm others may be prohibited legally, even when others consent, if their consent is not valid. This point is extremely important in connection with legislation governing medical experimentation. Consider, for example, the problem of experiments on children, where the experiments are not primarily intended to aid in their therapy and where there are potential hazards. Given that the consent of the children may not count if they are young enough, and given that the relevance of parental consent is unclear, Mill's principles could allow for enforcing some socially determined moral standards in this area. In fact, the 1993 U.S. regulations on research involving children enforce a very strict moral standard; the risks must represent only a minor increase over minimal risk, and the information must be of vital importance.

Third, this liberal position is not identical either with the English common-law tradition or with American constitutional law. Both have allowed for legal prohibitions that are unacceptable in the liberal framework. For example, the consent of the person killed in an act of voluntary euthanasia has been, at least until the early 1990s, no defense against a charge of murder in either legal system. Some of the language in the U.S. Supreme Court case *Cruzan v. Missouri Department of Health*

(1990) suggests that many judges are now prepared to say that the right of a competent adult to refuse life-preserving therapy is a protected constitutional right, a result that liberals would applaud. Nothing in the text of this decision, however, suggests the extension of that view to assisted suicide or voluntary active euthanasia.

Adherents of the liberal approach have in recent years expanded upon it and modified it in a number of ways. One question that has received considerable attention is determining whose consent is valid. The current understanding of mental illness makes it very difficult to accept a sharp dichotomy between those competent to consent and those incompetent, since there are many degrees of mental disturbance. Some (including Buchanan and Brock, 1989) have responded that the standard for competency must be more demanding when the decision is more momentous. Others (including Brody, 1988) insist that we must recognize that competent decisions may be overridden when the costs to the individual are great and the person's decision making is impaired, even if he or she is somewhat competent.

Another question that has received considerable attention is the extent to which society can legitimately use the law temporarily to prevent an individual from carrying out certain decisions, to see whether the individual will change his or her mind or whether the choice is truly voluntary. Within the liberal framework, could we legally require, for example, a period between a request for voluntary euthanasia and the implementation of that request? Following Joel Feinberg, many liberal authors have allowed for this form of weak or soft paternalism.

A third question that has received considerable attention is the legitimacy of legally imposing certain positive moral duties. Mill was primarily concerned with challenging the legitimacy of laws prohibiting immoral actions; it is unclear how he would have dealt with Good Samaritan laws—laws that would, for example, require trained medical personnel to come to the aid of accident victims. Would such laws that require positive actions, and not mere forbearances, be a legitimate legal enforcement of morality?

A final question that has received considerable attention is whether society can pass laws designed to prevent harm to animals. If it could, this would markedly change the liberal attitude toward laws governing experimentation on animals. Peter Singer (1979) and Tom Regan (1983) are two liberal authors who have advocated the extension of the liberal tradition in this way.

From its very beginning, the liberal tradition has had its critics. Writers in the natural-law tradition objected, of course, to the liberal presupposition that the moral and legal status of rules could be separated. But even some of those who agreed with positivism have argued that there is a wider scope for legislating morality than the scope allowed by Mill.

James Fitzjames Stephen (1829–1894), in his influential *Liberty, Equality, Fraternity* (1873), argued that one of the purposes of both the criminal and the civil law is to promote and encourage virtue while discouraging vice. Stephen conceded that certain areas of morality could not be dealt with by the law because the relevant laws could not be enforced without destroying privacy and individual rights; he claimed, however, that there are many areas of morality that should be treated by the law despite Mill's strictures. This point of view has been extended by Patrick Devlin, a distinguished English jurist. Devlin contends that the continued existence and strength of a society require a common moral code. There is, therefore, a social interest in the preservation of such a code, and it is at least sometimes appropriate to enforce part of the code through the use of the law. Devlin limits his conclusions to cases where this enforcement of morality will not violate human rights. He applied this approach to English abortion legislation in the 1960s. He argued that the severe punishment of the illegal abortionist cannot be justified on the grounds that such a person poses a threat to the health of the mother, since that threat exists primarily because the abortionist's activities are illegal. Instead, such laws can be explained and justified only as an attempt by society to protect its fundamental views on sexuality and on human life.

A number of recent authors (Bellah et al., 1985; MacIntyre, 1981; Sandel, 1982) have emphasized, in different ways, the importance of communities and a sense of community values, and they have seen this as standing in opposition to the liberal account. This new communitarianism no doubt has significant implications for the legislation of morality in areas related to bioethics, but those implications have not yet been studied systematically.

There are, then, a number of differing systematic approaches to the question of which aspects of morality should be enforced legally. In addition to those systematic approaches, various authors and courts have suggested additional considerations that must be weighed in deciding whether legally to enforce moral standards. Among the most prominent of the considerations are the following.

1. *Respect for differing views in a pluralistic society.* In the 1973 discussion of abortion statutes in *Roe v. Wade*, the U.S. Supreme Court suggested that legislation enforcing a moral viewpoint is inappropriate when those who are experts in the relevant area disagree as to the legitimacy of that viewpoint. This principle is in keeping with a wider movement against legislating disputed moral positions. A number of important considerations support this mode of thought. To begin with, people

seem to have a right to follow their own conscience rather than to be compelled to follow the conscience of the rest of society. Moreover, there are tremendous detrimental consequences for a society when many of its citizens feel that the law is being used to coerce them into following the moral views of others. Such considerations are even more important in societies where there are substantial moral disagreements among the citizens. One author who has particularly stressed the importance of respecting differing views in a pluralistic society is H. Tristram Engelhardt, Jr. (1986).

2. *Respect for privacy.* There are laws that cannot be enforced without infringing the privacy of the citizens involved. Following a long tradition that appealed to this point, the U.S. Supreme Court suggested (in *Griswold* v. *Connecticut,* 1965), that such laws are illegitimate because of the inability to enforce them in an acceptable fashion. For that reason, the Court declared unconstitutional a Connecticut law prohibiting the use (and not merely the production) of contraceptive devices. It has also been argued that laws regulating the patient-doctor relation are inappropriate because they can be enforced only by the state's entering into and examining a relation that must be private. Many authors have criticized the U.S. "Baby-Doe" law (P.L. 98-457, 1984), which limits on moral grounds the decision-making authority of parents and physicians with regard to severely disabled newborns, because it involves state intrusion into a private relation.

3. *The consequences of passing such a law.* It is sometimes argued that certain moral positions ought not to be enforced legally because the laws that codify them will be violated anyway, and their surreptitious violation will lead to many tragic results. Thus, it has been argued that laws prohibiting abortion only result in women's seeking unsafe, illegal, and very dangerous abortions. Again, it has been argued that laws prohibiting voluntary euthanasia or allowing to die only result in surreptitious acts of voluntary euthanasia and in informal decisions to "let the patient die," acts and decisions that can be abused. Many studies of such abuses (by, e.g., Bedell and Delbanco, 1984; Evans and Brody, 1985) led in the 1980s to more formal policies governing such decisions.

Considerations 1–3 are reasons why certain actions should not be illegal, whether or not they are immoral. Most authors would agree that these legitimate considerations must be balanced against others that argue for the criminalization of the acts in question. These include the extent of the harmful consequences of the actions in question and the extent to which they involve infringements of the rights of others.

There are, in addition, considerations for making actions illegal even if they are not immoral. Two deserve special notice:

4. *The difficulty of distinguishing between fraudulent and legitimate cases.* Suppose that there are no moral objections to voluntary euthanasia. Some have argued that it would will be wise legally to prohibit such killings because it is difficult to distinguish cases of honest requests from cases of consent obtained by subtle fraud or duress. Again, some have argued that despite the moral permissibility of experimenting upon consenting adults, there should be laws prohibiting experiments conducted upon prison inmates, because one cannot tell when the consent of such inmates is truly voluntary.

5. *Slippery-slope arguments.* It is often argued that legalizing certain morally acceptable actions would later lead to irresistible pressures for legalizing immoral actions, and that the only way to avoid sliding down this slippery slope is to prohibit even the acceptable actions. Thus, it has been argued that voluntary euthanasia should be illegal, even if morally acceptable, as a way of ensuring against the later legalization of involuntary euthanasia. Naturally, both of these factors must be weighed against the possible desirable results of legalizing the morally acceptable actions.

Conclusion

It is clear, then, that there are no easy answers to questions about the relation between law and morality. There are strong considerations favoring legal positivism, but there are other considerations favoring a natural-law doctrine. And even if one is a legal positivist, there are conflicting considerations that one has to weigh in deciding on the appropriate relation between one's moral code and society's legal code.

Baruch A. Brody

Directly related to this entry are the entries Rights, *article on* rights in bioethics; *and* Natural Law. *For a further discussion of topics mentioned in this entry, see the entries* Justice; Medical Ethics, History of, *section on* europe, *subsection on* ancient and medieval; *and* Paternalism. *This entry will find application in the entries* Public Health and the Law, *article on* legal moralism and public health; *and* Substance Abuse, *article on* legal control of harmful substances. *For a discussion of related ideas, see the entry* Ethics, *articles on* social and political theories, *and* religion and morality. *Other relevant material may be found under* Law and Bioethics.

Bibliography

Aquinas, Thomas. 1945. *Summa theologica,* I-II, 90–95. *Basic Writings of Saint Thomas Aquinas,* vol. 2, pp. 747–789. Edited by Anton C. Pegis. New York: Random House.

AUSTIN, JOHN. 1832. *The Province of Jurisprudence Determined.* London: J. Murray.

BEDELL, SUSANNA, and DELBANCO, THOMAS. 1984. "Choices About Cardiopulmonary Resuscitation in the Hospital: When Do Physicians Talk with Patients?" *New England Journal of Medicine* 310, no. 17:1089–1093.

BELLAH, ROBERT; MADSEN, RICHARD; SULLIVAN, WILLIAM; SWIDLER, ANN; and TIPTON, STEVEN. 1985. *Habits of the Heart: Individualism and Commitment in American Life.* Berkeley: University of California Press.

BRODY, BARUCH. 1988. *Life and Death Decision Making.* New York: Oxford University Press.

BUCHANAN, ALLEN, and BROCK, DAN. 1989. *Deciding for Others.* New York: Cambridge University Press.

CONGREGATION FOR THE DOCTRINE OF THE FAITH. 1987. *Instruction on Respect for Human Life in Its Origin and on the Dignity of Procreation: Replies to Certain Questions of the Day.* Vatican City: Author.

DEVLIN, PATRICK. 1965. *The Enforcement of Morals.* London: Oxford University Press.

ENGELHARDT, H. TRISTRAM, JR. 1986. *The Foundations of Bioethics.* New York: Oxford University Press.

EVANS, ANDREW, and BRODY, BARUCH. 1985. "The Do-Not-Resuscitate Order in Teaching Hospitals." *Journal of the American Medical Association* 253, no. 15:2236–2239.

FEINBERG, JOEL. 1984–1988. *The Moral Limits of the Criminal Law.* 4 vols. New York: Oxford University Press.

FRIEDRICH, CARL JOACHIM. 1958. *The Philosophy of Law in Historical Perspective.* Chicago: University of Chicago Press.

FULLER, LON L. 1964. *The Morality of Law.* Storrs Lectures on Jurisprudence, 1963. New Haven, Conn.: Yale University Press.

GIERKE, OTTO FRIEDRICH VON. 1957. *Natural Law and the Theory of Society, 1500 to 1800: With a Lecture on the Ideas of Natural Law and Humanity by Ernest Troeltsch.* Translated by Ernest Barker. Boston: Beacon Press.

GRISEZ, GERMAIN, and BOYLE, JOSEPH M. 1979. *Life and Death with Liberty and Justice: A Contribution to the Euthanasia Debate.* Notre Dame, Ind.: University of Notre Dame Press.

GROTIUS, HUGO. 1925. *De jure belli ac pacis.* Vol. 2, *The Translation.* Translated by Francis W. Kelsey. Oxford: At the Clarendon Press.

HART, HERBERT L. A. 1958. "Positivism and the Separation of Law and Morals." *Harvard Law Review* 71, no. 4: 593–629.

———. 1963. *Law, Liberty, and Morality: The Harry Camp Lectures.* Stanford, Calif.: Stanford University Press.

LOCKE, JOHN. 1960. *Two Treatises of Government.* Edited by Peter Laslett. Cambridge: At the University Press.

MACINTYRE, ALASDAIR. 1981. *After Virtue: A Study in Moral Theology.* Notre Dame, Ind.: University of Notre Dame Press.

MILL, JOHN STUART. 1859. *On Liberty.* London: J. W. Parker.

PACKER, HERBERT L. 1968. *The Limits of the Criminal Sanction.* Stanford, Calif.: Stanford University Press.

PASSERIN D'ENTRÈVES, ALESSANDRO. 1951. *Natural Law: An Introduction to Legal Philosophy.* London: Hutchinson.

Protection of Human Subjects. 45 CFR 46.

REGAN, TOM. 1983. *The Case for Animal Rights.* Berkeley and Los Angeles: University of California Press.

SANDEL, MICHAEL. 1982. *Liberalism and the Limits of Justice.* Cambridge: At the University Press.

SINGER, PETER. 1979. *Practical Ethics.* Cambridge: At the University Press.

STEPHEN, JAMES FITZJAMES. 1873. *Liberty, Equality, Fraternity.* London: Smith, Elder.

WILLIAMS, GLANVILLE. 1957. *The Sanctity of Life and the Criminal Law.* New York: Alfred A. Knopf.

LAW AND PUBLIC HEALTH

See PUBLIC HEALTH AND THE LAW.

LICENSING, DISCIPLINE, AND REGULATION IN THE HEALTH PROFESSIONS

Licensure is "the process by which an agency of government grants permission to persons meeting predetermined qualifications to engage in a given occupation"; certification is "the process by which a non-governmental agency or association grants recognition to an individual who has met certain predetermined qualifications specified by that agency or institution" (Welch, 1976, p. 179). The purpose of licensure, regulation, and discipline is to protect the public at large; the assumption that grounds these practices is that government and nongovernmental institutions are competent to judge how such protection will be accomplished.

Background

Public efforts to regulate the health professions, especially by imposing restrictions on those who shall be allowed to practice them, go back to the Babylonian emperor Hammurabi. Rules for medical practice existed in ancient Greece and tenth-century Baghdad. By the Middle Ages in Europe, it was customary for civil powers to demand a university education, examination, and experience as conditions for permission to practice medicine. In this period the first professional societies were founded, modeled on the merchant guilds (Gross, 1984, p. 51). University and guild combined to link education to licensing, government permission to practice.

The first licensing statutes were passed in the American colonies in the seventeenth century, although not until the eighteenth century did the statutes seek to restrict practice. Eliot Freidson (1970) claims that medicine did not emerge as a consulting, as opposed to a teaching, practice until the late nineteenth and early twentieth centuries. Throughout the two millennia since Hippocrates, the medical elite created by education and licensed by the state was supplemented by a vast number of unlicensed healers, mostly women (generally barred from medicine), who treated the common folk.

The trend to state regulation, endorsement, and protection of the health professions suffered a brief hiatus in the nineteenth century in the United States, a deliberate experiment in egalitarian deregulation following from a democratic belief that the common folk were as good as the educated elite in most matters. The experiment was abandoned later in the century, as Texas passed a medical practice act in 1873, California followed suit in 1875, and by 1905, thirty-nine states licensed physicians (Council of State Governments, 1952). Nurses formed a national professional association in 1896; by 1926 forty states required licenses of nurses.

The trend is not, however, universal. Professional recruitment, standard setting, and discipline can be carried out by professional groups and associations without the protection of the state. Typically, groups of serious practitioners band together, agree to set standards, and develop informal review procedures for adherence to standards—for members only. Professional ethics and oaths, including professional standards of education and compensation, can be enforced by the professional association alone, and in some cases (various psychological and holistic health professions, for example) the process goes no further. In several healing professions, there is no regulation beyond that of the voluntary association; the only penalty for professional wrongdoing, if it is discovered, is loss of membership in that association.

Regulation tends to be reserved for those health professions that are widely perceived to have powers the abuse of which can lead to public injury. At one time, only the profession of medicine was included in that category; now it has extended through dentistry, nursing, pharmacy, and others (close to fifty, on one count; Council of State Governments and National Clearinghouse on Licensure, Enforcement and Regulation, 1987), on a state-by-state basis (naturopathy, for instance, is regulated in some states but not in others). Licensure varies in kind as well as in range: As of 1973, nine states still had "permissive" licensing for nurses—an unlicensed nurse could practice without hindrance as long as she did not claim to be licensed. "Scope-of-practice statutes" ordinarily accompany licensure, defining the procedures for which the practitioner is licensed.

The limited competence of the state

Well established as the custom is, there is a certain awkwardness of fit between professional standards and state enforcement. The request by the health professions for state protection of their monopoly is not implausible: While the state can play little part in instructing or defining the work of the professions, it certainly has always

had as part of its police power the protection of the public from outright dangers to health, including health frauds—quacks, charlatans, and sincere professionals whose education was simply inadequate to their tasks (*Dent v. State of West Virginia*, 1889). But a profession is defined in large part by its esoteric knowledge: Only professionals can set professional standards, determine when they have been violated, and, by extension, determine the sanction that would be appropriate as a punishment.

The result is that the public ends up enforcing rules that only a private association can set, presumably for its own benefit as much as for the public good. Nor is it clear that licensing in general, especially in the context of rigid scope-of-practice statutes, is in the public interest. The costs of licensing will normally be passed along to the consumer in the form of higher costs, and the license requirement restricts entry into the profession to those who can afford the initial outlay. The scope-of-practice acts make sure that auxiliary professions, with less expensive preparation and lower fees, cannot perform certain procedures that they may in fact be perfectly competent to perform (Council of State Governments and National Clearinghouse on Licensure, Enforcement and Regulation, 1987). Built into the arrangement, if it is to be tolerable, is a strong presumption of altruism on the part of the professional and trust on the part of the public. Let either fail, and the system is in danger.

Professional exclusion: The Flexner report

One of the most worrisome aspects of that arrangement is its systematic historical exclusion of certain groups of health professionals, especially women. Until recently women have been the traditional healers in many cultures, and have had exclusive charge over pregnancy and childbirth. The systematic exclusion of the women by the organized men, regardless of the women's competence or empirical evidence of their effectiveness—especially the use of medical credentialing to discredit and restrict the activities of midwives—was a clear and blatant abuse of the system described here, and caused one of the more serious cracks in the edifice of trust (Gross, 1984).

In 1906 Abraham Flexner, an educator, obtained a grant from the Carnegie Foundation to review the quality of medical schools. When his report was published in 1910, it revealed wide discrepancies among the 155 schools studied, and produced a strong impetus to regulate education for the medical profession at the state and federal levels. Having no independent standards of their own, nor any idea of how to develop them, the states appealed to the American Medical Association's (AMA) Council on Medical Education, which set new standards for accreditation of the medical schools.

Physicians also staffed the state licensing boards. The consequence of this major public intervention in the health-care professions was that by the mid-1920s, the AMA had a virtual monopoly, guarding the gate to the medical profession at several levels: admission to medical school, choice of specialty, obtaining of license to practice.

Such a state-sponsored monopoly is clearly subject to abuse (one commentary on the process was aptly entitled *Of Foxes and Hen Houses* [Gross, 1984])—but it was widely imitated as succeeding levels of health professions sought and obtained state endorsement and protection. By tradition, the major regulatory role in the United States is played by the states, and the licensing laws are typically administered by state agencies and boards dominated by professionals.

Disciplinary procedures

Disciplinary procedures responding to charges of fraud, incompetence, or malpractice occur at several levels. A certain amount of discipline is carried out by the professional association and is entirely a private matter among the professionals. At the state level, the procedure for disciplining delinquent practitioners varies, but generally it requires that some aggrieved party—a dissatisfied patient, a cost-conscious insurance company, or the plaintiff's lawyer in a malpractice case—register a complaint with the disciplinary board of the state. The agency in charge of these matters will investigate the case, assemble evidence, schedule a hearing, make a finding, and recommend appropriate action. The action can range from dismissing the complaint or requiring some hours of community service, to removing a license. Increasingly, part of the decision is a refresher course in medical ethics.

The accused practitioner must consent to the penalty. Short of actual revocation of license, if the penalty is completed without further incident, the practitioner will be restored to good standing at the end of it. When the license is revoked, that fact is recorded and circulated through the National Practitioner Data Bank, where misconduct and malpractice findings are logged. The data bank is available to regulators in all fifty states. So far, only physicians and dentists are in the data bank; eventually it will include all the health professions and practitioners.

Consumers' protest

The federal government has been active in the regulation of health matters for most of the twentieth century. The Pure Food and Drug Act, under which all drugs are approved for sale in the United States, was passed in 1906; since then the federal government has taken an active role in protecting occupational health and public accountability. Early in the 1970s, corresponding to the general wave of public skepticism regarding professional and corporate claims of authority and trustworthiness, a citizen/consumer rebellion turned on the health professions. Seminal works by Eliot Freidson and others spearheaded a literature of public protest against professional privilege, and urged vigorous and vigilant oversight of the health professions, medicine in particular.

The protest tended to portray state legislatures as weak, ignorant, or pawns of the powerful professions, and urged a drastic widening of the federal oversight function. Such expansion was made possible by the passage of Medicare legislation (1965), followed by Medicaid and other programs that cast the federal government in the role of major funder of health care. A *Proposal for Credentialing Health Manpower* (Cohen, 1976) recommended that a national certification commission be established "to develop, evaluate and oversee national standards" for agencies that certify health-care personnel. The National Commission for Health Certifying Agencies was formed on that recommendation, charged with developing universal standards for credentialing health-care personnel. This effort was supported through the 1980s by the U.S. Department of Health and Human Services, through the Health Resources and Services Administration (Council of State Governments and National Clearinghouse on Licensure, Enforcement and Regulation, 1987).

The origins of consumerism are generally attributed to Ralph Nader, whose investigations of the safety of the American automobile alerted a generation to the possibility that the goods and services available from the trusted providers of the American marketplace might not be as good as they were claimed to be. A Nader offshoot, the Public Citizen Health Research Group of Washington, D.C., maintains that the disciplinary and regulatory powers and laws presently available to the American public are completely inadequate to the task. These groups have changed the broad direction of legislative action. In the era of consumerism, the people's authority exercised at the state or federal level now protects the consuming public from the professional provider instead of ranging itself with the professional against fraudulent competition.

In a return to the democratic assumptions of the nineteenth century, the mantle of legal and moral credibility as protector of the public has passed from the profession to the elected legislature: In the areas of technical expertise and professional wisdom, as well as in the areas of economic self-interest, the American voters are now assumed to be the best guardians of their own interests. Patients' autonomy vis-à-vis their physicians has been generalized to public autonomy vis-à-vis the profession as a whole.

Typical of consumerist initiatives in health care is congressional action requiring nationwide licensing of nurses' aides. The bill, put forward by Congressman Henry Waxman, was demanded by, among others, the American Association of Retired Persons, an interest group of the elderly with a strong stake in the conduct of nursing homes and chronic-care facilities heavily populated by elderly patients. Its passage at the federal level made it immune to the objections of state organizations of such facilities. Now the states must implement it.

Also typical are the regulations proceeding from the work of the National Commission for the Protection of Human Subjects of Biomedical and Behavioral Research, established by Congress in the 1970s in response to claims that patients were being abused by their physicians in pursuit of scientific research (and that aborted fetuses were being used for research). The commission's work resulted in an immense number of federal regulations to protect the rights of human subjects of clinical research, including the formation of institutional review boards in any institution where such research is carried on, charged with reviewing all research that receives any federal money (in effect, all research in the institution).

A third example of such initiatives is the Patient Self-Determination Act, passed as part of the Omnibus Budget Reconciliation Act of 1990, which requires that all health-care providers inform all adult in-patients of their rights to refuse treatment; to submit to the provider a document, generally known as a "living will," specifying their desires regarding treatment or nontreatment should they become terminally ill and unable to give consent to treatment on their own; and to appoint any adult to speak for them to ensure that the living will's instructions are carried out, should they become unable to speak for themselves.

The contrast between profession-oriented and consumer-oriented approaches can be seen in the norms governing confidentiality of investigations of professionals charged with incompetence or negligence. If government is to protect the profession, then the identity of credentialed professionals who are under investigation for wrongdoing must be kept secret until it is determined that they are unsalvageable in the profession, so as to maintain their good name and practice. Consumer advocate groups, on the contrary, demand that the names of accused professionals be made public as soon as the investigation begins, so that the public may take steps to protect themselves.

Rejoinders to consumerism in health care have come from diverse sources. One very influential reply, from the perspective of the medical profession, is Charles Bosk's account of a surgical training program, *Forgive and Remember* (1979). In the training of surgical residents, as chronicled by Bosk, supervision was strict, the patients' interests were paramount, and discipline was swift, although generally informal, and highly effective. Bosk found in place an unwritten but well-understood set of rules, rapidly internalized by all surgical

residents as a condition of success as surgeons, and regularly enforced at all levels. The suggestion that emerged, although not explicitly, was that bureaucratic regulations could not possibly be as effective as the present method of professional socialization in producing the surgeons we want and need—at least at the level of the elite practitioners. On the other side, regulation has been attacked by libertarian theorists, arguing that any regulation puts an artificial and uneconomic barrier in the free market.

Alternatives to licensing can easily be imagined: Gross (1984) outlines a system of state registration of unlicensed practitioners whose competence is determined by the consuming public on the basis of full disclosure of background and skills. Given full disclosure and the absence of coercion, on the principle of freedom of contract, any two persons of mature years should be free to make between themselves any contract for goods and services. The point is primarily theoretical but of very wide application: If accepted, this doctrine would abolish a few dozen federal agencies and all state licensing and disciplinary functions. Concretely, this doctrine has been invoked as primary in cases where patients request drugs not approved for distribution or sale, like Laetrile and other unproven cancer remedies, or the experimental drugs currently being tested for use against the acquired immunodeficiency syndrome (AIDS).

Problems

Notorious problems attend the disciplining of professionals for negligent, fraudulent, or otherwise unacceptable conduct. It is not the wealth or social status of the offenders that obstructs justice; we have no trouble trying these people for common crimes. But we bring conflicting expectations to professional discipline—that the profession will discipline itself; that the hospitals will take responsibility for the competence of the professionals on their staffs; that state agencies will police the health marketplace and arrest wrongdoers; and that the federal government will use its power to withhold Medicaid reimbursement to drive crooks and incompetents from the profession; and that since the contract between professional and patient is a private one, private litigation is the best protector of rights.

The end product of these conflicting expectations is a nightmare of overlapping jurisdictions. No one is clearly in a position to initiate action. But once a health professional has been accused of misconduct, every agency—federal, state, or professional—involved at all with the profession typically attempts to get into the case. Routine involvement in all cases is the only way they can ensure public perception of their importance and continued public support. Often public agencies are alerted to the possibility of professional (usually medical) incompetence by private lawyers preparing malpractice or negligence suits, since public citation will strengthen their case. When all the agencies take off after a physician at once—threatening loss of hospital privileges and/or the right to prescribe drugs, fines for incorrect billing of Medicaid and insurance companies, and devastating publicity for the whole affair—the result can be personally and professionally catastrophic, and quite unjust. On the other hand, complaints continue, occasionally on the front pages of our newspapers, that physicians work essentially without supervision, that it is very difficult for patients to criticize or check their work, and that bad physicians are practicing, able to evade all scrutiny.

Not all problems are technical or supervision problems. There are conflicting principles at the root of some of them. One of the most common is the conflict between patient autonomy and the protection of patient welfare. If adults regularly choose treatments or interventions that serve very little medical purpose (liposuction, cosmetic surgery or implants, or experimental drugs may serve as examples), who shall be held responsible for the undesirable outcomes? To what extent shall we forbid the medical profession, by law, to provide such services?

Another typical conflict is that between professional salvage and patient protection. A health professional's training is long, difficult, and expensive, and society cannot afford to lose the investment that it represents. There is good reason to try to rehabilitate a health professional who has mismanaged his or her practice. The problem lies in deciding which lapses are remediable and which are not. There is always a danger that the professional who has offended once will do it again, no matter how tight the supervision. The problem is compounded by the need, given the nature of the professional–client relationship in health care, to keep the professional's problems absolutely confidential. Typically, if the physician or other practitioner is "impaired"—psychologically incapacitated; found not guilty of a crime by reason of insanity; alcoholic; drug abusing; or otherwise unable to practice until a course of therapy has been completed—the records will be kept confidential while he or she undergoes therapy. Should he or she leave therapy or breach other agreements (by testing positive for controlled substances, for instance), the matter becomes one of "misconduct" rather than "impairment," and is no longer confidential.

The future

In the future, licensing, regulation, and disciplinary action will no doubt respond to greater consumer insistence on quality and cost control, thus limiting professional autonomy still further. Two major trends can be discerned.

First, higher and more public standards for certification can be expected. Even now, nonprofessional members have been added to licensing boards in most states (Council of State Governments and National Clearinghouse on Licensure, Enforcement and Regulation, 1987). It is likely that a requirement that health professionals be recertified at some point or at regular intervals in their careers will become part of the law. The public is acutely aware that the scientific foundations of health care are rapidly changing, and that professional education has a half-life of under ten years—five, in the case of certain medical specialties. Mandatory continuing-education requirements are already part of the licensing laws for medicine and nursing; it is not a large step from there to provisions for occasional retesting. Some sources foresee that "good moral character" requirements—already part of the licensing statutes in most states but undefined—will be made more precise and more vigorously enforced (Council of State Governments and National Clearinghouse on Licensure, Enforcement and Regulation, 1987).

Second, there will be a major trend in the direction of cost control. There is a widely held perception that health costs are too high and out of control. Major initiatives to limit them are expected, either by explicit rationing of public funds or by ingenious exclusion of sick people from private health insurance.

The United States entered the twentieth century with the assumption that only one consent was needed for medical treatment: that of the physician or other health professional. In the last decades we have realized that two consents are needed: the professional's and the patient's. As we head into the twenty-first century, and the next millennium, we may face an unprecedented restriction of access to health care, based on the realization that another consent must be obtained: Not only must someone agree to offer the treatment and someone agree to accept it, but someone must also agree to pay for it. That third consent may become much more problematic. Patients are also taxpayers. There is an increasing mandate to limit the amount of the national wealth that goes into health care, and there is no telling how far this new stringency will go in reshaping the health professions.

LISA H. NEWTON

Directly related to this entry are the entries PROFESSION AND PROFESSIONAL ETHICS; MEDICINE AS A PROFESSION; *and* NURSING AS A PROFESSION. *For a further discussion of topics mentioned in this entry, see the entries* FRAUD, THEFT, AND PLAGIARISM; MEDICAL CODES AND OATHS; MEDICAL MALPRACTICE; RESEARCH POLICY; *and* WOMEN, *section on* WOMEN AS HEALTH PROFESSIONALS. *This entry will find application in the entries* ALLIED

HEALTH PROFESSIONS; *and* IMPAIRED PROFESSIONALS. *For a discussion of related ideas, see the entries* AUTONOMY; HARM; TRUST; *and* VIRTUE AND CHARACTER. *Other relevant material may be found under the entries* MEDICAL EDUCATION; PUBLIC POLICY AND BIOETHICS; *and* SEXUAL ETHICS AND PROFESSIONAL STANDARDS. *See also the* APPENDIX (CODES, OATHS, AND DIRECTIVES RELATED TO BIOETHICS), SECTION II: ETHICAL DIRECTIVES FOR THE PRACTICE OF MEDICINE, *and* SECTION III: ETHICAL DIRECTIVES FOR OTHER HEALTH-CARE PROFESSIONS.

Bibliography

BOSK, CHARLES L. 1979. *Forgive and Remember: Managing Medical Failure.* Chicago: University of Chicago Press.
———. 1985. "Social Controls and Physicians: The Oscillation of Cynicism and Idealism in Sociological Theory." In *Social Controls and the Medical Profession,* pp. 31–51. Edited by Judith P. Swazey and Stephen R. Scher. Boston: Oelgeschlager, Gunn & Hain.
BOSTON WOMEN'S HEALTH COLLECTIVE. 1985. *New Our Bodies, Ourselves.* New York: Simon and Schuster.
COLLINS, RANDALL. 1979. *The Credential Society: An Historical Sociology of Education and Stratification,* New York: Academic Press.
COMMITTEE FOR THE STUDY OF CREDENTIALING IN NURSING. 1979. *The Study of Credentialing in Nursing: A New Approach.* Vol. 2. Kansas City, Mo.: American Nurses' Association.
COUNCIL OF STATE GOVERNMENTS. 1952. *Occupational Licensing Legislation in the States.* Chicago: Author.
COUNCIL OF STATE GOVERNMENTS and NATIONAL CLEARINGHOUSE ON LICENSURE, ENFORCEMENT AND REGULATION. 1987. *State Regulation of the Health Occupations and Professions: 1986–1987.* Lexington, Ky.: Authors.
Dent v. State of West Virginia. 1889. 129 U.S. 114.
FREIDSON, ELIOT. 1970. *Profession of Medicine: A Study of the Sociology of Applied Knowledge.* New York: Dodd, Mead.
FRIEDMAN, MILTON, and FRIEDMAN, ROSE. 1980. *Free to Choose: A Personal Statement.* New York: Harcourt Brace Jovanovich.
GRAD, FRANK P., and MARTI, NOELIA. 1979. *Physicians' Licensure and Discipline: The Legal and Professional Regulation of Medical Practice.* Dobbs Ferry, N.Y.: Oceana Publications.
GROSS, STANLEY J. 1984. *Of Foxes and Hen Houses: Licensing and the Health Professions.* Westport, Conn.: Quorum Books.
LARSON, MAGALI S. 1977. *The Rise of Professionalism: A Sociological Analysis.* Berkeley: University of California Press.
MOGUL, KATHLEEN M. 1985. "Doctor's Dilemmas: Complexities in the Causes of Physicians; Mental Disorders and Some Treatment Implications." In *Social Controls and the Medical Profession,* pp. 133–156. Boston: Oelgeschlager, Gunn & Hain.
U.S. PUBLIC HEALTH SERVICE. HEALTH MANPOWER COORDINATING COMMITTEE. SUBCOMMITTEE ON HEALTH MANPOWER. 1976. *A Proposal for Credentialing Health Manpower.* Washington, D.C.: Author.
WELCH, CLAUDE E. 1976. "Professional Licensure and Hospital Delineation of Clinical Privileges: Relationship to Quality Assurance." Chap. 9 in *Quality Assurance in Health Care.* Edited by Richard H. Egdahl and Paul Gurtman. Germantown, Md.: Aspen Systems.

LIFE

Like many of the concepts foundational to the field of bioethics, life is a subject about which there is both long-standing conviction and increasing uncertainty. The beginnings and endings of life, as well as its creation, have become subject to greater technological modification, particularly through the rise of the modern biological sciences and new reproductive and genetic technologies. In the late twentieth century, increasing technological control over the management, regulation, and production of life and lifelike systems, as well as the accelerating commodification of life forms, raise questions about the limits of what can or should be done to life itself. Hence, seemingly timeless and universal human attitudes toward life, such as mourning in the wake of its loss and joy in its creation, are today accompanied by profound ambiguities concerning the meaning, value, and definition of life.

Some commentators have claimed that even a few decades ago life was more often understood as an absolute value—for example, among medical professionals, for whom the protection of life was an unquestioned moral duty (Parsons et al., 1972). Related arguments hold that the technologization of life has produced a shift away from an understanding of life as an absolute value, and toward more relative assessments of the quality of life (Parsons et al., 1972, pp. 405–410). The appearance of an entry entitled "Life" in an encyclopedia of bioethics would support the position that life itself has become the object of increased management in the form of decision making.

In contrast to the urgent call for guidelines concerning the subject of life is the difficulty of defining this term. Neither philosophers, theologians, nor scientists can offer a clear understanding of life. This is in part due to the wide-ranging uses of the term. Not only does life have many meanings as a noun, it is a key term within a wide range of systems of thought from religion to science. In all of the many senses in which the word is used, definitions of it have varied historically in relation to changing social forces and cultural values. Contemporary moral, legal, theological, and scientific uncertainty attends the origins of life, the relative importance of human versus other forms of life, the beginnings and endings of life, the creation and destruction of life, and the nature of life. These and other concerns follow from the definitional issues, raised by the concept of life itself, that remain subject to dispute and ongoing transformation.

Historical and cultural variations

To be animate or vital is a condition for which cross-culturally and transhistorically there exists a range of modes of recognition. Broadly speaking, notions of life, or of a vital force, are often connected to beliefs about the supernatural, divinity, and sacredness. It is also generally the case that understandings of life are often made most explicit in relation to death (Bloch and Parry, 1982; Huntington and Metcalf, 1979). These features characterize both Judaeo-Christian and classical understandings of life, the two predominant sources of its definition in the Euro-American tradition prior to the rise of modern science.

According to the Judaeo-Christian tradition, life is interpreted and valued as a gift from God. The Old Testament relates that God created man (Adam) in his own likeness, with dominion over all living things. In the Garden of Eden, life was everlasting; and Adam and Eve's expulsion, through which they became mortal, was both a sign of divine displeasure and a partial rescinding of the gift of life. According to the New Testament, the gift of everlasting life was restored through the sacrifice of God's only begotten son, Jesus, and his resurrection to the kingdom of Heaven. Consequently, only those who believe in the resurrection of Christ have "life" in the Christian sense. When Jesus states "I am life" (or "I am the way, the truth, and the life"), it is the resurrection promised to believers in the life, death, and salvation of Christ that is invoked. The historian Barbara Duden notes:

> In most of the New Testament and in two thousand years of ecclesiastical usage, to "have life" means to participate as a believing Christian in the life of Christ. . . . Even the dead live in Christ, and only those who live in Christ can have life in this world. Of those who exist outside this relationship, the Church has consistently spoken of those who "live" under conditions of death. (Duden, 1993, p. 102)

Blood is a key symbol of life in the Christian tradition as well as in much secular culture, most notably medicine. To give the "gift of life" is more literally possible today than ever before in the context of organ donation, whereby a body part of a deceased person may "live on" in the body of another person, or a living donor may sacrifice a body part (such as a kidney) on behalf of a relative. The capacity to donate not only blood and vital organs but also egg and sperm cells, and the increasing availability of bodily tissues through a service sector and a marketplace, complicate the understanding of life as a "gift" (Parsons et al., 1972; Titmuss, 1971). The sacrificial importance of the body and the blood of Christ makes the exchange of body tissue a potent symbolic practice, as does the definition of kin ties in terms of "blood relations."

The association between the flow of blood and the flow of life anticipates the notion of germ plasm (the hereditary material of the germ cells) as the basis for heredity; this in turn gives rise to the modern scientific concept of the gene, which is today described as the essence of life. While the gene in some senses represents the triumph of mechanistic explanations of life itself, the most reductionist accounts of genes as "selfishly" reproducing entities defined by the attainment of their own inbuilt "ends" may seem not dissimilar from that of the most influential proponent of vitalism, Aristotle.

Aristotelian definitions of life were predominant for nearly two millennia, in part because Aristotle was among the few philosophers of antiquity to pay significant attention to the problem of defining life. According to Aristotle, life is defined by the possession of a soul, or vital force, through which an entity is rendered animate and given shape. The attainment of a predetermined end point is seen as the purpose of life in Aristotelian terms, a purpose that is contained in itself, independent of any external causal agent. This view is known as entelechy—a telos, an ultimate end that is self-defined as the achievement of a final form.

Although the Aristotelian view was based on close observations of the natural world and eschewed any notion of divine creation, it is strongly criticized by modern scientists for its teleologism (conflation of an endpoint with a cause) and essentialism (predeterminism), which are dismissed as metaphysical and therefore insufficiently empirical. Cartesian accounts of animation, which defined life in terms of the organization instead of the essence of matter, succeeded Aristotelian vitalism in the seventeenth century. From the perspective of mechanism, which explained motion or aliveness purely in terms of the articulation among parts of a whole (as in the ticking of a watch), Aristotelian vitalism came to be seen as mystical, nonobservable, and therefore unscientific.

The history of the concept of life in Western science, from which many of the most authoritative contemporary definitions of it are derived, underscores the importance of change and variation in the meanings of this term (Canguilhem, 1994; Schroedinger, 1956). Eighteenth-century natural historians employed a horizontal ordering strategy to classify diverse life forms into taxonomies of kind or type. A vertical ranking of the value of these life forms (known as the great chain of being, descending from God to humanity and thence to other living entities) was based on their proximity to the divine. According to this conceptual framework, "life" comprised a diverse array of animate entities classified epistemologically and ranked theologically in terms of proximity to God. The sacred act of divine creation that brought life into being was, in this schema, paralleled by the secular production by natural philosophers, such as Carolus Linnaeus (1707–1778), of a classification system through which life forms were named, defined, and ordered according to their perceived nature, which was seen to be immutable.

The stability of these vertical ranking and horizontal classifying axes was irrevocably shaken by the gradual acceptance of the evolutionary model of life, in particular the work of Charles Darwin, which, over the latter half of the nineteenth century, gained acceptance in Europe and America. With the rise of Darwinian theories of evolution came a radical new understanding of life: as an underlying connectedness of all living things. It was the evolutionary view of life as a distinct object of study in its own right that gave rise to the modern notion of "life itself"; not until this time could such a thing have been conceived. Many of the current dilemmas in bioethics demanding our attention came to be understood as a direct result of the emergence of this particular conceptualization of life.

As the historian Michel Foucault points out, life itself did not exist before the end of the nineteenth century; it is a concept indebted to the rise of the modern biological sciences.

> Historians want to write histories of biology in the nineteenth century; but they do not realise that biology did not exist then, and that the pattern of knowledge that has been familiar to us for a hundred and fifty years is not valid for a previous period. And that if biology was unknown, there was a very simple reason for it: *that life itself did not exist*. All that existed was living beings, which were viewed through a grid of knowledge constituted by natural history. (Foucault, 1970, p. 128; emphasis added)

Life, in the sense of life itself, is thus a concept linked closely to the rise of the modern life sciences, founded on notions of evolutionary change, the underlying connectedness of all living things, and a biogenetic mechanism of heredity through which life reproduces itself. As the foundational object of the modern life sciences, the concept of life itself does not exist as a thing, as something visible or tangible. Only its traces are accessible, through the forms in which life manifests itself. Like Newtonian gravity, Darwinian life is a principle or force subject to an orderliness decipherable by science,

such as the process of natural selection by which evolution is understood to proceed.

Life as defined by modern science

From the vantage point of the modern life sciences, life itself has come to be associated with certain qualities, including movement, the ability to reproduce and to evolve, and the capacity for growth and development. Other criteria for defining life as opposed to nonlife include the capacity to metabolize, in particular through the possession of cells. These characteristics of aliveness in turn comprise key areas in the study of life forms, and in the forms of connectedness and interrelatedness among them. Whereas the comparative anatomy or morphology of animals and plants was the definitive technique for the classification of life forms during the classical period of natural history, it is molecular biology that today provides the primary analytic perspective on the essence of life, which is seen to be DNA, or the genetic code. It is DNA, composed of nucleotide chains that guide the manufacture of essential proteins, that all living beings are said to have in common. Thus DNA is the substance and mechanism of heredity intrinsic to the neo-Darwinian notion of life itself. (For an historical account of Darwinian notions of life itself, see Jacob, 1973. For a contemporary view, see Pollack, 1994.)

The most definitive accounts of life itself today rely on evolutionary and genetic models. "The possession of a genetic program provides for an absolute difference between organisms and inorganic matter," claims the biologist Ernst Mayr, one of the great twentieth-century exponents of evolution as a unifying theme in modern biological thought (Mayr, 1982, p. 55). "Life should be defined by the possession of those properties which are needed to ensure evolution by natural selection," states John Maynard Smith, one of the leading evolutionary biologists in Britain (Maynard Smith, 1986, p. 7).

In addition to offering the most definitive accounts of life, the modern life sciences provide the most detailed and substantive information on the subject. In the article "Life" written for the *Encyclopaedia Britannica*, Carl Sagan notes: "A great deal is known about life. . . . Anatomists and taxonomists have studied the forms and relations of more than a million separate species of plants and animals." A range of biological specialties have together compiled "an enormous fund of information" on the origin, diversity, interaction, and complexity of living organisms and the principles that order their existence (Sagan, 1992, p. 985).

Yet even such definitive accounts of life from established scientific figures are often admittedly provisional. Both within and outside the scientific community there is considerable uncertainty about what is being studied when the subject is life itself. As Sagan notes perfunctorily, "There is no generally accepted definition of life" (Sagan, 1992, p. 985).

Problems in defining life

The definition of life is not only contested from within the scientific community; it is also troubled by the proximity of lifelike systems, especially those that are computer-generated, to the requisite features of animate existence. There may well be, as Stephen Levy notes in his account of artificial life, a "particular reluctance to grant anything synthetic or man-made the exalted status of a life-form" (1992, p. 6). Yet insofar as the biogenetic definition of life itself relies on an informational model, of DNA as a message or a code, the distinction between life and nonlife is readily challenged by complex informational systems that are to a degree self-regulating and that have the capacity both to replicate themselves and to evolve. If, as some have claimed (Oyama, 1985), information is the modern equivalent of form, then life is transformed from an absolute property into a receding horizon merging with artificial, synthetic, or virtual "life." (See also Langton, 1989, and Levy, 1992.)

Today, both the border between human and nonhuman life and the distinction between life and death are increasingly blurred. Genetic science offers the possibility of transspecies recombinations effecting a merging of human and animal body parts. Artificial-life scientists using information technology distinguish computer-generated organisms, which live, evolve, reproduce, and die, from the "wet" life forms they imitate (Levy, 1992). Health professionals distinguish degrees of death: dead (in the sense of brain-dead); double dead (respiratory failure); and triple dead (no body parts suitable for donation). Such distinctions indicate the increasing difficulties of establishing the parameters of life and death.

In sum, life itself may be charted along the course of its four-billion-year history to its estimated point of origin, and along this path may be classified and analyzed scientifically according to established principles, such as the operation of natural selection, and specific qualities, such as the possession of DNA. It is from the perspective of the modern life sciences that the most elaborate and definitive accounts of life are constructed, and from these in turn that the concept of life itself emerges. Yet the instability of these definitional parameters, like those of previous eras that they replaced, ensures their continued transformation.

Life as a moral issue

Despite the ubiquity and authority of biological definitions of life, they are also reductionist and materialist, relying upon mechanistic and objective terms that are ultimately most meaningful to professional specialists. Most people, when asked "What is life?" do not appeal to Darwinian principles.

Many of the more everyday definitions of life can be classed as processual or phenomenological, referring to the course of events comprising the life of an individual or other entity (including inanimate objects, as in the expression "shelf life"). Expressions such as *c'est la vie* ("that's life") invoke the fortuitous and inexplicable dimensions of life, very much in contrast to scientific accounts, which emphasize order and predictability even while admitting great uncertainty. Such expressions convey a sense of limits to the capacity for rational understanding, and especially prediction or control, in relation to the vicissitudes of life and living.

The lengthy debate in early modern science concerning mechanism (the presumption that animate and inanimate entities alike are composed of matter, which can be explained through inherent principles of structure and function) versus vitalism (the presumption of an inherently inexplicable vital force differentiating the quick from the dead) opposes the ancient association of lifelike properties with mystery and the sacred to their accessibility through instrumental reason (see Merchant, 1980). In relation to the moral questions concerning life—whether as a process, a possession, or a right—the vitalistic notion of life as something inexplicable and deserving of reverence and protection is far more prevalent than the more mechanistic and instrumental account dominant within science. In both secular and religiously derived accounts, life does not need to be fully explicated or rational to be seen as uniquely deserving of protection, especially human life.

The protection of life

In his discussion of abortion and euthanasia, two of the most controversial areas of debate concerning human life, philosopher Ronald Dworkin emphasizes the importance of recognizing that life is not exclusively or even primarily understood by many people in terms of scientific explanations, but rather in terms of a value more akin to sacredness. In relation to moral dilemmas, he claims, life does not present itself as a question of objective fact, but rather as a truth, or a "quasi-religious" principle held to be self-evident through "primitive conviction" (Dworkin, 1993).

Dworkin's approach thus differs from the more utilitarian arguments about the beginnings and endings of life propounded by philosophers and other commentators who use rights or interest-based approaches to questions of the meaning and value of life. In demarcating the value of life as a "quasi-religious" one, something essentially felt rather than reasoned, Dworkin returns the question of the value of life to an older, more traditional paradigm linked to notions of divinity or a vital force.

Social scientists have shown the value of life to be a key symbolic resource in struggles of many kinds, including both ways of life (as in the preservation of ethnic traditions or indigenous cultures) and life forms (such as endangered species). Anthropologist Faye Ginsburg's study of the abortion debate in a midwestern American community, for example, demonstrates the symbolic dimensions of life as a subject of dispute extending to notions of citizenship, nationalism, and the sexual division of labor (Ginsburg, 1989). Precisely because the preservation of human life may be seen as an absolute moral value, it proves readily amenable to the social function of grounding other beliefs and practices.

Abortion is one of the best-known arenas of controversy in which both definitions of life and the value of human life are paramount and explicitly formulated. Opponents of abortion argue that life begins at conception and therefore that the deliberate termination of a pregnancy is the taking of a human life, which is seen to be immoral or even comparable to murder. Proponents of a woman's right to control her own fertility, including the choice to terminate an unwanted pregnancy, often argue on the basis of consequentialism, that is, that the moral value of an act should be measured in reference to its outcome. Rights-based claims are used by both sides, antiabortionists stressing the right to life of the fetus, which they argue to be paramount, and pro-choice advocates stressing a woman's right to control her own reproduction, on which they, in turn, place primary importance.

Current legislation on abortion in many industrialized countries, including the United States, invokes a combination of rights-based arguments and biologically based distinctions. Hence, for example, the 1973 U.S. Supreme Court decision in *Roe v. Wade,* which currently determines abortion law in the United States, combines protection of the individual right to privacy with a biologically based definition of fetal viability as the determinant of the upper time limit for abortion. The same standard holds in Great Britain.

Both the notion of biological viability and the definition of the person to whom rights are ascribed invoke a particular construction of life. Viability, for example, is strictly biologically determined: it is measured by the ability of a fetus to survive biologically. The question of the social viability of a child's life, such as its likelihood of receiving adequate nurture, shelter, protection from disease, or sustenance is not considered part of the criteria valid in determining the morality of a decision to terminate a pregnancy.

Feminists have been prominent in the challenge to the notion of the person often used by antiabortionists on similar grounds. It is undeniably the case that an embryo is human, that it is a being, and that it is a form of life. That it is a living human being is therefore undeniable. Yet it is no more or less a living human being in this sense than an egg or sperm cell, or for that matter a blood cell, none of which is considered a person or seen as entitled to civil rights. Increasingly, antiabortionists have used biologically based arguments to support their position, even when it is derived from religious principles. Hence, it is the potential for an embryo—unlike an egg, a sperm, or a blood cell—to develop into a human being that is often stressed. This argument is based on an embryo's possession of a unique genetic blueprint, which some established theologians claim is evidence of ensoulment (see Ford, 1988).

Hence, arguments against abortion based on fetal viability, or those that stress the genetic potential of the fetus to develop into a person, are based on a particular model of life, according to which its sanctity may be represented in biogenetic terms. Historian Barbara Duden has called this historically recent turn toward biology as an arbiter of moral decision making the "sacralisation of life itself" (Duden, 1993). Life, in this sense, is not a biological fact but a cultural value, an essentialist belief, or even a fetish.

The geneticization of life itself

Similar claims have been made regarding the biogenetic definition of life as possession of a genetic blueprint. Critical biologists have argued against the genetic reductionism or genetic essentialism such definitions risk (see Hubbard, 1990). Social scientists also have warned of the dangers of eugenicism implicit in such a view (Nelkin and Lindee, 1995); other scholars have minimized such risks (Kevles, 1986).

Advocates of a "strong" genetic essentialism argue not only that genes are the essence of life but that life itself is consequently based on the selfish desire to reproduce itself. From this vantage point, humans are mere epiphenomena of a primordial genetic drive to self-replicate, and human moral or ethical systems are a complex admixture of altruism motivated by strategic sacrifice, which benefits one genetic trajectory or another (Dawkins, 1989).

The belief that life processes will one day be subject to much greater control through instrumentalized understandings of their genetic code is the basis for a major expansion in the biotechnology industry, and corresponding scientific research, since the early 1980s. International scientific projects such as the attempt to map the human genome, by sequencing all of the DNA in the twenty-three pairs of human chromosomes, reflect the increasing importance of genes and genetic processes to the understanding of life itself. (For a description of the Human Genome Project, see British Medical Association, 1992, and Cook-Deegan, 1994. For an account of the ethical dimension, see Kevles and Hood, 1992. For a critical account, see Hubbard and Wald, 1993.) In turn, increasing information about the role of genes in heredity will pose new choices and decisions, as well as dilemmas, for many. On the one hand, new diagnostic procedures utilizing genetic screening to detect severe, chronic, degenerative, and often terminal disorders caused by a single gene are claimed to offer greater reproductive choice and control, and the potential to alleviate human suffering and disease. On the other hand, the identification of gene "defects" poses worrisome questions, especially when linked to notions of individual predisposition, genetic selection, and the elimination of "undesirable" traits. Controversies such as that attending the putative discovery of a "gay gene" underscore the dangers of social prejudice wedded to genetic determinism in the name of greater reproductive choice and control.

Altering the genetic code of an individual entity, be it human, plant, or animal, is most controversial when the alteration has the potential to be replicated in subsequent generations, therefore resulting in irreversible and cumulative hereditary effects. Although a distinction is currently maintained between somatic cell gene therapy (genetic alteration of nonreproductive bodily tissue) and germ-line gene therapy (genetic modification of the egg or sperm cells, or the early embryo), this boundary is known to be unstable. Considerable ethical concern therefore surrounds the advent of human gene therapy, now practiced in both Great Britain and the United States. (For further discussion, see British Medical Association, 1992.) The release of genetically engineered organisms into the environment, largely in the form of plants and microorganisms, has also attracted controversy, in particular concerning the labeling of foodstuffs and the limits of acceptable risk.

It is the biogenetic definition of life, then, that informs many of the moral debates about the protection of life, whether human, animal, or environmental—the latter category denoting the ecosystem as a complex "living whole." (For a discussion of protecting life as "biodiversity," see Wilson, 1992; also Kellert and Wilson, 1993.) Confusions about when life begins, for example, as in debates about fetal rights, derive from a biogenetic definition of life, which is continuous: each life form has its origin in the lives of those preceding it, and their connectedness underscores the interrelation of life itself. Given such a definition of life, clear demarcations concerning the beginnings and endings of life,

of a life, or of life itself are understandably subject to dispute.

Artificial life

New techniques for technologically assisting the creation of life (e.g., assisted conception) and for prolonging life or redesigning life (genetic engineering) add to the difficulties of establishing a clear basis for decision making by health professionals, relatives, policymakers, or legislators. Technology now enables the production, extension, and even redesign of life forms, including humans, animals, plants, and microorganisms. Increasingly sophisticated medical technology has affected both the beginning and the ending of human life. Life-support technologies can artificially sustain human life in the context of severely restricted life functions both at the beginning of life (perinatal support) and toward the end of life, in cases where the individual becomes fully dependent on technology for respiration. Cases of prolonged "vegetative" human existence raise difficult questions as a result of the availability of technologically maintained biological viability. Insofar as a person is more than a biological life, difficult decisions concerning continued treatment for a person who is only minimally alive are the inevitable result of modern technology's capacity to sustain baseline survival functions indefinitely.

Technology also affects the creation of life itself. As medical scientists acquire ever greater command of genetic structure, the question of the ethical acceptability of the creation of life forms such as the Harvard "oncomouse," genetically engineered to develop cancer so it can be used in the design of new drugs for the treatment of human disease, must be addressed. The subject of a major patent dispute in the European Parliament, and removed from the market in 1993 by its manufacturer, DuPont, the oncomouse was among the first higher life forms to be defined as a technology, comparable to other forms of laboratory apparatus. As both a mammal and a scientific instrument, the oncomouse inhabits a domain subject to increasing ethical, commercial, and political controversy (Haraway, 1992).

Most significant, the oncomouse raises the question of ownership of life, which is established as an inviolable right for humans within the liberal democratic tradition and was described by humanist philosopher John Locke as "ownership of one's person." This principle, used in arguments favoring the emancipation of women and the abolition of slavery (both women and slaves being considered chattels), is more recently evident in disputes concerning body parts. In the landmark case of *John Moore v. California Regents*, conflict over the use of Moore's body tissue in the design of a drug, through production of an immortal cell line derived from his spleen cells, culminated in a U.S. Supreme Court decision prohibiting the individual ownership of bodily tissue. Ownership of human life in this case was declared not subject to extracorporeal extension.

The question is again different in the case of the "right to life" of the oncomouse, or the "geep," the transspecies hybrid of a goat and a sheep produced through genetic manipulation. Here, the question concerns the deliberate production of a life that brings great suffering to the resultant organism. Only the greater good to humans of such developments can justify their deliberate creation by scientists. But the basis for ethical decision making in such an instance remains indeterminate.

Conclusion

Many of the ethical questions addressed to life itself concern the degree of protection it requires. These questions in turn depend on how life is defined. Whether they concern the beginnings or endings of life, its creation, redesign, or sustenance under technological conditions, the underlying definition of life itself is a fundamental force shaping ethical decision making. Scientifically, life is defined according to the modern life sciences in a biogenetic idiom, which constructs it as a continuous and connected force unto itself, manifested by the self-replicating properties of DNA. In the liberal humanist tradition, human life is also seen as a possession, and the persistent association of life with sacredness is well established. The rights to life, the protection of life, and the quality of life are extended to some degree to other life forms, on the principle of avoiding cruelty and suffering. In none of these areas are definitive boundaries or limits available upon which to base ethical practice. Instead, as definitions of both life and death are subject to ongoing transformation, so are the ethical frameworks brought to bear on the creation, management, and protection of all life forms.

SARAH FRANKLIN

For a further discussion of topics mentioned in this entry, see the entries ABORTION; ANIMAL WELFARE AND RIGHTS, *article on* ETHICAL PERSPECTIVES ON THE TREATMENT AND STATUS OF ANIMALS; DEATH; DEATH, ATTITUDES TOWARD; DEATH, DEFINITION AND DETERMINATION OF; DEATH: ART OF DYING; DEATH AND DYING: EUTHANASIA AND SUSTAINING LIFE; EUGENICS; EVOLUTION; FERTILITY CONTROL; GENETICS AND RACIAL MINORITIES; HOMICIDE; HOSPICE AND END-OF-LIFE CARE; LIFE, QUALITY OF; *and* TECHNOLOGY. *For a discussion of related ideas, see the entries* DEATH EDUCATION; DEATH PENALTY; ETHICS, *article on* RELIGION AND MORALITY; EUGENICS AND RELIGIOUS LAW; FAMILY; FEMINISM; FETUS; GENE THERAPY; GENETIC ENGINEERING; GENETICS AND HUMAN BEHAVIOR, *article on* PHILOSOPHICAL AND ETHICAL ISSUES; NARRATIVE; NATIONAL SOCIALISM; ORGAN AND TISSUE PROCUREMENT; PATENTING ORGANISMS; PERSON; POPULATION ETHICS, *sections on* ELEMENTS OF POPULATION ETHICS, *and* NORMATIVE APPROACHES; REPRODUCTIVE TECHNOLOGIES, *articles on* ARTIFICIAL INSEMINATION, IN VITRO FERTILIZATION AND EMBRYO TRANSFER, *and* CRYOPRESERVATION OF SPERM, OVA, AND EMBRYOS; *and* RIGHTS. *Other relevant material may be found under the entries* ANIMAL RESEARCH, *article on* PHILOSOPHICAL ISSUES; ARTIFICIAL ORGANS AND LIFE-SUPPORT SYSTEMS; BIOMEDICAL ENGINEERING; BIOTECHNOLOGY; BODY; CRYONICS; DNA TYPING; GENETICS AND HUMAN SELF-UNDERSTANDING; HOMOSEXUALITY; JAINISM; PAIN AND SUFFERING; RACE AND RACISM; *and* UTILITY.

Bibliography

BLOCH, MAURICE, and PARRY, JONATHAN, P., eds. 1982. *Death and the Regeneration of Life.* Cambridge: At the University Press.

BRITISH MEDICAL ASSOCIATION. 1992. *Our Genetic Future: The Science and Ethics of Genetic Technology.* Oxford: Oxford University Press.

CANGUILHEM, GEORGES. 1994. *A Vital Rationalist: Selected Writings from Georges Canguilhem.* Translated by Arthur Goldhammer. Edited by Francois Delaporte. New York: Zone.

COOK-DEEGAN, ROBERT M. 1993. *The Gene Wars: Science, Politics, and the Human Genome.* New York: Norton.

DAWKINS, RICHARD. 1989. *The Selfish Gene.* New ed. Oxford: Oxford University Press.

DUDEN, BARBARA. 1993. *Disembodying Women: Perspectives on Pregnancy and the Unborn.* Cambridge, Mass.: Harvard University Press.

DWORKIN, RONALD M. 1993. *Life's Dominion: An Argument About Abortion and Euthanasia.* New York: HarperCollins.

FORD, NORMAN M. 1988. *When Did I Begin? Conception of the Human Individual in History, Philosophy and Science.* Cambridge: At the University Press.

FOUCAULT, MICHEL. 1970. *The Order of Things: An Archaeology of the Human Sciences.* New York: Vintage.

GINSBURG, FAYE D. 1989. *Contested Lives: The Abortion Debate in an American Community.* Berkeley: University of California Press.

HARAWAY, DONNA. 1992. "When Man Is on the Menu." In *Incorporations,* pp. 36–43. Edited by Jonathan Crary and Sanford Kwinter. New York: Zone.

HUBBARD, RUTH. 1990. *The Politics of Women's Biology.* New Brunswick, N.J.: Rutgers University Press.

HUBBARD, RUTH, and WALD, ELIJAH. 1993. *Exploding the Gene Myth: How Genetic Information Is Produced and Manipulated by Scientists, Physicians, Employers, Insurance*

Companies, Educators, and Law Enforcers. Boston: Beacon Press.

HUNTINGTON, RICHARD, and METCALF, PETER. 1979. *Celebrations of Death: The Anthropology of Mortuary Ritual.* Cambridge: At the University Press.

JACOB, FRANÇOIS. 1973. *The Logic of Life: A History of Heredity.* Translated by Betty E. Spillman. Princeton, N.J.: Princeton University Press.

KELLERT, STEPHEN R., and WILSON, EDWARD O., eds. 1993. *The Biophilia Hypothesis.* Washington, D.C.: Island.

KEVLES, DANIEL J. 1986. *In the Name of Eugenics: Genetics and the Uses of Human Heredity.* Berkeley: University of California Press.

KEVLES, DANIEL J., and HOOD, LEROY E., eds. 1992. *The Code of Codes: Scientific and Social Issues in the Human Genome Project.* Cambridge, Mass.: Harvard University Press.

LANGTON, CHRISTOPHER G., ed. 1989. *Artificial Life: Proceedings of an Interdisciplinary Workshop on the Synthesis and Stimulation of Living Systems, Held September, 1987, in Los Alamos, New Mexico.* Santa Fe Institute Studies in the Sciences of Complexity, vol. 6. Redwood City, Calif.: Addison-Wesley.

LANGTON, CHRISTOPHER G.; TAYLOR, CHARLES J.; FARMER, J. DOYNE; and RASMUSSEN, STEVEN, eds. 1992. *Artificial Life II: Proceedings of the Workshop on Artificial Life Held February, 1990, in Santa Fe, New Mexico.* Santa Fe Institute Studies in the Sciences of Complexity, vol. 10. Redwood City, Calif.: Addison-Wesley.

LEVY, STEPHEN. 1992. *Artificial Life: The Quest for a New Creation.* New York: Pantheon.

MAYNARD SMITH, JOHN. 1986. *The Problems of Biology.* Oxford: Oxford University Press.

MAYR, ERNST. 1982. *The Growth of Biological Thought: Diversity, Evolution, and Inheritance.* Cambridge, Mass.: Harvard University Press.

MERCHANT, CAROLYN. 1980. *The Death of Nature: Women, Ecology, and the Scientific Revolution.* San Francisco: Harper & Row.

NELKIN, DOROTHY, and LINDEE, SUSAN. 1995. *Supergene: DNA in American Popular Culture.* New York: W. H. Freedman.

OYAMA, SUSAN. 1985. *The Ontogeny of Information: Developmental Systems and Evolution.* Cambridge: At the University Press.

PARSONS, TALCOTT; FOX, RENÉE C.; and LIDZ, VICTOR M. 1972. "The 'Gift of Life' and its Reciprocation." *Social Research* 39, no. 3:367–415.

POLLACK, ROBERT. 1994. *Signs of Life: The Language and Meanings of DNA.* Boston: Houghton Mifflin.

SAGAN, CARL. 1992. "Life." In vols. 10 and 22 of *Encyclopaedia Britannica,* 15th ed., pp. 893 and 979–996. Chicago: Encyclopaedia Britannica.

SCHRODINGER, ERWIN. 1956. [1944]. *What is Life? and Other Scientific Essays.* New York: Doubleday.

TITMUSS, RICHARD M. 1971. *The Gift Relationship: From Human Blood to Social Policy.* New York: Pantheon.

WILKIE, TOM. 1993. *Perilous Knowledge: The Human Genome Project and Its Implications.* Berkeley: University of California Press.

WILSON, EDWARD O. 1992. *The Diversity of Life.* New York: Norton.

LIFE, QUALITY OF

I. QUALITY OF LIFE IN CLINICAL DECISIONS

Quality of life is one of the most important but controversial issues in clinical ethics. The contemporary development of the concept and its use as a normative criterion in clinical decision making date from the period after World War II, when advances in medical technology increased tremendously. Along with other ethical criteria—for example, a medical indications policy (Meilaender, 1982; Ramsey, 1978; U.S. Department of Health and Human Services, 1985); the ordinary–extraordinary means criterion (Connery, 1986; Johnstone, 1985; Reich, 1978a); or the reasonable person standard (Veatch, 1976)—quality of life is used in conflict situations to help make clinical decisions about whether or not to forgo or to withdraw medical treatment from patients.

Modern medicine has the capacity through the application of technology to save lives that until relatively recently would have been lost to acute disease or accident. As a consequence, some of these lives either are shaped by severe disabilities or chronic illness or continue to exist only at the biological level (for example, infants born with multiple congenital abnormalities; elderly patients who suffer chronic illnesses after recovery from an acute illness; and patients in a persistent vegetative state (PVS). Quality of life is frequently proposed as a criterion in making treatment decisions about these patients, whose lives might be saved only to be lived out in severely impaired conditions.

Quality-of-life considerations arise in several key areas of clinical ethics: termination or shortening of human life, including issues of abortion and euthanasia; limiting human reproduction, such as through contraception, sterilization, or abortion; interventions that alter the genetic and biological nature of humans, such as embryo cloning or eugenic engineering; and public policy areas, including economics, ecology, and cultural development (Reich, 1978a). This article will focus principally on the first issue.

Quality-of-life considerations raise a number of important questions that bear specifically on clinical ethics: (1) Given the tremendous advances in medical technology and the implicit imperative to use it, what are the goals and limits of medicine? (2) What is normatively human, and thus, what is it that we value about life? (3) Are quality-of-life judgments purely subjective, or are there objective criteria that guide them? (4) Can there be a life that is so burdened by pain or disability that it can be judged not worth living? (5) Who should decide to terminate treatment? (6) Is it morally legitimate to include considerations of the patient's prior medical condition in a decision about forgoing future medical interventions? and (7) Is it morally legitimate to include in treatment decisions the potential burdens on affected others who will have to care for a severely handicapped patient?

The following sections will provide some preliminary clarifications and conceptual frameworks for understanding quality of life; define quality of life and identify the spectrum of positions that come under the general heading of this normative criterion; articulate the evaluative status of life that is adopted in the various quality-of-life positions and compare the so-called quality-of-life ethic with the sanctity-of-life ethic; and analyze both the normative dimensions of quality-of-life judgments and the normative theories that justify these judgments.

Preliminary clarifications

Statements or claims about a "quality" or "qualities" of life can be either evaluative or morally normative (Reich, 1978a; Walter, 1988). Evaluative claims or statements indicate that some value or worth is attached either to a characteristic of the person (for example, capacity to choose) or to a type of life that is lived (for example, free of pain and handicap). Thus, evaluative statements assess that the quality, and by implication the life that possesses the quality, is desired, appreciated, or even considered sacred. These statements, however, do not establish whether an action to support or to terminate life is morally right or wrong, nor do they specify which action would be morally obligatory. On the other hand, morally normative or prescriptive claims about a quality of life always involve a moral judgment on the valued quality and, by implication, a judgment on the life that possesses the quality. These latter statements, then, not only presume that a quality—for example, cognitive ability—is valued, but they also entail judgments about whether, and under which conditions, one must or ought to protect and preserve a life that possesses the valued quality or qualities. Thus, one could

formulate a prescriptive claim that "any life that has cognitive abilities always ought to be given all medical treatment." Evaluative statements about quality of life do bear on clinical decisions, but the more important and controversial issues are concerned with the validity and use of the normative claims about quality of life, especially with regard to patients who lack any ability to participate in the clinical decision.

Many different perspectives could be used in establishing, defending, and assessing evaluative and normative claims in the area of quality of life. A feminist perspective could be used to analyze and critique an evaluative claim that proposes the discursive quality of rationality to be superior to a rationality based on the qualities of affectivity and caring (e.g., Gilligan, 1982; Sichel, 1989). A perspective from the elderly (Kilner, 1988) or the disabled community could be used to assess the normative claim that the qualities of youth, physical beauty, independence, and athletic ability—qualities that are extolled and prized in modern Western culture—are necessary for one to live well. Sociological perspectives could be used to study the cultural patterns of commitment to quality of life (e.g., Gerson, 1976), or legal perspectives to study the jurisprudential implications of these claims on the disabled (e.g., Destro, 1986). Each of these perspectives, and more, would be important to consult in adequately assessing both evaluative and normative claims about quality of life. However, the remainder of this article will use only the philosophical and theological perspectives that have been developed in the literature on quality of life vis-à-vis treatment decisions.

Definitions of quality of life

There is much ambiguity about what "quality of life" means, and consequently there is little agreement about the definition of this criterion. First, there is the word "life." It can refer to two different realities in this context: (1) vital or metabolic processes that could be called "human biological life"; or (2) "human personal life" that includes biological life but goes beyond it to include other distinctively human capacities, for example, the capacity to choose or to think. Anencephalic infants and PVS patients have biological life, but they do not possess human personal life.

Similarly, "quality" can refer to several different realities. Sometimes the word refers to the idea of excellence. So defined, its meaning is bounded only by the horizons of our imaginations and desires. It is difficult to discover any objective criteria to assess quality-of-life judgments under this definition. Consequently, one may fear that patients whose lives cannot achieve the expected level of imagined or desired excellence, such as the handicapped or the dying, will either not be offered any life-sustaining treatment or will be actively killed.

Another possible definition is to understand "quality" as an attribute or property of either biological or personal life. Most proponents of quality of life subscribe to this general definition. Some authors identify quality of life with a single valued property of life, while others identify it with a cluster of valued properties. Thus, this definition represents a spectrum of positions. At one end of the spectrum is the original position of Richard McCormick, who isolated only one quality or attribute to be considered as the minimum for personal life: the potential for human relationships (McCormick, 1974). For McCormick, a Down syndrome baby would possess the potential for human relationships, but an anencephalic infant would not. At the other end of the spectrum, Joseph Fletcher originally defined the indicators of "humanhood" by reference to fifteen positive qualities, among them self-awareness, concern for others, curiosity, and balance of rationality and feeling, and five negative properties, among them, that humans are not essentially parental (Fletcher, 1972). He believed that many, if not all, severely handicapped children would not possess the attributes necessary to live a life of quality. Between these two ends a number of "median" positions exist that identify quality of life with valued properties of life. For example, Earl Shelp has proposed minimal independence as the central property in his quality-of-life position. He includes in this basic property the abilities to relate to others, to communicate, to ambulate, and to perform the basic tasks of hygiene, feeding, and dressing (Shelp, 1986). From this perspective, many, but not all, Down syndrome children would possess the necessary attributes to live a life of quality.

James Walter has suggested that the word "quality" should not primarily refer to a property or attribute of either physical or personal life. Rather, the quality that is at issue is the quality of the relationship that exists between the medical condition of the patient, on the one hand, and the patient's ability to pursue human purposes, on the other. These purposes are understood as the material, social, moral, and spiritual values that transcend physical, biological life. The quality referred to is the quality of a relation and not a property or attribute of life (Walter, 1988). Thus, for patients to judge that they possess a quality of life means that the patients themselves would evaluate that, based on their medical condition, they are able to pursue values important to them at some qualitative or acceptable level.

Evaluative status of life

When quality of life is defined by reference to a property or attribute of physical life, then some basic questions are raised about the value of physical life itself. What is it that we value about our physical lives? Do we value biological existence in and for its own sake, or because of the presence of some property or attribute in that life, for example, cognitive ability? What theological or philosophical justifications can be offered for one's evaluations of life?

Many who define quality of life basically by reference to a property do not attribute intrinsic value to physical life. For example, in some of his writings McCormick has suggested that physical life does not possess inherent value but is a good to be preserved precisely as the condition of other values (McCormick, 1981, 1984). Based on his theological convictions that physical life is a created, limited good and that the ability to relate to others is the mediation of one's love of the divine, McCormick resists attributing to physical life itself the status of an absolute value. Kevin O'Rourke and Dennis Brodeur (1986) have stated that physiological existence as such is not a value if that life lacks any potential for a mental-creative function. Other quality-of-life proponents such as David Thomasma and his colleagues have described physical life as only a conditional value (Thomasma et al., 1986). According to these positions, what is valuable or worthwhile about physical life is either the properties that inhere in life or the values that transcend biological existence but whose pursuit is conditioned on the presence of physical life.

When quality of life is not defined as a property or attribute but rather as a qualitative relation between the patient's medical condition and his or her ability to pursue human values, then a different evaluative status is accorded to physical life. Walter (1988) has argued that physical life, as a created reality, is an ontic value, that is, a true and real value that does not depend on some property to give it value. He has tried to acknowledge that physical life is objectively a value in itself, though it may not always be experienced as such by some patients. Thus, physical life is not simply a useful or negotiable good; on the other hand, neither is it an absolute value that must be preserved in every instance.

Some commentators have attempted to address questions about the evaluative status of life by contrasting the quality-of-life ethic with the sanctity-of-life ethic (e.g., Johnstone, 1985; Reich, 1978b; Weber, 1976). Most proponents of a sanctity-of-life ethic (e.g., Connery, 1986; Johnstone, 1985; Meilaender, 1982; Reich, 1978a) do not argue that physical life itself is an absolute value. In this regard, at least, they agree with all proponents of the quality-of-life ethic. However, these authors frequently claim that when quality of life is understood as a property of life, either no value or only varying degrees of value is accorded to physical life. Possessing no intrinsic worth, physical life must receive its value based on whether it possesses one or more of the valued qualities, for example, neo-cortical function.

The sanctity-of-life position argues that this view is intolerable on several counts. First, quality of life does not acknowledge the equality of physical lives and the equality of persons because it assigns only relative or unequal value to physical lives and persons when certain valued qualities are only partially present or totally absent. Second, quality of life denies that all lives are inherently valuable, and so it leaves open the possibility that some lives can be deemed "not worth living." Finally, it is charged that the quality-of-life position adopts a two-level anthropology committed to protecting physical life only as an instrumental value (Reich, 1978b). Consequently, it is argued that the sanctity-of-life position is far superior because it affirms the equality of life on the basis that physical life is truly a value or good in itself. Life is not merely a useful or negotiable value, dependent on some other intrinsically valuable property.

In conclusion, it is not always clear how useful it may be to contrast sanctity of life with quality of life, as if each position could be represented by an individual and distinct "ethic." Because there are many positions that fit under each one of these "ethics," the terms and results of the comparison really depend on which two positions are selected.

Normative considerations of quality of life

The most important issues related to quality of life in clinical decisions are those concerned with the normative dimensions of the criterion. This level involves several considerations: (1) assessments about what is considered normatively human, or what reasons can be adduced to consider a certain trait or property of life decisive in making a clinical decision to treat or not to treat; (2) the normative moral theory that grounds and justifies moral obligations; and (3) the limits or exceptions to moral obligations to preserve life and the moral justifications for these limits or exceptions. The first issue is definitional in nature, although it also entails some normative features. The second issue relates to the debate over deontology, which determines the rightness of actions by reference to moral rules or the doing of one's duty, and teleology, which determines moral rightness by reference to the ends or consequences of actions. The third issue involves a discussion of the nature and degree of obligation in moral duties to preserve life.

Before turning to actual positions and their normative implications, it is important to distinguish cases where quality-of-life judgments are made by patients who possess decision-making capacity, and those cases where patients—for example, PVS patients, neonates or severely mentally handicapped adults from birth—lack the capacity to decide. Many issues need to be faced once patients with decision-making capacity are permitted to make treatment choices based on their own assessments of quality of life. However, these problems may pale in comparison to the application of the quality-of-life criterion to situations where a proxy or surrogate must make a decision to terminate treatment.

Some authors (e.g., Ramsey, 1978) argue that quality-of-life judgments should never be permitted in treatment decisions for patients who lack decision-making capacity. Only competent patients can make these judgments for themselves; no one may morally substitute his or her quality-of-life judgments for those of someone else. Thus, the moral criterion that applies in treatment decisions for patients who lack decision-making capacity is whatever is medically indicated. However, quality-of-life proponents argue that the medical indications policy could be devastating for these patients. If surrogates do not apply some measure of the quality-of-life criterion, these patients may be condemned to lives of pain, suffering, or burden that no person with decision-making capacity would reasonably choose (Hastings Center, 1987). Most of the following considerations will be concerned with the use of quality-of-life judgments in cases involving patients who lack decision-making capacity.

When some proponents of this criterion define quality of life as a property or attribute that gives value to physical life, they are either implicitly or explicitly defining what is normatively human, that is, how personhood ought to be defined. For example, when Fletcher originally defined the fifteen positive and five negative indicators of humanhood, he was defining the nature of personhood, and therefore, who is morally entitled to medical care. If a handicapped neonate or adult lacked a number of the indicators of humanhood but needed medical treatment to survive, in Fletcher's view (1972), the patient should not be treated.

The moral obligation to treat or not to treat patients is derived from the objective presence or absence of a valued property that gives worth and moral standing to the patient's life. When the properties that define humanhood are absent, the patient is not considered a moral subject who possesses any rights to health care. The moral theory that Fletcher adopts in his quality-of-life position is a form of teleology called consequentialism. In this theory, any moral claim about the value of a patient's life or any moral duty to provide medical treatment is almost entirely based on predictable qualitative consequences for the patient or for others whose interests are involved in the situation.

In a similar position on quality of life, Earl Shelp (1986) has sought to articulate the quality or property that defines the normatively human for handicapped neonates and the extent to which parents and the medical community have moral obligations to these never-competent patients. He adopts a quality-of-life position that corresponds to the main features of a property-based theory of personhood. A property-based theory, as opposed to a genetic-based theory, seeks to designate a desired quality or property that must be present before one can consider a particular human life to be an unqualified member in the moral community.

Shelp has argued that any neonate must possess the possibility of attaining a "minimal independence" before the child can be considered a person in a full sense. If the newborn will never have the capacity of minimal independence, even with the help of modern medicine, then the parents can decide on the basis of quality-of-life considerations that their child, who is in need of medical treatment, should not be treated.

The normative position that underlies Shelp's quality-of-life criterion is a type of a socially weighted calculus. Because he believes that no newborn, whether normal or impaired, is a full member of the moral community (person), he maintains that there is no compelling reason why a severely defective newborn's interests should take priority over those of the parents or siblings who are already persons in a moral sense. In fact, the interests of the ill newborn can be weighed against the independent interests of those whom the child will affect. Thus, if the burden imposed on others is unreasonable or disproportionate, then a decision to forgo or terminate all treatment for the imperiled child is morally legitimate.

What may be problematic in both Fletcher's and Shelp's versions of quality of life, and certainly what worries all opponents of quality-of-life positions, is that their views appear to define and prescribe the "good life" in terms of the quality or qualities necessary to live a minimal moral existence. Their positions then become entrapped within what William Aiken (1982) has called the "exclusionary" use of quality of life. The lack of certain valued qualities in a patient's life is a way of positively excluding potential patients from the normal standards of medical and moral treatment.

Other versions on the spectrum of quality-of-life positions do not limit the meaning of quality of life merely to a property of life and then establish moral obligations on the basis of the presence or absence of the property. In addition, these positions do not define the normatively human by reference to a valued attribute and then identify it with quality of life. For them, quality of life functions as a way to include what they believe are morally relevant factors in the clinical decision that are often excluded by other criteria. In other words, some proponents of this normative position hold that quality of life is a patient-centered way of discovering the best interests of a patient.

These authors (e.g., Sparks, 1988) argue that in the clinical situation for noncompetent patients, we should be trying to discover what is in their best interests. They recognize that other criteria, such as the ordinary–ex-

traordinary means criterion, have also been used to determine the patient's best interests, and that these criteria have been used to ground moral duties to patients in treatment decisions. However, they argue that these criteria often exclude some morally relevant factors needed to make an adequate and informed moral judgment, for example, the experienced burdens of the patient's prior medical condition in cases of spina bifida.

A comparison of the quality-of-life criterion with the ordinary–extraordinary means criterion might be helpful in illustrating the point that these authors are making. Those who subscribe to the ordinary–extraordinary means criterion argue that all ordinary means of preserving life are morally obligatory, but extraordinary means are morally optional. They do permit surrogates to use what could be called a limited version of the quality-of-life criterion. Surrogates can legitimately include quality-of-life considerations in their treatment decisions, but these considerations are only valid where the treatment itself would cause either excessive harm or leave the patient in a debilitated state (Connery, 1986; Reich, 1978b). For example, a surrogate could morally refuse quadruple amputation because the surgery itself would leave the patient with such an extremely low quality of life that the patient would have no duty to undergo the surgery.

All too often, however, the use of this criterion excludes all quality-of-life considerations that cannot be directly connected to the treatment itself or to its application. For example, the fact that a child who is born with Lesch-Nyhan syndrome will have a very poor quality of life is not considered relevant in the clinical decision to treat the child for a life-threatening condition. Lesch-Nyhan is an incurable genetic disease that causes its victims to suffer uncontrollable spasms and mental retardation. Once the young patients of this disease develop teeth, they gnaw their hands and shoulders, and they often bite off a finger or mutilate other parts of their bodies.

Some proponents of the quality-of-life criterion (e.g., McCormick, 1986; Sparks, 1988) identify this criterion with the category of "patient's best interests." They adopt what they believe is a patient-centered, teleological assessment of the best interests of the patient. If a patient in a life-threatening condition does possess at least a minimal ability to relate to others, then it can be presumed that the patient would want treatment; thus, treatment should be provided. This form of the quality-of-life criterion maintains that physical life itself is the ground of a prima facie duty to preserve it.

However, other factors—for example, the patient's prior medical condition, which might include permanent loss of all sentient and cognitive abilities, or the financial cost to the family and society of caring for these patients—also come to bear in determining the actual moral duty these patients have to preserve their own lives. Proponents of this version of the criterion argue that medical interventions to continue the lives of accurately diagnosed PVS patients and neonates born with anencephaly or hydranencephaly are unwarranted. These patients have reached the limits of their moral obligations to preserve their own lives, based on an assessment of their best interests. Any medical intervention to save their lives would only perpetuate a condition that most people who possess decision-making capacity would judge burdensome and intolerable. These authors do not judge that some patients' lives are not worth living; however, they do argue that the experienced burdens on patients' lives prior to treatment must be considered in determining the patient's best interests, and thus whether the patient himself or herself has a moral obligation to preserve life.

One of the more difficult questions involved in the debate over the use of quality-of-life judgments is whether one can include in the assessment of best interests of the patient any of the burdens that accrue to affected others. For example, when a family must face the tragic situation of financially and psychologically caring for a severely handicapped child, many would find such a lifelong commitment quite burdensome. Must one discount in treatment decisions the burdens experienced by the family and society in caring for these children, and focus only on the burdens imposed on the child either by the disease or by the treatments themselves? Or is it morally legitimate to include at least some of the burdens imposed on the family and society in assessing the patient's best interests? In other words, how broadly should one interpret the category of "best interests of the patient"? And finally, should the interests of others be considered in their own right? These are some of the questions that the proponents of quality of life regularly ask in clinical situations.

Richard Sparks (1988) is critical of any position that tries to understand the proportionality of benefits and burdens in a way that weighs a severely handicapped child's claims against the interests, claims, and rights of others who are affected, whether within the family or in society. He is also critical of quality-of-life proponents like McCormick, whom he sees as too narrowly defining the range of burdens in these cases. Sparks suggests the phrase "total best interests" as a way not only of including the burden experienced by the patient but also of including the broader social factors, for example, the financial cost, psychic strain, and inconvenience borne by others. He reasons that the patient's social nature must be taken into account, not only in calculating benefits (for example, the benefit to the patient derived from his or her ability to relate to others), but also in calculating burdens (for example, psychic strain to the family or financial cost to society).

Sparks's version of the quality-of-life criterion rejects a socially weighted calculus similar to the one Shelp adopts in determining the best interests of the patient. He judges that such a calculus denies the inherent worth of each individual patient, and that it weighs the benefits and burdens experienced by the patient against those of affected others. Although he argues that the burden to others should be included in assessing the total best interests of the patient, this burden is only one factor among many that must be considered. What is essential is that one not construe the burden to the patient and the burden to affected others as being in competition with one another when making decisions to terminate medical treatment.

By trying to construe the social burdens from the patient's perspective, Sparks believes one can avoid the competitive atmosphere that is part of the socially weighted position. His version of quality of life seems to imply that the child would not, and perhaps should not, want to be treated if it were an excessive social burden because the child's best interests would not be served if these burdens were placed on those who must care for him or her.

The spectrum of definitions and positions representing quality of life makes it difficult to identify any one quality-of-life ethic for analysis or critique. Though there are some shared features among the various positions, in the end it is necessary to assess the validity or invalidity of each position on its own merits.

JAMES J. WALTER

Directly related to this article are the other articles in this entry: QUALITY OF LIFE IN HEALTH-CARE ALLOCATION, *and* QUALITY OF LIFE IN LEGAL PERSPECTIVE. *For a further discussion of topics mentioned in this article, see the entries* ABORTION; AGING AND THE AGED; DEATH; DEATH AND DYING: EUTHANASIA AND SUSTAINING LIFE; ETHICS, *article on* NORMATIVE ETHICAL THEORIES; FAMILY; FEMINISM; HARM; HEALTH AND DISEASE, *article on* THE EXPERIENCE OF HEALTH AND ILLNESS; HUMAN NATURE; MENTALLY DISABLED AND MENTALLY ILL PERSONS; NATURE; OBLIGATION AND SUPEREROGATION; PAIN AND SUFFERING; *and* RIGHTS. *For a further discussion of related ideas, see the entries* ARTIFICIAL ORGANS AND LIFE-SUPPORT SYSTEMS; DEATH, ATTITUDES TOWARD; DEATH, DEFINITION AND DETERMINATION OF; DEATH: ART OF DYING; EUGENICS; FUTURE GENERATIONS, OBLIGATIONS TO; GENETIC COUNSELING; GENETICS AND HUMAN SELF-UNDERSTANDING; GENETIC TESTING AND SCREENING; HOSPICE AND END-OF-LIFE CARE; NATIONAL SOCIALISM; PATIENTS' RIGHTS; PROFESSIONAL–PATIENT RELATIONSHIP; UTILITY; *and* VALUE AND VALUATION. *Other relevant material may be found in the entries* AIDS; EUGENICS AND RELIGIOUS

Law; Health Care, Quality of; Infants, *article on* history of infanticide; Informed Consent; *and* Judaism.

Bibliography

Aiken, William. 1982. "The Quality of Life." *Applied Philosophy* 1 (Spring):26–36.

Connery, John R. 1986. "Quality of Life." *Linacre Quarterly* 53 (February):26–33.

Destro, Robert A. 1986. "Quality-of-Life Ethics and Constitutional Jurisprudence: The Demise of Natural Rights and Equal Protection for the Disabled and Incompetent." *Journal of Contemporary Health Law and Policy* 2: 71–130.

Fletcher, Joseph. 1972. "Indicators of Humanhood: A Tentative Profile of Man." *Hastings Center Report* 2, no. 6: 1–4.

———. 1974. "Four Indicators of Humanhood—The Enquiry Matures." *Hastings Center Report* 4, no. 6:4–7.

Gerson, Elihu M. 1976. "On 'Quality of Life.'" *American Sociological Review* 41:793–806.

Gilligan, Carol. 1982. *In a Different Voice: Psychological Theory and Women's Development.* Cambridge, Mass.: Harvard University Press.

Hastings Center. 1987. *Guidelines on the Termination of Life-Sustaining Treatment and the Care of the Dying: A Report.* Briarcliff Manor, N.Y.: Author.

Johnstone, Brian V. 1985. "The Sanctity of Life, the Quality of Life and the New 'Baby Doe' Law." *Linacre Quarterly* 52 (August):258–270.

Keyserlingk, Edward W. 1979. *Sanctity of Life; or, Quality of Life in the Context of Ethics, Medicine and Law: A Study.* Ottawa: Minister of Supply and Services.

Kilner, John F. 1988. "Age as a Basis for Allocating Life-saving Medical Resources: An Ethical Analysis." *Journal of Health Politics, Policy and Law* 13, no. 3:405–423.

McCormick, Richard A. 1974. "To Save or Let Die." *America* 131, no. 1:6–10.

———. 1978. "The Quality of Life, the Sanctity of Life." *Hastings Center Report* 8, no. 1:30–36.

———. 1981. *How Brave a New World? Dilemmas in Bioethics.* Washington, D.C.: Georgetown University Press.

———. 1984. *Health and Medicine in the Catholic Tradition: Tradition in Transition.* New York: Crossroad.

———. 1986. "The Best Interests of the Baby." *Second Opinion* 2:18–25.

Meilaender, Gilbert C. 1982. "If This Baby Could Choose . . ." *Linacre Quarterly* 49 (November):313–321.

O'Rourke, Kevin D., and Brodeur, Dennis. 1986. *Medical Ethics: Common Ground for Understanding.* St. Louis: Catholic Health Association of the United States.

Ramsey, Paul. 1978. *Ethics at the Edges of Life: Medical and Legal Intersections.* New Haven, Conn.: Yale University Press.

Reich, Warren T. 1978a. "Life: Quality of Life." In vol. 2 of *Encyclopedia of Bioethics,* pp. 829–840. Edited by Warren T. Reich. New York: Macmillan.

———. 1978b. "Quality of Life and Defective Newborn Children: An Ethical Analysis." In *Decision Making and the Defective Newborn: Proceedings of a Conference on Spina Bifida and Ethics,* pp. 489–511. Edited by Chester A. Swinyard. Springfield, Ill.: Charles C. Thomas.

Shelp, Earl E. 1986. *Born to Die? Deciding the Fate of Critically Ill Newborns.* New York: Free Press.

Sichel, Betty A. 1989. "Ethics of Caring and the Institutional Ethics Committee." *Hypatia* 4, no. 2:45–56.

Sparks, Richard C. 1988. *To Treat or Not to Treat: Bioethics and the Handicapped Newborn.* New York: Paulist Press.

Thomasma, David C.; Micetich, Kenneth C.; and Steineker, Patricia H. 1986. "Continuance of Nutritional Care in the Terminally Ill Patient." *Critical Care Clinics* 2, no. 1:61–71.

U.S. Department of Health and Human Services. 1985. "Child Abuse and Neglect Prevention and Treatment." *Federal Register* 50, no. 72:14887–14892.

Veatch, Robert M. 1976. *Death, Dying, and the Biological Revolution: Our Last Quest for Responsibility.* New Haven, Conn.: Yale University Press.

Walter, James J. 1988. "The Meaning and Validity of Quality of Life Judgments in Contemporary Roman Catholic Medical Ethics." *Louvain Studies* 13 (Fall):195–208.

Walter, James J., and Shannon, Thomas A., eds. 1990. *Quality of Life: The New Medical Dilemma.* New York: Paulist Press.

Weber, Leonard J. 1976. *Who Shall Live? The Dilemma of Severely Handicapped Children and Its Meaning for Other Moral Questions.* New York: Paulist Press.

II. QUALITY OF LIFE IN HEALTH-CARE ALLOCATION

Issues concerning quality of life in health-care allocation arise because of three factors. First, there is an important project that a society wants to undertake: in this case, to provide health care for all the people, especially for those who cannot do so on their own. Second, unlike the ordinary marketplace, where individuals purchase what they want for their own reasons and there is no need for anyone else's agreement about what to purchase, a society that collectively funds a community project must agree on what outcomes will count as fulfilling that goal. Third, resources are limited partly because taxpayers cannot be expected to forfeit an unlimited amount of their income, and partly because there are other important projects that command taxpayers' funds. Hence, we need assurance that expenditures will actually enhance health without wasting resources.

Prioritizing expenditures becomes urgent because health care is extraordinarily expensive, consuming some 15 percent of the gross domestic product of the United States in the early 1990s. The need is further dramatized by certain publicized cases, such as that of

Baby K, an anencephalic infant whose mother insisted on unlimited medical support, regardless of the cost, on the grounds that all life is infinitely precious (*Matter of Baby K*, 1994). Many observers deem it clearly wasteful to prolong the life of someone who will never be conscious while so many other social needs, from health care to education, are underfunded. More controversial examples point out the trade-offs between costly new technologies that benefit a few identified patients versus more routine kinds of care that benefit many more people whose identities may never be known (Eddy, 1992a, 1992b). Cases such as these raise the question whether it is permissible, and if so in what way, to consider "quality of life" in health-care resource allocation.

There are two ways to do so. Negatively, one might rule out certain kinds of expenditure on the grounds that they produce little or no benefit for their patient. This might be based on evidence that the treatment has not been shown to be effective, for example, when a treatment is highly experimental or when a patient is so close to death that no medical interventions can help. Positively, one might invoke quality-of-life judgments to give funding priority to health interventions that will produce the greatest overall benefit for the money spent. Since health care is intended to improve as well as prolong life, quality-of-life judgments would shape this quest for the greatest benefit.

It is important to identify some basic distinctions. To speak of the quality of life is not equivalent to making judgments about the value of that life. Persons suffering from a painful terminal illness might have a poor quality of life; their value and dignity as human beings, however, are every bit as precious as those of healthier persons. Similarly, the quality that someone's life has for himself or herself is not equivalent to the impact that the person has on another's quality of life. A patient suffering from advanced Alzheimer's disease or other dementia, for instance, might be content and free of suffering, while posing serious burdens and sorrow for family members. Finally, judgments about the quality of an individual's life might come from the individual himor herself, or from others. The most common instruments for measuring quality of life rely on views elicited from the public at large as they contemplate the life quality caused by certain illnesses or disabilities. However, these opinions may not match the views of people who actually experience these conditions.

A variety of instruments have been developed to measure the benefits of health-care interventions. The "human capital" approach, for instance, measures the value of saving or prolonging a life by projecting that person's future earnings. This method is not widely accepted, mainly because it looks only at market valuation of economic contributions, and not at broader features of the person's experiences and relationships.

A considerably more sophisticated instrument, the "willingness-to-pay" approach, hypothetically lets individuals determine what value they place on a prolongation or improvement of their lives by indicating how much they would actually be willing to pay in order to avoid a certain risk of mortality or morbidity, or to gain a chance at improving their lot. Though this approach permits individuals to make their own quality-of-life judgments, its main disadvantage is that it could reflect not personal preferences but wealth status, which may reflect factors such as social injustices (Brock, 1993).

An even more sophisticated approach does not try to translate morbidity and mortality directly into cash equivalents, nor to count lives saved or the number of years saved by a particular health-care intervention. Rather, it attempts to determine the effect that an intervention has on the quality as well as duration of life by computing Quality-Adjusted Life-Years (QALYs). Extending an extra year for a patient in a vegetative state, it is assumed, is not as worthwhile as adding a year of vigorous, healthy function. This approach estimates the quality of life that may accompany a particular set of circumstances before and after the intervention and how long the change is expected to last. The cost of that intervention can then be compared with other health-care interventions for their respective cost-effectiveness to identify which ones produce the greatest value.

Various instruments have been used to measure quality of life. The Quality of Well-Being (QWB) Index defines twenty-four health or functional states from perfect health to death. Through questionnaires and community surveys, each QWB state is given a weight, from 0 for death to 1 for perfect health (Kaplan, 1992, 1985; Kaplan et al., 1976). Other scales, such as the Quality of Life Index or the Sickness Impact Profile, evaluate quality of life according to factors such as ability to perform daily activities, feelings of satisfaction with one's health status, and the like (Brock, 1993; Zeckhauser, 1975; Zeckhauser and Shepard, 1976; Wenger et al., 1984).

The state of Oregon used the QALY approach in an effort to ensure, on the negative side, that it does not waste limited state dollars, and on the positive side, to maximize the good achieved by its Medicaid program by avoiding marginally valuable expenditures while expanding coverage to encompass numerous uninsured people. Initially, a series of town meetings and phone surveys elicited community opinions about the value of a variety of conditions, such as perfect health, feeling depressed and upset, being burned over large areas of one's body, and so on. The value system thus generated was then combined with physicians' estimates of the magnitude and duration of effects produced by various medical interventions for various conditions. After combining the QALY units derived for these treatment/condition pairs with their respective costs, a priority list was developed. Taking the prevalence and cost of treatment for each condition on that list, accountants were able to tell the legislature how much money would be required to fund the program as the next lower priority item was added. The legislature then set its Medicaid budget and identified a cutoff point: Eligible recipients would receive all services prioritized above that line, but not below it (Garland, 1992; Eddy, 1991; Hadorn, 1991; Kaplan, 1992). This first attempt yielded enough unexpected results that the priority list was significantly changed before the program was finally approved (Eddy, 1991).

The problems Oregon encountered illustrate the ethical challenges in using quality-of-life considerations in health-care allocation. They begin with methodological problems. Oregon's plan, and QALY approaches generally, are criticized for ignoring the wide variations of severity that can characterize any medical condition, from broken bones to lupus, and the equally varying results that any given treatment can have for a particular condition. Further, it is not clear whose values should be attached to these factual descriptions. Opinions solicited from the public at large may be based on a poor understanding of the medical condition at stake. A one-sentence summary on a questionnaire, for instance, is hardly sufficient for understanding what it is like to live as a paraplegic. Similarly, college students are not necessarily the best people to survey regarding the quality of retired persons' lives (Vaupel, 1976). Moreover, patients' views on their own quality of life cannot always be discovered. Advanced dementia, infancy, stroke retardation, and a host of conditions can prevent the individual from expressing his or her views or even, in some cases, from conceptualizing his or her quality of life. The Oregon plan, in particular, was criticized for eliciting values mainly from articulate, middle-class persons rather than from the poor and disabled, who would be most affected by the resulting distribution of health-care resources. These and other methogical criticisms (Morreim, 1986, 1992), are important, because even if one can on principle justify allocating health-care resources according to treatments' impact on life quality, it is morally more difficult to justify using measures that may not capture what they should.

Moral issues also concern the very idea of using quality of life as a basis on which to allocate care. Vitalists who believe that all life is infinitely valuable, regardless of its quality, simply reject the idea that interventions should be graded according to how well they enhance quality of life. Others would insist that it is wasteful, if not unconscionable, to spend limited resources sustaining the lives of permanently unconscious or imminently dying patients.

A corollary objection insists that the cost of treatment is no reason for restricting it. Individuals should not suffer needlessly just because their care is costly. Rather, costs should be contained in other ways, such as by eliminating wasteful expenditures. In reply, it is argued that needs are always greater than resources, rendering rationing inevitable, and that overt public decisions are preferable to covert priorities.

A further critique holds that maximizing QALYs, somehow reified as a good in themselves, ignores the justice of the distribution. This is a classic challenge to utilitarianism. Here, critics point out that a pure cost–benefit approach can ignore terrible suffering, simply because some other intervention may be cheaper and help larger numbers of people. The first listing of Oregon's priorities, for instance, ranked dental caps for pulp exposure higher than surgery for ectopic pregnancy, and splints for temporomandibular joints higher than appendectomies for appendicitis. Although some people might reply that only the methodology needs to be adjusted (Eddy, 1991), others would argue that this approach is inherently incapable of honoring the preciousness that attaches to the lives and well-being of individual people (Hadorn, 1991). Severely disabled persons may not be capable of enjoying as great a benefit as healthy persons snatched from the jaws of death, but their comfort and personhood are not necessarily less important.

Another controversy concerns whose values should shape estimates of life quality. If the purpose of medical interventions is to help individuals, should not patients be permitted to define what constitutes a benefit? Studies indicate that persons afflicted with a particular malady often rate their quality of life higher than observers do (Evans et al., 1985). Fairness might require recognition that sometimes individual preferences are costly and idiosyncratic and acknowledgment that the society paying for care should be permitted to use community values to determine monetary allocation (Morreim, 1986, 1992).

A related issue points out that the QALY approach inherently discriminates against the elderly and disabled, whose prognoses and initial quality of life are typically lower than average. In reply, it is argued that the elderly at least have had the opportunity to complete their life's biography (Callahan, 1987), and that while methods to value the comfort and improved function of the disabled can be developed, aggressive medical interventions may not serve the most severely compromised patients well.

The issues cannot be resolved here, but a few comments seem pertinent. First, society is not required to fund every expenditure that each citizen might find worthwhile. Vitalists should arguably be permitted to seek life support for permanently unconscious loved ones, but this does not entail that a society that does not share this belief must pay for their quest (Morreim, 1992). Second, the moral character of a society is at least partly reflected by the ways it treats its weakest members. The fact that someone is not useful to others does not entail that his or her sensibilities are insignificant or undeserving of help. Third, those obligations are not unlimited. There is a virtually endless variety of ways in which society can arrange its resource priorities, and none of them is the single morally correct approach. What is probably most important is the development of procedures that are fair and open to wide participation, are sensitive to varying viewpoints, and show a respect for citizens as persons (Brock, 1993; Engelhardt, 1992).

E. HAAVI MORREIM

Directly related to this article are the other articles in the entry: QUALITY OF LIFE IN CLINICAL DECISIONS, *and* QUALITY OF LIFE IN LEGAL PERSPECTIVE. *Also directly related are the entries* ECONOMIC CONCEPTS IN HEALTH CARE; UTILITY; HEALTH-CARE FINANCING; HEALTH-CARE RESOURCES, ALLOCATION OF; *and* HEALTH POLICY, *article on* POLITICS AND HEALTH CARE. *This article will find application in the entries* ARTIFICIAL HEARTS AND CARDIAC-ASSIST DEVICES; ARTIFICIAL ORGANS AND LIFE-SUPPORT SYSTEMS; DEATH AND DYING: EUTHANASIA AND SUSTAINING LIFE, *article on* ETHICAL ISSUES; GENETIC TESTING AND SCREENING; HOSPICE AND END-OF-LIFE CARE; *and* KIDNEY DIALYSIS. *Other relevant material may be found under the entries* HEALTH CARE, QUALITY OF; HEALTH AND DISEASE, *article on* THE EXPERIENCE OF HEALTH AND ILLNESS; PUBLIC POLICY AND BIOETHICS; *and* RIGHTS, *article on* RIGHTS IN BIOETHICS.

Bibliography

Baby K, In re. 1993. 832 F.Supp. 1022 (E.D.Va.); 16 F.3d 590 (4th Cir. 1994).

BROCK, DAN W. 1993. *Life and Death: Philosophical Essays in Biomedical Ethics.* Cambridge: At the University Press.

CALLAHAN, DANIEL. 1987. *Setting Limits: Medical Goals in an Aging Society.* New York: Simon and Schuster.

EDDY, DAVID M. 1991. "Oregon's Methods: Did Cost-Effectiveness Analysis Fail?" *Journal of the American Medical Association* 266, no. 15:2135–2141.

———. 1992a. "Clinical Decision Making: From Theory to Practice. Applying Cost-Effectiveness Analysis: The Inside Story." *Journal of the American Medical Association* 268, no. 18:2575–2582.

———. 1992b. "Clinical Decision Making: From Theory to Practice. Cost-Effectiveness Analysis: Is It Up to the Task?" *Journal of the American Medical Association* 267, no. 24:3342–3348.

ENGELHARDT, H. TRISTRAM, JR. 1992. "Why a Two-Tier System of Health Care Delivery Is Morally Unavoidable." In *Rationing America's Medical Care: The Oregon Plan and Beyond,* pp. 196–207. Edited by Martin A. Strosberg, Joshua M. Wiener, Robert Baker, and I. Alan Fein. Washington, D.C.: Brookings Institution.

EVANS, ROGER W.; MANNINEN, DIANE L.; GARRISON, LOUIS P.; HART, L. GARY; BLAGG, CHRISTOPHER R.; GUTMAN, ROBERT A.; HULL, ALAN R.; and LOWRIE, EDMUND G. 1985. "The Quality of Life of Patients with End-Stage Renal Disease." *New England Journal of Medicine* 312, no. 9:553–559.

GARLAND, MICHAEL J. 1992. "Rationing in Public: Oregon's Priority-Setting Methodology." In *Rationing America's Medical Care: The Oregon Plan and Beyond,* pp. 37–59. Edited by Martin A. Strosberg, Joshua M. Wiener, Robert Baker, and I. Alan Fein. Washington, D.C.: Brookings Institution.

HADORN, DAVID C. 1991. "Setting Health Care Priorities in Oregon: Cost-Effectiveness Meets the Rule of Rescue." *Journal of the American Medical Association* 265: 2218–2225.

KAPLAN, ROBERT M. 1985. "Quality-of-Life Measurement." In *Measurement Strategies in Health Psychology,* pp. 115–146. Edited by Paul Karoly. New York: Wiley.

———. 1992. "A Quality-of-Life Approach to Health-Resource Allocation." In *Rationing America's Medical Care: The Oregon Plan and Beyond,* pp. 60–77. Edited by Martin A. Strosberg, Joshua M. Wiener, Robert Baker, and I. Alan Fein. Washington, D.C.: Brookings Institution.

KAPLAN, ROBERT M.; BUSH, J. W.; and BERRY, CHARLES C. 1976. "Health Status: Types of Validity and the Index of Well-Being." *Health Services Research* 11, no. 4:478–507.

MORREIM, E. HAAVI. 1986. "Computing the Quality of Life." In *The Price of Health,* pp. 45–69. Dordrecht, Netherlands: D. Reidel.

———. 1992. "The Impossibility and the Necessity of Quality of Life Research." *Bioethics* 6, no. 3:218–232.

———. 1994. "Profoundly Diminished Life: The Casualties of Coercion." *Hastings Center Report* 24, no. 1:33–42.

VAUPEL, JAMES W. 1976. "Early Death: An American Tragedy." *Law and Contemporary Problems* 40, no. 4:73–121.

WENGER, NANETTE KASS; MATTSON, MARGARET E.; FURBERG, CURT D.; and ELINSON, JACK. 1984. "Overview: Assessment of Quality of Life in Clinical Trials of Cardiovascular Therapies." In *Assessment of Quality of Life in Clinical Trials of Cardiovascular Therapies,* pp. 1–22. Edited by Nanette Kass Wenger. New York: LeJacq.

ZECKHAUSER, RICHARD. 1975. "Procedures for Valuing Lives." *Public Policy* 23, no. 4:419–464.

ZECKHAUSER, RICHARD, and SHEPARD, DONALD. 1976. "Where Now for Saving Lives?" *Law and Contemporary Problems* 40, no. 4:5–45.

III. QUALITY OF LIFE IN LEGAL PERSPECTIVE

Law has addressed quality-of-life issues primarily in the context of the withholding or withdrawal of life-sustaining medical intervention. The legal dilemma arose when medical technology became capable of keeping alive persons with gravely debilitating and potentially fatal afflictions long beyond the point that most people would wish to live. The questions became, Under what circumstances is the removal of life support lawful? and, Can decisions to remove life support be grounded on quality-of-life factors?

Many sources contend that deteriorated quality of life—in the sense of a patient's prospective mental and physical debilitation—is a natural and inevitable element in shaping the bounds of medical intervention in the dying process. Most people, faced with a prolonged and debilitated dying process for themselves or a loved one, prefer that life support be withdrawn at some stage of deterioration. Decisions about life support for formerly vital people are therefore often grounded on factors like extreme mental dysfunction, immobility, and helplessness.

The opponents of using quality-of-life factors in ending people's lives cite numerous concerns. The most common is that judicial or legislative sanctioning of quality-of-life considerations will undermine the traditional focus of both criminal and tort law on preserving and protecting all human life, regardless of quality. One asserted hazard is that quality of life will be measured in terms of utilitarian elements such as cost of care, social productiveness of the patient, and burdens imposed upon the people caring for the patient. Such a utilitarian calculus would place the lives of the weak and vulnerable—the very young, the developmentally disabled, and the elderly—at particular risk (Destro, 1986).

Even if quality-of-life considerations are confined to factors that, from the patient's own perspective, make existence intolerable, some observers find moral hazards. If dismal quality of life focuses on physical and mental dysfunction, a concern is that the lives of disabled persons generally might be devalued and their morale eroded. Surrogate decision makers for incompetent patients might also be insensitive to the value of life as a disabled person, so that vulnerable populations would be endangered by arbitrary determinations. Some sanctity-of-life proponents prefer to protect and support all human existence even in the face of fatal afflictions and severe degeneration.

This tension between sanctity of life and quality of life has surfaced in a number of legal settings. Each of the following sections discusses the resolution of that tension in a particular legal context.

Patients competent to make their own decisions

Current law, rooted in concepts of self-determination and bodily integrity, establishes that competent patients are entitled to reject life-sustaining medical interven-

tion. The relevant cases recognize that patients can and often do base their rejection of life-sustaining treatment on quality-of-life factors. That fact emerges most clearly in cases involving severely disabled persons who reject treatment capable of preserving their existences for many years.

The typical situation involves a quadriplegic person dependent on mechanical life support who finds the debilitated existence so painful or demeaning that he or she orders the cessation of life-sustaining measures (*Thor v. Superior Court*, 1993; *McKay v. Bergstedt*, 1990; *State v. McAfee*, 1989; *Bouvia v. Superior Court*, 1986). Courts uniformly uphold the patient's decision. These courts recognize that patient self-determination encompasses personal values and preferences about whether a prospective medical state is intolerably painful or degrading—that is, constitutes an unacceptable quality of life. A California court explained:

> Since death is the natural conclusion of all life, the precise moment may be less critical than the quality of time preceding it. Especially when the prognosis for full recovery from serious illness or incapacity is dim, the relative balance of benefit and burden must lie within the patient's exclusive estimation: "That personal weighing of values is the essence of self-determination." (*Thor*, 1993, p. 384)

These same courts reject any notion that judicial acceptance of debilitated patients' fatal decisions weakens respect for life generally or devalues the lives of the disabled. The judges view their decisions as upholding individual autonomy and thereby promoting a critical element of human dignity, rather than as denigrating the sanctity of life.

Incompetent patients

Many medical patients lack the capacity to make their own decisions about life-sustaining treatment. A surrogate must then act on the patient's behalf. Some sources oppose the use of quality of life—determining whether a patient's life is "worth" preserving—in decision making for incompetent patients. Again, the concerns include use of utilitarian factors such as economic costs and social unproductivity of the patient. Beyond that, sanctity-of-life proponents fear arbitrary decisions by surrogates who are insensitive to the value of disabled persons' lives or motivated by self-interest.

In some instances, the now-incompetent patient has exercised personal autonomy by previously, when competent, having issued written or oral instructions about terminal medical care. Both courts and legislatures accept in principle this prospective autonomy (though some state legislatures have confined their endorsement of advance medical directives to situations in which the patient is in a "terminal" state). Through advance instructions, people can seek to discontinue medical intervention at a point when their existence becomes intolerable according to their own previously expressed definitions of quality of life.

The situation is more complicated when a now-incompetent patient facing a potentially fatal affliction has never articulated personal values and preferences about life-sustaining medical intervention. Courts in a few states disallow any terminal decision on behalf of an incompetent patient who has never issued advance instructions (*Westchester County Medical Center*, 1988; *Cruzan v. Harmon*, 1990; *Mack v. Mack*, 1993; *DeGrella v. Elston*, 1993). These courts express grave apprehension about allowing surrogates to determine that another person's life is not worth preserving. They insist either upon the patient's personal prior assessment of an intolerable quality of life or upon legislative guidance concerning what kinds of deteriorated existence are so undignified as not to be worth preserving.

Insistence upon clear-cut prior instructions as a prerequisite for withdrawal of life support from an incompetent patient disregards certain interests of people who have simply neglected to address the issue of terminal care (as well as those of people who have never been competent). The hazard is that such persons, once afflicted with debilitating medical conditions, will be indefinitely maintained in a status that the patients themselves would deem intolerably painful or demeaning, were they able to express their wishes. In the words of one judge, invariable preservation of life without regard to the incompetent patient's prospective deteriorated status "transforms human beings into unwilling prisoners of medical technology" (*Guardianship of L.W.*, 1992, p. 74). To avoid this unfortunate consequence, most courts that have spoken to the issue allow some surrogate decisions to reject life support even in the absence of prior instructions.

Courts subscribing to this position usually articulate a best-interests-of-the-patient standard to guide the surrogate decision maker (*Conroy*, 1985; *Guardianship of Drabick*, 1988). This normally means that in order to justify removal of life support, the "burdens" to the patient must clearly outweigh the "benefits," with irremediable physical suffering being the primary burden and pleasure being the primary benefit. The relevant cases carefully exclude "social utility" or "personal worth" as factors in the best interests calculus (*Conroy*, 1985, pp. 1232–1233). However, the role of quality of life (in the sense of a severely deteriorated and undignified patient status) is uncertain. Quality of life or dignity of the patient is often mentioned as an element within the best interests formula, but in application that factor has only been determinative in the context of permanently unconscious patients.

A few commentators have suggested that the concept of "medically inappropriate" or "futile" treatment ought to fix the bounds of life support for gravely debilitated patients (e.g., Jecker, 1991). Futile treatment, in the sense of medical intervention that cannot achieve a particular physiological goal, may be a meaningful and useful concept. However, when medical intervention can extend life, albeit debilitated life, the futility concept is much less helpful. A determination that life-sustaining medical intervention is futile really represents a judgment that the quality of life is so dismal that life support ought to be withdrawn as inconsistent with the best interests of the incompetent patient. That determination may be appropriate for surrogate decision makers (though the legal issue is still unresolved), but it cannot be the province of medical personnel alone (Cranford and Gustin, 1992; Veatch and Spicer, 1992).

Patients in a permanent vegetative state

A permanently unconscious patient cannot experience suffering or sense the bodily invasions that normally constitute "burdens" to be assessed under a best interests of the patient standard. At the same time, permanent unconsciousness represents a dehumanizing condition, with the patient indefinitely devoid of sensation, emotion, or human interaction. The vast majority of people contemplating such a status deem it so degrading that they would not want to be medically sustained in that insensate condition. (Some commentators even argue that the legal definition of death should be changed to include permanently vegetative beings, a suggestion that has not yet been adopted).

The clear majority of state court decisions regarding permanently unconscious patients has permitted surrogate decision makers to end life support. Still undecided is the precise legal rationale for this result and whether this line of cases represents use of quality of life as a determinative factor in surrogate decision making.

In some instances, the courts upholding removal of life support rely on prior expressions (whether written or oral) by the now unconscious patient. Those courts simply respect the patient's self-determination and accept the patient's own declaration of permanent unconsciousness as an unacceptable quality of life. These cases sometimes disclaim any surrogate's prerogative to define another person's quality of life as unacceptable (e.g., *DeGrella*, 1993).

Yet a number of cases uphold removal of life support from a permanently unconscious patient even in the absence of prior expressions. Some of these cases include never-competent patients, such as infants. None of the cases relies on the burdens placed upon society or surrounding family by care of the insensate patient. Rather, the judges articulate diverse rationales. Some courts use the substituted judgment rationale and accept that the patient, if competent, would have wanted removal of life support (*Guardianship of Jane Doe*, 1992). Other courts purport to apply a best interests standard, but rely on the patient's dismal existence without cognitive function as warranting removal of life support (*Guardianship of Crum*, 1992).

Most courts confronting the fate of permanently unconscious patients recognize, either explicitly or implicitly, that the patient's status is so dehumanizing that it represents what most people would regard as an unacceptable quality of life. These courts sometimes demand that the surrogate decision maker not rely on his or her personal views about the value of an unconscious person's life (*Guardianship of L. W.*, 1992). But they do allow for surrogates' reliance on the common judgment that most people wish to avoid a permanently unconscious state (because it lacks dignity and is devoid of value from the perspective of the unconscious patient), as long as the patient's ostensible preferences did not deviate from that norm.

By contrast, courts in a few jurisdictions have refused to endorse removal of life support from a permanently unconscious patient in the absence of prior expressions from that patient (*Cruzan*, 1990; *Westchester County*, 1988; *Mack*, 1993; *DeGrella*, 1993). These courts see the removal decision as a quality-of-life determination that should be made, if at all, pursuant to legislative directions. Some judges also fear that permission to remove life-sustaining medical intervention from the permanently unconscious would ultimately endanger vulnerable populations, such as the severely retarded (*Mack*, 1993; *Guardianship of Jane Doe*, 1992, dissent).

Infants and young children

Some congenital anomalies entail a foreshortened life span, as well as neurological impairment, physical incapacity, repeated bodily invasion, and suffering so severe that the affected infant is arguably better off dead than alive. As patient autonomy cannot function in this setting, the question becomes whether parents, in conjunction with medical sources, can withhold life support on the basis that the child's life would be so burdened or devoid of personal value that death is preferable. Some commentators oppose this surrogate option, fearing that decisions would be based on prejudice or ignorance about life as a disabled person or concern for parental burdens, rather than burdens upon the child (Field, 1993).

Only a small number of cases has been litigated and the legal picture concerning removal of infants' life support is murky. A few cases use a best-interests standard and rely on likely physical suffering to uphold parental decisions involving withholding of life-sustaining inter-

vention (*C.A.*, 1993; *Newmark v. Williams*, 1991). A few cases purport to apply a substituted judgment rationale (reasoning that the child, if competent, would choose death) in order to uphold removal of life support from a permanently vegetative child (*L.H.R.*, 1984; *Guardianship of Barry*, 1984).

The best-interests approach seems more plausible, allowing consideration of irremediable suffering and continuous bodily intrusions (Weir, 1984). An unresolved issue is the extent to which a dismal quality of life—in the sense of total helplessness and minimal potential for human relationships—can be used legitimately in this best-interests calculus. As a practical matter, it is hard for decision makers to exclude extreme debilitation in applying a best-interests standard. Extreme disability is commonly associated with hardship for the affected child. This element apparently emerges in decision making not only in the United States but also in Australia, Canada, and Great Britain (Charlesworth, 1993).

At the same time, stereotypes about disabled persons might prompt inappropriate terminal decisions. This happened in one case involving an infant afflicted with Down syndrome (*Baby Doe v. Hancock County*, 1982). One possible limitation appears in U.S. federal statutes and regulations prohibiting hospital discrimination against the disabled and requiring states to protect the interests of disabled infants (see *Baby K*, 1993; *Johnson v. Thompson*, 1993). The effect of these measures is still unclear. U.S. federal regulations purport to bar quality-of-life considerations in decisions about infants' medical treatment (Clark, 1993). However, decisions about medical treatment ineluctably involve consideration of the hardship and debilitation to be encountered by the patient after treatment. Where a patient's disability is intertwined with the contemplated medical service (as in spina bifida), a nontreatment decision cannot be deemed unlawful discrimination if the decision is grounded on a reasonable assessment of the suffering and hardship to be encountered by the affected individual. The disabled infant's fate is being determined by the same criteria—overall best interests—applicable to any child under treatment.

Conclusion

Diminished quality of life, in the sense of grievous bodily deterioration, is a frequent consideration in shaping the bounds of medical intervention in the dying process. The current challenge for law and medicine is to fix quality-of-life criteria for surrogate decision makers that avoid arbitrariness and abuse toward vulnerable, incapacitated patients. The key, for previously competent patients without advance instructions, should be assessment of which levels of deterioration the great majority of competent persons would consider (for their own dying processes) to be so undignified that they would prefer that life support be withdrawn.

By using this common-dignity guideline, decision makers will better replicate the likely wishes of now-incompetent patients, thus ultimately attaining results as consistent as possible with personal preferences. Empirical data for measuring common notions of dignity can be gleaned from public surveys as well as from scrutiny of patterns in advance medical directives. Anyone whose preferences diverge from common notions of dignity can provide individualized instructions reflecting those preferences.

NORMAN L. CANTOR

Directly related to this article are the other articles in this entry: QUALITY OF LIFE IN CLINICAL DECISIONS, *and* QUALITY OF LIFE IN HEALTH-CARE ALLOCATION. *For a further discussion of topics mentioned in this article, see the entries* DEATH AND DYING: EUTHANASIA AND SUSTAINING LIFE, *articles on* ETHICAL ISSUES, *and* ADVANCE DIRECTIVES; DISABILITY, *articles on* ATTITUDES AND SOCIOLOGICAL PERSPECTIVES, *and* LEGAL ISSUES; *and* PAIN AND SUFFERING. *For a discussion of related ideas, see the entries* ARTIFICIAL ORGANS AND LIFE-SUPPORT SYSTEMS; AUTONOMY; COMPETENCE; INFANTS, *article on* PUBLIC-POLICY AND LEGAL ISSUES; MENTALLY DISABLED AND MENTALLY ILL PERSONS, *article on* HEALTH-CARE ISSUES; *and* VALUE AND VALUATION. *See also the entries* LIFE; OBLIGATION AND SUPEREROGATION; *and* UTILITY.

Bibliography

Baby Doe v. Hancock County Bd. of Health. 1982. 436 N.E.2d 791 (Ind.).

Baby K, In re. 1993. 832 F. Supp. 1022 (E.D. Va.) aff'd 16 F.3d 590 (4th Cir. 1994).

Bouvia v. Superior Court (Glenchur). 1986. 225 Cal. Rptr. 297 (Dist. Ct. App.).

BUCHANAN, ALLEN E., and BROCK, DAN W. 1989. *Deciding for Others: The Ethics of Surrogate Decision Making.* New York: Cambridge University Press.

C.A., In re. 1992. 603 N.E. 2d 1171 (Ill. App.); *cert. denied,* 610 N.E. 2d 1264 (Ill. 1993).

CANTOR, NORMAN L. 1987. *Legal Frontiers of Death and Dying.* Bloomington: Indiana University Press.

———. 1990. "The Permanently Unconscious Patient, Non-Feeding, and Euthanasia." *American Journal of Law and Medicine* 15, no. 4:381–437.

CHARLESWORTH, MAX. 1993. "Disabled Newborn Infants and the Quality of Life." *Journal of Contemporary Health Law and Policy* 9:129–137.

CLARK, FRANK I. 1993. "Withdrawal of Life-Support in the Newborn: Whose Baby Is It?" *Southwestern University Law Review* 23 (Fall):1–46.

Conroy, In re. 1985. 486 A.2d 1209 (N.J.).

CRANFORD, RONALD, and GOSTIN, LAWRENCE. 1992. "Futility: A Concept in Search of a Definition." *Law, Medicine & Health Care* 20, no. 4:307–309.

Cruzan v. Harmon. 1990. 760 S.W.2d 408 (Mo. 1988), aff'd 497 U.S. 261.

DeGrella v. Elston. 1993. 858 S.W.2d 698 (Ky.).

DESTRO, ROBERT A. 1986. "Quality–of–Life Ethics and Constitutional Jurisprudence: The Demise of Natural Rights and Equal Protection for the Disabled and Incompetent." *Journal of Contemporary Health Law and Policy* 2 (Spring):71–130.

DRESSER, REBECCA S. 1990. "Relitigating Life and Death." *Ohio State Law Journal* 51 (Summer):425–437.

DRESSER, REBECCA S., and ROBERTSON, JOHN A. 1989. "Quality of Life and Non-Treatment Decisions for Incompetent Patients: A Critique of the Orthodox Approach." *Law, Medicine & Health Care* 17, no. 3:234–244.

FIELD, MARTHA A. 1993. "Killing 'the Handicapped'—Before and After Birth." *Harvard Women's Law Journal* 16 (Spring):79–138.

Guardianship of Barry, In re. 1984. 445 So. 2d 365 (Fla. Dist. Ct. App.).

Guardianship of Crum, In re. 1991. 580 N.E. 2d 876 (Ohio P. Ct. [Franklin County]).

Guardianship of Drabick, In re. 1988. 245 Cal. Rptr. 840 (Dist. Ct. App.), cert. denied, 488 U.S. 958.

Guardianship of Jane Doe, In re. 1992. 583 N.E.2d 1263 (Mass.); cert. denied sub nom. Doe v. Gross, 112 S. Ct. 1512.

Guardianship of L.W., In re. 1992. 482 N.W.2d 60 (Wis.).

JECKER, NANCY S. 1991. "Knowing When to Stop: The Limits of Medicine." *Hastings Center Report* 21, no. 3:5–8.

Johnson v. Thompson. 1992. 971 F.2d 1487 (10th Cir.); cert. denied, 113 S. Ct. 1255 (1993).

L.H.R., In re. 1984. 321 S.E.2d 716 (Ga.).

Mack v. Mack. 1993. 618 A.2d 744 (Md.).

McKay v. Bergstedt. 1990. 801 P.2d 617 (Nev.).

Newmark v. Williams. 1991. 588 A.2d 1108 (Del.).

RHODEN, NANCY K. 1985. "Treatment Dilemmas for Imperiled Newborns: Why Quality of Life Counts." *Southern California Law Review* 58, no. 5:1283–1347.

———. 1988. "Litigating Life and Death." *Harvard Law Review* 102, no. 2:375–446.

State v. McAfee. 1989. 385 S.E.2d 651 (Ga.).

Thor v. Superior Court. 1993. 855 P.2d 375 (Cal.).

VEATCH, ROBERT M. 1989. *Death, Dying and the Biological Revolution: Our Last Quest for Responsibility.* Rev. ed. New Haven, Conn.: Yale University Press.

VEACH, ROBERT M., and SPICER, CAROL M.. 1989. *Abating Treatment with Critically Ill Patients: Ethical and Legal Limits to the Medical Prolongation of Life.* New York: Oxford University Press.

———. 1992. "Medically Futile Care: The Role of the Physician in Setting Limits." *American Journal of Law and Medicine* 18, nos. 1–2:15–36.

WEIR, ROBERT F. 1984. *Selective Treatment of Handicapped*

Newborns: Moral Dilemmas in Neonatal Medicine. New York: Oxford University Press.

Westchester County Medical Ctr. (O'Connor), In re. 1988. 531 N.E.2d 607 (N.Y.).

YUEN, MICHELE. 1992. "Letting Daddy Die: Adopting New Standards for Surrogate Decisionmaking." *University of California at Los Angeles Law Review* 39, no. 3:581–632.

LIFE EXPECTANCY AND LIFE SPAN

See AGING AND THE AGED, *articles on* LIFE EXPECTANCY AND LIFE SPAN, *and* SOCIETAL AGING.

LIFE EXTENSION

See AGING AND THE AGED, *article on* THEORIES OF AGING AND LIFE EXTENSION.

LIFESTYLES AND PUBLIC HEALTH

The people of every nation would be healthier if they adopted healthier lifestyles. Ninety percent of those who die of lung cancer would not have contracted the disease if they had not smoked. Exercise, sensible diet, and compliance with treatment for high blood pressure can, and do, prevent countless episodes of cardiovascular disease. Practicing safe sex reduces the risk of contracting AIDS. Use of seat belts and motorcycle helmets lowers the chance of injury from accidents on the road.

The prospect of improving health and reducing illness through changes in living habits rather than through curative health care is attractive on a number of grounds. Since it is preventive, it avoids the distress of disease; side effects and iatrogenic consequences may be fewer; cost may be lower; and the healthier ways of living may be rewarding in their own right. For these reasons, any government that failed to promote healthy lifestyles could be faulted on ethical grounds.

Nevertheless, the encouragement of healthier lifestyles has drawn moral criticism in the literatures of bioethics and health policy. The chief concern is that governmental (and even private) attempts to bring about changes in living habits will encroach on personal liberty or privacy. A second complaint is that lifestyle-change programs may have the wrong motives, and may have undesirable social and psychological effects.

Health versus liberty

Intervention: What justification? Nearly everything we do affects health in some way, if only because the time spent could be devoted to exercise or other health-enhancing behavior. The notion of unhealthy lifestyles, however, is typically associated with a small number of habits. Smoking, the leading killer in the United States, always takes first place, closely followed by alcohol and other drug abuse, lack of exercise, and being overweight. Other risk factors affected by individual choice veer toward the medical, including behavioral change intended to control serum cholesterol and hypertension, perhaps including compliance with doctors' orders. Construed still more broadly, a "healthy lifestyle" would include living in a region not plagued by pollution or recurring natural disasters; avoidance of unsafe jobs; and purchasing the safest cars and appliances.

Attempts to change unhealthy behavior through education and exhortation are relatively unproblematic from the moral point of view. But these measures are less likely to be effective than programs that seek to influence behavior more directly through penalties, taxes, restrictions, or prohibitions. These, however, involve or border on coercion, and in some cases, as with sexual behavior, they necessarily intrude into a person's most private domains.

The fact that good health may be valued by every person does not by itself justify these interventions, since for some people the health risks seem to be less important than the benefits derived from the risk-taking behavior. Few would seriously assert that eating rich ice cream or smoking falls within the category of fundamental human rights, but each encroachment on individual autonomy is commonly regarded as standing in need of justification, especially in the United States, which has a cultural history marked by an ideology of individualism. Three kinds of justification have been offered for programs aiming to change lifestyles: (1) paternalist concern for the person's good; (2) protection of others from burdens involuntarily imposed by the risk-taking behavior; and (3) the public's stake in the nation's health.

Paternalist justifications. In the United States, paternalist justifications are rarely provided as such. Though exceptions and counterexamples abound, lip service is still paid to the tradition of John Stuart Mill's *On Liberty.* It is easier to argue for motorcycle helmet laws as a means of reducing the costs of medical care than as a means of protecting human life, despite the greater importance of the latter. When paternalism is explicitly defended, however, it is usually on the grounds that the choices the paternalistic policy prohibits are not fully voluntary ones: Bad habits, such as smoking and overeating, may be sustained by addiction or genetic predisposition. This "soft" paternalism avoids the need to argue for the "hard" paternalist view that even fully voluntary choices may be overruled if the state concludes that the individual might benefit.

For many unhealthy habits, the argument that the behavior is not fully voluntary is easy to make. The individual choice may be determined by chemical, psychological, or social causes. Once a person is addicted to nicotine, it is extremely difficult to stop smoking, as millions of unhappy smokers know; the same holds true for alcoholics and those addicted to legal or illegal drugs. The original decision to try cigarettes, alcohol, or drugs is often made during adolescence, when the individual's ability to resist peer pressure is typically weak.

Nevertheless, the soft paternalist argument faces a number of objections. Not all unhealthy choices are obviously involuntary. The decision to engage in unprotected sex, for example, may be the result of partner coercion, or inner compulsion or denial, but it may also stem from the individual's dislike of condoms or not having a condom. Moreover, even the person whose behavior is shaped by an addiction may be capable of deciding to seek professional help in breaking the addiction. The decision to forgo seeking help, a "second-order" choice about choice, is not necessarily rendered involuntary by the "first-order" addiction. In these instances, paternalistic intervention will be of the hard variety, which involves the authorities acting on the principle that their goals for the individual should be imposed on the individual's own goals.

Intervention aimed at altering lifestyle choices on paternalist grounds may overemphasize the goal of health at the expense of other goals. If the paternalist justification is strongest when the unhealthy choices are least voluntary, these may also be the occasions when the choices are most difficult to influence, and the degree of coercion required may be objectionable in itself. Smokers subjected to very high excise taxes, for example, may suffer from the taxes without giving up cigarettes. Finally, the behavior in question may be difficult to change without considerable meddling in the individual's culture and milieu, whether these champion "wine, women, and song," or risk taking and violence, or quiet (and unathletic) contemplation. The life of the fitness-loving moderate is not for everyone, even if it is most conducive to long life and good health.

Fair distribution of burdens. Mill's principle of liberty sought to limit intervention to the protection of others from the effects of one's own actions; "self-regarding" behavior is thus the domain of the individual, while others have a say in the regulation of "other-regarding" behavior. Critics have long noted that the boundary is indistinct; nearly everything we do has effects on others. Sexual behavior, the most private of acts, is not at all self-regarding in the era of the AIDS epidemic. And

since few people pay all their health-care bills out of pocket, any behavior that necessitates care will impose a financial burden on other parties.

If these behavioral choices are to be protected, they will have to find some shelter other than Mill's principle. In the case of AIDS, an argument might be made that intrusive regulation would violate a right of privacy, where "private" does not mean "self-regarding" (AIDS transmission is anything but that) but "intimate" or "personal." This right might not be defensible in light of the seriousness of the AIDS epidemic, however; and in any case, other unhealthy habits and choices—for example, smoking, which incurs risks to others through passive smoke inhalation—fall outside of this personal zone. Since there is no general right of liberty when our choices affect the lives of others, the individual's prerogative to maintain unhealthy practices must be decided on other grounds.

Paternalist arguments aim at justifying interventions that seek to curb unhealthy behavior. Arguments that point to the burden of unhealthy behavior for other people, however, may or may not share this aim. They may indeed seek to justify curbs on the behavior in order to forestall the imposition of burdens. But this can also be accomplished by requiring the individual to pay his or her own way, perhaps through excise taxes, without any diminution of the unhealthy behavior. Finally, the individual whose choices result in illness may be made to pay for his or her own health care, or to forfeit any claim on the resources of others, or, at the least, to be placed at the end of the line when resources are scarce.

These steps represent a particular understanding of distributive justice. They seek to impose the true costs of choices on the one who chooses, so that these costs will be taken into account at the moment of choice. Those who believe that the welfare state should assist its citizens in meeting their basic needs, in this view, should not regard all needs as equal. Unhealthy lifestyles create avoidable needs, and individuals should be held responsible for these choices. Those who refuse to take care of themselves, in this view, forfeit at least some of the liberties (to individual choice) and the entitlements (to help, on an equal footing, in time of need) that others deserve.

As with the paternalist justification for intervention in lifestyle choices, this argument concerning the fair sharing of burdens faces a number of objections. One might argue that distinguishing between patients with similar health-care needs on the basis of personal responsibility for illness introduces a concept of fault more at home in the legal world than in the system of health care. Treating all patients according to need, without regard to such factors as status, ability to pay, or fault, is a powerful way of affirming the importance of those aspects of people in virtue of which they are equal, relative to those that divide, distinguish, and rank us. This equality is important both to us as patients and to doctors and other health-care providers, whose first instinct should be compassionate response to human suffering.

On more technical grounds, the burden-sharing argument rests the case for intervention into unhealthy lifestyles on the outcome of an economic calculation: that the habit in question incurs a net cost. The problem is that those who die prematurely because of unhealthy habits avoid burdening others with the cost of maintaining them in their old age. Economists have long debated whether smokers burden others or relieve others of a financial burden of care; the answer may vary by country, depending on such variables as the cost of health care and the cost of living. If there are places in which smokers actually save society money, the burden-sharing argument would entail penalties for those who do *not* smoke.

Care must be taken, moreover, in stating the burden-sharing argument. Insurance, including health insurance, protects against risk, but it also can make risk taking less unwise. Those Americans who play football, for example, can regard America's health-care system as a partial safety net; the sport would be too dangerous for many without it. In this light, the burden-sharing argument might succeed in justifying special and higher insurance premiums for risk takers, but unless the risk takers refused to pay these fees, it would not justify curbs on the actual risk taking. Even the special fees would be unjustified if there were rough equivalence in the degree of risk taken by a large number of coinsureds, one person's motorcycle riding offsetting another's sedentary library dwelling.

Public health.   The third justification for intervention on behalf of healthier lifestyles points to the collective health of the public as a common good. In material terms, a healthy population enhances economic productivity and the nation's capacity to defend itself. General health also provides some degree of protection from the spread of infectious disease. Theorists of public health have contended, moreover, that the "public health," meaning the sum of each person's health, constitutes a further goal of public policy that can be distinguished from both the paternalist and the burden-sharing arguments.

Another feature of the public-health perspective is the "prevention paradox," the observation that many critical prevention policies affecting lifestyles produce large aggregate savings in lives but little demonstrable benefit to each individual. For example, seat-belt policies may save thousands of lives nationally but only marginally reduce the risk for each individual who drives. Similarly, changes in fat intake will strongly reduce the number who die prematurely from heart disease but affect the chances of each individual only slightly.

The prevention paradox thus arises from the fact that even small changes in the behaviors of tens of millions of individuals involved in low to moderate lifestyle risks avert thousands of deaths. The prevention paradox further underscores the emphasis in public health on rates of disease and deaths averted, and the difficulty of producing mass changes in behaviors through voluntary measures alone.

Far more important than the government's stake in a healthy work force is the centuries-old tradition of governmental responsibility to protect the health and safety of the public, construed as a public or common good. The public-health perspective is rooted in the democratic and constitutional tradition of assigning to elected officials and members of executive agencies responsibilities for protecting the common good, where this has been interpreted by courts as involving the protection of health and safety (and morals as well, which accounts for the long entanglement of public health and moralism). The public-health or regulatory power of government has long been justified on the grounds that reasonable restrictions on liberty and property, as weighed by the legislature, to promote the common good are the very essence of the regulatory power. This tradition is rooted in theories of government and the duties of citizens that antedate the rise of concerns with paternalism and Mill's famous essay.

Motives and effects of intervention programs

The preceding discussion of arguments for intervention in unhealthy lifestyles has taken the arguments at face value. Critics, however, have suggested that the real motivations for these policies are usually unannounced. The actual motivation, in this view, is moral—or, to be more precise, moralistic, proceeding from a rarely examined and rarely defended set of moral premises. Once these are made explicit, according to the critics, both the motive and the policies are rendered less attractive.

One sign that lifestyle intervention has a moralistic motive, according to critics, is the selectivity of targets. Many kinds of behavior have negative health effects that are not equally addressed. Promiscuity, lack of exercise, and overweight are merely the medieval vices of lust, sloth, and gluttony. These habits have negative effects on health, to be sure; but so do other kinds of behavior not viewed as vices. Childbirth, for example, presents a certain level of risk to every woman and a decided risk for some; but because it is socially approved, there is no thought of penalizing, taxing, or discouraging the behavior. The burden-sharing argument presents itself as a neutral act of accounting; but, in the critics' view, it is actually concerned with the costs of behavior deemed undesirable on moral grounds while it tolerates behavior of which it approves, no matter how costly.

The moral perspective from which lifestyle intervention is urged, moreover, has been criticized as "healthism," a parochial view that elevates health from a self-interested goal to a virtue. In this light, "personal responsibility for health" stems not from the need to avoid burdening others with the costs of one's care but from the conviction that healthy people (at least, those who choose health) are better people, morally speaking. This perspective is also said to be linked to an ideology that emphasizes the degree to which one's state of health is a function of choices one makes, rather than the whims of nature or the safety of one's environment and workplace.

One of the most frequent complaints about the lifestyle debate is that it is used to "blame the victim" and undercut the justification for collective action. Thus, those who wish to restrict in various ways the availability of alcohol or tobacco, to limit overall use of these risky products, meet counterclaims that these are not problems of regulation but of individual responsibility and education. The advocates for regulation, in effect challenging the motivation of this view, argue that their opponents do not really want to see a well-financed campaign against smoking and drinking but want no official action at all. Instead, they want wider acceptance of the view that these are problems that will be resolved only when people take more responsibility for their own health and safety.

Conclusion

Though this entry has dwelt on the difficulties in making a convincing case for intervening in unhealthy lifestyles, the collective weight of such lifestyles should not be exaggerated. Much of the bioethical literature on lifestyles indicates that the choices posing the greatest problem for public-health authorities are those which involve personal or intimate behavior, are entirely self-regarding, and represent fully voluntary behavior. Little in our behavioral repertoire falls in this narrowly defined category, however, and those who wish to pursue this promising avenue to health can enter the argument on an even footing.

DANIEL WIKLER
DAN E. BEAUCHAMP

Directly related to this entry is the entry PUBLIC HEALTH, *especially the articles on* DETERMINANTS OF PUBLIC HEALTH, HISTORY OF PUBLIC HEALTH, *and* PHILOSOPHY OF PUBLIC HEALTH. *For a further discussion of topics mentioned in this entry, see the entries* AIDS; AUTONOMY; ECONOMIC CONCEPTS IN HEALTH CARE; FREEDOM AND COERCION; HEALTH-CARE FINANCING; HEALTH-CARE RESOURCES, ALLOCATION OF; HEALTH OFFICIALS AND THEIR RESPONSIBILITIES; HEALTH POLICY; HEALTH

PROMOTION AND HEALTH EDUCATION; HEALTH SCREENING AND TESTING IN A PUBLIC-HEALTH CONTEXT; IATROGENIC ILLNESS AND INJURY; JUSTICE; PAIN AND SUFFERING; PATERNALISM; PUBLIC HEALTH AND THE LAW; RESPONSIBILITY; RISK; SUBSTANCE ABUSE; *and* UTILITY. *For a discussion of related ideas, see the entries* ADVERTISING; BEHAVIOR MODIFICATION THERAPIES; COMPASSION; GENETICS AND HUMAN SELF-UNDERSTANDING; LAW AND MORALITY; *and* PROSTITUTION.

Bibliography

BEAUCHAMP, DAN E. 1985a. "Community: The Neglected Tradition of Public Health." *Hastings Center Report* 15, no. 6:28–36.
———. 1985b. *The Health of the Republic: Epidemics, Medicine, and Moralism as Challenges to Democracy.* Philadelphia: Temple University Press. See especially chaps. 3 and 4.
FEINBERG, JOEL. 1986. *Harm to Self.* New York: Oxford University Press.
HODGSON, THOMAS A. 1992. "Cigarette Smoking and Lifetime Medical Expenditures." *Milbank Quarterly* 70, no. 1:81–125.
LEICHTER, HOWARD M. 1991. *Free to Be Foolish: Politics and Health Promotion in the United States and Great Britain.* Princeton, N.J.: Princeton University Press.
ROSE, GEOFFREY. 1985. "Sick Individuals and Sick Populations." *International Journal of Epidemiology* 14, no. 1: 32–38.
VEATCH, ROBERT M. 1980. "Voluntary Risks to Health: The Ethical Issues." *Journal of the American Medical Association* 243, no. 1:50–55.
WIKLER, DANIEL I. 1978. "Persuasion and Coercion for Health: Ethical Issues in Government Efforts to Change Lifestyles." *Milbank Memorial Fund Quarterly/Health and Society* 56, no. 3:303–338.

LIFE SUPPORT

See ARTIFICIAL ORGANS AND LIFE-SUPPORT SYSTEMS; *and* DEATH AND DYING: EUTHANASIA AND SUSTAINING LIFE. *See also* TECHNOLOGY, *article on* HISTORY OF MEDICAL TECHNOLOGY.

LITERATURE

Theoretical contexts

If dialogue—sophisticated, passionate, often angry dialogue—is the mark of a lively field of inquiry, then the study of creative literature has seldom been livelier than in the years since the first appearance of this encyclopedia in 1978. Central to the dialogue has been the question of the relation, if any, of literature to the world outside itself—that is, to the so-called real world of culture, politics, and ethics. Some of the most influential philosophers of literature (e.g., Derrida, 1972) have been warning readers that they can no longer go to the classics of literature to mine gold nuggets of knowledge about life. Ironically, all this has been happening at the same time that certain prominent ethicists have been rediscovering the moral value of literature while speaking of "virtue" (MacIntyre, 1981) and "narrative ethics" (Hauerwas and Burrell, 1989). Have literature and ethics passed each other in the night? This much is clear: Before anyone can speak responsibly of the relationship of bioethics to literature, it is necessary to understand the general terms of the literary professionals' fight about meaning.

Of course, the agitation is far more complicated than it will appear here in a nontechnical summary. But the commentators can fairly be divided into two loose groups called values-oriented and language-oriented theorists. This distinction is related to the ethics/aesthetics, art for life's sake/art for art's sake, and content/form divisions of the past in that the first term of each pair (values, ethics, life, content) encourages the use of literature as a tool for living a good life, and the second term (language, aesthetics, art, form) points to a view of literature as an important end in itself. But today's values/language debate, particularly the language side, is by no means strictly congruent with past positions. The values-oriented people can be taken to include those who believe that the relationship between literature and ethics can be richly productive of change in individuals and society; the language-oriented group includes those who believe that, given contemporary understandings of language, such a relationship is an illusion. Thus far, the language theorists have prevailed—if not in the classroom, then certainly in the scholarly conferences and journals as well as in the commercial reviews.

Values-oriented theories.   But the values side has been accorded intelligent attention, too. Using various technical terms for values in literature (e.g., "classic realism," "hermeneutics," "ethical criticism," and "moral imagination"), literary commentators have: (1) celebrated the death of critics interested primarily in moral values (Belsey, 1980); or (2) suggested that, in the words of Mark Twain, the reports of their death have been greatly exaggerated and would, in any case, be disastrous for both literature and society (Graff, 1979); or (3) proclaimed that moralists may very well have died but should be resurrected and readmitted, within certain limits, to the practice of criticism (Booth, 1988). Influential endorsement for the values-oriented position has also come from outside literature. Most notably, the philosopher Martha Nussbaum (1990) has insisted that literary narratives of ideas and emotions constitute an essentially—and, for her, sometimes the solely—adequate depiction of ethical dilemmas. And psychiatrist Robert Coles has championed the orthodox view of literature as balm for the human spirit (Coles, 1989).

The complete history of values-oriented critics must make space for the two towering figures who, in the first half of the twentieth century, took up the mantle of Matthew Arnold (1822–1888) to proclaim that a commitment to individual and social morality was the mark of supreme writers. F. R. Leavis wrote in *The Great Tradition* that the finest novelists "are all distinguished by a vital capacity for experience, a kind of reverent openness before life, and a marked moral intensity" (Leavis, 1967, p. 9). And Lionel Trilling, whose influence in the United States was once as widespread as Leavis's in England, said in *The Liberal Imagination*: "For our time the most effective agent of the moral imagination has been the novel of the last two hundred years" (Trilling, 1978, p. 209).

Today, the two men are ignored or reviled by many of the most famous critics of literature. To some of them, Leavis's and Trilling's classics-minded disciples share part of the blame for enthroning the traditional academic canon—largely produced, in the now infamous phrase, by "dead, white, male writers"—as opposed to a more flexible list that is open to writers of both sexes and multicultural origins. The followers of Leavis and Trilling are among those who have been tagged as "liberals" and "humanists" by self-proclaimed "radicals" of the Marxist, African-American, and feminist schools of literary criticism. But, if examined closely from the perspective of this entry, these arguments are all in the family—the family of literary critics whose guidelines promote discussions of values. So are the arguments of the so-called reader-response critics, such as Wolfgang Iser, who locate the meaning of literature in the interaction between the text and the reader, and, probably, even the "formalists" of various stripes (e.g., Mikhail Bakhtin), who emphasize form over—and occasionally at the expense of—content.

Language-oriented groups.   The true opposition to the values-oriented approach comes from the theorists who, under several different banners (most often "semiotics," "deconstruction," and, according to some definitions, "postmodernism"), deny that literary texts have an objective relationship to the world outside themselves. The founding father of these language-oriented thinkers is often said to be Ferdinand de Saussure, whose revolutionary book, *Course in General Linguistics*, was published in 1916 and is still being analyzed for its contributions to literary studies. Paul de Man, Roland Barthes, and Jacques Derrida are other influential writers whose theories undermine literature's direct contribution to ethics.

The basis of their position, which is introduced by Catherine Belsey (1980), is roughly this: Contrary to the empiricist-idealistic tradition that language, and therefore literature, is a reflection of the real world of facts, objects, and transcendent states of being, language is arbitrary and constructed solely by cultural convention. Language does not name things that are already in existence, but is, instead, responsible for our recognizing distinctions in what would otherwise be a blurred continuum. If, for instance, our language recognizes a difference between the color blue and the color green, we will see a line on the horizon over land. If there is no such distinction, the sky will melt into the earth. In other words, the language-oriented literary critics say, we cannot experience the world except through language; there is no reality except for language. In effect, we are prisoners of the languages we understand, for they structure our world.

None of these ideas is remotely startling anymore. But trouble arises when they are logically extended, for, with these ideas in place, it is foolish to speak of a literary text as possessing any "truth" about ethical matters or about an empirical world in which ethical matters must be considered. Language is not related directly to the world, but only to other language, texts only to other texts. Does this post-Saussurean conclusion leave any room for ethicists seeking help from literature? For the most extreme of the language theorists, the answer is "very little." They would grant that literature may portray people making moral decisions, or, at most, shame readers into feeling "a little ethical flutter, a little *frisson*" (Bly, 1988, p. xix). But they would add that since language by itself has no agency—that is, no power to bring anything about in the real world—then neither has literature.

There have been profound challenges to the language-oriented critics, and not only from their values-oriented opponents. Geoffrey Galt Harpham (1992), for one, manages to put the lie to the dichotomy, which, like most dichotomies, is useful mainly as a temporary device for clarification. Derrida himself has come to see that his theories oblige us to take a greater responsibility for inventing values in the midst of what he describes as a constantly shifting world. But for bioethicists, what is finally important about the maelstrom of contemporary literary/linguistic theory is that, first, whether they acknowledge it or not, people who think about bioethics and literature (e.g., Brody, 1987, 1992; Brock and Ratzan, 1988; Jones, 1987) generally derive their theoretical justification from the values-oriented thinkers, and, second, these ethicists are thereby ignoring the dominant literary epistemology of the past twenty-five years.

The ethics of literary form

To be sure, there are strong signs that the dominance of language-oriented theory is ending. In addition, there have always been routes through literature to ethics that circumvent the whole values/language debate. A number of these routes are a matter of form as opposed to content.

Chief among them is the form called "narrative" or "story." Narrative is not exclusively literary: Writers from nearly every academic discipline have asserted that human beings tend to perceive life not as isolated ideas, facts, or problems, but as stories—a series of plotted events involving characters and told from certain perspectives. In literature, the study of narrative form has become highly sophisticated (Martin, 1986), and literature-and-medicine scholars have participated in its development (Hunter, 1991). The so-called narrative ethicists use the narrative paradigm to counter, or at least to supplement, an ethics based solely on abstract principles (e.g., Reich, 1988). In other words, narrative ethics is an attempt to return ethical dilemmas to the messy, complicated lives from which they arose, and to plumb those narrated dilemmas with other stories that are coherent and meaningful.

Narrative ethics usually stops there, and it should not. Nor should anyone looking to literature for moral exempla think that the task is complete when they are found, for the narrative form itself may present—or, more commonly, mask—ethical problems. Most of them derive from questions about the adequacy and authority of what is called the "narrative point of view." Whether a story is oral or written, whether it is from life or art, we need to know the narrator's angle of perspective. That is, who is telling a particular story, and what constitutes his or her authority for doing so? Did the narrator witness the events related or is the report second-hand? Is the narrator deeply involved with the events, distant from them, or perhaps not able to understand them? T. Hugh Crawford reminds us to determine the narrator's social privilege, which, in the case of physicians, may be so great that the truth of their stories will go unchallenged (Crawford, 1992). An ethicist should also realize that the narrator always functions as an editor and therefore inevitably omits some elements of the imaginary "complete story" that may have a substantial moral impact. A second set of questions should concern the audience to whom the narrator directs the story, for the tale will be adjusted accordingly.

The questions become more complicated when a story is written, more complicated still when it is part of literary art. For instance, the narrator must not be unthinkingly identified with the real man or woman who composed the story, especially when the story is written in the first person, or even when authors use their own names for the narrators. The doctor who narrates the William Carlos Williams stories about patients in Rutherford, New Jersey, where the author practiced medicine, is not the same person as the Dr. Williams who made house calls or the Bill Williams who was Floss's husband; for the simple truth is that the author is never precisely the same as the narrator. Medical ethicists, writing about paternalism in Williams's famous short story "The Use of Force," do not always make this distinction, and their conclusions are thereby less precise. However, most literary narratives are written in the third person ("Sid was thinking that the surgeon seemed unresponsive"). It is an ethical, as well as an aesthetic, question to ask whether the narrator is positioned inside Sid's head, as it were, and therefore knows authoritatively only what Sidney knows, or whether the narrator also knows that "the surgeon was thinking about Sid's gall bladder," that outside "the wind was pushing the fall leaves around the parking lot," and that in the world at large "it was the worst of times." The first kind of narrator is technically a "concealed narrator" or "center of consciousness," the second an "omniscient narrator." Fashion in our century has favored the first kind for its epistemological and ethical qualities because the omniscient narrator's sweeping knowledge is suspect. In the United States, especially, we tend to balk at according anyone—a president, a spouse, a doctor, a narrator—that kind of power.

These sticky questions about narrators lie in wait for medical ethicists when they are using their favorite narrative form, the case history. When "participant-observer" David Barnard published an extended case history, his intentions were to broaden the social and temporal bases from which we make ethical decisions and to show that a given illness affects the caregivers as well as the patient. He achieved these goals, but the form of the case was challenged by literary critic Eric Rabkin, who asserted that Barnard-as-narrator and the physician, Valerie Walsh, had unconsciously produced "a story in which each could be the hero" (Banks et al., 1986, p. 52). The resultant furor, summarized by Barnard (1992), has helped to clarify the ethics of narrative form, but some aspects are still underexplored.

The study of narrative is only one of the important ways to understand how literary form affects ethics. In fact, an awareness of what genre a given work falls into—is it a story or a play, a comedy or a tragedy?—is almost always important for the ethicist. Since drama, for instance, is distinguished from other literary forms by virtue of its dialogue and conflict, perhaps ethical conflicts should be presented in dramatic form rather than in narrative case histories. Not only would the various positions on a problem be fully embodied in each "character's" own language, the format would encourage the greater objectivity for which drama has a reputation. An argument can also be made that great plays and their first cousins, films, ought to be studied by ethicists to sharpen their awareness, not only of dialogue and conflict, but also of such matters as role, costume, setting, set speeches, and audience reaction, for all of them change the moral climate of any scene from life. It would not matter whether the play chosen was specifi-

cally about bioethics or not. Any good play would serve the ethical goals (Banks, 1990).

Genre also affects more pervasively and subtly, for genres are, finally, forms that cultures select to convey their deepest values. For example, the form of Greek tragedy inevitably introduced certain ethical values. One of the most troublesome for modern individualists is the widespread attitude toward fate (often personified as the vengeful Erinys, or, in Rome, the Furies), whereby the Greeks believed that, once a sequence of events had been set into motion, human beings had no ability to prevent its outcome. Once Oedipus had unknowingly killed his father, he was destined to marry his mother. Furthermore, he had to be punished for these acts even though he had no evil intention. That is, in order for the good to triumph in the ultimate balance of the universe, all those who had done wrong, whether consciously or not, had to pay. Like all great artists, Sophocles lived in creative tension with what conventional form forced upon him: His Oedipus sees himself as free enough to be blamed and to inflict his own punishment by blinding himself. Nevertheless, a belief in what might be called the "Greek tragic plot" not only affected ethical decisions—in a sense, it precluded them. Though less confining, certain ethical perspectives are already inherent in modern authors' affinity for mixing the traditional genres, as in "tragicomedy" and "docudrama." We may be too sophisticated to separate the serious from the funny, the real from the make-believe; or—and here is the ethical issue—we may be too confused to understand the difference.

If literary form may thus limit ethics, form may also free it. George Bernard Shaw's *The Doctor's Dilemma* (1954) can serve as an efficient illustration of both capabilities. Next to Williams's "The Use of Force," Shaw's play is probably the most oft-cited example of medical ethics in literature (see, e.g., Brody, 1991, on teaching Shaw in an ethics class). Shaw, of course, was a first-rate comic writer: The pompous, ignorant, and fee-grabbing physicians in this play are squarely in the tradition of Molière's hilariously unethical doctors. But Shaw was also a playwright of great moral passion, an unabashed didact who mounted theatrical soapboxes to preach his ideas about social reform. The play form simply did not give this second Shaw enough room. Therefore, to most plays he published, he attached an essay of polemical prose that allowed him to go over much of the same material in a different literary form. In the case of *The Doctor's Dilemma*, this material was medical ethics.

The two forms, preface and play, dictate two startlingly different takes on the same ideas. Whereas the preface requires precision, the play requires ambiguity, or, more accurately, encourages it. In the play, Sir Colenso Ridgeon, who has recently discovered a successful treatment for tuberculosis, is forced by limited resources into deciding whom to treat and whom to allow to die.

Specifically, he must choose between a poor, worthy—and dull—doctor, and a poor, reprehensible—and uniquely brilliant—artist. The situation is complicated by Sir Colenso's amorous feelings for the artist's wife, whom he imagines as an available widow. That is the dilemma of the title. Sir Colenso resolves it by treating the doctor. His justification for this action is that since the artist has no moral integrity, he, Sir Colenso, is saving the wife from discovering her husband's deceit and killing herself, as she has threatened. When he reveals his reasoning to the wife, now the widow, she accuses him of murder. In reply, he justifies his actions by citing Arthur Hugh Clough's satiric poem, *The Latest Decalogue:* "Thou shalt not kill, but needst not strive/ Officiously to keep alive."

Shaw's play raises more questions than it answers. When he writes polemical prose, Shaw argues easily, logically, and from an unshakable moral perspective. But when he takes ethics into the personal realm of drama, he cannot manage equally clear conclusions. So the play, as distinct from the preface, reverberates with moral ambiguity. The central dilemma is soundly debated by Sir Colenso and an older, sensible physician—but no conclusion is drawn by Shaw. Similarly, Sir Colenso's decision is padded with ethical red herrings. When, with no apology, he recommends as a physician for the artist a man of eminent reputation but shameful ignorance, Sir Colenso is behaving in a superficially licit manner that serves to distract him from the ethical problem. What the playwright does face directly is that ethical decisions in medicine are difficult to sort out logically; that no physician alone, or even in consultation with other professionals, can make them on objective grounds; that the results, when allocating limited medical resources, will be a type of murder; and that these burdens are too much for one person to bear.

For Shaw the playwright, then, the dilemma of who shall live and who shall die cannot be answered without dishonor and tragedy. (He calls this play, and this play only, a tragedy.) For Shaw the political philosopher, the same question is answered in terms that, by contrast to the subtleties of the play, are chillingly clear. He asserts in the preface that "invalids, meaning persons who cannot, beyond reason, expect to be kept alive by the activity of others," must be allowed for social reasons to die. "The theory," Shaw concludes firmly, "that every individual alive is of infinite value is legislatively impracticable . . . the man who costs more than he is worth is doomed by sound hygiene as inexorably as by sound economics" (Shaw, 1954, pp. 86–87). And that's that.

Abortion and AIDS, among others

Shaw, Williams, Molière: These names are the beginning of a long, long list of first-rate creative writers who have narrated, dramatized, and, in general, illuminated specific topics of bioethics. Hundreds of other names and their works could be added. A partial roll call of the most useful would include Tobias Smollett's *Roderick Random* (1748), Herman Melville's *White-Jacket* (1850), Anthony Trollope's *Doctor Thorne* (1858), George Eliot's *Middlemarch* (1871–1872), Georg Büchner's *Woyzeck* (1879), Henrik Ibsen's *An Enemy of the People* (1882), Sinclair Lewis's *Arrowsmith* (1925), Albert Camus's *The Plague* (1948), Peter Nichols's *A Day in the Death of Joe Egg* (1967), Joyce Carol Oates's *Wonderland* (1971), and Peter Shaffer's *Equus* (1973).

In the basic bibliography of literature and medicine (Trautmann and Pollard, 1982), which annotates about 1,400 literary works from classical to contemporary times under thirty-nine categories, ethicists can check for information not only under "medical ethics," but also under "abortion," "euthanasia," and "evil doctors." The years since the bibliography's publication have, of course, added more authors, and many more works, to the inventory of resources. It is intriguing that the years have also changed the categories. Among the bibliography's topics, "age," "handicaps," "mental retardation," "plague," "suicide," "venereal disease," and "women as patients" have taken on extensive political, and therefore ethical, implications. New categories have emerged too. "Cross-cultural," for instance, must be clearly distinguished from the old "poverty and health"; "AIDS" deserves its own category, having grown beyond "plague" and "venereal disease" (which itself has developed into "sexually transmitted diseases").

To demonstrate precisely how literature illuminates bioethics, it might be helpful to go beyond the Trautmann and Pollard bibliography and to analyze, first, a traditional work on an established topic—in this case, abortion—and, second, a group of fiery works about a new topic—AIDS.

One of the most important recent novels on U.S. medical ethics is John Irving's *The Cider House Rules* (1985). Morality—the metaphorical "rules" of the title—is its central concern, specifically the morality of abortion before *Roe v. Wade*, the case that established abortion's constitutionality. One of the book's two main characters is Dr. Wilbur Larch, who performs illegal abortions at the orphanage he establishes in a remote area of Maine. He offers women a choice—an orphan or an abortion. The other character is Homer Wells, one of those orphans, who, as a young man, is an ardent antiabortionist, able to articulate arguments in opposition to Larch. But, in the end, breaking his own and society's rules, Homer assumes a medical identity that allows him to take over Dr. Larch's practice.

As is so often the case in life, Homer's position begins with an image rather than an idea. At the age of thirteen, Homer sees a dead, nearly nine-month-old entity, whom Dr. Larch wants to call a "fetus," but Homer feels compelled to call a "child." After that, any argument from Larch about "the products of conception" before the quickening are immediately linked by Homer to the image of the dead baby. Now the pictures of even the eight-week-old fetuses in Gray's *Anatomy* strike Homer as having an "expression," or, the narrator tells us, what other people call a "soul."

Nor is Dr. Larch initially won over to abortion by arguments. As a medical student, Larch sees for himself the damage inflicted on women by the alleyway butchers and poisonous aborticides. He stares into the dead face of a woman to whom he had refused an abortion. He witnesses the deprivations of orphans. Later, Dr. Larch adds reason to his emotions. He has a large array of arguments at his command, including, for instance, his disgust at someone "who cares more for the misgivings suffered in his own frail soul than for the actual suffering of countless unwanted and mistreated children" (Irving, 1985, p. 260). He presents another argument that finally convinces Homer. Written in a letter, it reads: "If abortions were legal, you could refuse—in fact, given your beliefs, you *should* refuse. But . . . HOW CAN YOU FEEL FREE TO CHOOSE NOT TO HELP PEOPLE WHO ARE NOT FREE TO GET OTHER HELP?" (Irving, 1985, p. 488).

These characters, these events, and these ethical concepts are all embedded in a form that must be described and its intimate connection to the ethical content made plain. Basically, the form is adapted from the nineteenth-century, realistic, English novel because it suits Irving's traditionalism—his sense that fiction has as its chief mission the examination of values. In that regard, his model is surely Charles Dickens. *The Cider House Rules* has Dickensian size. Like a Dickens novel, it is openly concerned with individual and social ethics. Every night, Homer reads Dickens's *David Copperfield* or *Great Expectations* to the boy orphans, who unquestioningly accept them as portals to morality.

To the girls, by the way, he reads Charlotte Brontë's *Jane Eyre*, whose orphan heroine is blatantly offered as a role model—and is sometimes blatantly rejected. Jane's sweet optimism is too much for one angry, world-weary orphan. In a vividly comic instance of what scholars like Booth and Nussbaum would be forced to call "ethical criticism," the hulking, teenaged orphan demonstrates the power of literature: "Even for me [chirped little Jane Eyre], life had its gleam of sunshine."

"'Gleams of sunshine'!" Melony shouted in violent disbelief. "Let her come here! Let her show *me* the gleams of sunshine!" (Irving, 1985, p. 84).

From the nineteenth century, too, comes the novel's narrative voice. It is omniscience, moving freely in and out of any character's mind and making such general observations as: "Society is so complex that even [the little town of] Heart's Haven had a wrong part to it" (Irving, 1985, p. 125). The narrator knows everything in this created world. If he (let us say) can build an aes-

thetically convincing world, readers may believe he knows a great deal about the real world, too. Irving has tried to buttress the authority of his novel's narrator by appending the scholarly apparatus of endnotes. Tied to certain pages and narrative "facts," these notes assert that Irving has researched his material. He has read medical texts, both old and modern. He has consulted with physicians, including one of the canonical authors in literature and medicine, Richard Selzer. All the evidence points to this author's being very serious about the real world, a values-oriented thinker as described earlier, rather than one for whom language is a closed system.

Irving writes tragicomedy. One distinguishing mark of an Irving novel (the most successful was *The World According to Garp* [1978]) is that, after much humor, someone innocent dies. This is Dickensian too: Think of Little Nell in *The Old Curiosity Shop*. As noted earlier, the mixed genre of tragicomedy is a favorite twentieth-century form, and cultural critics are still sorting out its implications. More and more, tragicomedy seems appropriate to the creative literature of medical ethics because the genre deals simultaneously with patients' tragic losses and caregivers' need to continue in spite of them. Tragedy ends something, but comedy always implies continuation, and the two are interdependent. Here is a literary lesson that bioethicists, whose "quandary ethics" proceeds from an exclusively tragic premise, have yet to learn. As that wily moralist, George Bernard Shaw, has Dr. Ridgeon say, "Life does not cease to be funny when people die any more than it ceases to be serious when people laugh" (Shaw, 1954, p. 185).

Literary writers have responded to AIDS faster and more often than to abortion. They have also tended to leap more aggressively from art to ethics. Taken as a group, the narratives, plays, poems, films, and critical essays about AIDS (see Nelson, 1992, for a bibliography) are fervently contesting the ethical boundaries of language itself. For a start, some of the creative writers and critics who write about AIDS are activists. Larry Kramer, author of *The Normal Heart* (1985), is still the best known of them. These activists insist that the first goal of AIDS literature must be to change the critical circumstances of the disease and its sufferers. They call for "stridently interventionist cultural practice" (Nelson, 1992, p. 8, citing Douglas Crimp). They say that to write about AIDS at all is automatically to be a moralist, for, in this battle, no sidelines exist. Demurrers about art for art's sake are irrelevant and themselves immoral. So one question about activist AIDS literature is, Does such work fit into the artistic genre called "social realism" or is it not art at all, but, instead, blatant propaganda whose first and last goal is social change? To the first category, literary historians have assigned, for instance, Ibsen's *An Enemy of the People*, which is an ardent piece about an idealistic doctor's crusade to warn tourists about his town's polluted public baths in the face of community pressure, as represented by his brother the mayor, to keep his mouth shut. The play is comparable to Kramer's *The Normal Heart,* in which another doctor battles to get money for AIDS research in a New York whose mayor seeks to prevent would-be tourists from knowing about the epidemic. But where do we draw the line between taking a stand and propaganda, wherein the end shapes, even justifies, the means?

What might any writer, activist or not, be excused for saying in order to bring about a desired end? What language—which images, which metaphors—may validly be used to inflame audiences with a just passion? One of the most common metaphors for the AIDS epidemic in the homosexual community is the Holocaust (e.g., Nelson, 1992), which is said to be recurring through the establishment's lack of a plan to prevent the genocide of gay men. Is this horrifying image apt? Is it logical? Alternatively, are these questions themselves out of place in view of the absolute primacy, for some people, of subjective data about illness—that is, "I have AIDS, and it feels as though I am living through another Holocaust. What do you know about it?"

The morality of metaphor is the territory famously covered by Susan Sontag in *Illness as Metaphor* (Sontag, 1978). There she argues that to substitute metaphors, especially negative metaphors, for the reality of bodily suffering is to impose a spurious meaning on illness and a sense of guilt on the patient. If cancer, in the common military metaphor, is a battleground, then the patient can be blamed for not winning. Sontag comes back to her point in *AIDS and Its Metaphors* (Sontag, 1989), where she contends that "plague," the most common metaphor for AIDS, implies judgment on a corrupt society. In her own story about AIDS, "The Way We Live Now" (Sontag, 1987), there are no metaphors for the illness. Moreover, in what would seem to be a further attempt to free AIDS from contaminating linguistic associations, she does not even name it.

Sontag's reasoned approach to this crisis is similar to the theories of the German playwright Bertolt Brecht (1898–1956). Unlike the AIDS plays, most of which are designed to be deeply cathartic, Brecht's plays aimed for the "alienation effect" in order to limit his audience's emotional involvement in the work. He used various devices to remind audiences that they were watching illusion, not reality—a play, not life. This distancing, he hoped, would free their minds to reason clearly that humanitarian action was needed in the world outside the theater. A former medical student, Brecht wanted to achieve the theatrical equivalent of clinical objectivity. His goal, like that of AIDS activists, was to change society, but, unlike some of them, he thought it unethical to reach minds by manipulating emotions.

In arguing against metaphor, Sontag seeks to chip away at the use of language as a shield to protect people from difficult experience. Given the symbol-making na-

ture of the human mind, she has chosen a position that finally may be impossible to defend. She seems to know that, and yet she thinks it eminently worthwhile to fight for the "thereness" of the human body, for the indisputable fact of its physical presence. So does James Morrison, who is worried that postmodernism (read: "language-oriented thinking") has infected criticism about AIDS literature. Defining allegory as "a series of metaphors arranged in sequence" (Nelson, 1992, p. 169), Morrison complains that the postmodern attraction to allegory—that is, to expressing experience as an abstract text that refers only to other language and not to the real world—has moved readers farther away from the actual experience of AIDS. In his eyes, allegories dictate that both AIDS and the person with AIDS be classified as "other"—something, at any rate, that cannot be approached without the intervention of elaborate figures of speech. The allegory to which he objects most vehemently is the series of metaphors that describe the body as text. When logically extended, he says, such an allegory would allow someone to "read," as it were, "the lesions of Kaposi's sarcoma as indexical signs" of the body-book (Nelson, 1992, p. 171). This he thinks a ludicrously unsympathetic way to approach the body in pain.

Morrison may not realize it, but his challenge implicitly goes out to the scholars in the interdisciplinary field of literature and medicine for whom the patient-as-text is both metaphor and method. He might just as well challenge every one of us, for the process of abstracting that he condemns in the case of literary criticism and AIDS seems to be a universal human phenomenon. The combined evidence of the writers examined here suggests that all of us are trapped between our suffering bodies and our symbolizing minds—that is, between a world whose existence we can prove simply by stubbing a toe and the engrossing stories that we are constantly creating about that world. It would appear to be nearly useless to ask which level of experience, the physical or the imaginative, is more real; or to look to one, at the exclusion of the other, for ethical insight.

In a sense, we are back to the values/language split with which this article began. In calling for a clear-sighted view of every specific person with AIDS, Morrison aligns himself with the values-oriented camp. He wants not only creative writers but also commentators on literature to write justly. So does Sontag. But, as she demonstrates in her own fictional works, language is a powerful and playful human trait that tends to seek its own ends, regardless of its possible relationship to the real world of ethical problems. Language, in fact, creates new worlds all the time. In short, the values/language dichotomy is more properly seen not as a true division but as a perpetual ethical tension.

JOANNE TRAUTMANN BANKS

Directly related to this entry are the entries NARRATIVE; INTERPRETATION; *and* METAPHOR AND ANALOGY. *For a further discussion of topics mentioned in this entry, see the entries* BIOETHICS; ETHICS; FEMINISM; VALUE AND VALUATION; *and* VIRTUE AND CHARACTER. *For a further discussion of related ideas, see the entries* ABORTION, *especially the section on* CONTEMPORARY ETHICAL AND LEGAL ASPECTS; AIDS; AUTHORITY; CASUISTRY; DEATH AND DYING: EUTHANASIA AND SUSTAINING LIFE; EUGENICS; HOMOSEXUALITY; NATIONAL SOCIALISM; *and* PATERNALISM.

Bibliography

BANKS, JOANNE TRAUTMANN. 1990. "Literature as a Clinical Capacity: Commentary on 'the Quasimodo Complex.'" *Journal of Clinical Ethics* 1, no. 3:227–231.

BANKS, JOANNE TRAUTMANN; BARNARD, DAVID; RABKIN, ERIC; and SMITH, DAVID H. 1986. "A Controversy About Clinical Form." *Literature and Medicine* 5:24–57.

BARNARD, DAVID. 1992. "'A Case of Amyotrophic Lateral Sclerosis': A Reprise and a Reply." *Literature and Medicine* 11:133–146.

BELSEY, CATHERINE. 1980. *Critical Practice.* New York: Routledge.

BLY, CAROL. 1988. "Foreword." In *Full Measure: Modern Stories on Aging*, pp. xv–xxiii. Edited by Dorothy Sennett. St. Paul, Minn.: Graywolf.

BOOTH, WAYNE C. 1988. *The Company We Keep: An Ethics of Fiction.* Berkeley: University of California Press.

BROCK, D. HEYWARD, and RATZAN, RICHARD M., eds. 1988. *Literature and Medicine* 7. Special issue, "Literature and Bioethics."

BRODY, HOWARD. 1987. *Stories of Sickness.* New Haven, Conn.: Yale University Press.

———. 1991. "Literature and Bioethics: Different Approaches." *Literature and Medicine* 10:98–110.

———. 1992. *The Healer's Power.* New Haven, Conn.: Yale University Press.

COLES, ROBERT. 1989. *The Call of Stories: Teaching and the Moral Imagination.* Boston: Houghton Mifflin.

CRAWFORD, T. HUGH. 1992. "The Politics of Narrative Form." *Literature and Medicine* 11:147–162.

DERRIDA, JACQUES. 1972. "Structure, Sign, and Play in the Discourse of the Human Sciences." In *The Structuralist Controversy: The Languages of Criticism and the Sciences of Man*, pp. 247–272. Edited by Richard Macksey and Eugenio Donato. Baltimore: Johns Hopkins University Press.

GRAFF, GERALD. 1979. *Literature Against Itself: Literary Ideas in Modern Society.* Chicago: University of Chicago Press.

HARPHAM, GEOFFREY GALT. 1992. *Getting It Right: Language, Literature, and Ethics.* Chicago: University of Chicago Press.

HAUERWAS, STANLEY, and BURRELL, DAVID. 1989. "From System to Story: An Alternative Pattern for Rationality in Ethics." In *Why Narrative? Readings in Narrative Theology.* Edited by Stanley Hauerwas and L. Gregory Jones. Grand Rapids, Mich.: William B. Eerdmans.

HUNTER, KATHRYN MONTGOMERY. 1991. *Doctors' Stories: The Narrative Structure of Medical Knowledge.* Princeton, N.J.: Princeton University Press.

IRVING, JOHN. 1985. *The Cider House Rules: A Novel.* New York: William Morrow.

JONES, ANNE HUDSON. 1987. "Literary Value: The Lesson of Medical Ethics." *Neohelicon* 14:383–392.

LEAVIS, FRANK RAYMOND. 1967. *The Great Tradition.* New York: New York University Press.

MACINTYRE, ALASDAIR C. 1981. *After Virtue: A Study in Moral Theory.* Notre Dame, Ind.: Notre Dame University Press.

MARTIN, WALLACE. 1986. *Recent Theories of Narrative.* Ithaca, N.Y.: Cornell University Press.

NELSON, EMMANUEL S., ed. 1992. *AIDS: The Literary Response.* New York: Twayne.

NUSSBAUM, MARTHA C. 1990. *Love's Knowledge: Essays on Philosophy and Literature.* New York: Oxford University Press.

REICH, WARREN THOMAS. 1988. "Experiential Ethics as a Foundation for Dialogue Between Health Communication and Health-Care Ethics." *Journal of Applied Communication Research* 16:16–28.

SHAW, GEORGE BERNARD. 1954. *The Doctor's Dilemma: A Tragedy.* Baltimore: Penguin.

SONTAG, SUSAN. 1978. *Illness as Metaphor.* New York: Farrar, Straus, Giroux.

———. 1987. "The Way We Live Now." In *The Best American Short Stories 1987*, pp. 1–19. Edited by Ann Beattie and Shannon Ravenel. Boston: Houghton Mifflin.

———. 1989. *AIDS and Its Metaphors.* New York: Farrar, Straus, Giroux.

TRAUTMANN, JOANNE, and POLLARD, CAROL. 1982. *Literature and Medicine: An Annotated Bibliography.* Rev. ed. Pittsburgh: University of Pittsburgh Press.

TRILLING, LIONEL. 1978. *The Liberal Imagination: Essays on Literature and Society.* Uniform ed. New York: Harcourt Brace Jovanovich.

LIVING WILLS

See DEATH AND DYING: EUTHANASIA AND SUSTAINING LIFE, *articles on* ADVANCE DIRECTIVES, ETHICAL ISSUES, *and* PROFESSIONAL AND PUBLIC POLICIES.

LONG-TERM CARE

I. Concept and Policies
    Rosalie A. Kane
II. Nursing Homes
    Jill A. Rhymes
    Laurence B. McCullough
III. Home Care
    Terrie Wetle

I. CONCEPT AND POLICIES

Long-term care (LTC) is an individualized mix of health-care, personal-care, and social services for persons whose functional impairments dictate that they receive help with tasks of everyday living (Kane and Kane, 1987). Clients may live in group residential settings such as nursing homes and board-and-care homes, but most live in their own homes and are candidates for community-based LTC programs including home care, adult day care, home-delivered meals, emergency assistance, and home renovation. LTC may be provided by paid workers, but most often it is provided voluntarily by family and friends. The need for LTC is assessed by evaluating the client's ability to perform activities of daily living (ADL), such as bathing, dressing, using the toilet, getting in and out of bed, eating, and performing household and other practical tasks including cleaning, cooking, shopping, money management, and transporting oneself. LTC services correspond directly to measured impairments in ADL performance and other functional impairments. People may choose to purchase similar services for convenience alone, but the service is defined as LTC only if a measurable disability prevents them from performing the tasks.

Most LTC clients are elderly and, indeed, are over seventy-five years old. But many younger persons also need and receive LTC. These include physically disabled adults with conditions such as multiple sclerosis, spinal-cord injuries, head injuries, and late-stage cancer; persons with late-stage acquired immunodeficiency syndrome (AIDS); technology-dependent, severely disabled children; and persons of all ages with developmental disabilities such as cerebral palsy. Anyone who needs and receives help with everyday functioning because of a disability may be seen as receiving long-term care. They may, of course, also receive preventive and curative acute medical care from time to time.

The goals of LTC may be multiple and often are ambiguous. Sometimes the goal appropriately includes rehabilitation or improvement of the client's functional abilities, but frequently the most reasonable goal is to enable clients to live as meaningfully as possible given their impairments, abilities, interests, and life-cycle stage and roles. Sometimes LTC providers treat the LTC services (e.g., the bath or the transfer assistance) as the actual goal of LTC. Other LTC programs promulgate ambitious goals, for example, that LTC clients should be well-satisfied with life and score well on absolute indicators of well-being or social adjustment. In either case, practitioners and policymakers struggle to attend to rehabilitation possibilities while avoiding grandiose or intrusive goals. Assuming responsibility for global outcomes of someone's life along with providing a necessary, routine service requires some hubris, and LTC professionals are perplexed about how comprehensively to cast their goals.

LTC is an enterprise in which the services are diverse though often ordinary, the providers are diverse (including professionals, paraprofessionals, and family members), the clientele is diverse, and the goals are often unclear. Add to this that much LTC, and most publicly subsidized LTC, takes place in nursing homes, where the functionally impaired client may have been involuntarily relocated, and that the high cost of LTC in residential settings and in the community is of concern to private and public payers. Finally, LTC is a woman's issue because the clients, the family caregivers who are pressed into service (Brody, 1985), and the paid caregivers are predominantly female. Of course, husbands give care to their wives as needed, but the typical long-term-care consumer is a widow and the typical family caregiver is a wife, a daughter, or a daughter-in-law.

Ethical themes in LTC

Intimacy of LTC. Whether it is provided in clients' own homes or in group residential settings, LTC is inextricably tied to daily routines. The way it is provided literally affects how long-term-care consumers live, where they live, whom they see, and how they spend their time. Ethical issues arise concerning the extent to which personal preferences and wishes should be honored, especially when they conflict with operating procedures of a caregiving organization or when they entail public costs. For example, should a person receiving home care be permitted to establish the timing for getting up and going to bed, even if this requires an attendant to visit late in the evening? Because LTC plans can be so comprehensive and intrusive, many believe that the client should be given as much choice and control as possible. Further, George Agich (1993) suggests that a legalistic ethic based narrowly on the right to noninterference ignores the existential reality of LTC. He argues that respect for autonomy must include provision of meaningful choices and maintenance of personal identity. Writing largely about nursing homes, Bart Collopy, Philip Boyle, and Bruce Jennings (1991) also argue for a view of autonomy that takes into account "the moral ecology" of LTC settings. A large ethnographic and anthropological literature offers insights into the complexity of this moral ecology, that is, the settings and arrangements of care (e.g., Gubrium, 1991).

With its focus on intimate, repetitive tasks and assistance with bodily functions that adults usually handle independently and privately, LTC can profoundly affect the dignity of the clients and alter their sense of personal identity and worth. Cognitively intact LTC clients may retain a keen sense of privacy concerning their bodies, their possessions, and even information about themselves. Assembly-line approaches to dressing, toileting, and bathing may be perceived as demeaning. Questions arise about how much energy LTC providers should be obliged to expend protecting the dignity of clients and helping them preserve their sense of identity. Even if clients are cognitively incapacitated and completely helpless physically, many believe it is wrong to subject them to procedures that are inherently undignified.

Dependency of LTC clients. Functionally impaired people are, by definition, dependent to some degree. Some people receiving care, though they may have the ability to conceive, plan, and choose actions, are virtually helpless to initiate or carry out actions. This creates a paradox: The more physically dependent the LTC client, the more he or she must depend on the help of others to exercise autonomy. Although providers taking a rehabilitation stance may strive to have clients do things for themselves, respect for the client's autonomy might dictate responsive fulfilling of requests. Striking the right balance between encouraging independence and providing help is an ethical issue for LTC providers.

Group-living settings. When LTC is provided in a collective, residential setting, the needs and interests of residents can collide. Residents in group settings are always expected to modify their individual wishes and behaviors to adjust to collective situations, and such expectations are usually well understood by all who enter such a setting. But it is unclear what rules of conduct and mutual expectations should govern a nursing home, an entity that is neither a hospital nor a housing unit. Typically, nursing homes accommodate, in multiple-occupancy rooms and close quarters, residents who are markedly varied in physical ability, cognitive ability, prognosis, age, social class, interests, and personal taste. To some degree, the facility's search for efficient routines defines permissible behavior and opportunities for nursing-home residents.

Family roles. LTC is inevitably a family affair. Most of the care given to people at home is provided by family members. Indeed, much paid home care is organized explicitly to give relief, assistance, or training to family members, who in turn are expected to do most of the work. Questions arise about what is right to expect of various family members, and even whether an older person should be forced to accept help from a family member against his or her will. One also wonders whether family anxiety for a relative's safety should send that relative into a nursing home. On the personal level, LTC evokes questions about the duties and rights of spouses, parents and adult children, and other relatives.

In practice, LTC providers, and especially case managers who coordinate and allocate care, sometimes view the whole family constellation as the client, especially if all the family members are elderly or if they live in the same household as the person getting care.

(Sometimes the needs and characteristics of the LTC client are interpreted by a family member who supplies most of the information.)

But family members' interests are not always identical to those of the clients, nor are their intentions always benign. Nursing-home staff often find that family members disagree with each other about the resident's care. They also sometimes note that the decisions of family members are motivated by an interest in minimizing the costs of care. Nursing-home personnel, who may themselves have a conflict of interest involving payment and money management, for example, when their recommendations entail more payment to the nursing home, often turn to the state's nursing-home ombudsperson to resolve such disputes. Home-care providers and state-designated case managers who purchase publicly subsidized home care also often disagree with family members about the type and amount of care needed and about whether a nursing-home admission is in the LTC client's best interest.

End-of-life issues. Death typically occurs during a period of LTC, either at the end of decades of care or after a relatively short episode. For this reason, many of the issues about death that confront acute-care providers also arise in long-term contexts, including the use of cardiopulmonary resuscitation, starting or stopping a respirator, or starting or stopping tube placement for nutrition and fluid intake. Issues of active or passive euthanasia also arise, which in turn evoke basic questions about the extent of the obligation of the health-care professional to preserve life on the one hand, and to avert suffering on the other. It is a challenge to give proper, systematic attention to end-of-life issues in LTC, while also giving weight to the everyday ethical matters that shape the quality of LTC clients' lives (Kane and Caplan, 1990).

Risks, risk aversion, and liability. Functionally disabled people are frequently unable to protect themselves against outside dangers such as fending off an intruder or escaping from a fire. Increased risks are associated with the simplest activities—walking to the bathroom, getting out of bed, boiling a pot of water. If the person's physical health is precarious, he or she may be at increased risk of a fall or of a sudden health incident, such as a stroke or heart attack, that needs immediate attention. If the LTC client suffers memory loss, the risks to safety because of forgetfulness or bad judgment increase. At the same time, supervision and surveillance exact a high price in both dollars and personal freedom.

In every type of LTC, questions arise about when it is right to leave a vulnerable person unprotected and subject to risk. The corollary question asked less often, is when it is right to force a functionally impaired person to accept protection and eliminate risks, even risks he or she prefers to take. The extreme example of restricting a person for his or her own protection is the use of physical restraints, which were formerly ubiquitous in nursing homes but have been curbed by regulatory changes following a highly publicized Institute of Medicine study on the quality of long-term-care settings (Committee on Nursing Home Regulation, 1986). Sedatives and psychoactive medications also have been used as a form of restraint and behavior control, presumably for safety reasons. On a less dramatic level, numerous organizational routines and professional practices and decisions designed to keep a client safe also restrict his or her freedom and may conflict with client preferences. Although attorneys point out that LTC providers have rarely been sued successfully for injuries sustained by a client while he or she was pursuing an expressed preference or choice, the fear of liability is pervasive in LTC industries (Kapp, 1987).

Professional standards and paraprofessional roles. It is a truism that ethical care must be competent care. The codes of ethics that govern health professionals generally require that health professionals act within the framework of correct and up-to-date scientific knowledge, and that they comply with the standards of adequate professional practice. Such judgments are easier to make about specific medical and nursing procedures than about the more amorphous and less specialized services of LTC, even when professionals are delivering the services. Without clear criteria for an adequate assessment of LTC needs or a competent care plan for a person with particular characteristics, it is difficult to promulgate standards or hold any one individual accountable.

One might argue that standards for care be set high and held to rigidly, to ensure safety. However, the more particular educational and other standards (e.g., caseload size) are mandated, the higher the cost of services. Professionals may unwittingly deny services to some older persons by advocating standards that inflate prices. Since professional self-interest usually accompanies concern for clients in advocacy for professional standards, this subject has ethical import. Also, the more rigid the standards, the less flexibility there is for clients to work out plans that suit their individual preferences.

The mainstays of LTC are the nursing assistants, home-health aides, homemakers, chore workers, and personal-care attendants who do the bulk of the difficult, labor-intensive, sometimes unpleasant work of LTC both in the community and in nursing homes. Little consensus has been reached about either the responsibilities of the paraprofessional LTC worker or the extent to which the worker should be expected to do independent problem solving. Little attention has been paid to the rights of the paraprofessional worker, who is typically paid a poor wage and sometimes faces substan-

dard working conditions in people's homes. The worker may also suffer verbal or physical abuse from clients or their family members. The care providers are often members of ethnic or racial minority groups serving a largely white, middle-class clientele.

Resource limitation. Decisions about what ought to be done must take costs into account, particularly when governments pay or subsidize payment of the bills. For each element of LTC services and programs, one can ask whether it is worth the money, compared to other good uses for the resources. Limited resources result in fewer staff to give care in residential facilities, poorly paid home-care attendants or limited hours of home care for each person, less space, less privacy, and less personal attention overall.

A scarce resource might be a single room in a nursing home or an extra half hour of attention at home. Without explicitly translating cost-consciousness into human terms—such as the numbers of baths or assisted trips to the toilet an LTC client is entitled to, or the number of minutes an LTC client should have to wait after a call button is pushed—authorities tacitly accept that the resources available are limited and that resource constraints will compromise the best care for functionally impaired persons.

Intergenerational issues. Finally, LTC forces consideration of what an ethical society should offer to older people. Older people—people over seventy-five—are by far the most numerous group needing LTC; however, the lifetime costs of LTC may be greater for a younger person. Some LTC planners ask whether the claims on society for care of a younger disabled person and an older one are different in kind, degree, or justification.

Although justifications are often made for caring for older people based on reciprocity across the generations, the elderly are given resources and encouraged to manage their own care less often than are younger disabled persons. Indeed, political action among younger disabled persons has led to changes for older people receiving community LTC. In the 1980s and early 1990s, several states restructured their LTC programs under Medicaid and state financing to comprise disabled adults of all ages. As a result, these administrators now need to determine how to allocate resources fairly among clients of widely different ages and circumstances. Advocacy groups representing younger disabled persons argue for a model of LTC that gives more power to the LTC client or his or her agent (Litvak et al., 1987). They prefer a social rather than a medical model of care that would, as much as possible, relegate to the client the prerogative of selecting, training, supervising, and firing those who provide personal care. A personal-care assistant who accompanies the client as needed is perceived as liberating, whereas home care was seen as restricting.

Authorities disagree about whether the personal-assistant model is desirable or feasible for the much larger group of elderly LTC clients.

Policy issues

As with acute care, LTC poses interrelated problems in access, quality, and cost. Access to care is uneven because of geographic variation in supply and price. Care is most available in the least-preferred nursing-home form, because that is the form that is publicly subsidized. Quality concerns are present for both nursing-home care and home care. Public and private costs are high. Reimbursement methods and levels for LTC often create perverse incentives. Flat-rate systems discriminate against those who need the most care. At the same time, "case-mix-adjusted" systems, which increase payment for persons with greater disabilities, provide clear incentives against rehabilitation (Kane and Kane, 1987).

Benefits and coverage.   Approximately 5 percent of the elderly population in the United States are among the 1.9 million nursing-home residents. However, it is estimated that an additional 10 percent of the elderly population have comparable functional impairments requiring LTC (Wiener et al., 1994). For every person in a nursing home, more than one equally disabled older person resides in the community. In contrast to many other industrialized countries, publicly funded LTC in the United States is available only to persons of low income. Moreover, also in contrast to other countries, the vast bulk of public LTC expenditures are for nursing-home care. Despite expectations that LTC costs be met first by the clients themselves, at least 50 percent of nursing-home costs in the United States are borne publicly (largely through the Medicaid programs), because private resources are quickly exhausted. The public share of the costs also increases because some older people divest their resources in the years before they expect a nursing-home admission in order to qualify for Medicaid. The extent to which divestment increases public costs is a matter of sharp debate. Publicly financed home-care benefits, though they became more widely available in the 1980s and 1990s, accounted for a relatively small outlay and were used by relatively few clients. Further, almost all publicly funded home care has been capped at a rate less than the rate of public reimbursement for nursing-home care for the same client in the same state.

Nursing homes are perceived negatively. People do not want to live in them, send their family members to them, or expend their life savings and deplete their estates to pay for them. If the LTC-service setting were less aversive in terms of unappealing settings, rigid routines, and high costs, presumably some who now depend on volunteered family help would use paid LTC. This consideration dampens the enthusiasm of officials for expanding home-care benefits; they fear that home care, rather than substituting for nursing-home care, would be received by people formerly receiving uncompensated care from families.

Private LTC insurance is financially viable for only a fraction of the group at risk (Rivlin and Wiener, 1988). Both private insurers and public policymakers worry that if benefits were more desirable, they would be heavily used. After all, some LTC services (e.g., cooking, housekeeping, laundry) are intrinsically desirable even for people without LTC needs. Moreover, despite earlier beliefs, research has conclusively shown that at certain disability levels home care is more expensive than nursing-home care (Carcagno and Kemper, 1988). Economies of scale are achieved when brief, intermittent services and protective oversight are offered in centralized locations.

When community-based LTC is financed through Medicaid or state appropriations, case managers, usually social workers or nurses, typically perform initial assessments, authorize payments for home care, and monitor the quality of care and its continuing appropriateness. The case-management role promotes equity and efficiency in the use of benefits across a population, but also creates a powerful agent, involved in the allocation of benefits, who may have no clear professional ethic, training, or authority. Home-health agencies often complain that interposing a case manager between them and their clientele is wasteful and interferes with client choice; state officials argue that case managers who are separate from service delivery provide a distinterested advocate for the client. Juggling the roles of advocate and gatekeeper creates ethical tension for the case manager (Kane and Caplan, 1993). Case managers often have difficulty reconciling these roles, but at a minimum, should disclose to clients the assumptions under which they work. In the early 1990s and before, informed-consent processes for case management were rudimentary.

Reimbursement issues are confounded by confusion about the extent to which LTC is a health program. In the United States, health care is considered a public responsibility (at least in part), whereas housing and social services are typically considered private responsibilities to be purchased with private income and with government subsidies for the poor. LTC includes social services and, when provided in nursing homes, housing. Policymakers have not determined whether they should extricate these components for financing purposes, or how to do so. Rosalie Kane and Keren Brown Wilson (1993) advocate development of assisted-living programs where functionally disabled, nursing-home-certifiable tenants have private apartments with kitchenettes, full baths, and doors that lock from the inside, but will also have three meals in a communal dining room, and housekeeping and personal care according to individual care plans. Such programs have been emerging in many states, most notably in Oregon, since 1989. They sometimes use home-care agencies to deliver services to assisted-living residents, and sometimes Medicaid reimburses the service component. This blurs the distinction between institutional care and home care. It also permits separating the financing of the room and lodging from that of the personal-care and nursing services, so the latter can be funded publicly and the former privately.

LTC costs and payment are also complicated by unclear boundaries with acute hospital care, primary health care, and post-acute care. Medicare, the universal health insurance for persons over sixty-five, covers rehabilitation, skilled nursing-home care, and skilled home care in the immediate aftermath of an acute illness. These types of services, known as "post-acute" or "sub-acute" care, fall in an ill-defined area between acute care and LTC. Efforts to save money in acute care and post-acute care—for example, through earlier hospital discharge or denial of Medicare claims for post-acute care—can result in higher LTC costs. Demonstration projects have paid a per capita rate to care providers who are then responsible for both acute care and LTC costs; the projects are meant to determine whether better or more efficient use can be made of the total dollars when acute care and LTC are integrated into a single program. The Social Health Maintenance Organization is one such model, and another is the Program of All-Inclusive Care for the Elderly (PACE), which was modeled on an innovative program in San Francisco's Chinatown that uses a day health-care center as a key feature.

Professionalization and regulation.   The more professional standards are exacted for LTC services and the more providers are regulated, the more expensive LTC becomes. Because family members provide much LTC, some state policymakers suggest that professional-practice acts in most states are unduly restrictive about requiring licensed nurses for many procedures routinely done by family caregivers. Others believe that vulnerable LTC clients need protection by high standards for professional practice and managed professional supervision of nonprofessionals. This issue is salient because many LTC clients would like to purchase cost-effective services. The break-even point, at which community services exceed the price of home-based services, can be reached rather quickly and is influenced not only by the disability levels of the client but also by the price of the services. These, in turn, are influenced by regulations governing professional practices and agency licensure.

Regulation of care providers such as nursing homes and home-care agencies through state licensure, quality inspection, and federal certification programs also drives up costs, stifling innovation and consumer choice. Protection of vulnerable adults and avoidance of politically damaging incidents fuel these efforts. Regulation of supply of nursing homes also occurs to stimulate community care and to save money (on the theory that a licensed bed will be used). This form of regulation has been criticized by those who believe that if market forces prevail, quality will improve.

Family policy.   Case managers make implicit and explicit decisions about the ability of family members to provide help before they allocate publicly funded service to LTC clients. LTC policymakers do not want to replace family care with public programs, but want to protect families from undue burden. Respite programs have been developed specifically to provide episodic or emergency assistance to family caregivers. Various forms of compensation for family members have been suggested, ranging from tax credits to direct payment. In some states, LTC clients have received cash payments, which they, in turn, can and often do use to pay relatives. Supporting these strategies, Nathan Linsk and his colleagues (1992) note the irony of paying strangers but not relatives. Direct payments to family caregivers are also seen as an income-transfer to poor families. Opponents of family payment cite the cost implications. A midway position argues for family payments only when the caregiver has left the labor force to provide care—disqualifying most retirement-age spouses—and only for low-income families.

LTC labor force.   Paraprofessional workers in nursing homes and, more particularly, in home care, may receive minimum wages and no benefits. The cost implications of paying the workers an adequate wage are enormous. Although advocates of greater LTC benefits for senior citizens historically ignored the situation for workers, in the 1990s groups such as the Older Women's League formally recognized the condition of care workers as an issue. The very persons who perform the hands-on LTC tasks—typically, persons with low wages and nonexistent benefits—will become at risk for LTC themselves, without any personal financial reservoir from which to draw.

With the aging of the population and the chronicity of disease, long-term-care policies may be expected to receive great attention beyond the 1990s. Many specific policies discussed here are in flux, and themes and policy changes may be expected in response to current debates. The nagging questions about how a society can meet the ordinary needs of people with functional impairments competently, efficiently, fairly, and without compromising the autonomy and quality of life of the clientele are likely to endure.

ROSALIE A. KANE

Directly related to this article are the other articles in this entry: NURSING HOMES, *and* HOME CARE. *Also directly related is the entry* CHRONIC CARE. *For a further discussion of topics mentioned in this article, see the entries* AGING AND THE AGED; ALLIED HEALTH PROFESSIONS; DEATH AND DYING: EUTHANASIA AND SUSTAINING LIFE; DISABILITY, *article on* HEALTH CARE AND PHYSICAL DISABILITY; FAMILY; HEALTH-CARE DELIVERY, *article on* HEALTH-CARE INSTITUTIONS; HEALTH-CARE FINANCING; HEALTH-CARE RESOURCES, ALLOCATION OF, *article on* MICROALLOCATION; PROFESSION AND PROFESSIONAL ETHICS; PUBLIC POLICY AND BIOETHICS; *and* WOMEN. *For a discussion of related ideas, see the entries on* AUTONOMY; JUSTICE; *and* PRIVACY IN HEALTH CARE.

Bibliography

AGICH, GEORGE J. 1993. *Autonomy and Long Term Care.* New York: Oxford University Press.

BRODY, ELAINE M. 1985. "Parent Care as a Normative Family Stress." *Gerontologist* 25, no. 1:19–29.

CARCAGNO, GEORGE J., and KEMPER, PETER. 1988. "The Evaluation of the National Long Term Care Demonstration: 1. An Overview of the Channeling Demonstration and Its Evaluation." *Health Services Research* 23:1–22.

COLLOPY, BART; BOYLE, PHILIP; and JENNINGS, BRUCE. 1991. "New Directions in Nursing Home Ethics." *Hastings Center Report* 21, no. 2:1–15.

COMMITTEE ON NURSING HOME REGULATION. INSTITUTE OF MEDICINE. 1986. *Improving the Quality of Care in Nursing Homes.* Washington, D.C.: National Academy Press.

GUBRIUM, JABER F. 1991. *The Mosaic of Care: Frail Elderly and Their Families in the Real World.* New York: Springer.

KANE, ROSALIE A., and CAPLAN, ARTHUR L., eds. 1990. *Everyday Ethics: Resolving Dilemmas in Nursing Home Life.* New York: Springer.

———, eds. 1993. *Ethical Conflicts in the Management of Home Care: The Case Manager's Dilemma.* New York: Springer.

KANE, ROSALIE, A., and KANE, ROBERT L. 1987. *Long-Term Care: Principles, Programs, and Policies.* New York: Springer.

KANE, ROSALIE, and WILSON, KEREN BROWN. 1993. *Assisted Living in the United States: A New Paradigm for Residential Care for Frail Older Persons?* Washington, D.C.: American Association of Retired Persons.

KAPP, MARSHALL B. 1987. *Preventing Malpractice in Long Term Care: Strategies for Risk Management.* New York: Springer.

LINSK, NATHAN L.; KEIGHER, SHARON M.; SIMON-RUSINOWITZ, LORI; and ENGLAND, SUZANNE E. 1992. *Wages for Caring: A Survey of Attendant Service Programs for People of All Ages with Disabilities.* New York: Praeger.

LITVAK, SIMI; ZUKAS, HALE; and HEUMANN, JUDITH E. 1987. *Attending to America: Personal Assistance for Independent Living: A Survey of Attendant Service Programs for People of All Ages with Disabilities.* Berkeley, Calif.: World Institute on Disability.

RIVLIN, ALICE M., and WIENER, JOSHUA M. 1988. *Caring for the Disabled Elderly: Who Will Pay?* Washington, D.C.: Brookings Institution.

WIENER, JOSHUA M.; ILLSTON, LAUREL H.; and HANLEY, RAYMOND J. 1994. *Sharing the Burden.* Washington, D.C.: Brookings Institution.

II. NURSING HOMES

The decision to enter a nursing home is the most wrenching outcome of long-term-care decision making. It changes almost every aspect of the life of an elder, who moves to new surroundings, may acquire a perfect stranger as a roommate, and must adhere to the nursing-home schedule. The either/or nature of the decision and the move to what has been described as a "total institution" (Lidz et al., 1992) marks the decision about nursing-home admission as a "nodal" decision (Agich, 1993).

A nursing home is an institution in which persons, usually elderly (65 years of age and older), live and receive nursing care and supervision. The provision of nursing care and supervision differentiates nursing homes from other senior residences; the lack of advanced medical and surgical services, and the fact that a nursing home is also a residence, differentiate it from a hospital. At any time, about 5 percent of those in the United States over sixty-five years of age are in nursing homes, many more than in acute-care hospitals. Over 40 percent of those over sixty-five will spend at least some time in a nursing home (Kemper and Murtaugh, 1991). Residents of nursing homes tend to be old, poor, and sick; younger patients, often with mental disorders or post-traumatic conditions, account for a relatively small number. Nursing-home residents are disproportionately female and white.

Most nursing-home residents have trouble performing normal daily activities, such as bathing and dressing. They often have multiple long-term problems, such as confusion or walking difficulties. Nursing homes are increasingly used to provide further care after hospital discharge (Densen, 1991).

Ethical problems in nursing homes differ in several ways from those seen in other settings. Decision making tends to be "temporally thick," involving many related decisions made over time. There are multiple participants. Family members are intimately involved. Many nursing-home residents are unable to make or communicate decisions, resulting in reliance on proxy decision makers. Institutional policies and practices act as powerful constraints on the autonomy of decision makers (Lidz et al., 1992; Kane and Caplan, 1990).

Demographic changes in developed countries that have led to an increased need for nursing homes include an increase in the aging population in both absolute numbers and percentage of the population, nuclear rather than extended families, and more women in the work force. The emphasis on autonomy and the fear of lawsuits on the part of health-care providers and institutions may be unique to the United States, but basic ethical conflicts between respecting personal autonomy and ensuring personal safety occur in nursing homes everywhere in the world.

Reimbursement

In the United States, nursing-home care is paid for almost entirely by Medicaid and "self-pay," with Medicare and long-term care insurance accounting for only a small percentage. Over two-thirds of those in nursing homes for more than six months are covered by Medicaid. Medicaid reimbursement is usually low, and nursing homes may react by raising the rates for other payers to subsidize the Medicaid population, maximizing the number of self-payers, or minimizing the amenities offered.

Asset management, in which assets are shielded or transferred while the elder becomes eligible for Medicaid, raises several questions. Is it ethically justified for relatively well-off elders to use programs meant for the poor? Alternatively, should those elders have to spend all their resources in the last few months or years of life? Several state programs have been developed in response to these questions, in which elders who purchase long-term care insurance are covered by Medicaid when their insurance runs out (Mahoney and Wetle, 1992).

Major questions regarding reimbursement remain. Who should bear the responsibility for the long-term care of elders? What are the ethically justified means of financing nursing-home care? What mix of long-term care settings should be offered as a matter of public policy? What incentives to improve care ought to be provided to those who care for nursing-home residents? In the United States, changes in health-care policy in the future may affect reimbursement for long-term care, including nursing-home care.

The admissions process

A sustained effort by families to keep elders at home or in other community settings usually precedes nursing-home admission. Problems leading to admission may include increasing confusion, decreasing ability to care for oneself, and collapse of social supports.

Pertinent questions concerning nursing-home admission include "Who is making the decision?" and "Who ought to participate in making the decision?" The circumstances in which decisions are made exert powerful influence. Thus, a hospital may put pressure on the physician and family to have the patient discharged to a nursing home after acute problems are resolved. Involved parties may have conflicting interests and obligations. For example, family members may be involved as overburdened caregivers, concerned relatives, and proxy decision makers. These factors should be identified to prevent ethical conflict in the decision-making process.

Many conflicts arise between respecting the elder's autonomy and protecting his or her safety. Participants may disagree about whether the elder's safety is actually threatened (elder: "I'm all right, I've just tripped once or twice"; versus family: "She falls all the time. I'm terrified she's going to break her hip"). They may also disagree about the relative safety of the nursing home. Health-care professionals and family members may perceive the nursing home as a safer environment than it is. Confusion, falls, and increased dependency are common sequelae of nursing-home admissions. However, those admitted to nursing homes are often very frail, and it is usually not clear whether they would have fared better at home.

The nursing home itself challenges the elder's autonomy. Lack of privacy, regimented schedules, and uniform treatment of residents without regard for their wishes or interests are common. Autonomy is also constrained by other factors, including mental and physical disorders that limit the ability to make and carry out decisions, the elder's obligations to respect the legitimate interests of caregivers and family members, and the lack of a stable public policy establishing the justice-based obligations of society to elders and of elders and their families to society (Jecker, 1991). The ethical complexity of long-term-care decision making throws into question the relevance of the acute-care model of decision making, with its emphasis on patient autonomy (Agich, 1993; Hofland, 1990). A distinctive ethic may be required for long-term care, perhaps based on mediation and negotiation of opposing views (Collopy et al., 1991; Moody, 1992).

Decision making in treatment

After admission to a nursing home, everyday issues such as phone access, roommate selection, and opportunity for spiritual growth must be addressed, requiring mediation among several concerns: respect for the elder's autonomy, the obligations of residents to each other, the institution's legitimate interests, and the family's role in decision making (Agich, 1993; Kane and Caplan, 1990, 1993). The task for nursing homes is to identify meaningful possibilities for the elder's exercise of everyday autonomy in the context of these legitimate constraints on autonomy.

Under the Patient Self-Determination Act (PSDA), implemented in 1991 in response to the case of Nancy Cruzan in Missouri, advance directives must be explained to the patient on admission. The impact of the PSDA on the current low rates of advance directives for nursing-home patients (Gamble et al., 1991) is not yet apparent. Issues requiring decision making that often arise in nursing homes include hospital transfers, artificial feeding, antibiotic use, amputation, and the use of restraints (Besdine, 1983).

Discussions of treatment choices should involve the resident, if he or she is able to participate, and family members or designated proxy decision makers, if the elder is unable to participate or desires their involvement. Although family members may not make the same choice the elder would make, many elders would still rather have family members make decisions for them (Menikoff et al., 1992). Demented patients may be able to make some decisions about their health care. Decision-making capacity should be assessed by the physician relative to the particular decision that must be made. For example, a patient with moderate dementia might be able to decide not to have a leg amputated, and yet be unable to remember to take her medications without being reminded.

Competent patients or surrogate decision makers have the well-established right to refuse any treatment, though there is debate about whether they have the right to demand any treatment (Brett and McCullough, 1986). Trying a therapy for a time to evaluate its effectiveness may be a better choice than simply using or not using a treatment. However, institutions and caregivers, who have traditionally been reluctant to stop a treatment once begun, must be flexible if this approach is to succeed. Before such a trial of therapy, specific goals (such as expected improvements in status) should be agreed upon.

Conflict between family members and staff is often exacerbated by serious illness. For example, a family member who has not previously been involved in the patient's care may demand inappropriately aggressive care (Molloy et al., 1991). When family members or staff members cannot reach a decision without significant disagreement, they may refer the matter to an ethics committee or consultant. Clerics may be helpful in addressing conflicts arising out of religious beliefs held by various participants. Legal proceedings are usually a last resort.

Many nursing-home residents with severe dementia who are not able to eat are kept alive with feeding tubes; many of these persons might not have wished to be kept alive under these circumstances. Legal decisions in U.S. courts in the 1980s and 1990s have treated the provision of nutrition and hydration as medical decisions and have recognized that artificial feeding is not always obligatory.

However, withholding of nutrition poses special problems for some because of the special standing of "food and water" in human life. Many nursing-home policies require the use of artificial feeding if the resident's weight or oral intake falls below specified guidelines, even if this is against the patient's or family's wishes. Such policies may not be legally supportable if challenged.

When nursing-home residents develop serious illness requiring treatment not available in the nursing home, transfer to the hospital becomes an issue. If a decision to limit medical intervention has been made, transfer may be unnecessary. Such decisions are best made well in advance of a crisis. Patients and surrogate decision makers should be asked their views on such transfers at the time of admission or when there is any major change in the resident's condition. When patients are transferred, advance directives written in the nursing home may not be sent to or considered valid by the hospital, and emergency services and other treatment unwanted by the elder or family may be given. Nursing-home administrators and physicians need to address this problem of the "portability" of advance directives.

Restraints

Restraints are commonly used in nursing homes to prevent falls and injuries to the patient and others, to prevent wandering, and for behavioral problems. Restraints can be physical (e.g., vests or wrist restraints) or chemical (e.g., drugs that alter behavior). Restraints may be used to protect the patient or for the convenience of the staff and can cause adverse physical and psychological outcomes, including death. Less use of restraints enhances the autonomy of nursing-home residents and several studies show either no change or a decrease in the risk of falls and injuries. However, restraint-free environments are often opposed due to inadequate staffing levels, fear of litigation, and the weight of traditional practice in the United States. The informed-consent process should address the benefits and risks of a restraint-free environment versus restraint use.

Research

Research in nursing homes (for example, into the treatment of urinary incontinence) may contribute to the quality of life of nursing-home residents. However, nursing-home research is complicated by problems of obtaining permission from nursing-home administrators to do such research, obtaining adequate informed consent or proxy consent in this vulnerable population, and ensuring privacy and confidentiality (High, 1992; Sachs and Cassel, 1990). Professionals should balance the protection of this vulnerable population with an accurate assessment of each elder's ability to give consent and should allow those who are able to consent to participate. Proxy decision makers should consider what is known about an elder's preferences as well as the benefits, risks, and need for the research.

Staff concerns

Nursing-home staff perform difficult, frustrating tasks and are usually poorly paid and poorly trained. Those who criticize them, whether clients, family members, or better-paid staff members, are not in their situation. Staff turnover is high in most nursing homes, affecting continuity of care and staff-elder relationships. Staff members are also often people of color, in contrast to nursing-home residents, which can lead to a mutual lack of understanding and, on occasion, to racist remarks and abuse from elderly residents or their families.

Staff members who provide regular personal care often develop strong emotional ties to residents; they are exposed daily to the outcomes of treatment choices and may disagree with patients or family members. Where staff members are de facto family members, sometimes with more emotional concern and contact time with the resident than actual family members, the nursing home may reasonably question whether the relatives should remain the proxy decision makers of first choice. Information from staff members about the patient's wishes should be considered by those responsible for the patient's care.

Local, state, federal, and accrediting requirements and regulations pose ethical challenges to administrators in allocating the scarce resource of staff time. Complying with these regulations absorbs significant staff time and resources, diminishing the time and energy staff can devote to the care of residents. The worst institutions are unlikely to be caught, and the best are likely to spend substantial amounts of time on paperwork that does not clearly contribute to care. In addition, regulatory overemphasis on the safety of residents may restrict the autonomy of elders (Lidz et al., 1992).

Death and dying

A common cause of death in nursing homes is an infection or another acute illness superimposed on a chronic or progressive illness. Often, patients or family members, together with physicians and nursing home staff, have decided not to treat such illnesses. Many terminally ill patients in nursing homes are eligible for the Medicare hospice benefit. Hospice care may ensure that these patients receive improved treatment of pain and other symptoms; it may also make it easier for the family and staff to accept less aggressive medical care, such as not treating pneumonia with antibiotics. Hospice units have been developed in nursing homes, and they may

provide hospice care for severely demented patients (Volicer et al., 1986).

Cardiopulmonary resuscitation (CPR) initiated in nursing homes or in seriously ill patients is rarely successful (Applebaum et al., 1990). Nursing homes may be justified in not offering CPR because of the very low probability of success. In any case, patients and family members should understand that CPR is only an attempt at resuscitation with little likelihood of success. "Do not resuscitate" (DNR) orders should not be equated with "do not treat" orders. Decisions about specific treatments should be discussed and well documented in advance.

When death is imminent, many nursing homes transfer the resident to a hospital or contact emergency medical services so that death can occur elsewhere. This may be contrary to the elder's and the family's wishes. Most emergency medical service protocols require cardiopulmonary resuscitation to be attempted, which may be traumatic to the staff and family.

Conclusion

The bioethics literature tends to typify ethical conflicts among people as involving a clash between beneficence and respect for an individual's autonomy. Nursing-home ethics is far more complex and subtle, both intellectually and practically; it includes the obligations of elders to family members, other residents, staff, and institutions; the management of scarce resources, especially in response to external constraints; the limits of caregiving obligations on the part of family members and nursing-home staff; and the anticipation and prevention of the ethical problems discussed in this article.

JILL A. RHYMES
LAURENCE B. McCULLOUGH

Directly related to this article are the other articles in this entry: CONCEPT AND POLICIES, *and* HOME CARE. *Also directly related is the entry* CHRONIC CARE. *For a further discussion of topics mentioned in this article, see the entries* ABUSE, INTERPERSONAL, *article on* ELDER ABUSE; AGING AND THE AGED; ALLIED HEALTH PROFESSIONS; DEATH AND DYING: EUTHANASIA AND SUSTAINING LIFE; FAMILY; HEALTH-CARE DELIVERY, *article on* HEALTH-CARE INSTITUTIONS; HEALTH-CARE FINANCING; HEALTH-CARE RESOURCES, ALLOCATION OF, *article on* MICROALLOCATION; HOSPICE AND END-OF-LIFE CARE; *and* MENTALLY DISABLED AND MENTALLY ILL PERSONS. *For a discussion of related ideas, see the entries* AUTONOMY; COMPETENCE; INFORMED CONSENT; PRIVACY AND CONFIDENTIALITY IN RESEARCH; *and* RIGHTS, *article on* RIGHTS IN BIOETHICS.

Bibliography

AGICH, GEORGE J. 1993. *Autonomy and Long Term Care.* New York: Oxford University Press.

APPLEBAUM, GARY E.; KING, JOYCE E.; and FINUCANE, THOMAS E. 1990. "The Outcome of CPR Initiated in Nursing Homes." *Journal of the American Geriatrics Society* 38, no. 3:197–200.

BESDINE, RICHARD W. 1983. "Decisions to Withhold Treatment from Nursing Home Residents." *Journal of the American Geriatrics Society* 31, no. 10:602–606.

BINSTOCK, ROBERT H.; POST, STEPHEN G.; and WHITEHOUSE, PETER J., eds. 1992. *Dementia and Aging: Ethics, Values, and Policy Choices.* Baltimore: Johns Hopkins University Press.

BRETT, ALLEN S., and MCCULLOUGH, LAURENCE B. 1986. "When Patients Request Specific Interventions: Defining the Limits of the Physician's Obligation." *New England Journal of Medicine* 315, no. 21:1347–1351.

COLLOPY, BART; BOYLE, PHILIP; and JENNINGS, BRUCE. 1991. "New Directions in Nursing Home Ethics." *Hastings Center Report* 2, no. 2:1–15.

DENSEN, PAUL M. 1991. *AHCPR Monograph: Tracing the Elderly Through the Health Care System: An Update.* Rockville, Md.: U.S. Department of Health and Human Services, Public Health Service, Agency for Health Care Policy and Research.

DUNKLE, RUTH E., and WYKLE, MAY L., eds. 1988. *Decision Making in Long-Term Care: Factors in Planning.* New York: Springer.

GAMBLE, ELIZABETH R.; MCDONALD, PENELOPE J.; and LICHSTEIN, PETER R. 1991. "Knowledge, Attitudes, and Behavior of Elderly Persons Regarding Living Wills." *Archives of Internal Medicine* 151, no. 2:277–280.

HIGH, DALLAS M. 1992. "Research with Alzheimer's Disease Subjects: Informed Consent and Proxy Decision Making." *Journal of the American Geriatrics Society* 40, no. 9:950–957.

HOFLAND, BRIAN F. 1988. "Autonomy in Long Term Care: Background Issues and a Programmatic Response." *Gerontologist* 28 (June, suppl.):3–9.

———, ed. 1990. *Generations* 14 (suppl.):1–96. Special issue, "Autonomy and Long-Term Care Practice."

JECKER, NANCY S., ed. 1991. *Aging and Ethics: Philosophical Problems in Gerontology.* Clifton, N.J.: Humana.

KANE, ROBERT A., and KANE, ROSALIE, eds. 1982. *Values and Long-Term Care: Factors in Planning.* Lexington, Mass.: Lexington.

KANE, ROSALIE A., and CAPLAN, ARTHUR L., eds. 1990. *Everyday Ethics: Resolving Dilemmas in Nursing Home Life.* New York: Springer.

———, eds. 1993. *Ethical Conflicts in the Management of Home Care: The Case Manager's Dilemma.* New York: Springer.

KEMPER, PETER, and MURTAUGH, CHRISTOPHER M. 1991. "Lifetime Use of Nursing Home Care." *New England Journal of Medicine* 324, no. 9:595–600.

LIDZ, CHARLES W.; FISCHER, LYNN; and ARNOLD, ROBERT M. 1992. *The Erosion of Autonomy in Long-Term Care.* New York: Oxford University Press.

MAHONEY, KEVIN J., and WETLE, TERRIE. 1992. "Public-Private Partnerships: The Connecticut Model for Financing Long Term Care." *Journal of the American Geriatrics Society* 40, no. 10:1026–1030.

MENIKOFF, JERRY A.; SACHS, GREG A.; and SIEGLER, MARK. 1992. "Beyond Advance Directives—Health Care Surrogate Laws." *New England Journal of Medicine* 327, no. 16:1165–1169.

MOLLOY, DAVID W.; CLARNETTE, ROGER M.; BRAUN, E. ANN; EISEMANN, MARTIN R.; and SNEIDERMAN, B. 1991. "Decision Making in the Incompetent Elderly: 'The Daughter from California Syndrome.'" *Journal of the American Geriatrics Society* 39, no. 4:396–399.

MOODY, HARRY R. 1992. *Ethics in an Aging Society.* Baltimore: Johns Hopkins University Press.

OUSLANDER, JOSEPH G.; OSTERWEIL, DAN; and MORLEY, JOHN. 1991. *Medical Care in the Nursing Home.* New York: McGraw-Hill.

SACHS, GREG A., and CASSEL, CHRISTINE K. 1990. "Biomedical Research Involving Older Human Subjects." *Law, Medicine, and Health Care* 18, no. 3:234–243.

VOLICER, LADISLAV; RHEAUME, YVETTE; BROWN, JUNE; FABISZEWSKI, KATHY; and BRADY, ROGER. 1986. "Hospice Approach to the Treatment of Patients with Advanced Dementia of the Alzheimer Type." *Journal of the American Medical Association* 256, no. 16:2210–2213.

III. HOME CARE

Home care is an almost limitless array of preventive, therapeutic, restorative, and supportive services delivered to persons living in their own homes or the home of another in the community. In the long-term care context, home care comprises home-based services delivered to chronically ill or impaired persons. Although this care may, and increasingly does, involve high-technology medical services, the majority of care is directed at functional support (Koff, 1988). Home-care services can be divided into those services considered "skilled," such as skilled nursing, rehabilitation, speech therapy, occupational therapy, and physician home visits; and those considered "unskilled," such as personal assistance with activities of daily living (like bathing or dressing), household maintenance, monitoring, supervision, and instrumental assistance (for example, shopping or financial management).

Until the twentieth century, virtually all medical care was provided in the home. As modern medicine developed more effective and technically sophisticated interventions, medical care shifted to hospitals and physicians' offices. However, by World War I, the steadily growing numbers of persons with chronic illness reignited interest in formal home-care services. During the 1940s, limitations in the ability of hospitals to meet the increased demand for inpatient services contributed to the development of hospital-based home-care services.

The 1965 amendments to the U.S. Social Security Act that created Medicaid and Medicare were intended, in part, to expand the supply of home care. Further amendments in 1967 made home care a mandatory benefit, and others in 1972 streamlined the terms of Medicare program participation for home-care agencies (Benjamin, 1993). By the mid-1980s, home care was described as the fastest-growing service under Medicare (Reilly et al., 1990).

Growth in the home-care industry has been attributed to several factors, including the preference of patients for care at home rather than in institutions such as nursing homes, the availability of informal caregivers, the increased number of users, the intensity of utilization, and the increase in public reimbursement of services. As of 1987, home-care services were provided to about 7.7 million persons of all ages in the United States, but almost three-fourths of these persons were over the age of sixty-five (Wieland et al., 1991). The elderly (over sixty-five) population in the United States is projected to increase by 40 percent by 2020, and the use of home care is expected to increase by 60 percent during that time (Rivlin and Wiener, 1988). Among the non-aged (under sixty-five) population, use of home-care services has been profoundly affected by the growth, in certain major cities, of the population of persons with acquired immunodeficiency syndrome (AIDS)—a 600 percent increase between 1984 and 1990 (Burbridge, 1993).

The increasing use of formal home-care services—those paid for directly or by third-party reimbursement, such as Medicare, Medicaid, or private insurance—has triggered concerns regarding the cost, quality, and availability of home care. The home-care "industry" has experienced increased competition, oversight, and regulation as well as growth of the for-profit sector. There has also been a steady "medicalization" of home-care services, driven to a great degree by third-party reimbursement (Estes and Binney, 1989).

About 85 percent of home care is provided by informal caregivers, usually unpaid family members, friends, or acquaintances, and a majority of both formal and informal caregivers are women (Stone et al., 1987). Care is provided in the most personal and intimate aspects of daily life to persons who may be vulnerable because of physical frailty and/or cognitive impairment. Several aspects of home care other than the location in which it is provided differentiate it from institutionally based long-term care. Because care is provided in the home of the client or of another individual, the client may have a stronger sense of autonomy and control, may be more comfortable, and may have the protection and security of others in the home. However, care at home raises concerns of quality assurance in unsupervised settings and the protection of the client from unscrupulous or abusive providers of formal and informal care.

Several concerns are shared in institutional and home-based long-term care. For example, problems arise in addressing autonomous decision making for persons with diminished cognitive function. There are also stresses involved in receiving intimate care from strangers. Many persons needing long-term care encounter serious limitations in the availability of services and in the funds to pay for them. Clear methods to ensure quality in both settings are lacking. And families experience stress whether care is provided at home or in institutions. There are, however, important differences. Autonomy is more strongly asserted by many home-care patients, but home-care patients may be more isolated and thus dependent on family caregivers (Young et al., 1988).

The remainder of this article considers ethical issues that pertain to the individual receiving home care, to families, to paid workers, and to the system of care more generally.

The home-care patient/client

Chronically impaired patients, particularly elderly patients, may be at "ethical risk" of being excluded from decisions regarding their care, of having their preferences disregarded, and of having no voice in social policy decisions that affect them. This risk may result from several factors, including ageism, negative stereotypes regarding disability, misinformation, well-meaning but misguided paternalism, or reactions to spiraling health-care costs driven in part by public spending for the old and disabled. The home setting itself may influence the nature and degree of ethical risk (Collopy et al., 1990).

Home care may enhance the opportunity to make autonomous decisions, but it may also constrain and influence decision making. The traditional view of autonomy assumes that action is intentional, self-initiated, and not influenced by others; in reality, however, we live in a complex web of influences, including those of family members, loved ones, acquaintances, and professional caregivers. Nowhere is this web more evident than in care provided at home. Family, friends, and neighbors, as well as formal care providers, may all have an interest in the decision-making process regarding the nature and scheduling of care, the selection of workers to provide the services, and even whether or not the client can be maintained safely at home.

Safety and the assessment of risk are major considerations in the provision of home care and contribute to some of the most perplexing ethical dilemmas for providers of care. Most people of any age prefer living at home, no matter how humble or risky, to entering an institution. This preference, combined with an overestimation by some clients of their own abilities and an underestimation of the risk of living at home, frequently results in an insistence to be at home despite substantial safety concerns on the part of family and professionals.

Determination of risk is an inexact science, and it is not unusual for family and professionals to underestimate or disregard the comparable risks of institutional life. Caregivers feel strong obligation to act in the best interests of clients or loved ones by protecting them from harm, and these feelings are compounded by fear of liability should harm come to the client. While some commentators argue that fears of lawsuit have been exaggerated, they remain a powerful force in evaluating the safety of a home-based care plan (Detzel and Kapp, 1992). An emerging model for addressing the question of risk involves "negotiating" what is an acceptable risk with the client and family by being clear about the nature of the risk and about their willingness to accept both the risk and the outcomes of negative events.

The level and nature of autonomy afforded the home-care client depends in part on the characteristics of the clients, such as their age or their cognitive or physical impairments. There are significant differences in the philosophy and organization of services for the elderly as compared to younger disabled persons (Simon-Rusinowitz and Hofland, 1993). Home health care for older persons tends to emphasize the avoidance of nursing home placement, to employ case management to coordinate services, and to use public regulation of providers to ensure quality of care (Eustis and Fisher, 1992). What is termed "personal assistance" in the support of the nonelderly disabled, however, evolved from the independent-living movement among working-age disabled persons who maintain that they are handicapped primarily by environmental barriers rather than by individual impairments or disabilities (DeJong et al., 1992). Personal assistance encompasses a broader array of services than is usually found in medically oriented programs; it aims to maintain the client's well-being, personal appearance, comfort, safety, and interaction beyond the home. To the extent possible, these services to the disabled nonelderly are user-directed, with consumers supervising their personal care when possible. By comparison, for older clients, despite an emphasis on client autonomy, decisions such as scheduling services and selecting caregivers are made primarily by agency personnel without significant attention to consumer preferences (Hofland and David, 1990).

Clients may be motivated in several ways to control formal and informal caregivers. Clients are, after all, living in their own homes, and they are accustomed to having tasks accomplished in specific ways. They have habits and routines, and they may be supported by family members who share their preferences. Caregivers, for their part, are prompted to provide care and perform tasks not just by the wishes of the client but by their own values, preferences, work styles, and competing demands—and for formal caregivers, by the rules and regulations of their agencies and payors. Harry Moody (1988) argues that a model of decision making that focuses on accommodating and reciprocating autonomies is most appropriate in addressing these multiple interests. By this, he refers to a negotiation among competing needs and preferences. For example, a home-care client may not be able to refuse all formal care and remain at home and engage in behavior that is dangerous and disturbing to other persons in the building. He or she may, instead, negotiate staying at home with unwanted services.

Family issues

Families are intimately involved in home care in several ways: They may be direct providers of informal services, may be involved in care decisions, or may live in the same home as the client and thus have their lives directly affected by formal care providers. While clients and their families might be expected to share values, preferences, and living styles, they often do not; sometimes, in fact, interests and values clash. For example, a family member may value safety and cleanliness more than the client does; the client may be more interested in preserving privacy and avoiding having a stranger "messing with my things." The relationship between formal and informal caregivers is poorly understood, raising concerns that the increased support of formal services may "erode" family caregiving (Hanley et al., 1991). Ethical concerns arise when "needs assessment" for formal services includes consideration of the availability of family caregivers, as is required by law in some U.S. states. This raises the question of whether clients with family members who might provide services should be considered less eligible for home care than those with no such family members.

Conflicts may also arise about what can reasonably be expected from informal caregivers. Most families do not "dump" disabled family members into institutions but rather struggle to maintain elders at home for as long as possible. Surveys of family caregivers document a variety of stress-related illnesses, such as heart disease, stomach ulcers, and sleep disturbance, as well as alcohol or drug problems and marital difficulties (Brody, 1985). Because women are more likely to be caregivers, they carry a disproportionate share of the burden. Many women find themselves "sandwiched" between the care needs of an older parent or grandparent and the needs of a spouse, child, or grandchild. Because the extent of filial obligations is unclear, family caregivers may feel guilt and shame for not "doing enough," and persons needing care may feel either that they have been abandoned or that they are asking too much. Stephen Post (1988) argues that there are limits to familial obligations, and that social policy should do more to support the family in meeting its obligations.

Although we speak of the moral obligations of "the family," it is usually an individual family member, either explicitly or implicitly designated, who bears most of the burden of caregiving. These caregivers are usually women, most of whom have been providing care for more than five years; 35 percent of them are over the age of sixty-five, and 80 percent provide assistance every day of the week (Stone et al., 1987). Women who provide home care to a parent, spouse, or other family member may do so at substantial personal cost, including personal health, lost professional and work opportunities, other personal interests, and other relationships. The interests of and burdens on caregivers should be considered when care plans are developed. If the care plan places heavy demands on an informal caregiver, it may justify constraints on client autonomy. Although "caregiver burden" is a well-recognized concept, Jaber Gubrium (1990) argues that we should hesitate to identify caregivers as "victims," noting that there are important factors that mitigate caregiver stress, including social supports, attitude toward caregiving prior to caregiving crises, personal well-being, a sense of mutuality between the caregiver and persons receiving care, and how prepared caregivers feel for the caregiving role (Archbold et al., 1990; Zarit et al., 1980).

Families differ in many ways that directly influence informal care and use of the formal system. While high levels of diversity exist within ethnic groups, differences among ethnic groups have been noted. Blacks and Native Americans have more widowed and divorced persons of both sexes than do whites, and they are somewhat more likely to live in extended family structures. There is also substantial home care provided by minority family members, attributable both to preference and to other factors, such as poverty, racial bias in the service system, and willingness to tend to young children in return for care (Brown, 1990; Cueller, 1990).

In health care, we tend to focus on the individual client; for most persons, however, there is a family context in which decisions are carried out. This context may constrain choices, but it also provides the individual with support and assistance that would otherwise be unavailable. Moreover, for clients whose capacity to make decisions is impaired, the family usually provides guidance in decision making (Nelson, 1992). This practice is supported in common law, and many states have enacted "family decision" laws that formalize this cus-

tom. The priority list is similar in most states: court-appointed guardians, spouse, adult children, parents, adult siblings, close friends, and extended family (Capron, 1992).

Although the family is usually viewed as a resource and source of support for the client, there are circumstances in which the family may perpetrate abuse and neglect. Protection of clients from abuse is difficult for several reasons. Abuse in the home may go undetected: The client may be unable or reluctant to report abuse due to extreme disability, fear of the caregiver, or shame. The client may be unwilling to act, preferring to stay in an abusive setting because alternatives are unknown, unavailable, or unattractive. Many states require that professional caregivers report suspected abuse of elderly persons via "elder abuse reporting laws," but responding to family failure in care is strategically difficult and ethically complex (Collopy et al., 1990).

The work force

The paid work force for long-term home services consists of both skilled professionals and "unskilled" aides and personal assistants. Workers may enjoy the relationships that develop with patients and families, the opportunity to help others, and some flexibility in hours. However, workers may also face difficult working situations, travel to unsafe or dangerous neighborhoods, homes that are unclean and sometimes hazardous, and close contact with clients and/or family members who may be unpleasant, noncompliant, and even abusive. For unskilled workers such as aides and assistants, these difficulties are compounded by fluctuating schedules and hours, limited benefits, minimal training in necessary skills, and limited opportunities for promotion. The majority of home-care workers, both paid and informal, are women.

The quality of care and the reliability of workers are heavily influenced by the nature of the work, which may be monotonous and unpleasant, and by difficulties in attracting quality workers for minimum wage. In some cities, workers are drawn heavily from immigrant and/or minority populations, sometimes resulting in cultural conflicts and language difficulties between workers and clients. Clients may be uncomfortable having unfamiliar persons in their house, and workers may be treated with suspicion or hostility and confronted with racist comments. Work-force difficulties are increasingly exacerbated by the entry of women (who would otherwise provide informal care) into the paid labor force. Increased competition for workers from other service industries has reduced the availability of home-care workers in some areas. The affordability of some home-care services has been based, in part, on the low wages and benefits paid to unskilled workers, who are mostly women; this fact raises concerns regarding the exploitation of persons unable to find employment elsewhere.

The health-care system

Despite legislation intended to increase home-care services, restrictive eligibility requirements, perverse reimbursement incentives, and gaps in the continuum of care impede the home-care system. Not-for-profit agencies, such as the Visiting Nurse Association, face increasing competition for "attractive" clients, that is, those who are eligible for sufficient reimbursement. Hospitals, responding to reimbursement incentives, discharge patients who require heavier and more complex care. Third-party care "managers" regularly review clients' needs and have expanded paperwork and administrative reporting.

Case management, which has become an integral component of the home-care system, involves assessment of clients, determination of eligibility for public funding or insurance benefits, development of a care plan, and monitoring the quality of services (Quinn, 1993). While case management is viewed by many policymakers as fulfilling necessary gatekeeping and quality assurance functions, many home-care agencies view case management as yet another layer of bureaucracy and an additional expense in the system. Most case management agencies seek to empower clients by assisting them in implementing decisions. In their role as client advocates, case managers may find themselves in conflict with home-care agencies or family members who do not agree that the plan of care is safe, or who argue for more services than the agency can "afford" to provide under spending limits for individual clients or budget caps for groups of clients. The ethical conflicts case managers face as they balance the roles of gate keeping, quality assurance, and client advocacy are just beginning to be explored (Kane, 1991; Wetle, 1992).

Conclusion

Home care involves a complex and growing industry that is intricately intertwined with family caregiving. Most persons would prefer to remain at home, even when their need for assistance is substantial. Many persons would also prefer to give and receive care within a family context. However, the demand for home-care services can overwhelm the ability of family members to provide care in the face of other, competing family and work demands. Emerging changes in the health-care system, including long-term-care insurance and public-health-care reform, may encourage increased reliance on home care for persons with chronic conditions and illnesses. While additional resources for home care would be welcomed, we must be vigilant to the ethical concerns and values, not only of the home-care client but also of family caregivers and the paid work force, particularly women and disadvantaged persons. Efforts should also be made to develop formal services that are culturally appropriate and that meet the special needs of persons from diverse cultures and racial minorities.

TERRIE WETLE

Directly related to this article are the other articles in this entry: CONCEPT AND POLICIES, *and* NURSING HOMES. *Also directly related is the entry* CHRONIC CARE. *For a further discussion of topics mentioned in this article, see the entries* ABUSE, INTERPERSONAL, *article on* ELDER ABUSE; AGING AND THE AGED; AIDS; DEATH AND DYING: EUTHANASIA AND SUSTAINING LIFE; DISABILITY, *article on* HEALTH CARE AND PHYSICAL DISABILITY; FAMILY; HEALTH-CARE FINANCING; HOSPICE AND END-OF-LIFE CARE; *and* WOMEN. *For a discussion of related ideas, see the entries* AUTONOMY; PATERNALISM; RACE AND RACISM; RISK; *and* TRUST. *Other relevant material may be found under the entries* ALLIED HEALTH PROFESSIONS; *and* MENTALLY DISABLED AND MENTALLY ILL PERSONS.

Bibliography

ARCHBOLD, PATRICIA G.; STEWART, BARBARA J.; GREENLICK, MERWYN R.; and HARVATH, TERESA. 1990. "Mutuality and Preparedness as Predictors of Caregiver Role Strain." *Research in Nursing and Health* 13, no. 6:375–384.

BENJAMIN, A. E. 1993. "An Historical Perspective on Home Care Policy." *Milbank Quarterly* 71, no. 1:129–166.

BRODY, ELAINE M. 1985. "Parent Care as a Normative Family Stress." *Gerontologist* 25, no. 1:19–29.

BROWN, DIANE ROBINSON. 1990. "The Black Elderly: Implications for the Family." In *Minority Aging: Essential Curricula Content for Selected Health and Allied Health Professions*, pp. 275–295. Edited by Mary S. Harper. Rockville, Md.: U.S. Department of Health and Human Services.

BURBRIDGE, LYNN C. 1993. "The Labor Market for Home Care Workers: Demand, Supply, and Institutional Barriers." *Gerontologist* 33, no. 1:41–46.

CAPRON, ALEXANDER MORGAN. 1992. "Where Is the Sure Interpreter?" *Hastings Center Report* 22, no. 4:26–27.

COLLOPY, BART; DUBLER, NANCY; and ZUCKERMAN, CONNIE. 1990. "The Ethics of Home Care: Autonomy and Accommodation." *Hastings Center Report* 20, no. 2 (suppl.): 1–16.

CUELLAR, JOSE B. 1990. "Hispanic American Aging: Geriatric Education Curriculum Development for Selected Health Professionals." In *Minority Aging: Essential Curricula Content for Selected Health and Allied Health Professions*, pp.

365–413. Edited by Mary S. Harper. Rockville, Md.: U.S. Department of Health and Human Services.

DeJong, Gerben; Batavia, Andrew I.; and McKnew, Louise B. 1992. "The Independent Living Model of Personal Assistance in National Long-Term Care Policy." *Generations* 16, no. 1:89–95.

Detzel, Joyce, and Kapp, Marshall. 1992. "Developing Alternatives to Plenary Guardianship: Overcoming Fear of Legal Liability." *Gerontologist* 32, no. 2:A131–A132.

Estes, Carroll L., and Binney, Elizabeth A. 1989. "The Biomedicalization of Aging: Dangers and Dilemmas." *Gerontologist* 29, no. 5:587–596.

Eustis, Nancy N., and Fischer, Lucy R. 1992. "Common Needs, Different Solutions? Younger and Older Homecare Clients." *Generations* 16, no. 1:17–22.

Gubrium, Jaber F. 1990. *The Mosaic of Care: Frail Elderly and Their Families in the Real World.* New York: Springer.

Hanley, Raymond J.; Wiener, Joshua M.; and Harris, Katherine M. 1991. "Will Paid Home Care Erode Informal Support?" *Journal of Health Politics, Policy and Law* 16, no. 3:507–521.

Hofland, Brian F., and David, Debra. 1990. "Autonomy and Long-Term Care Practice: Introduction." *Generations* 14 (suppl.):3–9.

Kane, Rosalie A. 1991. "Case Management in Long Term Care: It Can Be As Ethical and Efficacious As We Want It to Be." In *Ethics and Care Management: A Delicate Balance; Conference Proceedings 1989,* pp. 1–6. Philadelphia: Pennsylvania Care Management Institute.

Koff, Theodore H. 1988. *New Approaches to Health Care for an Aging Population.* San Francisco: Jossey-Bass.

Moody, Harry R. 1988. "From Informed Consent to Negotiated Consent." *Gerontologist* 28 (June, suppl.):64–70.

Nelson, James Lindemann. 1992. "Taking Families Seriously." *Hastings Center Report* 22, no. 4:6–12.

Post, Stephen. 1988. "An Ethical Perspective on Caregiving in the Family." *Journal of Medical Humanities and Bioethics* 9, no. 1:6–16.

Quinn, Joan. 1993. *Successful Case Management in Long-Term Care.* New York: Springer.

Reilly, Thomas W.; Clauser, Steven B.; and Baugh, David K. 1990. "Trends in Medicaid Payments and Utilization." *Health Care Financing Review* 11 (suppl.):15–33.

Rivlin, Alice M., and Wiener, Joshua M. 1988. *Caring for the Disabled Elderly: Who Will Pay?* Washington, D.C.: Brookings Institution.

Simon-Rusinowitz, Lori, and Hofland, Brian F. 1993. "Adopting a Disability Approach to Home Care Services for Older Adults." *Gerontologist* 33, no. 2:159–167.

Stone, Robyn; Cafferata, Gail L.; and Sangl, Judith. 1987. "Caregivers of the Frail Elderly: A National Profile." *Gerontologist* 27, no. 5:616–626.

Wetle, Terrie. 1992. "A Taxonomy of Ethical Issues in Case Management of the Frail Older Person." *Journal of Case Management* 1, no. 3:71–75.

Wieland, Darryl; Ferrell, Bruce A.; and Rubenstein, Laurence Z. 1991. "Geriatric Home Health Care: Conceptual and Demographic Considerations." *Clinics in Geriatric Medicine* 7, no. 4:645–664.

Young, Ann; Pignatello, Catherine H.; and Taylor, Marietta B. 1988. "Who's the Boss? Ethical Conflicts in Home Care." *Health Progress* 69, no. 11:59–62.

Zarit, Steven H.; Reever, Karen E.; and Bach-Peterson, Judy. 1980. "Relatives of the Impaired Elderly: Correlates of Feeling of Burden." *Gerontologist* 20, no. 6:649–655.

LOVE

Love is a disposition of the self that manifests in solicitude for the welfare of the other, and usually a delight in his or her presence. It is a curbing of the self-centered tendency and a transfer of interests to another for his or her own sake, on the basis of the other's positive properties or existence per se.

Love is not always distinguished from care, but such a distinction may be argued for. To care is to be neither indifferent nor unconcerned; something does matter and therefore cannot be treated apathetically (Ruddick, 1990; Gilligan, 1982). To love is to champion the other's interests with the anxiety of care deepened and intensified. Love does not necessarily require radical self-denial, but it may. Its controlling motive must always be the good of others, so that unselfishness replaces selfishness.

This article considers the foundational debates about love, and relevant issues in bioethics.

Foundational debates

A first debate distinguishes love based on some perceived positive attribute in the other from love based on value bestowed by the lover. The former love is reason dependent, that is, X can provide property-based reasons for loving Y. The attractive properties of the object account for the presence of love and determine its longevity (Soble, 1990). Critics of a strictly property-based love believe that it leaves love too insecure, since the properties for which X loves Y may disappear, or X may no longer perceive them as attractive. They therefore introduce a love of bestowal, or a nonappraising love. While a wholly nonappraisive love may be foreign to human nature, any love worthy of the word requires a security or commitment that goes beyond strictly appraisive categories (Singer, 1987).

A closely related debate concerns whether love is an acquisitive desire seeking the agent's good or a benevolent one seeking the other's good (Hazo, 1967). Acquisitive tendencies include desires for food, drink, possessions, and merely instrumental relations with others, such as, sexual relations without care or commitment. Some contend that strictly acquisitive love is not really love at all, because it implies indifference to the other's welfare except as a means to self-gratification, that is, as a means of acquiring a good for the self, with benevolence never a controlling motive. For love to be genuinely present, assisting and protecting the other must be the controlling motive. Love and indifference to the other's good are incompatible. Good for the self, while not controlling, can acceptably remain as a motive, for instance, personal satisfaction in caring, moral development, mutuality (as in friendship), gratification, or social recognition. Thus did the eighteenth-century British moralists such as Francis Hutcheson and Joseph Butler insist that benevolence is perfectly coincident with self-love. The property-based love considered above can be benevolent, as in the compassion of friendship.

A third debate concerns the desire for reciprocity. Giving and receiving love is characteristic of friendship, marriage, and other forms of companionate love. Søren Kierkegaard (1962), in order to test the selflessness of love's motivation, rejected these spheres of reciprocity, and stated that the highest form of love is love for the dead, since surely they cannot reciprocate. In contrast with Kierkegaard, mutuality of love, even if asymmetrical, can be viewed as essential for reliable expectations regarding the conduct of the others, as necessary for predictable relationships, and as reinforcing benevolence (Becker, 1986). Insofar as love involves giving as well as receiving, "Love lives not only from the ecstasy of fulfillment, but from a loyalty not yet fulfilled" (Daniel Day Williams, 1968, p. 14). Even love for the stranger, while it should not require a response in kind, should never refuse such response (Toner, 1968). Yet love can exist unrequited.

A fourth debate concerns the order of love (*ordo caritatis*), that is, the balance of love for friends and family (special relations) with love for the stranger. With respect to Christian ethics, for example, while Augustine could easily accept special relations in his order of love, "The agapic normative tradition represented by Outka and exemplified in the extreme by Kierkegaard is very uneasy about special relations" (Purvis, 1991, p. 19). Theological debate juxtaposes two opposing approaches: In the first, particular and special relations "function as a sign of and call toward a love more universal in scope"; In the second, we begin with "universal love—true charity—and justify particular loves, if at all, on the basis of Christian love in the fullest sense" (Meilaender, 1987, p. 22).

Bernard Williams (1973) has argued against the impartiality of utilitarianism, for it creates a rift between moral obligations and heartfelt personal commitments. He thinks this rift violates the "integrity" of the moral agent. In a number of religious and philosophical traditions, particular and exclusive forms of love are haunted by the requirement of radical universal love. But in re-

cent decades, "special relations" and reciprocities have increasingly been recognized in philosophical and religious ethics as having moral value. No moral calculus indicates the proper balance between love for those near and dear, and love for strangers. However, love for humanity should never be eclipsed by proximate ties.

Finally, there is debate about the extent to which love requires self-denial. Clearly love requires the abrogation of selfishness, but it is a mistake to confuse the valid ideal of unselfishness with selflessness, its invalid exaggeration (Saiving, 1979). Selflessness violates the reasonably reciprocal structures of most social existence, and obscures the extent to which self-concern or care for the self is necessary for love of the other to be sustained in commitment. Moreover, selflessness is questionable because it invites exploitation of the moral agent and fails to correct the other's harmful behavior (Outka, 1972). Feminism, psychology, philosophy, and theology increasingly converge on this point. Analysis of intermediate norms between self-preference and radical self-denial, such as parity, other-preference, and self-subordination is imperative.

Love and bioethics

Love for humanity. While some have suggested that love for humanity is an unrealistic ideal, or even a way of obscuring a failure to love those who are near (Camus, 1991), it remains a moral ideal in most traditions. Insofar as the moral idealism of universal love is absent from society, it may be true that love is relegated to the private sphere due to masculine thinking that associates public life with greatness in the form of self-assertion (Bologh, 1990). Love for humanity can be property based if grounded in some universal aspect of persons, such as the Stoic notion of reason or the Judaeo-Christian concept of the self as being in the image of God. It can also be interpreted as a love of bestowal, especially when human capacities dim.

Beginning with the Hellenistic age, Greek antiquity developed the norm of *philanthropia*, referring to a generous hospitality even to the stranger. One Hippocratic precept is "Where there is love of humanity [*philanthropia*], there is love of medical science." Influenced by the demands of Stoic ethics, the physician is to assist "even aliens who lack resources" (Temkin, 1991, p. 32). The ideal of love for humanity is found among the Stoics, Cynics, Pythagoreans, Hellenized Jews, and early Christian theologians, where *philanthropia* was often used interchangeably with *agape,* the New Testament Greek word for love of humanity (Ferguson, 1959). There is debate over the extent to which the Hippocratic notion of *philanthropia* is indebted to early Eastern Christianity, and vice versa.

It is not clear whether the commandment in Leviticus to "Love your neighbor as yourself" originally applied to Jews only or to non-Jews as well (Lev. 19:18). However, in medieval Judaism it was certainly applied to the non-Jew, as is clear in the writings of the rabbi-physician Moses Maimonides. "Love thy neighbor as thyself" is central to Jewish medical ethics (Green, 1982). In Christianity, building on Judaism, the practice of medicine was profoundly influenced by the story of the Good Samaritan, who assisted a wounded stranger by the roadside (Luke 10:33–34). After three centuries of persecution, Christians opened hospitals and made care of the sick an expression of love. Christians were unusually heroic in the leprosarium. It is argued that Christianity gave rise to a decisive change in attitude toward the sick, who now even assumed what may be described as a preferential position (Sigerist, 1943). Mother Teresa, awarded the Nobel Peace Prize in 1979, has devoted her exemplary life to love for the homeless and sick strangers on the streets of Calcutta. It has been suggested that a postmodern moral philosophy could gain much through a recovery of the saintly examples of "compassion, generosity, and self-sacrifice" (Wyschogrod, 1990). The story of the Good Samaritan continues to spur voluntary caring in American culture (Wuthnow, 1991).

The story of the Good Samaritan and the requirement that all Christians assist the sick and those in need disinterestedly (Matt. 25:35–46) deeply shaped Western medical culture. A classic expression of love ethics is that of the seventeenth-century physician Sir Thomas Browne, for whom the foundation of all medical virtue "is love for God, for whom we love our neighbor. For this, I think, is charity, to love God for Himself and our neighbor for God" (Browne, 1966, p. 98). Religious women in the United States, from the Sisters of Charity to the Sisters of Mercy, nursed the sick and opened numerous hospitals. During the Civil War and various nineteenth-century epidemics, the actions of these nurses won the respect of American society. Lutheran deaconesses and Episcopalian sisters also engaged in nursing ministry (Stepsis and Liptak, 1989). A contemporary physician writes that the virtue of charity, that is, "benevolent self-effacement," shapes "the whole of medical morals" (Pellegrino, 1989).

An ethics of love for humanity implies that health-care professions in the past were driven by moral idealism at least as much as by self-interest. Universal love generally does not require radical self-denial, nor an abandonment of familial and other proximate forms of love, although on some occasions it may. The health-care professional has a duty to be self-concerned, even as a necessary condition for being able to serve others. Since no exactness is possible in determining the right symmetry among self-love, neighbor love, and love for family and friends, considerable latitude must be allowed for individual conscience. A simple assertion of physi-

cian self-effacement without attention to some general symmetry and competing obligations is inadequate.

Universal love may imply justice according to need (Childress, 1985). A summary of the contemporary Protestant literature concludes that love requires "at least a basic provision of medical care" (Bouma et al., 1989, p. 162). Gene Outka (1974) contends that universal love overlaps with theories of justice according to need. Love may require that basic human needs be met, regardless of the recipient's productivity, merit, or contribution to society as measured by a utilitarian calculus. Human beings as such, regardless of their resources and achievements, deserve adequate health care to remove them as much as is possible from suffering.

Preferential love. One form of preferential love is romantic love. This includes an intense longing for union with the other, profound physiological arousal, aesthetic attraction, desire for reciprocity, degrees of benevolence, and some idealization of the beloved. There is a general condemnation of romantic love between physicians and patients. Leon Kass, drawing on the notion of purity in the Hippocratic oath and tradition, believes that the role of the physician is antithetical to that of the sensual lover, that "medical and erotic gazing" must be kept separate lest the patient be manipulated and abused in the midst of bodily exposure and vulnerability (1985). The weight of medical tradition supports this view, as does ethical concern with respect for patients. The American Medical Association concurs: "Sexual or romantic interactions between physicians and patients detract from the goals of the physician–patient relationship, may obscure the physician's objective judgment concerning the patient's health care, and ultimately may be detrimental to the patient's well-being" (1992, p. 40).

Kant noted that in romantic love and sexual relations, the "appetite for another human being" can be harmful, for through sexual appetite one human being often plunges another into "the depths of misery," casting him or her aside "as one casts away a lemon which has been sucked dry" (1963, p. 163). Similarly, feminists have long regarded romantic love with moral suspicion. At the end of the eighteenth century, Mary Wollstonecraft wrote that girls are inculcated with the coercive assumption that their happiness and fulfillment depend on romantic love, love that is inevitably fleeting and that diverts women's attention from education and other, more lasting goods. After a man falls out of love, a woman has little to depend on professionally, and no self-reliance (Wollstonecraft, 1975). Wollstonecraft described preoccupation with delicacy and beautification as slavishness. Germaine Greer writes in the tradition of Wollstonecraft: "Love, love, love—all the wretched cant of it, masking egotism, lust, masochism, fantasy under a mythology of sentimental postures . . ." (1971,

p. 165). Psychoanalyst Karen Horney (1934) writes of the obsession with romantic love that hinders women's self-realization in work and achievement, resulting in an emptiness that increases with age. Feminist literary critics have condemned fairy tales that present figures, such as Sleeping Beauty, fulfilled through the romantic kiss of a prince.

A more sympathetic interpretation is that romantic love has allowed women to become the objects of devotion, thus providing them with "an inherent value that had not existed in the ancient world," as well as a degree of equality and a freedom to love the man of choice (Singer, 1987, p. 12). Romantic love can be viewed positively as a context for compassion and benevolence, and as a precursor to what psychologists call companionate love. Elaine Hatfield maintains that romantic love often evolves into companionate love, "the affection we feel for those with whom our lives are deeply entwined" (1988, p. 205). Irving Singer holds that the romantic "falling in love" can lead to the more stable "being in love," followed by companionate or marital love. Psychiatrists have interpreted romantic love both negatively, as delusional overvaluation and the result of the self's inadequacies, and positively, as a source of meaning in life (Frankl, 1984). Willard Gaylin (1986) and others who find such meaning are highly critical of any theorists who justify sex without love, or who reduce sex to discussions of technique.

Another form of preferential love is companionate love. It is associated in the psychological literature with enjoyment, acceptance, commitment, trust, respect, mutual assistance, confiding, understanding, and spontaneity. A study of couples married fifteen years or more indicates that the most common explanation of longevity is "My spouse is my best friend" (Davis, 1985). The word "companion" derives from the Latin ("with bread"), referring to the fellowship between those who share a meal. Companionate love can include marital love, friendship, and the affection between those bound together by common experiences. It differs from universal love because it is preferential and directed only toward those who are known. In moral philosophy the importance of friendship has been rediscovered. Friendship has been interpreted as a locus for the expression of sympathy, compassion, and a willingness to sacrifice that goes beyond ordinary expectations (Blum, 1980).

American medical ethics since the 1970s has tended to devalue companionate love as a model for the physician–patient relationship. The more adversarial approach may be partly explained by the beginnings of contemporary medical ethics in concern over abusive human experimentation (Rothman, 1991). If that is true, American medical ethics has roots in the image of physicians at their worst, which leads directly to the assumption that patients must be protected from their doctors. In many cases patients need protection, especially from those who might want to justify unjustifiable coercion with an appeal to "friendly" motives.

The modern health-care system treats the patient anonymously, and allows little opportunity for the trust of friendships to develop. But more centrally, the friendship model is suspect on the grounds that it inherently threatens patient autonomy, that is, has paternalistic tendencies (Veatch, 1985). The friendship model is judged "psychologically oppressive," and the satisfaction of even authentic patient desire for friendship is wrong because "its satisfaction would diminish autonomy" (Illingworth, 1988).

In contrast with many American medical ethicists, the Spanish historian of medicine and ethics Pedro Laín Entralgo highlights the central importance of friendship for the physician–patient relationship: "Rather than a provision of technical help, rather than diagnosis and therapy, the relation between doctor and patient is—or ought to be—friendship, *philia*. For the ancient Greeks, this *philia* was the basis of the relationship" (1969, p. 17). Laín Entralgo suggests that *philia*, which has its roots in benevolence, is distinct from *eros*, with origins in visual pleasure: The art of hearing characterizes friendship, while sight is appropriate for *eros*. His conclusion is that "medical *philia*," characterized by attentive hearing and communication, should continue to define the physician–patient relationship. James F. Drane provides an American model of "medical friendship" as follows: "The affective dimension of the doctor/patient relationship has all the generic notes of an ordinary friendship: There is pleasure in one another's company, confidences are shared, and there is an exchange of benefits" (1988, p. 85). Care, confidentiality, beneficence, honesty, respect, and forgiveness have been traditionally understood as aspects of friendship.

Parental love.   The traditional physician–patient relationship has been widely condemned as paternalistic—or, to use a nonsexist word, parentalistic. Parental love is subject to a series of criticisms. As a general rule, physicians have over the centuries assumed an authoritarian parental role over patients, whose submission is akin to filial piety. Much of Enlightenment Anglo-American political thought emerged from John Locke's necessary refutation of Sir Robert Filmer's patriarchalism, that is, of fatherhood writ large so as to justify the absolute power of kings. Daughters and daughters-in-law have been manipulated by some parents into coerced roles as filial caregivers. The broad arguments against parental love include the temptation to play savior, wielding inordinate power to "protect" others, denying initiative and autonomy, and establishing unhealthy dependencies.

Outside of bioethics, the ideal of parental love is undergoing a recovery. Theologian Sally McFague warns against the potential oppression of the parental metaphor but adds, "Nevertheless, in spite of these qualifications, the maternal metaphor is so powerful and so right for our time that we *should* use it" (1989, p. 139). In an age of nuclear and ecological threat, McFague claims that a metaphor emphasizing nurture and "life as a gift" is necessary, for parental love "nurtures what it has brought into existence, and wants it to grow and be fulfilled." She holds that the ethical task is to "universalize parenthood." Paul Ramsey saw in parental love a divine likeness: "We procreate new beings like ourselves in the midst of our love for one another, and in this there is a trace of the original mystery by which God created the world . . ." (1970, p. 38). Nel Noddings views parental affection as the wellspring of all human caring and moral behavior. "The caring attitude that lies at the heart of all ethical behavior is universal," she argues. Noddings does not think that the starting point for ethics should be an analysis of moral judgment and moral reasoning but, rather, "our earliest memories of being cared for" (1984, p. 5). It is a well-established psychological fact that children who are uncared for will themselves never be able to care.

But any ethic of parental love must attend deeply to the respect for freedom and individuality that love requires. Outka includes respect for freedom as one of the three purposes of love (1972). James F. Childress stresses that a love ethic has the tendency to become paternalistic, and that more attention in theological ethics should be given to this problem (1982). Concern with respect for freedom is imperative.

Bioethics needs to reflect systematically on the meaning and value of parental love. In order to further interpret such phenomena as surrogate mothering, reproductive technologies, adoption, infanticide, and the fate of congenitally imperiled newborns, the field of biomedical ethics might gain from an in-depth analysis of parental love with respect to its natural or cultural foundations, and the extent to which such love can be expected to shoulder sometimes onerous burdens. Numerous issues in human reproduction finally must be related to the meaning of parenthood and its relationship to human nature. Raymond M. Herbenick (1975), for example, argues that infertile couples have a right to experience parenthood and parental love, so that abortion should be legally proscribed, in order to procure infants for adoption. Many would find such a suggestion highly oppressive of women.

STEPHEN G. POST

Directly related to this entry are the entries CARE; *and* PROFESSIONAL–PATIENT RELATIONSHIP. *For a further discussion of topics mentioned in this entry, see the entries* FAMILY; FEMINISM; FRIENDSHIP; MARRIAGE AND OTHER DOMESTIC PARTNERSHIPS; PASTORAL CARE; *and* VIRTUE AND CHARACTER. *This entry will find application in the entries* HOSPICE AND END-OF-LIFE CARE; SEXUAL ETHICS; *and* SEXUAL ETHICS AND PROFESSIONAL STANDARDS. *For a discussion of related ideas, see the entries* AUTONOMY; BENEFICENCE; COMPASSION; EMOTIONS; FREEDOM AND COERCION; JUSTICE; METAPHOR AND ANALOGY; PAIN AND SUFFERING; PATERNALISM; TRUST; *and* UTILITY.

Bibliography

AMERICAN MEDICAL ASSOCIATION. COUNCIL ON ETHICAL AND JUDICIAL AFFAIRS. 1992. *Code of Medical Ethics: Current Opinions.* Chicago: American Medical Association.

BECKER, LAWRENCE C. 1986. *Reciprocity.* London: Routledge & Kegan Paul.

BLUM, LAWRENCE A. 1980. *Friendship, Altruism, and Morality.* London: Routledge & Kegan Paul.

BOLOGH, ROSLYN W. 1990. *Love or Greatness: Max Weber and Masculine Thinking—A Feminist Inquiry.* London: Unwin Hyman.

BOUMA, HESSEL; DIEKEMA, DOUGLAS; LANGERAK, EDWARD; ROTTMAN, THEODORE; and VERHEY, ALLEN. 1989. *Christian Faith, Health, and Medical Practice.* Grand Rapids, Mich.: William B. Eerdmans.

BROWNE, SIR THOMAS. 1966. [1642]. *Religio medici.* Edited by Frank L. Huntley. New York: Appleton-Century-Crofts.

CAMUS, ALBERT. 1991. [1957]. *The Fall.* Translated by Justin O'Brien. New York: Vintage Books.

CHILDRESS, JAMES F. 1982. *Who Should Decide? Paternalism in Health Care.* New York: Oxford University Press.

———. 1985. "Love and Justice in Christian Biomedical Ethics." In *Theology and Bioethics: Exploring the Foundations and Frontiers,* pp. 225–243. Edited by Earl E. Shelp. Dordrecht, Netherlands: E. D. Reidel.

DAVIS, KEITH E. 1985. "Near and Dear: Friendship and Love Compared." *Psychology Today* 19, no. 6:22–28.

DRANE, JAMES F. 1988. *Becoming a Good Doctor: The Place of Virtue and Character in Medical Ethics.* Kansas City, Mo.: Sheed and Ward.

FERGUSON, JOHN. 1959. *Moral Values in the Ancient World.* New York: Barnes and Noble.

FRANKL, VIKTOR E. 1984. *Man's Search for Meaning: An Introduction to Logotherapy.* Rev. ed. New York: Washington Square Press. First published in 1946.

GAYLIN, WILLARD. 1986. *Rediscovering Love.* New York: Penguin.

GILLIGAN, CAROL. 1982. *In a Different Voice: Psychological Theory and Women's Development.* Cambridge, Mass.: Harvard University Press.

GREEN, RONALD M. 1982. "Jewish Ethics and Beneficence." In *Beneficence and Health Care,* pp. 109–125. Edited by Earl E. Shelp. Dordrecht, Netherlands: E. D. Reidel.

GREER, GERMAINE. 1971. *The Female Eunuch.* New York: McGraw-Hill.

HATFIELD, ELAINE. 1988. "Passionate and Companionate Love." In *The Psychology of Love,* pp. 191–217. Edited by

Robert J. Sternberg and Michael L. Barnes. New Haven, Conn.: Yale University Press.

HAZO, ROBERT. 1967. *The Idea of Love.* New York: Praeger.

HERBENICK, RAYMOND M. 1975. "Remarks on Abortion, Abandonment, and Adoption Opportunities." *Philosophy & Public Affairs* 5, no. 1:98–104.

HORNEY, KAREN. 1934. "The Overvaluation of Love: A Study of a Common Present-Day Type." *Psychoanalytic Quarterly* 3:605–638.

ILLINGWORTH, PATRICIA M. L. 1988. "The Friendship Model of Physician/Patient Relationship and Patient Autonomy." *Bioethics* 2, no. 1:22–36.

KANT, IMMANUEL. 1963. [1780]. "Duties Toward the Body in Respect of Sexual Impulse." In *Lectures on Ethics,* pp. 162–168. Translated by Louis Infield. Indianapolis: Hackett.

KASS, LEON. 1985. *Toward a More Natural Science: Biology and Human Affairs.* New York: Free Press.

KIERKEGAARD, SØREN. 1962. [1857]. *Works of Love.* Translated by Howard Hong and Edna Hong. New York: Harper & Row.

LAÍN ENTRALGO, PEDRO. 1969. *Doctor and Patient.* Translated by Francis Partridge. New York: McGraw-Hill.

McFAGUE, SALLY. 1989. "Mother God." In *Motherhood: Experience, Institution, Theology,* pp. 138–143. Edited by Anne Carr and Elisabeth Schussler Fiorenza. Edinburgh: T. and T. Clark.

MEILAENDER, GILBERT. 1987. *The Limits of Love: Some Theological Explorations.* University Park: Pennsylvania State University Press.

NODDINGS, NEL. 1984. *Caring: A Feminist Approach to Ethics and Moral Education.* Berkeley: University of California Press.

OUTKA, GENE. 1972. *Agape: An Ethical Analysis.* New Haven, Conn.: Yale University Press.

———. 1974. "Social Justice and Equal Access." *Journal of Religious Ethics* 2:11–32.

PELLEGRINO, EDMUND D. 1989. "*Agape* and Ethics: Some Reflections on Medical Morals from a Catholic Christian Perspective." In *Catholic Perspectives on Medical Morals: Foundational Issues,* pp. 277–300. Edited by Edmund Pellegrino et al. Dordrecht, Netherlands: Kluwer.

PURVIS, SALLY B. 1991. "Mothers, Neighbors, and Strangers: Another Look at Agape." *Journal of Feminist Studies in Religion* 7, no. 1:19–34.

RAMSEY, PAUL. 1970. *The Patient as Person: Explorations in Medical Ethics.* New Haven, Conn.: Yale University Press.

ROTHMAN, DAVID J. 1991. *Strangers at the Bedside: A History of How Law and Bioethics Transformed Medical Decision Making.* New York: Basic Books.

RUDDICK, SARA. 1990. *Maternal Thinking: Toward a Politics of Peace.* New York: Ballantine Books.

SAIVING, VALERIE. 1979. "The Human Situation: A Feminine View." In *Womanspirit Rising: A Feminist Reader in Religion,* pp. 25–42. Edited by Carol Christ and Judith Plaskow. New York: Harper & Row.

SIGERIST, HENRY. 1943. *Civilization and Disease.* Ithaca, N.Y.: Cornell University Press.

SINGER, IRVING. 1987. *The Nature of Love: The Modern World.* Chicago: University of Chicago Press.

SOBLE, ALAN. 1990. *The Structure of Love.* New Haven, Conn.: Yale University Press.

STEPSIS, URSULA, and LIPTAK, DOLORES, eds. 1989. *Pioneer Healers: The History of Women Religious in American Health Care.* New York: Crossroad.

TEMKIN, OWSEI. 1991. *Hippocrates in a World of Pagans and Christians.* Baltimore: Johns Hopkins University Press.

TONER, JULES. 1968. *The Experience of Love.* Washington, D.C.: Corpus Books.

VEATCH, ROBERT. 1983. "The Physician as Stranger: The Ethics of the Anonymous Patient-Physician Relationship." In *The Clinical Encounter: The Moral Fabric of the Patient-Physician Relationship,* pp. 187–207. Edited by Earle Shelp. Dordrecht, Netherlands: E. D. Reidel.

WILLIAMS, BERNARD. 1973. "A Critique of Utilitarianism." In *Utilitarianism: For and Against,* pp. 77–150. Edited by J. J. C. Smart and Bernard Williams. Cambridge: At the University Press.

WILLIAMS, DANIEL DAY. 1968. *The Spirit and the Forms of Love.* New York: Harper & Row.

WOLLSTONECRAFT, MARY GODWIN. 1975. [1792]. *A Vindication of the Rights of Woman.* New York: W. W. Norton.

WUTHNOW, ROBERT. 1991. *Acts of Compassion: Caring for Others and Helping Ourselves.* Princeton, N.J.: Princeton University Press.

WYSCHOGROD, EDITH. 1990. *Saints and Postmodernism: Revisioning Moral Philosophy.* Chicago: University of Chicago Press.

LOYALTY AND FIDELITY

See FIDELITY AND LOYALTY.

LUXEMBOURG

See MEDICAL ETHICS, HISTORY OF, *section on* EUROPE, *subsection on* CONTEMPORARY PERIOD, *article on* THE BENELUX COUNTRIES.

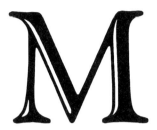

MALAYSIA

See MEDICAL ETHICS, HISTORY OF, *section on* SOUTH AND EAST ASIA, *article on* SOUTHEAST ASIAN COUNTRIES.

MALPRACTICE

See MEDICAL MALPRACTICE. *See also* LICENSING, DISCIPLINE, AND REGULATION IN THE HEALTH PROFESSIONS.

MARRIAGE AND OTHER DOMESTIC PARTNERSHIPS

Marriage is the legally recognized union of a man and woman as husband and wife. It endures until terminated by annulment, divorce, or the death of either spouse. As an institution, marriage provides a social structure for sexual relations, procreation, and the sharing of familial property. Marriage creates particular moral rights and duties between partners; some religious groups believe that marriage has spiritual significance. Domestic partnerships are other types of sexual relationships that endure over a period of time, include a shared domestic life, and involve some public acknowledgment by the partners of that shared life. Domestic partnerships may be heterosexual or homosexual.

This entry focuses on the history of moral ideas concerning marriage and domestic partnerships in Western civilization. Throughout much of Western history these influential ideas were articulated primarily by educated males. Thus, most statements concerning the role of wife, concubine, or lesbian partner describe that role from the male perspective. Moreover, this entry concentrates on normative views; the life experience of married couples and domestic partners is a different matter. Finally, these ideas often reflect the perspective of the educated, upper classes; the historical reality for the majority of couples who were poor may have differed from these ideal statements.

Over time the primary moral meanings of marriage have changed, but ideals whose roots are in earlier periods of history still influence our thinking and practice today. Marriage and domestic partnerships are crucial human relationships. Assumptions about and structures surrounding both marriage and domestic partnerships have important bioethical implications for matters such as reproductive issues, domestic violence, proxy decision making, and health-care access.

The moral end in marriage

According to both Plato and Aristotle the main purpose of marriage, in the upper classes, was the begetting of the male children who would become good citizens for the polis, or Greek city-state. Aristotle advised that marriages should be arranged so that a couple's prime reproductive years coincided, because high-quality offspring were the main good of marriage. Thus, in the *Politics* he suggested the marriage of a man about thirty-seven years old to a woman about eighteen years old.

Among the ancient Hebrews, the patriarchal family was the root of communal stability and well-being. Marriage channeled sexuality for the sake of the extended family and the people of Israel. Procreation was a chief good of marriage, especially the birth of male heirs. A wife's sexuality and fertility were family assets belonging exclusively to her husband. Polygyny and concubinage were permitted for wealthy, powerful males.

In rabbinic and later Judaism, men and women were expected to marry and bear children who would perpetuate the covenant. Procreation is a *mitzvah*, or a religious obligation, for the husband. The assumption is that his wife will cooperate, but procreation is not a moral command for her. Marriage also allows Jewish men and women to handle sexual desire in a stable, orderly way.

Augustine (354–430 C.E.) determined the view of Christianity for many centuries when he declared that the ends of Christian marriage were procreation, sexual fidelity, and *sacramentum*, marriage's function as a sign of the enduring love between Christ and the church. A Christian marriage must be indissoluble to function as *sacramentum*.

After the Roman Empire disintegrated, Christian leaders struggled to control marriage and its termination in order to promote marital indissolubility. Converts to Christianity from Germanic tribes were accustomed to concubinage and to divorce initiated by either the husband or the wife. It was centuries before church officials gained social control over the formation and annulment of marriages (Glendon, 1989).

During the Middle Ages, Christian theologians emphasized the voluntary exchange of marriage vows by the partners. The church refused to recognize marriage based on a betrothal promise exchanged by families. Thus, the church protected the free choice of the spouses in a social context in which marriage for the landed classes was a crucial economic and, at times, political decision of the family.

The Protestant theologians who led the Reformation accepted the traditional ends of Christian marriage: conception of children and avoidance of sexual sins. However, leaders of the Anglican church articulated explicitly a third purpose for marriage: mutual support, solace, and companionship. The Puritans recognized, as a primary good, the love that developed between spouses within marriage. Some Puritans advised that a child be allowed to refuse a potential partner selected by the parents, if the child felt that it would be impossible to learn to love the spouse *after marriage*.

The development and distribution of reliable means of birth control and a secular birth-control movement challenged the centrality of procreation as a basic good of marriage. In the twentieth century, mainstream Protestant churches decided that it was morally acceptable for spouses to limit procreation for the good of the family while remaining sexually active. Even the Roman Catholic magisterium explicitly acknowledged the moral worth of conjugal relations as a unique expression of love and mutual self-giving between spouses, as well as a means of procreation. By the late twentieth century, loving sexual intimacy was highly valued in its own right, and procreation was no longer viewed by many as the principal moral purpose for marriage. Thus, a serious question arose: "Is the moral distinction between marriage and other committed, sexually intimate relationships still valid, if marriages are no longer understood primarily as unions for the purpose of procreation?"

Celibacy and the value of Christian marriage

Throughout early and medieval Christian history, the value of marriage was relativized by admiration for religiously committed celibacy. The apostle Paul favored celibacy as a means to focus one's entire energies on the impending Kingdom of God. Still, Paul accepted marriage for most Christians as a necessary alternative to sinful sexual behaviors (1 Cor. 7:8–9, 29–35). Paul viewed celibacy as a charism granted by God only to some (Countryman, 1988).

From the second through the fourth centuries C.E., the Mediterranean world turned toward asceticism. Marriage with its sexual passion and its reproduction of corruptible bodies needed religious justification. The Christian church fathers were increasingly attracted by religious virginity, a vow by one not yet sexually experienced to forgo all sexual activity in order to devote herself or himself to God's service. Still, these Christian thinkers affirmed the fundamental goodness of marriage and procreation as aspects of God's good creation.

In Western Christianity by the fourth century, a lengthy ethical controversy arose over the widespread practices of clerical marriage and concubinage. During the eleventh and twelfth centuries, church reformers made a major effort to require clerical celibacy, culminating with the First Lateran Council's decrees in 1123.

The Protestant reformers challenged the view that committed celibacy was superior to marriage. Martin Luther (1483–1546) esteemed marriage as a divinely ordained institution. He emphasized one's duty to God in the midst of worldly activities and, hence, offered a positive evaluation of the demanding household activities of husband and wife. Luther believed that very few persons received the divine grace to remain celibate. The Reformers extolled chaste marriage as the vocation of almost all adult Christians.

The ideal relationship between husband and wife

Throughout Western history it has been difficult for male thinkers to imagine women as equal marital partners. One exception is Plato's depiction of the relationships among men and women in the group he called the "guardians," who constituted the ruling strata in his ideal republic. Male and female guardians would have radically equal lives with respect to both procreation and public service. The guardians should practice communal marriage, child rearing, and property holding. Otherwise, Plato feared, the governing class would act to advance the interests of particular households, established by monogamous marriage with particular heirs, instead of promoting the welfare of the entire polis. Plato offered *Republic* as an intellectual ideal. In his more realistic treatment of community life, contained in *Laws,* Plato recommended a traditional, patriarchal family structure.

Aristotle asserted that upper-class males are naturally suited to rule in marriage and the polis. There is a type of friendship between husband and wife, but it is a friendship of unequals in which the husband, as the superior party, should gain superior benefits. For example, it is morally appropriate for the wife to love her husband more than he loves her (*Nicomachean Ethics,* VIII).

Among the Hebrew people, the relationship between Adam and Eve served as the paradigm of human sociality. It is not good for human beings to be alone (Gen. 2:18). Men valued marriage to a faithful wife enough to use it as a metaphor for the community's relationship with God. God is a benevolent husband and Israel ought to be a faithful wife. Similarly, in Ephesians 5:22–32, a loving, but male-dominated, marriage served as a key religious analogy. The husband is to the wife as Christ is to the church. Therefore, the wife ought to be submissive to her husband, and the husband ought to have a self-giving love for his wife.

Actually Jesus, as presented in the gospels, took little interest in the patriarchal family, which was a central social institution in his culture. For Jesus, faithful commitment to the Kingdom of God was crucial, even if it threatened to disturb family bonds (Luke 14:26). Jesus' statements concerning adultery and divorce implicitly undermined key social privileges of the patriarchal husband. When questioned about marriage, Jesus advocated lifelong, reciprocal sexual fidelity (Mark 10:2–12; Matt. 19:3–9).

For the rabbis, loving companionship was a boon experienced in a fortunate marriage. The Talmud proclaims "any man who has no wife lives without joy, without blessing, and without goodness" (Yebamoth 62b). Sexual intercourse ought to be enjoyed by the married couple. Indeed, a husband is bound by *onah,* a duty to provide sexual satisfaction for his wife. Many rabbis have held that the Sabbath, the holiest day of the week, is an especially appropriate time for spouses to make love. Yet, sexuality has its moral limits, even within marriage. Among the most important limits are the laws of *niddah,* the family purity laws that restrict sexual contact with a menstruating wife.

Augustine held that between man and woman there is the possibility of a friendly companionship based on the rule of the husband and the obedience of the wife (*De bono conjugali,* I). According to Thomas Aquinas (1225–1274), men enter into marriage for the sake of procreation, since a man can have a more satisfying partnership with another man in any other endeavor (*Summa Theologiae,* I.92.1). Nevertheless, he acknowledged that a husband and wife may experience a unique friendship as a result of their sexual relationship and joint domestic activity (*Summa Contra Gentiles,* III, II, 123). Yet, Aquinas believed that the more rational husband rightfully served as head of the household.

Luther held that God willed that wives be subject to their husbands. Yet, a virtuous wife was a valued helpmate in all things, and she established a relationship of deep mutual respect with her husband. According to Luther, marital love that desired union with the spouse as a full partner was "the greatest and purest of [human] loves" (*Sermon on the Estate of Marriage*). Despite the greater Puritan appreciation of the value of companionship in marriage, beloved wives were still not full equals of their husbands. Rather, ministers taught that both nature and God had given the husband dominion over the wife; and the good wife accepted the authority of her husband.

John Stuart Mill (1806–1873) acknowledged the injustices done to women in patriarchal marriage. In nineteenth-century England, married women's wages and property were largely controlled by their husbands, and child custody was controlled by the father. Mill said that real friendship in marriage was subverted by social practices that subordinated women to men. He insisted that husband and wife can share familial authority. Unfortunately, Mill undermined his own demands for sexual equality when he declared that a traditional division of labor—husband as breadwinner, wife as housekeeper and nurturer—was best for most families. Nevertheless, Mill recognized: "The moral regeneration of mankind will only really commence, when the most fundamental of the social relations [marriage] is placed under the rule of equal justice . . ." (Mill, 1988, p. 103).

The later twentieth-century feminist movement forced ethicists to grapple with the unequal power dynamics within heterosexual relationships, particularly within marriage. Ethicists have confronted the high incidence of sexual abuse and domestic violence in marriages and domestic partnerships. As a result, religious ethicists began to articulate a new norm for marriage and domestic partnerships: just love. This norm entails both fair treatment of the spouses/partners and just, institutional patterns that safeguard the equal human dignity of both spouses/partners. When a norm of just love is employed, marriages marred by abuse or domination are judged morally deficient. Domestic partnerships characterized by tenderness, a mutual commitment to the well-being of the partner, reciprocal fairness, and a struggle to achieve social equality are judged morally laudatory.

Marriage, community, and individual freedom

Since the Enlightenment, there has been a greater emphasis on personal autonomy and a greater reliance on contracts as a mechanism to structure moral obligations. Both these trends have subtly influenced marriage. In a number of countries, the power to regulate marriage and divorce has been taken away from the churches. In the eyes of the state, marriages have become a matter of civil contract.

Immanuel Kant (1724–1804) taught that a voluntary, juridical marriage contract granting the spouses reciprocal, exclusive sexual access to each other's bodies tempered the inherently exploitative character of sexual passion. He asserted that, outside of marriage, people are apt to treat their sex partners as things to be used and discarded. Marriage alone safeguards the personal dignity of the sexual partner. In marriage, people can preserve the species without debasing their partners (Kant, 1930).

For Georg Wilhelm Friedrich Hegel (1770–1831), marriage was a basic human institution that allowed persons to reconcile their being in community with their freedom as individuals. However, Hegel was able to harmonize individuality and community within marriage partly by assuming that women had a unique nature that was fulfilled precisely by working at home to promote family happiness. According to Hegel, a united family was appropriately represented in the marketplace and the state by its male head (Hegel, 1942).

While for Hegel the complementarity of heterosexual partners was conducive to marital unity, marriage still required that both spouses restrain their individuality for the sake of the relationship. Ironically, marriage began with a contract in which the individual parties agreed to transcend, through marriage, the individuality that was a prerequisite for making any contract. Paradoxically, however, through self-surrender in marriage, both husband and wife deepened their selfhood.

Theorists from Mary Wollstonecraft (1992) to Susan Okin (1989) have criticized the injustices suffered by women within the institution of male-dominated marriage. Simone de Beauvoir (1908–1986), in particular, explored the history of marriage as a social mechanism for the control of women's sexuality, reproductive power, and domestic services. Beauvoir observed the contradictions inherent in marriage as a permanent commitment between radically free moral actors. According to Beauvoir, an erotic relationship should involve a willing surrender to desire with a partner recognized as another free subject of desire; it should not be a marital duty. Ultimately, Beauvoir asserted that women's economic, political, and cultural equality are a necessary precondition for an egalitarian marriage, a freely chosen commitment made by self-sufficient subjects (Beauvoir, 1953).

Domestic partnerships: Some historical reflections

Heterosexual domestic partnerships outside of marriage have been recognized and sometimes tolerated in Western history. Concubinage was a practice in which the community acknowledged the long-lasting domestic and sexual relationship between a man and a woman, but did not grant the woman and her children the same legal protections afforded through marriage. In the early centuries, the Christian church accepted concubinage, if the partners were monogamous. During the Middle Ages, Christian clerics disparaged sexual relationships outside of marriage and sought to discourage concubinage, particularly clerical concubinage, through social penalties. Finally, in the Roman Catholic church, concubinage for any believer was condemned at the Council of Trent (1545–1563). In some jurisdictions, two people living together as husband and wife, but without a marriage ceremony, created a legally recognized bond—a common-law marriage.

Homosexual activity has been known throughout European-American history. However, it was not until the late nineteenth century that experts theorized that some persons have a permanent erotic orientation toward others of the same sex. Therefore, most of the thinkers discussed here probably could not even have imagined that same-sex couples might create long-lasting relationships in which domestic activity and companionship were shared along with sexual intimacy.

For example, Plato extolled highly the total relationship—sexual, intellectual, and spiritual—between a younger man and his older, more virtuous mentor/lover. Still, Plato expected male citizens to establish households with wives. In contrast, John Chrysostom (d. 407 C.E.) denounced homosexual activity, because, if sexual desire could be satisfied with the same sex, men and women would have less motivation to establish harmonious marriages (*Ad Romanos*, iv).

In rabbinic Judaism, a Talmudic saying advised against two men sleeping together under a shared blanket, for fear of homosexual contact (M. Kiddushin 4:14). Other rabbis considered strict observance of this rule too scrupulous, specifically because they claimed that homosexuality was virtually unknown among Jewish men. Lesbian acts were disparaged, but since these did not involve a "spilling of the [male] seed," they were considered not a serious moral evil. Still, Moses Maimonides (1135–1204) cautioned husbands and fathers to control their wives' and daughters' friendships, lest the women engage in lesbian sexual activity.

There is limited historical material documenting relationships akin to contemporary homosexual domestic partnerships. In 342 c.e., the Theodosian Code of the Byzantine Empire condemned the passive male partners in homosexual marriages, although no punishment was prescribed. However, historians disagree about whether the term "marriage" was used descriptively or facetiously. This ban on homosexual marriage was reiterated when medieval law codes were reformed in conformity with ancient Roman models.

One arena in which intense same-sex relationships—some genital, some not—might have flourished were monasteries and convents. (There are many, often exaggerated, criticisms of perverse monastic homosexual practices.) When monasteries and convents were closed in Protestant territories during the Reformation, a socially approved way to concentrate on same-sex relationships was foreclosed.

In some localities in the United States, couples can register with a designated municipal office as domestic partners. Legal status as domestic partners carries a variety of property and other rights that vary from jurisdiction to jurisdiction. A growing number of public and private employers are providing health-care coverage for dependent domestic partners on a basis comparable to spouses. In some cases, benefits are offered to all domestic partners. In other cases, benefits are restricted to homosexual partners, since heterosexual partners have the option to marry.

Contemporary bioethical issues

Today, marriage is esteemed as a unique opportunity to experience emotional intimacy and self-fulfillment, including sexual self-fulfillment. But many persons, particularly committed religious persons, hold an ideal of marriage as a solemn promise to share the life destiny of the spouse until death. There is a potential conflict in marriage and other committed domestic partnerships between a relationship contingent on experiencing self-fulfillment and a promise to remain with the partner during difficult times. For example, does a person have a special obligation to care for a spouse/partner suffering a protracted illness, even if the relationship is no longer "self-fulfilling"? Is the obligation to continue to care weightier for those who exchange marriage vows?

Many persons view marriage as the socially preferred location in which to conceive and rear children. Another potential ethical tension exists between marriage/

domestic partnerships, which make a moral claim on each partner only as long as intimacy and self-fulfillment are provided, and long-term, responsible child rearing (see Blustein, 1982). For example, when a child suffers from a severe illness, the consequences for the adult caregivers' marriage/partnership can be devastating.

In addition, the moral preference accorded to child rearing within marriage is disputed. Some unmarried persons, including some gay men and lesbians, request technological assistance with reproduction. Should medical services to facilitate conception be restricted to heterosexual, married couples? Or are other domestic partners capable of equally reliable, loving nurture of children?

In the modern period, love has become the primary norm for marriage. A naive expectation that love animates marriage might contribute to social blindness toward domestic violence. In addition, the tradition that viewed the husband as responsible for order in the household has been used to legitimate husbands' use of physical force to control their wives. Thus norms about love and authority in the family have played a part in medicine's overly slow realization that domestic violence is a leading cause of injury to women.

Ethical rhetoric that praised the companionship of husband and wife while simultaneously prescribing wifely subordination showed that love as a moral value was not synonymous with equality. Society has been challenged to forge a new ethic of equality for heterosexual partners. This has become a crucial ethical task for society, because it is in the male-dominant household that children learn that relationships of dominance and subordination are morally acceptable.

Throughout much of history, marriage has been understood as a social institution essential to the fundamental welfare of society. Moral support from the community contributes to the stability of many marriages. There is dispute about whether society ought to offer moral support for long-term, committed homosexual relationships, for example, through social customs, legal recognition, or religious ceremonial affirmation.

There has been limited ethical attention to marriage and domestic partnerships as economic relationships. Questions of economic justice between spouses/partners, particularly when a relationship is terminated, have not been adequately addressed. It is most often the female partner who suffers serious economic disadvantages when a long-term heterosexual relationship ends. Among the economic harms suffered by such women is diminished access to, or quality of, health care for themselves and their children.

In industrialized welfare states, routine provision of medical insurance coverage to the spouses of workers is an important entitlement. With major restructuring of the U.S. health-care system in prospect, it is difficult to discuss how marital status influences access to health care. Still, there are questions of justice that need to be considered. Under health-care reform, will innovative health-insurance benefits for domestic partners be eliminated, retained, or even extended to more people?

Society accords many privileges to marriage partners. Domestic partners do not always receive the same social recognition of their central, shared-life relationship. In medical settings, married people customarily receive such benefits as credit for spouses' blood donation, special visitation opportunities, and routine participation in discharge planning. In health-care matters, there is a legal presumption that one is the proxy decision maker if one's spouse becomes incompetent. Health-care proxy documents, for those who have them, allow domestic partners to make medical decisions for a partner who becomes incompetent. Still, if love, an intimate knowledge of the patient's values, and a paramount concern for the well-being of the patient are what is presumed to qualify marriage partners as proxy decision makers, other domestic partners should qualify morally as substitute decision makers on similar grounds.

Marriage and domestic partnerships are central life relationships with complex, disputed moral meanings. There are many complicated ethical questions about one's responsibilities to self, spouse/partner, children (if any), and society. Our moral assumptions about marriage and domestic partnerships will influence our bioethical judgments in many situations.

BARBARA HILKERT ANDOLSEN

Directly related to this entry is the entry FAMILY. *For a further discussion of topics mentioned in this entry, see the entries* ABUSE, INTERPERSONAL, *article on* ABUSE BETWEEN DOMESTIC PARTNERS; ETHICS, *article on* RELIGION AND MORALITY; FEMINISM; FRIENDSHIP; HEALTH POLICY, *article on* POLITICS AND HEALTH CARE; HOMOSEXUALITY; JUDAISM; LOVE; PROTESTANTISM; ROMAN CATHOLICISM; *and* WOMEN, *especially the article on* HISTORICAL AND CROSS-CULTURAL PERSPECTIVES. *This entry will find application in the entries* DEATH AND DYING: EUTHANASIA AND SUSTAINING LIFE, *article on* ETHICAL ISSUES; REPRODUCTIVE TECHNOLOGIES; *and* SEXUAL ETHICS. *Other relevant material may be found under the entries* CHILDREN, *especially the article on* CHILD CUSTODY; *and* FERTILITY CONTROL.

Bibliography

BAILEY, DERRICK SHERWIN. 1955. *Homosexuality and the Western Christian Tradition.* Hamden, Conn.: Archon.

———. 1959. *Sexual Relation in Christian Thought.* New York: Harper and Brothers.

BEAUVOIR, SIMONE DE. 1953. *The Second Sex.* Translated by Howard Madison Parshley. New York: Alfred A. Knopf.

BLUSTEIN, JEFFREY. 1982. *Parents and Children: The Ethics of the Family.* New York: Oxford University Press.

BOSWELL, JOHN. 1980. *Christianity, Social Tolerance, and Homosexuality: Gay People in Western Europe from the Beginning of the Christian Era to the Fourteenth Century.* Chicago: University of Chicago Press.

BROWN, PETER R. 1988. *The Body and Society: Men, Women, and Sexual Renunciation in Early Christianity.* New York: Columbia University Press.

CAHILL, LISA SOWLE. 1985. *Between the Sexes: Foundations for a Christian Ethics of Sexuality.* New York: Paulist Press.

COOKE, VINCENT M. 1991. "Kant, Teleology, and Sexual Ethics." *International Philosophical Quarterly* 31, no. 1:3–13.

COUNTRYMAN, LOUIS WILLIAM. 1988. *Dirt, Greed, and Sex: Sexual Ethics in the New Testament and Their Implications for Today.* Philadelphia: Fortress.

DUBERMAN, MARTIN BAUML; VICINUS, MARTHA; and CHAUNCEY, GEORGE, JR., eds. 1989. *Hidden from History: Reclaiming the Gay and Lesbian Past.* New York: NAL Books.

FARLEY, MARGARET A. 1990. *Personal Commitments: Beginning, Keeping, Changing.* San Francisco: Harper.

FELDMAN, DAVID M. 1974. *Marital Relations, Birth Control, and Abortion in Jewish Law.* New York: Schocken.

GLENDON, MARY ANN. 1989. *The Transformation of Family Law: State, Law, and Family in the United States and Western Europe.* Chicago: University of Chicago Press.

HEGEL, GEORG WILHELM FRIEDRICH. 1942. *Hegel's Philosophy of Right.* Translated by Thomas Malcolm Knox. Oxford: At the Clarendon Press.

KANT, IMMANUEL. 1930. *Lectures on Ethics.* Translated by Louis Infield. New York: Century.

MILL, JOHN STUART. 1988. *The Subjection of Women.* Edited by Susan Moller Okin. Indianapolis, Ind.: Hackett.

NELSON, JAMES B. 1978. *Embodiment: An Approach to Sexuality and Christian Theology.* Minneapolis, Minn.: Augsburg.

OKIN, SUSAN MOLLER. 1989. *Justice, Gender, and the Family.* New York: Basic Books.

STONE, LAWRENCE. 1977. *The Family, Sex, and Marriage in England, 1500–1800.* London: Weidenfeld and Nicolson.

WOLLSTONECRAFT, MARY. 1992. *Vindication of the Rights of Women.* New York: Knopf.

MATERNAL–FETAL RELATIONSHIP

I. MEDICAL ASPECTS

During the last decades of the twentieth century, perinatal medicine has made tremendous advances in scientific knowledge and in the successful application of this knowledge toward improving pregnancy outcomes. These advances have also brought a dramatic change in medicine's conceptualization of the fetus. No longer is the fetus defined predominantly as a part of the pregnant woman, but rather as a distinct entity that can be the independent focus of diagnostic tests and individual therapies: "A second patient with many rights and privileges comparable to those previously achieved only after birth." It is the widely shared view of obstetricians that the fetus is a patient to whom they owe ethical duties. The purpose of this article is to delineate the medical advances that have brought about this change in fetal identity and to discuss the impact of these changes on pregnant women and the obstetrical decision-making process.

Pregnancy and maternal health

Maternal morality in pregnancy fell dramatically in the United States from more than one in 200 in 1935 to less than one in 10,000 in 1994. Most of this reduction was accomplished earlier in this century through improved surgical techniques and increased access to safe blood products, antibiotics, intravenous fluids, and improved prenatal care.

Despite these improvements, pregnancy still poses the risk of serious illness and, in rare cases, death. It has been calculated that the risk of mortality in pregnant women is 179 times that of the risk of death among women using the safest method of birth control. The major causes of maternal death are hypertensive disorders of pregnancy, pulmonary embolism, uterine hemorrhage, and sepsis. The risks of pregnancy are proportional to the age of the pregnant woman and to her underlying state of health. Women with medical illness may note worsening of their disease during pregnancy, sometimes with serious long-term consequences. But even women who begin a pregnancy in excellent health may find themselves suddenly confronting the morbidity and mortality risks associated with cesarean section (23.5% of all U.S. deliveries in 1990), postpartum hemorrhage (4–8% of all deliveries), or pre-eclampsia (a pregnancy-related condition that can lead to seizures, strokes or death in the pregnant woman) (5% of all pregnancies).

Pregnant women may experience preterm labor (U.S. incidence is 10%), the development of premature contractions that if not stopped can result in delivery of the fetus before adequate development has occurred. Preterm delivery poses significant risk of disability and death for the fetus. While preterm labor itself does not pose a health risk to the pregnant woman, many of the treatments recommended for its treatment have significant maternal side effects. The three drugs commonly used to treat (attempt to stop) preterm labor have serious side effects ranging from nausea, vomiting, dizziness, flushing, tremor, and jitteriness to life-threatening risks of pulmonary edema (fluid in the lungs), alterations in blood chemistries (hypokalemia, hyperglycemia), heart rate abnormalities (tachycardia, arrhythmias), hypotension, respiratory depression, and cardiac arrest.

For all women, pregnancy is a complex physiologic process; almost every organ system undergoes adaptation to support the maternal–fetal unit. It is important to appreciate the range of symptoms experienced by many pregnant women due to these physiologic changes. These include nausea, vomiting, fatigue, syncope (fainting), round ligament pelvic pain, backache, heartburn, hemorrhoids, constipation, urinary frequency, carpal tunnel syndrome (numbness and tingling of the hands), pedal edema, and sciatica (hip and leg nerve pain). Thus, while pregnancy is described as a normal physiologic process, it is not without common discomforts and the potential for serious illness. Most pregnant women willingly assume these sacrifices for their developing fetus.

Pregnancy and fetal therapies

Perinatal technologies have benefited the fetus by increasing the understanding of normal fetal development as well as improving prenatal diagnostic capabilities and therapeutic interventions. The fetus can be visualized with ultrasound, its well-being assessed with fetal heart-rate monitoring, and its diseases diagnosed with chorionic villus sampling, amniocentesis, and fetal blood sampling. Increases in diagnostic capabilities have been accompanied by the development of techniques to treat the fetus directly in utero. Our increasing ability to act on behalf of the fetus has made its claims to our care more compelling.

Prenatal technologies designed to benefit the fetus range from the simple to the complex, with differing risks and benefits for both the pregnant woman and her fetus. The most commonly used technology with the intention of improving fetal outcome is electronic fetal monitoring (EFM). EFM was introduced in the United States in the early 1970s with the promise that it would enable early detection of fetal hypoxia in labor and alert the physician to perform an immediate delivery, preventing the serious consequences of oxygen deprivation, including brain damage and stillbirth. Its use rapidly expanded from high-risk pregnancies to all pregnancies; in 1978, it was estimated that two-thirds of all U.S. pregnancies were monitored. Unfortunately, the wide acceptance of this technology occurred before adequate studies had been done to assess its efficacy and safety. There have now been six prospective randomized trials of EFM that have been unable to demonstrate a decrease in intrapartum fetal death or better newborn health in low-risk pregnancies. However, the use of EFM was shown to double the C-section (cesarean-section) rate for the indication of fetal distress, thus exposing more women to the increased morbidity and mortality risks of C-section without the promised fetal benefit.

A C-section entails a greater risk of maternal morbidity and mortality than does a vaginal delivery. The mortality rate associated with C-section is between two and four times that associated with a vaginal delivery. Maternal morbidity is also more frequent and usually more severe with a C-section. The common causes of morbidity associated with C-sections are infection, injury to the urinary tract, and hemorrhage with the possible risk of transfusion. Even an uncomplicated C-section requires a much longer recovery period for the mother at a time when she is experiencing increased physical and emotional demands.

The simplest fetal therapies are medications given to a pregnant woman for the benefit of her fetus. A well-accepted treatment of a woman who develops mild diabetes during pregnancy is to give her insulin until delivery. This practice benefits the fetus by preventing its excessive growth and associated birth trauma and by avoiding the potential neonatal difficulties of an infant of a diabetic mother. While insulin is not essential for the pregnant woman's health, it may be beneficial by reducing her risk of C-section delivery and the potential harms of a mildly elevated glucose to her own organ systems. Digoxin is a medication administered to pregnant women for the benefit of a fetus with cardiac arrhythmia. Unlike insulin, digoxin offers no benefit to the health of the pregnant woman. The risks to the pregnant woman of ingesting insulin or digoxin are minimal if administered appropriately. In summary, these pharmacologic fetal therapies confer benefit upon the fetus and are minimally invasive; one offers some benefit for the pregnant woman; the other solely benefits the fetus.

An accepted but more invasive therapy of sole benefit to the fetus is a fetal blood transfusion for isoimmunization from Rh disease (a condition in which the immune system of the pregnant woman destroys the blood cells of the fetus resulting in fetal death if severe and untreated). The most common technique is cordocentesis, in which a needle is placed through the maternal abdominal and uterine wall into the umbilical blood vessel for the purpose of transfusing blood into the fetus. This technique is not without its risks for both the fetus and the pregnant woman. This procedure poses a 2 percent chance of fetal death. It also increases the risk of fetal bradycardia (a dangerous lowering of the heart rate), a condition that mandates an emergency C-section for the safety of the fetus. All the maternal risks of C-section delineated above are increased in an emergency C-section, with the addition of the increased risk of death from general anesthesia. Cordocentesis is an example of an accepted fetal therapy that is potentially beneficial for the fetus and invasive for the pregnant woman, with significant risks to her in complicated cases.

The most invasive fetal therapy is in utero fetal surgery. Several operations are being investigated. One example is the surgical removal of a lung mass in the fetus. The rationale for the surgery is that without prenatal removal, the fetal lungs will be unable to grow sufficiently to support survival after birth. The pregnant woman must undergo a major abdominal operation and take medications to prevent the preterm labor that might be caused by the surgery. The surgery entails the usual risks associated with a C-section but at a higher rate because of the type of uterine incision, the thickness of the uterine wall, and the need for general anesthesia. Because of the type of uterine incision necessary for this fetal surgery, the woman must have a C-section in this pregnancy, even if her fetus is stillborn, as well as in all future pregnancies. Due to the experimental nature of this procedure, the long-term benefit is yet to be established.

Neonatal advances and obstetrical decision making

Simultaneous advances in neonatology have had a significant impact on obstetrical knowledge and care. The gestational age at which survival is possible in the modern intensive care nursery has been pushed back continuously over the past few decades to the age of twenty-four to twenty-five weeks (fifteen to sixteen weeks premature). Many fetuses/babies who in the past would have been considered nonviable now survive and develop normally. However, the cost of this success is measured in hundreds of thousands of dollars per premature infant and in the potential for severe lifelong impairments.

This improved neonatal survival has had two significant influences on the perspective of obstetrical providers. Most have seen or participated in the care of very premature babies; thus fetuses in utero from twenty-four weeks on possess a very concrete human image for those who care for them. In addition, the possibility of survival beginning at twenty-four gestational weeks creates an argument for aggressive obstetrical management at earlier and earlier stages of pregnancy. The lower the gestational age at birth and the lower the birth weight, the lower the chance of survival and the higher the risk of severe physical and mental impairment. Between twenty-four to twenty-eight weeks the likelihood of survival increases from 20 percent to 90 percent, with a 20 percent incidence of severe neonatal impairment in the survivors. Complicating this situation is the inaccuracy of techniques to estimate gestational age and fetal weight. The inability to predict with certainty before birth either the survival or the likelihood of impairment creates legitimate divergent perspectives on what to do in individual pregnancies and ensures difficult decision making for obstetricians and pregnant women.

Formerly, a woman who developed preterm labor at twenty-five weeks would have been allowed to deliver vaginally and comforted regarding the certain death of her baby. Today, that pregnant woman will be faced with the option and probable recommendation that the fetus be monitored in labor and delivered by C-section if needed for fetal benefit. A C-section at this gestational age is riskier for her than one at term and because the type of uterine incision required commits her to C-section delivery of future pregnancies. The chance of the infant's survival is between 30 and 50 percent depending on its weight (which is difficult to predict prior to delivery). If the infant does survive, there will be a significant chance of neurologic or physical impairment. Some women will choose to take any risk for a slim possibility of fetal benefit, and accept aggressive obstetrical management. Other women decide that the risk of C-section in this and future pregnancies combined with the potential suffering for their premature infant is not worth the slight chance of being able to take home a normal or mildly impaired child. They choose to let "nature take its course," and hope that their next pregnancy will be free of complications. For the obstetrician faced with this clinical dilemma, the uncertainty of prognosis (this fetus might do well), the availability of technologic intervention (C-section), the desire to do something, and the legal fear of doing nothing may prompt him or her to advocate intervention as the baby's only hope. This is a persuasive argument for most pregnant women, especially if alternatives are not presented as legitimate.

The beneficial effects of fetal therapies and neonatal advances are impressive when successful: Babies previously at high risk of stillbirth, birth trauma, hypoxia, and neonatal death now have a greater chance of being born safely and having a near normal development. However, some babies who would have died now survive but with significant handicaps and at a significant cost to the physical, emotional, and financial well-being of the mother, her child, and her family. Some therapies are recommended with hope of fetal benefit but without good scientific evidence and with known maternal risks of death and morbidity. Pregnant women must be able to choose the best medical option based upon accurate

scientific knowledge and an honest appraisal of the uncertainties involved in medical science.

Pregnancy and fetal development

Increased understanding of fetal development has allowed identification of environmental factors that can promote or impair the development of a healthy fetus. The placenta was once felt to operate as a barrier allowing only those substances beneficial to the fetus to pass. Now it is known that the placenta is an efficient transporter of many substances to the fetus, regardless of their toxicity, including both therapeutic and recreational drugs. Media coverage has focused on the rising incidence of crack cocaine use by pregnant women. It has been estimated that 11 percent of pregnant women use an illegal drug during their pregnancies and that 75 percent of these women use cocaine. While there are methodologic shortcomings in the studies of cocaine's effect on pregnancy, many serious sequelae of using this drug have been suggested, including an increased spontaneous abortion rate; suspected cardiac, genitourinary, facial, and limb abnormalities (though these may be alcohol-related); growth retardation; and in utero strokes. Obstetrical complications include preterm delivery, abruption (placental separation), and fetal distress. Newborns who have been exposed to cocaine in utero experience withdrawal symptoms, making them more irritable and less able to bond with caregivers. Many believe that cocaine-exposed babies will be more likely to experience learning disabilities.

Alcohol is a well-known danger to the developing fetus. Fetal alcohol syndrome has been identified in the offspring of women who consumed excessive alcohol during their pregnancy; it is defined by a triad of symptoms: gross physical retardation; central nervous system dysfunction, including mental retardation; and characteristic facial abnormalities. Fetal alcohol effects are more common; they include cardiac, genitourinary, skeletal, and muscular anomalies; hypoxia; irritability; and hyperactivity. While excessive alcohol use during pregnancy has clearly been documented to cause significant fetal harm, no minimum safe level of consumption has been established. Many experts have recommended total abstinence from alcohol during pregnancy as the only way to avoid all possible harm.

Smoking has significant effects on pregnancy outcome. Approximately 30 percent of U.S. women of childbearing age smoke. Cigarette smoking results in reductions in birthweight, length, and head circumference. It has been estimated that between 20 and 40 percent of all low birthweight births in the United States can be attributed directly to smoking. Smoking has also been associated with higher rates of spontaneous abortion, preterm birth, perinatal mortality, and deficits in later physical, intellectual, and emotional development. A comparison of the known perinatal dangers of alcohol, smoking, and cocaine consumption illustrates that the legal substances a pregnant women may ingest are no less medically harmful than the illegal ones.

Public policy aimed at improving perinatal outcomes by reducing the use of fetotoxic substances by pregnant women must be grounded in medical knowledge. Recreational drug use by most pregnant women is an addiction; they do not consume the drug to harm the fetus but to satisfy an acute physical or psychological need. To address the problem of addiction, comprehensive and supportive programs designed to enlist the individual in her own recovery are necessary. There have been documented successes in programs that emphasize early identification of women at risk for substance abuse and that utilize comprehensive education, prenatal care, psychological intervention, and social services. However, there are very few substance abuse programs available to pregnant women. In one notable case of criminal prosecution of a woman for drug use during her pregnancy, the accused woman had sought drug treatment during her pregnancy without success.

Punitive approaches to addictive disease are generally ineffective. They have the potential to drive the addicted individual away from the very care that could be beneficial. Because the developing fetus is so vulnerable to uterine exposure to toxins, it is critical that pregnant women not be deterred from care. Prenatal care alone, in the presence of continuing drug use, can improve perinatal outcome for the drug-exposed fetus.

Obstetrical decision making

While a pregnant woman and her fetus may be conceptualized as two independent patients, they are in fact intimately interdependent, and actions taken to benefit one may pose a risk to the other. A pregnant woman may suffer from a serious illness that requires a treatment that will itself pose risk to her fetus; premature delivery to improve maternal health and chemotherapy for maternal cancer are two examples. Alternatively, treatment for the benefit of the fetus (C-section delivery, treatment of preterm labor, fetal surgery) may pose a risk to the pregnant woman. In addition, a medical treatment for presumed fetal benefit may interfere with the nonmedical needs of the pregnant woman.

These situations have been described by many as maternal–fetal conflict when they more accurately might be described as maternal–physician conflict. When an obstetrician agrees with the pregnant woman's choice and underlying values, no conflict ensues, even in the presence of potential fetal risk. The disagreement that does occur often is based on differing views of what is beneficial for the pregnant woman and her fetus and what are acceptable maternal risks to achieve obstetrical goals.

Obstetricians have a predominant focus on the current pregnancy. Appropriately, they emphasize the medical health of their patient and the fetus, give expert advice to improve pregnancy outcome, and urge women to follow this advice as a priority in their lives. However, medical recommendations are at times influenced by the fear of malpractice, research interests, a reluctance to give up, and a provider's own personal values.

A pregnant woman's values may differ from those of her providers and she may place a different value on the physician's medically based goals. Like other adults, a pregnant woman must and does make decisions about her prenatal activity within the broader context of her life. Her obligation to her fetus is sometimes weighed against her obligations to her other children, her parents, her partner, or others with whom she has a special relationship. Her decision may be influenced by religious or other strongly held personal beliefs.

Some have argued that pregnant women should be forced to undergo certain treatments if the benefit to the fetus would be substantial and the risk to the woman would be minimal or low. Medical uncertainty and medical practice make this a difficult policy to administer rationally or fairly. As delineated above, perinatal medicine is limited by diagnostic and prognostic uncertainty. This is best illustrated by a legal case in which a judge ordered a woman to undergo a forced C-section. In seeking the court order, the obstetrician testified that without delivery by C-section, the fetus had a 99 percent chance of dying and the pregnant woman had a 50 percent chance of mortality. However, the pregnant woman fled the court's jurisdiction and had an uneventful vaginal delivery. The ability to predict fetal distress in labor is frequently inaccurate. Because of this uncertainty, a policy of enforcing obstetrical recommendations would allow obstetricians to make the wrong decisions sometimes but would never allow a pregnant woman to be wrong or right about decisions that profoundly affect her life.

The problem of precisely defining fetal risk is matched by the complex task of delineating what constitutes an acceptable risk of harm for the mother. Risks, no matter how small in the medical context, may take on a different meaning within the context of an individual's life. The small risk of maternal death from a C-section may be very significant to a single woman who is the sole supporter of her children. Bed rest for the prevention of preterm labor may mean the loss of work and health insurance for her whole family. A Jehovah's Witness who is forced to receive blood may believe she is condemned to eternal damnation and may undergo significant stress or rejection within her religious community.

If obstetricians are given the authority to force pregnant women to follow their recommendations, this force may be used in a very arbitrary way. Not only is there variation in obstetrical diagnostic and prognostic accuracy, there are obstetrical debates about the appropriate management of various conditions. The medical justifications in the reported cases of requests for court-ordered C-sections have included breech presentation, prior C-section, and rupture of membranes for twenty-four hours without signs of febrile morbidity. Many obstetricians would disagree with each of these indications for C-section. Furthermore, the women who have been subjected to court orders have been shown to be more likely subjects of other forms of discrimination. In one study of forced C-sections, 81 percent of the women belonged to a minority group and 24 percent did not use English as their first language, and all requests for the court orders involved women who received care at a teaching hospital or who were receiving public assistance.

If the use of force by doctors against pregnant women were to be legitimized, it would have negative implications for their therapeutic relationship. The relationship would become less cooperative and supportive and more adversarial; compromise in situations of disagreement would become less and less possible. Under these circumstances of care, some women might lie about their behaviors or symptoms, fearing that their obstetrician would use this information to force upon them unacceptable treatment. Others might avoid prenatal care completely. The adversarial climate created by the use of force would decrease the effectiveness of obstetricians in improving maternal and fetal health.

Conclusion

Perinatal advances have dramatically improved the perinatal survival and well-being of fetuses/babies, fulfilling the obstetrical goals of prenatal providers and the personal goals of pregnant women. Increased understanding of the developing fetus and improved technologies have given the fetus an enhanced human identity and status as a direct patient of the obstetrician. The new therapeutic options with their maternal risks have created difficult ethical decisions for the pregnant woman and her obstetrician. A discussion regarding the legitimate use of force against pregnant women for fetal benefit has begun. The resolution of this debate must take into account the implications of the uncertainty inherent in medicine, the maternal risks associated with fetal therapies, the inevitable influence of an obstetrician's personal values upon his or her medical recommendations,

the harmful influence of force in any therapeutic relationship, and the ethical and constitutional rights of all parties, including pregnant women.

Nancy Milliken

Directly related to this article are the other articles in this entry: ETHICAL ISSUES, *and* LEGAL AND REGULATORY ISSUES. *Also directly related is the entry* FETUS. *For a further discussion of topics mentioned in this article, see the entries* HEALTH SCREENING AND TESTING IN THE PUBLIC-HEALTH CONTEXT; INFORMED CONSENT; LIFESTYLES AND PUBLIC HEALTH; PATIENTS' RESPONSIBILITIES; PROFESSIONAL–PATIENT RELATIONSHIP; RIGHTS, *article on* SYSTEMATIC ANALYSIS; SUBSTANCE ABUSE; *and* WOMEN, *articles on* HISTORICAL AND CROSS-CULTURAL PERSPECTIVES, *and* HEALTH-CARE ISSUES. *For a discussion of related ideas, see the entries* AUTONOMY; COMPETENCE; CONFLICT OF INTEREST; HARM; LOVE; PATERNALISM; RESPONSIBILITY; *and* VIRTUE AND CHARACTER. *Other relevant material may be found under the entries* ABORTION; *and* FEMINISM.

Bibliography

CHASNOFF, IRA J.; BURNS, WILLIAM J.; SCHNOLL, SIDNEY H.; and BURNS, KAYREEN A. 1985. "Cocaine Use in Pregnancy." *New England Journal of Medicine* 313, no. 11: 666–669.

CHASNOFF, IRA J.; LANDRESS, HARVEY J.; and BARRETT, MARK E. 1990. "The Prevalence of Illicit Drug or Alcohol Use During Pregnancy and Discrepancies in Mandatory Reporting in Pinellas County, Florida." *New England Journal of Medicine* 322, no. 17:1202–1206.

CHERVENAK, FRANK A., and McCULLOUGH, LAURENCE B. 1985. "Perinatal Ethics: A Practical Method of Analysis of Obligations to Mother and Fetus." *Obstetrics and Gynecology* 66, no. 3:442–446.

COUNCIL ON SCIENTIFIC AFFAIRS. 1989. *Fetal Effects of Maternal Alcohol Abuse.* Chicago: American Medical Association.

CREASY, ROBERT K., and RESNICK, ROBERT, eds. 1989. *Maternal Fetal Medicine: Principles and Practice.* 2d ed. Philadelphia: Saunders.

FREEMAN, ROGER. 1990. "Intrapartum Fetal Monitoring: A Disappointing Story." *New England Journal of Medicine* 322, no. 9:624–626.

GABBE, STEVEN G.; NIEBYL, JENNIFER R.; and SIMPSON, JOE LEIGH. 1986. *Obstetrics: Normal and Problem Pregnancies.* New York: Churchill Livingstone.

KOLDER, VERONIKA E. B.; GALLAGHER, JANET; and PARSONS, MICHAEL T. 1987. "Court-Ordered Obstetrical Interventions." *New England Journal of Medicine* 316, no. 19:1192–1196.

NELSON, LAWRENCE J., and MILLIKEN, NANCY. 1988. "Compelled Medical Treatment of Pregnant Women: Life, Liberty, and Law in Conflict." *Journal of the American Medical Association* 259, no. 7:1060–1066.

PRITCHARD, JACK A.; MACDONALD, PAUL C.; and GANT, NORMAN F. 1985. *Williams Obstetrics.* 17th ed. Norwalk, Conn.: Appleton-Century-Crofts.

RHODEN, NANCY K. 1987. "Informed Consent in Obstetrics: Some Special Problems." *Western New England Law Review* 9, no. 1:67–88.

ROBERTSON, PATRICIA A. 1992. "Neonatal Morbidity According to Gestational Age and Birth Weight from Five Tertiary Care Centers in the United States, 1983 Through 1986." *American Journal of Obstetrics and Gynecology* 166, no. 6 (pt. 1):1629–1641.

SCHULMAN, JOSEPH, ed. 1986. "Fetal Therapy." *Clinical Obstetrics & Gynecology* 29, no. 3:481–614. Special issue.

U.S. CONGRESS. COMMITTEE ON GOVERNMENTAL AFFAIRS. 1989. *Missing Links: Coordinating Federal and Drug Policy for Women, Infants, and Children: Hearings.* Washington, D.C.: Author.

II. ETHICAL ISSUES

Only since the 1960s has it been recognized that the fetus in utero can be harmed by a range of maternal behaviors. Now that it is known that drinking, smoking, and using drugs during pregnancy can harm the unborn child, the question of what moral obligations a pregnant woman has to the fetus she carries has become a significant issue in biomedical ethics. When conflicts arise between what a pregnant woman wants to do or believes is right to do, on the one hand, and what may be best for the fetus, on the other, how and on what basis should those conflicts be resolved? And who should be involved in resolving them?

This article attempts to provide a conceptual framework for thinking about maternal–fetal conflicts. Whether one believes that women have moral obligations to their fetuses in utero depends largely on one's view of the moral status of the fetus—possibly the central issue in the abortion debate. The debate over whether (and at what developmental stage) fetuses can be harmed is a heated one. Pro-lifers think that fetuses can be harmed, and base their opposition to abortion on the ground that being killed is the ultimate harm. They also oppose behavior on the part of pregnant women that is likely to have less severe effects on the fetus. By contrast, many pro-choicers deny that fetuses (or at least early gestation fetuses) can be harmed. However, even if the pro-choice view of the fetus is the correct one, it does not follow that pregnant women are free to drink, smoke, or use drugs during pregnancy, if they are planning to have the baby. For if the pregnant woman does not abort but goes to term, her behavior during pregnancy can have lasting, destructive effects on the born child. Concern for the born child is a common ground that unites all people, regardless of their stance on abor-

tion. This distinction between the fetus per se and the fetus-who-will-be-born differentiates maternal–fetal conflicts from the issue of abortion. Yet these conflicts are not entirely unrelated to the problem of abortion, because both issues concern justifications for restricting or controlling women's behavior during pregnancy.

The moral status of the unborn

One of the thorniest issues in bioethics is the moral status of the fetus. (Here, the term "fetus" is used to refer to the unborn during all stages of pregnancy.) One view is that fetuses are merely potential children who do not have full-fledged moral rights, or perhaps any rights at all. According to this view, attempts to limit reproductive choices or coerce behavior during pregnancy violate very basic moral rights to bodily self-determination.

A different view is that fetuses are "pre-born children," with all the rights of born children. Someone who regards the fetus in this way will think that a pregnant woman has the same moral obligations to protect her fetus from harm as she has to protect her born children. In keeping with this view of the fetus, some states have adopted "fetal rights" legislation, for example, making behavior during pregnancy that puts the fetus at risk of damage or death a form of child abuse.

Those who differentiate morally between fetuses and children tend vigorously to oppose "fetal rights" legislation, often seeing it as part of a larger political agenda to make abortion illegal. Even apart from the abortion question, many people are concerned that any attempts to control women's behavior during pregnancy violate their rights to privacy and self-determination. At the extreme, the position taken by some feminists and civil libertarians is that whatever a woman does during her pregnancy is her own business. They have opposed even noncoercive measures, such as a bill requiring the posting of signs warning pregnant women of the dangers of alcohol consumption (Sack, 1991).

However, if a woman decides not to abort, but to carry to term, then her behavior during pregnancy may have an adverse effect not only on the fetus but also on the child who is born. Whatever one's position on the moral standing of fetuses, born children clearly have moral status and rights.

The right not to be injured is one of the most basic moral and legal rights. To extend this right to prenatal injury requires only the recognition that a person can be injured by events that occurred before his or her birth—indeed, even before conception. Here is an example of preconception injury: In the 1940s, diethylstilbestrol (DES) was sometimes prescribed to prevent miscarriage. Not only was the drug ineffective, it sometimes resulted in damaged reproductive systems in the female children of women who used it. When these girls grew up, their reproductive abnormalities sometimes led to miscarriages and premature births. Prematurity can cause cerebral palsy. Thus, a child might be born with cerebral palsy due to a premature birth ultimately caused by her grandmother's ingestion of DES years before her own conception (*Enright by Enright* v. *Eli Lilly & Co.*, 568 N.Y.S.2d [Ct.App. 1991]). The legal right to recover for injuries negligently inflicted during pregnancy has been widely recognized in the United States since the landmark case of *Bonbrest* v. *Kotz* (65 F. Supp. 138 [D.D.C. 1946]). Courts have been much more reluctant to accept a right to recover for preconception injuries, primarily out of a concern to confine liability within manageable limits.

The important point for bioethics is that recognition of a moral right to be free from injuries inflicted before birth is not based on recognition of the fetus as having the moral status of a person. The concern is not primarily for the fetus but for the surviving child. At the same time, attempts to protect children from prenatal injury can be accomplished only through the body of the pregnant woman. As a result, some women have been subjected to forced cesareans (Annas, 1982; Rhoden, 1986, 1987; Nelson and Milliken, 1988). With the development of new fetal therapies and surgery, women could be asked, or even required, to undergo possibly painful and risky procedures for the sake of the not-yet-born child (Robertson, 1982). Thus, if the focus is exclusively on the prevention of harm to the future child, there is a risk of forgetting that the pregnant woman is a person in her own right, not merely a "fetal container" (Annas, 1986). The moral question, then, is how to balance the interests and rights of the pregnant woman against those of her not-yet-born child.

Most women who are expecting a child voluntarily adapt at least some of their behavior to protect their babies. But what if the woman is an alcoholic or a crack addict? What if, for religious or other reasons, she refuses a cesarean section her doctor thinks is necessary to prevent serious damage to her nearly born baby? Such cases "pit a woman's right to privacy and bodily integrity . . . against the possibility of a lifetime of devastating disability to a being who is within days or even hours of independent existence" (Rhoden, 1987, p. 118). How should such conflicts be resolved? What moral obligations do women have to prevent harm to the children they intend to bear?

Conceptualizing maternal–fetal conflict

People have moral obligations to other people, both those existing today and those who will exist in the future. The mere fact that people do not now exist is no reason to discount the interests they will have when they come into existence. If people today do nothing about the national debt, if they allow the ozone layer to be depleted, if they pollute the air and water, then actual (as opposed to possible or potential) individuals, living in the future, will be harmed by what is done, or is not done, today. There is a responsibility to these actual, though future, people not to destroy the world they will live in. That they do not now exist does not obviate present obligations to them. Similarly, women have moral obligations to their future children, that is, the ones they will bring into the world.

In the United States, as in most societies, the primary responsibility for protecting the interests of children belongs to their parents. Although parents have a great deal of discretion in deciding how to care for and raise their children, they do not have absolute freedom. In industrialized nations, at least, it is widely accepted that parents are not only morally but also legally obligated not to inflict injury on their children, to feed and clothe them, to provide them with necessary medical care. It would seem, then, that pregnant women who intend to complete their pregnancies have comparable moral obligations to avoid harming their not-yet-born children. However, preventing prenatal harm is not the only morally relevant consideration. The woman's own interests count, too. How are conflicts between the interests of the future child and the interests of the pregnant woman to be resolved?

Some object to the very notion of "maternal–fetal *conflict.*" They regard this as being misleadingly adversarial, pitting pregnant women against the children they will bear, when in most cases their interests are inseparably intertwined. A less adversarial framework stresses that what is good for pregnant women, such as better prenatal care, is also good for fetuses. While this is undeniable, some women want to do things, such as smoking or using drugs or alcohol, that risk harming their unborn children. Admittedly, behavior that endangers the fetus often endangers the health of the pregnant woman, but this does not necessarily make their interests identical. What if the woman is willing to risk her own health for the enjoyment the tobacco or alcohol or cocaine brings? She may decide—perhaps irrationally, perhaps not—that use of the substance is in her own interest, all things considered. That does not mean it is in the interest of her as-yet-unborn baby. It is wishful thinking to pretend that the possible harmful effect on the pregnant woman prevents the possibility of conflict.

Others object to characterizing the conflict as one between mother and fetus. In the so-called obstetrical cases (e.g., forced cesareans), the conflict may not be between mother and fetus. Rather, it is between mother and doctor, who disagree about what is best for both mother and child. In one case, doctors sought a court order because the fetus's umbilical cord was wrapped around its neck, a clear indication for an emergency cesarean. The woman, who had nine children, refused surgery out of concern for her own health, a belief in "natural childbirth," and an intuition that the delivery would turn out fine, despite the doctors' dire predictions. She delivered vaginally, and the child was fine (Rhoden, 1986).

Attempts to prevent prenatal harm often impose risks or burdens on pregnant women, particularly when an intervention, such as a cesarean section or blood transfusion, is deemed necessary to protect the unborn child. The moral question then becomes how much risk, burden, or sacrifice a woman must undergo for the sake of her future child.

Moral obligations to the not-yet-born

It is important to distinguish the question of moral obligation and responsibility from legal obligation. Only the most extreme legal moralist would advocate compelling people to do whatever they morally ought to do. Claims that women have moral obligations to their future children should not be construed as advocating legal coercion.

Thinking about moral obligations to future children in the context of general parental obligations to children prevents sentimentalizing pregnancy and the imposing of especially stringent obligations on pregnant women, or thinking that pregnant women are morally required to subordinate all their interests to their fetuses. After all, parents are not morally required to avoid any and all risks to their children's health. The obligation is, rather, to avoid *unreasonable* risks of *substantial* harm.

With a few notable exceptions (King, 1979; Robertson, 1982; Shaw, 1984), most commentators have argued that a pregnant woman should not be forced to undergo medical treatment even when this is judged necessary to preserve the life or health or her fetus (Annas, 1982; Gallagher, 1987; Johnsen, 1986; Nelson and Milliken, 1988; Rhoden, 1986, 1987). Cesarean sections are major surgery and, while generally very safe, are associated with higher rates of maternal mortality, morbidity, and increased pain than occur with vaginal delivery. Requiring a woman to undergo a cesarean requires her to risk her own life and health for the sake of her not-yet-born child. This is contrary to our legal tradition, which forbids the forced use of the body of one person to save another. In one widely cited case, *Shimp v. McFall* (10 Pa. D. & C.3d 90 [1978]), a court refused to order David Shimp to donate bone marrow to his cousin, Robert McFall, who was dying of aplastic anemia. The court emphasized that there is no legal duty to rescue others. It would seem to follow that compelling a pregnant woman to undergo medical treatment for the sake of the fetus, when this is not required of other potential rescuers, violates equal protection.

There are compelling arguments against the government's using coercive and punitive measures to regulate women's actions in order to promote healthy births. Most people do not want to live in a society in which they can be compelled to undergo surgery or to sacrifice body parts, even if it would be morally incumbent on them to do so. Placing limits on what can be demanded of citizens, especially where bodily integrity is involved, is essential to a free society. This helps to justify the conviction that people are not legally obligated to donate parts of their bodies, even if others need them for life itself.

The situation is different when we consider people's moral obligations. While an absolute ban on forced donation seems the correct legal response, a balancing approach seems more appropriate from a moral perspective. Whether one has a moral obligation to donate a body part, or undergo invasive surgery, depends on the degree of risk and sacrifice incurred, balanced against the need of the endangered individual. Perhaps people are morally required to donate replenishable body parts, such as blood, to others who need it. Blood donation takes only an hour, has no lasting effects, and causes only slight discomfort to most donors. Where a special relationship exists between the potential donor and the needy person, there may be a moral obligation to incur greater risks and sacrifices. Parents may be thought to have a moral obligation to donate blood and bone marrow, and perhaps even nonreplenishable body parts, such as kidneys, to their children, because of their duty to protect and care for their children, and because parents are supposed to love their children. Certainly a parent who refused to give a kidney to a dying child, saying, "It's my body, and I do not feel like donating," would be rightly regarded as morally deficient.

What are the implications for women whose doctors advise a cesarean section for fetal indications? Most women, faced with the possibility of a stillbirth or having a baby born with cerebral palsy, readily consent to the treatment their doctors recommend. Occasionally, however, a woman rejects a physician's recommendation. The moral justifiability of her refusal depends largely on her reasons for refusing. Typically, women who refuse cesareans do so out of religious objections, concern for their own health, or belief that a vaginal birth is best for the baby, and they disagree with the doctors' assessment of the risk. These are not selfish or unimportant reasons. Refusing a cesarean for such reasons is not obviously immoral. By contrast, it would be immoral for a woman to refuse a cesarean, and risk having her nearly born child die or suffer permanent disability, for a trivial reason, such as wanting to avoid a scar in order to be able to wear a bikini. One can morally condemn such a refusal, even if one thinks that she should not be compelled to submit to a cesarean.

"Lifestyle cases," where the risk to the child comes from nonessential behavior, such as drinking alcohol, smoking tobacco, or using drugs, present a different situation. In lifestyle cases, the welfare of the future child appears paramount. If the woman forgoes these substances, the only harm done to her is loss of pleasure and choice—in fact, abstention is likely to benefit her physically—while the potential harm to the child is serious. On the other hand, when the risk to the fetus is slight, the obligation of the pregnant woman is less clear.

Consider, for example, drinking during pregnancy. Heavy drinking during pregnancy can cause fetal alcohol syndrome (FAS), which is typically marked by severe facial deformities and mental retardation. One study showed that even moderate drinking—defined as one to three drinks daily—during early pregnancy can result in a lowering of IQ by as much as five points (Streissguth et al., 1989). Perhaps most important, there is no established "safe" level of alcohol consumption. While there is no evidence that a rare single drink during pregnancy does damage, there is no guarantee that it does not. The safest course is therefore total abstention. But is the safest course the morally obligatory one? We do not require this standard of parents regarding their already born children. Having a single drink occasionally in pregnancy is arguably morally permissible, primarily because the risk of causing harm is very low (perhaps nonexistent), but also because the nature of the harm (loss of a few IQ points) is not so serious as to justify moral condemnation. For a child of normal intelligence, the loss of five IQ points is not devastating. (At the same time, five IQ points can mean the difference between a mildly and a severely retarded child.)

If the occasional drink should be considered a matter of individual discretion, binge drinking, which has a 35 percent chance of subjecting a baby to full-blown FAS, clearly qualifies as an unreasonable risk to the health of a baby. So does smoking crack cocaine. Whether women have a moral obligation not to drink heavily or smoke crack during pregnancy is profoundly complicated by the fact that these behaviors are often the product of addictions. They are less than fully voluntary—some would say they are not voluntary at all. If a woman cannot modify her behavior, then she cannot have a moral obligation to do so.

But is it true that someone who is addicted cannot modify his or her behavior? The distinction should be drawn between being able to stop doing something at will, and not being able to stop at all. Although it is difficult to get over addictions, many smokers, alcoholics, and drug users do manage to change their behaviors. We can recognize that it may be very difficult for some women to fulfill their moral obligations to the babies they intend to bear, and acknowledge that they will need help to do so, without denying that they have such obligations.

Should drug or alcohol treatment be imposed on addicted pregnant women? Perhaps—if it could be shown that coerced treatment works, and therefore protects babies from prenatal harm. However, discussion of the justifiability of coerced treatment seems premature when there are not enough treatment programs for pregnant addicts who want to get over their addictions. Many inpatient alcohol rehabilitation programs exclude pregnant women, largely due to a fear of liability. The situation is even worse for pregnant drug addicts (Chavkin, 1990); sudden withdrawal of drugs can be as damaging to the fetus as continued exposure. As a result, a few treatment programs are able or willing to treat pregnant addicts. Even in areas where there are such treatment programs, there are not nearly enough spaces for all who want help. The absence of treatment programs makes it virtually impossible for substance abusers to fulfill their moral obligations to the children they intend to bear, even with the best will in the world.

To summarize, all women who intend to bear children have moral obligations to protect those children from the serious risk of substantial harm. Heavy smoking, binge drinking, and use of drugs such as crack cocaine and heroin constitute such risks. However, the moral wrongness of engaging in such behaviors during pregnancy is affected by the woman's ability to stop. A woman who is not addicted to cocaine, but who goes on using it during her pregnancy (perhaps on the weekends, because she enjoys it), fully aware of the risks she imposes on her future child, acts very wrongly indeed, and is properly blamed. It would be inappropriate similarly to condemn the pregnant woman who wants what's best for her baby and tries to get help with her addiction, only to be turned away because of the dearth of drug programs. Such a woman is trying to do the right thing; blame properly belongs with society for failing to help her. Nevertheless, if her baby is born damaged due to her drug use, she will—and should—feel moral regret at the harm caused by her drug habit, even if she should not be blamed.

The intention to bear a child

Some people object to making the future child, rather than the fetus, the locus of moral obligation, on the grounds that the existence of the future child depends entirely on the pregnant woman's decision. These critics find it unacceptable that a woman can avoid her obligations to her not-yet-born child by ensuring that it not be born (that is, by aborting it). Moreover, a woman may decide to abort, but later change her mind and continue the pregnancy. During the period when she thought she would have an abortion, she may have continued to smoke and drink. As long as she did not intend to bring a child into the world, there was no one for whose sake she should abstain; continuing to smoke or drink seems morally acceptable in this light. Yet if she changes her mind and continues the pregnancy, she may have harmed the child she bears. Is she now morally blameworthy for the harm she causes?

Two responses can be made. The first is to recognize that moral responsibility for outcomes can extend beyond harms knowingly risked, to harms unintentionally caused. The fact that a woman did not intend to continue a pregnancy at the time she engaged in heavy drinking or used drugs does not entirely absolve her from blame. Even though she does not intend to have a baby at the time of the risky behavior, the failure to consider the possibility that she might change her mind may be negligent, and thus blameworthy. The second response concerns the futility of crying over spilt milk. It says that there is nothing a woman can do about her past behavior, and that if she changes her mind and decides to carry the pregnancy to term, she should focus on what she can do to ensure her baby's health. For example, giving up smoking in the second or third trimester gives the not-yet-born child a better chance than continuing to smoke throughout the pregnancy. If, despite her efforts, the baby is born damaged (a fairly unlikely result), the woman does not completely escape responsibility, but her blameworthiness is mitigated by the fact that she acted rightly once she decided to continue the pregnancy.

Another objection to making "the child she intends to bear" rather than the fetus the object of the pregnant woman's moral obligation is that often women do not "intend" to bear children. Drug addicts, in particular, may regard pregnancy as something that "happens" to them, often as a result of bartering their bodies for drugs, rather than something they intend. Nor do they necessarily choose to give birth: They may not be able to afford an abortion, or it may not be available in a particular geographical area. For some women, abortion is not a morally or culturally acceptable option. Do restrictions on the choice of whether to bear a child affect the woman's moral obligations to the child she bears? It can be argued that these restrictions do not affect how the woman ought to act, but they may affect how much she is to be blamed if she acts wrongly.

Consider a woman who deliberately gets pregnant, intending to have a baby. If she goes on drinking and smoking and using recreational drugs, knowing of the possible effects on her baby's health and making no effort to stop, she acts very wrongly indeed. By contrast, consider a woman who has no responsibility for becoming pregnant (she was raped), in a jurisdiction that prohibits abortion. She is the victim of two grave injustices, first in being raped and second in being denied an abor-

tion. Still, that would not justify behavior likely to inflict severe damage on the child she will perforce bear. Ideally, she should behave as if the pregnancy were chosen, since she is prevented from terminating the pregnancy. That is, she should stop smoking, drink moderately or not at all, and so on. However, her failure to do so is certainly less blameworthy than the failure of a woman who has chosen to conceive and bear a child. Most cases will fall somewhere in between the extremes of deliberate conception and forced childbirth. In general, the fewer options a woman has regarding pregnancy and childbirth, the less she deserves blame for failing to fulfill her obligations to her future child. However, women are not relieved of moral responsibility simply because they do not see pregnancy as a choice.

Conclusion

Deciding to have a baby carries with it certain moral responsibilities. Children have a moral right to be protected from harm, whether inflicted post- or prenatally. This right to be free from harm imposes obligations on those in a position to protect children, including their mothers during pregnancy. Yet a single-minded focus on the risk of harm to the future child ignores the impact on the pregnant woman. She is not a "fetal container" but an individual in her own right, one whose interests must be considered in determining morally permissible options.

Another factor in determining the moral obligations of pregnant women to their future children is the degree of risk and the nature of the harm. Just as parents are not morally required to avoid any and all risks to their born children, neither are pregnant women morally obligated to curtail their own interests to avoid even the slightest risk of harm.

Distinct from the question of the obligations women have to their future children is the issue of their blameworthiness for failing to fulfill those obligations. In general, blameworthiness is mitigated by the inability to have done otherwise. Such factors as addiction and the degree of control over reproductive ability must be considered in assessing morally the conduct of pregnant women.

BONNIE STEINBOCK

Directly related to this article are the other articles in this entry: MEDICAL ASPECTS, *and* LEGAL AND REGULATORY ISSUES. *Also directly related is the entry* FETUS. *For a further discussion of topics mentioned in this article, see the entries* ABORTION; FREEDOM AND COERCION; FUTURE GENERATIONS, OBLIGATIONS TO; HARM; PROFESSIONAL–PATIENT RELATIONSHIP, *article on* ETHICAL ISSUES; RESPONSIBILITY; *and* SUBSTANCE ABUSE. *For a discussion of related ideas, see the entries* FEMINISM; *and*

PATIENTS' RESPONSIBILITIES. *Other relevant material may be found under the entries* AUTONOMY; BEHAVIOR CONTROL; HEALTH PROMOTION AND HEALTH EDUCATION; JUSTICE; LAW AND BIOETHICS; LAW AND MORALITY; OBLIGATION AND SUPEREROGATION; PATERNALISM; RIGHTS; *and* WOMEN, *article on* HEALTHCARE ISSUES.

Bibliography

ANNAS, GEORGE J. 1982. "Forced Cesareans: The Most Unkindest Cut of All." *Hastings Center Report* 12, no. 3:16–17, 45.

———. 1986. "Pregnant Women as Fetal Containers." *Hastings Center Report* 16, no. 6:13–14.

BAYS, JAN. 1990. "Substance Abuse and Child Abuse: Impact of Addiction on the Child." *Pediatric Clinics of North America* 37, no. 4:881–904.

CHAVKIN, WENDY. 1990. "Drug Addiction and Pregnancy: Policy Crossroads." *American Journal of Public Health* 80, no. 4:483–487.

CHERVENAK, FRANK A., and McCULLOUGH, LAURENCE B. 1991. "Justified Limits on Refusing Intervention." *Hastings Center Report* 21, no. 2:12–18.

GALLAGHER, JANET. 1987. "Prenatal Invasions & Interventions: What's Wrong with Fetal Rights." *Harvard Women's Law Journal* 10:9–58.

JOHNSEN, DAWN. 1986. "The Creation of Fetal Rights: Conflicts with Women's Constitutional Rights to Liberty, Privacy, and Equal Protection." *Yale Law Journal* 95:599–625.

KING, PATRICIA A. 1979. "The Juridical Status of the Fetus: A Proposal for Legal Protection of the Unborn." *Michigan Law Review* 77:1647–1687.

"Maternal Rights and Fetal Wrongs: The Case Against the Criminalization of 'Fetal Abuse.'" 1988. *Harvard Law Review* 101:994–1012.

MATHIEU, DEBORAH. 1991. *Preventing Prenatal Harm: Should the State Intervene?* Dordrecht, Netherlands: Kluwer.

MOSS, KARY L. 1990. "Substance Abuse During Pregnancy." *Harvard Women's Law Journal* 13:278–299.

MURRAY, THOMAS H. 1987. "Moral Obligations to the Not-Yet Born: The Fetus as Patient." *Clinics in Perinatology* 14, no. 2:329–343.

NELSON, LAWRENCE J., and MILLIKEN, NANCY. 1988. "Compelled Medical Treatment of Pregnant Women: Life, Liberty, and Law in Conflict." *Journal of the American Medical Association* 259, no. 7:1060–1066.

RHODEN, NANCY K. 1986. "The Judge in the Delivery Room: The Emergence of Court-Ordered Cesareans." *California Law Review* 74, no. 6:1951–2030.

———. 1987. "Cesareans and Samaritans." *Law, Medicine & Health Care* 15, no. 3:118–125.

ROBERTSON, JOHN A. 1982. "The Right to Procreate and In Utero Fetal Therapy." *Journal of Legal Medicine* 3, no. 3:333–366.

SACK, KEVIN. 1991. "Unlikely Union in Albany: Feminists and Liquor Sellers." *New York Times*, April 5, p. B1.

SHAW, MARGERY W. 1984. "Conditional Prospective Rights of the Fetus." *Journal of Legal Medicine* 5, no. 1:63–116.

STEINBOCK, BONNIE. 1992. "Maternal-Fetal Conflict." In her *Life Before Birth: The Moral and Legal Status of Embryos and Fetuses,* pp. 127–163. New York: Oxford University Press.

STREISSGUTH, ANN P.; BARR, HELEN M.; SAMPSON, PAUL D.; DARBY, BETTY L.; and MARTIN, DONALD C. 1989. "I.Q. at Age 4 in Relation to Maternal Alcohol Use and Smoking During Pregnancy." *Developmental Psychology* 25:3–11.

III. LEGAL AND REGULATORY ISSUES

The intimate relationship between a woman and a fetus developing within her body has long given rise to vital questions of morality, religion, science, medicine, law, and public policy. The United States in the early 1980s witnessed a new strand of legal and public policy issues—separate from the issue of abortion—concerning the maternal–fetal relationship when women continue pregnancy and give birth. Courts, legislatures, and state prosecutors increasingly sought to compel women to behave in ways deemed likely to promote the birth of healthy babies. Women faced pregnancy-related restrictions and penalties, including civil suit, criminal prosecution, and court-ordered surgery, aimed at a wide range of conduct: driving an automobile, failing to follow a doctor's advice, drinking alcohol, and taking prescription and illegal drugs, among others. This article describes the status of such efforts and explores the implications for children's well-being and women's liberty.

Biological aspects of the maternal–fetal relationship

Beliefs about the independent moral and religious status of the fetus vary widely among Americans. The physical status, however, is clear: A fetus cannot exist apart from a particular woman prior to "viability," which occurs at approximately twenty-four to twenty-eight weeks' gestational age. Only the pregnant woman can sustain a fetus's growth and meet its needs. That a fetus does not and cannot exist wholly apart from a woman makes the maternal–fetal relationship unique.

During pregnancy, a woman and the fetus developing within her body profoundly affect each other. A fetus makes unparalleled physical and psychological demands on a woman, subjecting her body to tremendous physical adjustments and creating significant risks for even the healthiest woman. Concomitantly, with the fetus completely dependent upon and entirely within a particular woman's body, her actions, experiences, and physical health during and even prior to pregnancy substantially affect fetal development and the health of her child at birth. Throughout their reproductive lives, women inevitably confront innumerable decisions, large and small, that create varying probabilities of harm or benefit to fetal development.

The biological realities of the maternal–fetal relationship may not dictate any particular social response, but they highlight the need to scrutinize the impact on women of any law or policy aimed at fetuses. If not formulated with care, governmental policies adopted to promote healthy births can substantially and unnecessarily intrude on women's fundamental liberties and ability to decide how to live their lives, and may in fact decrease the likelihood of healthy births.

Law versus morality

In general, women have a strong interest in giving birth to healthy children and go to great lengths to increase the likelihood that they will do so. Widespread consensus exists that a woman who chooses to bear a child has a moral obligation to consider the effects her actions will have on her future child. Current public policy recognizes a role for the government in supporting women's ability to have the healthy pregnancies they desire. Existing programs seek to help women overcome obstacles such as poverty and dangerous addictions by providing prenatal care, food, housing, and drug and alcohol treatment, though the adequacy and appropriate scope of such programs is hotly debated.

Far more controversial are the rare instances when governmental action coerces rather than supports, and seeks to compel women to change their behavior. Should the government use punitive measures to regulate women's actions in an effort to promote healthy births? Should the government thereby transform women's moral obligations into legally required standards of conduct?

The current U.S. legal system generally deems the pregnant woman the proper person to make decisions during pregnancy and does not recognize competing fetal rights that would provide a basis for overriding her decisions. Women retain the freedom to make their own judgments and to balance their obligations to their future children against other responsibilities, such as to family and to work. This approach is consistent with women's constitutional rights to liberty, privacy, and equal protection, guaranteed by the U.S. Constitution as well as by state constitutions.

Beginning in the early 1980s, however, some commentators called for greater regulation of women's actions during pregnancy (Shaw, 1984; Robertson, 1983). Arguing that fetuses, as future children, deserve legal protection from their mothers, they advocate that women be held liable for actions during pregnancy that may be harmful to fetal development. Many more commentators have opposed adversarial approaches, arguing that they not only infringe on women's freedoms but also

are ineffective, even counterproductive, in promoting healthy births (Johnsen, 1986, 1992; American Medical Association [AMA], 1990; Annas, 1987; Gallagher, 1987). The remainder of this article examines some particular forms of pregnancy-related restrictions aimed at women, including exclusionary employment policies, civil suits for prenatal injuries, criminal prosecution, loss of child custody, and court-ordered surgery.

Exclusionary employment policies

The U.S. Supreme Court has not directly considered the constitutionality of a governmentally imposed pregnancy-related restriction. The Court, however, has reviewed the legality of a private employer's exclusion of all fertile women from employment viewed as potentially harmful to fetal development (*International Union, United Auto Workers* [UAW] v. *Johnson Controls*, 1991). The Supreme Court ruled in March 1991 that a policy prohibiting fertile women from working in positions where they would be exposed to lead discriminated against women on the basis of pregnancy, in violation of a federal antidiscrimination law. Although a private employer's policy was at issue, some of the reasoning of the Supreme Court and the lower appellate court applies equally to governmental attempts to regulate women's decisions and actions for the sake of the health of their future children.

The Supreme Court acknowledged that "[e]mployment late in pregnancy often imposes risks on the unborn child," but found that "Congress made clear that the decision to become pregnant or to work while being either pregnant or capable of becoming pregnant was reserved for each individual woman to make for herself." The Court implied that the individuals most directly affected, rather than a court or employer, are best situated to balance competing factors and make such decisions: "Decisions about the welfare of future children must be left to the parents who conceive, bear, support, and raise them rather than to the employers who hire those parents" (*International Union, UAW* v. *Johnson Controls*, 1991, pp. 205–206).

Two lower court opinions in the case highlight the difficulties and dangers of allowing anyone other than the woman directly affected to make these judgments. Judge Frank Easterbrook noted: "How does the risk attributable to lead compare, say, to . . . driving a taxi? A female bus or taxi driver is exposed to noxious fumes and the risk of accidents, all hazardous to a child she carries. Would it follow that taxi and bus companies can decline to hire women? That an employer could forbid pregnant employees to drive cars because of the risk accidents pose to fetuses?" (*International Union, UAW* v. *Johnson Controls*, 1991, p. 917). Judge Richard Cudahy asked: "What is the situation of the pregnant woman, unemployed or working for the minimum wage and unprotected by health insurance, in relation to her pregnant sister, exposed to an indeterminate lead risk but well-fed, housed, and doctored? Whose fetus is at greater risk? Whose decision is this to make?" (*International Union, UAW v. Johnson Controls*, 1991, p. 902).

Civil suits for prenatal injuries

The same issues of personal autonomy are implicated by proposals to subject women to civil liability if they fail to comply with prescribed standards of behavior during and even prior to pregnancy—by creating, for example, legally enforceable "prenatal duties" (Shaw, 1984, p. 83) or a "duty to bring the child into the world as healthy as is reasonably possible" (Robertson, 1983, p. 438). The only appellate court to adopt such a standard, a Michigan appellate court, ruled in 1980 that a child could sue his mother for prenatal injuries if she failed to comply with the standard of a "reasonable" pregnant woman (*Grodin v. Grodin*, 1980). The only state supreme court to consider the issue, the supreme court of Illinois, ruled in 1988 that a child could not sue her mother for prenatal injuries allegedly caused when the woman was in an automobile accident while she was pregnant. In rejecting the girl's request to recognize a legal right to begin life with a sound mind and body, the Illinois court noted the serious ramifications that would result for women: "[M]other and child would be legal adversaries from the moment of conception until birth" (*Stallman v. Youngquist*, 1988, p. 359). Any one of a woman's many decisions that could affect fetal development might later be scrutinized by a judge or jury acting with the benefit of hindsight.

In this arena, women rarely face an isolated decision for which there is a clear "right" answer. Rather, women make inherently complex judgments that balance competing interests and are fraught with uncertainty as to the likely effects on fetal development. Courts, legislatures, and private employers are not better situated than the woman whose life and liberty are at issue to make the judgments—whether and where to work, when to take what medication, whether to spend limited resources on prenatal care or food for herself or her children—that necessarily vary from case to case according to each woman's circumstances.

Criminal prosecutions for actions during pregnancy

The most common form of adversarial governmental action against women for engaging in behavior viewed as harmful to fetal development has been criminal prosecution. State prosecutors have relied on laws that clearly were not intended to create special restrictions on women's actions during pregnancy, including laws prohibiting child abuse, distributing drugs to a minor, or murder.

Several prosecutions have been based on women's otherwise lawful actions. One of the first occurred in 1986, when a California woman was prosecuted for allegedly causing her infant son to be born severely brain damaged, and ultimately to die, as a result of her own excessive loss of blood during delivery. The prosecution claimed that, by waiting a number of hours before obtaining medical care when she went into labor and began bleeding vaginally, the woman had violated a statute that required parents to provide their children with clothing, food, shelter, and medical care. Other prosecutions have involved alcohol use during pregnancy. A Massachusetts woman who suffered serious injuries in a car accident, including a miscarriage, was prosecuted for involuntary manslaughter of the fetus because she allegedly caused the accident by driving while intoxicated. In another reported case, a pregnant woman in Wyoming who notified the police that her husband had physically assaulted her was arrested for child abuse when they detected she had been drinking. The charges were ultimately dismissed in all three of these cases (Johnsen, 1992).

In many more cases, women have been prosecuted for using illegal drugs while pregnant. Of course, a woman's pregnancy does not immunize her from prosecution under generally applicable laws prohibiting the use or possession of drugs. In some cases, however, women were subjected to special prosecutions and greater penalties for the express reason that they were pregnant at the time they used drugs. Although some pleaded guilty in return for reduced sentences, women have prevailed in the overwhelming majority of cases where they challenged the prosecution because the statutes were not intended to apply to prenatal behavior (Johnsen, 1992).

Both of the two high state courts that have considered such a case ruled that the statute had been misapplied. In 1992, the supreme court of Ohio dismissed an indictment for child endangerment against a woman who allegedly used cocaine while pregnant (*Ohio v. Gray*, 1992). Also in 1992, the supreme court of Florida reversed a woman's conviction under a statute prohibiting the distribution of a controlled substance to a minor and imposing a penalty of up to thirty years' imprisonment. In holding that the statute was not intended to apply to prenatal behavior, the court rejected the "State's invitation to walk down a path that the law, public policy, reason and common sense forbid it to tread" (*Johnson v. State*, 1992, p. 1297).

Loss of child custody for actions during pregnancy

States have attempted to deprive women of custody of their children based solely on women's actions during pregnancy, rather than on the customary determination of the current ability of the woman and other family members to care for the child. While most cases involved a woman's use of illegal drugs during pregnancy, several courts have based custody decisions on activity that was lawful but seen as detrimental to fetal development. For example, in 1987 a Michigan woman temporarily lost custody of her infant and was charged with child abuse because while pregnant she had taken Valium without a prescription to relieve pain from injuries she suffered in a car accident (*In re J. Jeffrey*, 1987).

The first high state court to consider this issue, the supreme court of Connecticut, ruled in 1992 that state law did not allow the termination of parental rights based on a woman's use of cocaine during pregnancy. The court concluded that the legislature had determined that the threat of loss of custody of their children would cause women to avoid prenatal care and substance abuse treatment and "would lead to more, rather than fewer, babies being born either without adequate prenatal care or damaged by prenatal drug abuse, or both" (*In re Valerie D.*, 1992, p. 764).

Although the use of illegal drugs during pregnancy may at first glance seem to be the strongest justification for punitive governmental action such as the imposition of enhanced criminal penalties or deprivation of child custody, these approaches have been widely repudiated. The government clearly has a strong interest in preventing pregnant women from using dangerous drugs. Commentators, however, have with remarkable consistency agreed that this interest is best pursued through programs that help women overcome drug and alcohol dependencies and obtain prenatal care. Entities such as the U.S. General Accounting Office (GAO) and the AMA have argued that fear of prosecution and loss of custody of their children will discourage women from seeking care and increase the number of unhealthy births (GAO, 1990; AMA, 1990). As the Florida Supreme Court noted: "Rather than face the possibility of prosecution, pregnant women who are substance abusers may simply avoid prenatal care or medical care for fear of being detected. Yet the newborns of these women are, as a group, the most fragile and sick, and most in need of hospital neonatal care" (*Johnson v. State*, 1992, pp. 1295–1296).

Court-ordered cesarean sections

Courts in at least eleven states have ordered women against their wishes to give birth by cesarean section rather than vaginal delivery (Kilder et al., 1987). The severe bodily intrusion of this court-ordered surgery contrasts sharply with our legal system's general refusal to order invasive medical procedures or to force one person to assume any personal risk to save the life of another. Although judicial opinions are rare in these time-pressured cases, three published appellate court decisions illustrate both the motivations behind and the harm caused by such court orders.

In the first published appellate court decision, the supreme court of Georgia in 1981 declined to lift a court order authorizing the performance of a cesarean section against a woman's religious objections where the examining physician found a "ninety-nine percent certainty" that the child would not survive a vaginal delivery and a 50 percent chance the woman would die (*Jefferson v. Griffin Spalding County Hospital Authority*, 1981, p. 459). With no analysis of the constitutional and policy implications, the court granted "temporary custody" of the fetus to the state and gave it full authority to make all surgical decisions concerning the birth. In the end, a court-ordered cesarean section was not performed; despite the physician's predictions, the woman gave birth by vaginal delivery to a healthy baby without adverse effects.

Both appellate courts that have considered the constitutionality of a coerced cesarean section declared it unconstitutional (*In re A.C.*, 1990; *Baby Boy Doe*, 1994). In the first, a District of Columbia court ordered a woman who was twenty-six weeks pregnant and terminally ill with cancer to undergo the surgery. The woman did not consent to the cesarean and her husband, parents, and attending physicians all opposed it on the ground that the woman's health and comfort should be the first priority. The cesarean section was performed nonetheless. The fetus was not viable and did not survive. The woman died two days after the cesarean section. After the woman's death, a three-judge panel of the D.C. Court of Appeals issued an opinion explaining why it had affirmed the order. The Court acknowledged, ". . . [w]e well know that we may have shortened [her] life span," but found that, because she was likely to die soon of cancer, the value of the woman's life was outweighed by the fetus's admittedly "slim" chance of survival (*In re A.C.*, 1987, pp. 613–614).

The full D.C. Court of Appeals reversed the decision of the three-judge panel, ruling that "in virtually all cases the question of what is to be done is to be decided by the patient—the pregnant woman—on behalf of herself and the fetus" (*In re A.C.*, 1990, p. 1237). The court found that a court order compelling a woman to have a cesarean section violates her rights to bodily integrity and to refuse medical treatment, protected under both common law and the U.S. Constitution. The court graphically described the violent bodily intrusion that would be required to enforce an order against a woman who resisted: "[She] would have to be fastened with restraints to the operating table, or perhaps involuntarily rendered unconscious by forcibly injecting her with an anesthetic, and then subjected to unwanted major surgery. Such actions would surely give one pause in a civilized society . . ." (*In re A.C.*, 1990, p. 1244, n.

8). Indeed, in another case a court-ordered cesarean section was performed by tying the woman to the operating table and forcibly removing her husband from the room (Gallagher, 1987).

An Illinois appellate court similarly ruled in 1994 that ordering a woman to give birth by cesarean section would violate her constitutional rights. Citing *In re A.C.*, the court held that "a woman's competent choice in refusing medical treatment as invasive as a cesarean section during her pregnancy must be honored, even in circumstances where the choice may be harmful to her fetus" (*Doe*, 1994, p. 330). The woman's physician had testified that the chances that the fetus would survive a natural labor were close to zero. In fact, the woman vaginally delivered a healthy baby three weeks after the state unsuccessfully sought the court order (*Doe*, 1994).

A number of medical and public-health organizations have opposed court orders overriding a pregnant woman's decision concerning medical treatment. The AMA is among the organizations that has endorsed respect for women's constitutional right to bodily integrity: "[D]ecisions that would result in health risks are properly made only by the individual who must bear the risk. Considerable uncertainty can surround medical evaluations of the risks and benefits of obstetrical interventions. Through a court-ordered intervention, a physician deprives a pregnant woman of her right to reject personal risk and replaces it with the physician's evaluation of the amount of risk that is properly acceptable" (AMA, 1990, p. 2665). The practice of seeking court orders not only violates women's right to evaluate the risks and uncertainties involved in their medical care, it is counterproductive to the goal of promoting healthy pregnancies and births because it causes women to distrust physicians. Citing a case in which a woman left the hospital to avoid a court-ordered cesarean section, the AMA expressed concern that "women may withhold information from the physician. . . . Or they may reject medical or prenatal care altogether . . ." (AMA, 1990, pp. 2665–2666).

Gender and racial disparities

Pregnancy-related restrictions and penalties directed at women raise serious concerns about gender discrimination. As the Supreme Court noted in the 1991 *Johnson Controls* case, the company's justification for excluding women from jobs for the good of their future children echoed the nineteenth-century rationale for restricting women's ability to work outside the home or participate in political or civic affairs. Virtually all attempts to impose special behavioral restrictions in order to improve infant health have been targeted solely at women, even where evidence suggests that the activity at issue can cause damage to sperm, as is the case for exposure to lead, smoking, drinking alcohol, and using certain drugs.

Significant evidence reveals that pregnancy-related restrictions also have been imposed in a racially discriminatory manner. A 1987 survey of court-ordered cesarean sections published in the *New England Journal of Medicine* found that 80 percent of the women against whom orders were sought were African-American or Asian (Kolder et al., 1987). A 1990 study, also published in the *New England Journal of Medicine*, found that African-American women were ten times more likely than white women to be reported to health authorities when they tested positive for illegal drug use during pregnancy (Chasnoff et al., 1990). Another 1990 survey of forty-seven women prosecuted for behavior during pregnancy found that 80 percent of the prosecutions were against women of color (Paltrow, 1992).

Conclusion

Attempts to impose special pregnancy-related restrictions or penalties on women have been relatively rare and typically have been invalidated by courts and opposed by interested organizations and most commentators. The threat of criminal prosecution, loss of custody of children, and court-ordered medical interventions would likely deter the women who are most at risk of poor birth outcomes from seeking prenatal care and drug and alcohol treatment.

The government can, however, do a great deal to improve the health of children by helping women to have healthy pregnancies. For example, experts agree that the high rate of infant mortality in the United States can be drastically cut by providing prenatal care to the approximately one-third of American women who receive inadequate or no prenatal care. Drug treatment programs routinely turn away pregnant women, and the few that will treat women during pregnancy have long waiting lists. Government studies have shown that expending the funds necessary to provide these services would actually save taxpayers three to four times as much in reduced infant health-care costs.

While creating legal conflicts between a woman and the fetus within her is ineffective and even counterproductive, laws and policies that respect women's rights can effectively promote the healthy pregnancies and births that are in the interests of all.

DAWN E. JOHNSEN

Dawn E. Johnsen is Deputy Assistant Attorney General, Office of Legal Counsel, United States Department of Justice. The views expressed here do not necessarily reflect the positions of the Department of Justice of the United States.

Directly related to this article are the other articles in this entry: MEDICAL ASPECTS, *and* ETHICAL ISSUES. *Also directly related to this article is the entry* FETUS. *For a further discussion of topics mentioned in this article, see the entries* ABORTION; ABUSE, INTERPERSONAL, *article on* CHILD ABUSE; AUTONOMY; BEHAVIOR CONTROL; FAMILY; FREEDOM AND COERCION; FUTURE GENERATIONS, OBLIGATIONS TO; HARM; OBLIGATION AND SUPEREROGATION; RACE AND RACISM; SEXISM; SUBSTANCE ABUSE; SURGERY; *and* WOMEN, *especially the articles on* HISTORICAL AND CROSS-CULTURAL PERSPECTIVES, *and* HEALTH-CARE ISSUES. *For a discussion of related ideas, see the entries* BODY; CHILDREN; CONFLICT OF INTEREST; DOUBLE EFFECT; ETHICS, *article on* RELIGION AND MORALITY; FERTILITY CONTROL; GENETIC COUNSELING; GENETIC TESTING AND SCREENING; OCCUPATIONAL SAFETY AND HEALTH, *article on* ETHICAL ISSUES; PATERNALISM; PATIENTS' RESPONSIBILITIES; PERSON; REPRODUCTIVE TECHNOLOGIES; *and* RIGHTS.

Bibliography

A.C., In re. 1990. 573 A.2d 1235 (D.C.) (en banc), *reversing,* 533 A.2d 611 (D.C. 1987).

AMERICAN MEDICAL ASSOCIATION BOARD OF TRUSTEES. 1990. "Legal Interventions During Pregnancy: Court-Ordered Medical Treatments and Legal Penalties for Potentially Harmful Behavior by Pregnant Women." *Journal of the American Medical Association* 264, no. 20:2663–2670.

ANNAS, GEORGE J. 1987. "Protecting the Liberty of Pregnant Patients." *New England Journal of Medicine* 316, no. 19:1213–1214.

Baby Boy Doe v. Mother Doe. 1994. 260 Ill. App. 3d 392, 632 N.E.2d 326 (Ill. App.).

CHASNOFF, IRA J.; LANDRESS, HARVEY J.; and BARRETT, MARK E. 1990. "The Prevalence of Illicit-Drug or Alcohol Use During Pregnancy and Discrepancies in Mandatory Reporting in Pinellas County, Florida." *New England Journal of Medicine* 322, no. 17:1202–1206.

GALLAGHER, JANET. 1987. "Prenatal Invasions and Interventions: What's Wrong with Fetal Rights." *Harvard Women's Law Journal* 10:9–58.

Grodin v. Grodin. 1980. 301 N.W.2d 869 (Mich. App.).

International Union, United Auto Workers (UAW) v. Johnson Controls. 1991. 499 U.S. 187, 113 L Ed 2d 158, Ill S Ct 1196, *reversing,* 886 F.2d 871 (7th Cir. 1989).

Jefferson v. Griffin Spalding County Hospital Authority. 1981. 274 S.E.2d 457 (1981) (per curiam).

J. Jeffrey, In re. 1987. No. 99851 (Mich. Ct. App. April 9).

JOHNSEN, DAWN E. 1986. "The Creation of Fetal Rights: Conflicts with Women's Constitutional Rights to Liberty, Privacy, and Equal Protection." *Yale Law Journal* 95, no. 3:599–625.

———. 1992. "Shared Interests: Promoting Healthy Births Without Sacrificing Women's Liberty." *Hastings Law Journal* 43, no. 3:569–614. Symposium issue on "Substance Use During Pregnancy: Legal and Social Responses."

Johnson v. State. 1992. 602 So. 2d 1288 (Fla.).

KOLDER, VERONICA E. B.; GALLAGHER, JANET; and PARSONS, MICHAEL T. 1987. "Court-Ordered Obstetrical Interventions." *New England Journal of Medicine* 316, no. 19:1192–1196.

Ohio v. Gray. 1992. 584 N.E.2d 710 (Ohio).

PALTROW, LYNN M. 1992. "Criminal Prosecutions Against Pregnant Women: National Update and Overview." New York: Reproductive Freedom Project, American Civil Liberties Union Foundation.

RHODEN, NANCY K. 1986. "The Judge in the Delivery Room: The Emergence of Court-Ordered Cesareans." *California Law Review* 74, no. 6:1951–2030.

ROBERTS, DOROTHY E. 1991. "Punishing Drug Addicts Who Have Babies: Women of Color, Equality and the Right of Privacy." *Harvard Law Review* 104, no. 7:1419–1482.

ROBERTSON, JOHN A. 1983. "Procreative Liberty and the Control of Conception, Pregnancy, and Childbirth." *Virginia Law Review* 69, no. 3:405–464.

SHAW, MARGERY W. 1984. "Conditional Prospective Rights of the Fetus." *Journal of Legal Medicine* 5, no. 1:63–116.

Stallman v. Youngquist. 1988. 125 Ill. 2d 267, 531 N.E.2d 355 (Ill. 1988), *reversing,* 152 Ill. App. 3d 683, 504 N.E.2d 920 (1st Dist. 1987).

UNITED STATES. GENERAL ACCOUNTING OFFICE. 1990. *Drug-Exposed Infants: A Generation at Risk—Report to the Chairman, Committee on Finance, U.S. Senate.* Washington, D.C.: Author.

Valerie D., In re. 1992. 223 Conn. 492, 613 A.2d 748.

MEDIA AND BIOETHICS

See COMMUNICATION, BIOMEDICAL, *article on* MEDIA AND BIOETHICS.

MEDIA AND MEDICINE

See COMMUNICATION, BIOMEDICAL, *article on* MEDIA AND MEDICINE.

MEDICAID

See HEALTH-CARE FINANCING, *article on* MEDICAID.

MEDICAL ANTHROPOLOGY

See MEDICINE, ANTHROPOLOGY OF.

MEDICAL CODES AND OATHS

I. History
> *Robert M. Veatch*

II. Ethical Analysis
> *Robert M. Veatch*

I. HISTORY

The following is a revision and update of the first-edition article "Codes of Medical Ethics: History" by Donald Konold. Portions of the first-edition article appear in the revised version.

In the ethics of health care, explicit statements of ethical standards have been formulated for physicians and members of the other health professions, for persons conducting medical experiments involving human subjects, for administrators, and for patients and other laypeople who make health-care decisions. These have often been written by members of the relevant practitioner group, but they may also be written by members of religious, cultural, national, or international bodies. While codes of ethics have long been regarded as the classic expression of these directives, various principles and rules have also been stated in the form of prayers, oaths, creeds, institutional directives, and statements. Prayers state a very personal commitment of duty; oaths publicly pledge the oath taker to uphold specified responsibilities; and codes provide more comprehensive standards to guide the practicing health practitioner, patient, or other decision maker. Each form of ethical statement implies a moral imperative, either to be accepted by the individual personally or to be enforced by a practitioner organization, religious community, or governmental body.

While practitioner bodies have often assumed responsibility for writing their own codes of ethics for their members, governmental, religious, and cultural bodies have also claimed authority to articulate the moral norms of conduct in health care. Disputes over who has the authority to articulate codifications of ethical duties in the medical sphere reveal important controversies over who can legitimately claim moral authority in determining what these duties are. This article first examines prayers, oaths, and codes written by health providers or practitioner groups, and then examines those written outside the profession.

Documents created by practitioners

Medical prayers. Health-care providers in all ages have composed prayers expressing gratitude for divine blessings and asking for divine inspiration in their practitioner conduct. Such prayers signify that the writer stands within a religious tradition and grounds medical duties in that religion's moral framework.

An ancient Greek poem that has the quality of a prayer or a hymn was found inscribed on a monument in a sanctuary of Asclepias, originally on the south slope of the Acropolis. According to the poem, the physician should be "like God: savior equally of slaves, of paupers, of rich men, of princes, and to all a brother, such help he would give" (Etziony, 1973, p. 21).

Likewise, ancient Jewish sources include texts extolling the physician's healing. An early Jewish prayer was written by the early-twelfth-century Spanish poet, philosopher, and physician Yehuda Halevi (Etziony, 1973). The most widely acclaimed Jewish example is the Daily Prayer of a Physician, once ascribed to the Jewish physician and philosopher Moses Maimonides (1135–1204) but now believed to be the work of the eighteenth-century German Jewish physician Marcus Herz (Rosner, 1967). In the manner of most medical prayers, the Daily Prayer asks for courage, determination, and inspiration to enable the physician to develop skills, meet responsibilities, and heal patients. It commits the physician to place duty to patients above the physician's own concerns and places the physician's healing in clear subordination to divine authority.

Many examples of Christian prayers of physicians exist from ancient and medieval times. More modern prayers sometimes reflect more eclectic, nondenominational perspectives. The theology expressed in the prayers of these physicians, who, theologically, are laypeople, is sometimes not an authoritative reflection of the tradition in which they stand.

Oaths for physicians. In the ancient world physicians often expressed their ethical commitments in the form of oaths, which were an integral part of the initiation ceremony for medical apprentices. Like many medical prayers, ancient oaths reflect the physician's belief that success in the healing profession required an alliance with the deity in the treatment of disease. The ancient oaths often beseech the deity to inspire physicians to fulfill their moral obligations, reward those who honor their sacred trust, and punish those who violate it.

One of the oldest of these oaths, a medical student's oath taken from the *Charaka Samhita* manuscript of ancient India, contains concepts that had pervaded Indian ethical thought for many centuries before their inclusion in the oath at about the beginning of the common era (Menon and Haberman, 1970). Pledging the medical student to live the life of an ascetic and a virtual slave of his preceptor in accordance with Indian custom for apprenticeships, the path requires personal sacrifice and commitment to duty from the student comparable to the physician's responsibilities to patients. By the terms of the oath, the student physician is to place the patient's needs above personal considerations, serving day and night with heart and soul; abstaining from drunkenness, crime, and adultery; and scrupulously observing practitioner secrecy.

In sharp contrast to the medical ethics of the Western world, the Indian oath obliges the physician to deny services to enemies of his ruler, evildoers, unattended women, and those on the point of death. Ancient Indian thought condemned aid to anyone who was immoral or was involved in any circumstance that might suggest illicit sexual contact; it also condemned interference with the process of dying. Despite these differences, the oath of the Indian student reveals significant parallels between the medical ethics of India and those of the Western world, which may suggest a diffusion of ideas, probably from India to the West.

The most enduring medical oath of Western civilization is the Oath of Hippocrates. Despite its renown, its origin is obscure. It is a part of the Hippocratic Collection, which was catalogued and edited by a group of Alexandrian librarians sometime after the fourth century C.E. Copies of these writings available to modern scholars, however, date from the tenth to the fifteenth centuries C.E. and do not preserve the original text with verbal accuracy. None of the manuscripts in this collection can be positively verified as genuine works of the great Greek physician, and clearly the documents are the products of many contributors, with the earliest predating the latest by at least a century.

Twentieth-century scholars, especially Ludwig Edelstein (1943), have suggested that the oath conforms closely to the teachings of Pythagoras (fourth century B.C.E.). He noted the similarities with the principal ethical beliefs of the Pythagoreans, which included reincarnation, avoidance of shedding of blood, prohibition on taking of life, and commitment to sexual purity and secrecy. Edelstein held that the oath was composed by a group of Pythagoreans who practiced the healing arts. More recent historians of medical ethics have argued over whether the dependency is as close as Edelstein maintained, suggesting that the influence of other philosophical/ethical traditions may also be present (Carrick, 1985). Nevertheless, some degree of affinity of Hippocratic with Pythagorean thought is generally conceded. The oath, in accord with Pythagorean ethics, proclaims a more strict morality for physicians than was established by Greek law, Platonic or Aristotelian ethics, or common Greek medical practice.

The Oath of Hippocrates consists of two parts, the first serving as a contractual agreement between pupil and teacher and the second constituting an ethical code. The opening sentences pledge the novice physician (invariably a male) to become an adopted member of his teacher's family, to help support his teacher and his teacher's children in case of need, and to instruct his teacher's children free of charge. The oath forbids sharing the precepts and medical knowledge with anyone who has not taken the oath. Since familial bonds between teacher and pupil implied careful selection of those admitted to the family group, the covenant enabled physicians to prevent unworthy persons from entering the profession and to keep tight control on knowledge transmission.

The ethical code contained in the Oath of Hippocrates places restrictions on the medical techniques of the physician and defines relations with the patient's family. One who takes the oath pledges, "I will apply dietetic measures for the benefit of the sick according to my ability and judgment; I will keep them from harm and injustice" (Edelstein, 1943, p. 3). He also agrees to refuse to dispense poisons or abortive remedies, and to leave surgery (including lithotomy or removal of a stone from the urinary bladder) to those trained in that art. He makes the commitment that "whatever houses I may visit, I will come for the benefit of the sick, remaining free of all intentional injustice" (Edelstein, 1943, p. 3). The taker of the oath swears to abstain from sexual relations with all those in the houses the physician enters. Regarding confidentiality, in an ambiguously qualified way, the physician promises not to disclose that "which on no account one must spread abroad." The oath ends with a plea for reward that is unusually self-serving for a code of ethics: that if the physician keeps the oath he be "honored with fame among all men for all time to come." If he transgresses it, "may the opposite of all this be my lot" (Edelstein, 1943, p. 3).

The oath's provisions contrast sharply with what is otherwise known about ancient Greek medical practice, which permitted physicians to abet suicide and infanticide and to perform surgery. They introduced an element of respect for slave as well as freeman and, even though the secrecy requirement is qualified, it is extended outside the practitioner relationship. These precepts, though they represent the thought of only a small group of medical practitioners, extended their influence beyond the importance of the Hippocratic school of medicine in the ancient world.

For centuries following the appearance of the Hippocratic oath, the practitioners of the medical art showed no inclination to accept it. Hellenistic physicians ignored its injunctions without compunction. It is sometimes held that the rise of Christianity, which had certain ethical positions similar to Hippocratic ethics, is responsible for the ascendancy of the Hippocratic oath (Edelstein, 1943; Carrick, 1985). There is, however, very little evidence of early Christian interest in the Hippocratic oath; increasingly there is emphasis on important ethical differences between the Hippocratic and Christian traditions (Veatch and Mason, 1987). Medical historian Owsei Temkin has identified considerable tension between Hippocratic and Christian medicine and their ethical commitments (Temkin, 1991). One exception to this generalization is the fourth-century Christian figure Jerome, who explicitly mentions the Hippocratic oath, but in doing so he points out that the Christian physician's obligation is even more stringent.

Precisely what happened to bring the oath into prominence during the Middle Ages is uncertain. Perhaps the early post-Constantinian Christian culture found similarities between Christian and Hippocratic views, as has been suggested. A strong case can be made, however, that although there were significant differences between Graeco-Roman and Christian medical ethics, lay physicians were simply not sufficiently schooled in Christian theology to perceive them. One way or another, increased attention to the oath led to renewed interest in it. Modifications were introduced in order to bring it somewhat more into harmony with Christian ideological concepts and practices. This could be taken either as evidence to support the convergence hypothesis or to support the contrary claim that the oath had to be corrected significantly to bring it into harmony with Christian thought.

The earliest of these extant revisions, entitled "From the Oath According to Hippocrates Insofar as a Christian May Swear It" (dating from the tenth or eleventh century), substitutes a statement of Christian adoration of God for the references to the Greek deities in the original oath and replaces its covenant with a statement of teaching responsibilities based on Christian brotherhood, pledging the physician to teach the medical art to whomever wants to learn it (Jones, 1924; Leake, 1927). The injunction against surgery does not appear in this version of the oath. No reason is known for its omission, but later Christian versions do contain it. The appeal for reward and honor for the physician should he follow the oath is abandoned, probably because it is inconsistent with Christian views of grace.

The Oath of Asaf, from the seventh-century *Sefer Asaf* manuscripts of the oldest Hebrew medical work, reveals Hippocratic influences in its injunctions against administering poisons or abortifacient drugs, performing surgery, committing adultery, and betraying practitioner confidences (Rosner and Muntner, 1965). Like the medieval Christian oaths, it is consistent with Talmudic ethics and instructs physicians to give special consideration to the poor and needy, a concern absent from the Hippocratic oath. A revision of the Oath of Hippocrates also appeared in medieval Muslim literature, where the only significant changes replaced references to Greek gods with statements in harmony with Islamic theology. The oath in its original form was also known to Christian and Muslim scholars; however, among the Christian church fathers, only rare mention is made of it. The texts that do refer to the oath reveal a perception of a difference between Hippocratic and Christian medicine.

Following the transition from medieval to modern Western civilization, the Oath of Hippocrates apparently continued to be a model for ethical pledges by physicians. Its legacy is ambiguous. On the one hand, it repudiates exploitation of the sick, often the most vulnerable. On the other hand, it locates all authority about what constitutes a benefit in the physician's "ability and judgment." In this way, the oath has sanctioned a medical paternalism throughout the ages that is in conflict with the modern assertion of the right of patients to determine for themselves the benefits they seek from medical care.

Western medical schools in the eighteenth and nineteenth centuries, seeking to impart high ethical ideals to their students, administered oaths to their graduates. It is unclear whether or how often the Hippocratic oath itself was used, but certainly the typical oaths, such as that of the great medical school of Montpellier, incorporated Hippocratic ideas (Etziony, 1973).

Our knowledge of professional medical ethics in the early modern period is very limited. Historians have not done enough specific research in European and American medical schools and professional societies to know what local religious, philosophical, and political influences helped shape medical education. Additional research is underway. The received tradition holds that Western medical schools, seeking to commit their students to the pursuit of high ethical ideas, continued a tradition begun in the Middle Ages of incorporating Hippocratic concepts in oaths for their graduates, especially the covenant's requirement for the physician to instruct his teacher's children and the ethical injunctions for secrecy and against administering harmful drugs. During the nineteenth century, some medical schools in the United States required their graduates to take the Hippocratic oath in its original form, and that continued to be a common practice in the twentieth century, even though many of the oath's provisions were archaic or offensive to some of the students. A study published in 1991 found that sixty of 141 U.S. medical schools administered the Hippocratic oath (Dickstein et al., 1991).

A document patterned after the Oath of Hippocrates appeared in 1948, when the newly organized World Medical Association adopted the Declaration of Geneva. In 1991 forty-seven U.S. medical schools used it (Dickstein et al., 1991). (Of the remainder, fourteen schools used the Prayer of Maimonides or more recently written oaths.) The declaration attempts to make the original oath applicable to modern conditions of medical practice and diverse cultural, religious, and ethnic groups in the world community. In doing so, it raises serious questions of how any one single ethical text could be made appropriate for a wide range of religious and cultural groups that clearly have fundamental differences, not only about significant medical ethical controversies, but also about the very foundations and meanings of ethical propositions. The Declaration of Geneva is a secular oath that contains no reference to religious tenets or loyalties, thus appealing to secular physicians while perhaps offending those who continue to ground their ethics in some particular religious framework.

Although the claim is made that the Declaration of Geneva simply updates the Hippocratic oath, the reformulation clearly involves significant differences. The declaration commits the physician to make the patient's health his or her first consideration, a provision reminiscent of the Hippocratic oath's pledge to use dietetic measures for the benefit of the sick. But in addition to the secularization of the declaration by the removal of the religious references, the 1948 text deletes the pledge to refuse to reveal information to those who have not taken the oath. The loose Hippocratic pledge of confidentiality is replaced with an exceptionless pledge, one that conflicts with the increasingly recognized necessity of disclosing in order to protect third parties from serious threats of harm, as well as with the more paternalistic exceptions seen in many modern interpretations of the oath. The oath's surgical restriction is also omitted from the declaration, as is the injunction against sexual contact with those in the patient's household.

The physician of the declaration vows not to let considerations of religion, nationality, race, party politics, or social standing interfere with his duty to his patient. Obviously, those who conceived and adopted the declaration found united support for clearer condemnation of these prejudices than the original oath provided. In sharp contrast, however, the declaration's statement of the physician's responsibility regarding suicide, mercy killing, and abortion is obscured in generalities that conceal modern controversy on these matters among physicians and laypeople alike. The physician of the declaration pledges only to maintain respect for human life from the time of conception and not to use medical knowledge in ways that are contrary to the laws of humanity. While the Declaration of Geneva has found some acceptance among medical professional groups, it has not been endorsed by significant national professional associations, and it certainly conflicts with the ethical precepts of many secular and religious groups in both East and West.

Practitioner codes. Physicians of the modern world have not been content with the spiritual inspiration of prayers and the moral commitments of medical oaths. The large medical institutions of urban society have required complex relationships among medical personnel who demand detailed procedures to prevent embarrassing ethical controversy and disruption of services. Lengthy treatises on medical subjects, which had enlightened physicians on ethical matters since the earliest times, were not easy to cite by paragraph and line and frequently concealed ethical instruction in needless verbiage. Reducing these essays to lists of rules, proponents of practitioner control produced elaborate ethical codes.

A code is an ordered collection of injunctions and prohibitions, usually created by an authoritative body and adopted as a statement of ideals and rules for a group or organization. The modern idea of codes derives ultimately from the Renaissance ideal of rationalizing Roman law, putting the diverse parts into some order and stating briefly and clearly the essence of the rule. Sometimes individually authored documents, such as the work of Sun Szu-miao and Thomas Percival discussed below, have taken on the status of systematic codifications.

One of the earliest codes of medical ethics appeared in China, where the Oath of Hippocrates never made a significant impression. From the seventh century, an indigenous Chinese tradition in medical ethics developed in works by Sun Szu-miao. Generally regarded as Taoist, his writing stresses the importance of preserving life and the subordination of self-interest to compassion for the patient. It reflects the differentiation of an elite group of physicians referred to as "great physicians" and marks the emergence of a group claiming special medical authority (Unschuld, 1979). A Confucian response authored by Lu Chih (754–805) attacks this elitist trend, indicating medicine should be the responsibility of all persons (Unschuld, 1979). This tradition received clear expression in the Five Admonitions and Ten Maxims listed by Ch'en Shih-kung in a seventeenth-century treatise on surgery (Unschuld, 1979). Along with much guidance for social intercourse, Ch'en's precepts instruct physicians to give equal treatment to patients of all ranks, to keep expenses modest, and to treat the poor without charge, providing the same services regardless of the amount of payment. Above all, the physician is to know the principles of Confucianism. The key Confucian virtues are compassion and "applied humaneness," terms that do not enter Western medical ethics until the twentieth century.

These instructions continue to characterize Chinese medical ethics in modern times, but they have had little influence elsewhere. Although they bear some resemblance to ethical concepts in Western medicine, there are significant differences and little evidence of cross-fertilization.

In the West, the Royal College of Physicians provides an interesting example of a professional code. In the first Statutes of the College in 1555, and in the revision of 1647, there is a section entitled, *De statutis moralibus seu penalibus*. This contains precepts requiring good behavior in the meetings of the college, regular attendance and, in addition, proper etiquette between several physicians called into consultation. They admonish physicians not to disparage or accuse one another in public, but only before the college. They also prohibit physicians from telling their patients and the public the names and composition of medicines, "lest the people be harmed by abuse of them" (Clark, 1964, p. 384).

A treatise published in 1803 by Thomas Percival, an eminent physician of Manchester, England, strongly influenced the development of codes of medical ethics (Leake, 1927; Baker et al., 1993; Baker, 1993). Originally prepared in 1794 to mediate a dispute among surgeons, physicians, and apothecaries in Manchester, and expanded in 1803 to include physicians in general practice, *Medical Ethics; or, A Code of Institutes and Precepts Adapted to the Professional Conduct of Physicians and Surgeons* expresses standards of morality and etiquette that were in sharp contrast to the quarrelsome conduct of British practitioners of that era. Percival's treatise places emphasis on the professional relationships of physicians to one another; to hospital personnel, apothecaries, and others engaged in the care of the sick; and to the law.

In its advice to physicians to treat patients with the eighteenth-century virtues of "tenderness, steadiness, condescension, and authority," it conveys the attitudes of the English gentleman philanthropically bestowing benefits on patients who are expected to show proper gratitude. Percival's *Medical Ethics* stands in the Hippocratic tradition, but begins to acknowledge obligations of physicians to the society as well as to patients. Unlike the Hippocratic oath, Percival holds both surgery and medicine as acceptable practices.

As befits a volume having its origins in a local dispute among professions, a principal concern of Percival's *Medical Ethics* is with the etiquette of professional conduct. It offers elaborate procedures for consultation among physicians in difficult cases and for preservation of distinction of rank in relationships between junior and senior physicians on hospital faculties and in consultations. It cautions physicians to display respect for one another, to avoid criticizing the practice of their colleagues, to conceal professional differences from the public, and not to steal patients from one another. In justifying these procedures, Percival reasoned that criticism of the profession was usually unfounded and always degrading both to the doctors criticized and to the profession. In most of its provisions, Percival's *Medical Ethics* suggests a modified utilitarian philosophy, calling for individual physicians to conduct themselves in a manner that would enhance public respect for the entire medical profession.

Among the earliest American writings in physician-authored ethics were those by Columbia University phy-

sician Samuel Bard and revolutionary patriot Benjamin Rush; early codes were also prepared by the medical associations of the cities of Boston and Baltimore and the state of New York. When the American Medical Association was organized in 1847, it adopted a code of ethics drawn from Percival's *Medical Ethics* as well as these other sources. The code of ethics made no mention of etiquette for hospital staff and barely referred to the relations of physicians with pharmacists and courts of law, but it expanded and elaborated the principles for physicians in private practice, even presuming to include a statement of obligations of patients and the public to physicians.

The medical profession in the United States faced a crisis in public confidence in 1847. Medical licensure laws in most states had been repealed with the result that uneducated practitioners and charlatans had begun to compete for patients with educated physicians. In addition, a vigorous debate raged between various schools of medical science over which was the correct or orthodox system. Proponents of the code of ethics hoped that the public would cooperate with allopathic physicians in establishing standards for medical practice that would reinstate public respect for the medical profession.

The code of ethics contained a variety of restrictions on open competition among physicians. It branded as quacks all medical practitioners who lacked orthodox training, claimed special ability, patented instruments or medicine, used secret remedies, or criticized other practitioners. In doing so, it also became a weapon in the internal dispute among physicians of different schools, particularly challenging the homeopaths. The requirement of orthodox training made outcasts of physicians who belonged to medical sects such as the homeopaths, the eclectics, the Thomsonians, and later the osteopaths and chiropractors. Since each sect claimed superior results from its form of treatment, practitioners with sectarian designations were guilty of claiming superior ability as well as handicapped by their incomplete education.

Charging that these offenses resulted from selfishness and efforts to discredit rivals, the code of ethics also demanded that reputable physicians avoid any appearance of soliciting the patient of another doctor. Although these provisions united the profession against heterodoxy and quackery, the prohibition on claims of special ability produced conflict between general practitioners and aspiring specialists. This ethical rule ceased to cause dissension only after the establishment of specialist organizations to certify the credentials of their members and after specialization won sufficient acceptance to permit physicians to restrict practice to their specialties.

The code of ethics provided orthodox physicians with one means of exposing those undeserving of confidence. It stated that physicians should not consult professionally with anyone who lacked a license to practice or was not in good professional standing. Since professional standing was determined by the local medical societies, this provision had the effect of substituting a collective professional judgment for that of individual physicians and patients, thus superseding the Hippocratic oath's focus on the individual physician's judgment. In those cases where the patient insisted on inviting a consultant who was not approved by the local medical organization, the attending physician would have to retire from the case in order to retain professional standing. While physicians argued that they could not fulfill their obligation to patients if they admitted a right for fraudulent practitioners to advise in any capacity, their ethics required that they withdraw, thus giving full charge of the case to the allegedly unqualified practitioner. Moreover, the majority of physicians found the consultation restriction a useful means for excluding many qualified physicians from association with the dominant organization. Thus the codes served a monopolistic function as instruments for restraint of trade. Before 1870, regular medical societies excluded from membership and forbade consultations with female physicians and Negro physicians and, throughout the latter half of the century, with physicians who adopted a sectarian designation, even if they were certified by licensing boards. Because of mounting criticism, the consultation restriction was eliminated from the code of ethics in 1903, but its spirit was revived by a 1924 resolution of the American Medical Association forbidding voluntary association of its members with cultists. In effect, the AMA code, so vociferously debated in the nineteenth century was double edged: It did state, in Percivalian terms, certain ideals of good practice, but at the same time, it was an instrument to create a monopoly.

Establishment of the World Medical Association in 1948 encouraged physicians to develop international standards of medical ethics. The new organization adopted an International Code of Medical Ethics (International Code) in 1949, which attempted to summarize the most important principles of medical ethics. Since 1900, certification laws had reduced the prevalence of unqualified medical practitioners, and scientific advances had increased the effectiveness of trained physicians. By mid-century, physicians were directing their attention more to the actual treatment of patients and less to the formality of relations between one doctor and another, or between doctor and patient. The International Code reflects these new concerns in a shift away from the detailed regulations of the preceding 150 years. In place of elaborate etiquette for consultations and other medical confrontations, it recommends only that physicians behave toward colleagues as they would have colleagues behave toward them, that they call specialists in difficult cases, and that they not entice each other's patients. It warns against the profit motive and prohibits unauthorized advertising, medical care plans that deprive the physician of professional independence, fee splitting or rebates with or without the patient's knowledge, and refusal to treat emergency cases. It also commits physicians to honor professional secrecy in an unqualified way, an obligation that continues after the death of the patient, according to an amendment to the code adopted in 1968.

The International Code only hints at the ethical problems of abortion and euthanasia by asserting the physician's responsibility to preserve life. It does, however, warn specifically against any action that would weaken the patient's resistance without therapeutic justification. Applicable to the dying patient and experimental subject alike, this standard requires the physician to consider the patient's well-being above all else. The International Code also recognizes the need for adequate testing of innovations by urging great caution in publishing discoveries and therapeutic methods not recognized by the profession.

Using the International Code of Ethics as an example, the American Medical Association reduced its elaborate code to ten one-sentence Principles of Medical Ethics in 1957 (Ten Principles). This was intended as an epitome rather than a reduction. ("Every basic principle has been preserved," according to the Council that submitted the draft.) It retained the essentially Hippocratic focus on benefit of the patient, but added that the responsibilities of the physician extend also to the society.

Most of these principles had been anticipated in the International Code, but there are a few noteworthy exceptions. Reflecting a continuing distrust of sectarian practitioners by regular physicians in the United States, the 1957 principles warn against professional association with unscientific practitioners. They also oblige physicians who are AMA members to expose the legal and ethical violations of other doctors. Instead of warning against premature publication of discoveries, the 1957 principles urge physicians to make their attainments available to patients and colleagues. Finally, while reaffirming the principle of confidentiality, the 1957 principles authorize physicians to violate this principle when required by law or to advance the welfare of the individual or the community. This provision suggests more discretionary authority for the physician than do the codes of most nations and the World Medical Association, which emphasize the inviolability of professional secrecy.

By the late 1970s, there was again dissatisfaction with the principles. A special committee was appointed to prepare a new draft that would clarify and update the language, eliminate reference to gender, and seek a "proper and reasonable balance between professional standards and contemporary legal standards in our changing society" (American Medical Association, 1989, p. viii). The report submitting the new version acknowledged the increasing recognition of laypeople's role in defining the moral terms of the patient–physician relation. Nevertheless, the new code was prepared and adopted by a group made up entirely of members of the association. The new principles affirm the virtues of compassion and respect for human dignity. It, for the first time, shifts to the use of the language of "rights," saying that "a physician shall respect the rights of patients, of colleagues, and of other health professionals" (p. ix). It generally removes the traditional Hippocratic paternalistic authorization for physicians to act for the benefit of the patient according to the physician's judgment. For example, it permits breaking confidentiality only "within the constraints of the law" (p. ix).

Scientific advances and changing social standards in recent decades have raised ethical questions in a number of areas that are not adequately covered by existing general codes. The Council on Ethical and Judicial Affairs of the American Medical Association regularly issues opinions that elaborate (and occasionally contradict) the principles adopted by the AMA's legislative body, the House of Delegates. In recent years, other medical organizations, such as the American College of Physicians, have prepared and issued codes of ethics for their members.

Codes from outside the profession

Governmental codes. In the twentieth century, a number of national governments have incorporated ethical codes into legal statutes governing the medical profession, to be enforced by an official, publicly appointed medical board. The precepts in these codes sometimes accord with the broader principles of the Percival tradition, but many provisions deal with problems of recent origin and reflect a modern concern for both public and individual welfare.

Some of these codes deal with single subjects. For example, the Nuremberg Code, which is the product of international law, deals with medical research on human subjects. In the United States, the federal government's regulations on the same subject function as a code of conduct as does the Belmont Report, a set of ethical principles on research developed by the National Commission for the Protection of Human Subjects of Biomedical and Behavioral Research (1978).

Underlying the development of these codes is a fundamental issue of ethics: Is the professional group or the general public responsible for deciding what the ethical norms of the lay–professional relation should be? Even if the profession is deemed the proper authority for determining what constitutes ethical conduct, it is not clear exactly who should have the authority to speak for the profession and what the content of the codes should be. Some functions of the codes are clearly more for public relations and control of competition rather than for articulation of ethical norms. Many provisions that clearly are normative in content are still controversial. It is increasingly doubtful that the organized professional associations should have the authority to speak even for the profession as a whole (including the large numbers of physicians who are not members of the organizations) and that these groups should have any authority to speak on ethical matters that affect laypeople.

While modern medical ethics has often presumed that the profession should define its own code of conduct, this has not always been the case. Religious as well as governmental groups have sometimes claimed this prerogative. Increasingly, professional groups as well as laypeople are insisting that judgments about ethics are not the exclusive province of the professions and that the norms of lay–professional relations should be grounded in cultural, philosophical, or religious commitments.

A government-sponsored medical oath was adopted in the former Soviet Union, where its Presidium approved the Oath of Soviet Physicians in 1971. Modeled after an oath that had been used at the University of Moscow since 1961, the Soviet oath pledged the physician to conduct himself in accordance with communist principles and to order his responsibility to the Soviet government. This commitment to political creed and government was unique among medical oaths. The Soviet oath did not neglect other moral obligations, however; it instructed the physician to honor professional secrets, constantly improve knowledge and skill, always be available to calls for medical care or advice, and dedicate all knowledge and strength to professional activities. Like other recent oaths, the Soviet oath voiced virtually the same ideal of humanitarian duty to individual patients that appears in the earliest medical creeds, but it also pledged the physician to serve the interests of society.

Postcommunist Russia is undergoing a major reassessment of its health-care policies, including its medical ethics (Tichtchenko and Yudin, 1992). In November of 1991, the Russian Supreme Soviet adopted the Declaration of Rights and Liberties of Citizens, which includes the principle of voluntary consent for participation in medical experiments and declares a right of every citizen to qualified medical care in the state health-care system.

The Russian Medical Academy has developed a "Solemn Oath" (1993) to replace the Oath of the Soviet Physician. The new oath is a modernized revision of the Hippocratic oath. Approved by the Minister of Health in 1992, it is an official government document, not merely the product of a professional medical association.

Nongovernmental groups. Throughout history, codes, prayers, and oaths dealing with medical ethics have also been sponsored by private groups, religious bodies, and consumer groups that do not represent the medical profession.

For centuries, the Catholic church has articulated moral views about medical matters including abortion, euthanasia, and fertility control. These have appeared, at least since the medieval era, in systematic theological treatises, cases of conscience (collections analyzing morally perplexing cases), and in the theology manuals of the early modern era (Kelly, 1979; Griese, 1987). Formal codes of medical ethics, such as the Ethical and Religious Directives for Catholic Health Facilities prepared by the United States Catholic Conference (1975; Griese, 1987), are not only considered binding on Catholics but also affect non-Catholics who are associated with Catholic health facilities and others who find their reasoning persuasive.

The statements of the directives on secrecy, consent, organ transplantation, and terminal care closely resemble those of other codes. It prohibits abortion, except when justified by the principle of double effect, that is, when it is an unintended result of a procedure employed to protect the mother. It prohibits both male and female sterilization except in the treatment of a serious pathological condition, and it prohibits artificial insemination. Thus, the directives articulate the Vatican's "Instruction on Respect for Human Life" (Sacred Congregation for the Doctrine of the Faith, 1987).

The modern consumer movement has also influenced the ethics of medical practice. As hospitalization became a major consumer service, consumers increasingly demanded the right of patients to minimum standards of care and respect. In 1972, the American Hospital Association responded to consumer pressure and adopted A Patient's Bill of Rights, which pertains primarily to hospitals but involves physicians with several responsibilities to patients ("Statement," 1973). A physician who subscribes to the bill of rights is obligated, with limited exceptions, to keep the hospitalized patient informed of diagnosis, treatment, and prognosis, to instruct the patient fully regarding possible consequences and alternatives before obtaining consent for medical procedures, to honor a patient's refusal to consent to treatment to the extent permitted by law, to protect the patient's right to confidentiality and privacy from physicians and staff not involved in his or her case, and to instruct the patient of his or her care require-

ments after discharge. These standards represent a significant departure from the traditional paternalism prevailing in the patient–physician relationship.

Still, the Patient's Bill of Rights was generated by a professionally dominated group. On some issues, such as informed consent, it actually incorporates traditional paternalistic exception clauses that might be rejected by those emphasizing the rights of patients. Other bills of rights have been developed such as those for nursing home patients, the mentally retarded, children, and other vulnerable groups. It is not clear how the statements of these documents are to be sanctioned, since no mechanisms of enforcement are specified.

Conclusion

The difficulties that confront professional leaders, patients, surrogates, and public policymakers who undertake the establishment of ethical standards on new issues reflect the conflicts in fundamental values inherent in diverse views of medical ethics. The traditional professional ethics of physicians places great emphasis on the virtue of benevolence and the physician's responsibilities to serve the patient. This tradition honors the individuality of the patient–physician relationship, professional secrecy, and the physician's duty to promote the patient's welfare. In these and other matters, ethical formulations by physicians have been paternalistic, making the physician the dominant party in determining which action will best further both the physician's and the patient's interests. Codes prepared by interests outside the medical profession (including those written by religious and governmental bodies) have advanced other philosophical tenets as foundations for medical ethics. Some of these codes have focused on justice or equity in allocating resources. This has resulted in mounting ethical confusion as physicians become subject to competing ethical authorities with conflicting standards.

Responsibility for the development of ethical guidelines relative to the physician–patient relationship may be shifting from the physician to the society as a whole. In those contingencies not anticipated by accepted guidelines, the responsibility for ethical criteria rests partly with the individual physician, partly with patients, and partly with society's general ethical standards. Future success in the use of codes to control medical practice may well depend on an accommodation of the ethical norms of physicians with those of the larger society.

ROBERT M. VEATCH

Directly related to this article is the companion article in this entry: ETHICAL ANALYSIS. *For a further discussion of topics mentioned in this article, see the entries* ABORTION; ADVERTISING; ALLIED HEALTH PROFESSIONS; CONFIDEN-

TIALITY; DEATH, DEFINITION AND DETERMINATION OF; DEATH AND DYING: EUTHANASIA AND SUSTAINING LIFE; DOUBLE EFFECT; INFORMED CONSENT; JUDAISM; LIFE; PATIENTS' RIGHTS; PROFESSIONAL–PATIENT RELATIONSHIP; PROFESSION AND PROFESSIONAL ETHICS; PROTESTANTISM; PUBLIC POLICY AND BIOETHICS; RACE AND RACISM; RESEARCH, HUMAN: HISTORICAL ASPECTS; ROMAN CATHOLICISM; SURGERY; *and* UNORTHODOXY IN MEDICINE. *For a discussion of related history, see the entry* MEDICAL ETHICS, HISTORY OF, *section on* NEAR AND MIDDLE EAST, *article on* ANCIENT NEAR EAST; *section on* SOUTH AND EAST ASIA, *article on* INDIA, *and subsection on* CHINA, *article on* PREREPUBLICAN CHINA; *section on* EUROPE, *subsections on* ANCIENT AND MEDIEVAL, RENAISSANCE AND ENLIGHTENMENT, *and* NINETEENTH CENTURY, *and subsection on* CONTEMPORARY PERIOD, *article on* RUSSIA; *and section on* THE AMERICAS. *For a discussion of related ideas, see the entries* AUTHORITY; PATERNALISM; RESPONSIBILITY; *and* UTILITY. *See also the* APPENDIX (CODES, OATHS, AND DIRECTIVES RELATED TO BIOETHICS), SECTION I: DIRECTIVES ON HEALTH-RELATED RIGHTS AND PATIENT RESPONSIBILITIES; SECTION II: ETHICAL DIRECTIVES FOR THE PRACTICE OF MEDICINE; SECTION III: ETHICAL DIRECTIVES FOR OTHER HEALTH-CARE PROFESSIONS; *and* SECTION IV: ETHICAL DIRECTIVES FOR HUMAN RESEARCH.

Bibliography

[*The bibliography for this article and its companion article can be found following the companion article.*]

II. ETHICAL ANALYSIS

The following is a revision and update of the first-edition article "Codes of Medical Ethics: Ethical Analysis" by the same author.

Codes, oaths, and prayers of medical ethics have emerged over the centuries from disparate sources, representing disparate societies, time periods, organizations, and perspectives. It is not surprising that they differ significantly in style and content. This article will examine systemically the ethical content of this divergent collection of documents from the earliest to contemporary times. In the Appendix, the reader will find the texts of codes and additional bibliography of codes and commentaries on codes for ethics of the medical and other health professions.

Ethical analysis of the codes of medical ethics creates problems. Such codes are not fully developed, systemic theories of medical ethics. On the other hand, the codes, at least the modern ones, are normally the product of much discussion, debate, and review. These codes, along with the historical documents that have had lasting significance, can reasonably be expected to reflect the basic ethical views of the organizations that have endorsed them.

When one turns to the substance of the codes, especially the codes written by physicians, one can identify what might be called a central ethical obligation, a basic principle that provides the physician with a core moral stance for resolving ethical dilemmas. Striking features are the presence of contradictions among the codes and the controversial nature of these central ethics.

Hippocratic oath

Modern Western medical ethics has reiterated the central ethic of the Hippocratic oath into the twentieth century. The core ethic of the Hippocratic oath is the physician's pledge to do what he or she thinks will benefit the patient. This is repeated twice in the oath, once as applied to matters of diet, and once when referring to visits to the homes of patients.

The principle that the physician's first obligation is to do what the individual physician thinks will benefit the sick person is picked up in the Declaration of Geneva, where the physician swears, "The health of my patient will be my first consideration," and in the International Code of Medical Ethics of the World Medical Association (WMA), which proclaims, "A physician shall owe his patients complete loyalty and all the resources of his science." Likewise, the postcommunist Russian oath has the physician pledge, in Hippocratic fashion, to work always for the patient's good (Solemn Oath of a Physician of Russia).

The Hippocratic oath's individualism. The first characteristic of the Hippocratic ethic is that it is individualistic; it concentrates only on the benefit to the individual patient. In contrast, classical utilitarian ethics of the tradition of Jeremy Bentham (1748–1832), John Stuart Mill (1806–1873), and G. E. Moore (1873–1958) would consider such a narrow focus on consequences for the patient to be ethically unjustified, unless it would serve the greater good of the greater number in the long run. They would consider benefits to all persons and to society as a whole. There is no evidence that the Hippocratic authors or their twentieth-century counterparts had such an indirect utilitarianism in mind. Rather, they seem to hold that the physician has a special ethical obligation to benefit his or her patient, independent of the net consequences for others who are not patients. The real test comes in cases in which the physician believes that one course will produce the most good in total, but another course will most benefit the patient. A physician who feels required to choose the course most beneficial to the patient is faithfully following the oath and rejecting the utilitarian alternative.

The American Medical Association (AMA), in its 1957 Principles of Medical Ethics, did not accept the Hippocratic individualism. It instructs the AMA physician that "the principle objective of the medical profession is to render service to humanity." The tenth principle made this interpretation unambiguous:

> The honored ideals of the medical profession imply that the responsibilities of the physician extend not only to the individual, but also to society where these responsibilities deserve his interest and participation in activities which have the purpose of improving both the health and the well-being of the individual and the community.

This focus on the community continued in the major revision of 1980. The last principle of that version is, "A physician shall recognize a responsibility to participate in activities contributing to an improved community" (American Medical Association, 1989, p. ix).

Here the AMA is closer to the now-abandoned Soviet physicians' oath of 1971 than to the Oath of Hippocrates. The Soviet physician more boldly swore "to work conscientiously wherever the interests of society will require it" and "to conduct all my actions according to the principles of the Communistic morale, to always keep in mind the high calling of the Soviet physician, and the high responsibility I have to my people and to the Soviet government." By contrast, the postcommunist Russian oath reverts to the pure Hippocratic focus on the good of the individual patient, abandoning any reference to the interests of the community or state (Solemn Oath of a Physician of Russia). The Criteria for Medical Ethics of the Ministry of Health of the People's Republic of China (1989) are actually closer to the postcommunist Russian oath and its Hippocratic ancestors by focusing on the interests of the patient. It lacks any appeal to the duty of the physician to the community that is seen in the AMA and the Soviet oaths.

The Hippocratic oath's paternalism.   The central ethic of the Hippocratic tradition is also paternalistic. The physician is to benefit his or her patient "according to my ability and judgement" (Edelstein, 1943, p. 3).

Addressing the meaning of the injunction to protect the patient from mischief and injustice, Edelstein concludes that the oath means that "the physician must protect his patient from the mischief and injustice which he may inflict upon himself if his diet is not properly chosen" (Edelstein, 1943, p. 24).

This paternalism is also seen in the provision of the Hippocratic oath that medical knowledge is to be kept secret and not disclosed to people outside the Hippocratic group. A similar provision is seen in a sixteenth-century Japanese medical code called the Seventeen Rules of Enjuin, which actually required that, if a suc-

cessor trained in the School of Enjuin could not be found upon retirement or death, the medical books of the school had to be returned to the school.

Physicians, according to Percival (1740–1804) (who also shared in this Hippocratic paternalism), should study not only tenderness and steadiness but also "condescension and authority, as to inspire the minds of their patients with gratitude, respect, and confidence" (Leake, 1927, p. 71). The AMA principles of 1957 and the 1959 British Medical Association (BMA) codes held that medical confidences could be broken if, in the judgment of the physician, it was in the patient's interest for them to be broken.

The Hippocratic oath's focus on consequences.   Finally, one sees the controversy of the Hippocratic patient-benefiting ethic when it is contrasted with other theories that can be called nonconsequentialist, that is, ethical theories in which certain principles are taken to be simply inherently right-making or where certain claims are taken to be "inalienable rights." Holders of views in which there are certain characteristics of actions that make them inherently tend toward being right (other things being equal) or holders of the view that certain things, such as life, liberty, and the pursuit of happiness, are "inalienable rights" would have to reject the ethic of doing what one thinks will benefit the patient. At least they would reject patient benefit in cases where benefiting the patient will be at the expense of fulfilling prima facie duties or respecting basic rights of the patient.

There may be a paradox in the Hippocratic oath. The physician is to do what he or she thinks will benefit the patient but is not to give an abortive remedy or a deadly drug and is not to "use the knife, not even on sufferers from stone." What is the physician to do who believes that giving a deadly drug or an abortifacient remedy, or using the knife, will benefit the patient? Perhaps this apparent contradiction is resolved by the belief of the Pythagorean physician that such actions can never be beneficial to the patient. In that case, the oath simply spells out some rules that guide the physician in deciding what will be beneficial. More likely, however, these actions are seen as inherently wrong even if they might be of benefit. If so, then the Hippocratic ethic abandons its consequentialism, at least for these cases.

Codes written by groups outside the medical profession

Many of the more recent codes written by governmental and religious groups have not shown these characteristics of individualism, paternalism, and consequentialism. The Nuremberg Code (1947), one of the first codes relevant to medical ethics emerging in international law, could have addressed the problem of abuse of human subjects in medical research by retreating to Hippocratic individualism, thus making all use of subjects for purposes of gaining knowledge immoral (because, by definition, doing something for the pursuit of general knowledge is not acting for the purpose of benefiting the patient). It did not. Instead it acknowledged the legitimacy of physician participation in efforts to benefit society by doing research on human subjects. It introduced protections for those subjects by abandoning the exclusive focus on consequences—on producing benefits and avoiding harms—and replacing it with an ethic that speaks in terms of duties and responsibilities, including the duty to ensure that the subjects give their informed consent.

Other codes coming from governmental and religious sources adopted the language of rights as a way of signaling their break with the professional medical ethical traditions that focus exclusively on consequences. This focus on rights is influenced heavily by the tradition of the liberal political philosophy of John Locke, Thomas Hobbes, Jean Jacques Rousseau, and the authors of the Bill of Rights of the United States Constitution. It is a moral tradition significantly different from that of the traditional, professionally written medical codes.

The focus on rights and duties includes an emphasis on the right to give informed and voluntary consent not only for research but for all clinical, medical treatments. Consent, grounded in the moral principle of autonomy and the legal notion of self-determination, is totally absent from the classical codes written by medical professional groups. The introduction of the perspective of rights and duties, and the underlying moral notion of respect for persons (including the principle of autonomy), signals a rejection of both traditional Hippocratic paternalism and consequentialism. It also provides a way of moving away from pure individualism, incorporating a more social ethic without lapsing into a social utilitarianism that would completely subordinate the individual to the aggregate social good.

The first health-care association that used the language of rights was the International Council of Nurses' Code for Nurses (1973, reaffirmed 1989). Still using gender-specific language, it nevertheless signaled a revolution in the philosophical orientation of professional codes when it said, "Inherent in nursing is respect for life, dignity and rights of man." This use of "rights" language also appeared in the American Nurses' Association (ANA) code revision in 1976, when it proclaimed (with more gender-neutral language), "Each client has the moral right to determine what will be done with his/her person" (American Nurses' Association, 1976). By making self-determination of clients its first principle, the ANA announced it was the first organization of health-

care professionals to abandon Hippocratic paternalism and exclusive focus on consequences. However, ambivalence persists; after announcing that self-determination is its first principle, it says that "the nurse's primary commitment is to the health, welfare, and safety of the client" (American Nurses' Association, 1985, p. 6). At this juncture, the nursing profession seemed unable to decide whether to abandon Hippocratic paternalism in favor of respect for rights of self-determination or remain Hippocratic.

The AMA followed this pattern in its 1980 revision. It begins to use rights language saying, "A physician shall respect the rights of patients, of colleagues, and of other health professionals" (American Medical Association, 1989, p. ix). It commits the physician for the first time to deal honestly with patients, reversing the longstanding, more paternalistic approach in which physicians were expected to withhold information when they believed it might harm the patient. Yet, it still proclaims the Hippocratic notion that the AMA's ethical statements are developed "primarily for the benefit of the patient," and not, apparently, to protect the patient's rights.

Specific ethical injunctions

The strictures against abortion, euthanasia, and surgery in the Hippocratic oath are examples of specific injunctions that occur from time to time in the codes and oaths of medical and physician ethics. Code-by-code comparison of these injunctions reveals interesting differences. The conflict among the codes on the question of confidentiality is perhaps the most dramatic.

Confidentiality. The Hippocratic injunction on breaking confidentiality is sometimes taken to forbid breaking medical confidences. The text is really much more ambiguous. It says, "Whatever I may see or hear in the course of treatment in regard to the life of men, which on no account one must speak abroad, I will keep to myself holding such things shameful to be spoken about." The individual physician, however, is left with the question of just which things he or she hears "on no account must be spoken abroad." Possibly physicians are to use the "patient-benefiting" criterion for deciding when breaking the confidence is appropriate. That was the explicit principle in the 1959 version of the BMA code, which said:

> The complications of modern life sometimes create difficulties for the doctor in the application of this principle of confidentiality, and on certain occasions it may be necessary to acquiesce in some modification. Always, however, the overriding consideration must be the adoption of a line of conduct that will benefit the patient, or protect his interests.

The World Medical Association's International Code of Medical Ethics (1949, amended 1968 and 1983) and the Declaration of Geneva (1948, amended 1968 and 1983) both close any such patient-benefiting loophole in the confidentiality principle. They simply require "absolute secrecy," much as did the ancient Jewish Oath of Asaph. No exception is considered even in a case where the physician has learned that the patient is about to commit mass murder. The Ethical and Religious Directives for Catholic Health Facilities (1975) is almost as blunt. It requires that

> professional secrecy must be carefully fulfilled not only as regards the information on the patient's charts and records but also as regards confidential matters learned in the exercise of professional duties.

In keeping with their more social commitment to the welfare of others as well as the patient, the now outdated 1957 American Medical Association Principles (1957, revised 1971), and the American Psychiatric Association's (1973), which were based on them, were quite explicit in providing three exceptions to the general principle of confidentiality:

> A physician may not reveal the confidences entrusted to him in the course of medical attendance, or the deficiencies he may observe in the character of his patients, unless he is required to do so by law or unless it becomes necessary in order to protect the welfare of the individual or of the society.

Confidences could be broken not only when the physician thought it would benefit the patient but also when he or she thought it would benefit society or when it was required by law, for example, informing the police of a bullet wound incurred in a crime. The ethical problem of such broad exceptions, of course, is not only the paternalism of the patient-benefiting exclusion but also the potential subordination of the patient's interests and rights to the interests of the society.

The BMA was confronted by a particularly difficult case in which the physician disclosed to the parents of a sixteen-year-old that she was taking birth-control pills. He defended the breaking of the confidence on the grounds that he thought it was for her benefit. Since this was explicitly permitted by the BMA code at the time, the General Medical Council acquitted him of the charge of unprofessional conduct. After that case, the BMA in 1971 amended its confidentiality principle and became the first to recognize the patient's right to confidence in cases where the patient and the physician disagreed. The new position stated that "if, in the opinion of the doctor, disclosure of confidential information to a third party seems to be in the best medical interest of the patient, it is the doctor's duty to make every effort to allow the information to be given to the third party, but where the patient refuses, that refusal must be respected."

However, in the years that followed, the BMA's position seems to have reverted to a modified version of the old policy permitting disclosures "if it is in the patient's own interest that information should be disclosed but it is either impossible, or medically undesirable in the patient's own interest, to seek his consent" (British Medical Association, 1988, p. 21). The BMA also has added a provision permitting disclosure for social purposes when it is necessary to safeguard the national interest or when the doctor has an "overriding duty to society."

Abortion. On the controversial subject of abortion, groups authoring codes have followed the ethical stances of their subcultures. The Hippocratic oath follows the Pythagorean prohibition on abortion, even though abortion was not considered unethical in the broader Greek culture (Edelstein, 1943). In the Oath of Asaph, the early medieval Jewish medical initiate is instructed, "Do not prepare any potion that may cause a woman who has conceived in adultery to miscarry." The 1975 Ethical and Religious Directives for (U.S.) Catholic Health Facilities follow, consciously and precisely, a traditional, theological explanation of official church teaching, devoting seven of forty-three principles to the subject. Directly intended termination of pregnancy before viability is never permitted nor is the directly intended destruction of a viable fetus. Treatments not intended to terminate a pregnancy but which nonetheless have that effect are permitted, provided there is a proportionately serious pathological condition of the mother and the treatments cannot be safely postponed until after the fetus is viable.

When the cultural base of the group writing the code is very broad, the code is predictably less specific about the ethics of abortion. The Declaration of Geneva said, "I will maintain the utmost respect for human life from the time of conception," without directly prohibiting abortion. Its 1983 revision softened the position even further, changing "from the time of conception" to "from its beginning" (Declaration of Geneva, 1948, amended 1968 and 1983). The WMA's International Code in its draft, but not in its finally adopted form, stated, "Therapeutic abortion may only be performed if the conscience of the doctors and the national laws permit." The American Nurses' Association (ANA), which also represents individuals with a wide variety of viewpoints, similarly avoids direct comments. In its code, revised in 1968 and in effect prior to the 1976 revision, the ANA says that "the nurse's respect for the worth and dignity of the individual human being extends throughout the entire life cycle, from *birth* to death" (italics added). The implication may be that fetal life is not included. A 1966 statement approved by the ANA Board of Directors recognizes "the right of individuals and families to select and use such methods for family planning as are consistent with their own creeds and mores," again appealing to individual conscience. Is the combined implication a toleration of the nurse's participation in abortion?

Euthanasia. An explicit obligation to preserve life is strikingly absent from the codes of ethics, both professional and public. In light of a widely held view that the duty, or one of the duties, of the physician is to preserve life, one would expect to find this duty emphasized. The only explicit, well-known reference is the weak formulation in the International Code (1949, amended 1968 and 1983), which says that "a physician shall always bear in mind the obligation of preserving human life." This obligation to "bear in mind" rather than explicitly attempt to preserve life is a very soft injunction, especially when combined with the patient-benefiting principle the code emphasizes.

Proscribing active killing is much more common in the codes, as might be expected from the general ethical prohibition on active killing, even for mercy, in many cultures and subcultures. The Hippocratic oath's formula is, "I will neither give a deadly drug to anybody if asked for it, nor will I make a suggestion to this effect." Interpretation of this prohibition is controversial. Some take it to forbid any criminal, malevolent homicide. What seems more likely, however, is a prohibition against merciful killing or assisting in suicide. While suicide, especially in the face of medical suffering, was not uncommon in ancient society, it was forbidden by the Pythagorean cult. This fact is cited by Edelstein in his defense of the hypothesis that the Hippocratic oath is a Pythagorean document (Edelstein, 1943). According to the Caraka Samhita, acts "causing another's death" were one of the few things the Indian medical student should not do at his teacher's behest. The oath of Asaph instructs the Jewish medical student to "take heed that you not kill any man with a root decoction."

In the professionally written codes or those of the Catholic church, however, the prohibition against assisting in an act of killing has never been extended to apply to cooperating in withdrawal from treatment. The distinction between active killing and withdrawal of certain treatments is clear in the Ethical and Religious Directives for Catholic Health Facilities, according to which "the directly intended termination of any patient's life, even at his own request, is always morally wrong," and "euthanasia ('mercy killing') in all its forms is forbidden." The directives go on, however, to say that while "failure to supply the ordinary means of preserving life is equivalent to euthanasia . . . neither the physi-

cian nor the patient is obliged to use extraordinary means." Nor is it considered euthanasia "to give a dying person sedatives or analgesics for the alleviation of pain, when such a measure is judged necessary, even though they may deprive the patient of the use of reason, or shorten his life."

The AMA states in its Judicial Council Opinions that "the physician should not intentionally cause death" (American Medical Association, 1989, p. 13). At the same time, it acknowledges the legitimacy of forgoing life-sustaining treatment in accord with the preferences of the patient or surrogate. The postcommunist Russian oath, following the original Hippocratic language, commits the Russian physician never to give a deadly drug.

The distinction between active killing and forgoing treatment is made clearer when rights language is used, as in A Patient's Bill of Rights (1973), written under the auspices of the American Hospital Association. That document proclaims that "the patient has the right to refuse treatment to the extent permitted by law," presumably even if the result will be the death of the patient. However, there is clearly no corresponding right to drugs that will actively hasten death.

Truth-telling. One conspicuous conflict between the patient-benefiting principle and the more deontological ethical theories is over the question of what one ought to tell a dying patient. Historically, many of the professional codes are simply silent, presumably expecting the patient-benefiting principle to apply. The Indian oath of the Caraka Samhita is explicit: "Even knowing that the patient's span of life has come to its close, it shall not be mentioned by thee there, where if so done, it would cause shock to the patient or to others." The 1847 version of the AMA code instructs: "A physician should not be forward to make gloomy prognostications . . . but he should not fail, on proper occasions, to give to the friends of the patient timely notice of danger, when it really occurs; and even to the patient himself, if absolutely necessary." The violation of confidentiality in communicating to family or friends before informing patients either is not noticed or is justified on patient-benefiting grounds. Using the patient-benefiting principle as a basis for withholding the truth is traditional in professional physician ethics. The 1847 code makes the grounding explicit: "It is, therefore, a sacred duty . . . to avoid all things [that] have a tendency to discourage the patient and to depress his spirits."

The latent paternalism that justifies withholding information from patients for their own good is retained even in the period after 1980 when the AMA principles themselves pledge unqualified honesty. In the AMA Council on Ethical and Judicial Affairs' interpretation, an exception can be made to the requirement of informed consent "when risk-disclosure poses such a serious psychological threat of detriment to the patient as to be medically contraindicated" (American Medical Association, 1989, p. 32).

Even the authors of A Patient's Bill of Rights seem to yield to the paternalistic patient-benefiting principle when it conflicts with the patient's right to know. The bill first states that "the patient has the right to obtain from his physician complete current information concerning his diagnosis, treatment, and prognosis in terms the patient can be reasonably expected to understand." But it then qualifies this by stating, "When it is not medically advisable to give such information to the patient, the information should be made available to the appropriate person in his behalf." The potential conflicts of such an exception with the right to privacy or the right to receive information necessary for informed consent are not discussed. By contrast, U.S. courts and many codes generated outside the Hippocratic tradition insist that information be adequate for the patient to make a self-determining choice, even if that information is potentially upsetting.

Justice in delivering health care.   Many of the codes of physician and other medical ethics have some reference to the duty to deliver health care justly or equitably. The Hippocratic oath uses a term, *adiki'e*, often translated into English as "justice," but it really means "wrongdoing" more generally; it does not refer to equality of treatment or equitable distribution of benefits. The statement in the Hippocratic oath that physicians must abstain from sexual relations with males and females, free and slave, during a medical visit is as close as the text comes to a pledge of equal treatment.

The ancient Chinese medical ethical codes are much more far-reaching in emphasizing equal treatment of rich and poor. The commandments written by Chen Shi-Kung, a seventeenth-century physician, include the explicit commitment that "physicians should be ever ready to respond to any calls of patients, high or low, rich or poor."

Equality of access seems generally recognized as an ideal in many modern codes even if it is absent in the Hippocratic original. The twentieth-century Declaration of Geneva holds forth this ideal: "I will not permit considerations of religion, nationality, race, party politics, or social standing to intervene between my duty and my patient." The American Nurses' Association code declares, "The nurse provides services with respect for the dignity of man, unrestricted by considerations of nationality, race, creed, color, or status." The AMA recognizes that society must make decisions regarding the allocation of limited health-care resources and urges that they be allocated on the basis of "fair, socially acceptable, and humane criteria." At the same time, it empha-

sizes that the physician's duty is "to do all that he can for the benefit of his individual patient" (American Medical Association, 1989, p. 3). The postcommunist Russian oath, by contrast, pledges never to deny medical assistance to anybody and to provide care with equal diligence to patients regardless of means or national or religious affiliation.

The ethics of professional relations

In contrast with the lay or public codes or bills of rights, virtually all professional codes devote significant attention to relationships among professionals. The Hippocratic oath begins with a covenant by which the new physician pledges "to hold him who has taught me this art as equal to my parents and to live my life in partnership with him, and if he is in need of money to give him a share of mine, and to regard his offspring as equal to my brothers in male lineage and to take them this art— if they desire to learn it—without fee and covenant." It includes a pledge to keep secrets, much as any initiation ritual into a cult might.

The longest of the three sections of the AMA code of 1847 is devoted to "the duties of physicians to each other and to the profession at large." Since many of the codes emerged at a point historically when the profession was separating itself from others claiming to offer treatments and cures, there is often, even to modern times, strong language forbidding association with those not properly members of the group. The American Osteopathic Association, for instance, requires that a physician "shall practice in accordance with the body of systemized knowledge related to the healing arts and shall avoid professional association with individuals or organizations which do not practice or conduct organization affairs in accordance with such knowledge."

In terms of the sociology of the professions, it has been suggested that restraints on advertising, rules structuring referral of patients, instruction on the ways of handling an incompetent member of the profession, or exclusion of those not properly initiated into the profession have important functions in maintaining the professional monopoly. Apart from their role in protecting professional interests, however, it is also pertinent to analyze them as sets of ethical obligations.

Three different kinds of ethical arguments may underlie the detailed formulations of professional obligations to other professionals. First, such duties to one's colleagues may be defended on what could be called "universal" grounds. That would be the case if the ethical principles claimed as the foundation of such intraprofessional obligations are principles generally recognized by all persons. For instance, the AMA code of 1847 states detailed rules regarding professional consultation prohibiting "exclusion from fellowship" of duly licensed practitioners and requiring punctuality in visits of physicians when they hold consultations as well as secrecy and confidentiality so that the patient will not be aware of consultants' disagreements. These standards for consultation are defended on the grounds that "the good of the patient is the sole object in view." Although it is not generally argued, there is a presumption that rational patients should accept this principle. We have seen, however, that the principle of patient benefit is quite controversial when put up against competing ethical principles.

A second foundation for intraprofessional duties might be a special ethic for a special group, which nonmembers would not be expected to share or even understand. This would be the case, for example, if the profession is viewed as a kind of club or fraternity that invents its own norms and applies them only to its own members. The ethic of a profession is in part the ethic of fraternal loyalty, of special obligation to one's adopted brothers. The professional obligation may be seen deriving from the professional nexus rather than from some more universal source. It is a special ethic of a special cult.

The ethic of the AMA's 1847 code, like the ethic of the code written by Percival, is an ethic of dignity and honor among gentlemen: "There is no profession, from the members of which greater purity of character and a higher standard of moral excellence are required, than the medical." The discussion of duties of physicians to each other begins with the admonition that "every individual, entering the profession, as he becomes thereby entitled to all its privileges and immunities, incurs an obligation to exert his best abilities to maintain its dignity and honor, to exalt its standing, and to extend the bound of its usefulness." The text goes on to entreat the physician to avoid "all contumelious and sarcastic remarks relative to the faculty, as a body; and while by unwearied diligence, he resorts to every honorable means of enriching the science, he should entertain a due respect for his seniors, who have, by their labors, brought it to the elevated condition in which he finds it."

This gentlemanly ethic of honor and purity (the Hippocratic phrase is "purity and holiness") gives rise to special ethical burdens for the medical profession that the layperson cannot be expected to grasp. Professional "courtesy" (gratuitous services for practitioners, their wives, and their children) should probably be understood in these terms. "Courtesy" is an ethical expectation for members of the brotherhood.

A third possible foundation confounds the two. It could be that professional duties are defended as being in the public interest (or in some other manner consistent with a more universal ethic), but that only members of the profession can be expected to understand this

to be so. Advertising, for instance, could be attacked, as it is in the AMA's 1847 code, as "derogatory to the dignity of the profession," but it is defended as necessary to separate the profession from "the ordinary practices of empirics." The authors might well hold that it is really in the public interest that the separation be made, but also concede that only members of the profession could see the necessity of that separation.

If there are special ethical obligations for members of the profession that in principle cannot be recognized from outside the professional group, it follows that there are likely to be conflicts between the profession's formulation of its ethical obligation and the broader public's formulation. The issue is not the existence of different ethical responsibilities attaching to different roles, but rather a disagreement between the profession and the broader public over what constitutes the proper behavior of the professional in his or her specific professional role. Even if a profession agrees that it has a special duty to preserve life or limit advertising, it is still an open question whether the public wants physicians always to act on that norm. If the professional group holds that there is a special professional source of norms, then conflict is predictable.

A specific example of such conflict involves the ethics of advertising. Many professional codes, in the manner of the 1847 AMA code, prohibit or restrict advertising by members of the profession. The 1957 Principles of Medical Ethics of the AMA claim that "this principle protects the public from the advertiser and salesman of medical care by establishing an easily discernible and generally recognized distinction between him and the ethical physician." While such prohibitions on advertising might be seen as the behavior of a cartel restraining price competition, it is also possible that physicians really believe that they are engaged in a service that must not be peddled as a commodity. Whether the medical profession sees such advertising as unethical or not, the public may see restraint on advertising as unethical. At stake are not only two different perceptions of ways to maximize benefits to potential patients, but also two sources of ethical norms—one from within the professional nexus and the other from the broader society. In this regard, an important transition occurred when the committee responsible for the 1980 revision of the AMA principles acknowledged that increasingly the public will be determining the norms for moral conduct in the lay–professional relationship.

Conclusion

The codes, oaths, prayers, and bills of rights derive from disparate contexts, representing differing professional groups, public agencies, and private, lay organizations such as churches and patients' groups. It is not surprising that radically different ethical conclusions are reached and that they are based on radically different fundamental ethical theories and methods of ethical reasoning.

One critical problem faced by health professionals as well as laypeople is what ethical directives should be decisive when an individual professes identification with more than one group. A health professional may also be a member of a religious or cultural group that has an ethical framework relevant to the moral problems faced by the individual. For example, if the ANA position can be interpreted as endorsing the nurse's tolerance of a woman's right to choose abortion, what is the Catholic nurse to do, or what is a nurse who works in a Catholic health facility to do if he or she believes in the right of the individual to select methods for family planning? These conflicts for individuals who are simultaneously members of more than one group, each of which has authored a code, arise for many ethical issues in health care. Moreover, individuals may reach conclusions of conscience that fail to conform to any codes of ethics whether written by health-care professions or by religious, cultural, or governmental groups. An active understanding of the ethical differences among these codes is needed to begin developing a response.

ROBERT M. VEATCH

Directly related to this article is the companion article in this entry: HISTORY. *Also directly related are the entries* BENEFICENCE; AUTONOMY; PATERNALISM; AUTHORITY; PROFESSION AND PROFESSIONAL ETHICS; MEDICINE AS A PROFESSION; *and* HEALTH OFFICIALS AND THEIR RESPONSIBILITIES. *For a further discussion of topics mentioned in this article, see the entries* ABORTION; CONFIDENTIALITY; DEATH AND DYING: EUTHANASIA AND SUSTAINING LIFE; INFORMATION DISCLOSURE; *and* INFORMED CONSENT. *Other relevant material may be found under the entries* BIOETHICS EDUCATION, *articles on* MEDICINE, *and* NURSING; COMPETENCE; ETHICS, *article on* NORMATIVE ETHICAL THEORIES; PROFESSIONAL–PATIENT RELATIONSHIP; RESPONSIBILITY; RIGHTS; UNORTHODOXY IN MEDICINE; *and* WHISTLEBLOWING. *For a discussion of the development of medical ethics in general, see the various articles in the entry* MEDICAL ETHICS, HISTORY OF. *See also the* APPENDIX (CODES, OATHS, AND DIRECTIVES RELATED TO BIOETHICS), SECTION II: ETHICAL DIRECTIVES FOR THE PRACTICE OF MEDICINE; *and* SECTION III: ETHICAL DIRECTIVES FOR OTHER HEALTH-CARE PROFESSIONS.

Bibliography

[*This bibliography refers to secondary literature on codes, oaths, and prayers dealing with medical ethics. For references to primary documents, see the Appendix in Vol. 5.*]

BAKER, ROBERT. 1993. "The History of Medical Ethics." In *Companion Encyclopedia of the History of Medicine*, pp. 852–887. Edited by W. F. Bynum and Roy Porter. London: Routledge & Kegan Paul.

BAKER, ROBERT; PORTER, DOROTHY; and PORTER, ROY, eds. 1993. *The Codification of Medical Morality: Historical and Philosophical Studies of the Formalization of Western Medical Morality in the Eighteenth and Nineteenth Centuries*. Dordrecht, Netherlands: Kluwer Academic Publishers.

CARRICK, PAUL. 1985. *Medical Ethics in Antiquity: Philosophical Perspectives on Abortion and Euthanasia*. Dordrecht, Netherlands: D. Reidel.

CLARK, GEORGE. 1964. *A History of the Royal College of Physicians of London*. Oxford: At the Clarendon Press.

DICKSTEIN, EMIL; ERLEN, JONATHAN; and ERLEN, JUDITH. 1991. "Ethical Principles Contained in Currently Professed Medical Oaths." *Academic Medicine* 66, no. 10: 622–624.

EDELSTEIN, LUDWIG. 1943. "The Hippocratic Oath: Text, Translation, and Interpretation." *Bulletin of the History of Medicine*, supp. 5, no. 1:1–64.

———. 1956. "The Professional Ethics of the Greek Physician." *Bulletin of the History of Medicine* 30, no. 5: 391–419.

ETZIONY, M. B. 1973. *The Physician's Creed: An Anthology of Medical Prayers, Oaths, and Codes of Ethics Written by Medical Practitioners Through the Ages*. Springfield, Ill.: Charles C. Thomas.

GRIESE, ORVILLE. 1987. "Origin and Development of a Catholic Hospital Code of Ethics, 1921–1971." In *Catholic Identity in Health Care: Principles and Practice*, pp. 1–19. Braintree, Mass.: Pope John Center.

JAKOBOVITS, IMMANUEL. 1975. *Jewish Medical Ethics: A Comparative and Historical Study of the Jewish Religious Attitudes to Medicine and Its Practice*. New ed. New York: Bloch.

JONES, WILLIAM H. S. 1924. *The Doctor's Oath: An Essay in the History of Medicine*. Cambridge: At the University Press.

KELLY, DAVID F. 1979. *The Emergence of Roman Catholic Medical Ethics in North America: An Historical-Methodological-Bibliographical Study*. New York: Edwin Mellen Press.

LEAKE, CHAUNCEY D., ed. 1927. *Percival's Medical Ethics*. Baltimore: Williams and Wilkins.

MENON, I. A., and HABERMAN, H. F. 1970. "The Medical Students' Oath of Ancient India." *Medical History* 14, no. 3:295–299.

NATIONAL COMMISSION FOR THE PROTECTION OF HUMAN SUBJECTS OF BIOMEDICAL AND BEHAVIORAL RESEARCH. 1978. *The Belmont Report: Ethical Principles and Guidelines for the Protection of Human Subjects of Research*. Washington, D.C.: U.S. Government Printing Office.

ROSNER, FRED. 1967. "The Physician's Prayer Attributed to Moses Maimonides." *Bulletin of the History of Medicine* 41:440–454.

ROSNER, FRED, and MUNTNER, SUSSMAN. 1965. "The Oath of Asaph." *Annals of Internal Medicine* 63, no. 2:317–320.

SACRED CONGREGATION FOR THE DOCTRINE OF THE FAITH. 1987. "Instruction on Respect for Human Life in Its Origin and on the Dignity of Procreation." *Origins* 16, no. 40:698–711.

TEMKIN, OWSEI. 1991. *Hippocrates in a World of Pagans and Christians.* Baltimore: Johns Hopkins University Press.

TICHTCHENKO, PAVEL D., and YUDIN, BORIS G. 1992. "Toward a Bioethics in Post-Communist Russia." *Cambridge Quarterly of Healthcare Ethics* 1, no. 4:295–303.

UNSCHULD, PAUL ULRICH. 1979. *Medical Ethics in Imperial China: A Study in Historical Anthropology.* Berkeley: University of California Press.

VEATCH, ROBERT M., and MASON, CAROL G. 1987. "Hippocratic vs. Judeo-Christian Medical Ethics: Principles in Conflict." *Journal of Religious Ethics* 15, no. 1:86–105.

MEDICAL DECISION MAKING

See MEDICINE, ART OF. *See also* LIFE, QUALITY OF, *article on* QUALITY OF LIFE IN CLINICAL DECISIONS.

MEDICAL EDUCATION

When this subject was addressed in the first edition of this encyclopedia, the paucity of systematic analyses of the ethical issues peculiar to medical education was underscored (Pellegrino, 1978). In recent years, this deficiency has gradually been redressed, so that today, a considerable body of literature is available. This entry is therefore a substantial revision of the first. The emphasis has shifted from underlying values to more specific, normative issues, particularly in clinical education.

Ethical issues arise in medical education because of the special societal role of medical schools, the necessary intermingling of patient care with education, and the conflicts that may arise because of the obligations among students, patients, faculty members, and society. Similar ethical issues are present in the education of nurses, dentists, and the allied health professions.

The social mandate of medical schools

Medical schools occupy a unique moral position in society. They are mandated to meet society's need for a continuous supply of competent practitioners who can care for the sick and promote the public's health. For this reason, medical schools are supported as loci for the advancement and transmission of medical knowledge and are granted authority to select who shall study medicine, what shall be studied, and what standards of performance shall be established.

To achieve these goals, medical schools require certain special privileges, for example, to dissect human bodies, to provide "hands on" practical experience for students in the care of sick people, and to conduct human experimentation. These practices would be criminal were they not socially mandated for a good purpose.

When medical schools, students, and faculty avail themselves of these privileges, they enter an implicit covenant with society to use them for the purposes for which they are granted.

To fulfill this social covenant, medical schools and their faculties must perform a tripartite function with respect to medical knowledge: 1) they must preserve, validate, and expand it by research; 2) transmit it to the next generation by teaching; and 3) apply it by practice in the care of the sick. However, these three functions have different aims. The aim of research is truth that requires dedication to objectivity, freedom of inquiry, rigorous design, as well as peer review and publication. The aim of teaching is learning that requires dedication to student welfare, competent pedagogy, and opportunities for students to practice their skills. The aim of practice is the welfare of the patient that requires dedication to compassion, competence, and ethical concern for the vulnerability, dignity, and autonomy of the sick person.

In the past, these three functions were less often in conflict with each other than they are today. This conflict is the result of several factors in the evolution of medical education since the late nineteenth century. The first factor is the realization of the power of the physical and biological sciences to advance medical knowledge and their integration into medical education. Second is the incorporation of teaching hospitals into medical schools for the clinical education of medical students (Flexner, 1910). Third is the increasing reliance on practice income to support salaries of medical teachers. Previously, teachers had been self-supporting practitioners from the community, while only a few were university-funded full-time teachers. Today's "tenure track" clinical faculty member is expected to excel in research, to support himself or herself financially through practice and overhead cost recovery from grants, and to teach at the bedside. Each function has its own legitimacy, but taken together, these functions conflict with each other.

Ethical obligations of medical schools

The ethical obligations of medical schools as societal entities are defined in terms of the constituencies they serve: society, faculty, student body, and patients (Pellegrino, 1976).

Medical schools have been granted a virtual monopoly over the number of students they admit and the number of training places in the various specialties in teaching hospitals. Medical schools are the sole portal into the practice of the profession and, as a result, medical schools incur a responsibility to match the kind and number of physicians they produce with the needs of society. This requires a socially responsive appraisal by medical schools of the way resources are used and curricula are designed, as well as how faculty rewards are distributed. Societal aims sometimes can, and do, conflict with a medical school's pursuit of esteem among its peers, which usually comes not through renown in teaching or the quality of practitioners it produces, but excellence in producing research and academic leaders.

Another important obligation of medical schools is to ensure that graduates are competent to enter postgraduate training and are free of obvious traits of character that would make them dangerous practitioners. Today, most of those admitted to medical school graduate and obtain licenses. Few fail, particularly in the clinical years. This places an obligation on medical schools to evaluate not only a student's knowledge and skill, but some facets of his or her character as well. Close supervision by clinical teachers is mandatory if dubious character traits are to be detected. Educators must balance fairness in their evaluations of students against their obligations to protect future patients from unsafe or dishonest practitioners.

Another societal responsibility of medical schools is to ensure equal opportunity for admission to all qualified students. Despite early progress, there is recent evidence of retrenchment in the support, financial and otherwise, available for minority student recruitment in the United States and in Great Britain (Hanft and White, 1987; Esmail and Everington, 1993). Subtle forms of discrimination probably still exist in the interview process where it is difficult to detect and prove (Connolly, 1979). Gender discrimination and sexism are no longer legally tolerable, but remain a persistent social problem (Hostler and Gressard, 1993). Academic administrators and faculty members are morally obliged to ensure equitable treatment of all applicants and must assume collective responsibility for inequities and injustice. In doing so, medical schools must thread their way carefully through an ethical maze of competing claims for preferential treatment and reverse discrimination.

Ethical obligations exist in the relationship between medical schools and faculty members. Faculties are owed freedom of inquiry in research and teaching, justice in hiring, tenure, promotion, compensation, and redress for injury or grievances. Faculty members in turn are morally responsible for the quality of their instruction, for fairness in the evaluation of students, and for properly apportioning their time and effort between teaching and personally remunerative activities such as clinical practice and consultation. Imbalance among these activities compromises the societal responsibilities of a medical faculty.

Faculty and administration are therefore obligated to detect inadequate teachers and to rehabilitate and reassign them or terminate their appointments when necessary. Tenure is among the most privileged benefits of academic life. The obligation to use it responsibly rests squarely on faculty members and administrators.

Incidents of scientific fraud, abuse of consulting and travel privileges, and conflicts of interest are cause for legitimate public concern. While the number is small, such abuses by faculty members invite external limitations and regulation of privileges that can interfere with the educational mission. The ethics of medical academia cannot be a private matter since the moral behavior of academics affects students, patients, the use of public funds, and the quality of fulfillment of the medical school's covenant with society.

Some ethical issues peculiar to clinical education

The ethical issues outlined thus far are particular only in part to medical education. What is unique is the medical school's engagement in clinical education, i.e., in providing "hands on" experience for students in the actual care of patients. It is here that serious conflict may arise between patient care and student learning.

Physicians since Hippocrates have taught their students from actual cases. Usually, this was accomplished by preceptorship with a practicing physician or by case demonstrations to entire classes of students. In the mid-nineteenth century, it was a rare school that incorporated more intimate involvement in the care of patients in its teaching (Ludmerer, 1985). Toward the end of the same century, William Osler involved students more directly as clinical clerks at the Johns Hopkins Hospital, where they ". . . lived and worked . . . as part of its machinery, as an essential part of the work of the wards" (Osler, 1943, p. 389). This practice lagged in other schools until the reform of education in 1910 (Ludmerer, 1985). Since then, however, it has become standard pedagogic practice.

Today, clinical education centers on practical experience under supervision at every level, from medical school through postgraduate specialty training to lifelong continuing education. Until recently, the merits of this training have been so much taken for granted that the ethical conflicts inherent in the process have been neglected (Fry, 1991; Pilowski, 1973).

Clinical education by its nature unavoidably puts the aims of caring for patients into potential conflict with the aims of teaching and learning. The involvement of medical students, interns, and residents in patient care slows the process of care, increases its discomforts and fragmentation, and, at times, poses significant danger to the patient. With close supervision by experienced clinical teachers, these potential conflicts are tolerable. The clinical teacher therefore carries a double responsibility for balancing the quality of his or her pedagogy with the quality of patient care.

The moral status of medical students is ambiguous. They are physicians in utero, that is, in a developmental state of competence to provide care. When they enter medical school they are laypersons. When they graduate they are physicians, still in need of further training before they can become safe and competent practitioners. During this process, they take on progressive degrees of responsibility associated with the privilege of caring for patients, although their capacity to fulfill that responsibility is limited.

Patients come to university hospitals primarily to receive optimal treatment, not to be subjects of teaching. They may understand in a general way what being in a teaching hospital means. This in no way suggests, as some assume, that patients give implicit consent to become "teaching material." Patients in teaching hospitals preserve their moral right to know the relative degrees of competence of those caring for them. They have a right to give informed consent to any procedures and to know whether an untrained or partially trained person will perform that procedure. When unskilled students participate in procedures, patients are owed appropriate supervision by someone of significantly greater competence who can protect their safety.

Medical students, therefore, should disclose the fact that they are students to avoid the attributions of knowledge and trust patients still associate with anyone bearing the title "doctor" (Greer, 1987; Ganos, 1983; Brody, 1983; Liepman, 1983). They should be introduced as students by their supervisors before procedures like spinal taps and chest taps are performed. For their part, students as well as their supervisors must thoroughly acquaint themselves with the procedures in question and must observe a sufficient number performed by experienced clinicians. Students are under an obligation to refrain from conducting a procedure until these requirements are met and to resist the "see one, do one" philosophy of some clinical teachers. They must also receive instruction on how to obtain a morally and legally valid consent (Johnson et al., 1992).

Students must also be sensitive enough to discontinue even the simplest procedures, such as a venipuncture, if their efforts cause discomfort (Williams and Fost, 1992). These injunctions are particularly important in highly personal and sensitive situations such as learning to do vaginal or rectal examinations (Bewley et al., 1992; and Lawton et al., 1990).

Medical students also face problems of personal ethical integrity with respect to abortion, treating patients with acquired immunodeficiency syndrome (AIDS), and attitudes toward the poor (Christakis and Feudtner, 1993; Dans, 1992; Crandall et al., 1993; Currey et al.;

1990; Holleman, 1992). They may observe unethical or unacceptable behavior of teachers or colleagues (Morris, 1992). The extent of their responsibility and the real possibility of punitive treatment if students "blow the whistle" is a difficult, unresolved, but genuine ethical issue. Students may cheat on exams or see others do so (Rozance, 1991; Stimmel, 1990). By virtue of their presence at the bedside as members of the "team," they may be drawn prematurely into advising about the ethics of other colleagues. Helping students to deal with these moral dilemmas poses a new challenge to students and to their clinical teachers. This is a crucial part of the ethical maturation of the student (Drew, 1992; Andre, 1992; Wiesemann, 1993).

Two final examples of recently debated ethical dilemmas center on the moral status of dead human bodies and of animals of other species similar to humans. To what extent may recently dead human bodies be used to teach intubation, resuscitation, and tracheostomy? Who can, or should, give permission? May it be presumed? Is it necessary at all (Benfield et al., 1991; Iserson, 1993)? Are the moral rights of other animal species to be considered so that they never or rarely should be used in teaching or research? Do computer models or tissue and cell preparations adequately replace animal experimentation?

Conclusion

Despite the sanction society gives to clinical education, there are important ethical obligations that limit this privilege. In no sense can learning by practice be a "right" of medical students or medical schools no matter how high the tuition or the degree of social utility. The privileges of clinical education cannot be bought at any price by the student, or granted even for good purpose by the medical school. Only a social mandate can legitimize the invasions of privacy a medical education entails.

The ethical issues of clinical education have just begun to receive the ethical scrutiny they deserve. Fundamental conceptual issues like the moral status of medical students, dead bodies, and animals are coupled with very practical issues regarding student–faculty and student–patient relationships. Clearer guidelines are needed to deal with the ethical issues characteristic of clinical education. We can expect the literature on this topic to expand in size, sophistication, and importance in the immediate future.

EDMUND D. PELLEGRINO

Directly related to this entry is the entry BIOETHICS EDUCATION, *especially the article on* MEDICINE. *For a further discussion of topics mentioned in this entry, see the entries*

ACADEMIC HEALTH CENTERS; ALLIED HEALTH PROFESSIONS; ANIMAL WELFARE AND RIGHTS, *article on* ETHICAL PERSPECTIVES ON THE TREATMENT AND STATUS OF ANIMALS; CLINICAL ETHICS; CONFLICT OF INTEREST; DENTISTRY; FAMILY; FRAUD, THEFT, AND PLAGIARISM; INFORMED CONSENT; NURSING ETHICS; RACE AND RACISM; SEXISM; UTILITY; VIRTUE AND CHARACTER; *and* WHISTLEBLOWING. *For a discussion of related ideas, see the entries* AUTHORITY; COMPETENCE; HARM; HEALTH CARE, QUALITY OF; IATROGENIC ILLNESS AND INJURY; MEDICINE, ANTHROPOLOGY OF; PROFESSIONAL–PATIENT RELATIONSHIP; RISK; *and* TEAMS, HEALTH-CARE.

Bibliography

ANDRE, JUDITH. 1992. "Learning to See: Moral Growth During Medical Training." *Journal of Medical Ethics* 18, no. 3:148–152.

BENFIELD, D. GARY; FLAKSMAN, RICHARD J.; LIN, TSUN-ASIN; KANTAKI, ANAND D.; KOKOMOOR, FRANKLIN W.; and VALLMAN, JOHN H. 1991. "Teaching Intubation Skills Using Newly Deceased Infants." *Journal of the American Medical Association* 265, no. 18:2360–2363.

BEWLEY, SUSAN. 1992. "Teaching Vaginal Examination." *British Medical Journal* 305, no. 6849:369.

BRODY, HOWARD. 1983. "Deception in the Teaching Hospital." In *Difficult Decisions in Medical Ethics: The Fourth Volume in a Series on Ethics and Humanism in Medicine*, pp. 81–86. Edited by Doreen L. Ganos, Rachel E. Lipson, Gwynedd Warren, and Barbara J. Weil. New York: Alan R. Liss.

CHRISTAKIS, DMITRI A., and FEUDTNER, CHRIS. 1993. "Ethics in a Short White Coat: The Ethical Dilemmas that Medical Students Confront." *Academic Physician* 68, no. 4:249–254.

CONNOLLY, PAUL H. 1979. "What Are the Medical Schools Up To? Abortions and Admissions." *Commonwealth* 105, no. 17:551–552.

CRANDALL, SONIA J.; VOLK, ROBERT J.; and LOEMKER, VICKI. 1993. "Medical Students' Attitudes Toward Providing Care for the Underserved: Are We Training Socially Responsible Physicians?" *Journal of the American Medical Association* 269, no. 19:2519–2523.

CURREY, CHARLES J.; JOHNSON, MICHAEL; and OGDEN, BARBARA. 1990. "Willingness of Health-Professions Students to Treat Patients with AIDS." *Academic Medicine* 65, no. 7:472–474.

DANS, PETER E. 1992. "Medical Students and Abortion: Reconciling Personal Beliefs and Professional Roles at One Medical School." *Academic Medicine* 67, no. 3:207–211.

DREW, BARBARA L. 1992. "What If the Whistle Blower Is a Student? The Advisory Role of the Instructor." In *Ethical Dilemmas in Contemporary Nursing Practice*, pp. 117–127. Edited by Gladys B. White. Washington, D.C.: American Nurses Publishing.

ESMAIL, A., and EVERINGTON, S. 1993. "Racial Discrimination Against Doctors from Ethnic Minorities." *British Medical Journal* 306, no. 6879:691–692.

FLEXNER, ABRAHAM. 1910. *Medical Education in the United States and Canada: A Report to the Carnegie Foundation for the Advancement of Teaching*. Birmingham, Ala.: Classics of Medicine Library.

FRY, SARA T. 1991. "Is Health Care Delivery by Partially Trained Professionals Ever Justified?" *Journal of Clinical Ethics* 2. no. 1:42–44.

GANOS, DOREEN L. 1983. "Introduction: Deception in the Teaching Hospital." In *Difficult Decisions in Medical Ethics: The Fourth Volume in a Series on Ethics and Humanism in Medicine*, pp. 77–78. Edited by Doreen L. Ganos, Rachel E. Lipson, Gwynedd Warren, and Barbara J. Weil. New York: Alan R. Liss.

GREER, DAVID S. 1987. "To Inform or Not to Inform Patients About Students." *Journal of Medical Education* 62, no. 10:861–862.

HANFT, RUTH S., and WHITE, CATHERINE C. 1987. "Constraining the Supply of Physicians: Effects on Black Physicians." *Milbank Quarterly* 65 (suppl. 2):249–269.

HOLLEMAN, WARREN LEE. 1992. "Challenges Facing Student Clinicians." *Human Medicine* 8, no. 30:205–211.

HOSTLER, SHARON L., and GRESSARD, RISA P. 1993. "Perceptions of the Gender Fairness of the Medical School Environment." *Journal of the American Medical Women's Association* 48, no. 2:51–54.

ISERSON, KENNETH V. 1993. "Postmortem Procedures in the Emergency Department: Using the Recently Dead to Practice and Teach." *Journal of Medical Ethics* 19, no. 2:92–98.

JOHNSON, SHIRLEY M.; KURTZ, MARGOT E.; TOMLINSON, TOM; and FLECK, LEONARD. 1992. "Teaching the Process of Obtaining Informed Consent to Medical Students." *Academic Medicine* 67, no. 9:598–600.

LAWTON, FRANK G.; REDMAN, CHARLES W. E.; and LUESLEY, DAVID M. 1990. "Patient Consent for Gynaecological Examination." *British Journal of Hospital Medicine* 44, no. 5:326, 329.

LIEPMAN, MARCIA K. 1983. "Deception in the Teaching Hospital: Where We Are and Where We've Been." In *Difficult Decisions in Medical Ethics: The Fourth Volume in a Series on Ethics and Humanism in Medicine*, pp. 87–94. Edited by Doreen L. Ganos, Rachel E. Lipson, Gwynedd Warren, and Barbara J. Weil. New York: Alan R. Liss.

LUDMERER, KENNETH M. 1985. *Learning to Heal: The Development of American Medical Education*. New York: Basic Books.

MORRIS, MARK. 1992. "When Loyalties Are Divided Between Teachers and Patients." *Journal of Medical Ethics* 18, no. 3:153–155.

OSLER, WILLIAM. 1943. *Aequanimitas: With Other Addresses to Medical Students, Nurses, and Practitioners of Medicine*. 3d ed. Philadelphia: Blakiston.

PELLEGRINO, EDMUND D. 1976. "Medical Schools as Moral Agents." *Transactions of the American Clinical and Climatological Association* 88:54–67.

———. 1978. "Medical Education." In vol. 2 of *Encyclopedia*

of Bioethics, pp. 863–870. Edited by Warren T. Reich. New York: Macmillan.

PILOWSKI, I. 1973. "The Student, the Patient and His Illness: The Ethics of Clinical Teaching." *Medical Journal of Australia* 1, no. 17:858–859.

ROZANCE, CHRISTINE P. 1991. "Cheating in Medical Schools: Implications for Students and Patients." *Journal of the American Medical Association* 266, no. 17:2453, 2456.

STIMMEL, BARRY. 1990. "Cheating in Medical Schools: A Problem or an Annoyance?" *Rhode Island Medical Journal* 73, no. 9:413–416.

WIESEMANN, CLAUDIA. 1993. "Eine Ethik des Nichtwissens." *Ethik Med* 5:3–12.

WILLIAMS, CHARLES T., and FOST, NORMAN. 1992. "Ethical Considerations Surrounding First Time Procedures: A Study and Analysis of Patient Attitudes Toward Spinal Taps by Students." *Kennedy Institute of Ethics Journal* 2, no. 3:217–231.

MEDICAL ETHICS, HISTORY OF

I. NEAR AND MIDDLE EAST

A. ANCIENT NEAR EAST

In its conventional sense the term "ancient Near East" includes a diverse range of cultures. This article limits its coverage to Mesopotamia from the Sumerian period (beginning ca. 3100 B.C.E.) through the Babylonian period (ending with the Persian conquest in 539 B.C.E.), Egypt from about 3100 B.C.E. to its conquest by Alexander the Great (332 B.C.E.), and Israel from the Exodus (variously dated from 1446 B.C.E. to 1280 B.C.E.) to the destruction of Jerusalem by the Romans in 70 C.E.

In both Mesopotamia and Egypt thriving medical professions existed throughout the period under consideration. In Israel a distinct medical profession appears to have developed very late (second century B.C.E.). If anything that could be called medical literature was produced in Israel, it was at the very end of our period. By contrast a large body of medical literature, some of which has survived, existed in both Mesopotamia and Egypt.

Conceptual observations

No writer in the ancient Near East appears to have addressed what we call medical ethics as an area of specific discussion. No one seems to have written even on that weak precursor of medical ethics known as medical etiquette. Nevertheless, medical ethics existed as much in the ancient Near East as in any other culture. The medical ethics of any society is generally congruous with that society's moral perceptions. As a subset of its ethical values, medical ethics will be as simple or as complex as any culture is monolithic or pluralistic. An ethical framework exists for the practice of medicine wherever those who treat disease, even in a magico-religious form, administer healing. In seeking to reconstruct the medical ethics of any society, one must understand the broad cultural framework within which healers function in order to appreciate the ethical considerations that directly or indirectly govern the practice of their art. This picture may be supplemented by the incidental illumination of relevant aspects of medical practice gleaned from medical and other literature, as well as by evidence of legal constraints upon the activities of practitioners of the healing arts.

J. V. Kinnier Wilson remarks that "Medically, as in other respects, Egypt, Mesopotamia, and Palestine were three quite different worlds. Each developed along independent lines of thought and was of its own kind"

(1982, p. 337). While this statement is essentially correct, Mesopotamia and Egypt are sufficiently similar when contrasted with Israel that they may be considered together, while Israel, because of its unique religious and moral outlook, merits separate treatment.

Mesopotamia and Egypt

The understanding of disease and the role of physicians. In Egypt and Mesopotamia all aspects of life were molded by religions that were naturalistic and polytheistic, based on the worship of cosmic forces, and steeped in magic. Health and physical wholeness were perceived as being present so long as life remained in harmony with the forces of deified nature, while illness reflected a dissonance between the individual and his or her total environment. It was imperative to identify the cause of sickness in order that the appropriate treatment might be given for the restoration of health. Edwin Yamauchi isolates

> four main sources of illness, which were not mutually exclusive: (1) a divine source which sent illness as a punishment for sin; (2) a demonic source which indwelt or tormented the individual; (3) a magical source sent from a sorcerer or practitioner of black magic; and (4) a natural source as discerned by experience. The modes of treatment would include: (1) prayer, sacrifice and repentance; (2) the exorcism of demons; (3) countermagic; and (4) empirical applications of medicine, drugs, or surgery. Quite frequently different kinds of treatment were combined. (1986, p. 99)

In both Mesopotamia and Egypt the treatment of disease attributed to divine, demonic, or magical sources fell within the purview of a class of healers different from those who treated disease attributed to natural causes. In Mesopotamia the latter class (the *azu* or *asû*) appears to have emerged much earlier than the former (the *āšipu*). According to Kinnier Wilson, "In Sumerian times—as it would seem—the *azu* was the only doctor who was prominent in society. It is only at a later period, in Babylonia, that one meets the *āšipu*, a specialist in incantations and a kind of medical 'diviner,' capable of reading the 'signs' of suffering or of divine punishment" (1982, p. 349). The two professions were functionally and ideologically distinct, and only the *āšipu* was a priest. Similarly, in Egypt, the *seynu* (or *swnw*), like the Mesopotamian *asû*, was concerned with the treatment of physical conditions, whether sicknesses or injuries, for which a proximate, natural causality was evident; the *heri-ha'ab*, the equivalent of the Mesopotamian *āšipu*, was essentially a magician or exorcist (Kinnier Wilson, 1982). In a third category was the *wabw*, the priest of Sekhmet, lion-headed goddess of war, who both caused and cured epidemics. The *wabw* often combined features of both the *seynu* and the *heri-ha'ab*. Although each constituted a distinct profession, any two or even all three might be combined in the same practitioner.

Medical ethics.   The ethics of healers reflected an environment in which the understanding and explanation of reality were thoroughly religious: All aspects of life, including sickness and healing, received their meaning from religion (see Amundsen and Ferngren, 1982). The therapeutics employed by the *asû* and the *seynu* in dealing with acute diseases and injuries seem rational when compared with the predominantly magico-religious techniques of the *āšipu* and the *heri-ha'ab*. But the words of Owsei Temkin are cogent here:

> To be historically comprehensive, medicine cannot be defined as a science or the application of any science or sciences. Medicine is healing (and prevention) based on such knowledge as is deemed requisite. Such knowledge may be theological, magic, empirical, rationally speculative, or scientific. The fact that medicine in our days is largely based on science does not make other forms less medical—though it may convince us that they are less effective. (1977, p. 16)

Those ancient Near Eastern practitioners who seem to have been more rational than their magico-religious colleagues were not more ethical. Theirs were complementary, not competitive, professions. We do not have here a case of medical rationalism vying with superstition. Within their cultures neither approach was more or less rational than the other. Both perceived the causality of disease within an epistemological context in which spiritual, magical, and natural categories were not clearly distinguished. Hence, in this environment, the ethical obligations of healers must be appreciated in terms of their role as interpreters of sickness and healing within the broader cosmological realities and social values of their community. Within this general framework we can glean from the primary sources some specific, although fragmentary, aspects of medical ethics of the ancient Near East.

To treat or not to treat.   The Egyptian physician, as revealed by the medical papyri, made a prognosis before undertaking treatment. If the prognosis was favorable, the physician's comment was "an ailment that I shall treat"; if it was uncertain, "an ailment that I shall combat"; and if the prognosis was unfavorable, "an ailment not to be treated." The Edwin Smith Papyrus (a sixteenth-century B.C.E. copy of an earlier text that was probably written between 3000 and 2500 B.C.E.) contains the record of fifty-eight examinations, each followed by either treatment or a decision not to treat (Breasted, 1930). The author recommends treatment in forty-two cases and leaves sixteen untreated. In three of the hopeless cases (6, 8a, and 20), some alleviating treatment is indicated. In the Papyrus Ebers (Ebbell, 1937), which dates from roughly the same period, a

small number of cases are regarded as untreatable (e.g., cols. 108–110), and in one hopeless case there is an attempt to relieve the patient. That specific alleviatory instructions are given only in a minority of hopeless cases does not necessarily indicate a lack of compassion. Incidental remarks in these papyri suggest that physicians carefully and gently treated their patients and showed kindness to the ill, injured, and maimed.

In Mesopotamia *āšipus* were prognosticators whose medical repertoire consisted mostly of incantations and charms, occasionally supplemented by ointments and purgatives. They did not hesitate to withdraw from cases that they regarded as hopeless. Their colleagues, the *asûs*, who administered medicines, performed some surgery, and seldom used incantations, seem only rarely to have refrained from treating hopeless cases, but continued with treatment to the end. This difference may be due in part to the fact that the *āšipu* treated primarily chronic illnesses, while the *asû* usually dealt with acute diseases and injuries (Ritter, 1965).

Euthanasia and abortion.   There is no direct evidence pro or contra regarding the ethics of euthanasia. It appears that in both Mesopotamia and Egypt those who committed suicide were regarded as having cut themselves off from the gods. A touching dialogue between a man contemplating suicide and his *ba* (soul), survives from Egypt, dating from the end of the third millennium B.C.E. (Pritchard, 1969). Although the man is not considering suicide owing to illness, the psychological struggle portrayed reveals a culture in which suicide was not accepted simply as a personal option without moral and religious compunctions, although the text suggests that it was not uncommon. Whether physicians assisted in suicide or viewed active euthanasia as opprobrious is unknown.

Prescriptions for induced abortion are found in the Egyptian medical papyri, but its legality remains unclear. In Mesopotamia, Middle Assyrian laws (fifteenth century B.C.E.?; Pritchard, 1969) stipulate that if a woman has an abortion by her own act, whether or not she survives the ordeal, she is to be impaled on a stake and left unburied. The purpose here (as in much other ancient law prohibiting abortion) is not to protect the fetus but to protect the husband's right to have the child he fathered. There is no mention of the involvement of physicians in abortion.

Regulation of the medical professions and legal protection of patients.   The first recorded attempt to protect the patient from the incompetent physician is from Babylonia, in the Code of Hammurabi (ca. 1750 B.C.E.; Pritchard, 1969). There it is specified that if a physician performs a major operation with a bronze lancet on a member of the nobility that results in the patient's death, or an operation with a bronze lancet on his or her eye that results in its loss, the physician's hand will be cut off. If an operation with a bronze lancet results in the death of a commoner's slave, or if the operation causes the loss of the slave's eye, the physician is to pay half the slave's value in silver. No punitive regulations are extant governing medical procedures other than surgery. This is understandable, particularly in a culture permeated by magical beliefs. The unsuccessful use of incantations or sympathetic magic (the administration of medicinal herbs may be included in this category), in which the healing role of the practitioner is nearly passive because of the supernatural agents at play, stands in marked contrast to the active immediacy of the physician in surgery. The Code of Hammurabi also establishes fees for surgery. The amount is determined by the social status of the patient, indicating the intention of the legislator to peg medical fees to the patient's economic means.

Little is known about the regulation of healers in Egypt. Although there appears to have been no system of medical licensure, medical procedure became rigidly prescribed over the centuries. A Greek historian, Diodorus Siculus (first century B.C.E.), whose material on Egypt was derived from the sixth-century B.C.E. Greek geographer Hecataeus, writes that Egyptian physicians gave treatment in accordance with ancient written procedures. If their patients died, the physicians were absolved from any charge. If they deviated from traditional methods in any way, they were subject to the death penalty, on the assumption that few physicians could be wiser than the physicians of old. In the *Politics*, Aristotle describes a slightly more flexible situation in Egypt, in which physicians could alter their prescriptions after four days; if they altered them earlier, they did so at their own risk.

Little evidence exists from the ancient Near East regarding experimentation with novel procedures. In a letter to the Assyrian king (seventh century B.C.E.?), a physician suggests that a particular prescription be tested on members of the domestic staff before being administered to a member of the royal family. While cesarean section is known to have been performed in Mesopotamia in the second millennium B.C.E. as a last resort to save the infants of dying women, the evidence suggests that the procedure was used only on slaves. These examples suggest the fear of risk involved in novel procedures. But there were other hindrances to therapeutic experimentation: the tendency of empirical physicians to rely on traditional procedures; the existence of a written tradition of medical knowledge and procedures in both Mesopotamia and Egypt; and the fact that medicine was often allied ideologically with religion. These factors are likely to have inhibited innovation that deviated from accepted practice even in late Egyptian medicine. Although evidence is lacking for Mesopota-

mian attitudes to novel procedures, they are not likely to have been more positive.

Ancient Israel

The basic difference between the worldview of the Hebrews (ca. 1300 B.C.E.–70 C.E.) and that of their ancient Near Eastern neighbors was one of religious outlook. Israel's religion was monotheistic, while that of its neighbors was polytheistic, focused on the worship of natural forces, particularly those associated with fertility. In the Hebrew Scriptures, the cosmos is perceived as being under Yahweh's direction. Although there is a personal force of evil (Satan), he is subordinate to Yahweh and poses no significant challenge to his authority. While polytheism imposed no absolute moral standards, the ethical beliefs of Israel were grounded in the character of Yahweh, who was regarded as the transcendent creator and sustainer of the world. Religion and ethics were inseparable, since both were derived from Yahweh, who was holy and required holiness of his people. Yahweh's absolute character gave authority to his revelation to Israel, and his holiness provided the ethical basis of Israel's laws. The law of Israel, the Torah, grew out of Yahweh's covenant with the Hebrews, which made them his special people. As a requirement of maintaining the covenant, Israel was to reflect the moral character of Yahweh in its national life.

The Hebrew understanding of disease and healing. In the Hebrew scriptures illness is viewed in its moral and spiritual dimensions rather than as a merely physical phenomenon. A close relationship between sin and illness was believed to exist at two levels: (1) Physical evil, including illness, entered the world as a consequence of sin; and (2) illness was sometimes visited upon both individuals and nations because of their sin. Hence disease and injury were a consequence of sin, but they were also within the realm of God's control. Yahweh says, "I kill and I make alive; I wound and I heal" (Deut. 32:39). Disease, as a manifestation of God's wrath against sin, could be seen on both an individual (e.g., Num. 12:9–12; 2 Kings 5:25–27; 2 Chron. 21:11–18) and a national level (e.g., 1 Sam. 5:6–12). Yahweh promises health and prosperity to his covenant people if they are faithful to him, and disease and other suffering if they spurn his love (e.g., Exod. 15:26; Lev. 26:14–16; Deut. 28:21–22, 27–28, 59–61; Ezek. 14:21; Hos. 6:1).

Passages often considered messianic offer the hope of healing, physical as well as spiritual (e.g., Isa. 53:4–5; Mal. 4:2). When the Messiah comes, "No one in Jerusalem will say 'I am sick'; the people who dwell there will be forgiven their iniquity" (Isa. 33:24). The mental and physical anguish that accompanies the guilt of a person smitten and disciplined by Yahweh for sin is spoken of repeatedly in the Psalms (e.g., Ps. 38:3, 5, 8), while to acknowledge and repent of sin is said to bring healing (Ps. 32:3–5). Forgiveness and consequent healing were not viewed as the result of appeasing a hostile deity through ritual and offerings (see, e.g., Ps. 51:16–17). Suffering in general, and sickness in particular, represented Yahweh's chastisement of his people, which was corrective rather than retributive. This theodicy, however, did not make suffering easier to endure for those who searched their hearts but could find no specific sin to be confessed (e.g., Ps. 88; Job, passim). The righteous sufferer must acknowledge God's inscrutable ways and ultimate goodness (e.g., Ps. 94:12; Prov. 3:11–12).

Physicians and medicine. The judgment upon King Ahaziah for consulting the god of Ekron concerning his illness (2 Kings 1:2–4) resulted from the same kind of sin for which Asa, king of Judah, was condemned. Asa was seriously ill, "yet even in his disease he did not seek the Lord, but sought help from physicians. And Asa slept with his fathers" (2 Chron. 16:12–13). Asa is not condemned for resorting to secular medicine as such but, rather, for consulting physicians who were probably Mesopotamian or, less likely, Egyptian. The procedures practiced by these physicians, even if empirical, would have been magico-religious. There is no evidence that priests functioned as physicians or surgeons in Israel. Their only involvement in matters pertaining to health was in the enforcement of a highly developed code of personal and social hygiene (Lev. 12, 13, 15, 21). Were there healers in Judah whom Asa could have consulted, whose practices would not have violated Jewish religious scruples? This question cannot be answered with certainty since there is no evidence in the Hebrew scriptures of the existence of a distinct medical profession.

The Hebrew word for healer or physician is the participle of the verb *rapha,* the original meaning of which appears to be "one who sews together" or "one who repairs." Its first participial occurrence is found in Gen. 50:2, where Egyptian physicians are said to have embalmed Jacob. The verb itself is often used literally in the sense of healing from disease or injury (e.g., Gen. 20:17; Num. 12:13; 2 Kings 20:5–8). When Jeremiah (ca. 645–ca. 575 B.C.E.) writes, "Is there no balm in Gilead? Is there no physician there?" (Jer. 8:22), although he is speaking metaphorically, he attests the existence of both balm, as a therapeutic substance, and some kind of healers. The Israelites, of course, had knowledge of the rudimentary treatment of wounds and of herbs that could be used to treat various ailments traceable to natural causes. The Torah stipulates that if a person injures another in a quarrel and the injured party survives, the assailant is to be held financially liable "for the loss of his time, and shall have him thor-

oughly healed" (Exod. 21:18–19). This passage implies that the expense both for medicines and for healers to dispense or apply them was to be borne by the guilty party. Several incidental references suggest the existence of binders of wounds (Isa. 3:7), knowledge of the setting of fractures (Ezek. 30:21), and the use of various therapeutic substances (Isa. 1:6; Jer. 51:8).

Although the Hebrew scriptures represent Yahweh as the only healer (e.g., Exod. 15:26) and command Israelites to refrain from resorting to magical or pagan healing practices (see, e.g., Ezek. 13:17–23), the use of natural or medicinal means is not discouraged, but is resorted to even in ostensibly miraculous healings (e.g., 2 Kings 20:7). Medical knowledge may have been limited to folk remedies, however, and there probably were no systematized therapeutics, much less medical practitioners who were distinctively Hebrew. Not until the second century B.C.E. is there evidence of a Jewish medical profession. Contact with Greek civilization in the Hellenistic age provided Jews with something that neither Mesopotamia nor Egypt could contribute: a religiously neutral theoretical framework for a rational understanding of disease and healing that allowed the coexistence of both divine explanations of ultimate causality and natural processes of proximate causality within Yahweh's created order.

The earliest mention of a Jewish medical profession is in the Wisdom of Jesus Ben Sira (also known as Ecclesiasticus), composed in Palestine early in the second century B.C.E. Ben Sira urges his readers to honor the physician as a servant of God, who gives him his skill. Dependence upon God is essential for the patient, because it is God who heals. The physician, too, must depend upon God, "for also he supplicates God that he may make his diagnosis successful and his treatment to save your life" (38:1–15, Noorda's translation [1979]). In spite of an occasional critic like Philo Judaeus (an Alexandrian Jew of the early first century C.E.), who scathingly condemned fellow Jews who trusted in medicine without reference to God and turned to him only as a last resort (Temkin, 1991), Hellenistic Jews accepted rational medicine based on the Greek model as fully compatible with their faith. Apart from the available medical resources, which were limited, healing could come only from Yahweh by confession of sin, supplication, and prayer (e.g., Job 33:19–30).

Medical ethics. Central to understanding Hebrew and Jewish medical ethics is the concept of the image of God (*imago Dei*). In the Genesis account of creation, Yahweh is depicted as having created man and woman in his image (Gen. 1:26–27). Endowed with rationality, self-consciousness, and volition, the human personality in Hebrew thought was represented as mirroring Yahweh's image. Persons are spiritual beings, created to have communion with God, and responsible for their own moral actions. The concept of the *imago Dei* had implications for the protection of human life, which was believed to possess intrinsic value, and hence to be sacred. Even human beings with physical defects are said to bear God's image. Yahweh asks Moses, "Who has made man's mouth? Who makes him dumb, or deaf, or seeing, or blind? Is it not I, the Lord?" (Exod. 4:11).

As a result of the Hebrew view of humanity as possessing intrinsic worth, the Torah exhibits a greater humaneness than other codes of the ancient Near East (e.g., the Code of Hammurabi). There are, for example, provisions that protect the rights of the blind and the deaf (e.g., Lev. 19:14). The fetus was regarded as having been created by Yahweh and designed for a specific purpose (Ps. 139:13–16; Jer. 1:5; Isa. 49:1). Yet abortion was not explicitly forbidden by either the Torah or later rabbinic Judaism. In fact, in the Talmud it was permitted in some circumstances. Whether the practice was acceptable in the pre-Christian era is disputed. The accidental destruction of the fetus was not a capital offense, but required monetary compensation (Exod. 21:22–25). The newborn child, however, was regarded as fully human and deserving of the same protection as an adult. Infanticide, a common practice in the surrounding Canaanite culture, was expressly prohibited (Lev. 18:21, 20:2), and the exposure of newborn children was also condemned (see Exod. 1:17–21; Ezek. 16:5). Castration, sometimes practiced by Canaanites for religious purposes, was also forbidden, and eunuchs were excluded from Hebrew religious life (Deut. 23:1).

The Hebrew scriptures provide no information regarding the behavior expected of Jewish physicians. Mesopotamian and Egyptian physicians had an enormously varied repertoire of religious and magical techniques of propitiation and manipulation, as well as of natural therapeutics, from which to choose. They also had the freedom to be imaginative, active participants in processes in which the lines between what we call the natural and the supernatural were blurred. By contrast, Jewish physicians, working with and through natural means and processes, and eschewing any techniques involving magic or the demonic, were, along with their patients, to depend upon the Creator, from whom alone all true and licit healing came (Deut. 32:39). Given the emphasis in the Hebrew scriptures on the compassionate nature of the God who heals, and the importance that Ben Sira assigns to the physician as an agent of God, it would be surprising if Jewish physicians were not encouraged to emulate the divine compassion in their treatment of the ill. This attitude would be especially compatible with the new emphasis on the meritorious nature of charity that is found in the Apocrypha (Jewish religious writings dating from third century B.C.E. to about 100 C.E. that were not included in the Hebrew scriptures). It is in the postexilic period (after 605–582 B.C.E.), too, that one begins to see a tradition of caring for the ill that makes the sick person no longer an object of stigmatization (e.g., Job 19, esp. 13–20; Ps. 42:4–10), but a person deserving of special care, like widows and orphans (e.g., Sirach 7:35; 2 Macc. 8:28). This specific concern for the sick within the community of Israel is a theme that is extended and developed in the Talmud.

DARREL W. AMUNDSEN
GARY B. FERNGREN

While the other articles in this entry are relevant, see especially the other articles in this section: IRAN, TURKEY, CONTEMPORARY ARAB WORLD, *and* ISRAEL. *For a further discussion of topics mentioned in this article, see the entries* ABORTION; ALTERNATIVE THERAPIES; DEATH AND DYING: EUTHANASIA AND SUSTAINING LIFE; ETHICS; HEALING; HEALTH AND DISEASE; MEDICAL CODES AND OATHS, *article on* HISTORY; MEDICINE, ANTHROPOLOGY OF; MEDICINE, SOCIOLOGY OF; PROFESSION AND PROFESSIONAL ETHICS; RIGHTS; SURGERY; *and* UNORTHODOXY IN MEDICINE. *Other relevant material may be found under the entries* JUSTICE; RESPONSIBILITY; *and* VALUE AND VALUATION.

Bibliography

AMUNDSEN, DARREL W., and FERNGREN, GARY B. 1982. "Medicine and Religion: Pre-Christian Antiquity." In *Health/Medicine and the Faith Traditions: An Inquiry into Religion and Medicine*, pp. 53–92. Edited by Martin E. Marty and Kenneth L. Vaux. Philadelphia: Fortress.

BIGGS, ROBERT. 1969. "Medicine in Ancient Mesopotamia." *History of Science* 8:94–105.

BREASTED, JAMES HENRY, trans. 1930. *The Edwin Smith Surgical Papyrus: Published in Facsimile and Hieroglyphic Transliteration, with Translation and Commentary.* 2 vols. Chicago: University of Chicago Press.

EBBELL, BENDIX, trans. 1937. *The Papyrus Ebers: The Greatest Egyptian Medical Document.* Copenhagen: Levin and Munksgaard.

FERNGREN, GARY B. 1987. "The *Imago Dei* and the Sanctity of Life; The Origins of an Idea." In *Euthanasia and the Newborn: Conflicts Regarding Saving Lives*, pp. 23–45. Edited by Richard C. McMillan, H. Tristram Engelhardt, Jr., and Stuart F. Spicker. Dordrecht, Netherlands: D. Reidel.

GHALIOUNGUI, PAUL. 1963. *Magic and Medical Science in Ancient Egypt.* London: Hodder and Stoughton.

HOGAN, LARRY P. 1992. *Healing in the Second Temple Period.* Göttingen: Vandenhoeck and Ruprecht.

JACOB, IRENE, and JACOB, WALTER, eds. 1993. *The Healing Past: Pharmaceuticals in the Biblical and Rabbinic World.* Leiden: E. J. Brill.

KINNIER WILSON, J. V. 1982. "Medicine in the Land and Times of the Old Testament." In *Studies in the Period of David and Solomon and Other Essays: Papers Read at the International Symposium for Biblical Studies, Tokyo, 5–7 December, 1979*, pp. 337–365. Edited by Tomoo Ishida. Winona Lake, Ind.: Eisenbrauns.

NOORDA, SIJBOLT J. 1979. "Illness and Sin, Forgiving and Healing: The Connection of Medical Treatment and Religious Beliefs in Ben Sira 38, 1–15." In *Studies in Hellenistic Religions*, pp. 215–224. Edited by Maarten Jozef Vermaseren. Leiden: E. J. Brill.

OPPENHEIM, A. LEO. 1962. "Mesopotamian Medicine." *Bulletin of the History of Medicine* 36, no. 2:97–108.

PREUSS, JULIUS. 1978. *Julius Preuss' Biblical and Talmudic Medicine*. Translated by Fred Rosner. New York: Hebrew Publishing.

PRITCHARD, JAMES BENNETT, ed. 1969. *Ancient Near Eastern Texts: Relating to the Old Testament*. 3d ed. with suppl. Princeton, N.J.: Princeton University Press.

REINER, ERICA. 1964. "Medicine in Ancient Mesopotamia." *Journal of the International College of Surgeons* 41, no. 1:544–550.

RITTER, EDITH K. 1965. "Magical-Expert (= Āšipu) and Physician (= Asû): Notes on Two Complementary Professions in Babylonian Medicine." In *Studies in Honor of Benno Landsberger on His Seventy-fifth Birthday; April 21, 1965*, pp. 299–321. Chicago: University of Chicago Press.

ROSNER, FRED. 1977. *Medicine in Bible and the Talmud: Selections from Classical Jewish Sources*. New York: Ktav.

SEYBOLD, KLAUS, and MUELLER, ULRICH B. 1981. *Sickness and Healing*, pp. 16–96. Translated by Douglas W. Stott. Nashville, Tenn.: Abingdon.

SIGERIST, HENRY ERNEST. 1951. "Ancient Egypt." In *Primitive and Archaic Medicine*, pp. 215–373. Vol. 1 of his *A History of Medicine*. New York: Oxford University Press.

———. 1951. "Mesopotamia." In *Primitive and Archaic Medicine*, pp. 377–397. Vol. 1 of his *A History of Medicine*. New York: Oxford University Press.

TEMKIN, OWSEI. 1977. *The Double Face of Janus*. Baltimore: Johns Hopkins University Press.

———. 1991. "The Almighty God." In his *Hippocrates in a World of Pagans and Christians*, pp. 86–93. Baltimore: Hopkins University Press.

WILSON, JOHN A. 1962. "Medicine in Ancient Egypt." *Bulletin of the History of Medicine* 36, no. 2:114–123.

YAMAUCHI, EDWIN. 1986. "Magic or Miracle? Diseases, Demons and Exorcisms." In *The Miracles of Jesus*, pp. 99–110. Edited by David Wenham and Craig Blomberg. Vol. 6 of *Gospel Perspectives: Studies of History and Tradition in the Four Gospels*. Edited by R.T. France and David Wenham. Sheffield, U.K.: JSOT.

B. IRAN

The following is a revision and update of the first-edition article "Medical Ethics, History of: II. Near and Middle East and Africa: 2. Persia" by Rahmatollah Eshraghi.

Iran, a vast country in Southwest Asia, was long called Persia by Europeans until, in 1935, its government requested that the common indigenous name, Iran, identifying the nation as the "land of the Aryan people," be used internationally. The extensive Iranian Plateau and surrounding lands have been the site of many powerful political regimes during its long history, beginning with the empire of Cyrus the Great, the first Achaemenid emperor, in 549 B.C.E. Located along a highway for the movement of people and ideas from the prehistoric period on, its indigenous Aryan culture has been an important link between Hellenic, Indic, and Semitic intellectual and religious traditions. Within the limits of this article, the history of Persian medicine cannot be traced; only the ethics characteristic of that history will be treated.

Prehistoric period

Little is known about the healing practices or beliefs of the earliest inhabitants of Iran. An epic poem, *Shāhnāmah* (Book of Kings), written in the tenth century C.E., relates ancient myths, legends, and stories that may reveal something of the ancient past. Surgery is mentioned in the tales of the superhuman exploits of the heros Rustam and Isfandyar. Rustam himself is said to have been delivered by an operation much like that now known as a cesarean section, while his mother was anesthetized with wine. Abortifacients were known. The Elamite civilization, centered around Susa in southern Iran from the third to the first millennium, had cultural contact (and often political enmity) with Babylon, and it is likely that the medicine of the Mesopotamian world was known by the Elamites (Sigerist, 1951). The Code of Hammurabi, ruler of Babylon (ca. 1750 B.C.E.), which contains strict injunctions and penalties regarding surgical practice and malpractice, is known primarily from a stela found at Susa in 1902.

The Aryan period (ninth–fourth century B.C.E.)

The nomadic Aryan peoples migrated from Central Asia, north and east of the Caspian Sea, to the Iranian Plateau around the seventeenth century B.C.E. By the ninth century, they dominated the region, and in 549 B.C.E., Cyrus consolidated rule over its inhabitants and established the Achaemenid dynasty, the first Persian empire. He and his successors, Cambyses, Darius, and Xerxes, extended the boundaries of Persian rule from the Ionian Sea in the west to the Indus River in the south. During this period, Persian medicine was undoubtedly in contact with Greek medicine. A story related in ancient texts tells of an invitation from Persian King Artaxerxes to Hippocrates, on the advice of a Persian physician, to become physician to the Persian army during a plague; Hippocrates refused, saying, "I have no right to share the wealth of the Persians or to liberate from disease barbarians who are enemies of the Greeks" (Pseudepigrapha 3; see Temkin, 1991).

In the seventh century, the mysterious religious figure Zoroaster appeared in eastern Persia. Very little is known of his life, and the writings attributed to him are brief. However, by the first century B.C.E., a defined cosmogony and theology attributed to his influence had been collected in the vast literature called *Avesta,* of which his own *Gathas,* or hymns, are a small part. The doctrine is basically constructed around a cosmic duel between good and evil, of which light and darkness, life and death are the material symbols. The powerful spirit of good and light, Ahura Mazda, the wise and greatest god, battles Ahriman (or Angra Mainyu), spirit of evil and darkness, and the world is the battlefield. Humans participate in the battle through their free choices. As individuals, humans are to maintain purity of life through moral goodness, pursuit of truth and physical cleanliness, and avoidance of pollution by the dead and unclean substances. As members of society, humans are to assure justice between social classes.

The *Avesta* also contains the elements of a theory of health and disease. Diseases, created by Ahriman, come from dirt, stench, cold, heat, hunger, thirst, and anxiety, although magical causes are also recognized. Medicinal plants are the creation of Ahura Mazda. Rules of healthful living are prescribed; cupping and bleeding are recommended to reduce hot blood. The destruction of life is prohibited for theological reasons; it would contribute to the victory of Ahriman over Ahura Mazda. Thus, abortion is forbidden, and both men and women are punished as willful murderers. Special rules are laid down for the care of pregnant females (both human and animal). Surgery is recognized and strictly regulated; one ancient law requires that a surgeon have three successful cases before being licensed to practice.

Three kinds of healers are mentioned: healers with herbs, with knives, and with holy words (the latter, one text notes, being the most efficacious). There were also persons (*durustpat,* masters of health) trained to remove the causes of disease by purifying earth, air, water, and food. These physicians were often drawn from the noble and priestly classes. A modern Parsi (the contemporary Zoroastrians of India) scholar describes what he believes would have been the ideals of the Avestan physicians of ancient times:

> The first indispensable qualification of a physician was that he should have studied well the science of medicine. He should hear the case of his patient with calmness. He should be sweet-tongued, gentle, friendly, zealous of honour of his profession, averse to protracting illness out of greed and God fearing. An ideal healer heals for the sake of healing. . . . He should carefully

watch the effect of medicine that he prescribes . . . visit the invalid daily at a fixed hour, labour zealously to cure him, and combat the disease of the patient, as it were his own enemy (Elgood, 1951, p. 13).

Hellenistic period (330 B.C.E.–224 C.E.)

In 330 B.C.E. Alexander of Macedon brought down the Achaemenid empire. For the next five centuries, the Greek culture that had long flourished on the Ionian frontier of the Persian empire dominated Persian ideas and institutions. Although the historical record is meager, it may be assumed that Greek medicine and Hippocratic ethics were included in this general influx of Hellenic culture. The Zoroastrian faith languished during that era, but it would not be unlikely that Avestan ideals that had permeated the culture survived.

Sassanid period (224–632)

The Sassanid dynasty, after victories over Roman and Parthian armies in the mid-third century, ruled Persia for four centuries, restoring the traditions, law, and culture of ancient Iran and, above all, reforming and fostering the Zoroastrian faith. In the earliest years of the Sassanid era, an event of great importance for the history of medicine occurred. In the mid-250s, King Shāpūr I, son of the founder of the dynasty, defeated the Roman emperor Valerian and sacked the city of Antioch. The king invited many of the Antiochean scholars, including physicians, to a new city, Gondishapur, that he established in 260. His son enlarged the city and founded a university that in time became the center of scholarly work in Persia.

To Gondishapur in the late fifth century came a group of Persian Christians of a denomination called Nestorian. These Christians had originally dwelt in and around the Persian city of Nisibis, then moved to the Byzantine city of Edessa, where in 363 they established a school of theology. After certain of their theological beliefs were repudiated and their leader, the patriarch Nestorius, excommunicated by the Catholic church at the Council of Ephesus (431), the Persian Christians accepted an offer of asylum at Gondishapur from the Persian king Qubād. They brought with them not only works of theology but also an extraordinary library including Syriac translations of the Hippocratic corpus and of Galen.

Another scholarly migration entered Gondishapur in 529 when the Sassanid king Anūshīrvān the Just welcomed the Neoplatonists exiled from Athens, at the urging of his chief minister Buzurgmehr, who according to legend was himself a physician and philosopher. He is quoted as having said, "I read in medical books that the best physician is one who gives himself over to his profession. . . . I exerted myself in the treatment of patients, those whom I could not cure I tried to make their suffering more bearable. . . . From no one whom I treated did I demand any sort of fee or reward" (Elgood, 1951, p. 52).

The king also sent missions to India to procure the arts and sciences of Hindu culture, including the works of Ayurvedic medicine. By his order, a massive work on poisons was compiled, and many Greek and Indian books were translated into Pahlavi (ancient Persian). He convened what may have been the first medical convention, summoning the physicians of Gondishapur to debate the major medical questions of the day. During his long reign, Gondishapur became a leading center of scholarship; within its walls Greek, Jewish, Nestorian, Persian, and Hindu ideas were exchanged and enriched, and Islamic, Christian, and Zoroastrian ethical ideas mingled. The art of translation of the classic texts from Greek, Latin, and Syriac into Pahlavi and Arabic was fostered. The school of medicine existed for five centuries, creating from many sources the medical science generally known as Arabic or Islamic, and its great hospital, Bimaristan (House of the Sick), was the model for the Muslim hospitals of Baghdad, Damascus, and Cairo and the Christian hospitals of Jerusalem and Acre (Whipple, 1936).

Islamic period (636–)

The victory of Arabian Muslim armies at al-Qādisiyah in 636 inaugurated the era of Islamic rule and culture in Iran. The distinctive ethic of Islam entered and eventually predominated in the rich mix of Persian life. Gondishapur continued to flourish under Arab rule and became more influential as its scholars, teachings, and books spread through rapidly expanding Islam, carrying Greek and Arabic medicine across Africa and, through Sicily and Spain, into western Europe. The new Muslim rulers summoned scholars from Gondishapur to their capital at Baghdad, where they established a new center of medical science. Studies in biology, human anatomy, and pathology were encouraged. The caliphs in Baghdad, Damascus, and Cairo organized public-health administrations, staffs of public-health doctors, public hospitals, and a public examiner of physicians, responsible for their skills and their ethical standards.

Some of the greatest names of medical history were Persian: Ṭabarī, Rhazes (known as the Galen of Islam), Haly Abbas, Avicenna (Ibn Sīnā), all of whom flourished in the tenth and eleventh centuries. Their scientific work was renowned. (Avicenna's *Canon of Medicine* was used as a text in many European schools as late as the seventeenth century.) All of these distinguished physicians wrote treatises on the ethical qualities of physicians. The text of one of these, *Advice to a Physician*, by Haly Abbas, reflecting Hippocratic and Islamic

sentiments, can be found in the Appendix of this encyclopedia. A book by the eleventh-century Iranian philosopher–physician Ibn-Hindū praises the nobility and criticizes physicians who use medicine only to win wealth and reputation, recalling the story that Hippocrates, when summoned by the Persian ruler, disdained to give his service only for gain (Mohaghegh, 1992). Another scholar of the next century, Niẓāmī 'Arūḍī, summarized the moral principles that should guide a physician:

> A physician should be of tender disposition and wise nature, excelling in acumen, this being a nimbleness of mind in forming correct views, that is, a rapid transition to the unknown from the known, and no physician can be of tender disposition if he fails to recognize the nobility of the human soul; nor of wise nature unless he is acquainted with logic, nor can he excel in acumen unless he be strengthened by God's aid, and he who is not acute in conjecture will not arrive at a correct understanding of any ailment (Elgood, 1951, p. 234).

Modern period

For many centuries medicine in Iran was more or less as has been described. The foundation of Dār-ul-Funūn (the Polytechnic School) in Tehran in 1852 changed the situation. At first it was a military academy, but it soon began to develop into a university. The foundation of the Faculty of Medicine was laid by a number of excellent European and Iranian teachers. The school curriculum at first was a combination of Iranian and Western medicine, and the ethical point of view was influenced by Iranian tradition.

Iranian students had been sent to Europe for medical studies for several decades before the founding of the medical school at Dār-ul-Funūn. With the return of these physicians and scientists and the establishment of a modern hospital in Tehran in 1868, the curriculum of Dār-ul-Funūn and the practice of medicine were gradually westernized. Also, during the nineteenth century, a number of Western physicians resided in Iran, the most famous being a Frenchman, Charles Fourier, physician to Shah Nāṣir al-Dīn.

Since the period of Reza Shah (1923–1941), the program of the medical school of the modern University of Tehran has been based completely on modern medicine; medical ethics and the history of the medical tradition are both taught. Graduates of the Tehran medical school are asked to take an oath, an excerpt from which follows:

> Now that I . . . have been found eligible to practice medicine, in the presence of you, the board of judgment of my thesis and others here present, I swear by God and the Holy Book of Koran and call to witness my conscience that in my profession I will always be abste-

mious, chaste, and honest and, as compared with the glory of the art of medicine, I will hold in contempt all else—silver, gold, status, and dignity. I promise to help the afflicted and needy patient and never divulge patients' secrets. I will never undertake dishonest work such as producing abortion and recommending a fatal drug.

What I do, I will try always to be approved by God and be known for my uprightness.

In the Islamic Republic of Iran, founded in 1979, the interest in vivifying Islamic tradition and law touches medical ethics as well. Issues related to bioethics are sometimes treated in works dealing with Islamic religious law, the *shar'ia*. However, the premodern *shar'ia* contains little that can directly guide conscience and conduct in morally troublesome cases, such as the permissibility or prohibition of medical treatments. Muslim jurists have undertaken to provide new rulings, the most prominent of which states the rights of the patient in determining which modes of treatment are compatible with his or her religious and moral beliefs. These scholars are also grappling with the medical technology developed in the Western secular culture, technology that has altered conventional understandings of life and death and has posed perplexing questions for a new, religiously aware generation of Iranian physicians and their "believing" patients.

Some recent works in medical ethics, such as *Fiqh va tibb* (Islamic Jurisprudence and Medicine) and *Qānūn dar tibb* (Law in Medicine), reflect a change in the attitude of Muslim physicians, who have become increasingly aware of the role religion plays in the lives of Iranian men and women. Whereas in the early days of modernization and secularization, Iranian physicians, not unlike their counterparts in other Third World countries, "played God" in attempting to save and restore human health, the 1980s and 1990s are characterized by a growing concern about the religious and cultural values of the society. Thus, for instance, an important issue in Islamic law is the recommended segregation of females and males, which has implications for medical ethics. The ethical issue is whether it is permissible for a physician to treat a member of the opposite sex. While responses have varied among the Muslim jurists, there is a consensus that since a physician should never sexually abuse his or her patients, it is strongly recommended that a physician examine patients of the opposite sex only in the presence of a third person, as a safeguard. This applies to both male and female doctors. However, under special circumstances, when no doctor of the same sex as the patient is available and there is an urgency in treating the condition, the law permits male doctors to treat female patients and female doctors to treat male patients.

Advances in biomedical technology raise issues that challenge Islam to provide concrete and relevant solutions. A group of Muslim jurists and philosophers has begun to develop guidelines for dealing with ethical issues that confront the medical profession. Leaders in both secular and religious education have begun to prepare textbooks on medical ethics. Two of these works are especially significant: *Akhlāq-i pizishkī* (Medical Ethics), prepared and published under the supervision of the Ministry of Health in 1991, and a book with the same title, written by Mansūr Ashrafī and published by the Medical Faculty of the Open University of Tabriz in 1988. The former includes chapters dealing with the juridical decisions by major Iranian religious leaders, including Ayatollah Khomeini, on issues related to what is known in the West as bioethics. The latter work is based more on the Western secular discussion of bioethical issues without any reference to Islamic or other religious views. Both are used as textbooks in the Iranian schools of medicine.

Major obstacles persist for those who work to solve the problems created when medical technology is brought into a culture steeped in religion. The most serious problem that confronts Muslims in general, and Iranians in particular, is denial of the ethical problems stemming from technicalization of the society and its adverse impact on interpersonal relationships. A striking example is acquired immunodeficiency syndrome (AIDS). To date, the Muslim ethical response to AIDS has characterized the disease as God's curse on those who engage in illicit sexual behavior. In this direct or indirect critique of the moral decadence of the West, important issues are overlooked, including the cause of the disease and its prevalence in the Muslim world, as well as guidelines for treatment of those affected.

Muslim jurists in Iran have not yet formulated relevant responses to some of the most complex ethical issues—those that arise because of human endeavors to improve health and extend life. The highly cherished religious value of compassion has been overshadowed by the language of condemnation for moral failure of humanity.

ABDULAZIZ SACHEDINA

While all the articles in this entry are relevant, see especially the section on EUROPE, *subsection on* ANCIENT AND MEDIEVAL, *article on* GREECE AND ROME, *and the other articles in this section:* ANCIENT NEAR EAST, TURKEY, CONTEMPORARY ARAB WORLD, *and* ISRAEL. *Directly related to this article is the entry* ISLAM. *For a further discussion of topics mentioned in this article, see the entries* ABORTION; ALTERNATIVE THERAPIES; ETHICS, *especially the article on* RELIGION AND MORALITY; HEALING; HEALTH AND DISEASE; MEDICINE, ANTHROPOLOGY OF; MEDICINE, SOCIOLOGY OF; *and* SURGERY. *Other relevant material may be found under the entries* JUSTICE; LIFE; *and* VALUE AND VALUATION. *See also the* APPENDIX (CODES, OATHS, and Directives Related to Bioethics), section ii: ethical directives for the practice of medicine, oath of a muslim physician *of the* islamic medical association of north america, *and the* islamic code of medical ethics *of the* islamic organization for medical sciences.

Bibliography

Ackerknecht, Erwin Heinz. 1968. *A Short History of Medicine.* 2d. rev. ed. Translated by Sula Wolff. New York: Hafner.

al-Akhavaynī al-Bukhārī, Abū Bakr Rabī ibn Ahmad. 1965. *Hidāyat al-muta 'allimīn fī al-tibb.* Edited by Jalāl Matīnī. Dānishgāh Intishārāt no. 9. Meshed, Iran: Meshed University Press.

al-Tūsi, Nasīr al-Dīn, Muhammad ibn Muhammad. 1964. [13th century]. *The Nasirean Ethics.* Translated and edited by G. M. Wickens. UNESCO Collection of Representative Works: Persian series. London: Allen & Unwin.

'Amili, Ja'far Murtada. 1989. *Akhlāq-i pizishkī dar Islām.* Tehran: Ministry of Health.

Aqili Alavī, M. H. 1870. [1770]. *Khulāsat al-Hikmah.* Tehran.

Ashrafi, Mansur. 1988. *Akhlaq-i pizishki.* Tabriz: Open University.

Avicenna (Abū 'Alī al-Husayn ibn 'Abdullah ibn Sīnā). 1966. [11th century]. *The General Principles of Avicenna's "Canon of Medicine."* Edited and translated by Mazhar H. Shah. Karachi, Pakistan: Naveed Clinic.

Browne, Edward Granville. 1921. *Arabian Medicine: Being the Fitzpatrick Lectures Delivered at the College of Physicians in November 1919 and November 1920.* Cambridge: At the University Press.

Clendening, Logan, ed. 1942. *Source Book of Medical History, Compiled with Notes.* New York: Paul B. Hoeber.

Davis, Nathan Smith. 1903. *History of Medicine, with the Code of Medicine.* Chicago: Cleveland Press.

Elgood, Cyril Lloyd. 1951. *A Medical History of Persia and the Eastern Caliphate from the Earliest Times Until the Year A.D. 1932.* Cambridge: At the University Press.

———. 1976. *Safavid Medical Practice; or, The Practice of Medicine, Surgery, and Gynaecology in Persia Between 1500 and 1750 A.D.* London: Luzac.

Eshraghī, R. 1969. *Akhlaq-i pizishki.* Meshed, Iran: Meshed Medical School.

Haly Abbas ('Alī ibn al-'Abbās al-Majūsī al-Arrajānī 1492. [10th century]. *Liber regalis disposito nominatus ex arabico.* Translated by Stephen of Antioch. Edited by Antonius Vitalis Pyrranensis. Venice: Bernardinus Ricius.

Iran. Ministry of Health. 1991. *Akhlāq-i pizishkī.* Tehran: Author.

Jurjānī, Ismā'īl ibn al-Hasan. 1960. [11th century]. *Zakhī-rah-i-khwārazmshāhī.* 5 vols. Tehran: Tehran University Press.

Levey, Martin. 1967. *Medical Ethics of Medieval Islam: With Special Reference to al-Ruhavi's Practical Ethics of the Physician.* Philadelphia: American Philosophical Society.

Mohaghegh, Mehdi, trans. 1992. "Ibn Hindū: The Key to Science of Medicine and the Student's Guide to Study." *Medical Journal of the Islamic Republic of Iran,* suppl. 6: 29–37.

Mokhtar, Ahmed Mohammed. 1969. "Rhases contre Galenum: Die Galenkritik in den ersten zwanzig Büchern des Continens von Ibn ar-Razi." Ph.D. diss., University of Bonn. Text in Arabic and German.

Nizāmī-'Arūdī-i-Samarqandī, Ahmad ibn 'Umar ibn 'Alī. 1936. [12th century]. *Chahār maqālā.* Tehran: Elmi Bookstore. Translated by Edward Granville Browne under the title *Revised Translation of the 'Chahár Maqála' ("Four Discourses") of Nizāmī-i 'Arú-dī of Samarqand, Followed by an Abridged Translation of Mírzá Muhammad's Notes to the Persian Text.* E. J. W. Gibb memorial series, vol. 11, no. 2. London: Cambridge University Press, 1921.

Plessner, Martin. 1974. "The Natural Sciences and Medicine." In *Legacy of Islam,* 2d ed. Edited by Joseph Schacht and C. E. Bosworth. Oxford: Clarendon Press.

Rahman, Fazlur. 1989. *Health and Medicine in the Islamic Tradition: Change and Identity.* New York: Crossroad.

Rhazes (Abū Bakr Muhammad ibn Zakariyā al-Rāzī). 1955–1971. [9th century]. *Kitāb al-Hāwī fī al-tibb.* 25 vols. Edited by the Osmania Oriental Publications Bureau. Hyderabad-Deccan: Dāiratu'l-Ma'ārif-il-Osmania.

Said, Hakim Mohammed. 1975. "Traditional Greco-Arabic and Modern Western Medicine: Conflict or Symbiosis." *Hamdard: The Organ of the Institute of Health and Tibi Research* 18, nos. 1–6:1–76, especially Appendix C, "Ethical Basis of Medicine," pp. 71–76.

———. 1976. *Al-Tibb al-Islami: A Brief Survey of the Development of Tibb (Medicine) During the Days of the Holy Prophet Mohammed (p.b.u.h.) and in the Islamic Age.* Karachi, Pakistan: Hamdard National Foundation. See especially "Muslim Medicine and Iran," pp. 80–82.

Siddiqi, Muhammad Zubair. 1959. *Studies in Arabic and Persian Medical Literature.* Calcutta: Calcutta University Press.

Sigerist, Henry Ernest. 1951. *Primitive and Archaic Medicine.* Vol. 1 of his *A History of Medicine.* New York: Oxford University Press.

Temkin, Owsei. 1991. *Hippocrates in a World of Pagans and Christians,* chap. 6. Baltimore: Johns Hopkins University Press.

Whipple, Allen O. 1936. "The Role of the Nestorians as the Connecting Link Between Greek and Arab Medicine." *Annals of Medical History* 8:313–323.

Wilcocks, Charles. 1965. *Medical Advance, Public Health, and Social Evolution.* Commonwealth and International Library, Liberal Studies Division. Oxford: Pergamon Press.

C. TURKEY

The modern nation of Turkey is situated on the continents of Europe and Asia, with the majority of its landmass occupying the vast Anatolian peninsula of Asia Minor. Surrounded by three seas, the Mediterranean and the Aegean seas on the west and south, and the Black Sea on the north, its territory has been the home of many nations and civilizations. It was ruled by the

Hittite and Phrygian kingdoms of the second and first millennia B.C.E., followed by the Persian, Hellenic, and Roman empires. In 330 C.E., the capital of the Roman Empire was moved to Byzantium, which was renamed Constantinople. In 1453, Mehmet II, the sultan of the Ottoman Turks, a people who during the previous century had invaded a great part of the deteriorating Byzantine Empire, captured Constantinople and established the Ottoman Empire over Asia Minor (and, in the course of time, over much of the Islamic world, from the Crimea to Morocco and the Balkan peninsula). The Ottoman Empire lasted from 1299 to 1922, and in 1923 it became a republic under the leadership of Mustafa Kemal. Turkey's medicine and its ethics bear the marks of this long history.

The Turkic peoples, dwelling from time immemorial in Central Asia, migrated into China, India, the Caucasus, and Persia. The earliest Turkic religion was a shamanistic animism marked by totems and magic. Contact with the spirit world was mediated by male and female shamans, called *kam*, who healed the sick with magic and charms and music. Other healers, called *otacı*, are mentioned in various sources, and archeological findings related to *otacı* exist as early as the eighth century C.E. *Otacı* were described as wise people informed of the causes of illness, advising about healthy living and treating mainly with herbs, as well as by bone-setting, massage, acupuncture, moxa, branding, etc. *Otacı* joined in a guild of healers called *kutu*. They were, according to the sources, in frequent debate with exorcists, who taught that illness was caused by evil spirits and driven out by charms. This conflict was especially emphasized following the conversion of many of the Turkic peoples to Islam in the tenth century.

In Turkistan, where Turkic peoples were in contact with Chinese Buddhism, monks functioned as healers (*otacı bakshy* in Old Turkish). Although supernatural healing powers were often attributed to them, they practiced medicine without remuneration as a way of achieving Buddhahood. Monasteries were places of hospitality and healing. A medical literature in Uighur Turkish began to appear in the eighth century. During this period there was considerable mingling of Chinese, Indian, and Persian medical concepts. Although healers were no longer believed to have supernatural powers, the attitude of holding them in high esteem was part of the Islamic culture.

From the sixth to the thirteenth century, Turkish tribes formed kingdoms throughout Central Asia and the Near East. In the tenth century, many Turkic tribesmen who were employed in the armies of the Abbasid caliphs were converted to Islam (some tribes adopted Buddhism; others, Manichaeanism; and some followed Nestorian Christianity or Judaism). Following the rise and fall of several significant pre-Islamic and Islamic Turkic king-

doms, one tribe, the Seljuks, became the most powerful force in Anatolia. They extended their rule into Iraq, Iran, and Syria, and during the eleventh and twelfth centuries they created the first major Turkish state, which fostered a rich literary, artistic, and scientific civilization. In 1066, Nizamul Mulk, vizier of the Seljuk ruler Alp Arslan, founded the Nazamiye University in Baghdad. The first state university known in history, it included a hospital. The Nureddin Hospital, founded by the Seljuk Atabeg Nurredin Zenagi in Damascus in 1154, educated many famous physicians, such as Ibn Abi Usaibia, Ibn al-Nafis, and Ibn al Qutt, and was the center of medicine at that period. The curriculum of the medical schools in the Seljuk period was demanding; after training and the presentation of their theses, the graduates were examined in the course of medical practice by the *muhtasib*, a high-ranking public official, and then swore an oath to practice medicine with competence and virtue.

During the reign of the Anatolian Seljuks, the nobility founded charity hospitals: In Kayseri, the Gevher Nesibe Hospital was established by Princess Gevher Nesibe in 1206, and the Divriği Hospital in 1228 by Princess Turan Melik; both are still standing. The hospital and medical school founded at Sivas in 1217 also remains; and the original charter, still extant, shows that the staff consisted of physicians, surgeons, ophthalmologists, nurses, and pharmacists. All persons in need, Muslim and non-Muslim, were accepted for treatment in these institutions. Although a rich medical terminology had existed in the Turkish languages in the eleventh century, medical literature in Arabic and Persian flourished during the Seljuk era and hundreds of Arabic and Persian works were written by Turks. Turkish cities—Ferghana, Tashkent, Samargand, Bokhara, Khwarizm, Balkh, Maraghah, Kashgar, Farab, and others—were the birthplace of many famous Islamic scientists, including Ibn Sina, Ibn Turk, Biruni, Farabi, and Harezm, and were also the important centers of Islamic culture.

Medical literature in the Turkish language began to flourish again in the fourteenth century. After the conquest of Constantinople, the Ottoman Empire continued to promote care for the needy sick and to further medical science and education. It was common for the large complexes built around mosques throughout the land to have a hospital attached for the sick poor, whether Muslim or not. Sultan Mehmet II opened a hospital in his new capital in 1470. A great hospital and a medical school were established within the complex of the Süleymaniye Mosque (1536). According to the founding documents, the professor of medicine was expected to be a faithful Muslim, virtuous, charitable, self-confident, courageous, gifted with intuition and keen senses, and educated in the subtleties of logic and medicine. He was required to teach students both medicine and the virtues and duties of the physician. Those who sought admission to medical school were to have graduated from the *medresse*, or university. (The Ottoman *medresse* not only provided necessary services of religion, science, and instruction; it also trained administrative and judicial personnel to meet the needs of the bureaucracy.) Medical school applicants were required to be persons of high moral character, and to be faithful Muslims. All received scholarships from charitable endowments. The professor as well as the students were supervised by a dean.

A chief court physician was the minister of health; he was responsible for public health, for the proper training of physicians and the administration of examinations, as well as for the safety of drug preparations. Physicians employed in the palace and hospitals outside were paid by the state, and their income increased in relation to their skill and rank. Still, there were more physicians practicing medicine in their special offices than employed by the state. Pharmacists, trained in an apprentice system, worked in hospitals and palace pharmacies. A school for surgeons and ophthalmologists existed in the sultan's palace.

Women were admitted to the practice of medicine during the Ottoman period, particularly for the care of women. The Topkapi Palace in Istanbul had a well-appointed infirmary for women in the harem, as well as an infirmary for royal pages. Renowned female physicians were summoned to care for women of the harem when necessary. Nurses were employed in the palace infirmaries as well as in hospitals outside the palace and were expected to be gentle, dedicated, and devoted to their patients. Midwives were respected and given official recognition after an apprenticeship. Women prepared and sold herbal extracts, and women inoculated against smallpox. Women were also influential in the founding of hospitals and the support of charitable works.

The ethics of Turkish medicine were formed by Islamic morality, Turkish mores, and the Hippocratic ideas inherited from Greek medicine. Many medical manuscripts from the thirteenth to the nineteenth centuries state these values in chapters generally titled "Advice for the Physician." Chief among the qualifications required of the Ottoman physician was good character, which included mercy, generosity, honesty, modesty, and an even temper. Physicians were expected to be clean and properly attired, and never to exaggerate. Such virtues were said to have a positive effect upon the sick person. Advice was also given about preserving confidentiality, charging fair prices, and serving the poor without charge. Physicians were warned not to make definitive statements about prognosis, since the course of disease is not predictable with certainty. Medicine made from unknown herbs, folk remedies, and experimental treatments were not to be used. Administering poisons and abortion, except for a therapeutic purpose, were strictly forbidden. In general, as the eminent fifteenth-century Ottoman surgeon Sabuncuoğlu noted, the conscience of the physician should prevail over his desires and passions.

Physicians and surgeons were held responsible for injuries that resulted from their ignorance, incompetence, or use of unorthodox methods. Islamic law required that patients give personal permission, in the presence of a judge and witnesses, before undergoing surgery. Many records of the religious courts bear testimony to this practice. Edicts were often issued to bar quacks from practice, and, in order to ensure that only qualified practitioners served the sick, examinations for medical licensure were frequently repeated and only the licenses of the successful renewed.

Although Turkish medicine had been in contact with European medicine since the sixteenth century (inoculation against smallpox was originally introduced into Europe from Turkey at the beginning of the eighteenth century) (Ünver, 1958), European medicine became influential with the founding, by Sultan Mahmud II, of a school of medicine in 1827 and a school of surgery in 1832; these schools were combined in 1836 and moved, three years later, to Galatasari, then a suburb of Constantinople. Although it was primarily a military school, civil students were admitted, too; all students were given scholarships by the state. European physicians joined the Ottoman instructors on the faculty, and from 1839 to 1870 the language of instruction was French. A vigorous flow into Turkey of faculty members from the European medical centers and a flow of students and specialists from Turkey to Europe marked nineteenth-century medical education. An Ottoman professor, Nahabed Roussignan, lectured on ethics in 1876–1877 at the University of Constantinople School of Medicine. The course was continued for many years by Professor Hovsep Nouridjan, who published his lectures as *Précis de déontologie medicale,* one of the earliest books on this subject printed in Europe. In 1933, the first department of medical history and ethics was founded by Süheyl Ünver in Istanbul University. Doctorates in medical ethics are now awarded, and as of 1994, ten of the twenty-eight Turkish medical schools had departments of ethics and such courses were given in all schools of medicine.

After establishment of the Turkish Republic in 1923, new laws and regulations were passed regarding health care, public health, and the duties of physicians. A successful fight was waged against epidemic diseases, and many municipal and state hospitals were founded all over Turkey. The Turkish Medical Association was founded in 1929, and the current version of the medical ethics code appeared in 1960; it comprises rules dealing with patient–physician and physician–physician relationships, confidentiality, advertising, human research, termination of pregnancy, malpractice, truth-telling, consultation, fees, and organization of practice. This code has juridical standing. Provincial medical associations have disciplinary authority over physicians who violate the code. Dentists and pharmacists have formed associations in recent years and also have codes of ethics. A National Congress on Medical Ethics was organized by the Medical Faculty of the University of Istanbul in 1977. It opened discussion of many topics, such as organ transplantation, determination of death, reproductive technologies, and military medicine. A second such congress was held in 1994.

A law on organ transplantation was passed in 1979. It specifies procedures for consent, donation, and determination of death, and prohibits advertising and commercialization of organs. Regulations dealing with the education and duties of those who provide family-planning services, including abortion and sterilization, appeared in 1983. Abortion, available on demand for any reason if there is no medical contraindication for the mother, is permitted up to the tenth week of gestation, and therapeutic abortion after that time; married women must have permission of their husband, and minors, of their parents. Married persons seeking sterilization must have consent of their spouse. Centers providing assisted reproduction must be licensed by the Ministry of Health. Embryos are not to be used for purposes other than reproduction and cannot be sold. A professional committee has been established for the oversight of assisted reproduction.

The Turkish Medical Association endorses the Nuremburg and Helsinki declarations. In 1993, a state regulation governing research with human subjects required review committees in research hospitals, and a Central Ethics Committee was established in the Ministry of Health. Local review committees sometimes function as ethics committees as well. In 1992, the Turkish Human Rights Association, the Turkish Medical Association, and the Torture Victims International Rehabilitation Council sponsored the Fifth International Conference on Torture and the Medical Profession in Istanbul. This conference issued a declaration against torture and specifically against any physician's involvement.

NIL SARI

While all the articles in this entry are relevant, see especially the other articles in this section: ANCIENT NEAR EAST, IRAN, CONTEMPORARY ARAB WORLD, and ISRAEL. Directly related to this article are the entries ISLAM; HOSPITAL, article on MEDIEVAL AND RENAISSANCE HISTORY; and VIRTUE AND CHARACTER. For a further discussion of topics mentioned in this article, see the entries ABORTION; FERTILITY CONTROL; LICENSING, DISCIPLINE, AND REGULATION IN THE HEALTH PROFESSIONS; MEDICAL CODES AND OATHS; ORGAN AND TISSUE TRANSPLANTS; RESEARCH METHODOLOGY; *and* RESEARCH POLICY. *Other relevant material may be found under the entries* ALTERNATIVE THERAPIES; BENEFICENCE; COMPASSION; HEALTH AND DISEASE; *and* MEDICAL EDUCATION.

Bibliography

ESIN, EMEL. 1981. "'Otacı': Notes on Archaeology and Iconography Related to the Early History of Turkish Medical Science." In *Uluslararası Türk-islam Bilim ve Teknoloji Tarihi Kongresi 14–18 Eylül 1981,* vol. 5, pp. 11–22. Istanbul: Istanbul Teknik Üniversitesi.

KIYAK, YAHYA. 1987. *Lectures on Medical Ethics.* Istanbul: Marmara University.

SARI, NIL. 1988. "Educating the Ottoman Physician." *Tip Tarihi Araştırmaları. History of Medicine Studies* 2:40–64.

———. 1989. "A View on the Dealers with Health in the Turkish Medical History." *Tip Tarihi Araştırmaları. History of Medicine Studies* 3:11–33.

ÜNVER, A. SÜHEYL. 1958. *Turki nizam-i-tib ki tarikh..* Lahore: Avicanna Society.

D. CONTEMPORARY ARAB WORLD

The Arab world comprises the twenty-one Arabic-speaking countries extending from the south of Iran westward to the coast of the Atlantic. Not all the people in these nations are descendants of the Semitic Arabs of the Arabian Peninsula, but the spread of Islam outward from Arabia in the seventh century led to widespread adoption of Arabic, the language of the Qur'an, Islam's scripture. Islam is the religion of 95 percent of the inhabitants of the Arab world. Of the world's nearly one billion Muslims, some 20 percent are Arab. Classical Arabic has been preserved through the constant standard in the Qur'an (the Islamic scripture that Muslims believe is God's very words received verbatim by Muhammad); colloquial dialects are used regionally but are easily understood by all.

Despite religion and language, the Arab world is not politically, socially, or economically homogeneous. Some countries are ruled by hereditary monarchies; others, by revolutionary military or quasi-military governments. Democracy is, on the whole, lacking, although it is the aspiration of the masses. Some countries are affluent (usually due to oil wealth), while others are poor; some are overpopulated and others sparsely populated. Currently the Arab world is categorized as belonging to the Third World. The average birth rate is 38.3 per 1,000, and the average infant mortality rate (first year of life) is about 68.2 per 1,000 (United Nations, 1992).

A characteristic of the region is the religious orientation of its people and the influence of religion on their lives. Islam recognizes both Judaism and Christianity as religions that come from God; all three religions hold generally the same prevailing moral values and thus have a unified ethical base. Society (of all religious backgrounds) tends to be conservative, sanctifying family integrity and family ties, upholding moralities prescribed by religion(s), averse to unchecked liberalism, and falling back on religion to categorize social trends and new lifestyles as acceptable or unacceptable.

Islam has a comprehensive framework of a legal system based on the Qur'an and tradition, covering all aspects of life, that serves as the source of legislation and the derivation of ethical rulings. And yet the great majority of the Arab world is not ruled by Islamic law, most of the governments being practically secular. One area has uniquely remained under the jurisdiction of Islamic law: that of family law. It is in this area that the bulk of medical ethics resides. Although many non-Muslims are physicians and patients in Arab countries, there is little dispute about medical ethics among them, since many common positions are shared by Islam, Christianity, and Judaism.

The medical profession is highly esteemed in the Arab world, and the physician is still called "the wise man," a centuries-old nomenclature. The physician is very highly regarded, and the doctor–patient relationship, based on trust and confidence, tends to be paternalistic.

Seeking medical help when one is sick is a religious duty. Muhammad said, "Your body has a right over you," and "Seek treatment, for God has created a cure for every illness; some already known and others yet to be known." The establishment of the medical profession is a religious duty of the community, which should designate some of its members to study medicine and should provide for the needs and requirements of medial education. A doctor should be appropriately qualified, for Muhammad said, "Whoever practices medicine without the appropriate knowledge is liable to pay compensation [if harm comes to the patient]."

It is not uncommon for medical practitioners who enjoy the confidence of their community to be consulted on nonmedical problems faced by families or individuals. People tend to accept that therapeutic ability is not absolute, and as long as the doctor has done his (or her) best, there is a willingness to accept and even forgive undesired outcomes. Insurance against professional liability is nonexistent, and the judicial system heeds this fact; unless it is a clear case of neglect or inexcusable ignorance, the physician is rarely held responsible for damages.

Medical education has deep historical roots in the major capitals (Baghdad, Cairo, and Damascus) since the era of Islamic civilization (eighth to sixteenth centuries). Modern schools have emerged since the nineteenth century, and many are as recent as the oil boom late in the twentieth century. With one or two exceptions, all Arab countries have one or more medical schools, Egypt, as many as thirteen.

English is the common language of education, with French or Arabic used in exceptional cases. Conversion to Arabic is under debate. Medical education and practice are open to both sexes and all religions without discrimination. Coeducation is the rule except in a few schools. There is no ban on examining the opposite sex. Dissection of the human body and postmortem examination are permitted; some schools, however, have to import cadavers from abroad to satisfy the need for teaching anatomy.

Medical ethics

The Arab world has known medical ethics since the writings of Imhotep of Egypt (3000 B.C.E.) and the Code of Hammurabi of Babylon (about the same time). The Oath of Hippocrates (ca. 460–355 B.C.E.) later took over, and since the ninth century various Islamic adaptions of it, as well as treatises and books on medical ethics, have been contributed by Al-Rahawi, Ibn Rabban, Avicenna (Ibn Sīnā), and many others.

In modern times, medical ethics has been taught as part of the curriculum of various disciplines, but since the 1940s it has become a separate course in the majority of medical schools, whether as a part of forensic medicine, community medicine, history of medicine, or on its own.

Although Islam is the principal source of medical ethics, the increasing complexity of biomedical discoveries and technological achievements during the latter half of the twentieth century have made it difficult for religious scholars to comprehend the issues and formulate rules on ethical acceptability from an Islamic point of view. There has been need for a forum in which religious scholars join with biomedical scientists and specialists in relevant disciplines such as law and sociology, policymakers, economists, and civic leaders of both sexes, to discuss specific issues in order to develop an Islamic consensus. To continue this collaboration, institutions have come into being since the early 1980s: the Islamic Organization of Medical Sciences (IOMS, Kuwait), the Islamic Research Congress (Egypt), and the Fiqh Congress of Makka (Saudi Arabia). The rulings of these government-approved agencies have a high moral weight and almost fill the legal gap that results because legislation usually lags behind new developments. These agencies have significantly contributed to Islamic medical ethics, addressing a number of issues that will be surveyed briefly.

An important milestone was the formulation of the Islamic Code of Medical Ethics (IOMS, 1981), ratified by the First International Conference on Islamic Medicine (held in Kuwait, January 1981) and endorsed by many Arab and Islamic countries. This code comprises eleven chapters: Definition of Medical Profession; Characteristics of the Medical Practitioner; Relations Between Doctor and Doctor; Relations Between Doctor and Patient; Professional Confidentiality; Doctor's Duty in Wartime; Responsibility and Liability; Sanctity of Human Life; Doctor and Society; Doctor and Biotechnological Advances; and Medical Education. All topics were authenticated by sources in the Qur'an and Islamic law. The code also includes the latest version of the Islamic Medical Oath, which reads (roughly translated):

> I swear by God: To regard God in practicing my profession; To respect human life in all stages, under all circumstances, and to do my best to rescue it from death, malady, pain and anxiety; To uphold people's dignity, cover their privacy, and keep their secrets; To be an instrument of God's mercy to near and far, virtuous and sinner, and friend and enemy; To pursue knowledge and to harness it for the benefit, not the harm, of humankind; to revere my teachers, teach my juniors, and cherish the fraternity with my colleagues; and to live my faith in private and in public . . . and God is my witness to this oath.

Derivation of Islamic medical ethics

The totality of Islamic law, called the Shari'a, is drawn from the Qur'an, the verbal teachings of Muhammad, followed by analogy and consensus. The Shari'a is expressed in a code of moral behavior that states what is sinful and what is not, as well as a body of laws that states what is legal and what is not. These two systems need not coincide. (An example is a person who commits adultery in the privacy of a closed room. Such a person has committed a sin but not a legal crime, since Islamic law requires four witnesses in order to establish the legal charge of adultery. The fate of such a sinner is left entirely to God, who will punish or forgive upon the perpetrator's repentance and appeal for mercy.) When ruling on the admissibility (or inadmissibility) of an issue, jurists take into consideration a number of rules such as "Necessities overrule prohibitions," "Choose the lesser of two evils if both cannot be avoided," "Public interest outweighs individual interest," and, especially in matters not specified in the primary sources of Shari'a, "Wherever welfare goes, there goes the statute of God." Examples of applying some of these will follow later.

Sanctity of human life

Human life should never be violated except in situations explicitly specified in the penal code and observing the rigorous criteria it establishes. Commenting on the killing of Abel by his brother Cain (the two sons of Adam), the Qur'an states: "On that account We ordained for the Children of Israel that if anyone killed a soul, unless it be for murder or mischief in the land, it would be as if he killed the whole people. And if anyone saved a life, it would be as if he saved the life of the whole people" (5:32). This principle has been invoked when ruling on abortion and euthanasia.

Abortion

In general terms abortion is legally prohibited and punishable. However, some physicians perform abortions illicitly, mainly in the private sector. In some countries, if abortion is done to avoid tarnishing the family name (pregnancy of the unmarried is a great shame in the Arab world), this circumstance is considered a mitigating factor if the case ever goes to court. Tunisia has gone a step further and legalized abortion after the third child, thus allowing it to be considered a form of family planning.

Among the religious community, various views on abortion have been held over the centuries. The writings of early scholars differed according to their perception of the beginning of life, and their views continued to be followed by generations of their adherents. On the belief that life started when the mother felt the movements of the fetus inside her (quickening, usually at the end of four months), some thought that abortion before then entailed no aggression on life. Others maintained that the fetus attained its human form at the end of the seventh week, and aborting it at or beyond this date would be unlawful. The majority, however, espoused the views of the great jurist Al-Ghazālī (eleventh century c.e.), who believed that life started with the fusion of the male and female seeds, and that it proceeded through an occult phase to the palpable phase felt by the mother. This view of the beginning of life therefore outlaws abortion and makes it reprehensible at any stage of pregnancy.

Modern juridical opinion has put an end to the historical diversity of opinion and settled for Al-Ghazālī's, following a number of conferences in the 1970s and 1980s (see, e.g., Gindi, 1989b) at which religious scholars met with medical scholars and a full account of the process of conception and early development was illustrated by ultrasound and cinematographic recordings of the fetus in utero. Five criteria were collectively acknowledged as signifying the beginning of life: (1) it is a fairly clearly defined event; (2) it exhibits the phenomenon of growth; (3) such growth, unless interrupted, leads to the known subsequent stages of life; (4) it contains the genetic package characteristic both of humanity and of a unique individual; and (5) it is not preceded by any stage combining the first four criteria (Gindi, 1989a).

Abortion is permitted if the continuation of pregnancy poses a serious threat to the life of a sick mother (the choice of the lesser of the two evils if both cannot be avoided). In Shari'a the mother is the root and the fetus the offshoot, and it is lawful to sacrifice the latter if it is the only way to save the former.

Selective abortion for the sake of sex selection is doubly unlawful, being an aggression on life as well as discrimination against the female (almost invariably the unwanted sex). The Qur'an severely rebuked pre-Islamic Arabs (up to seventh century C.E.) for practicing female infanticide (16:59). Sex selection by means not entailing embryocide, to suit the wishes of individual families, has been debated. There is consensus that its admissibility would eventually lead to an upset of the sex ratio in favor of male preponderance, which could lead to grave social consequences.

Euthanasia, suffering, and care of the elderly

Euthanasia and suicide are completely unacceptable in Islam. There are no euthanasia proponents, and therefore there is no debate. Suicide and complicity thereto are legal crimes, but the problem is of minute dimensions. The Prophet Muhammad told about a man who took his own life due to an illness that taxed his endurance, upon which God said, "My subject has himself forestalled Me; I have forbidden him Paradise" (narrated by Al-Bukhari). Resort to medical or surgical means for alleviation of pain is lawful, but the taking of life is a matter of God's sovereignty.

Patience in the face of unavoidable pain or adversity is an important value, and the Prophet teaches that through such patience a person's sins are washed away by God, like a tree shedding its leaves. The right to die is therefore not recognized because humans do not own life; they are only entrusted with it. The same applies to the "duty to die," recently proposed for human beings who, through age or infirmity, become consumers but not producers. Caring for a growing group of old and disabled can be very costly, as modern budget figures show, but under Islamic law society has to meet this need by rearranging expenditure priorities rather than allowing euthanasia. Care of the old is a principal value in Islam, especially with regard to one's parents: "Your Lord has decreed that you worship none but Him and that you be kind to your parents. . . . whether one or both of them attain old age in your life, say not to them a word of contempt nor repel them, and lower to them the wing of humility out of compassion, and say: 'My Lord, bestow on them your mercy even as they cherished me in childhood'" (Qur'an 17:23, 24).

However, it is generally agreed that in his or her defense of life, the doctor is well advised to realize the limitation of medical efforts. It is the process of life that the doctor aims to maintain, not the process of dying.

When treatment holds no promise, it ceases to be mandatory and withholding or discontinuing the artificial means is justified. No active intervention, however, shall be made to terminate life.

Death

Under ordinary circumstances the time-honored recognition of death based on cessation of heartbeat and respiration is workable, followed by a waiting period of two hours before the death certificate is issued. Nevertheless, advances in transplant surgery and the occasional need for a fresh heart for transplantation have called for a more sophisticated definition of death. Such a heart can usually be procured from a trauma victim whose brain—including brain stem—is dead and who therefore has been pronounced dead although artificial means are employed to maintain the functions of respiration and circulation.

The issue was discussed in a number of conferences bringing together high-ranking religious scholars and medical scientists (see, e.g., Gindi, 1989a). An old juridical rule, "The movement of the slain," was reviewed. Centuries ago it was ruled that if an aggressor stabbed a victim in the abdomen and the bowel extruded, this was considered a fatal injury; although the victim could still move, his or her prospects for life were practically nil. "The movement of the slain" was the descriptive term given to the death throes. If a second aggressor finished the victim off, the first aggressor would still be charged with murder for having dealt the fatal injury; and the second aggressor would be punished, but not for murder. Realizing that abdominal trauma with extrusion of the bowel is no longer considered a fatal injury by contemporary surgical standards, the scholars removed it from the category of "the movement of the slain." In its stead, the condition of brain death including the brain stem fulfills the description, since the victim has practically departed from life without the prospect of return and, in spite of the signs of life (circulation, respiration, etc.), is subject to the rulings governing the dead, including taking the heart for transplantation into a needy recipient, without the death of the patient being legally or morally attributed to the surgery. The disconnection of artificial life-support apparatus from such patients would be permissible.

Transplant surgery

Transplant surgery is practiced in many Arab countries, and some have excellent units. The Qur'anic saying "And whoever saves a life, it is as though he has saved all the people" (5:32) is the basis of considering organ donation as an act of charity. It is a religious duty of the community to provide necessary donors, in analogy with the decree of Umar (the second caliph) that if a person dies due to lack of sustenance, the society should pay legal reparations as if they killed him. The human body is honored whether living or dead, but its surgical violation to procure a needed organ is ruled permissible by invoking the juridical rule of "choosing the lesser of the two evils," for the alternative would be the death of the prospective recipient. Bodily organs should not be offered for sale, but if purchase is the only source, then buying is permissible under the rule "Necessities overrule prohibitions." In reality, however, apart from close relatives, most donors receive a price under the pressure of poverty. The need is felt for a governing authority to regulate the process, lest an exploitative market be created and patients with limited means be excluded. Donation should be purely and truly voluntary through consent of the living donor, bequeathed in a will or with the consent of the next of kin.

Transplantation of fetal suprarenal medulla to the brain to ameliorate certain diseases is lawful, although abortion performed specifically to obtain that tissue remains unlawful. The anencephalic fetus may be used as a donor, and its maintenance by artificial means for that purpose is acceptable, but removal of organs is permitted only after its natural death, without artificially terminating its life. Transplantation of sex glands to provide sex cells (ova or sperm) is unlawful because the prospective fetus would have been formed by elements not bound by a marriage contract. Sterile sex glands providing only hormones are devoid of that objection, but obviously their use is not medically feasible (Gindi, 1989c).

Hygiene and preventive health care

"Cleanliness is part of the faith," Muhammad said. Ritual ablutions are necessary before prayers several times daily, including a full bath (tuhr) after sexual intercourse, menstruation, and the puerperium. Muhammad forbade overindulgence in food and drink, and enjoined physical fitness. Circumcision of male children is required by Islam. Female circumcision, not an Islamic commandment, has been practiced in Sudan and Egypt since pre-Islamic times, and is now waning.

Preventive health care is well heeded. One of Muhammad's pertinent teachings is "If there is pestilence in a locality, do not enter it, and if you are already in it, do not go out." Alcohol is categorically forbidden by Islam (as are stupefying drugs, in order to protect mind and health). Nevertheless, the law in many Arab countries allows the sale and consumption of alcoholic beverages. Currently, there is widespread objection to the practice, and steps have even been taken to avoid alcohol in medicinal preparations. Extramarital sex is forbidden in Islam, although it certainly takes place in a clandestine manner. The virginity rate of girls at the

time of marriage approaches 100 percent. The sexual revolution and its sequelae in the West since 1960 have not erupted in the Arab world, although the powerful influence of communications markets the Western model and at the same time evokes a strong reaction expressed in a revival of religious values.

Care of the environment is emphasized in Muhammad's teachings, but unfortunately poverty, overcrowding, and unbridled movement from rural to urban regions with limited and failing infrastructure have led to a gap between the real and the ideal in many Arab cities. Muhammad taught, "Faith has many branches, including the removal of dirt from the street," and "Beware of the triple curse of polluting water resources, shady spots, and trodden roads." On water conservation he instructed those expending much water while making the ritual ablution: "Economize, even if you are at a flowing river." Encouraging agriculture, he said, "Whoever farms land will be rewarded by God every time a person eats from its crop, even if a thief steals and eats from it." Another of his recommendations is "If the end of the world comes and you have a little shoot in your hand to plant, then plant it if you can."

Kindness to animals is a religious dictate. They should not be overburdened or worked to exhaustion or tortured, and they should not be killed except for food. Muhammad spoke of God's pleasure with a man who, encountering a thirsty dog unable to reach water in a well, filled his shoe with water and offered it to the dog, and—conversely—God's anger with a woman who imprisoned a cat. These concepts were borne in mind when discussing the ethics of animal experimentation. Although it is approved when necessary for medical research, due care and humaneness should be shown in keeping and handling the animals.

Contraception

Contraception is lawful provided both husband and wife agree. Contraceptive measures are easily available and in some countries are subsidized by the state to curb overpopulation. Family planning should not be directly or indirectly imposed; the method should not be harmful; it should not entail abortion. Governmental and voluntary agencies use propaganda and education to promote family limitation in overpopulated countries, whereas incentives for a larger family are given in the underpopulated, affluent countries. However, family limitation policies are often attacked by some religious elements for a variety of reasons (Hathout, 1989), including the accusation that they are "imperialistic" designs against poor countries (see The Information Project for Africa, 1990). The use of the intrauterine contraceptive device has been controversial for fear that it acts by inducing abortion, but its use is widespread.

The 1987 World Health Organization announcement that its mechanism of action was contraceptive and not abortifacient was welcomed by religious authorities.

Breast-feeding is highly recommended in the Islamic tradition; the Qur'an says: "The mothers shall give suck to their offspring for two whole years, for those who desire to complete the term of lactation" (2:233). This would have been a potent measure for wider spacing of pregnancies at the level of the society at large, being associated with a high rate of ovulation suppression (of course it would not be a reliable prescription for contraception for the individual family). Unfortunately, the growing number of women joining the labor force does not work in its favor. Surgical sterilization (both male and female) is frowned upon except for pressing medical indications or at an advanced age (nearing menopause) for the highly parous woman.

Reproductive interventions

The quest for fertility is legitimate, and treatment of infertility by medical or surgical means is lawful and available within the Shari'a. Artificial insemination is permitted only if the husband's semen is used; donor semen is forbidden (by religion and by law) because it is outside the marriage contract. Since legitimate marriage is the only approved venue for reproduction, in vitro fertilization technology is permitted only if it involves a married couple and is carried out during the span of their marriage. No alien "element" should be involved, be it donated sperm, donated ovum, donated embryo, or surrogate uterus. When the wife is widowed or divorced, she is no longer the wife of her husband, and she can no longer be impregnated by his semen that had been preserved in a semen bank, for the marriage contract has come to a conclusion. Surrogacy is outlawed, and contracts for surrogate pregnancy are null and void.

Alternative family structures, not based on legitimate marriage, have no place in Arab societies.

HASSAN HATHOUT

While the articles in the other sections of this entry are relevant, see especially the other articles in this section: AN-CIENT NEAR EAST, IRAN, TURKEY, *and* ISRAEL. *For a further discussion of topics mentioned in this article, see the entries* ABORTION, *section on* RELIGIOUS TRADITIONS, *article on* ISLAMIC PERSPECTIVES, *and section on* CONTEMPORARY ETHICAL AND LEGAL ASPECTS; ANIMAL WELFARE AND RIGHTS, *article on* ETHICAL PERSPECTIVES ON THE TREATMENT AND STATUS OF ANIMALS; BODY, *article on* CULTURAL AND RELIGIOUS PERSPECTIVES; CIR-CUMCISION; DEATH, *article on* EASTERN THOUGHT; DEATH, ATTITUDES TOWARD; DEATH, DEFINITION AND DETERMINATION OF; ENVIRONMENT AND RELIGION; ETHICS, *article on* RELIGION AND MORALITY; EUGENICS; EUGENICS AND RELIGIOUS LAW, *article on* ISLAM; FERTILITY CONTROL; ISLAM; MEDICAL CODES AND OATHS; MEDICINE, ANTHROPOLOGY OF; MEDICINE, SOCIOLOGY OF; POPULATION ETHICS, *section on* RELIGIOUS TRADITIONS, *article on* ISLAMIC PERSPECTIVES; *and* WOMEN, *articles on* HISTORICAL AND CROSS-CULTURAL PERSPECTIVES, *and* HEALTH-CARE ISSUES. *Other relevant material may be found under the entries* AUTHORITY; BENEFICENCE; BIOETHICS EDUCATION; COMPASSION; DEATH AND DYING: EUTHANASIA AND SUSTAINING LIFE, *article on* ETHICAL ISSUES; FAMILY; HEALTH PROMOTION AND HEALTH EDUCATION; OBLIGATION AND SUPEREROGATION; ORGAN AND TISSUE PROCUREMENT; PATERNALISM; RESPONSIBILITY; SUICIDE; *and* TRUST. *See also the* APPENDIX (CODES, OATHS, AND DIRECTIVES RELATED TO BIOETHICS), SECTION II: ETHICAL DIRECTIVES FOR THE PRACTICE OF MEDICINE, OATH OF HIPPOCRATES, *and* ISLAMIC CODE OF MEDICAL ETHICS.

Bibliography

GINDI, A. R. AL-, ed. 1989a. *Human Life: Its Inception and Its End as Viewed by Islam.* Translated by A. Asbahi. Kuwait: Islamic Organization of Medical Sciences and Kuwaiti Foundation for the Advancement of Science.
————. 1989b. *Human Reproduction in Islam.* Translated by A. Asbahi. Kuwait: Islamic Organization of Medical Sciences and Kuwaiti Foundation for the Advancement of Science.
————. 1989c. *The Islamic Vision of Some Medical Practices.* Translated by A. Asbahi. Kuwait: Islamic Organization of Medical Sciences and Kuwaiti Foundation for the Advancement of Science.
HATHOUT, HASSAN. 1988. *Islamic Perspectives in Obstetrics and Gynecology,* pp. 95–100. Cairo: Alam al-Kutub.
————. 1989. "On Ethics and Human Values in Family Planning." In *Proceedings of 12th CIOMS Conference, on Ethics and Human Values in Family Planning.* Edited by Z. Bankowski, José Barzelatto, and Alexander Capron. Geneva: Council for International Organizations of Medical Sciences.
INFORMATION PROJECT FOR AFRICA, INC. 1990. Summary analysis of "National Security Study Memorandum 200—Implications of Worldwide Population Growth for U.S. Security and Overseas Interest. Dated Dec. 10, 1974—Classified. Declassified July 3, 1989. Released/U.S. National Archives, June 26, 1990." Washington, D.C.: Author.
Islamic Code of Medical Ethics: Kuwait Document. 1981. Kuwait: International Organization of Islamic Medicine.
UNITED NATIONS. 1992. *Demographic Yearbook 1990.* New York: Author.
WORLD HEALTH ORGANIZATION. 1987. *Mechanism of Action, Safety and Efficiency of Intrauterine Devices: A Report of a WHO Scientific Group.* WHO Technical Report Series no. 153. Geneva: Author.

E. ISRAEL

Medicine in Israel, like the country itself, is a blend of contrasts and contradictions, of compromises between tradition and modernity, between myth and reality. Israel, a tiny country made up of a dominant religion and culture (18 percent of the population are non-Jewish), is neither homogeneous nor monolithic. Over fifteen political parties are represented in the Knesset (parliament), and many Israelis are concerned about an ever-impending Kulturkampf between religious and secular factions.

Like all else in Israel, health care has been shaped by diverse inputs from a variety of lands of origin, and by the dialectic between the Mosaic and rabbinical tradition and modern Western secular humanism. Each of these major streams is itself heterogeneous. Lip service is paid to myths violated in practice, while traditions overtly denied and rebelled against often provide the spiritual sustenance in which rebels' values are rooted.

The ties that bind Jews to medicine are powerful and deeply rooted. Rabbinic leaders in the Middle Ages often practiced medicine for their livelihood, Maimonides being perhaps the best known in this tradition. In almost every society, Jews have been disproportionately represented in medicine. The most recent example is the 2.5 to 3 percent of Jewish immigrants to Israel from the former Soviet Union who are physicians, a ratio ten to fifteen times higher than that encountered in developed Western countries. The extraordinary value that Judaism places on human life explains in part the attraction of Jews to medicine. The Talmudic statement "He who saves a single life is regarded by the Scripture as if he saved an entire world" (Babylonian Talmud, Sanhedrin 37a) has led to the useful myth that life is of infinite value and to the "sanctity of life" concept that so permeates Jewish tradition.

The foundations of health care in modern Israel were laid by Zionist pioneers several decades before the creation of the State of Israel. These individuals were largely secularist, socialist ideologues with deep roots in the social justice ethos of Judaism and in the value placed on human life. Workers in 1912 created a "sick fund" for mutual assistance and health-care insurance, similar in many ways to the *Krankenkasse* of Central Europe from which they had emigrated. But the principles underlying this Jewish institution were derived no less from the traditional principles of *gemilut hadisim* (loving charity or mutual aid) so clearly spelled out in the Torah, whose rituals the pioneers had often discarded or drastically modified. All were to be equal in the receipt of health care, and money was not to be collected from a person in time of need and distress. This nongovernmental Histadrut labor union sick fund continues to be the major health-care provider in Israel today. It is both

an insurer and a provider of health care, owning and operating hospitals and community clinics, and insuring about 80 percent of the population. Smaller sick funds, also funded by mandatory employee and employer contributions, cover the rest of the population.

During the last few years, as health-care financing has become problematic worldwide—with citizens often placing a higher priority on such personal amenities as choice of physician and attractive waiting rooms than on the concept of equality—the egalitarian foundations of the health-care system in Israel have been threatened. Gaps in the public sector are being met by a growing fee-for-service private sector. Nevertheless, Israel has managed to maintain both a respectably high level of health care and reasonably equal availability of this care, in spite of a relatively low national expenditure. Israel currently spends about 7.5 percent of its gross national product on health care, but since its GNP is considerably smaller than those of most Western European countries, the absolute per capita expenditure is modest.

Manifestations of the strong ethos for saving human life at all costs include the relatively high renal dialysis rates in Israel and the intense efforts made by the military medical corps to provide physician coverage virtually at the battle line, in order to enhance every possible chance to save soldiers' lives. Public appeals by private individuals regularly raise tens of thousands of dollars to send patients abroad for complex surgical procedures that are not performed in Israel.

Yet, simultaneously, there is much evidence that the myth of the infinite value of human life is often shattered in the face of economic realities. Open-heart surgery is rarely offered to those over eighty, and long waiting periods for critical surgical procedures are not uncommon because of limited resources. The distribution of physicians and facilities is not even, with development towns and Arab villages sometimes at a disadvantage compared with the major metropolitan areas. The continued public tolerance of preventable deaths due to smoking and traffic accidents also exposes the mythical nature of the commitment to human life "at all costs." Recently, however, there has been improvement in all these areas.

Consonant with the high priority given to life, the Jewish tradition, unlike Anglo-Saxon law, requires the physician to respond to a patient's call for help. This requirement to render assistance to someone in distress is not confined to the physician; it obligates any individual to come to the aid of a fellow human being. To refuse would fall under the prohibition "Neither shalt thou stand idly by the blood of thy fellow" (Lev. 19:16). A physician who does not respond to a sick patient's request is regarded as one who spills blood. This attitude is incorporated into Israeli secular law, under which a citizen's failure to render assistance at the scene of an accident is a criminal act. Just as the physician is obligated to render care, so is seeking of care by the patient mandatory. The reason for this obligation is that in Judaism, human beings do not possess full title to life or body. Humans are but the stewards of the divine possession they have been privileged to receive. The terms of that stewardship are not of human choice but are determined by the Almighty's commands. Jewish law forbids suicide and requires that all reasonable steps be taken to preserve life and health. When beneficence conflicts with autonomy, the former is given precedence by Jewish tradition, a view clearly in conflict with the modern Western consensus (Beauchamp and Childress, 1983).

While such a violation of autonomy for the patient's good is not enforceable in modern pluralistic societies, it is sanctioned in the Jewish tradition; and were Jewish courts fully empowered, they might force medical treatment on a patient if it were indisputably indicated. In modern Israel, in contrast with most Western countries, the courts have not always decided unequivocally for autonomy over beneficence. There has been at least one case where the Israeli Supreme Court permitted a surgical procedure against the expressed will of the subject in order to prevent danger to his life (*Kortam* v. *State of Israel* 40 [III] P.D. 673–698).

Several medical ethical issues have attracted public attention in Israel over the years and provide interesting insights into the dynamics of Israeli society. For several decades, the issue of postmortem examinations and the laws regulating them were a major public and political issue (Glick, 1985). Judaism emphasizes respect for the human body in death as well as in life, and mandates early burial with integrity of the body preserved. Autopsies are permitted only if the information may contribute directly to the saving of a human life. With the creation of the first Israeli medical school, the rabbinate reached an agreement with the medical profession whereby autopsies would be permitted if three physicians attested that the cause of death was unknown. This exclusion of the deceased person's family from decision making and the subsequent frequent performance of postmortem examinations, even over strenuous family objections, turned the issue into a source of festering conflict. Subsequently, with a change in the political constellation that gave more power to religious parties, the law was changed radically as part of a backlash against the previous "liberalism." Not only is family consent now required, but other provisions, such as veto power for any member of the family, have led from one extreme to another. In all likelihood, the last word has not yet been said on the subject.

In spite of the religious limitations on postmortem examinations, the use of organs from the dead for lifesaving transplants is religiously acceptable and even mandated. For many years, the hesitation of the rabbi-

nate to accept brain death as the end of human life created difficulties for heart and liver transplants. After careful study, Israel's Chief Rabbinate in 1986 officially permitted heart transplants when donors' total brain death can be assured. This view has not been accepted by all rabbinical authorities, but religious objections now play a relatively minimal role in the limitations on organ transplantation.

Another area of conflict, as in most Western countries, has been abortion policy. Many factors lead to a restrictive policy in Israel. The Jewish tradition accords major rights to the fetus. The demographic and geopolitical situation of the Jewish people, particularly after the Holocaust, would seem to favor a strongly pronatal and antiabortion approach. Yet the Israeli public is quite permissive sexually, and its youth is very much a part of Western society.

The Israeli compromise, meant to satisfy all parties, includes a law forbidding abortions except for a "valid" medical or social reason, as determined by a hospital committee. These indications are liberally interpreted. Abortions performed outside this framework are illegal, thus satisfying religious sentiments. But no physician has ever been prosecuted for such illegal activities, thereby soothing the libertarians. This precarious balancing characterizes many of Israel's solutions to such conflicts.

Israel has a national committee appointed by the minister of health that advises the minister on many of the more complex and controversial areas in medical ethics, such as in vitro fertilization, genetic engineering, and the like. The committee, called the Supreme Helsinki Committee, is an outgrowth of a committee originally charged with the regulation of research in human subjects according to the Helsinki Declaration. It includes physicians, nonmedical scientists, jurists, philosophers, and clergy. It prefers to work by consensus rather than by vote, and makes every effort to weave its way through the maze of potential legal, religious, and sociopolitical conflicts. In the area of reproduction, the problems are great, since—unlike most areas of law that are adjudicated by the secular courts—marriage, divorce, and family law are largely in the hands of rabbinical courts (Shapira, 1987, pp. 12–14). Permissive decisions in the area of new reproductive technologies, unacceptable under religious law, might label the offspring of such practices as bastards, with serious consequences for them in their attempts to marry.

Israeli medical schools now have courses in medical ethics. Most provide the largely secular students with philosophical as well as religious approaches. The Israel Society for Medical Ethics serves as a forum for discussion, for the issuing of position papers, and for raising the consciousness of health-care professionals regarding medical ethics.

Some militant secular Israelis, chafing under the restrictions of Jewish tradition, have taken a number of bioethical issues to the courts in attempts to force rulings in favor of their position. Cases pressing the right to die have been brought before the courts without clear-cut resolution. Similar suits have been brought with respect to the restrictions placed on surrogate motherhood. These and other court decisions may bring about changes that legislators have been reluctant to press because of their hesitance to upset the "status quo"—which, in this case, refers to a freezing of the situation regarding the influence of the Jewish religion within Israel's public life prior to statehood.

In summary, Israel is a relatively young country that sees itself as part of the modern Western world, yet is the heir to an ancient and wise cultural tradition dating back thousands of years. Jewish tradition is characterized by a strong duty ethic, with emphases on both physician and patient responsibility; a high value on human life; and a strong sense of justice. Time will tell how successful Israeli society will be in distilling and blending the best of both these worlds.

SHIMON M. GLICK

While all the articles in the other sections of this entry are relevant, see especially the companion articles in this section: ANCIENT NEAR EAST, IRAN, TURKEY, *and* CONTEMPORARY ARAB WORLD. *Directly related to this article is the entry* JUDAISM. *For a further discussion of topics mentioned in this article, see the entries* ABORTION, *section on* RELIGIOUS TRADITIONS, *article on* JEWISH PERSPECTIVES; BENEFICENCE; BIOETHICS EDUCATION; BODY, *article on* CULTURAL AND RELIGIOUS PERSPECTIVES; DEATH, *article on* WESTERN RELIGIOUS THOUGHT; DEATH, ATTITUDES TOWARD; ETHICS, *article on* RELIGION AND MORALITY; HEALTH-CARE RESOURCES, ALLOCATION OF; KIDNEY DIALYSIS; MEDICINE, ANTHROPOLOGY OF; MEDICINE, SOCIOLOGY OF; ORGAN AND TISSUE PROCUREMENT; ORGAN AND TISSUE TRANSPLANTS; PATERNALISM; PATIENTS' RESPONSIBILITIES; *and* POPULATION ETHICS, *section on* RELIGIOUS TRADITIONS, *article on* JEWISH PERSPECTIVES. *Other relevant material may be found under the entries* AUTHORITY; AUTONOMY; FREEDOM AND COERCION; JUSTICE; LIFE; *and* OBLIGATION AND SUPEREROGATION.

Bibliography

Babylonian Talmud, Sanhedrin 37a. 1969. London: Soncino Press.

BEAUCHAMP, TOM L., and CHILDRESS, JAMES F. 1983. *Principles of Biomedical Ethics.* 2d ed. New York: Oxford University Press.

GLICK, SHIMON M. "Health Policy Making in Israel—Religion, Politics and Cultural Diversity." In *Health Policy, Ethics and Human Values: An International Dialogue,* pp. 71–74. Edited by Z. Bankowski, John H. Bryant, and Robert Veatch. Geneva: Council of International Organizations of Medical Science.

JAKOBOVITS, IMMANUEL. 1959. *Jewish Medical Ethics: A Comparative and Historical Study of the Jewish Religious Attitude to Medicine and Its Practice.* New York: Bloch.

Kortam v. State of Israel. 40 (III) P.D., pp. 673–698. (In Hebrew.)

SHAPIRA, AMOS. 1987. "In Israel, Law, Religious Orthodoxy and the Reproductive Technologies." Hastings Center Report 17 (supp.): 12–14.

II. AFRICA

A. SUB-SAHARAN COUNTRIES

The geographic region of sub-Saharan Africa includes all the African countries immediately below the Sahara Desert, together with all the associated island states but excluding the Republic of South Africa. Although the latter is within the region, it is excluded from this text in view of the heavy influence that apartheid exerted on indigenous African cultures. All the countries considered are bound by the Tropic of Cancer on the north and the Tropic of Capricorn on the south. In addition to a multitude of indigenous languages, the majority of the countries are either Anglophone or Francophone; five are Lusophone (Portuguese-speaking).

Medical ethics in sub-Saharan Africa is extremely complicated and cannot be considered homogeneous in any sense. This is because the vast geographic area (almost 23 million square kilometers, or about nine million square miles) contains forty-three independent countries with innumerable sociocultural groupings. Many of the countries are nation-states only superficially, since their borders enclose ethnic groups that have little in common with their fellow citizens, being more closely affiliated with groups in other countries. Quite apart from the matter of indigenous cultures, these countries were under the domination of European colonial powers that sought to impose their cultures upon local cultures. Some countries gained political independence only in the 1980s, and in some supposedly independent countries (Angola, Mozambique, Sudan) civil strife based on ethnic differences has raged throughout most of their independent period. The interaction between an externally introduced culture and a local one is more complicated in the field of medicine than in any other. The differences in urban-center development in East Africa and West Africa demonstrate the role that colonial power had in influencing cultural and ethical values (Larson, 1989).

Traditional and scientific methods

Some of the countries have had contact with scientifically based European medicine for less than 50 years, and others for little more than 100 years. The development of medical ethics in all the African countries has therefore tended to follow the existing European ethical values, principally those of France and Great Britain, the two dominant colonial powers. European medical professionals, faced with traditional African medical practice, took the position that all such medical practices and values, as well as their practitioners, were bad. Traditional African healers were considered no more than quacks and deceivers and therefore were either ignored or actively persecuted. Even the traditional midwives or "birth attendants," as they are now known, who from time immemorial have provided help to women at a most difficult time, were looked upon with disfavor. To a certain extent such attitudes were underwritten by the beliefs and practices of the colonizers' religion, Christianity. Since much of traditional healing relied on the intervention of gods and spirits, which Christians found abhorrent, the practice of traditional healing was strongly discouraged. Furthermore, European medical ethics required that European doctors not associate with practitioners whose training and beliefs differed from their own.

With the rise of black consciousness and the acceptance of the notion that blackness is not a sign of inferiority, African peoples have begun to reappropriate the medical knowledge gained over centuries by traditional medicine and medical practice. In some countries laws have been passed recognizing traditional medical practice as legal and effective. This process has been very slow. Many African medical schools still do not offer any instruction in traditional medicine, and where interest exists, it is only at a research level. Financial grants have been made for research into the methods and preparations of traditional medicine. In a few instances medical scientists are actively involved with traditional practitioners.

This new collaboration between traditional and imported medical practice is likely to be furthered by the indigenization of African churches and the improvement of the quality of their leadership. Previously, priests and ministers in the majority of churches had been inadequately trained, and they tended to assume a patronizing approach to their congregants. Now, a growing number can be considered well educated; some can even be viewed as theologians who are able to help formulate the churches' views on subjects of such crucial importance as the conflict between traditional and modern medical practice.

Medical professionals in the majority of countries now feel relatively free to develop new ways of practice and to work with traditional birth attendants, herbalists, and other healers without fear of losing either the respect or the comradeship of colleagues in Europe.

Traditional and Western practices are seeing crossover training in the areas of psychiatry, childbirth, and grass-roots education. Much of traditional medicine touches on the realm of psychiatry. Involvement of traditional practitioners in psychiatric treatment makes for a more humane treatment and much better integration of patients into society (Lambo, 1971). Among other efforts that may be cited is the involvement of the University of Ghana Medical School in training programs for traditional birth attendants. In many countries the medical schools (Makerere University in Uganda, University of Nairobi in Kenya, and University of Yaounde in Cameroon, for example) are striving to identify relevant practices within their own societies, such as use of peer groups to educate members of their societies on health-related issues. These medical schools are, therefore, embarking on programs that identify and preserve traditional practices considered valuable (Jelliffe and Bennett, 1960). In these programs, traditional practices considered harmless or beneficial are to be permitted, and those practices considered truly harmful are to be eliminated.

Standards for medical practice

Most English-speaking countries have general medical councils or boards responsible for registration, accreditation, and supervision of medical practice. In most of these countries the boards of control are generally quite distinct from the ministries of health (Kenya Government, 1977). Many of these medical councils or boards, however, have fashioned policies more responsive to western European norms and needs than to African ones. These boards have had little time to devote to the development of ethical guidelines relevant to social and cultural conditions peculiar to life within African countries. Some principles remain fundamental, however: Privacy of the patient is respected, and so is confidentiality, although here and there disclosure is required by the government for various reasons, including payment for medical service, granting of sick leave by employers, and mandatory registration of births and deaths.

Health-care service

There are very few scientifically trained medical personnel in Africa. The ratio of scientifically trained doctors to population ranges from 1:3,000 in such better-off cities as Dakar (Senegal), Accra (Ghana), and Nairobi (Kenya) to 1:200,000 in some poorer rural areas, such as most of the Northern Region of Nigeria and all of the immediate sub-Saharan countries including Mauritania, Mali, Burkina Faso, Niger, and Chad, which are sometimes referred to as the Sahel. There are countries within which there may not be a single specialist in any recognized field of medicine. This immediately raises the issue of what kind of medicine is most suitable in such conditions.

European medicine has developed and gained the reputation of being "one-on-one" medicine, and it also has concentrated more on curative than on preventive medicine. In Africa, on the other hand, the practice of one-on-one medicine, if it is accepted as the ideal, means excluding 80 to 90 percent or more of the population, who have no access to Western-oriented medical facilities. Such medical practice also places an inhuman load on the few medical practitioners and quickly reduces them to no more than purveyors of drugs and injections. Fendall (1972) sees this as the "quantity versus quality" dilemma, although not all agree with his view.

Doctors in Africa are now being asked to view their role in light of certain priorities—the first being promotive and preventive health services and the second being curative—in terms of individual patient treatment in offices or hospitals. In attempting to respond to the first priority, many have pointed out that not much can be done until medical practice is so arranged that the community is both the consumer and the provider of its own health care. This can be done only if delegation of health care to nonphysician personnel, such as traditional birth attendants and community leaders, is done on a basis of genuine need. The debate will continue, but almost all the new medical schools have agreed that doctors' training should be responsive to the needs of the community and to the organization and priorities set by ministries of health.

Many African countries depend on the use of paramedical personnel in the running of health services at the level of primary health care. Paramedics are often the only health-care personnel available at this level. They include clinical officers, laboratory technologists, public-health technicians, environmental health officers, and various kinds of nurses. They are usually trained at medical training colleges, which are non-university, diploma-awarding institutions established in countries including Zambia, Kenya, and Tanzania. Apart from the nurses, who take an oath at graduation, paramedical personnel are not subject to any ethically binding oath. This cadre of personnel has on occasion been the source of breaches of confidentiality.

Pharmacies and pharmacists, too, have presented new dilemmas to medical practice in Africa. The regulation of the drug supply has been the prerogative of the ministries of health and their relevant licensing bodies. In keeping with the increased number of university-trained pharmacists, there is increased licensing of private pharmacies, especially in Zaire, Kenya, Cameroon, and Nigeria. Pharmacists regard themselves as trained "doctors" and dispense drugs without prescription, including drugs that have previously required doctors' prescriptions. Pharmacies also may dispense inactive drugs or drugs that have no relevance to the patient's illness (World Health Organization, 1992).

The ethics of educating and remunerating doctors

Medical education has had to contend with the issue of "excellence versus quantity" in the training of doctors. Most African medical schools have felt it necessary to enroll students of the highest possible scientific caliber and to train them to internationally accepted standards. (These students are chosen based on their national high school final examination results.) The result has been that very few doctors can be graduated in any given year; but much more important, in many countries the best and sometimes the only available scientific skills are channeled into medicine, depriving other socially important areas of potential contributors. This is an ethical issue of considerable importance. In the end, many of the doctors produced choose to become specialists who can practice medicine only where they find quite sophisticated support facilities and services. Frequently they serve existing hospital needs rather than those of preventive medicine. The frustration and wastefulness of this situation underscore one of the major ethical issues on the African medical scene.

Doctors' fees have been the subject of debate in many African countries. Poverty is a major socioeconomic problem in all the countries of sub-Saharan Africa. Civil wars, political instability, ethnic violence, drought, and famine have transformed millions of already poor individuals into refugees who have fled across borders. In the midst of extensive poverty, charging fees for care raises serious ethical questions. In most of these countries, physicians are employed by the government and are not supposed to charge fees for their services. However, government pay schedules have not kept up with the cost of living, and many government doctors engage in private practice to supplement their salaries. In the late 1980s, the Kenya Medical Association considered fee schedules that would charge standard amounts for various services, without waivers or reductions for the poor. Objections were raised, and the schedule was not adopted. In Ghana, attempts have been made to adjust doctors' salaries to costs of living. In general, the costs of physicians' services, drugs, and hospitalization amid such serious deprivation deserve serious ethical scrutiny.

Population, family planning, and abortion

Population control as advocated in the Western world unfortunately has blurred the issues of family planning and led to a debate that should have been completely unnecessary. There are two basic concepts in family planning. The first is to regulate total family size to a level that can be comfortably maintained using the available resources. The second is to space the intervals between pregnancies in order to promote the health of both mothers and children (King, 1966). Many African countries rightly consider themselves underpopulated. Some, such as Gabon, Cameroon, and the Central African Republic, want much larger populations. All feel that they need development for the benefit of their people; but with very few exceptions, they refuse to admit that curbing population growth is relevant to the need for increased development.

Unfortunately, some doctors have failed to recognize the doctor's role in articulating relevant issues in family planning. Many doctors seem not to understand the medical importance of postponing pregnancies until a woman is biologically most prepared and of helping to stop reproduction when biological factors are no longer in a woman's favor. They also fail to recognize that spacing of births—which used to be practiced in Africa based either on sexual abstinence or on a geographic separation of husband and wife—is necessary to ensure the health of both mother and child. The excessive mortality in childbirth for women fourteen to forty-five years of age has not been fully appreciated by most of the medical profession in Africa (World Health Organization, 1975). Even where this situation is recognized, continued adherence to inappropriate laws and practices imposed from Europe often means that family-planning services are withheld from the majority of the population in need. The Catholic church, through its influence in the French-speaking countries, did much to prevent medical leadership in family planning. French laws passed in 1920 prohibiting contraception are still on the statute books of many French-speaking African countries, despite their repeal by France and Mali in 1972 (Wolf, 1978).

In the field of contraception, the major ethical question the doctor faces is, therefore, whether he or she should encourage free provision of contraceptives by non-medical personnel, knowing that Europe and the United States, which are the sources of these supplies, require that they be dispensed almost exclusively by doctors. The doctor must weigh the possibility of breaking outdated laws against the results of withholding such supplies from populations that have no other source.

Other serious ethical questions are raised in providing contraception to women who are not married, according to the traditional norms prevailing in their locality, or who want to practice contraception without the knowledge of their regular partner. Yet so tenuous are some of the marital relationships, so difficult is it to get some husbands into a hospital or family-planning clinic, that insistence on consent by both parties might, in the end, do an injustice to the woman. Physicians must resolve this ethical dilemma within their own national frontiers.

African societies generally do not accept abortion because they value highly the continuity of lineage; the unborn child, for example, may be a reincarnation of an ancestor. However, it would be untrue to say that abortions were not known in Africa before the arrival of white colonizers. In many African cultures, pregnancies resulting from taboo relationships or from adultery are terminated generally by women—and the men are kept in the dark.

The question of abortion is now debated seriously. Many of the abortion laws in Africa are based on those of England and France, which repealed them in 1967 and 1974, respectively. However, in the majority of former British and French possessions the old laws are still on the statute books. The increasing number of illegal abortions, with their consequent mortality, morbidity, and sterility, have still not prompted the collective conscience of medical practitioners to have the laws reviewed. Zambia did review its laws and amend them in 1973, but stipulations within the new law, particularly one that the approval of two medical practitioners is required, make it unlikely to serve the majority of those in need. The Africa Regional Conference on Abortion held in Accra, Ghana, in 1973 agreed to call for a review of the laws, but little has been done.

The doctors' dilemma regarding abortion is twofold. Despite the law, increasing numbers of women risk their lives by recourse to back-street abortionists. At the same time there are so few doctors to respond to such a wide range of needs that to make abortion laws more liberal may mean increasing the load on doctors still further. Given these problems, it is difficult to understand the view of some doctors in African countries that education, information, and services for fertility regulation should be limited.

Health care and research in the era of AIDS

The acquired immunodeficiency syndrome (AIDS), first recognized in 1981, has had the most profound impact on health care in Africa. Major concerns in health-care provision are related to confidentiality, informed consent, counseling, research, drug therapy, serotesting, and care of the sick.

When AIDS was first identified as a major public-health problem and a rapidly spreading epidemic in Africa, many African governments reacted with violent denials. This behavior, which was attributed in part to the claim that AIDS originated in Africa, received support from some physicians and ministries of health. The early rapid spread of AIDS in Africa was partly a result of the fact that it was not acknowledged as a major public-health problem and thus received only slow governmental response (Ndinya-Achola, 1991).

Confidentiality and counseling are two components in AIDS-control programs that have received, at best, lip service in Africa. Counseling is an extension of preventive educational campaigns. At population levels these campaigns use information, education, and communication as their basic tools, and public-health officials as their main promoters. Counseling deals directly with the individual. The personal interaction between counselor and patient enables individuals to better understand their personal risks, to make informed decisions, and to take appropriate action.

Under ideal conditions, counseling is provided on a one-to-one basis and each case is dealt with on its own merit. Counseling also involves providing facilities that respond to the physical and emotional needs of the affected individuals and their loved ones. In Africa, AIDS counselors began to be trained in 1988; the needs of the society far exceed the number of counselors available. Much of the counseling that is provided is done by individuals who have no training. In many instances it amounts to informing an individual that he or she is infected with the AIDS virus; the health-care provider is faced with the ethical question of whether to withhold information about the illness because there are no facilities to cater to individual needs.

Even where conditions are adequate and counseling facilities are available, confidentiality is a major issue because some of the trained counselors are not ethically bound to keep confidentiality. In particular, confidentiality is lacking in Africa for individuals diagnosed with AIDS. Counselors, however, are not the only health-care providers ignoring confidentiality. Information regarding AIDS diagnosis often is leaked by hospital laboratory and other care staff.

Biomedical research

Care for those with AIDS and drug therapy are two additional areas of major ethical concern. In many African settings the diagnosis of AIDS results in patient neglect because of the stigma attached to the disease. AIDS is a stigmatized disease in Africa mainly because the earliest information linked it to homosexuality, which is regarded as antisocial behavior in many parts of Africa. After it was ascertained that AIDS was being transmitted primarily by heterosexual contact, the homosexual stigma of AIDS lessened; but then AIDS became further stigmatized because of the rapid spread among heterosexuals by means of multiple sex partners and increased promiscuity. AIDS educational programs also had the inappropriate but true message that death is the final outcome. For these reasons, AIDS has had a negative impact on social interactions. Many people fear to be associated with a person with AIDS. This fear is evident even among professionals. Nurses have been a little more ethical in their approach to care of AIDS patients than physicians, perhaps because the nurses' increased contact with the patients makes them more sympathetic to the patients' plight.

During the early years of the AIDs epidemic, researchers from all over the world quickly identified populations in Africa for epidemiological studies (Van de Perre et al., 1987; Kreiss et al., 1986; Piot et al., 1987). Clinical studies on drugs and vaccines are also being done. This research brings to the fore ethical questions about biomedical research in African countries that predated the AIDS epidemic: Should Western scientists do studies on populations that may never benefit from the results? Can appropriate informed consent be obtained in cultures that have different values? These questions are much debated within Africa and abroad (IJsselmuiden and Faden, 1992). Standards of research have been improved: Some medical journals, such as *East African Medical Journal*, insist that proof of informed consent be provided before articles are accepted; granting agencies in Europe and the United States require local ethical review before funding is provided; and local review boards are becoming quite strict.

One of the important contributions of biomedical research in AIDS is the development of antiretroviral drugs for treating infection caused by human immunodeficiency virus (HIV), the causative agent of AIDS. Although the available drugs do not currently offer a cure, some of them have been shown to prolong life significantly. These drugs are far too expensive for African populations. The same research groups that solicited funds for epidemiologic studies should be persuaded to do the same in order to make anti-AIDS drugs affordable for African populations.

The first ten years of the AIDS epidemic has had profound social, cultural, economic, and health impacts in sub-Saharan Africa. These effects, which include loss of social structure, orphaned children, reduced productivity, and severe depletion of health-care budgets, no doubt will significantly increase over the next decade. Even if medical care or a vaccine were made available immediately, the already large number of infected individuals will continue to burden the society. Health-care standards will be influenced by the AIDS epidemic for a long time. The decade of the 1990s is the right time for African health-care services to review their programs and put in place relevant practices and resources without compromising their ethics in caring for people with AIDS. It would be heartening to see African countries taking a lead in the care of people with AIDS.

Conclusion

Significant improvements are continually being made in medical training and standards of health care throughout sub-Saharan Africa. These improvements, however, are still not matched by proportionate improvement in medical ethics. Many African medical schools' curricula do not include ethics. Where it is included, the subject is still accorded very little time (usually a one-hour lecture). In order to sensitize doctors and other health-care personnel on issues related to medical ethics, African medical schools and medical training colleges should be encouraged to develop curricula on ethics. It may also be necessary to sensitize populations on the subject along the same lines that disease prevention has been brought to the community level through health education.

JECKONIAH O. NDINYA-ACHOLA

While all the articles in this entry are relevant, see especially the companion article in this section: SOUTH AFRICA. *Directly related to this article is the entry* AFRICAN RELIGION. *For a further discussion of topics mentioned in this article, see the entries* ABORTION, *section on* CONTEMPORARY ETHICAL AND LEGAL ASPECTS; AIDS; ALTERNATIVE THERAPIES; BIOETHICS EDUCATION; CONFIDENTIALITY; EPIDEMICS; FERTILITY CONTROL; HEALING; HEALTH CARE, QUALITY OF; HEALTH-CARE RESOURCES, ALLOCATION OF; HEALTH PROMOTION AND HEALTH EDUCATION; INFORMATION DISCLOSURE; INFORMED CONSENT; MEDICINE, ANTHROPOLOGY OF; MEDICINE, SOCIOLOGY OF; MEDICINE AS A PROFESSION; NURSING ETHICS; PHARMACEUTICS, *article on* ISSUES IN PRESCRIBING; PHARMACY; POPULATION ETHICS; POPULATION POLICIES; PROFESSION AND PROFESSIONAL ETHICS; PUBLIC HEALTH; RACE AND RACISM; SEXISM; UNORTHODOXY IN MEDICINE; UTILITY; *and* WOMEN. *Other relevant material may be found under the entries* ETHICS; FAMILY; FREEDOM AND COERCION; JUSTICE; OBLIGATION AND SUPEREROGATION; PRIVACY IN HEALTH CARE; PROTESTANTISM; RESPONSIBILITY; ROMAN CATHOLICISM; *and* VALUE AND VALUATION.

Bibliography

BRYANT, JOHN H. 1969. *Health and the Developing World.* Ithaca, N.Y.: Cornell University Press.

FENDALL, N. R. E. 1972. *Auxiliaries in Health Care: Programs in Developing Countries.* Baltimore, Md.: Johns Hopkins University Press.

GRANT, J. P. 1989. "The Bamako Initiative." In *UNICEF: The State of the World's Children.* Oxford: Oxford University Press.

IJSSELMUIDEN, CAREL B., and FADEN, RUTH R. 1992. "Research and Informed Consent in Africa: Another Look." *New England Journal of Medicine* 326, no. 12:830–834.

INSTITUTE OF MEDICAL ETHICS WORKING PARTY ON THE ETHICAL IMPLICATIONS OF AIDS. 1992. "AIDS, Ethics,

and Clinical Trials." *British Medical Journal* 305, no. 6855:699–701.

JELLIFFE, D. B., and BENNETT, F. J. 1960. "Indigenous Medical Systems and Child Health." *Journal of Paediatrics* 57, no. 2:248–261.

KENYA GOVERNMENT. 1977. The Medical Practitioners and Dentists Act, Cap 253. *Kenya Gazette.* Nairobi: Government Printer.

KING, MAURICE H. 1966. "Family Planning." In *Medical Care in Developing Countries.* Edited by Maurice H. King. Nairobi: Oxford University Press.

KREISS, JOAN K.; KOECH, DAVY; PLUMMER, FRANCIS A.; HOLMES, KING K.; LIGHTFOOTE, MARILYN; PIOT, PETER; RONALD, ALLAN R.; NDINYA-ACHOLA, JECKONIAH O.; D'COSTA, LOURDES J.; ROBERTS, PACITA; NGUGI, ELIZABETH N.; and QUINN, THOMAS C. 1986. "AIDS Virus Infection in Nairobi Prostitutes: Spread of the Epidemic to East Africa." *New England Journal of Medicine* 314, no. 7:414–418.

LAMBO, T. ADEOYE. 1971. "The African Mind in Contemporary Conflict." *WHO Chronicle* 25:343–353. Jacques Parisot Foundation Lecture.

LARSON, A. 1989. "Social Context of Human Immunodeficiency Virus Transmission in Africa." *Review of Infectious Diseases* 11, no. 5:716–731.

NDINYA-ACHOLA, JECKONIAH O. 1991. "A Review of Ethical Issues in AIDS Research." *East African Medical Journal* 68, no. 9:735–740.

PIOT, PETER; KREISS, JOAN K.; NDINYA-ACHOLA, JECKONIAH O.; NGUGI, E. N.; SIMONSEN, J. N.; CAMERON, D. W.; TAELMAN, H.; and PLUMMER, F. A. 1987. "Heterosexual Transmission of HIV." *AIDS* 1:199–206.

SYNDER, FRANCIS G. 1974. "Health Policy and the Law in Senegal." *Social Science and Medicine* 8, no. 1:11–28.

VAN DE PERRE, PHILLIPE; CLUMECK, NATHAN; CARAEL, MICHEL; NZABIHIMANA, ELIE; ROBERT-GUROFF, MARJORIE; DEMOL, PATRICK; FREYENS, PIERRE; BUTZLER, JEAN-PAUL; GALLO, ROBERT C.; and KANYAMUPIRA, JEAN-BAPTISTE. 1987. "Female Prostitutes: A Risk Group for Infection with Human T-Cell Lymphotropic Virus Type III." *Lancet* 2, no. 8454:524–527.

WOLF, BERNARD. 1973. *Anti-contraception Laws in Sub-Saharan Africa: Sources and Ramifications.* Laws and Population Monograph Series, no. 15. Medford, Mass.: Fletcher School of Law and Diplomacy, Law and Publication Program.

WORLD HEALTH ORGANIZATION. 1975. *World Health Statistics Annual, 1972.* Vol. 1, *Vital Statistics and Causes of Death.* Geneva: Author.

———. 1992. "Safe Drugs for Everyone." *World Health,* March–April, pp. 4–6.

B. SOUTH AFRICA

The histories of medicine and of medical ethics in South Africa are intimately linked to political, social, and economic aspects of that country's development, dominant components of which include racial discrimination and social segregation. A brief review of some key political events will provide an illuminating backdrop to a description of the evolution of medical services and the ethics of medical practice in this controversial country, which typifies in microcosm many of the world's diverse human problems and arguably poses the most challenging contemporary opportunity to demonstrate human ability to resolve conflict peacefully.

Political background

During the period of the Dutch settlers (1652–1820) the indigenous Khoi-Khoi (pastoral people) and the San (hunter-gatherers) were treated with the arrogance and paternalism that for subsequent centuries epitomized European domination over blacks and exploitation through enslavement and colonial/cultural imperialism. These attitudes, together with warfare and the introduction of new diseases (e.g., smallpox in 1713), led to the decimation and destruction of the organized cultures of these indigenous peoples (Burrows, 1958; Laidler and Gelfand, 1971).

British annexation of the Cape (1795) and the arrival of British immigrants in Algoa Bay were followed by ninety years of conflict that included devastating wars between rival black tribes, the freeing of slaves (1833), the "importation" of Indians to work in the cane fields of Natal (1860), the first Anglo-Boer War (1880), several wars against the Zulus, and the bitter second Anglo-Boer War (1899–1902), during which twenty-six thousand Afrikaner women and children died in British concentration camps.

The British Parliamentary Act of Union (1910), which gave whites the right to self-determination, and the subsequent failure of the British to exercise their veto powers to restrain the Union Parliament from enacting oppressive racial laws (Native Land Act of 1913, depriving blacks of their land, and the Native Administration Act of 1927, depriving them of their right to self-determination), set the scene for the growth of Afrikaner political and economic dominance. The rise to power of the Nationalist Party in 1948 was followed by proliferation of apartheid policies, relentlessly entrenched through legislation that oppressed and dehumanized the black people of South Africa.

Black opposition evolved from powerless peaceful protest into a politically powerful process of potentially peaceful progress. It was hampered, however, by a growing culture of individual and group violence, fueled by brutal elements within the state security forces and by internal sources of conflict that horrified the world (Schlemmer, 1992).

Intensification of black resistance, more clearly articulated demands for human rights globally, and changing foreign policy agendas progressively isolated South Africa from its previous friends and from international markets. By the 1980s economic decline, rapid population growth, urbanization, destabilization in the neighboring states, and collapse of communism in eastern Europe and the Soviet retreat from regional conflicts constituted the matrix from which arose the Nationalist Party's acceptance of the need to seek, with the black opposition parties, a negotiated settlement as a step toward developing a democratic South Africa (Benatar, 1992).

Legislative changes since the "unbanning" of the black opposition movements in February 1990 have included repeal of the 1913 Native Land Act, the 1927 Native Administration Act, the 1950 Population Registration Act, and the 1950 Group Areas Act, which together formed a powerful core of statutory discriminatory policies. While the transition period abounds with ironies and ambiguities, optimism that peaceful and constructive pathways to progress could and would be found followed the December 1991 Convention for a Democratic South Africa (CODESA) Conference and the March 1992 referendum. It is against this background that the history of medicine and medical ethics in South Africa can now be briefly reviewed.

History of medicine

The first manifestation of any formalized medical service was the erection of hospital tents following a smallpox epidemic introduced by a visiting fleet in 1713. Further episodes of smallpox (1751 and 1755) led to the construction of two rudimentary hospitals, one for poor Europeans and the other for slaves, the well-to-do being treated at home.

Medical practice developed in two directions: a private commercial venture predominantly for those who could afford to pay, and a public service for the poor, to which the mission medical service (introduced by the Missionary Society of London) made a major contribution in rural areas for well over a century. Concern for public health, stimulated by the 1918 influenza epidemic, generated decades of successful research on infections in close collaboration with the World Health Organization. Public health services of a high standard were developed through the creation of medical schools with public teaching hospitals open to all—on a segregated basis; ostensibly separate but equal.

The developing systems of medical practice and of medical education mirrored the diverse characteristics of South African society. Undisputedly high standards of medical education in the Western tradition, dedication of generations of practitioners to high standards of medical practice and patient care, considerable goodwill between doctors and patients of all races, extensive public-health facilities—including teaching centers of excellence and well-funded private medicine—reflect the successes. Privileged access to medical education; fragmentation and duplication of health services; lack of planning; wide disparities in health and in access to health care (predominantly on a racially discriminatory and unequal basis); focus on curative hospital-based medicine; paucity of preventive, promotive, and rehabilitative services; paternalistic attitudes to patients; and dismissive attitudes to African traditional medicine reflect the racist and oppressive aspects of a system doomed to failure through its institutionalized neglect of civil and social justice (Van Rensburg and Benatar, 1992).

Deficiencies in the health-care system were clearly articulated in the 1940s, and the case for reform toward a unitary health service has been the subject of intense debate since the 1980s (Benatar, 1986, 1990b, 1991). Traditional African medicine continues to be practiced, particularly in rural areas. While black Africans have increasingly accepted Western medicine, they eclectically choose varying combinations of modern and traditional medical advice (Edwards, 1986).

Medical ethics

The South African Medical and Dental Council (SAMDC), a statutory body, was established in 1929 with the primary purpose of protecting the public through maintenance of high professional (including ethical) standards of practice and with a view to serving the interests of the medical and dental professions—insofar as these interests are compatible with high standards. The wide range of powers vested in SAMDC included the power to institute inquiries into any complaint, charge, or allegation of improper or disgraceful conduct of its members and to exercise disciplinary power over them.

As in most other Western countries in the first sixty years of the twentieth century, discussions on medical ethics in South Africa largely took place within the framework of the authoritarian, paternalistic behavior expected of professionals supposedly adhering to the Hippocratic Oath and similar codes. The first South African text on medical ethics (Elliott, 1954) was limited to discussion of ethical codes, professional secrecy, advertising, the conduct of consultations, fees and financial matters, and upholding the "traditions" of medicine, with only brief reference to abortion and sterilization, and to the ethics of investigative medicine. This text, based on Guy Elliott's experience of deliberations on ethical matters by the Medical Association of South Africa (MASA) and the SAMDC, provides a succinct

outline of accepted medical ethics in South Africa (and in many Western countries) in the first half of the twentieth century.

Issues of bioethics have usually been stimulated by the widespread application of technological advances in everyday medical practice, the social changes that challenge many traditional professional values, cost considerations, uncertainty regarding the effectiveness of innovative treatments, and increasing concern for individual autonomy and shared decision making in the United States and Europe.

The pace of social change, and of change in medicine and bioethics in South Africa (a middle-income country—per capita GNP less than one-tenth that in the United States and falling), has been much slower. Expenditure on health has increased only marginally and, despite their high profile, modern lifesaving medical treatments are available only on a limited scale. Public and even professional debates on ethical issues in medicine have been very limited in a repressive, authoritarian society lacking a patients' rights movement and unaccustomed to public discourse on civil and political liberties (Benatar, 1988).

As in the United States, theologians have played a pioneering role in reawakening interest in bioethics; several conferences were held in South Africa (in the 1960s and 1970s) under church or theological auspices. The first, stimulated by the historic heart transplant in Cape Town (December 1967), was on the ethics of tissue transplantation (Oosthuizen, 1972). Others followed on abortion (Oosthuizen et al., 1974), euthanasia (Oosthuizen et al., 1978), professional secrecy (Oosthuizen et al., 1983), and clinical experimentation (Oosthuizen et al., 1985). These provoked little ongoing public or professional debate. In the 1980s some medical schools began developing modern bioethics education programs, but progress has been slow and the programs remain (1) in a fledgling state, (2) dependent on enthusiastic physicians who have heavy professional responsibilities and minimal formal training in philosophical ethics, and (3) without the financial and institutional support to develop formal programs with committed support from other disciplines (e.g., philosophy, law). One medical faculty has published the proceedings of four symposia on bioethics (Benatar, 1985, 1986, 1988, 1992). These have encompassed theological, philosophical, and sociological debates on death and dying; resource allocation; the doctor/patient relationship; abortion and in vitro fertilization; research on humans; principles of biomedical ethics; moral reasoning; withholding and withdrawing treatment; health care of detainees; hospital ethics; the right to health care and the structure of health services; ethical considerations in relation to acquired immunodeficiency syndrome (AIDS); and teaching medical ethics. These proceedings reflect progressive movement toward the views being popularized in bioethics debates in the United Kingdom and the United States. By retaining a degree of "cultural sensitivity" they endeavor to avoid the pitfalls both of "ethical imperialism" and of "ethical double standards."

A milestone event in the history of medical ethics in South Africa was the inadequate SAMDC and MASA responses to the unethical manner in which state-employed medical practitioners provided professional attention to prominent black activist Steve Biko prior to his death during detention without trial in 1977. Failure of SAMDC to exercise its duty to protect the public by acknowledging the unethical behavior of Biko's doctors and taking appropriate disciplinary action against them, and MASA's response to SAMDC's deficient protection of the public met with resounding criticism nationally and internationally (Nightingale et al., 1990). The sequence of events through which the efforts of a small group of rank-and-file members of the profession led to a Supreme Court injunction against SAMDC, which resulted in a reversal of its previous decisions and the imposition of disciplinary action, is well documented. The National Medical and Dental Association (NAMDA), formed in 1982 as a result of discontent with MASA's actions following the death of Steve Biko, has received international acclaim for its outspoken advocacy against discriminatory practices. MASA, which came under considerable criticism for its inadequate reactions to the Biko affair, has, to its credit, taken some sincere steps in an attempt to rectify its previous shortcomings. Its statements are now clearly on public record, and the challenge ahead is to ensure their further implementation in practice. Greater attention to ethical responsibilities toward prisoners, detainees, and hunger strikers has been a gratifying response to the Biko case (Benatar, 1990a; Kalk and Veriava, 1991). The public confession of guilt by the district surgeon who bore major responsibility for Biko's medical care, emphasizes the need to maintain professional independence in the face of state security and other coercive pressures.

Professional institutional responses intended to stimulate higher standards of ethical practice include the MASA and the Medical Research Council (MRC) guidelines on professional ethics and the ethics of medical research, respectively (both currently under further revision), and the publication by the College of Medicine of South Africa of its Credo. The long-standing requirement by some universities that all proposals for human and animal experimentation need approval by institutional ethics committees is spreading to other universities, and such prior approval has now become a requirement for all funding applications to the South African Medical Research Council.

Conclusion

In a period characterized by national economic attrition, real per capita expenditure on health of less than one-twentieth of what is spent in the United States, burgeoning population growth, rapid erosion of financial support for academic medicine, and political liberation with rapidly escalating human expectations, development of the discipline of bioethics in South Africa has been initiated and sustained more as a hobby by a few enthusiasts than as an integral component of medical education and practice. The need to include formal teaching of bioethics and clinical ethics in professional schools, which has gained widespread acceptance in the developed world, remains to be achieved in South Africa, as in other developing countries. Who should teach, what should be taught, how teaching of this discipline can be made most effective, and the ways in which such teaching can enrich medical and social education and practice are, as in any new discipline, matters of ongoing debate. If South Africa can learn from the developments in other countries and, with international support, use these lessons to build a national bioethics program and a better health-care system in South Africa, this could contribute toward restructuring a new South Africa that could play a vital role in helping to rehabilitate southern Africa.

SOLOMON R. BENATAR

While all the articles in this entry are relevant, see especially the companion article in this section: SUB-SAHARAN COUNTRIES. *Directly related to this article is the entry* AFRICAN RELIGION. *For a further discussion of topics mentioned in this article, see the entries* ALTERNATIVE THERAPIES; HEALTH-CARE RESOURCES, ALLOCATION OF; MEDICAL CODES AND OATHS; MEDICINE, ANTHROPOLOGY OF; MEDICINE, SOCIOLOGY OF; *and* RACE AND RACISM. *Other relevant material may be found under the entries* OBLIGATION AND SUPEREROGATION; PATERNALISM; PROFESSION AND PROFESSIONAL ETHICS; *and* PUBLIC HEALTH. *See also the* APPENDIX (CODES, OATHS, AND DIRECTIVES RELATED TO BIOETHICS), SECTION II: ETHICAL DIRECTIVES FOR THE PRACTICE OF MEDICINE, OATH OF HIPPOCRATES.

Bibliography

BENATAR, SOLOMON R. 1986. "Medicine and Health Care in South Africa." *New England Journal of Medicine* 315, no. 8:527–532.

———. 1988. "Ethics, Medicine and Health Care in South Africa." *Hastings Center Report* 18, no. 4 (suppl.): 3–8.

———. 1990a. "Detention Without Trial, Hunger Strikes and Medical Ethics." *Law, Medicine and Health Care* 18, no. 1–2:140–145.

———. 1990b. "A Unitary Health Service for South Africa." *South African Medical Journal* 77, no. 9:441–447.

———. 1991. "Medicine and Health Care in South Africa—5 Years Later." *New England Journal of Medicine* 325, no. 1:30–36.

———. 1992. "Transition Towards a New South Africa." *South African Medical Journal* 81, no. 6:295–298.

———, ed. 1985, 1986, 1988, 1992. *Ethical and Moral Issues in Contemporary Medical Practice: Proceedings of an "In House" Conference Faculty of Medicine, University of Cape Town.* Cape Town: University of Cape Town.

BURROWS, EDMUND H. 1958. *A History of Medicine in South Africa.* Cape Town: A. A. Balkema.

EDWARDS, STEPHEN D. 1986. "Traditional and Modern Medicine in South Africa: A Research Study." *Social Science and Medicine* 22, no. 11:1273–1276.

ELLIOTT, GUY A. 1954. *Medical Ethics.* Johannesburg: Witwatersrand University Press.

KALK, W. JOHN, and VERIAVA, YUSUT. 1991. "Hospital Management of Voluntary Total Fasting Among Political Prisoners." *Lancet* 337, no. 8742:660–662.

LAIDLER, PERCY W., and GELFAND, MICHAEL. 1971. *South Africa: Its Medical History 1652–1898: A Medical and Social Study.* Cape Town: C. Struik.

NIGHTINGALE, ELENA O.; HANNIBAL, KARI; GEIGER, JACK; HARTMAN, LAWRENCE; LAWRENCE, ROBERT; and SPURLOCK, JEAN. 1990. "Apartheid Medicine: Health and Human Rights in South Africa." *Journal of the American Medical Association* 264, no. 16:2097–2102.

OOSTHUIZEN, GERHARDUS C. 1972. *The Ethics of Tissue Transplantation.* Cape Town: Howard Timmins.

OOSTHUIZEN, GERHARDUS C.; ABBOTT, G.; and NOTELOVITZ, MORRIS. 1974. *Great Debate: Abortion in the South African Context.* Cape Town: Howard Timmins.

OOSTHUIZEN, GERHARDUS C.; SHAPIRO, HILLEL; and STRAUSS, SYBRAND A. 1978. *Euthanasia.* Cape Town: Oxford University Press.

———. 1983. *Professional Secrecy in South Africa: A Symposium.* Cape Town: Oxford University Press.

———. 1985. *Attitudes to Clinical Experimentation in South Africa.* Johannesburg: Hodder and Stoughton.

SCHLEMMER, LAWRENCE. 1992. "Violence—What Is to Be Done?" *South Africa International* 23:60–64.

VAN RENSBURG, HENDRICK C. J., and BENATAR, SOLOMON R. 1993. "The Legacy of Apartheid in Health and Health Care." *South African Journal of Sociology* 24, no. 4:99–111.

III. SOUTH AND EAST ASIA

A. GENERAL SURVEY

The articles that follow deal with the complex and varied traditions of medical ethics and practice in east, south, and Southeast Asia. In many respects these three areas have always represented very different cultural and geographical entities. The Indian subcontinent derived its cultural and linguistic influences from central and western Asia, but produced in Hinduism and Jainism its own religious, cultural, and intellectual forms, shaping attitudes toward disease and the ethics of medical practice. Concepts of human life and disease evolved quite independently in east Asia, where an agrarian society grew up isolated from other Asian peoples both by steep mountains and by what were for the early Chinese equally impenetrable oceans. Chinese society developed its own characteristic political and social practices—particularly its this-worldly religion, and orientation toward its ancestors. Early Japanese attitudes toward nature differed from the Chinese as the conceptions of an island people dependent on the seas for a living differed from those of plains-dwelling farmers. Nonetheless, significant interaction between China and Japan from about the seventh century C.E. infused Confucian ideas into early Japanese foundations. Southeast Asia, today comprising Vietnam, Laos, Thailand, Malaysia, and Indonesia and vividly characterized by Anthony Reid in *The Lands Beneath the Winds,* also evolved from independent social origins. As Reid writes: "Fundamental social and cultural traits distinguish Southeast Asia as a whole from either of its vast neighbors—China and India. Central among these are the concepts of spirit or 'soul-stuff' animating living things; the prominence of women in descent, ritual matters, marketing and agriculture; and the importance of debt as a determinant of social obligation" (Reid, 1988, p. 6).

Despite their very different cultural orientations, these societies are treated here as a group because they offered in traditional times a common contrast to Western medical practice and ethics, and have had throughout their histories a common influence from Buddhism. In more recent periods, the societies of east Asia have faced the common problem of reconciling the possibilities of Western medical technology with their own social goals. These common themes are explored here, by way of introduction to the more specialized articles that follow.

In traditional times, the societies of Asia had in common the fact that they never adopted the exclusively biological conception of disease that has become the norm in modern Western societies. In traditional Indian Ayurvedic medicine, as Desai Prakash argues, physicians classified the etiology of disease in three categories: external or invasive diseases caused by foreign bodies or possession states; internal diseases caused by disturbances of humors brought about by lapses in discretion; and a third category of disease brought about by the inexorable workings of karma. In ancient China, the metaphors were different but the origins of disease were equally complex, with health and illness deriving from the baneful or benevolent influence of departed ancestors, or the influence of demons. In Japan, the apprehension of human beings' relation to the sacred world of *kami*, and the southeast Asian conception of the relation of magic, religion, and health, allowed the possibility of social as well as strictly organic origins of disease.

These views of disease may reflect a general tendency in Asia to view the human order as more fully integrated with the natural and social orders than in the West. But it is probably as useful to view the differences between traditional Asian and modern European conceptions of disease as underlining the uniqueness of the European, perhaps Promethean, notion that the human world could understand, analyze, and ultimately control the natural order. Whatever the nature of the differences between Europe and Asia in the conception of disease, the Asians' more complex vision of disease had important consequences for the relationship of the medical practitioner and his patient. Since disease could arise from a variety of sources, the Asian medical practitioner addressed a wider spectrum of issues in a patient's life than did his Western counterpart. Moreover, the Asian patient might be free to consult many different types of practitioners than the European counterpart. Hence varied traditions of medical practice existed side by side, with no single system of medicine having an exclusive legitimacy.

In part, this pluralism of Asian medical practice made it possible for Buddhist practitioners to spread throughout Asia, beginning in about the second century C.E. The notion of loving friendship, and its institutional expression in the establishment of charitable hospitals, dispensaries, and comfort stations on the way to famous shrines and temples, was one of the concepts Buddhist monks carried with them as they made their way across the trade routes of central Asia from India to China between the second and the seventh centuries C.E. Once in China, Buddhist monks found a social environment quite different from the one they had left, for although the Chinese intellectual world was open to Buddhist doctrines, Chinese society was not as open to monastic life with its implied rejection of family and ancestors. In China, Mahayana or devotional Buddhism developed, which stressed the activities that the believer could perform while remaining within the realm of family and community. Thus, in China, Buddhist healing practices not only were carried out within charitable institutions formally run by the Buddhist establishment but also came to merge with folk medicine and healing practices from other traditions.

By the early part of the fifth century, Chinese immigrants had carried Buddhism of both the monastic and devotional varieties to Korea and Japan, and formal belief in Buddhism grew rapidly in Japan following the conversion of Prince Shotoku, who became regent for the Japanese emperor in 593. The spread of Buddhism to Southeast Asia was more complicated, with monastic and devotional Buddhism gradually making their way through Burma to Cambodia and the rest of Southeast Asia. In the eleventh and twelfth centuries, when a people of Mongol origin conquered the area now known as Thailand, they adopted monastic Buddhism as a state religion, and began to enforce it militarily on their neighbors in Cambodia and Laos.

By about the thirteenth century, the spread of Buddhism throughout Asia had provided a unity to traditional medical practice that had not existed previously. But it was at best a loose unity, in which Buddhist medical ideas came to coexist alongside traditional healing practices and institutions. When Western medicine came to Asia in more recent times, it experienced a similar fate. The importation of Western medicine to Asia was largely a product of colonial times; the earliest Western medical practitioners in Asia were often missionaries supported by European and American political or religious establishments. Twentieth-century Asian governments, consciously or unconsciously aware that Western medical technology could provide the same control over life and disease that Western military and social technology provided over political affairs, often vigorously pursued Western medical techniques. The Minister of Education of the government of Nationalist, or Guomindang, China declared in 1914 that he had "decided to abolish traditional Chinese medicine." Similarly, in 1874, the Meiji government in Japan decreed that all Japanese physicians had to have Western medical training.

Despite the vigorous efforts of Asian governments to promote Western medical education and practice, Western medicine has failed to supplant traditional medical practices in any of the countries under consideration, for several reasons. In part, the problem has been the absence of trained medical professionals: In China, for instance, despite the commitment of the government of the People's Republic to scientific medical practice, a realistic assessment of resources dictated that medical workers trained in traditional as well as modern Western techniques be employed. Possibly because of the paucity of trained personnel throughout Asia, Western medical practice has been and remains a largely urban and elite phenomenon. In part as well, traditional medical practices have proved their value as effective and inexpensive treatments for many of the maladies of modern life. As Pinit Ratanakul notes in the article on Southeast Asian countries, "This traditional method of healing may be especially suitable today for Southeast Asians, who, living in societies with increased urbanization and industrialization, need physical, psychological and spiritual care to enable them to cope with such change and the strains and stresses of modern life." Today, then, as in the past, different disciplines of medical treatment, each with its own ethical standards and requirements, exist side by side throughout much of Asia.

If modern Western medicine has not fully supplanted traditional medicine in Asia, the power and technology of modern medicine has in almost every country posed new ethical dilemmas. In some instances, as in the case of reproductive medicine, Western medicine has made accessible courses of action more radical than traditional medicine permitted. Abortion, though known and disapproved of in traditional Chinese and Indian medicine, has become much more common throughout Asia as population control has become an accepted political goal. Amniocentesis to determine the sex of a fetus has become a common practice in India, with female feticide often the consequence of the traditional religious imperative to produce a male heir.

In other areas of medicine, Western technology has fostered new and rather ominous practices in Asia. In China in the late 1980s debate arose about the merits of sterilization of the mentally retarded and other types of genetic experimentation. Sadly, as well, Asian practitioners of Western medicine have proved somewhat more willing to engage in experimentation on human subjects than have their Western counterparts. Wartime experimentation by Japanese doctors in Manchuria has, of course, been condemned not only in the West but also in Japan. Unfortunately, such experimentation has also been carried out in contemporary Southeast Asia, though such action is increasingly condemned by Southeast Asian and Western governments. As a result of the new ethical dilemmas posed by Western medical technologies, medical ethics has become both a heated issue throughout contemporary Asia and the subject of frequent international conferences and journal articles.

R. KENT GUY

While all the articles in this entry are relevant, see especially the other articles in this section, which discuss INDIA, CHINA, JAPAN, *and* SOUTHEAST ASIAN COUNTRIES. *For a further discussion of topics mentioned in this article, see the entries* ALTERNATIVE THERAPIES; BUDDHISM; CONFUCIANISM; EUGENICS; FRIENDSHIP; HEALTH AND DISEASE, *articles on* SOCIOLOGICAL PERSPECTIVES, *and* ANTHROPOLOGICAL PERSPECTIVES; HINDUISM; JAINISM; LOVE; POPULATION ETHICS, *section on* ELEMENTS OF POPULATION ETHICS, *and section on* RELIGIOUS TRADITIONS, *articles on* HINDU PERSPECTIVES, *and* BUDDHIST PERSPECTIVES; PROFESSIONAL–PATIENT RELATIONSHIP; RESEARCH, HUMAN: HISTORICAL ASPECTS; *and* RESEARCH, UNETHICAL.

Bibliography

REID, ANTHONY. 1988. *Southeast Asia in the Age of Commerce, 1450–1680: The Lands Below the Winds.* Vol. 1. New Haven, Conn.: Yale University Press.

B. INDIA

In this article, India refers to the entire Asian subcontinent south of Afghanistan and the Himalayan range, including the modern nations of India, Pakistan, Bangladesh, and Nepal (often referred to as the "Indic" region) as well as the island nation Sri Lanka. In the third millennium B.C.E. there flourished a civilization in and around the Indus Valley known as the Harrapan city culture. Gradually, from the second millennium, the subcontinent was infiltrated by Indo-European tribes from Central Asia. These people formed the classical culture that survives to modern times with many transformations. In the eighth century, Muslim invasions began in the north, culminating in the powerful Mogul empire of the fourteenth and fifteenth centuries. Historic India is the home of two of the world's major religions, Hinduism and Buddhism, as well as of Jainism, and host to Islam, now the majority religion in Pakistan and Bangladesh, as well as to ancient Christian and Jewish communities in the south. From the interaction of Hinduism and Islam grew another religion in India, the Sikh faith. In the sixteenth century, India's cultural and religious influence extended into China and Tibet, as well as to the lands of Southeast Asia.

The origins of medicine in India stretch back to antiquity. The urban architecture of the earliest civilization, in the cities of the Indus Valley, demonstrates knowledge of sanitary techniques. One of the Vedas, the sacred lore of the early Indo-Europeans (ca. 1500–1000 B.C.E.), contains chants to ward off disease, and lists of herbal medicines. The ancient texts extolled by the *bhesaj,* persons skilled in the medicinal uses of herbs. Priest-physicians prescribed prayers and fasts, as well as herbal medicines. Out of this text, the *Atharvaveda,* and other systems of philosophical speculations developed a system of medicine based upon a theory of bodily humors and a therapeutic regimen of herbs and plants. The term "Ayurveda," meaning knowledge of vitality and long life, designated this classical Indian medicine that is widely practiced in India today.

Ayurvedic medicine developed in the fifth century B.C.E.; its earliest classical treatise, *Carakasamhita,* can be dated to the first century C.E. The oldest known Sanskrit medical manuscripts, discovered in a Buddhist monastery in China and dating from about 450 C.E., reveal a developed medical system, mentioning elixirs for long life (including garlic), eye lotions, enemas, aphrodisiacs, and ways of caring for sick children. The text mentions Indian physicians of renown, including the most famous, Sushruta (second century C.E.). After the adoption of Buddhism by King Ashoka (273–232 B.C.E.), Buddhist monks, who were not bound by the rigorous Hindu laws of purity and pollution, were free to mingle with common people and to invite them into their monasteries, thus bringing their medical skills to the needy and hospitality to the sick. They also seem to have brought Ayurvedic medicine to Tibet and China. Monks of the Jain tradition, which arose about the same time as the Buddhist tradition, also contributed to the development of the medical system. Early medical speculations and observations about the body, mind, and illness were consistent with tenets of all three major religions.

There appears to have been a flowering of medicine during the first millennium C.E. (Jolly, 1977; Winternitz, 1967). In the course of time, six classic texts of Ayurveda were recognized. Two of these, *Sushruta-samhita* and *Carakasamhita*, are named after the most famous physicians of the tradition, Sushruta and Caraka (first century C.E.); it is suggested that the word "caraka," which also means "one who moves about," refers to the itinerant Buddhist monks; Sushruta was a physician to a Buddhist king. The other four—*Ashtangahridaya*, attributed to the physician Vagbhatta; *Madhavanidana*; *Sarangadharasamhita*; and *Bhavaprakasha*—date from the eighth, ninth, thirteenth, and sixteenth centuries, respectively. The latter two reveal the influence of Arabic medicine, and the last mentions *phirangi roga*, the disease of the Franks (the Portuguese who came to India in 1498), probably syphilis. The use of opium as a therapeutic agent is prescribed in these later texts.

Assumptions of Ayurveda

Ayurveda is deeply rooted in the great religious and philosophical traditions of India, whose visions of human nature and the universe informed medicine and, in turn, were enriched by the concepts formed in medical practice (Dasgupta, 1975). Ayurvedic constructs of the self and the body, concerns central to the medical enterprise, grew in tandem with the faith traditions. Ayurvedic physiology and pathophysiology rest on a doctrine of humors (*doshas*) and bodily substances (*dhatus*). The principal humors are wind (*vata*), bile (*pitta*), and phlegm (*kapha*), representing movement, heat, and moisture in the body, respectively. The primary body substance, *dhatu*, is "organic sap" (*rasa*) derived from food, transformed in various ways as it moves through the body, stored in various reservoirs, and excreted as waste. Sap is first transformed into blood, then into flesh, fat, bone, marrow, and semen, the last being the purest product of the transformation.

Health is a state of balance of bodily humors and substances (*dhatusamya*); illness is disequilibrium. The body is affected by external factors, such as food and climate, as well as internal influences, such as anger and jealousy; social experiences, such as praise or scorn, also affect bodily states. Each of these may cause disease or restore health. This interactive universe of substances blurs the boundaries between inside and outside, and makes for a constant flux. The body is in dynamic relationship with the cosmos, whose elements of wind, fire, and water are reflected in the body; similarly, the body is seen as a reflection of the mythic cosmogony, in which the primordial person arises from chaos and is differentiated into multiple forms. Breath (*prana*) is the supreme force that unites bodily parts and becomes the definition of life (*jiva*): "People say of a dead person, that his limbs have become unstrung," say the *Upanishads* (ancient religious discourses). Ayurvedic medicine visualizes the sick person as in a state of fragmentation; his or her bodily components must be taken apart, cleansed, and put together again (Desai, 1989). Breath also becomes equated with the narcissistic and metaphysical components: *ahamkara* and *atman*. Ahamkara, "I-ness," literally the saying of the word "I," is the perishable self; and *atman*, cognate with the Greek *atmos*, is visualized as a self beyond death, without properties, pure consciousness, and transcendental. Although Hindu, Buddhist, and Jain traditions have differing notions of the self, they share common beliefs about the transience of the perishable body, often a source of pain, and the consubstantiality of the body with the universe.

The theory of *gunas* (literally "strands" or "qualities") is an aspect of *samkhya* and an important foundation of Hindu ethics. Inherent and substantial, *sattva* (goodness), *rajas* (vitality), and *tamas* (inertia) are found in all material substances in various combinations and determine the overall constitutional disposition of persons, foods, activities, bodily substances, and so forth. Physically *sattva* is cool and light; *rajas*, hot and active; and *tamas*, heavy and dull. Psychologically they are calmness, passion, and lethargy or stupidity, respectively. In character they are purity or virtue, happiness or sorrow, and darkness or evil, respectively. Contemplation, meditation, silence, devotion, and fasting promote goodness; love, battle, attachment, pleasure seeking, and emotionality enhance vitality; sloth, sleep, and idleness increase inertia. In the hierarchy of values, the *sattva* categories tend to reign supreme and become less material and closer to the idea of *sat* (truth or essence); in Ayurvedic discourses they are understood to be the same as the mind or the self. The ethical aim, therefore, is to transform physical and mental dispositions from inertia to activity to goodness. Such transformations are promoted by ingestion of foods and performance of activities that are conducive to the higher strand. Therapeutic aims are also to transform the self and the body to higher levels of functions: from imbalance to equipoise, from idleness to activity, from agitation or pleasure seeking to calmness and contemplation.

The physician

An Ayurvedic physician, called a *vaidya*, is one of the quartet (the physician, the drugs, the attendant, and the patient) responsible for amelioration of diseases. Although esteemed for their powers to bring about health and disease-free states ("the cause of virtue"), physicians were regarded with mixed feelings in ancient India; anxiety concerning disease and death was displaced onto them. Physicians contracted impurity from their handling of body products, lesions, and corpses, and through their "democratic practice of mingling with the common people" (Chattopadhyaya, 1977). Religious texts enjoined people not to receive food from physicians and to avoid them at religious ceremonies. Taboos concerning touching caused palpation to fall into disuse as a diagnostic tool.

The Ayurvedic texts demand that a physician excel in theoretical knowledge, have extensive practical experience, be dextrous, and observe the rules of cleanliness. A physician began his education as an apprentice, teacher and pupil choosing each other. A good teacher was free from conceit, greed, and envy; the student was calm, friendly, and without physical defects. The physician must be compassionate, virtuous, of high lineage, devoted to learning, rational, and always ready to act. The *Carakasamhita* regards the profession as suitable to the upper castes: Brahmins (for the welfare of all living beings), Kshatriyas (for their own protection), and Vaishyas (for livelihood). The *Sushrutasamhita* also permits the Shudras, the lowest caste, to be physicians. Later the vaidyas became a caste, an occupational division, and the profession passed from father to son. In modern India, physicians, Ayurvedic or otherwise, may be from any caste.

Carakasamhita contains an extensive ethical treatise in the form of an initiation oath to be sworn by one entering the practice of medicine. Among its injunctions are these:

> Day and night, however you may be engaged, you shall strive for the relief of the patient with all your heart and soul. You shall not desert or injure your patient even for the sake of your life or your living.
>
> You shall be modest in your dress and appearance and speak words that are gentle, pure, righteous, pleasing, worthy, true, wholesome, and moderate.
>
> When entering a patient's house, you shall be accompanied by a man who is known to the patient and who has his permission to enter. Having entered, your

> speech, mind, intellect, and senses shall be entirely devoted to no other thought than that of being helpful to the patient, and of things concerning him only. The peculiar customs of the patient's household shall not be made public.
>
> Though possessed of knowledge, you should not boast very much about it. Most people are offended by the boastfulness of even those who are otherwise good and knowledgeable.
>
> There is no limit at all to which knowledge of Ayurveda can be acquired, so you should apply yourself to it with all diligence. The entire world is the teacher of the intelligent and the foe of the unintelligent. Hence, knowing this well, you should listen and act according to the words of instruction of even an unfriendly person when they are worthy and such as to bring fame and long life to you, and are capable of giving you strength and prosperity. (Menon and Haberman, 1940, pp. 295–296)

Sushrutasamhita describes procedures that include an ingenious method of making a new nose when the original has been cut off (a form of humiliation that was a common punishment for criminals and unfaithful wives). The text also contains directions for dissection of the cadaver. However, dissection for purposes of teaching and study was not normally practiced. The objection to dissection was based on the deep-seated Indian taboo on contact with dead matter of any kind. The doctrine of *ahimsa* (nonviolence), which was taught by Buddhism and Jainism, did not prevent dissection of a dead body, provided the body was not deliberately killed for that purpose; but *ahimsa* did act as a check on vivisection of any creature.

Care of animals such as cows, horses, elephants, and even birds formed an integral part of the prevailing religious beliefs. Mention is made in the literature of hospitals for sick and wounded birds. Although ancient Indian physicians were taught the care and treatment of animals, there were also veterinarians who cared only for animals.

Quacks and charlatans were unequivocally condemned. They were known by their loose tongues, superficial knowledge, pretense, and arrogance. When the patient worsened, they abandoned him. The fate of their patients was worse than death; one can survive a thunderbolt, says *Carakasamhita*, but not the medicine prescribed by quacks. A physician, on the other hand, was to hold his tongue, not enter into needless debates, and apply himself continuously to new learning. He was to avoid women who belong to others, not to enter the house of a patient without the presence of a person known to the family, to maintain confidentiality, and never to mention a patient's approaching death.

Modern Indian physicians, especially those trained in Western medicine under the British, took the Hippocratic oath. The Indian Medical Council promulgated its code of ethics in 1970. The code directs physicians to serve humanity without regard to religion or race, social or political affiliation. A physician must provide *pro bono* services, maintain confidentiality, and hold teachers in esteem with a sense of gratitude. An adulterous relationship with a patient or with a patient's family member is considered a breach of ethical principles (Medical Council of India, 1980).

The origin of life

The origin of life is a major concern of the authors of traditional medical texts. An embryo is formed through the union of the woman and the man when both have appropriate humoral dispositions and appropriate nourishment. The life principle is thought either to enter at the moment of conception or to be a latent property of the seeds; the latter is comparable to fire in the rays of the sun becoming manifest on passing through a lens, or the combining of male and female germinal substances. At other times the moment of quickening or the descent of the fetus in the womb is seen as a moment of independent life or viability. Defective germinal substances, "unnatural" coitus, failure of nourishment or inappropriate nourishment, and weakness or disturbance in humors explain the unexpected, such as multiple pregnancies and infertility. Initially the fetus is visualized as genderless and becomes male or female in the third to fourth month of pregnancy. Among the rites of passage, *samskaras,* there is one that is performed at this stage of pregnancy to promote the development of a male child.

Having a male child is a Hindu religious obligation, for the performance of funerary rites by a son secures passage to the land of the forefathers. In this rite of passage, the son symbolically reconstitutes the body of the dead father and reunites him with his lineage. Therefore, a man must have a son; if necessary, he must take another wife to beget a son, invite his younger brother or a Brahmin of good conduct to impregnate his wife (a custom called *niyoga*), choose another willing woman, or otherwise adopt, procure, or purchase a son. The epic *Mahabharata* provides examples of *niyoga*—the birth of the father of Pandavas, the protagonists, and of the Kauravas, the antagonists of the epic—and of in vitro fertilization—the development of embryos in pots, as in the case of the Kauravas. The birth of the last liberated sage of the Jain tradition, Mahavira, provides an example of embryo transfer from one womb to another, as does the birth of an older sibling of Lord Krishna (Desai, 1988). In light of these traditions, modern forms of surrogacy or new technologies present few problems.

Contraception and abortion also have precedents in Indian tradition. The medical texts dwell upon ways of enhancing the possibilities of conception through ma-

nipulation of a number of variables; the same variables can be manipulated to retard the chances of conception. In practice, sexual congress outside the Hindu religious Law was not prohibited for men, but women were scorned if found lacking in virtue—especially widows, who were forbidden to remarry—and means had to be sought to prevent unwanted pregnancies. *Bhavaprakasha,* a sixteenth-century medical text, provides a list of oral contraceptives. Modern methods of contraception have been introduced in India, and a massive family-planning campaign includes male and female sterilization. Research work on antipregnancy vaccine and depot preparations (large doses suspended in oil so that they are slowly released over a long period of time) of hormones is ongoing.

Medical texts, especially the *Sushrutasamhita,* describe various forms of arrested fetal development, fetal death, stillbirth, and obstructed deliveries, and the treatments for them that consist of induction of labor and/or destruction of the fetus. The text cautions against hasty action and requires royal permission to induce abortion and extraction of the fetus in case of danger to maternal life. Although early religious texts consider abortion to be a sin, equal to the killing of a Brahmin, by the seventeenth century Ayurvedic physicians were advising the use of an herb, administered vaginally, for the induction of labor, "a useful remedy for pregnant women in poor health, widows, and women of liberal morals" (as quoted from Vaidya Jeevanamin Chandrashekar, 1974, p. 45).

In colonial India abortions were governed by English law; in 1972 the government of India legalized abortion, mainly to prevent illegal abortions and to give further impetus to family planning. Abortions in the first trimester, and under special conditions in the second trimester, are available on demand. More recently, RU-486, "the morning after" pill, has been introduced in India on an experimental basis.

Amniocentesis has become extremely popular in India. Overwhelming preference for boys, permissive abortion laws, and the crushing burden of dowries have led parents to seek to ascertain the sex of the fetus, so that a female can be aborted. A vigorous debate, both for and against using the new technology for sex selection, has ensued, one camp arguing in effect that feticide is better than infanticide and the other decrying the culture's age-old cruelties against women (Desai, 1991).

Disease, death, and the laws of karma

Karma is the operative principle of Hindu ethics and has come to mean that every action has a consequence: "As you sow, so shall you reap." Karma has explanatory power for questions like "Why me?" and encourages action for future rewards. The cycle of birth, death, and rebirth, as well as that of health and disease, is governed by the laws of karma. The laws of karma also have dominated Buddhist and Jain ethics.

The ancient physicians classified the etiology of diseases into three categories. External or invasive diseases were caused by foreign bodies, war injuries, possession, or infestation. Internal diseases were disturbances of humors brought about by lapses in discretion, which included faulty diets, overexertion, sloth, sexual indulgence, and mental disturbances. The third category was reserved for the workings of karma, fruits of action from past deeds or previous lives. Some disease states were also seen as the workings of time, as in aging. The unseen hand of karma was invoked in all diseases, a schema that brought ordinary actions like dietary habits and seasonal observances under the umbrella of ethics. Mental illnesses also arose from these etiologies: possession by spirits, disturbances in humors, and lapses in discretion. Like other conditions that defy easy explanations, epidemics and natural disasters were thought to be caused by the collective misdeeds of a population or of a ruler. Physicians of the era of Caraka and Sushruta paid homage to the principle of karma but argued that passivity on part of a physician who assumed predetermination of disease or death made the whole medical enterprise meaningless. Human effort was always a factor in the workings of karma, and the human body was the object of physicians, who held alleviation of diseases and restoration of health as their primary objectives.

On the other hand, there were incurable diseases. It was prudent of physicians to be wary of heroic efforts to prevent the inevitable, which not only brought loss of income but social censure and ignominy as well. If the physician knew that a case was hopeless, he was to do no more than sustain the nutrition of a dying patient. Thus, prolonging life with artificial means is not always acceptable. Those who have led a full life must, like ripened fruits, fall from the tree; untimely death of the young is another matter. Yet, death is not the opposite of life; it is simply the other end, the opposite of birth. Those who are born must die.

Debates in the West on the issues of aging, the care of the terminally ill, and euthanasia have prompted a reexamination of medical ethics in the East. Not surprisingly the Hindu, the Jain, and the Buddhist views converge and have a place for a "willed death" or, more correctly, "hastened death" (Young, 1989; Desai, 1991; Bilimoria, 1992; Fujii, 1991). Shrinivas Tilak (1989), after examining Hindu and Buddhist texts, concluded that aging represents points in a life cycle, indicating both growth and maturity as well as eventual decline and loss; at the end point it is an indicator of ultimate dissolution of life. Hindu texts bemoan the inevitability of death, and the Buddhist texts point to pain and unhappiness as inherent in life. In the face of approaching or inevitable death or debilitating and painfully long suffering, traditional ethics provides "permission to leave" voluntarily. Also, the anxiety occasioned by the uncertain timing of death is to be mastered by death that is willed; choosing the moment of death is permitted to ascetics or otherwise superior and elevated souls. Each of the three traditions provides for taking a vow to gradually refrain from taking food and water (and medications, when relevant); thus one ultimately starves to death. The early discourses do not regard this as suicide, which is a death brought upon oneself in a state of desperation and imbalance, and therefore belongs to a different category. The three traditions, which uphold *ahimsa* as central to the view of sanctity of all life, find little difficulty with death that is hastened by starvation. A telling episode in the life of Mahatma Gandhi illustrates this debate (Parekh, 1989). A calf that had no hope of surviving and was suffering was put to death with Gandhi's consent. Gandhi rejected the view that killing was never justified and always represented violence. He said that there is violence when the intention is to cause pain; otherwise it is simply an act of killing. When confronted by his critics, especially the Jain merchants of Gujarat, with the problem of euthanasia, Gandhi gave the following response:

1. The disease from which the patient is suffering should be incurable.
2. All concerned have despaired of the life of the patient.
3. The case should be beyond all help or service.
4. It should be impossible for the patient in question to express his or her wish.
5. So long as even one of these conditions remains unfulfilled, the taking of life from the point of view of *ahimsa* cannot be justified.

Although Gandhi believed that he had arrived at his position independently, he was building on the position advanced by ancient medical authorities.

Other systems of medicine

Yoga philosophy and the related tantra have enriched the Indian medical system on the periphery. In classical yoga thought, the *Yogasutra* of Pantanjali, the aim is to bring the mind to focus by inhibiting its waywardness, through successive disciplines of body and thought and by regulation of body functions. Thus body and mind are yoked and come into correct conjunction. Later elaborations have included arduous physical practices and other forms of meditation. Modern relaxation techniques and biofeedback, popular in the West, owe their origin to the discipline of yoga.

Yogic thought visualizes the body in concentric layers, proceeding from the less important outside to the vital inside, from gross to subtle, from hard to soft, and from more material to less material. The body is penetrable and its boundaries permeable; only the innermost self, which must be realized through yoga, is an adamantine core of permanent joy and bliss.

Other forms of yoga, especially the kundalini yoga, advance a concept in which the spine is a vertical axis along which are chakras (wheels or lotuses), centers of energy and impulses. The lower chakras represent vegetative functions (e.g., genitoexcretory, digestive, circulatory, and respiratory); the higher ones, centers of thought and emotion. In this dualism, kundalini, the spiritual aspect of a person, lies dormant in the lowest chakra at the base of the spine; it must be awakened through yogic exercises and made to travel up the spine, activating other chakras on the way and finally uniting with the highest chakra, where the principle of consciousness resides. The regulation of breath is critically important in these exercises, for the breath is the source of energy and must travel through the chakras into the various nerves or channels (nadis). The left-handed form, tantra, is a fringe discipline emphasizing esoteric sexual practices. The feminine powers are invoked and sought for the purpose of incorporating them in the self of the practitioner. The way to accomplish this is literally to reverse the flow of sexual fluids from men to women. Ultimately the enriched semen will be forced up the spinal axis to repose in the head as a collection of the most vital and purified energy.

Another Indian medical system is the siddha tradition, practiced mainly in southern India. Based on the Ayurvedic principles, it favors the Greek pharmacopoeia, especially the metallic oxides. The use of astrology in diagnosis and treatment, including the wearing of precious and semiprecious stones, is quite common in India. There is also a rich tradition of folk medicine, including exorcists, bonesetters, snakebite curers, and those who use mantras for cure.

The Yunani or Arabic system of medicine was brought to India by the Muslim invaders. Accepted by the rulers, it began to displace the older Ayurvedic practice to the periphery but also interacted with it. Its humoral thinking, based on Galenic principles, was congenial to Ayurveda. The examination of the radial pulse became a central feature of Ayurvedic diagnosis, and whereas the Ayurvedic pathophysiology had until then been exclusively humoral, the liver and blood were now implicated in folk pathophysiology. Muslim rulers patronized the system and founded publicly funded hospitals and dispensaries. Hakims, the practitioners of Arabic medicine, enriched the Ayurvedic herbal apothecary with their metallic oxides. They often specialized in the treatment of male sexual dysfunctions. This system is especially patronized by the Muslim population of the subcontinent.

"Allopathy" is the term by which modern Western medicine is known in India. European missionaries, especially from Portugal and France, brought it in the fifteenth century, and the British introduced the system in the delivery of care of their own personnel, later founding hospitals and medical schools in the major Indian cities. Allopathy pushed Ayurveda and Yunani to the periphery of medical practice. Today in India all systems are patronized, allopathy more in the cosmopolitan areas and the indigenous systems more in the rural. Patients often move from one to the other, depending on their own explanatory system or the success or failure of one or the other. The indigenous systems are more often chosen for the treatment of chronic conditions, which by definition have failed to be cured by modern methods. Although antibiotics have changed the epidemiology of acute conditions, they are seen as heavy and harmful with many side effects, in contrast to the gentler herbal preparations. Preparations for internal use have to meet the test of culturally constructed theory of inputs and fluxes. The most significant impact of modern antibiotics has been on maternal and infant morbidity and mortality.

In the 1990s most hospitals are staffed by practitioners of allopathic medicine. There are over 100 allopathic medical schools, over 500,000 hospital beds, and over 300,000 licensed medical practitioners. About 100 Ayurvedic colleges exist, and over 250,000 practitioners, but they have only 20,000 hospital beds. Research in Ayurvedic and Yunani medicine has been organized under central institutes.

Surgery, for which ancient India was famous, has passed into the domain of modern Western medicine. With anesthesia, asepsis, and blood transfusion, modern surgical practice has totally excluded the traditional forms. Organ transplants are becoming common, since traditional beliefs about construction of the body from discrete parts allows for removal and replacement. However, extreme poverty has created a widespread and unregulated market in which poor people offer corneas and kidneys for sale to the wealthy.

A fragmented, either commercialized or bureaucratic system of care that is neither easily accessible nor affordable is the major ethical problem of India. Emigration of physicians and nurses to the West has not helped. Multinational drug cartels and fly-by-night Indian drug firms with little regulation in manufacture or prescription form a lethal combination with diagnoses made by divination or without examination. The cultivation of public health and prevention points a way out of the current problems.

PRAKASH N. DESAI

While all the articles in this section and the other sections of this entry are relevant, see especially the GENERAL SURVEY *and other articles in this section, which discuss* CHINA, JAPAN, *and* SOUTHEAST ASIAN COUNTRIES. *For a further discussion of topics mentioned in this article, see the entries* ABORTION, *section on* CONTEMPORARY ETHICAL AND LEGAL ASPECTS, *and section on* RELIGIOUS TRADITIONS, *article on* ISLAMIC PERSPECTIVES; ALTERNATIVE THERAPIES; ANIMAL WELFARE AND RIGHTS; BODY, *article on* CULTURAL AND RELIGIOUS PERSPECTIVES; BUDDHISM; DEATH AND DYING: EUTHANASIA AND SUSTAINING LIFE, *articles on* HISTORICAL ASPECTS, *and* ETHICAL ISSUES; DEATH, *article on* EASTERN THOUGHT; DEATH, ATTITUDES TOWARDS; FERTILITY CONTROL; HEALTH AND DISEASE; HINDUISM; ISLAM; JAINISM; JUSTICE; MEDICAL CODES AND OATHS; MEDICINE, ANTHROPOLOGY OF; MEDICINE, SOCIOLOGY OF; OBLIGATION AND SUPEREROGATION; PAIN AND SUFFERING; POPULATION ETHICS, *section on* ELEMENTS OF POPULATION ETHICS, *article on* HISTORY OF POPULATION THEORIES, *and section on* RELIGIOUS TRADITIONS, *the* INTRODUCTION *and articles on* HINDU PERSPECTIVES, ISLAMIC PERSPECTIVES, *and* BUDDHIST PERSPECTIVES; PROFESSION AND PROFESSIONAL ETHICS; REPRODUCTIVE TECHNOLOGIES, *articles on* IN VITRO FERTILIZATION AND EMBRYO TRANSFER, SURROGACY, *and* CRYOPRESERVATION OF SPERM, OVA, AND EMBRYOS; SIKHISM; SOCIAL MEDICINE; SURGERY; SUSTAINABLE DEVELOPMENT; UNORTHODOXY IN MEDICINE; VALUE AND VALUATION; VIRTUE AND CHARACTER; *and* WOMEN, *article on* HISTORICAL PERSPECTIVES. *See also the* APPENDIX (CODES, OATHS, AND DIRECTIVES RELATED TO BIOETHICS), SECTION II: ETHICAL DIRECTIVES FOR THE PRACTICE OF MEDICINE, OATH OF HIPPOCRATES, *and* OATH OF INITIATION.

Bibliography

Primary texts

Bhavaprakasha. 1981. Translated by Gaurishankar Mayashankar Shastri. Ahmadabad, India: Sastu Sahitya Vardhak Karyalaya. In Gujarati.

Brihadāraṇyaka Upaniṣad. 1962. Translated by F. Max Muller in *The Upanishads,* pt. 2. New York: Dover.

Carakasamhita. 1981–1985. [1884]. Translated by Priyavrat Sharma. 3 vols. Varanasi, India: Chaukhambha Orientalia.

Mahābhārata. 1973. Translated by Johannes Adrianus Bernardus Van Buitenen. 3 vols. Chicago: University of Chicago Press.

Sushrutasamhita. 1980. Translated by Vaidya Jadavji Trikamji Acharya and Narayana Ram Acharya. Varanasi, India: Chaukhambha Orientalia.

Secondary sources

BILMORIA, PURUSHOTTAMA. 1992. "The Jaina Ethic of Voluntary Death." *Bioethics* 6, no. 4:331–335.

CHANDRASHEKAR, SRIPATI. 1974. *Abortion in a Crowded World: The Problem of Abortion with Special Reference to India.* London: George Allen and Unwin.

CHATTOPADHYAYA, DEBIPRASAD. 1977. *Science and Society in Ancient India.* Calcutta: Research India Publications.

DASGUPTA, SURENDRANATH. 1975. [1922]. *A History of Indian Philosophy.* 5 vols. Delhi: Motilal Banarsidass.

DESAI, PRAKASH. 1988. "Medical Ethics in India." *Journal of Medicine and Philosophy* 13, no 3:231–255.

———. 1989. *Health and Medicine in the Hindu Tradition: Continuity and Cohesion.* New York: Crossroads.

———. 1991. "Hinduism and Bioethics in India: A Tradition in Transition." In *Theological Developments in Bioethics: 1988–1990.* Vol. 1 of *Bioethics Yearbook,* pp. 41–60. Edited by Baruch A. Brody, B. Andrew Lustig, H. Tristram Engelhardt, Jr., and Laurence B. McCullough. Dordrecht, Netherlands: Kluwer.

FUJII, MASAO. 1991. "Buddhism and Bioethics." In *Theological Developments in Bioethics. 1988–1990.* Vol. 1 of *Bioethics Yearbook,* pp. 61–68. Edited by Baruch A. Brody, B. Andrew Lustig, H. Tristram Engelhardt, Jr., and Laurence B. McCullough. Dordrecht, Netherlands: Kluwer.

JOLLY, JULIUS. 1977. [1901]. *Indian Medicine.* Translated by Chintamani Ganesh Kashikar. New Delhi: Munshiram Manoharlal.

MEDICAL COUNCIL OF INDIA. 1980. *Code of Medical Ethics.* Supplement to *Christian Medical Association of India Journal* (June).

MENON, A., and HABERMAN, HERBERT FREDERICK. 1970. "Caraka Samhita." *Medical History* 14:295–296.

PAREKH, BHIKHU C. 1989. *Colonialism, Tradition and Reform: An Analysis of Gandhi's Political Discourse.* New Delhi: Sage Publications.

TILAK, SHRINIVAS. 1989. *Religion and Aging in the Indian Tradition.* Albany: State University of New York Press.

WINTERNITZ, MORIZ. 1967. [1913, 1920]. *History of Indian Literature.* Translated by Subhadra Jha. 3 vols. Delhi: Motilal Banarsidass.

YOUNG, KATHERINE K. 1989. "Euthanasia: Traditional Hindu Views, and the Contemporary Debate." In *Hindu Ethics: Purity, Abortion, and Euthanasia,* pp. 71–130. Edited by Harold G. Coward, Julius J. Lipner, and Katherine K. Young. Albany: State University of New York Press.

C. CHINA

1. PREREPUBLICAN CHINA

The following article has been retained from the first edition, with minor revisions by the original author.

The cultural history of China, as reflected in its literature, shows that for at least two thousand years the Confucian worldview, an ideology concerned with the structure of social life, dominated Chinese society until the collapse of the empire early in the twentieth century. Although less obvious, the philosophy of Taoism exerted a strong influence on Chinese society in the same period. A third major influence in ancient China, that of Buddhism, was introduced from India about the first century C.E. Buddhism exerted its greatest impact on social life and scholarship in China from about the sixth to the early ninth century. Subsequently some of its metaphysical concepts were integrated into Confucianism, its worldly assets were secularized, and its teachings continued mostly on the level of a folk religion. Medical ethics in China, as a consequence of the parallel existence of these three major ways of life, reflects some of the values of all of them.

This article will focus on the history of explicit medical ethics in prerepublican China. By "explicit medical ethics" is meant those norms allegedly present in interactions between medical practitioners and their clientele. The historian has no way of investigating whether norms, as they were expounded by various groups providing health care in China, actually formed the basis of these groups' actions; it is a well-documented fact that explicit ethics are usually far more rigid than the norms actually followed. One can only infer, then, the ethical norms proposed as an appropriate basis of the actual relationship between individual practitioner and patient in prerepublican China. Evidence of appeals to a code of ethics is extant only with respect to a few individuals. One cannot infer from the explicit ethics of a few practitioners the ethics of the whole group. Professional organizations of medical practitioners that might have attempted to enforce a single code of ethics were unknown in prerepublican China.

Historical sources allow for an understanding of the values regarding life and death contained in various ideologies propagated in China. These values, of course, have their immediate bearing on norms regarding the provision of health care and medical services.

The historical sources further make possible an understanding of the relationship among various practitioner groups and between these groups and the general public. In addition, the historical material forces one to distinguish between traditional explicit medical ethics and modern explicit medical ethics. The former was characteristic of a period in history during which no group of independent practitioners achieved a place in the top ranks of the respective culture's social hierarchy; values dominant in society concerning life and death seem to have been quite stable during this epoch. One purpose of traditional explicit medical ethics, then, may be understood as an attempt by the medical group expounding it to demonstrate its continuous adherence and conformity to fixed, well-defined values.

Modern explicit medical ethics, in contradistinction, results from technologically based advances in Western medicine during recent decades. It represents an attempt to transform values into norms for new situations. The age-old values regarding life and death cannot simply be extended to the consequences of recent developments in health care. In contrast to the past, medical scientists in all modern societies work at the forefront of medical progress, and new norms, often representing differing values, have had to be created to cope with situations that formerly were inconceivable, for example, organ transplantation, allocation of scarce primary medical resources, and the maintenance of physiological functions in the terminal patient.

Although statements about medical practice and practitioners are found early in various branches of Chinese literature, the first lengthy and explicit statement on medical ethics of physicians, that of Sun Ssu-miao, appeared in the seventh century. The probable causes for the emergence of such statements at that time demand closer investigation.

Medical practice, in whatever form it is carried out, represents a basic necessity for survival not only of the individual but also of the society. Although communities are known that severely restrict, or even totally deny, medical practice, on grounds of the religious beliefs they follow, one otherwise finds an active acceptance in all cultures known so far.

The utilization and the improvement of available primary medical resources (i.e., medical knowledge and skills, drugs and medical technology, medical equipment and facilities) may be viewed as an integral part of most cultures. The problematic variable is which segment of society utilizes and controls these primary medical resources.

At the beginning of the Confucian era in China, about two thousand years ago, several groups already participated in the utilization and control of the primary medical resources then available. These resources included preventive and curative therapeutic strategies that derived from separately conceptualized understandings of health and illness. These included a metaphysical perspective concerning the origin of health and illness, which identified the influence of ancestors and demons as responsible for illness, and a naturalistic concept that focused on the relationship between humankind and its physical environment.

The ancestral paradigm is the earliest known conceptual response in China to the experience of illness and early death. It is documented in inscriptions on oracle bones dating back to the Shang dynasty (approximately from the eleventh century B.C.E. on). Even though this perspective lost its dominant position as an explanation of illness and for the design of strategies to prevent or cure illness by the middle of the first millennium B.C.E., it has survived in China until the present. Ancestral healing places living humans in a community with their ancestors, who, although dead, continue to exist. The ancestors guarantee the health of the living as long as the latter adhere to certain norms, and they send individual illness or social catastrophe when they notice a departure from these norms by an individual or society. Prayers and sacrifices by the living may cause the ancestors to withdraw their wrath and restore health or social harmony.

The ancestral paradigm was superseded during the period of the Warring States, in the middle of the first millennium B.C.E., by a belief in the power of demons (i.e., metaphysical entities not directly related to a living human being) to cause illness. Demons, it was assumed, will cause harm to a person regardless of that person's lifestyle; protection is achieved not by adherence to specific moral tenets but by alliances with the forces of stronger metaphysical entities, especially those of sun, moon, the stars, or thunder. Spells and talismans served to demonstrate these alliances and scare away demons in the lesser ranks of the supernatural hierarchy.

When in the early 1970s, a tomb sealed in 167 B.C.E. was unearthed near Changsha in the Chinese province of Hunan, the artifacts found included numerous texts related to health care and therapy. These manuscripts offer the earliest available evidence of the development, in ancient China, of a broad gamut of empirical therapeutic strategies, ranging from minor surgery and massage, dietary concerns and recommendations concerning sexual intercourse, to cauterization and, most prominently, elaborate pharmacotherapy. The resort to herbal, animal, and mineral drugs, as well as man-made substances, to cure and prevent illness remained the most important strategy in Chinese medicine until the twentieth century. Most of traditional Chinese medical literature consists of a long series of ever more comprehensive and sophisticated herbals discussing all possible facets of drug lore, and an even greater number of prescription collections, ranging from specialized treatises focusing on one problem to encyclopedic works. Inherent in the use of drugs against illness is an ontological notion that derives from demonologic beliefs. If they did not serve to cure symptoms such as pain or diarrhea, fever, and cough, drugs could kill intruders causing trouble in the organism.

At about the time China was united in the second century B.C.E., a further approach to understanding health and illness found its way into medical literature: the ideology of systematic correspondence. Based on a dualistic paradigm of yin-yang and on a scheme of five phases, the entirety of observed phenomena in the human organism and its environment was seen as a system of interrelated, and hence corresponding, items and processes. A person remained healthy as long as he or she was able to live in accordance with the underlying laws of this system; departure resulted in illness. Health care on the basis of these ideas was not so much focused on the treatment of manifest diseases as on prevention and on intervention at the earliest signs of change from a perceived status of normalcy. This system of health care

did not rely on drugs but on an application of needles meant to exert stimuli that serve to regulate imbalances. Nevertheless, the medicine of systematic correspondence also included strong ontological notions. On a more abstract level, if compared with pharmaceutics, the medicine of systematic correspondence harbored as one of its central notions an idea of "evil" entering the organism from the outside or being generated inside. This "evil" could be transmitted inside the body through a complicated system of conduits and network vessels, and had to be located in order to be purged or eliminated.

The theoretical framework and the terminology of the medicine of systematic correspondence closely paralleled the basic tenets and the language of the social theory of Confucianism. Health of the individual body was achieved by the same means as harmony of the social organism, that is, by adherence to specific moral rules. Deviance resulted in illness or social disorder. Just as no enemy was believed to be able to disturb society from within or to enter from outside as long as these rules were upheld, no illness could emerge in the body or be stimulated by an intrusion from the outside as long as an individual followed a specific lifestyle.

For this reason one may call the medicine of systematic correspondence "Confucian medicine." Confucian medicine, into which the utilization of drugs was integrated in the twelfth century C.E., was successfully challenged as the officially sanctioned healing system only with the downfall of the imperial society early in the twentieth century.

At the beginning of the Confucian era in the second century B.C.E., medical practice appears to have been in the hands of a variety of practitioners following the principles of the different known medical sciences. In addition there were practitioners, such as a mother treating her child or a neighbor, who possessed and utilized primary medical resources regarded as empirically effective. One has to keep in mind, then, that there was no group with any degree of professionalism practicing medicine in China at that time. In other words, no group of medical practitioners can be said to have been close to having control over all primary medical resources that were available in China almost two thousand years ago.

While it may readily be assumed that the motivation for some people to practice medicine was to help a family member or friend, there is no way to investigate the motives and the actual ethical bases of those persons who chose medicine over any other occupation to earn a living or to exert a social impact. Chinese texts concerned with medical ethics, however, clearly indicate that the desire for control over secondary medical resources (i.e., material and nonmaterial rewards that accrue from medical practice, such as financial wealth or social influence) was a major determinant of the way in which medicine was practiced. At the beginning of the Confucian era, medical practitioners had little control over secondary medical resources. The evaluation of their practice depended on public opinion, that is, on the satisfaction of the laity.

During the following twenty centuries, various groups attempted to reach higher levels of professionalization, that is, to increase the proportion of their control over available primary and secondary medical resources at the expense of the public. One of the important means employed to achieve this end was the appeal to medical ethics (Unschuld, 1979).

Prior to the seventh century C.E., outside of the imperial court in China, no systematic attempt to teach practitioners in medical schools or similar institutions is known. In the first half of the seventh century, the establishment of medical teaching institutions both in the capital of the empire and in the most important provincial cities was decreed. This may be interpreted as an attempt by Confucian decision makers to preserve control over medical resources for the ruling class, the gentry-bureaucracy.

The founding of these medical institutions reflects a basic tenet of Confucian ethics, the prevention of the accumulation by any one group in society of control over primary and secondary resources of any kind, which might result in a shift of power and possibly a social crisis or even change.

The underlying principle of many political decisions made in Confucian China was the suppression of emerging groups that had been able to gain control over specific resources. Medical resources were obviously recognized by Confucian decision makers as potential sources of power if accumulated and controlled by specific groups. Several political measures were undertaken to prevent the emergence of socially accepted, influential groups of practitioners. One was to emphasize the unethical character of practicing medicine for a livelihood by pointing out the evil practices employed by those doing so. It was urged that every educated man should possess sufficient medical knowledge to be able to care for his relatives. Another means was to place all extrafamilial care in the hands of civil servant physicians who were representatives of the Confucian class. Thus, it is not surprising that the education of medical officers in the seventh century was designed to supplement the common basic Confucian education. This tendency was further strengthened during later centuries.

The first noteworthy text of medical ethics appeared during the period when the first medical schools began to produce graduates. The author, a noted physician named Sun Ssu-miao (581–682?), was heavily influenced by both Buddhist and Taoist thought. Despite the fact that he was also well versed in Confucian scholarship, he refused on several occasions to accept calls to serve at the court. Sun Ssu-miao may well be called an outstanding representative of free-practicing physicians outside the Confucian group. By "free-practicing physicians" we mean those practitioners who traveled or stayed at home and treated all kinds of patients, in contradistinction to those physicians who had acquired their knowledge solely to assist family members or friends in need, or to serve as civil servants on medical assignments. The fact that Sun Ssu-miao's explicit medical ethics appeared at the same time as the establishment of the medical schools might suggest that it was a well-timed presentation designed to expound to the public the medical ethics of the group he represented.

In his voluminous medical work Ch'ien-chin fang (The Thousand Golden Prescriptions), Sun Ssu-miao chose the heading "On the Absolute Sincerity of Great Physicians" for the chapter devoted to medical ethics. The selection of the term ta-i (great physician) implied on the one hand that Sun Ssu-miao did not intend to speak for all medical practitioners of his time, but only for those whom he regarded as "great." It is a common characteristic of medical professionalization in East and West that at some time or other a few individuals form an elitist group that attempts to distinguish itself from the mass of its colleagues through the demonstration of its exclusive possession of superior primary medical resources. It should also be noted that Sun Ssu-miao's choice of the term ta-i was meant to imply that his group had a status similar to that of the most highly regarded imperial court physicians, or t'ai-i. The Chinese characters for these two terms are closely related in structure and meaning. Considering the low-ranking social position officially accorded to free-practicing physicians in Confucian China, the use of this title represented a bold demand for the social elevation of their elitist group of practitioners.

Sun Ssu-miao's treatise was meant to serve two purposes. First, by laying stress on the evaluation of treatment procedures rather than on the outcome of treatments, as was common at the time, he provided a measure of protection for the practitioner in instances where prognosis was unfavorable or outcome unsuccessful. The second purpose was to imply that his "great physicians" should be trusted more than was usually the case.

As an introduction to his explicit medical ethics, Sun Ssu-miao provided his readers with a framework of the healing system he and other great physicians allegedly adhered to. It was based on the same theories and concepts that underlay the Confucian-supported medicine of systematic correspondence. Other writings of Sun Ssu-miao reveal, though, that he also favored demonic medicine, a healing system persistently repudiated by Confucians. In his explicit medical ethics, Sun Ssu-miao chose not to mention this aspect of his medical beliefs. He laid a great emphasis on thorough training for those who wish to practice medicine successfully and thus aspire to the title "great physician." Such tactics were important at that time, because the medical practitioners approved for governmental service were being institutionally trained in official medicine and were thus calling into question the background of free-practicing physicians.

It is characteristic of explicit medical ethics, as propounded by individuals who strive for a higher level of professionalism for their group, to incorporate the basic social values of the dominant groups in society. Therefore, Sun Ssu-miao's explicit ethics frequently stresses certain values central to Confucian and Buddhist thought, such as *jen* (humane benevolence) and *tz'u* (compassion). Furthermore, certain maxims are emphasized, for example, the obligation to maintain life and to treat human beings regardless of their status, origin, appearance, or the kind of disease they have.

Sun Ssu-miao seems to have grasped some important psychological aspects of the patient-physician relationship. He apparently realized that in order to gain the confidence of patients, and thus unlimited access to secondary medical resources, the physician must appear neutral and above normal human emotions, uncorrupted by even the most tempting worldly rewards.

One recognizes as well Sun Ssu-miao's sense of belonging to the larger group of medical practitioners when he points out the inappropriateness of abusing physician-colleagues in public. The detrimental effects of such shortsighted behavior, directed toward individual gain, have been recognized by the best minds of the East and West as impeding group professionalization. Thus, from the very beginning of explicit ethics in medicine, elements were incorporated that seem to have little to do with the actual performance of medical treatment and may be regarded as beneficial solely to the medical practitioners.

Finally, Sun Ssu-miao touched on the problem of remuneration. Greed seems to have been one of the gravest complaints raised by the public against practicing physicians. Many statements, promulgated by Confucian interests, expressed this view. If the public were to be convinced that at least the "great physicians" did not intend to cheat their patients, then another system of equitable remuneration had to be elaborated. Sun Ssu-miao referred to a saying of Lao-tzu (604–? B.C.E.), the founder of Taoism, to the effect that good deeds would certainly be rewarded by fellow humans and that evil practices would induce retaliation from the spirits. Thus Sun Ssu-miao approached both the Confucian

ideal of virtue as its own reward in the continuation of one's name or fame in posterity and the Buddhist idea of reward or retaliation through supernatural forces, in either this or a later life (if not in another world).

The history of explicit medical ethics in China in the centuries following Sun Ssu-miao very much resembles a debate among three main groups. These were the free-practicing physicians (including Buddhists, Taoists, and others) in whose interest Sun Ssu-miao had spoken, the orthodox Confucians, and a group within Confucianism consisting of ordinary scholars (and at least part-time medical officials) who practiced medicine as a paid profession.

About 150 years after Sun Ssu-miao had published his ethics, Lu Chih (754–805), a well-known scholar from the top ranks of the Confucian bureaucratic hierarchy, made some statements on medical ethics that might be regarded as a direct answer to Sun Ssu-miao. He elaborated on the idea that medical knowledge, and the ability to practice medicine, must be regarded as open to everyone. The implication is that practitioners who specialized in medicine would become superfluous. Lu Chih also chastised those who practiced medicine for living in a manner characterized by greed and evil, and noted that they did so without suffering any kind of retaliation. This observation put Sun Ssu-miao's system of retribution in question. However, Lu Chih also pointed out that those who had practiced medicine without undue concern for material gain but, rather, as an obvious consequence of their concern for humanity had been rewarded one or two generations later, through the happiness and prosperity enjoyed by their children and grandchildren. Lu Chih closed his remarks with an open critique of Taoist and magical practitioners, among whom Confucian historians counted Sun Ssu-miao.

At the beginning of the thirteenth century a Confucian scholar-physician named Chang Kao published twelve short stories concerning medical ethics. While decrying the non-Confucian practitioners as "common physicians," Chang Kao recognized the need to allay the fears of orthodox Confucians, who were always suspicious of attempts to gain control over specialized resources.

In his stories, entitled "Retribution for Medical Services," Chang Kao conspicuously resorted to Buddhist concepts of reward and retaliation by forces of another world. These stories center on four major dimensions of medical ethics: greed vs. altruism; exploitation of sexual opportunities; conscientiousness in medical practice; and the problem of abortion.

The last is of special interest because other medical authors showed little concern over the practice of abortion. Relevant prescriptions are frequently provided in major collections. During the reign of the Mongol Yuan dynasty (1260–1367) an official decree prohibited unqualified women from performing abortions. Chang Kao's exceptional handling of this problem was certainly based on his adherence to Buddhist principles. The structure of his entire message seems highly psychological. In the first story, Chang Kao extolled the use of primary medical resources as an appropriate way to gain merit by giving assistance to others. In the second story, he recounted an example of very laudable behavior of a Confucian scholar-physician designed to reinforce confidence in that group. The third through the tenth stories portrayed the decay of morals and depicted examples of many "evil" practices (among them abortion) performed by physicians and others who openly practiced for money with the ulterior motive of cheating the patients. All of these characters received their proper punishment through the actions of gods, spirits, or demons. The last two stories again helped to create confidence in the group to which Chang Kao belonged.

About one century later Ko Ch'ien-sun (fl. 1348), a free-practicing physician, made an ethical statement that was somewhat different from others. In contrast to Confucian ethics, which stressed the study of literature, he emphasized the necessity of gathering clinical knowledge at the bedside as a prerequisite of the well-versed practitioner. Ko Ch'ien-sun departed even farther from official medicine in stating that the origin of his miraculously effective prescriptions rested with a supernatural being who had handed them to him and they were not, in fact, derived from concepts and theories of nature underlying Confucian medicine. Ko Ch'ien-sun is mentioned here as only one example of the vast heterogeneity often overlooked in Chinese traditional medicine.

Most interesting in Ko Ch'ien-sun's statements was the emphasis placed on the outcome of his own practice and the paucity of details concerning his treatment procedure. His reversion to outcome evaluation and other such evidence reminds one that ethical statements found in the literature cannot be taken as representative of the medical group as a whole. It must be assumed that they represent the views of a progressive minority, where "progressive" means an intention to increase professional control over the resources available in society.

In 1522, Yü Pien wrote an interesting modification of the orthodox Confucian claim that everyone ought to possess medical knowledge. Speaking for the group of practicing physicians, he stated that not everyone needed to have medical abilities but that those who called on "common physicians" for assistance could not be regarded as showing sufficient filial piety, and added that medical knowledge was imperative for those who wished to assist their relatives. This very cautious, almost paradoxical, statement may be interpreted as an attempt to legitimize free-practicing Confucian physicians and at the same time to discourage the public from

resorting to practitioners outside the Confucian sphere of influence.

New dimensions were incorporated into medical ethics by Kung Hsin, who lived around 1580, and by his son Kung T'ing-hsien (fl. 1625), both of whom had been imperial court physicians. Kung Hsin explicitly rejected patient solicitation, a practice common in China in his time and later. Patient solicitation implies that a particular physician may be better than at least some of his peers. The awareness of differences in standards of performance necessarily leads to public distrust of the group as a whole and, therefore, constitutes an obstacle to further professionalism. Only where the notion predominates that all members of the practitioner group are alike in their standards of performance will there be confidence among potential clientele.

Kung T'ing-hsien, the son, wrote short treatises entitled "Ten Maxims for Physicians" and "Ten Maxims for Patients." In the first of these he underlined the mastery of Confucian knowledge as a prerequisite for medical practice, a point his father had not explicitly mentioned. In his ethical prescriptions for patients, Kung T'ing-hsien demanded that they resort only to "enlightened physicians," willingly take their medicines, start treatment early, avoid sexual intercourse, refrain from belief in heterodox medical resources (i.e., not Confucian-sanctioned), and not worry over medical expenditures. This last point was underscored with the familiar rhetorical question "I ask you what is more valuable to you: your life or your property?"

Ch'en Shih-kung (fl. 1605) also belonged to the free-practicing group of Confucian physicians. He was the first known Chinese physician to suggest that such persons as prostitutes could be treated without risking defamation. Ch'en Shih-kung also offered his colleagues what may be the first investment counsel for physicians when he advised them to invest excess capital in real estate and not to spend money in unethical places like wine houses. His profound sense of belonging to a larger group led Ch'en Shih-kung to urge his peers not only to avoid open criticism of each other but also actively to display benevolent loyalty among themselves despite differences in training and opinion. Finally, he elaborated upon the prohibition of patient solicitation. He counseled that it was inappropriate for physicians to give extravagant presents or costly dinner invitations to other people. His remarks represent a most pragmatic view of medical ethics (Lee, 1943).

The progress in professionalization that becomes evident through the claims made in explicit medical ethics reached its peak at the end of the era of imperial China. Hsü Yen-tso (fl. 1895), the last author to be cited in this regard, followed the trend when he offered advice to both physicians and patients. He held that in order for a practitioner to maintain a proper level of morality, he was obliged to treat anyone who requested help, regardless of social or financial status; to provide conscientious treatments; to show extreme sincerity; and to respond to any call as soon as possible. In a statement regarding the patient-physician relationship he reminded his colleagues that patients await the arrival of the practitioner as if he were a supernatural being, like the Buddha himself. From this perspective it is not surprising that he asked patients to place themselves entirely in the hands of the practitioners. He demanded that patients have no secrets; that they bind themselves permanently to the physician, not only temporarily in case of an emergency; and that they be isolated from their normal social environment during treatment. The last stricture was possibly meant to prevent discussion of the case and the treatment provided, and had the effect of precluding criticism or interference from outsiders. Thus, at the end of the era of Confucianism, control by a specialized group over medical resources had progressed to a stage incompatible with the original Confucian maxims.

PAUL U. UNSCHULD

While all the articles in this section and the other sections of this entry are relevant, see especially the companion article in this subsection: CONTEMPORARY CHINA. *For a further discussion of topics mentioned in this article, see the entries* ALTERNATIVE THERAPIES, *article on* SOCIAL HISTORY; BUDDHISM; CONFUCIANISM; ENVIRONMENT AND RELIGION; EUGENICS; EUGENICS AND RELIGIOUS LAW, *article on* HINDUISM AND BUDDHISM; HEALTH AND DISEASE; INFANTS, *article on* HISTORY OF INFANTICIDE; MEDICINE, ANTHROPOLOGY OF; MEDICINE, SOCIOLOGY OF; PROFESSIONAL–PATIENT RELATIONSHIP; *and* TAOISM. *Other relevant material may be found under the entries* BENEFICENCE; COMPASSION; FAMILY; HEALING; HEALTH-CARE RESOURCES, ALLOCATION OF; LITERATURE; PATERNALISM; *and* VALUE AND VALUATION. *See also the* APPENDIX (CODES, OATHS, AND DIRECTIVES RELATED TO BIOETHICS), SECTION II: ETHICAL DIRECTIVES FOR THE PRACTICE OF MEDICINE, FIVE COMMANDMENTS AND TEN REQUIREMENTS.

Bibliography

HARPER, DONALD. 1990. "The Conception of Illness in Early Chinese Medicine as Documented in Newly Discovered 3rd and 2nd Century B.C. Manuscripts (Part I)." *Sudhoffs Archiv* 74, no. 2:210–235.

LEE, T'AO. 1943. "Medical Ethics in Ancient China." *Bulletin of the History of Medicine* 13:268–277. A partial translation of Li T'ao's original article in Chinese (see below). Most aspects of medical ethics in ancient China that, from a current point of view, might cast a negative light on the practices of Chinese physicians are omitted (but are included in the Chinese original).

NEEDHAM, JOSEPH. 1970a. "China and the Origin of Qualifying Examinations in Medicine." In his *Clerks and Craftsmen in China and the West: Lectures and Addresses in the History of Science and Technology,* pp. 379–395. Cambridge: At the University Press.

———. 1970b. "Medicine and Chinese Culture." In his *Clerks and Craftsmen in China and the West: Lectures and Addresses in the History of Science and Technology,* pp. 263–293. Cambridge: At the University Press.

QIU, REN-ZONG. 1988. "Medicine—The Art of Humaneness: On Ethics of Traditional Chinese Medicine." *Journal of Medicine and Philosophy* 13:277–300.

UNSCHULD, PAUL U. 1979. *Medical Ethics in Imperial China: A Study in Historical Anthropology.* Berkeley: University of California Press. Presents a comprehensive selection of texts on medical ethics from ancient China, written by prominent and less well-known physicians and Confucian thinkers. The period covered ranges from the seventh to the nineteenth century. Original sources for all Chinese citations in this article are in this book.

———. 1985. *Medicine in China. A History of Ideas.* Berkeley: University of California Press.

———. 1986. *Medicine in China. A History of Pharmaceutics.* Berkeley: University of California Press.

WARE, JAMES, ed. and trans. 1966. *Alchemy, Medicine, Religion in the China of A.D. 320: The Nei Pan of Ko Hung (Paopu tzu).* Cambridge, Mass.: MIT Press.

YÜ, YING-SHIH. 1964–1965. "Life and Immortality in the Mind of Han China." *Harvard Journal of Asiatic Studies* 25:80–122.

2. CONTEMPORARY CHINA

Republican period (1912–1949)

In January 1912, after decades of social upheaval and a failed struggle to achieve a constitutional government, the Qing dynasty, which had ruled China since 1644, collapsed and the Republic of China was inaugurated, with Sun Yat-sen (1866–1925) as its first president. Although the Republic was enmeshed in constant political and social turmoil, a strong movement of visionary intellectuals pressed for the modernization of Chinese life in all its aspects. While many reformers called for the wholesale abolition of Chinese culture and customs, others sought to blend Western political forms and scientific technology with what they saw as "the essence of Chinese culture." The Chinese attitude toward medicine during most of the twentieth century has been formed by these conflicts.

Western medicine had achieved recognition, principally among the elite but to some extent in the general population, during the latter decades of the nineteenth and first years of the twentieth centuries, largely due to the influence of Christian missionary physicians and nurses, and the hospitals they maintained. The effectiveness of the Northern Manchuria Plague Prevention Service, organized along Western lines to combat the

1910–1911 epidemic of pneumonic plague in Manchuria, heightened the prestige of Western medicine, particularly in its preventive and public-health aspects. (It was on the occasion of this epidemic that two practices abhorrent to Confucian morality, cremation and autopsy, were permitted by imperial edict.) This service was the first, and the prototype, public-health service in China (Wu, 1959). Peking Union Medical College, founded in 1915 with support from the Rockefeller Foundation, became the center of medical science and education in the Western mode. Although only a tiny segment of China's doctors practiced Western medicine, they attained positions of influence in government, education, and circles of intellectual reform. In 1914, Minister of Education Wang Daxie told a delegation of traditional physicians, "I have decided to abolish Chinese medicine" (Croizier, 1968, p. 69). In the next few decades, eighty-nine Western-style medical schools were established, and thousands of Western-trained students graduated. Although this development was frequently interrupted by wars and civil unrest, the values of modern medicine gradually took root in the Chinese soil, where they grew in uneasy association with traditional values.

The abolition of traditional medicine, however, much desired by reformers and government, was not a simple matter. Three times the Republican central government attempted to abandon traditional medicine and prohibit its practice, but each time it met with strong resistance. In 1913, the central government promulgated regulations that excluded the teaching of traditional medicine from the curriculum. In reaction, some intellectuals insisted that traditional medicine could be made more scientific and even integrated with Western medicine. They also noted that traditional doctors were likely to be the only sources of care for most people for many years to come. In 1929 Yu Yan, a physician and an official of the Ministry of Health, outlined administrative measures to curb and eventually abolish the practice of traditional medicine: traditional doctors were to be reeducated and were not allowed to organize schools or to advertise. Traditional doctors responded by organizing the first national association, the Institute for National Medicine (1931), with the goal of protecting and promoting traditional medicine. Even this group, however, affirmed that traditional medicine must be made more scientific, advocating research on the pharmacological basis of the thousands of drugs used in Chinese medicine.

Nevertheless, during the 1930s almost all Western-trained physicians refused to compromise and adamantly rejected traditional medicine. Westernizing authors, physicians and nonphysicians alike, argued that traditional medicine was unscientific, as different from Western medicine as astrology from astronomy, geomancy from geometry, alchemy from chemistry. Efforts to make traditional medicine more scientific or to ally the philosophical views of traditional medicine to the scientific principles of modern medicine were repudiated as nothing more than another example of the reactionary conservativism that had harnessed Chinese life for centuries. Such proposals were called "ignorant, nonsensical, blind, babbling." In the harsh words of one prominent physician, "Why should modern medicine accept this marriage proposal from such a lazy, stupid wife with bound feet wrapped in yards of smelly bandages?" (Croizier, 1968, p. 107). In 1933, the president of the Executive Department of the central government, Wang Jingwei, declared any discussion of yin yang or the five elements without anatomical dissection scientifically untenable, and the therapeutic efficacy of unanalyzed drugs doubtful. With his support, licensing authority over all physicians, Western or traditional, was located in the modernized Ministry of Health, thus holding traditional practitioners to standards they could hardly meet. Even so, attempts to abolish the practice of traditional medicine failed in the end. In 1949, 65 percent of all physicians practiced traditional medicine. The uneasy relationship between Western and traditional medicine would continue into the era of the People's Republic.

Medical ethics. *Ethics of Medical Practice* (1933), by the Western-trained physician Song Guo-Bin (1893–1956), might be called the first modern book on Chinese medical ethics. The author sought to integrate Western medical ethics with traditional ethics drawn from Confucianism. Ethics is the *tao*—path or way and, by extension, principle or reality—of practicing medicine, and is constituted by the Confucian concepts of humaneness and righteousness. Song defined humaneness as the Western concept of fraternity, and righteousness as what is appropriately done in compliance with humaneness. Physicians should have a spirit of love for people and a zeal to do good. The principle of humaneness requires physicians to treat poor patients at no charge when necessary; the principle of righteousness requires physicians to be competent, not to do harm, not to take advantage of the patient's vulnerability for their own benefit, not to experiment uselessly, and not to practice favoritism. On the moral character of physicians, Song followed his predecessors, emphasizing the right ordering of one's thoughts and feelings and the right ordering of one's world: the physician who is not ordered in body and spirit can hardly order the body and spirit of his patient. The physician should have the virtues of diligence, devotion, warmheartedness, and dignity. The responsibility of the physician to the patient is to treat disease, promote health, and relieve suffering. Song was the first Chinese medical ethicist to argue systematically for the obligation of confidentiality, although he recognized that this obligation is not unconditional. The patient's consent to disclosure, possible harm to others, or the legitimate needs of criminal justice release the physician from confidentiality. Among colleagues, physicians should respect self and others, and should maintain a friendly feeling and a modest attitude. The obligation of the physician to the state and society is prevention of disease and death, applying remedial measures, research on the cause of death, and the support of public charities. Song rejected contraception and abortion as immoral. Although Song's volume was known principally within the academic world, it was acknowledged as the standard statement of ethics for modern Chinese medicine.

In contrast to Song's ethical idealism, the life of the woman physician Yang Chongrui (1891–1956) represents ethics in practice. After graduating from Peking Union Medical College in 1917, she went to the countryside as one of the first Chinese physicians to bring modern medicine to the peasants, in accord with her personal maxim, "Sacrifice in order to benefit the people." She established the first school of midwifery in China and, at the end of her life, was chief of the Bureau of Maternal and Child Health. She is one of the heroines of Chinese medicine and is often cited as the ideal physician.

People's Republic period (1949–)

On October 1, 1949, the People's Republic of China came into being, a "people's democratic dictatorship" based on Marxist principles as interpreted for China by Mao Zedong. This event marked a radical break with Chinese tradition, which, based on Confucianism, had long been in decline and was considered by the new rulers to be incompatible with progress in a revolutionary society. Medicine and health care were to be thoroughly modernized, first on the Soviet model and later in harmony with indigenous practices. Medical ethics was to be reformulated to serve politico-ideological work performed by health-care providers.

The availability of health care to the whole Chinese population was a major goal of the People's Republic, and remarkable successes were achieved, given the resources available. From the beginning, Chairman Mao took a personal interest in policies that would improve personal and public health. Statistics for life expectancy for the population as a whole and for newborns in particular were greatly improved over those of other Third World countries, and approached the statistics of developed countries. Many endemic infectious diseases, such as cholera, smallpox, and plague, as well as many nutritional diseases, were brought under control.

Health care in rural areas. The first national conference on health care was held in August 1950. Policies that would govern health care were announced: they were designed to respond to the needs of workers, peasants, and soldiers; to emphasize prevention; to effect cooperation between Western and traditional medicine. Soon thereafter, the policy of mass movements was added, that is, highly organized and rapid campaigns to eradicate filth and pests and to instill habits of good health and exercise. For the first time in Chinese history, affordable and competent health care became available to millions of laboring people and peasants.

In June 1964, Mao Zedong issued "Instruction on Putting Stress on the Rural Areas in Health Care," in which he criticized the existing health-care system for its elitist and urban orientation. Urban practitioners, even scientific researchers, were sent to the countryside to practice and to train the public-health workers known popularly as "barefoot doctors." The implementation of this instruction did much to promote health care in the rural areas; nevertheless, at the end of the twentieth century, much remains to be done and, indeed, some deterioration has occurred. At the same time, these policies were detrimental to medical education and to scientific advances in medicine and health care.

Traditional and modern medicine. In the early years of the People's Republic, Marxist thought clearly favored modern scientific medicine and labeled traditional medicine as reactionary. Western medicine, however, was viewed as capitalist and imperialist. A realistic assessment of the need for health care made it clear that all available resources, including traditional medicine, had to be engaged in the vast work of bringing care to the masses. Mao Zedong issued "An Instruction on the Work of Traditional Chinese Medicine" (1954) ordering the integration of traditional and Western medicine into a unified new medicine. In research, education, and care, efforts were made to bring these two forms of medicine together. In "united clinics," both sorts of practice were encouraged, Western-trained physicians were required to study traditional techniques, and many large hospitals had sections for Western and for traditional treatment. A document of 1958 stated, "The objective is . . . a new type of doctor, versed in both Chinese and Western medicines, and one who has acquired communist consciousness under the leadership of the Party committees" (Croizier, 1968, p. 185). The ancient practice of acupuncture, for example, was applied to surgical anaesthesia. Reports of this experiment stimulated great interest in acupuncture throughout the world (Risse, 1973).

Official policy now favors the coexistence and competition between traditional Chinese medicine and modern or Western medicine, and the integration of these two into a new medicine (Qiu, 1982). Now the debate focuses on whether traditional medicine should be taught in its pure form, which would make it difficult to attract young people, or whether it should be modernized, leaving an uncertainty about what it would then offer. By 1987, the number of traditional physicians had declined to 279,000, while the number of modern physicians had risen to 1,132,000, 80 percent of all physicians. A 1986 survey showed that only 7 percent of respondents depended exclusively on traditional physicians.

Human experimentation.   Traditional medicine had no place for human experimentation in the modern sense; research came to China with Western medicine. In the 1950s, the government revealed that during the 1930s and 1940s, some foreign and Chinese physicians at Peking Union Medical College had used poor patients as experimental subjects without their informed consent. One such experiment, done by the American physician Richard Lyman in 1936, involved filming drug-induced seizures of healthy rickshaw drivers, who had been paid the equivalent of two U.S. dollars. This film was shown publicly with sensational effect during the "Ideological Transformation" of 1951–1952 and again during the Cultural Revolution. Since that revelation, many health officials and members of the public have been hostile to human experimentation. As a result, some insufficiently developed or inefficacious therapies became widely available without adequate human testing. In the 1950s, for example, during the movement known as "Learning from the Soviet Union," Vladimir Filatov's tissue therapy, in which human or animal tissues were inserted under the skin as a "biogen" for the cure of a great variety of diseases, was widely used with some fatal results. At the same time, some medical researchers used themselves as subjects for herbal medicines or new drugs and died of poisoning. After 1980, the method of clinical pharmacological trials was introduced into China, together with the principle of informed consent. Institutional review boards to provide oversight began to be set up at the request of foreign groups sponsoring research in China, although as of 1993 there is no universal governmental regulation of research.

Medical ethics.   During the early years of the People's Republic, Mao Zedong's writings were required reading for every Chinese. In the field of health care all medical personnel were required to read his essays "In Memory of Dr. Norman Bethune" and "Serve the People," in which Chairman Mao urged the people to cultivate their moral character in terms of the values of life and death. When one died for the people, he argued, it was a worthy death, weightier than Tai Mountain; otherwise, it was lighter than a feather of the wild goose, as Chinese ancient historian Sima Qian put it. Mao held up as an exemplar for health-care workers the Canadian physician Norman Bethune (1888–1939), who dedicated himself to the care of Chinese soldiers and civil-

ians during Japan's war against China (1937–1945), praising him as a virtuous person, selflessly committed to those in need, conscientious in his work, warmhearted toward all people, and continually improving his skills. The essay on Bethune was viewed as an incomparable formulation of medical ethics during the Maoist era.

Contemporary Chinese bioethics can be dated from 1979, when a conference on the philosophy of medicine, sponsored by the Chinese Society for Dialectics of Nature and the China Association of Science and Technology, was held in Guangzhou. Philosophers, physicians, and health administrators who attended this conference focused on two issues in medical ethics: the concept of death and the justifiability of euthanasia, and the delivery of health care without discrimination. The latter problem arose because the Cultural Revolution's emphasis on serving workers, peasants, and soldiers led to discrimination in health-care services against persons labeled "capitalists" and "bourgeois reactionaries," and to deaths of well-known persons as the result of negligence (Cai, 1980).

Until the 1980s, the discussion of medical ethics was confined to academic circles, specialized journals, and conferences on philosophy of medicine. Two journals, *Medicine and Philosophy* and *Chinese Journal of Medical Ethics,* appeared in the early years of the decade. In 1986 and 1987, however, two legal cases, one on active euthanasia and the other on artificial insemination by donor (AID), drew the attention of lawyers, journalists, policymakers, legislators, and the general public. The first two National Conferences on Philosophy of Medicine and Medical Ethics, devoted to social, ethical, and legal issues in euthanasia and in reproductive technology, were held in July and November 1988. The Chinese Society for Medical Ethics was established in 1988 and affiliated with the Chinese Medical Association. During the decade, most medical universities and colleges, as well as nursing schools, instituted required or elective courses on medical ethics. The curriculum includes study of the moral tradition, medicine in society, the patient–physician relationship, euthanasia, genetics, experimentation, reproduction, and health policy. Dozens of books on medical ethics were published, including Zhi-Zeng Du's *An Outline of Medical Ethics* (1985) and Ren-Zong Qiu's *Bioethics* (1987). Teachers of medical ethics, drawn from philosophy and medicine faculties, were trained in doctoral and master's programs and in special workshops.

Death and euthanasia.   During the Cultural Revolution, the concept of brain death was criticized as "bourgeois, capitalist and reactionary," created by "Western doctors . . . to unscrupulously open up a source for organ transplantation" (Jiang et al., 1977, p. 225). In fact, the problem of brain death arose not so much because or organ transplantation, which is not widespread in China, but because respiratory support was increasingly being employed for terminally ill persons. This was considered both futile for the individual and wasteful of health resources. At the 1988 conference on euthanasia, all participants, including physicians, ethicists, and lawyers, endorsed the concept of brain death, following guidelines widely accepted in Western countries, such as the Harvard criteria (Qiu, 1982). As of 1993, however, no administrative or legislative rules legalize the definition of death by brain criteria.

As modern techniques for life support, such as ventilation, dialysis, and artificial nutrition, have become more common, particularly in urban hospitals, the problem of their appropriate ethical use has been noted. Academic discussion of euthanasia has centered on how it might be identified as a special modality of death differentiated from natural death, accidental death, suicide, murder, and manslaughter. Ancient Chinese physicians were aware of the limits of medicine and asserted that when disease attacks the vital organs, it is beyond cure. Passive euthanasia for the terminally ill, long a part of traditional Chinese medicine, has been extended without qualm to the irreversibly comatose, seriously defective newborns, and very-low-birth-weight infants. At the 1988 conference, ethicists argued for the justifiability of euthanasia on the basis of the principles of beneficence, respect for autonomy, and justice. In the resolution passed at the conference, participants endorsed the right of terminally ill persons to choose the way of dying and encouraged the use of living wills. These principles and practices, while borrowed from U.S. bioethics, are compatible with the Confucian concept of "humaneness." Other deeply embedded Chinese attitudes influence thought on this subject. For example, euthanasia for the defective newborn is rendered more acceptable in view of Buddhist beliefs that such an infant must have failed in virtue in a previous life, while Confucian filial piety often causes reluctance to allow one's parents and the elderly to die (Qiu, 1980).

Active euthanasia, however, remains a subject of debate. In 1986, in Hanzhong, Shaanxi Province, two children of a comatose woman suffering from liver cirrhosis asked physicians to end her life by an overdose of morphine, without informing their siblings. The legal case brought against them evoked widespread media discussion. After their conviction on murder charges, they appealed to the Supreme Court, which in 1991 ruled that the defendants were not guilty since the harm to the decedent was minor in view of her inevitable death. Several surveys in 1986 and 1988 showed that the majority of respondents accept passive euthanasia, and even active euthanasia in certain circumstances.

Reproductive technology. Under the influence of the Confucian view of the importance of having a male successor to carry on the ancestors' lineage, infertile couples experience heavy psychological and moral pressure. In a traditional family, the woman is often blamed for the infertility of the couple and stigmatized or abused. Eagerness for offspring is stimulating the development of reproductive technology that replaces the traditional customs of "wife borrowing" and, among the wealthy, concubinage. At the 1988 conference on social, ethical, and legal issues in reproductive technology, artificial insemination by husband (AIH) and by donor (AID) were asserted to be widely practiced among the population. Sperm banks existed in eleven provinces, most of them without procedures to address ethical and legal issues. Except for a few centers in large cities, AID is undertaken without policies relating to the selection of donors and recipients, and the legal status of the child remains unresolved. The clash of traditional values and modern society was manifested in the first legal case involving reproductive technology, in which a Shanghai family refused to accept a baby boy conceived by donor sperm. In some clinics, prenatal sex selection has been practiced. The participants in the 1988 conference argued against it on the grounds that it could worsen the sex imbalance and cause negative social consequences. In the following year, the Ministry of Health prohibited the practice. In vitro fertilization (IVF) is limited to a few centers.

Family planning. In the early years of the People's Republic, China's enormous population and its prospect for continuous growth were recognized as a serious threat to all the social and economic gains expected from the modernization. During the 1950s, limitations on childbirth were encouraged by mass propaganda and contraceptive education. In 1980 the government announced an official policy of "one couple, one child" (the census of 1982 showed China's population had surpassed 1 billion people). This policy has caused thorny ethical problems. Although there is widespread agreement that control of population growth and limitation of reproductive freedom are ethically justifiable in view of China's vast and growing population, argument continues over whether "one couple, one child" is the best policy and over the means employed to implement it. Not only does it conflict with the traditional value that associates more children with better fortune; it also imposes significant hardships on families in rural areas, where labor needs and the care of elderly parents require several children. A 1979 survey by the Chinese Society of Sociology found that a majority of peasants in the villages near cities want two or more children, whereas the majority of respondents in cities are satisfied with one child. The one-child policy is implemented by intensive contraceptive education, by economic incentives and penalties, by sterilization (sometimes compulsory), and by abortion (sometimes coerced). Although population-control programs are officially designed as programs of incentives, education, and persuasion, the line between persuasion and coercion is not always clear, and the efforts of zealous officials in some places have clearly crossed the line. Again, the policy is most burdensome on dwellers in rural areas, where contraceptive services are often inadequate and local officials, under pressure from above, may employ abusive means. In recent years, reports of compulsory sterilization and coerced abortion have convinced certain international agencies and foreign governments to withhold financial support for population-control efforts in China.

Traditionally abortion has not been seen as a serious ethical issue in China. Most Chinese would agree with the ancient sage, Xun Kuang (286–238 B.C.E.), who argued that human life begins at birth; abortion (and contraception) were rarely discussed in pretwentieth-century medical literature, even in treatises on gynecology. Today, however, repeated and late abortions do arouse concern among health-care workers and ethicists. Unmarried women who become pregnant often seek a late abortion. Late abortion puts physicians in a dilemma, since it involves a conflict between obligation to the health of the patient, due to the dangers of late abortion, and obligation to the society to limit births. Finally, the socially imposed limits on reproduction and the desire for male offspring have encouraged some, especially in rural areas, to revive the ancient practice of female infanticide. This practice, long judged immoral by many commentators, such as the great philosopher Han Fei (third century B.C.E.), has always been abetted by the widespread and deep poverty of the peasants, for whom a girl child was a burden rather than a benefit. Condemned as criminal by the Law Protecting Women's Rights passed by the National People's Congress in 1992, this practice remains difficult to detect and to prosecute.

Reform of the health-care system. Since the founding of the People's Republic in 1949, the health-care system of China has consisted of four main components: workers' health care in state-owned factories or institutions; public medical service; free preventive immunization; and rural cooperative medical service. In all but the free preventive service, the costs of care are funded by the government, by employer/cooperative contributions, and by a small registration fee (typically less than the equivalent of ten cents per visit, although the fee can be graduated up to about one dollar if the patient wishes to see a professor in an academic hospital). The self- or privately employed must pay the full cost of their care. These programs have extended health care far more widely than ever before in China's history and have significantly improved the health of the population. Throughout most of China, patients have access to well-organized health services, provided by many levels of professionals at little cost.

Despite such progress, however, programs have faced major problems: the demand for treatment always exceeds the supply; ordinary people often receive less adequate care than officials; and almost all hospitals suffer large deficits, making renovation and replacement of equipment impossible. Since the implementation of a 1980 policy to dismantle the cooperative farms, the rural medical services have deteriorated and, in some poor rural areas, health care is not accessible to villagers. The government's most recent efforts to reform the health-care system involve implementing the contract system that has proven successful in agriculture. In this way, hospitals can supplement their government budget by increasing fees for registration, tests, and drugs, after approval from the local Bureau for Prices. A portion of these increases will be paid by the patient and the remainder by the factories and institutions for which they work. Since 1988, economists, ethicists, health administrators, and officials of the Ministry of Health have argued over whether it is ethically justifiable to consider health care a market commodity.

Professional ethics code. In December 1988, the Ministry of Health promulgated an ethics code for medical personnel that consists of seven articles: (1) rescue the dying and heal the injured, carry out socialist humanitarianism, always keep the patient's interest in mind, treat disease and relieve suffering by every possible means; (2) respect the patient's person and rights, treat patients as equals without discrimination on the basis of nationality, sex, position, social status, and financial situation; (3) serve patients conscientiously and politely, deport oneself in a dignified manner, speak to patients in a refined manner, be amiable, care for patients with compassion, concern, and solicitude; (4) be honest in performing one's duties, conscientiously observe discipline and law, do not serve selfish interests with medicine; (5) maintain confidentiality for patients, saying nothing that would harm the patient or reveal the patient's secrets; (6) deal properly with the relationship between colleagues and coworkers, learning from each other and holding each other in respect; (7) be rigorous and dependable in work, vigorous in spirit and eager to make progress, endeavor to improve professional proficiency, continuously renew knowledge, and increase technical competence.

This is the first code of ethics promulgated in the People's Republic of China, although the Chinese Medical Association had published a very brief seven-article "Doctor's Creed" in 1937 (Wang, 1944). While the new code is quite similar to medical codes around the world, it should be noted that "respect for the patient's person and rights" does not directly translate into the Western concepts of autonomy and informed consent. While it is now much more common to inform patients fully and to allow them to choose the course of therapy, older paternalistic practices, such as refraining from telling patients their diagnosis and depending on families and even work units for decisions about a patient's care, still prevail. In China, "informed consent with the aid of family and community" might more accurately express the ethical standard.

Compulsory sterilization of the mentally retarded.   A regulation for compulsory sterilization of the severely mentally retarded, promulgated in Gansu Province in 1988, specified that mentally retarded persons are to be sterilized when (1) retardation is caused by familial genetic factors, inbreeding, or other congenital factors; (2) the IQ is below 49; and (3) there is behavioral disability in language, memory, orientation, and thinking. Persons who meet these criteria are permitted to marry only after they have been sterilized. Women who meet the criteria and are pregnant must undergo abortion and be sterilized (Lei et al., 1991). Other provinces, following Gansu's lead, drafted similar regulations on compulsory sterilization, while others were more cautious, incorporating sterilization into their comprehensive regulations on family planning. Proponents of such regulation argue that the proportion of mentally retarded persons in the population is too high, that the burden to support them is too heavy, and that the heavy burden has seriously impeded social development and will influence future generations.

At a 1992 national workshop on ethical and legal issues in limiting procreation, participants pointed out that genetic factors play only a minor role in the epidemiology of mental retardation and that data on the incidence, prevalence, and etiology of the mentally retarded population are of variable reliability and subject to widely differing interpretations. Conference participants argued that if the goal is to reduce the mentally retarded population, only those whose mental retardation is known to be caused by genetic factors should be selected for sterilization—a policy requiring an adequate number of medical geneticists to perform genetic tests and identify the causal factors of mental retardation. The effort to reduce the incidence of mental retardation should focus on improving perinatal care and maternal and child care, developing prenatal diagnosis and genetic counseling, preventing inbreeding, and implementing programs of community development. When sterilization is recommended, it should be in the best interest of the retarded person, as a contraceptive measure that reduces personal misfortune; proxy consent should be obtained. Also, it was argued that the relatively high proportion of mentally retarded persons is not a cause of economic underdevelopment, but an effect of it. From the legal perspective, compulsory sterilization infringes upon some civil rights laid down in the Constitution and other Chinese laws, such as the right to inviolability of the person and the right to guardianship for the incompetent. The considerations raised by the 1992 workshop were delivered to the government

and apparently have impeded the expansion of compulsory laws. However, existing laws have not been repealed or revised, and there is no strong public protest against them.

Controlling the spread of sexually transmitted diseases.   As a result of a major health campaign in the early years of the People's Republic, the incidence of sexually transmitted diseases in the Chinese population was drastically reduced through a combination of medical, educational, and social policies (sometimes quite harsh, particularly against prostitutes). After three decades of dormancy, sexually transmitted diseases (STD) began to rise in the 1980s: from 1980 to 1992, some 700,000 cases of STD were reported (the actual number is probably much higher), including about 1,000 persons who have tested positive for infection with human immunodeficiency virus (HIV). Countermeasures have been taken in recent years to check the epidemic of STD, and several laws, ranging from management and surveillance to prohibition of drug trafficking and prostitution, have been enacted. However, programs for controlling STD are inhibited by several factors. One is the revival of an ancient concept in which disease is seen as punishment for misbehavior instead of being caused by a particular microorganism. Sexually transmitted disease is sometimes called "Heaven's punishment for moral deterioration." The Chinese National Expert Committee on acquired immunodeficiency syndrome (AIDS) attempts to counter this view in "An Open Letter to Medical Care Workers," asserting, "The disease is not the punishment to an individual, but a common enemy to the whole of mankind. . . . Every medical-care worker ought to be full of love in the heart, and help our compatriots who are threatened by AIDS with our hands and knowledge" (National Expert Committee, 1990, p. 1). The second factor is discrimination against patients and infringement upon their individual rights. HIV-positive persons have been expelled from their jobs or schools; AIDS patients have been refused admission to hospitals. Many medical workers have expressed reluctance to care for AIDS patients. A Health Department requirement that doctors fill out an STD patient card and send it to the public health office drives patients away from care, sacrificing the opportunity for education and treatment. The third factor is the lack of legitimate and effective policy to change at-risk behavior such as drug use, prostitution, and unsafe sexual behavior. In 1992, some cities set up hot lines to provide counseling and to protect patients' rights to confidentiality and privacy.

Conclusion

Since the new policy of reform and openness initiated at the end of the 1970s, China has been undergoing yet another fundamental change. Marxism faces challenges from internal pressures and from Western ideas and economics. Confucianism is still deeply engraved in the Chinese mind, but Buddhism, Taoism, Islam, and Christianity are experiencing a revival. Tension and conflict are inevitable as diverse and often incompatible values come to the fore at this historical juncture. Many fields, including medicine, face new challenges, and in this environment the field of medical ethics is flourishing as never before in China. As in many other nations, scholars have delved into problems, published articles, initiated courses, and formed organizations devoted to bioethics.

The word "ethics" is now translated into Chinese as *lun li*, two characters signifying "hierarchical human relationships" and "principle" or "pattern." Combined, these two characters designate guidelines for interpersonal relationships. In Chinese thought, ethics, or the guide for interpersonal relationships, blends with the laws that govern the universe. Thus, traditional Chinese philosophy, particularly Confucian, has a predilection for ethics, teaching how to be human within an orderly human community. In the last two centuries, Western influence in ideas and commodities has introduced an individualism not native to Chinese thought. Since the late nineteenth century, Chinese scholars have studied Western science and philosophy, with a particular interest in philosophical pragmatism. Marxist philosophy pays relatively little attention to ethics as such, since ethics is considered to be formulated by political ideology. Despite Western and Marxist influence, traditional Chinese ethics still weighs powerfully in the Chinese mind and in Chinese society.

The current interest in bioethics in China has been stimulated and influenced by American bioethics. Several leaders in Chinese bioethics are familiar with the American literature and participate in international bioethics activities. Also, since Western scientific medicine has long prevailed in China, Western ethical concerns are readily recognized, particularly as medical technologies are diffused. Thus, the principles of American bioethics—beneficence, nonmaleficence, autonomy, and justice—are frequently cited in Chinese discussions. However, these principles are not simply foreign imports: they correspond to significant Chinese values. Beneficence corresponds to the paramount Confucian virtue, *ren*, translated "benevolence" or "humaneness," which traditional Chinese medicine proposed as the primary virtue of the physician. It requires compassion and help for the sick, and the duty to avoid harm, as well as the obligation to care for the poor without charge (Qiu, 1988). Respect for autonomy, while not a traditional virtue in Chinese thought or medicine, which was strongly paternalistic, does correspond to the aspirations for personal freedom and social emancipation that marked the powerful current of modernization, sometimes known as the May 14th Movement, that be-

gan in the early twentieth century and continues to influence Chinese intellectuals (Spence, 1982). While not encouraged in the culture of the People's Republic, personal autonomy plays a real, if limited, part in modern thought about bioethical issues. Finally, justice in health care corresponds to the socialist ideal that a health-care system accessible to all persons, regardless of social class or economic status, is best realized by a centrally controlled, nonentrepreneurial service system (Sidel and Sidel, 1973). This ideal prompted the vast extension of health services in the 1950s and inspires debates over contemporary plans to reorganize those services. Thus, while Chinese bioethics may occasionally speak in terms similar to Western bioethics, its spirit and ideas are properly Chinese: it is a blend of traditional, modern, and socialist Chinese thought, created in the unique conditions of an evolving great nation.

REN-ZONG QIU
ALBERT R. JONSEN

While all the articles in this section and the other sections of this entry are relevant, see especially the companion article in this subsection: PREREPUBLICAN CHINA. *Directly related to this article are the entries* ALTERNATIVE THERAPIES, *and* VIRTUE AND CHARACTER. *For a further discussion of topics mentioned in this article, see the entries* CARE; CONFIDENTIALITY; CONFUCIANISM; DEATH, DEFINITION AND DETERMINATION OF; DEATH AND DYING: EUTHANASIA AND SUSTAINING LIFE; EUGENICS; FERTILITY CONTROL; HEALTH-CARE DELIVERY; MEDICAL CODES AND OATHS; POPULATION POLICIES; PUBLIC HEALTH; REPRODUCTIVE TECHNOLOGIES; *and* RESEARCH, UNETHICAL. *For a discussion of related ideas, see the entries* AUTONOMY; BENEFICENCE; INFORMED CONSENT; *and* PATERNALISM. *Other relevant material may be found under the entries* LICENSING, DISCIPLINE, AND REGULATION IN THE HEALTH PROFESSIONS; MEDICAL EDUCATION; RESEARCH, HUMAN: HISTORICAL ASPECTS; RESEARCH METHODOLOGY; *and* RESEARCH POLICY.

Bibliography

BOWERS, JOHN Z., and PURCELL, ELIZABETH, eds. 1974. *Medicine and Society in China.* New York: Josiah Macy, Jr., Foundation.

CAI, GEN-FA. 1980. "A Preliminary Approach to the Problem of Medical Ethics." *Medicine and Philosophy* 2:44–48.

CHEN, C. C., and BUNGE, FREDERICA M. 1989. *Medicine in Rural China: A Personal Account.* Berkeley: University of California Press.

CROZIER, RALPH C. 1968. *Traditional Chinese Medicine in Modern China: Science, Nationalism and Tensions of Cultural Change.* Cambridge: Harvard University Press.

DU, ZHI-ZHENG. 1985. *An Outline of Medical Ethics.* Nanchang: Jiangxi People's Press.

Fox, Renée C., and Swazey, Judith P. 1982. "Critical Care at Tianjin's First Central Hospital and the Fourth Modernization." *Science* 217, no. 4561:700–705.

———. 1984. "Medical Morality Is Not Bioethics—Medical Ethics in China and the United States." *Perspectives in Biology and Medicine* 27, no. 3:336–360.

Henderson, Gail E., and Cohen, Myron S. 1984. *The Chinese Hospital: A Socialist Work Unit.* New Haven, Conn.: Yale University Press.

Horn, Joshua S. 1969. *"Away with All Pests . . ."*: *An English Surgeon in People's China.* London: Hamlyn.

Jiang, Yu. 1977. "Criticize the Bourgeois Medical View—Grab the Transplantation Organs from Brain Dead Patients." *Exchange of Medical Information* 4:225–228.

Lei, Zhen-Hua; Guo, Ze-Zhong; He, Guan-Xin; Liu, Cai-Hong; and Liu, Yun-Hua. 1990. *Handbook for Family Planning.* Lanzhou: Lanzhou Xinhua Press.

National Expert Committee on AIDS/HIV Prevention and Control (China). 1990. "Open Letter to Chinese Medical Personnel." *Health Newspaper*, Dec. 1, p. 1.

Qiu, Ren-Zong. 1980. "Concept of Death and Euthanasia." *Medicine and Philosophy* 1:77–79.

———. 1982. "Philosophy of Medicine in China (1930–1980)." *Metamedicine* 3, no. 1:35–73.

———. 1987. *Bioethics.* Shanghai: Shanghai Peoples Press.

———. 1988. "Medicine—The Art of Humaneness: On Ethics of Traditional Chinese Medicine." *Journal of Medicine and Philosophy* 13, no. 3:277–299.

———. 1991a. "The Fiduciary Relationship Between Professionals and Clients: A Chinese Perspective." In *Ethics, Trust and the Professions: Philosophical and Cultural Aspects*, pp. 247–259. Edited by Edmund D. Pellegrino, Robert M. Veatch, and John Langan. Washington, D.C.: Georgetown University Press.

———. 1991b. "Morality in Flux: Medical Dilemmas in the People's Republic of China." *Kennedy Institute of Ethics Journal* 1, no. 1:22–27.

Risse, Günter B., ed. 1973. *Modern China and Traditional Chinese Medicine: A Symposium Held at the University of Wisconsin, Madison.* Springfield, Ill.: Charles C. Thomas.

Sidel, Victor W., and Sidel, Ruth. 1973. *Serve the People: Observations on Medicine in the People's Republic of China.* New York: Josiah Macy, Jr., Foundation.

Siven, Nathan. 1988. *Traditional Medicine in Contemporary China: A Partial Translation of Revised Outline of Chinese Medicine (1972): With an Introductory Study on Change in Present Day and Early Medicine.* Ann Arbor: Center for Chinese Studies, University of Michigan.

Song, Guo-Bin. 1933. *Ethics of Medical Practice.* Shanghai: Guoguang Bookstore.

Spence, Jonathan D. 1982. *The Gate of Heavenly Peace: The Chinese and Their Revolution, 1895–1980.* New York: Penguin.

———. 1990. *The Search for Modern China.* New York: W.W. Norton.

Wang, J. 1944. "The New Document of Medical Ethics." *Chinese Medical Journal* 30:39–40.

Wu Lien-Te. 1959. *Plague Fighter: The Autobiography of a Modern Chinese Physician.* Cambridge: W. Heffer & Sons.

Zhou, Yimou, ed. 1983. *Chinese Physicians on Medical Morality.* Changsha: Hunan Press of Science and Technology.

D. JAPAN

1. JAPAN THROUGH THE NINETEENTH CENTURY

The following is a revision of the first-edition articles on (1) the same subject by the same author, and (2) "Traditional Professional Ethics in Japanese Medicine" by Takemi Taro. Portions of the first-edition articles appear in the revised article.

The history of Japanese medical ethics must be seen in the context of the stratified development of Japanese culture. In each of the four layers discussed here, particular attention will be paid to medicine and ethics and the ways they were constituted with respect to changes in law, religion, custom, tradition, and social and political institutions.

Early Japan

The earliest layer of Japanese cultural stratification is the magico-religious universe of the ancient Japanese people, which persisted in subsequent periods (often submerged under later cultural layers and foreign traditions). From archaeological evidence, early mythic narratives, and poetry, we surmise that the ancient Japanese worldview was based on a mythic mode of apprehending the origin and nature of human beings, *kami* (usually translated as "deities"), the world, and the cosmos. This indigenous Japanese religion was later called Shintø or the "way of the *kami*." Early Shintø understood life to be essentially good and beautiful; evil was simply that which was unclean, ill omened, or inferior. Even the term *tsumi* (often translated as "sin") meant defilement or lack of beauty—for example, sickness, disaster, and error, all due to the influence of evil spirits and removable by ablution and lustration. The early Japanese believed that there were numerous *kami* and *mono* ("spirits," especially those of the fox, snake, badger, and other animals), which could possess humans and cause sickness. As a result, people depended on diviners, shamans, healers, and magicians to deal with physical and mental problems, to prevent disasters or sicknesses, and to avoid pollution. For example, early writings refer to medicinal fruits and plants as well as to common practices to avoid pollution, such as avoiding contact with sick people, menstruating women, and death. The early Japanese resorted to herbal infusions, hot-spring baths, frequent bathing, or gargling for prevention and healing. These practices are mentioned in the eighth-century *Kojiki*, a compilation of Japanese mythology, and even in fourth-century Chinese chronicles that describe Japan.

Socially, early Japan was organized by *uji* (a lineage group often translated as "clan"); the Yamato kingdom, an old designation for Japan, which emerged around the third or fourth century, was in effect a confederation of semiautonomous *uji*-groups under the nominal political authority of the chieftain of the leading *uji*, later known as the imperial household.

The Ritsuryō system

In the wake of the political changes on the Asian continent in the sixth and seventh centuries, Japan acquired a second cultural layer, with the heavy influx of Chinese civilization through Sinified Korea, including Confucianism, Taoism, and the Yin-Yang school, as well as law, medicine, philosophy, ethics, and various sciences and technologies and Buddhism. Stimulated by the unification of China, Japanese leaders made a serious attempt to unify Japanese culture and society. The Ritsuryō system—an important and early synthesis of religious, cultural, social, and political ideas—is the concrete embodiment of this second layer of Japanese culture. Its basic principles, especially the doctrine of the mutual interdependence of Shintō-, Confucian-, and Taoist-inspired imperial ideology and Buddhism, survived until the sixteenth century. Thanks to the emerging synthetic cultural matrix, the Japanese learned that it was possible to apprehend a universal structure governing the world of nature and the human body. Especially noteworthy was the popularization of an East Asian tradition of medicine much later called *kampō-i*, or "Chinese-style medicine." As early as 602, a prominent Korean Buddhist monk, Kwalluk, brought to Japan a series of books on diverse subjects, including astronomy, medicine, and magic. From that time on, with active support from the Yamato court, Chinese medicine was spread rapidly throughout Japan by émigré Korean and Chinese physicians, pharmacologists, and Buddhist priests, who utilized their medical knowledge for healing as a part of their religious activities. Many Japanese physicians were especially attracted by the medical theories of the Chinese scholar Sun Ssu-mo (581–682?).

In the main, Chinese medicine combined an emphasis on the prevention and healing of disease with a concern for "ethical behavior," in the belief that the body is not an individual's own possession but a gift from one's parents, and that one's health depends on the harmonious interaction of the negative (*yin*) and the positive (*yang*) principles. Thus it was one's filial duty to maintain one's health by maintaining harmony with the environment, inasmuch as sickness was believed to arise from imbalance at the physiological, psychological, or cosmological level. Chinese medicine also encouraged acupuncture (*hari*), massage (*amma*), moxa treatments (*akyu* or moxibustion, the application of plants as counterirritants, set on key acupuncture points and burned slowly), and herbal medicine. Chinese medicine did not stress anatomical studies and surgery, largely because of the Confucian emphasis on the sacredness of the human body.

Significantly, Buddhist leaders in Japan affirmed that what one learned from the Chinese medical-ethical tradition was in complete harmony with the fundamental Buddhist principle of compassion. In keeping with this principle, when Prince Regent Shōtoku (573–621) built a temple in what is today Osaka, he provided an asylum, a hospital, and a dispensary on the temple grounds. Following his example, pious monarchs and aristocrats sponsored medical and philanthropic works. Buddhism introduced to Japan not only the savior deity Amida (Amitâbha), and the bodhisattva of great compassion, Kannon (Avalokitesvara), but also the Buddha of Healing, Yakushi-nyorai (Bhaisajya-guru). The Chinese-inspired Taihō Code, promulgated in 702, stipulated the establishment of a Ministry of Health, to be staffed by ten physicians, who were massage specialists, herbalists, and magicians. Judging from the records of the imperial storehouse, the Shōsō-in, built in the mid-eighth century in the capital city of Nara, the Yamato court imported a variety of continental herbal medicines. Another subdivision of the government, the On-myō-ryo ("*Yin-Yang* bureau") was staffed by specialists in divination, astrology, and calendar making; its main task was to combine magico-religious features (e.g., geomancy, divination techniques, fortune-telling, and exorcism) and the semiscientific art of observing planetary movements.

During the seventh and eighth centuries the imperial government supported the officially sanctioned Buddhist schools but also strictly controlled the activities of their clerics by enforcing the Sōni-ryo ("law governing monks and nuns"). The government also made a serious effort to (1) discourage the popularity of the unauthorized Buddhist clerics—the rustic shamans, magicians, and healers who came under the nominal influence of Buddhism and wandered from village to village, offering divination, magic and healing; and (2) confine legitimate monks and nuns to monastic quarters, keeping them from exercising black magic and practicing medicine. On both accounts, the government failed miserably. The unauthorized clerics, called *ubasoku*, continued their preaching, philanthropic, magical, and healing activities among the lower strata of society, which were all too often ignored by official Buddhist schools. On the other hand, some of the officially sanctioned Buddhist monks, notably Genbō (d. 746) and Dōkyo (d. 772), were reputed to have miraculous healing and incantational powers, and they wielded great influence in court circles.

During the Heian period (781–1191), two new Buddhist schools, Tendai and Shingon, were introduced from China, bringing with them new forms of magic, incantations, and cosmological speculation, all of which greatly facilitated the blending of indigenous Japanese (Shintō), Chinese, and Buddhist traditions. Similar eclectic tendencies appeared in medicine and ethics, as exemplified by the thirty-volume medical work *Ishimpo*, compiled in 984 by Tanba Yasuyori. This work integrated native Japanese insights into the T'ang Chinese medical framework and coupled this with ethical exhortations. From the Heian period on, the term *kampō-i* ("Chinese-style medicine") was used in Japan to refer to this hybrid system comprising Buddhist, Confucian, *Yin-Yang*, and Japanese beliefs and practices, and covering a wide range of subjects: acupuncture, herbalism, moxibustion, massage, cures for the diseases of various internal organs, nutrition, dermatology, hygiene, pediatrics, obstetrics, and so forth. It was also during the Heian period that the government actively promoted its health service and the training of physicians.

For the most part, however, medical services were monopolized by the upper strata of society. The masses had no recourse except to traditional, indigenous folk or popular practices, for example, moxibustion and massage coupled with talismans and incantations. Ironically, the Heian period also witnessed, among both the elites and the masses, the popularity of native as well as Chinese forms of omen lore, demon lore, directional taboos, and exorcism. In this situation, even though learned Buddhist leaders expounded the lofty themes of the compassionate Buddha Amida, their teaching was easily transformed into a "*nembutsu* [recitation of Amida's holy name] magic" by the peasantry.

During the Kamakura period (1192–1333), the Japanese polity was split between the courtier-based Kyoto court and the samurai-based feudal regime (*bafuku* or shogunate) in Kamakura, not far from present-day Tokyo. Understandably, the Ritsuryō ideology declined, as did the Heian government-inspired health service. In its place a new class of professional physicians emerged who charged fees for their services. The thirteenth century witnessed an unusual heightening of Buddhist spirituality, which added luster to outstanding medical and philanthropic activities by saintly Buddhist monks. One monk, named Ninshō, of the Ritsu school, is credited with having cared for 46,800 patients in his medical relief station in Kamakura, and with having established a leprosy sanatorium in Nara. Among the many dedicated priest-physicians of the Kamakura period, mention must be made of Kajiwara Shozen, the compiler of two important medical works—the *Tan-i-shō*, a fifty-volume work in Chinese, and the *Man-an-pō*, a sixty-volume Japanese work.

During the Muromachi period (1338–1578), a semblance of the feudal regime under the Ashikaga dynasty was maintained even as the social order steadily broke down. Toward the end of this period, three strongmen—Oda Nobunaga (d. 1582), Toyotomi Hideyoshi (d. 1598), and Tokugawa Ieyasu (d. 1616)—terminated the moribund Ritsuryō religious, cultural, social, and political synthesis. During the later Muromachi period, the various schools of Buddhism were unable to exert signif-

icant spiritual influence, the only exception being Zen, which inspired art, culture, and learning, and was instrumental in transmitting the syncretistic Neo-Confucianism of Sung Dynasty China (960–1279), as well as legal, philosophical, and medical classics of the Yüan (1276–1368) and Ming (1368–1644) dynasties. During the Muromachi period a number of Japanese physicians (both secular and clerical) studied in China, and able Chinese physicians migrated to Japan. Warfare among warrior families, especially the devastating Onin War of 1467–1477, promoted interest in surgery. Many prominent surgeons of this period were military men who combined medicine, Zen, and the martial arts.

The Muromachi period is also uniquely important in the history of Japanese medicine because of the coming of European medicine with the arrival of Portuguese traders and Roman Catholic missionaries. In the mid-sixteenth century, Jesuit missionaries established clinics, hospitals, dispensaries, and leprosy sanatoriums in Japan. One of the famous medical missionaries was Luis de Alameida, a successful surgeon-turned-Jesuit. For the most part, the European missionary-physicians admired the high quality of *kampō-ijutsu* (Chinese-style, mostly "internal" medicine) then available in Japan, and they contributed new knowledge and techniques in surgery, which were badly needed in the war-torn nation. After 1560, when the Society of Jesus terminated its medical activities, Japanese physicians who had been trained by European missionary-physicians carried on their work until the feudal regime decided to exterminate all traces of Catholic missionary influence from Japan in the mid-seventeenth century. Although the tradition of Namban (literally, "Southern Barbarian") medicine was short-lived, its scientific approach, coupled with an altruistic spirit and ethical imperative, left a significant imprint on the history of Japanese medicine and medical ethics.

The Tokugawa era

In 1603, Tokugawa Ieyasu, one of the three strongmen mentioned above, inaugurated a shogunate that lasted until 1867, when the last Tokugawa shogun returned the prerogative of ruling the nation to the young Emperor Meiji. A different synthesis of religious, cultural, social, and political elements developed during the Tokugawa period. The Ritsuryō system discussed above tried to subsume two "universalistic" principles—*tao* ("the way"; *michi* in Japanese) of Confucianism and *dharma* ("the law"; *hō* in Japanese) of Buddhism—under the indigenous tradition represented by Shintō and the imperial system. The Tokugawa synthesis of religious, cultural, social, and political elements (the third layer of Japanese stratification) was based on "universalistic" Neo-Confucian principles of immutable natural laws and natural norms implicit in the human social and political order, grounded in the Will of Heaven (*t'ien; ten* in Japanese).

Ironically, it was the Confucian thrust that stimulated the nativist *kokugaku* ("national learning") movement, which in turn fostered the resurgence of Shintō as the guiding principle for restoration of an imperial regime in 1868, inaugurating Japan's "modern period."

From the perspective of medical history, the Tokugawa period was rich in variety, propelling the development of Chinese (classical Confucian and Neo-Confucian) and nativistic Japanese medicine, and the return of Western medical science. During the Tokugawa period, following the regime's policy in favor of Neo-Confucianism, Japanese medicine separated from its Buddhist underpinning and sought a new foundation in Neo-Confucian metaphysics, physics, psychology, and ethics. Under Neo-Confucian influence, *idō* (the "way or ethics of medicine") was summed up in the phrase *i wa jin nari* ("the practice of medicine is a benevolent art"). Significantly, the first systematic treatises on medical ethics written in Japan, the *Ibyo-ryogan* and the *Byoi-mando*, by Takenaka Tsuan, as well as the *Yojo-kun* ("Instruction on Hygiene"), by Kaibara Ekken (d. 1714), were published in the early Tokugawa period. About that time, among the physicians of *kampō-i* ("Chinese style medicine"), a group called *gosei-ha* ("school of later centuries") taught an intricate fusion of medicine and Neo-Confucian philosophy and became quite influential.

One of the most influential works on health care was the *Yojo-kun* ("how to live well"), by the samurai and physician Kaibara Ekken. A Neo-Confucianist scholar, Kaibara wrote widely on various subjects for the edification of people in all walks of life. His lifelong dedication to the cause of health care is summarized thus: "Medicine is the practice of humanitarianism. Its purpose should be to help others with benevolence and love. One must not think of one's own interests but should save and help the people who were created by Heaven and Earth." This represents the view that human beings are created by the union of Heaven and Earth, that is, the parents. Since medicine is an art that can make the difference between life and death, it is a profession of utmost importance. This means that physicians must be culturally and intellectually accomplished. Kaibara urged physicians to be conversant with the best medical books, to think logically and precisely, and to acquire important theories, practicing "lifelong education." He proposed an ideal image of the physician, who excels in qualities of character and scholarship, in contrast to the "inferior physician," who serves his own interests rather than saving others. At the end of his treatise Kaibara lists eight requirements for the physician: (1) to have a high goal in life; (2) to be cautious; (3) to acquire scholarship of broad knowledge; (4) to make the medical profession a full-time pursuit; (5) to be thirsty for new and ever greater knowledge; (6) to be humble; (7) to be clean at all times; and (8) to be magnanimous.

Meanwhile, in the latter part of the seventeenth century two interesting phenomena developed: (1) the emergence of "ancient studies" (*kogaku*) within the Japanese Confucian tradition, which encouraged *kampō-i* ("Chinese-style medicine") physicians to react against the Neo-Confucian orientation and to return to classical Chinese medicine; and (2) the emergence of the Japanese "national learning" school (*kokugaku*), inspired by Confucian *kogaku*.

Clearly, the "ancient studies" school was a reaction among Japanese Confucianists against the regime-sponsored Neo-Confucian orthodoxy that involved advocating a return to ancient Confucian sages. "Ancient studies" precipitated the rise of a school of medicine called *koihō-ha* ("school of ancient medicine") among Japanese *kampō-i* physicians, who advocated a return to ancient (i.e., Han dynasty, 206 B.C.E.–220 C.E.) Chinese medicine and, more specifically, tried to retrieve the medical work of a Han physician, Chan Ching-chung. For example, Chan's book on fevers and their remedies, the *Shokan-ron*, became widely read in Japan.

Paradoxically, the philological-philosophical approaches of *kogaku* inspired some nativists to apply its scholarly method to the study of ancient Japanese classics, thus developing the school of "national learning" (*kokugaku*), which soon grew into an influential movement and eventually joined with other nativists in the anti-Tokugawa and pro-royalist movement. One of the leading theoreticians of this school, Motoori Norinaga (1730–1801), was a physician. We are told that in his youth he studied both Neo-Confucianism and the Neo-Confucian-inspired *gosei-ha* tradition of medicine, but gradually discarded Neo-Confucianism in favor of national learning and repudiated the *gosei-ha* medical orientation, turning to the *koihō-ha* tradition. Other "national learning" scholars, such as Ueda Akinari (1734–1809) and Hirata Atsutane (1776–1843), were also physicians. Hirata attached great importance to mental therapy and excelled in taking his patients' psychosomatic conditions into account.

Western medicine, briefly introduced by the Jesuits, returned to Japan under Dutch influence. In order to exterminate Catholic influence, the Tokugawa feudal regime had proclaimed the policy of national seclusion in 1639, terminating all contacts with Western powers. It had allowed only non-Catholic Holland to maintain a small trading post in Nagasaki. Through this minimal contact, Dutch medical supplies and surgical methods continued to influence the Japanese medical profession. As early as the mid-seventeenth century a Dutch physician, Casper Schambergen, spent nearly a year at Nagasaki, teaching Dutch medicine. His influence greatly enhanced cosmopolitan (Westernized) medicine, especially surgery, then called the *aranda-ryu geka* ("Dutch surgical school"). This school became popular through a translation of the *Tavel Anatomia* (*Kaitai-shinsho*) by Mayeno Ryotaku, Sugita Gempaku, Nakagawa Jun'an, and Katsuragawa Hoshu in 1774. In 1823–1828, Philip Franz von Siebold, a German physician and scientist attached to the Dutch trading post in Nagasaki, was permitted to operate a clinic and an academy that attracted a number of able Japanese medical students. He revisited Japan in 1859–1862. Those Japanese students who studied Dutch learning had been well grounded in Confucian learning, which to them was essential for moral cultivation, whereas Dutch (and later, other Western learning in general) was considered practical learning. Hence the famous motto "Eastern ethics and Western science."

The Meiji synthesis and modern Japan

The once powerful Tokugawa feudal regime was exhausted politically when the last Tokugawa shogun surrendered feudal power in 1867. It was succeeded by the Meiji-era synthesis of religious, cultural, social, and political ideas that survived until the end of World War II in 1945. Unlike the Tokugawa regime, which authenticated its policy and culture in terms of "universalistic" Neo-Confucian principles, the Meiji regime reverted to "particularistic" Shintø and imperial traditions reminiscent of the Ritsuryō synthesis of the seventh century, notwithstanding the Meiji emperor's Charter Oath to the effect that "uncivilized customs of former times shall be abolished" and "knowledge shall be sought throughout the world." (Understandably, the basic contradictions of the Meiji synthesis have haunted modern Japan until our own time.)

In the modern period Japan welcomed Western knowledge and technology, which inspired, among other things, modern Westernized law, philosophy, ethics, and medicine. In medicine, the Japanese government officially adopted the German system of medical education in 1869. In 1873, there were slightly over five hundred Westernized physicians and twenty-three thousand traditional *kampō* doctors (or *kampō-i*). From 1876 on, the government required all physicians to study Westernized medicine, although *kampō* medicine, which never lost its official recognition, continued to flourish throughout the nineteenth century and into the twentieth. In retrospect it becomes evident that from early times to the modern period, through all the cultural layers, Japanese medicine and ethics—nurtured by Sino-Korean culture, Buddhism, and Western influences—never completely lost its ancient, indigenous orientations, including magico-religious beliefs and practices.

JOSEPH MITSUO KITAGAWA

While all the articles in this section and the other sections of this entry are relevant, see especially the companion article in this subsection, CONTEMPORARY JAPAN, *and the* GENERAL SURVEY *and other articles in this section:* INDIA, CHINA, *and* SOUTHEAST ASIAN COUNTRIES. *For a further discussion of topics mentioned in this article, see the entries* ALTERNATIVE THERAPIES; BENEFICENCE; BODY, *article on* CULTURAL AND RELIGIOUS PERSPECTIVES; BUDDHISM; COMPASSION; CONFUCIANISM; ENVIRONMENT AND RELIGION; HEALTH AND DISEASE; MEDICINE, ANTHROPOLOGY OF; MEDICINE, SOCIOLOGY OF; MEDICINE AS A PROFESSION; PROFESSION AND PROFESSIONAL ETHICS; SURGERY; TAOISM; WARFARE, *article on* MEDICINE AND WAR; *and* WOMEN, *article on* HISTORICAL AND CROSS-CULTURAL PERSPECTIVES. *Other relevant material may be found under the entries* DEATH, *article on* EASTERN THOUGHT; ETHICS; HEALING; HEALTH-CARE RESOURCES, ALLOCATION OF; JUSTICE; ROMAN CATHOLICISM; *and* VALUE AND VALUATION.

Bibliography

BARTHOLOMEW, JAMES R. 1989. *The Formation of Science in Japan: Building a Research Tradition.* New Haven, Conn.: Yale University Press.

EBISAWA, ARIMICHI. 1944. *Kirishitan no shakai katsudo oyobi Namban igaku.* Tokyo: Fuzanbō.

GRAF, ÒLAF. 1942. *Kaibara Ekken: Ein Beitrag zur japanischen Geistesgeschichte des 17. Jahrhunderts und zur chinesischen Sungphilosophie.* Leiden, Netherlands: E. J. Brill.

HATTORI, TOSHIRŌ. 1955. *Heian jidai igakushi no kenkyū.* Tokyo: Yoshikawa Kobunkan.

———. 1971. *Muromachi Azuchi Momoyama jidai igakushi no kenkyū.* Tokyo: Yoshikawa Kobunkan.

ISHIDA, ICHIRŌ. 1983. *Kami to Nihon-bunka.* Tokyo: Perikansha.

KAIBARA, EKKEN. 1974. *Yojokun: Japanese Secret of Good Health.* Tokyo: Tokuma Shoten.

LOCK, MARGARET M. 1980. *East Asian Medicine in Urban Japan: Varieties of Medical Experience.* Berkeley: University of California Press.

LOEWE, MICHAEL; BLACKER, CARMEN; and LAMA CHINE RAMA, RINPOCHE, eds. 1981. *Oracles and Divination.* Boulder, Colo.: Shambala.

PHILIPPI, DONALD L., trans. 1959. *Norito: A New Translation of Ancient Japanese Ritual Prayers.* Tokyo: Kougakuin University. Reprinted under the title *Norito: A Translation of Ancient Japanese Ritual Prayers.* Princeton, N.J.: Princeton University Press, 1959.

TUCKER, MARY EVELYN. 1989. *Moral and Spiritual Cultivation in Japanese Neo-Confucianism: The Life and Thought of Kaibara Ekken, 1630–1740.* Albany: State University of New York Press.

UNSCHULD, PAUL U. 1986. *Medicine in China: A History of Pharmaceutics.* Berkeley: University of California Press.

YAMAKAMI, IZUMO. 1981. *Miko no rekishi: Nihon shukyo no botai.* Tokyo: Yuzankaku.

YAMAZAKI, TASUKU. 1953. *Edoki-zen Nihon iji hōsei no kenkyū.* Tokyo: Chugai Igakusha. LL.D. diss., Nihon University, 1950.

2. CONTEMPORARY JAPAN

Dramatic changes in Japanese social, political, and economic life have occurred since the 1860s, due in part to Japan's conscious desire to modernize and to rapid developments worldwide in science and technology. In urbanized post–World War II Japan, the traditional nationalistic ethos of the Japanese people, based on a legally endorsed *kazoku-seido* (family system) as the social fabric of a *kokka* (state, literally, state-family) under the inviolable power of the emperor (Fukutake, 1981), has disappeared almost completely as a political system and faded as a social ideal. Some uniquely Japanese elements remain, however, especially in the realm of human relationships—for example, in the mentality of *amae* (dependency or relatedness), resulting in a typically deferential and obedient response to seniors or those in authority; the striving for harmony (*wa*) with other people; and the socially reinforced mentality of thinking of oneself as a member of a group rather than as an individual (Doi, 1971; Hall and Hall, 1987). This article will discuss the contemporary Japanese approach to various issues and problems of bioethics, in light of the social, cultural, and historical milieu from which it arose. The account of bioethics in contemporary Japan will be chronological, highlighting events in what Rihito Kimura has interpreted as the three stages of development for bioethics in modern Japan.

It is important to note that owing to the character of Japanese society and its distinctive historical understanding of medicine and the role and responsibilities of the physician, it was not until the 1960s that the bioethical and sociolegal concerns about the practice of medicine began to be deliberately reflected in Japanese society, and only during the 1980s that the notions of autonomy and rights in medicine, and of bioethics in general, became gradually influential (Kimura, 1979, 1987). In the long tradition of Japanese medical practice, the Confucian notion of *jin* (benevolence) has been one of the most important ethical elements; medicine itself is known as *jinjyutsu* (the art of *jin*). Physicians, as conduits of *jin*, were required to act with benevolence toward their patients, and were responsible for the welfare of patients in a fiduciary (trust) relationship (Kimura, 1991a). It was obligatory to use medicine, a gift of benevolence, for the good of others even without payment. Physicians fulfilled their responsibility toward their patients and the patients' family members by acting in a paternalistic and authoritative way; the Japanese, nurtured in the Confucian ethos to respect law, order, authority, and social status, acquiesced without murmur to the superior knowledge of the physician.

Traditionally, the mentality of *amae* (which Japanese psychiatrist Takeo Doi has explained as having some analogy to children's feelings of dependence on their parents; Doi, 1971) dictated this response—the patient's relationship to the physician was analogous to that between a child and the parent who acts to do what is best for the child. Rihito Kimura interprets the impact of *amae* in bioethics as a notion of "related-autonomy" or the making of decisions in relationship. This relatedness extends to all living beings and to one's bond with the environment. These notions of *jin* and *amae*, along with that of *wa*, which will be discussed later, form the backdrop for the development of bioethics in modern Japan.

Confucian virtues in a paternalistic medical tradition (1868–1937)

In the early seventeenth century, the Tokugawa Shogunate closed Japan to foreigners. One small Dutch trading post in Nagasaki was tolerated, but, until the end of the Edo era (1840s–1860s), contact with foreigners was prohibited and the influence of Dutch medicine remained very minor, while traditional Japanese and Chinese medicine continued to flourish. However, as the era drew to a close, restrictions were eased and Japanese physicians sought out texts on Western medicine, training themselves in Dutch methodology and practice (*Rangaku*) using texts available through the Dutch trading post and questioning its resident physicians.

To this end, a document by Christoph Wilhelm Hufeland, originally published in Berlin under the title *Enchiridion Medicum* (1836), was translated from German into Dutch by Hermann H. Hageman (1838) and became influential among the Ranpo-I or Dutch School physicians (those trained in Dutch medical techniques). An 1849 translation, *Ikai* (Medical Admonition), by Seikyo Sugita, of Hufeland's chapter on physicians' responsibilities, which asserted that physicians have a duty to take care of all patients regardless of their social or economic status, was widely read and accepted by Japanese physicians (Sugimoto, 1992). A thirty-volume translation of Hufeland's writing completed in 1861 by Kōan Ogata, a great forerunner of Japanese modern medicine, established this thinking more firmly among Japanese physicians. In 1859, a book traditionally known to Japanese physicians as *Ishimpō* (Heart of Medicine), the oldest extant medical encyclopedia in Japan, was reprinted by the Tokugawa government and made more widely available. This popular Ansei-era edition, originally written on thirty scrolls in 982 C.E. by Yasuyori Tamba, stated in its preface that physicians should embody the spirit of *Daiji-Sokuin*—*Daiji*, the great mercy of Buddha, from the Buddhist scripture, and *sokuin*, meaning sympathy or benevolence (also expressed as *jin*), from Confucian teaching.

In 1868, feudal samurai in particular *han* (local provinces), such as Satsuma, Chōshū, Tosa, and Hizen, initiated the restoration of political power to Emperor Meiji after the Tokugawa shogunate's reign of 265 years (1603–1867). The Confucian ethical teaching, dominant among the samurai during the Tokugawa shogunate, was integrated into *Kyoiku Chokugo* (the Educational Edict of the Emperor, 1890) as the basis for moral teaching in the elementary school curriculum; the classes were compulsory. (This edict was not abolished until 1948.) Confucian ethics, as embodied in this edict, attributes great mercy and benevolence to the emperor and affirms the importance of virtues such as loyalty to the emperor as the head of the "state-family," and filial piety and respect for parents. It also emphasizes the importance of brotherhood and sisterhood, obedience to law and maintenance of order, the necessity of education, and devotion to the state (exemplified for men in military service). Grass-roots movements for liberty and civil rights in the political process (*jiyuu-minkin undo*) were increasingly popular but were suppressed by the emperor's proclamation of the Meiji constitution in 1889, which consolidated political power in the hands of the emperor and established the Diet (Parliament) in his name. Modern Japanese medical ethics cannot be isolated from this social and political milieu. The strong paternalistic nature of Japanese medical practice is the natural outcome of Confucian teaching, which calls for respect of the master and for his authority as a source of unquestionable wisdom and truth.

As Japan became more open to the West, the Dutch ceased to be the sole source of Western culture and other nationalities replaced them. The process of modernizing Japan began in the second half of the nineteenth century and continued into the twentieth century, aided by *oyatoi gaikokujin* (foreign advisers) from Western countries, hired by the Japanese government to provide development advice in industry, education, government, finance, science, technology, and medicine. Japan, seeking models for modernization, was drawn to the German approach because of the success and progress of German science and technology, and the similarity of the German authoritarian political system under the Prussian kaiser to its own under the emperor. Official acceptance of Western, particularly German, medicine guided the development of Japanese policy on medical administration and education and set the course for the future (Oshima, 1983).

German physicians left a legacy of authoritarianism in medical education and practice that had far-reaching effects on the majority of the Japanese medical community. This approach, combined with the Confucian self-righteousness in rendering benevolence to the patient, undermined the development of any notion of patients' rights. Research became the supreme interest at many university hospitals, and patients who presented interesting cases were treated as research material. All of these influences can be seen in the *Isei* (seventy-six guidelines for medical administration) drafted by Sensai Nagayo in 1874. Traditional Japanese (*wahou*) and Chinese medicine (*kanpou*) have been out of the mainstream of medical science in Japan since the adoption of *Isei*, although acupuncture and moxibustion (quick, light heat from an ignited powder of medicinal leaves at key points of the body, called *tsubo*) have remained as folk medicine with popular support among the public (Otsuka, 1976).

As capitalism became established in Japan, the serious social and economic inequities exacerbating the health problems (e.g., widespread tuberculosis, malnutrition) of factory workers, miners, farmers, and fishery workers became evident, particularly in the Taisho Era (1912–1926). Even though the socially privileged physicians' group was not eager to address these health issues through social reform, some young physicians and medical students working for the settlement movement, introduced into Japan from England at the turn of the century, provided medical care in the slum areas of big cities such as Tokyo, Osaka, and Kobe in the 1920s. In 1919, the Medical Cooperative Movement (Iryo Seikyo Undo), which sought to establish community medical centers offering equal access, found great support among many Japanese (Seikyo, 1982).

During this period, Japanese medical ethics, guided by the two powerful influences of Confucian teaching and German authoritarianism, was generally understood simply to govern a physician's personal attitude in providing medical service to patients within the traditional model of a paternalistic trust relationship. It is important to note that during this time the eminent Japanese medical historian Yu Fujikawa asserted that physicians were bound by special obligations and responsibilities, and must develop a special ethical consciousness in their daily practice. His advice was not accepted by Japanese medical experts, who were obedient to the military regime during the following war years.

Medical loyalty to state and authority (1938–1968)

Increasing concern about the health of the Japanese population led to the establishment of Kōseishō, the Ministry of Health and Welfare, in 1938. The National Health Act and additional laws protecting factory workers were promulgated during the same year. Many young radical physicians dealing with serious health problems among the population, such as tuberculosis, raised questions of justice and equitable distribution of resources, but concerns associated with the war with China (which began in 1937) now dominated. In reality, one of the government's main purposes in establishing the Kōseishō was to strengthen the health of the nation to wage war. Similarly, the National Eugenic Law (1940), promulgated ostensibly for the health of the people, reflected the government's desire for increased family size and the elimination of genetically transmitted diseases and defects. To achieve the latter goal, it authorized the use of a "eugenic operation"—voluntary or involuntary sterilization of individuals with mental illness or retardation and those thought to be at risk of transmitting genetic diseases or physical deformities to offspring. (Although this law was abolished and replaced by the National Eugenic Protection Law in 1948, sterilization continued under the new law. Between 1955 and 1967, 418,178 women and 13,571 men were sterilized, 407,910 women and 9,608 men involuntarily. Data from the early 1990s show that, although far greater numbers of females than males continue to be sterilized, involuntary sterilization is almost nonexistent. In 1992, for example, 38 males and 5,601 females were sterilized, but only one operation on a female was reported to be nonvoluntary [Statistics and Information Department, 1993].) With the approach of war, the traditionally authoritarian, yet basically well-intentioned, practice of medicine came under the control of a militaristic state regime; this had dreadful repercussions for medicine and medical ethics in modern Japan.

At this point in time, the traditional purview of medical ethics in Japan did not extend to issues of human experimentation. Several horrible and unethical human experiments performed during World War II were uncovered after the war. The similarity of response to state authority exhibited by Japanese physicians and by Nazi physicians has been viewed with dismay. German defendants accused of committing crimes against humanity were put on trial at Nuremberg; and the medical atrocities and experiments there recounted led to the development of the Nuremberg Code in hope of preventing such practices in the future. However, Japanese medical experts serving in Unit 731, officially called the Water Supply and Epidemiological Disease Prevention Corps, who carried out and supervised experiments on Manchurian Chinese captives using bacteriological infections, frostbite, and mustard and poison gases, were not prosecuted by the international military court (Powell, 1980; Williams and Wallace, 1989).

Official classified documents exchanged between the United States and U.S. General Headquarters in Ja-

pan, now available at the U.S. National Archives, show that the U.S. military decided not to bring this case to trial. The interrogation task force of the occupation forces in Japan granted immunity to members of Unit 731, including General Ishii, chief of this corps, on the condition that all related medical records and specimens be handed over to the United States. The matter was regarded as highly important to national security because the United States wanted to prevent transfer of the medical knowledge gained through these experiments to the Communist governments in China and the Soviet Union (U.S. National Archives, 1949). The Soviets held their own military trial at Khabarovsk for members of Unit 731 they had captured. Based on documentation and the testimony of witnesses, the accused were found guilty (Ivanov and Bogach, 1989).

The Kyushu University Medical School vivisection case also serves as an example of unethical experimentation. Eight American bomber pilots were captured in Japan after an air raid on Tokyo in 1945; some of them were sentenced to death by the local unit of the Japanese Imperial Army, but instead were used as objects of medical experimentation. To avoid prosecution by the Yokohama District Military Tribunal, one key person involved in this experimentation committed suicide; full details may never be known (U.S. National Archives, 1949). The case served as the basis for a popular novel by Shūsaku Endō, titled Umi to dokuyaku (1960), in which he dramatically depicted the quandary of a medical scientist tempted by unethical but very interesting experimentation. Endo's novel forced consideration of the meaning and place of ethics and medicine in Japanese society—which, he argued, lacked a standard of absolute value.

Justified by state authority, professional experts in Japan sometimes lose critical consciousness and judgment. The Japanese national character nurtured during the Tokugawa era, and by an authoritarian government since the Meiji Restoration, demands absolute obedience to the state and to authority. As Endo points out in his novel, such pressure often creates serious problems when individuals must make independent, and individual, ethical decisions. As a member of a group—such as a family, corporation, or community—and as a citizen, the individual Japanese tends to follow what other people do. Harmony (wa), or getting along with others, is an important element of the Japanese ethos for maintaining good relationships. To insist on individual opinions is regarded as egoistic and arrogant. Suppressing oneself in order to cope with other people is a daily practice in every aspect of life for the Japanese. This has serious ethical implications, especially in terms of weakening critical consciousness necessary in professional experts. The majority of Japanese medical experts and the lay public are not interested in drawing serious lessons from the horrible wartime human experiments because they reason that such actions are performed only in "abnormal war settings by abnormal people."

Orders from the occupation forces led to large-scale changes in medical and nursing education, as well as in public-health policy and hospital management. An irreversible and radical shift in medical practice from the German orientation, dominant since the Meiji Restoration, to an American orientation occurred during this time. One of the first pieces of legislation implemented after the defeat of Japan was the Eugenic Protection Law of 1948. Unlike the National Eugenic Law (1940) that it abolished and the Japanese Criminal Code (1907), Chapter 29, Article 212-16, which still holds that abortion is illegal, the 1948 law permitted abortion for medical, and later for social and economic, reasons. Under the Japanese Criminal Code, abortion for other reasons remains a prosecutable offense. However, due to vigorous opposition from advocates for the disabled, it did not provide legal justification for the abortion of a genetically defective fetus. The endorsement of this abortion law by the General Headquarters of General Douglas MacArthur aroused adverse reactions from religious bodies in Japan and the United States (Kimura, 1987). MacArthur defended the policy, saying that it had arisen from and was implemented by the Japanese Diet. The law was still in effect in the 1990s.

The way survivors of the atomic bombs dropped at Hiroshima and Nagasaki were treated by the Atomic Bomb Casualty Commission (composed of U.S. medical and genetic experts) is one of the historical sources of the development of Japanese bioethics because of its significance in discussions about the relationship between human beings and science, technology, and research. Individuals suffering from the effects of radiation came seeking treatment, but instead became material for research on radiation and collection of genetic data. This situation raised the serious issue of the researcher's responsibility to obtain fully informed consent for research. At that time, no government regulation or review boards existed to deal with the situation. The implications of this research are only beginning to be studied in Japan.

In 1951, the Japan Medical Association (JMA) issued a statement on physicians' ethics. This action clearly ushered in a new epoch in medical practice in Japan and signaled a return to the prewar state of medical ethics. Article I explicitly reaffirmed the fundamental and central place of the ancient principle of *jin*, the benevolence of Confucian teaching, in medical practice and asserted that physicians, as the elite of society, must embody the spirit of *jin*, always thinking about the welfare of the patient and the benefit of the treatment. Fur-

ther, in cooperation with other professionals, physicians should take the initiative in social reform and, as ethically oriented people, should exercise great self-discipline (JMA, 1951).

In 1968, a series of consultations and presentations by scholars on ethical issues in medicine was held under the direction of Taro Takemi, then president of the JMA, in an attempt to update the 1951 statement. The publication of *Ishi rinri ronshū* (1968) was the outcome of this research, but no new ethical code was issued. During his twenty-five-year tenure, Takemi developed an interdisciplinary study project titled "Raifu saiensu no shimpu," which has focused attention on bioethical issues such as the allocation of medical resources, applications of high-tech medicine, and ethical problems. However, its professional orientation effectively excluded the lay public. Professional autonomy and authoritative decision making that excluded patients continued to be the model.

The Japanese Constitution, which became effective in 1947, guaranteed the right to health care and social security. Article 25 provides that "all people shall have the right to maintain the minimum standards of wholesome and cultural living. In all spheres of life, the State shall use its endeavors for the promotion and extension of social welfare and security, and of public health." The effort to implement national health insurance for all Japanese, originally begun in 1938, was finally realized in 1961. Since then, all Japanese "whoever, whenever, and wherever" they are, have had access to medical treatment for all illnesses. Treatment costs are covered by the government or by government-controlled systems, except 10 percent coinsurance for insurees and 30 percent for their family members.

Medical care for the elderly, once completely free as a result of the Health Care for the Elderly Act of 1973, now requires a payment of about 20 percent of the total fee (through a 1986 cost-containment amendment). Private medical insurance systems, once almost nonexistent, have sprung up to cover the gap between the actual cost of medical treatment and the amount covered by government insurance. Such coverage is particularly needed for chronic diseases, terminal illnesses, and cancer treatments, although a high-cost medical treatment assistance system was introduced in 1973. As of 1993, the assistance system covers all expenses beyond 33,600 yen/month for low-income families and 60,000 yen/month for average-income families.

Even Japan felt the effects of the worldwide trend in the 1960s of questioning established authority. Revolts occurred in many universities as dissatisfied medical students stood up against the traditionally paternalistic and authoritarian medical faculty they felt was exploiting them. Special legislation eased the unrest, but this first and radical challenge of the medical establishment, a very politically powerful group, had permanent ramifications for Japanese society and moved it into a new era.

Communal involvement in medical decision making (1969–1990s)

In the 1960s, numerous social issues competed for attention in Japan. Problems of air and water pollution; concerns about food additives, iatrogenic diseases, the revival of *kanpo* (traditional Chinese medicine), and increased emphasis on health became common concerns. The growing number of older people focused attention on the need for health care for the elderly. At present, Japan is one of the most successful countries in decreasing the birthrate, and life expectancy in 1991 was the longest in the world, eighty-two years for women and seventy-six years for men. Advances in medical technology and health care have raised additional issues for the Japanese medical profession and society in general. This time period has seen increased lay involvement in discussions about medical treatment and a strong desire to establish guidelines to protect the patient.

Organ transplantation.   Progress in organ-transplant technology created a demand to regulate and endorse cornea transplantation. A special law to this effect was enacted in 1958; in 1979 it was combined with a law governing kidney transplantation. Kidney transplantation from live donors is quite common (approximately 73 percent of all kidney transplants; Kimura, 1991b), and there have been approximately 100 cases of segmental liver transplantation from live donors.

The most vigorous public debate on bioethical issues was generated by the first heart transplant in Japan (1968), in which a heart was taken from a drowning victim and transplanted to a patient in heart failure. The patient died after eighty-three days. A surgeon at Sapporo Medical College, Jurō Wada, was accused of mishandling the surgery on both the donor and the recipient, and questions arose about the justification for the transplant and about the criteria used to determine death; but Wada was never formally prosecuted. However, the aftermath of this case gave rise to strong criticism of high-tech medical applications on ethical grounds. Concerns focused on the use of brain-based criteria of death, organ transplantation from brain-dead bodies, and the need to develop ethical guidelines to control the behavior of individual physicians who might seek fame through ill-prepared and drastic use of medical technology supposedly to benefit the patient.

This incident spawned the Patients' Rights Declaration in 1970 (Wada, 1970). This short, spontaneous expression of feelings, stating that the Wada case was a violation of the human rights of the patient and an example of the corruption of medicine and ethics, occurred in the public meeting at which Wada was accused of violating the donor's right to life. Repercussions from the Wada case were so great that almost three decades later, there have been no heart transplants in Japan and the brain-death criteria have not yet been accepted as public policy. However, corneas and kidneys are transplanted from brain-dead bodies—the heart is avoided because its removal clearly will cause the death of the donor.

Criteria for death.   Leading objections to brain-death criteria are the fear that organs will be removed prematurely and that transplants will be performed in unacceptable circumstances (Kimura, 1991b). In Japan, transplantation of vital organs from dead bodies is rare because of a concern about causing the death of the donor. To a limited degree, anencephalic infants have been used as sources for donor organs because they will die anyway, and because it is believed that they do not possess the fundamental consciousness necessary to be a human being. Declaration of death in the cases reported has ostensibly been based on the total cessation of heartbeat. However, the use of organs from anencephalics has stopped, owing to clinical concerns about the condition of the organs from such donors and public concerns about the appropriateness of such practices.

Resistance to hastening death and harvesting organs also comes from the traditional Japanese image of human beings as completely integrated mind–body units, rather than distinct and separate units of mind, body, and spirit. This unit continues after death, so that removing an organ from a cadaver is seen as disturbing this spiritual and corporeal unity, not merely altering the physical body. It also explains why autopsies are abhorred in Japan (Fujita, 1980). According to the Buddhist and Shinto ways of thinking, this unity extends beyond the individual to all living things. To the Japanese, death disturbs the rhythm of all living things and therefore should not be hastened. Also, Confucian teaching places strong emphasis on family relationships and filial piety. There is a strong prohibition on harming one's body, because it is derived from one's parents (Kimura, 1991b).

In addition, in accepting the reality of human mortality, some Buddhists would regard the extension of life by accepting organs from another individual's body as unnatural and unethical, since the procurement of those organs depends on the death of another person. Such an expectation of the death of someone else for the purpose of egoistic extension of life is not acceptable. Also, the totality of life should be supported by the notion of *arayashiki* (*alaya-vijnana*) (the fundamental consciousness within each individual being). This Buddhist notion holds that consciousness is not located solely in the brain; therefore the cessation of any one part or one organ (including the brain) of the individual does not extinguish consciousness, and consequently cannot be regarded as the death of the individual person (Tamaki, 1993; Fujii, 1991). Therefore, the basis for the uneasiness in accepting brain criteria for death and organ transplantation comes from both Confucian and Buddhist thought, which incorporate some ideas from Japanese traditional folk religions and Shintōism.

In 1990 an ad hoc research commission on brain death and organ transplantation was established under the Prime Minister's Office. Chaired by Michio Nagai, former minister of education, science, and culture, the commission made final recommendations in January 1992. The final report endorses brain-based criteria for death (the irreversible cessation of the function of the entire brain) and the permissibility of organ transplantation. However, the document also respects the traditional clinical criteria (absence of heartbeat, circulation, pulse, and respiration) as the basis for declaration of death, and permits the family and individual to choose between the two criteria (Prime Minister's Ad Hoc Committee). The opposing minority opinion, which was part of the document, was signed by four out of eighteen consultants and committee members; thus the decision was not unanimous. Even though public hearings were held in Hokkaidō, Kantō, Kansai, and Kyūshū, the committee meetings were closed to the public and no mechanism existed to ensure incorporation of public input. Almost two years after the final report of the committee, there were yet no organ transplantations from brain-dead cadavers. Draft legislation regarding these issues was presented to the Diet by the Inter-Party Committee in early 1994.

Truth-telling and death education. A complicating factor in obtaining permission for organ transplantation from terminal patients is that Japanese physicians normally withhold information about diagnosis and prognosis from patients, particularly in the case of cancer, and many Japanese hospices and palliative-care units make it a customary rule not to tell patients that they are dying, although there are some exceptions. Several studies examining the patient–physician–nurse relationship have been published, and several more, to examine the Japanese way of telling the truth to the patient, are proposed (JMA, 1990, 1992). Hospice care in Japan was initiated by Christian hospitals in the 1970s. Hospice units based on Buddhist beliefs were established in the 1980s, while the Japanese government began to endorse such palliative care only in 1990. As of December 1993, there were approximately twenty hospice-care systems, including ten palliative-care units, that were officially endorsed by the Ministry of Health and Welfare. There are a number of groups focusing on the study of death and dying. One of them, organized by a leading expert on death education, Alfons Deeken of Sophia University in 1982, has been expanding its network throughout Japan.

Euthanasia. Media coverage has made euthanasia one of the most debated topics in Japanese bioethics. The Japanese Euthanasia Society was established in 1976, and the first international conference on euthanasia was held at Tokyo in the same year. As of August 1993, the society, now called the Japanese Society for Dying with Dignity (JSDD), had a membership of 60,000. The Ninth International Conference of the World Federation of Right to Die Societies was organized by JSDD at Kyōto in 1992. No legally established procedure exists in Japan, but as in many other countries, the use of elevated doses of narcotics to relieve suffering and pain is acceptable even at the risk of hastening death (Murakami, 1979). According to Buddhist thought, the prolongation of life and suffering is not absolutely necessary, and ending the life of a dying, suffering patient might be regarded as a merciful act (Murakami, 1979).

A 1962 precedent-setting decision by the Nagoya High Court, which accepted the idea of euthanasia in principle, involved the case of a son who prepared poisoned milk as a result of his terminally ill father's repeated requests to die; the glass of milk was found by the man's wife, who, not knowing it was poisoned, gave it to her husband. Although the court found this case to involve unacceptable mercy killing, it established six criteria for allowable mercy killing: (1) the patient's condition must be terminal and incurable, with no hope of recovery, and death must be imminent (as determined by modern medical knowledge and technology); (2) the patient's pain must be so severe that no one should be expected to endure it; (3) the purpose of the act must be solely to relieve the patient's suffering; (4) a sincere request and permission are required from competent patients; (5) in general, this act should be performed only by physicians; and (6) only an ethically acceptable method must be used. Since the 1962 decision, no case that has come before the courts has been found to meet the criteria established for acceptable mercy killing, although the case of a doctor accused of the euthanasia of a patient in 1991 was still undecided as of 1994.

Treatment of the mentally ill. The Japanese Mental Health Act was passed in 1950 to prevent private home confinement of the mentally ill in violation of an identified right to be cared for in institutional situations. However, in the 1980s, disclosures of violations of rights of psychiatric patients led to serious questioning of the routine admittance and institutional treatment of the mentally ill. In 1987, an important amendment to this act, which adopted more rigorous procedures for involuntary hospitalization of the mentally disabled and established rehabilitation and treatment centers to protect the rights of patients with mental disabilities, passed after a nationwide campaign in its favor by the mass media and a strong recommendation for its passage by a special investigative mission of the International Commission of Jurists in Geneva. The commission's involvement underscores the importance and necessity of international cooperation on bioethical issues, especially those related to patients' rights.

Education of the public in bioethics.   Bioethical issues raised in the 1960s caught the attention of much of Japanese society, and in the 1970s concerned citizens formed bioethics study groups in Tokyo, Kyōto, and Nagoya. By the 1980s, these groups participated as bioethics volunteers in medical service organizations. The nationwide concern with health and medical services in Japan led to the new declaration of patients' rights (1984) issued by a group of patients, lawyers, physicians, and journalists (Kanjya, 1992). While this document carried no official authorization, it was more systematic than its 1970 precursor and showed the impact of discussions in other countries. The General Assembly of Japanese Medical Cooperatives, an official medical service organization of the Japanese Association of Life Cooperatives Union with 250 hospitals and clinics and a membership of 1.5 million individuals, endorsed its own version of a patients' bill of rights in May 1991—the first such action by a medical organization (Kanjya, 1992). The Patients' Rights Legislation Movement, largely initiated by medical malpractice lawyers and other members of the lay public, began in 1991 to urge passage of a statute on informed consent and respect for patient autonomy in medical decision making.

Ethics committees: Reproductive interventions.   The first medical ethics committee in Japan was established at Tokushima University Medical School in 1982 in order to review in vitro fertilization (IVF) technology and its application to infertile women. In Japan, a great deal of social and familial pressure exists to have children, so there is a great demand for IVF research. Artificial insemination by donor and artificial insemination by husband have been used since the early 1950s. The *Yomiuri* newspaper (April 15, 1993) reported that there were 199 registered clinics (registration is not required), and that the number of children born as a result of IVF seems to be increasing steadily. As of 1992, each of the eighty medical schools finally had its own medical ethics committee reviewing cases such as segmental liver transplantation, gene therapy, and IVF. Owing to a lack of national legislation regarding these committees, each has a different composition, although the majority of members are from the same medical faculty and are male (Kimura, 1989b). In 1991 the Greater Tokyo Metropolitan Government established the first hospital ethics committee with membership of nonmedical practitioners and opened all their meetings to the public. This committee serves as a policymaking body for the fourteen hospitals operated by the Tokyo Metropolitan Government.

Bioethics organizations.   Since the mid-1980s, medical professionals and government organizations have been involved in the study of bioethical issues. In 1984, the Ministry of Health and Welfare set up the Special Advisory Board on Life and Ethics; it published an official report in 1985, after a series of research conferences, then ceased activity. The JMA also set up the interdisciplinary Bioethics Council, consisting of medical experts and professionals from philosophy, anthropology, biochemistry, law, and industry. The council dealt with topics related to technological applications in clinical settings such as IVF (1986), sex selection of the fetus (1987), brain death and organ transplantation (1989), and explanation and informed consent (1990).

The Japanese Association for Bioethics, established in 1987, publishes a journal and a newsletter, and has more than eight hundred members who attend the annual national meeting and international meetings. The Japanese Association for Philosophical and Ethical Research in Medicine, the Japanese Society of Ethics, and the Japanese Society of Medical Law are also concerned with bioethical issues as they affect their respective disciplines. In addition, the members of the Japanese Diet participate in a study group called the Diet Members' Federation of Bioethics. Proceedings of the study meetings, including texts of lectures by guest speakers, and questions and answers relating to issues such as brain death, organ transplantation, anatomical gift of the body, aging, and allocation of medical resources are published and publicly available.

Bioethics education and publications.   In 1987, bioethics became a compulsory course in the Japanese higher education system, at the newly established School of Human Sciences at Waseda University. This course, team-taught by professionals from medicine, biology, and law, covered the beginning and end of life, the quality of life, and environmental problems. Increasing numbers of medical schools include courses in bioethics or medical ethics with their clinical curriculum, although there are very few faculty members who teach only this subject. There are now four research institutions in Japan that focus on bioethics: Kitasato University, Kanagawa; Kyōto Women's University, Kyōto; Waseda University, Tokyo; and the Eubios Ethics Institute, Tsukubu.

Beginning in the early 1980s, several books have influenced the thinking of the Japanese public and biomedical professionals on a range of ethical issues. They include Hisayuki Omodaka's *I no rinri* (1971), based on his teaching experiences at Osaka University's medical school as chair of the "General Introduction to Medicine" as well as full-time professor of philosophy; a book with the same title (1977) by Omadaka's successor, Yonezō Nakagawa, a leading scholar in medical humanities; and Takeshi Kawakami's book *Seimei no tameno kagaku* (1973), which criticized the medical establishment's cooperation with the bureaucratic health-policy planning of the local and central governments, and touched on issues of patients' rights and the ethical tasks in medical service. Clinical physician Shigeaki Hinohara, clinical pharmacologist Shigeichi Sunahara, biochemist Shunichi Yamamoto, bacteriologist and medical historian Yoshio Kawakita, medical law expert Koichi Bai, anatomist Kazumasa Hoshino, and lawyer and bioethicist Rihito Kimura write books and give lectures on bioethics in Japan (Kajikawa, 1989).

Concluding remarks

The contemporary discussion of bioethics in Japan started as a movement among the lay public in the late 1970s. This fact remains symbolic and important in many respects, as evidenced by the increased degree of individual decision making about desired medical treatment, as well as all areas of daily life. Optimistic attitudes toward science and technology enabled Japan to move toward the successful achievement of modernization since the Meiji Restoration. However, the devastating aftermath of the atomic bomb and the focus on economic and technological success after World War II exacted an enormous human toll in terms of pollution, health problems, and *karoushi* (sudden death from overwork). Because of this history, the Japanese people have a negative memory of rapid, uncontrolled, professionally oriented science and technology and its misuse, and quite naturally express a desire to have a more cautious process of social adaptation and application of science and technology. The Japanese public's fear of unwanted and unwarranted medical practices, both before birth and after death, has led to greater control of the medical profession and a serious demand for the information necessary to make informed medical decisions about the beginning and end of life.

Japan continues to struggle to recognize bioethics as integral to all spheres of life and to discuss public policy and the environment, as well as to deal with the tension between Western values and its traditional cultural practices. In Japan, bioethics is increasingly recognized as a suprainterdisciplinary endeavor embracing all traditional academic disciplines in equal partnership, for the valuable exchange of ideas and criticism each field has to offer. In Japan there are specific cultural values and customs that are distinctive and non-Western in pattern, but there is heterogeneity, too, and in any case, ethical values change, particularly among the younger generations. We need to ask: What kind of future do we want to construct? We are and will be seeing a globalization of values. In this age of global community it would be naive to overemphasize the uniqueness of a particular cultural heritage in human, family, and social relations. It is true that different cultural and ethical values should be respected, such as key concepts of the dignity of each human person, the importance of the family unit, and community life. But justification of any act or behavior against human dignity and the rights of the person for the sake of cultural tradition is not acceptable.

It may be that in the international community of the twenty-first century, with a globalization of values focusing on a universally accepted notion of fundamental human rights, the reality of limited resources and the increasing necessity of mutual cooperation, the notion of "related-autonomy" and the Japanese principle of *wa* may find greater voice in bioethics.

RIHITO KIMURA
WITH THE ASSISTANCE OF
LAURA BISHOP

While all the articles in this section and the other sections of this entry are relevant, see especially the companion article in this subsection: JAPAN THROUGH THE NINETEENTH CENTURY. *Directly related to this article are the entries* AUTHORITY; BUDDHISM; CONFUCIANISM; PATERNALISM; *and* TRUST. *For a further discussion of topics mentioned in this article, see the entries* ABORTION; AGING AND THE AGED; BENEFICENCE; BIOETHICS EDUCATION; COMPASSION; DEATH, DEFINITION AND DETERMINATION OF; EUGENICS; HEALTH-CARE DELIVERY; HEALTH-CARE FINANCING; HOSPICE AND END-OF-LIFE CARE; INFORMATION DISCLOSURE; LOVE; MEDICAL CODES AND OATHS; MENTAL HEALTH; MENTAL ILLNESS; NATIONAL SOCIALISM; ORGAN AND TISSUE TRANSPLANTS; PATIENTS' RIGHTS; PROFESSIONAL–PATIENT RELATIONSHIP; PUBLIC HEALTH; REPRODUCTIVE TECHNOLOGIES; RESEARCH, HUMAN: HISTORICAL ASPECTS; RESEARCH, UNETHICAL; RESEARCH ETHICS COMMITTEES; and VIRTUE AND CHARACTER. See also the entry* MEDICAL ETHICS, HISTORY OF, *section on* EUROPE, *subsection on* NINETEENTH CENTURY, *article on* EUROPE; *and subsection on* CONTEMPORARY PERIOD, *article on* GERMAN-SPEAKING COUNTRIES AND SWITZERLAND. *Other relevant material may be found under the entries* COMPASSION; FREEDOM AND COERCION; JUSTICE; *and* RIGHTS.

Bibliography

ASYOA, MASAHIKO. 1993. *Tāminaru kea to Shinto no seishi kan.* Heiwa to Shūkyō.
BAI, KOICHI, ed. 1987. *I no rinri.* Tokyo: Nippon Hyōron Sha.

BOWERS, JOHN Z. 1965. *Medical Education in Japan: From Chinese Medicine to Western Medicine.* New York: Hoeber.

COMMITTEE FOR THE INVESTIGATION OF ISSUES IN ORGAN TRANSPLANTATION. JAPANESE ASSOCIATION OF INDIAN AND BUDDHIST STUDIES. 1990. "Report of the Committee." *Journal of Indian and Buddhist Studies* 39, no. 1:291–301. In Japanese.

DOI, TAKEO. 1971. *Amae no kōzō.* Tokyo: Kobundo. Translated by John Bester under the title *The Anatomy of Dependence.* Tokyo: Kōdansha International, 1973.

ENDO, SHUSAKU. 1960. *Umi to dokuyaku.* Tokyo: Bungei Shunju Sha. Translated by Michael Gallagher under the title *The Sea and Poison.* Tokyo: Charles E. Tuttle, 1973.

FUJII, MASAO. 1991. "Buddhism and Bioethics." In *Theological Developments in Bioethics: 1988–1990,* pp. 61–68. Edited by B. Andrew Lustig. Bioethics Yearbook, vol. 1. Dordrecht, Netherlands: Kluwer.

FUJIKAWA, YU. 1941. *Nippon Igakushi.* Tokyo: Nissin Shoin.

FUJITA, SHINICHI. 1980. *Seito shi no mirai.* Tokyo: Asahi Shimbun-sha.

FUKUTAKE, TADASHI. 1981. *Nihon shakai no kōzō.* Tokyo: University of Tokyo Press. Translated by Ronald P. Dore under the title *The Japanese Social Structure: Its Evolution in the Modern Century.* Tokyo: University of Tokyo Press, 1982.

GOMER, ROBERT; POWELL, JOHN W.; and RÖLING, BERT V. A. 1981. "Japan's Biological Weapons: 1930–1945." *Bulletin of the Atomic Scientists* 37, no. 8:43–53.

HALL, EDWARD T., and HALL, MILDRED R. 1987. *Hidden Differences: Doing Business with the Japanese.* New York: Anchor.

HARDING, T. W. 1985. *Human Rights and Mental Patients in Japan: Report of a Mission.* Geneva: International Commission of Jurists.

HINOHARA, SHIGEAKI. 1981. *Sei no sentaku.* Tokyo: Nippon YMCA Syuppan.

HOSHINO, KAZUMASA. 1992. "Bioethics in Japan: 1989–1991." In *Regional Developments in Bioethics: 1989–1991,* pp. 379–397. Edited by B. Andrew Lustig, Baruch A. Brody, H. Tristram Engelhardt, Jr., and Laurence B. McCullough. Dordrecht, Netherlands: Kluwer.

HUFELAND, CHRISTOPH W. 1836. *Enchiridion Medicum: Der Anleitung zur medizinschen Praxis.* Berlin: Jonas Verlagsbuchhandlung. Original German.

———. 1838. *Enchiridion Medicum: Handleiding tot de geneeskundige praktijk. Erfmaking van eene vijftigjarige ondervinding.* Translated by Hermann H. Hageman. 2d ed. Amsterdam: Santbergen.

———. 1849. *Enchiridion Medicum.* Partially translated by Seikyo Sugita under the title *Ikai.* Tokyo: Suharaya, 1949. Reprinted Tokyo: Shakaishiso Sha, 1972.

IVANOV, N., and POGACH, V. 1989. *Unlawful Weapon: Who Speaks of Bacteriological Warfare.* Khabarovsk: Khabarovsk Publishing House. Translated into Japanese by Keisuke Suzuki and Kuniko Nakanishi under the title *Kyofu no Saikinsen.* Tokyo: Kobunsha Co., Ltd., 1991.

JAPAN MEDICAL ASSOCIATION (JMA). 1951. *Physicians' Ethics.* Tokyo: Author.

———, ed. 1968. *Ishi rinri runshu.* Tokyo: Kanehara Shuppan.

———, ed. 1974. *Raifu Saiensu no Shinpo,* no. 1.

———. 1990. *Setsumei to Dōi.* Tokyo: Author.

———. 1992. *Makki Iryo ni nozomu Ishi no arikata nitsuiteno Hōkoku.* Tokyo: Author.

KAJIKAWA, KIN-ICHIRO. 1989. "Japan: A New Field Emerges." *Hastings Center Report* 19 (spec. suppl., July-August): 29–30.

KAWAKAMI, TAKESHI. 1973. *Seimei no tameno kagaku.* Tokyo: Ohtsuki Shoten.

KAWAKITA, YOSHIO. 1989. *Seimei, Igaku, Shinkō.* Tokyo: Shinchi Shobo.

KIMURA, RIHITO. 1979. "Seimeisosajidai no Shogeki-baioeshikkusu no susume." *Fukuin to Sekai* 34, no. 11:26–32.

———. 1987a. *Inochi o kangaeru: Baioeshikkusu no susume.* Tokyo: Nippon Hyōron Sha.

———. 1987b. "Bioethics as a Prescription for Civic Action: The Japanese Interpretation." *Journal of Medicine and Philosophy* 12, no. 3:267–277.

———. 1989a. "Anencephalic Organ Donation: A Japanese Case." *Journal of Medicine and Philosophy* 14, no. 1: 97–102.

———. 1989b. "Ethics Committees for 'High-Tech' Innovations in Japan." *Journal of Medicine and Philosophy* 14, no. 4:457–464.

———. 1991a. "Fiduciary Relationships and the Medical Profession: A Japanese Point of View." In *Ethics, Trust, and the Professions: Philosophical and Cultural Aspects,* pp. 235–245. Edited by Edmund D. Pellegrino, Robert M. Veatch, and John P. Langan. Washington, D.C.: Georgetown University Press.

———. 1991b. "Japan's Dilemma with the Definition of Death." *Kennedy Institute of Ethics Journal* 1, no. 2: 123–131.

———. 1991c. "Jurisprudence in Genetics." In *Ethical Issues of Molecular Genetics in Psychiatry,* pp. 157–166. Edited by S. Bulyzhenkov, Radim J. Sram, V. Bulyzhenkov, L. Prilipko, and Y. Christen. Berlin: Springer-Verlag.

———. 1993. "Asian Perspectives: Experimentation on Human Subjects in Japan: Bioethical Perspectives in a Cultural Context." In *Ethics and Research on Human Subjects: International Guidelines,* pp. 181–187. Edited by Z. Bankowski and Robert J. Levine. Geneva: Council for International Organizations of Medical Sciences.

LOCK, MARGARET, and HONDE, CHRISTINA. 1990. "Reaching Consensus about Death: Heart Transplantation and Cultural Identity in Japan." In *Social Science Perspectives on Medical Ethics,* pp. 99–119. Edited by George Weisz. Philadelphia: University of Pennsylvania Press.

MINAMI, HIROKO. 1985. "East Meets West: Some Ethical Considerations." *International Journal of Nursing Studies* 22, no. 4:311–318.

MITCHELL, DOUGLAS D. 1976. *Amaeru: The Expression of Reciprocal Dependency Needs in Japanese Politics and Law.* Boulder, Colo.: Westview.

MURAKAMI, KUNIO. 1979. *I no rinri,* pp. 97–106. Tokyo: Nōsan-gyoson Bunka Kyōkai.

NAKAGAWA, YONEZŌ. 1977. *I no rinri.* Tokyo: Tamagawa University Press.

OGATA, KŌAN. 1857–1861. *Fushi keiken ikun.* Tokyo: Author.

Ohkura, Koji, and Kimura, Rihito. 1989. "Ethics and Medical Genetics in Japan." In *Ethics and Human Genetics: A Cross-Cultural Perspective*, pp. 294–316. Edited by Dorothy C. Wertz and John C. Fletcher. Berlin: Springer-Verlag.

Ohnuki-Tierney, Emiko. 1984. *Illness and Culture in Contemporary Japan: An Anthropological View.* New York: Cambridge University Press.

Oki, Taneo, ed. 1993. *The Living Will in the World.* Tokyo: Japan Society for Dying with Dignity.

Omodaka, Hisayuki. 1971. *I no rinri.* Tokyo: Seishin Shobo.

Oshima, Tomoo. 1983. "The Japanese-German System of Medical Education in the Meiji and Taisho Eras (1868–1926)." In *The History of Medical Education: Proceedings of the 6th International Symposium on the Comparative History of Medicine—East and West*, pp. 211–235. Edited by Teizo Ogawa. Tokyo: Saikon.

Otsuka, Yasuo. 1976. "Chinese Traditional Medicine in Japan." In *Asian Medical Systems: A Comparative Study*, pp. 322–340. Edited by Charles M. Leslie. Berkeley: University of California Press.

Powell, John W. 1980. "Japan's Germ Warfare: The U.S. Cover-up of a War Crime." *Bulletin of Concerned Asian Scholars* 12, no. 4:2–17.

Powell, Margaret, and Anesaki, Masahira. 1990. *Health Care in Japan.* New York: Routledge.

Prime Minister's Ad Hoc Research Commission on Brain Death and Organ Transplantation. General Affairs Office. Health Policy Bureau. Ministry of Health and Welfare. Government of Japan. 1992. *Important Issues Relating to Brain Death and Organ Transplantation (Recommendations).* Tokyo: Ministry of Health and Welfare.

Seikyo Iyōbukai. 1982. *Iryo Seikyo no Rekishi to Tokucho.* Tokyo: Iryo Seikyo.

Social Insurance Agency. Government of Japan. 1992. *Outline of Social Insurance in Japan.* Tokyo: Japan International Social Security Association.

Statistics and Information Department. Minister's Secretariat. Ministry of Health and Welfare. Government of Japan. 1993a. *Health and Welfare Statistics in Japan.* Tokyo: Health and Welfare Statistics Association. In English.

———. 1993b. *Heisei 4-nen yusei hogo tokei hokoku.* Tokyo: Kosei Tokei Kyokai.

Sugimoto, Tsutomu. 1992. *Edo ranpol kara no messeiji.* Tokyo: Perikansha.

Sunahara, Shigeichi. 1974. *Rinsho iryo no ronri to rinri.* Tokyo: Tokyo University Press.

Tamaki, Kōshiro. 1993. *Seimei Towa Nanika.* Kyōto: Hozokan.

U.S. National Archives. December 1947–June 1949. *Trial Case No. 394: Volume I, Record of Trial in the Case of United States vs. Kajuro Aihara, et 29.* Record Group 331. Record of General Headquarters, Supreme Commander of the Allied Powers. Box 1331, Folders nos. 3 and 4. Suitland, Md.: Author.

———. 1949. *Interrogation of Certain Japanese by Russian Prosecutor, August 1, 1947,* and *Enclosure: Interrogation of Certain Japanese by Russian Prosecutor—The Problem, May 2, 1947.* Record Group 165. Records of the War Department, General and Special Staffs. Reference SWNCC 351/2/D. Suitland, Md.: Author.

Wada Shizōishoku o Kokuhatsu suru Kai. 1970. *Wada shinzo shoku o kokuhatsusuruigaku no shinpo to byosha no jinken.* Tokyo: Hoken Dojin Sha.

Williams, Peter, and Wallace, David. 1989. *Unit 731: Japan's Secret Biological Warfare in World War II.* New York: Free Press.

Yamamoto, Shunichi. 1992. *Shiseigaku no susume.* Tokyo: Igaku Shoin.

E. SOUTHEAST ASIAN COUNTRIES

Southeast Asia is part of the continent where the major faiths arose; it is still a melting pot of different religious traditions and cultural beliefs, including animism and magic. Despite the rapid social change Southeast Asia has been undergoing, these religious and cultural beliefs remain vital, conditioning people's perceptions, values, attitudes, and behaviors in health and all other areas. An understanding of these beliefs is imperative for the implementation of projects in medicine and public health, and for the maintenance and improvement of public welfare.

This article will first analyze the different types of traditional medicine in Southeast Asian countries, particularly Thailand, the Philippines, Malaysia, and Indonesia, their concepts of health and disease, methods of healing, their practitioners, and their ethics. Second, it will discuss some central biomedical issues in the practice of modern medicine, and the current efforts to teach the new medical ethics at medical schools in these countries. Finally, it will argue as a matter of great urgency the need to promote and strengthen bioethical education and research in Southeast Asia, in order to enable its medical community to cope with the new ethical and moral dilemmas, challenges to its traditional morality and religion.

Magic, religion, and naturalism

Medical systems in Southeast Asian countries may be classified into two types, traditional medicine and modern (scientific) medicine. Traditional medicine in turn can be very broadly grouped into three general types, depending on whether it is dominated by magic, religion, or naturalism. Beliefs concerning health, disease and its treatment, and preventive measures are in accord with the type of traditional medicine practiced. When magic is the focus, disease is believed to be caused by sorcery, and countersorcery and other spells are used as medical remedies. Similarly, when religion predominates, disease is attributed to supernatural forces, which must be appealed to or propitiated. When it is dominated by naturalism, disease is defined in terms of natural processes and the imbalance of elements or opposing forces in the body, and a judicious equilibrium is the basis of medical practice.

These traditional medical systems are often a blend of two or more types. Traditional Chinese medicine in Singapore, for example, is largely secular or naturalistic but includes magico-religious elements. Traditional Thai and Malay medicine is mainly magico-religious but is also permeated by elements of naturalistic medicine.

Healers, shamans, and mediums

Traditional medicine is integrated into a complex of beliefs and values comprising the worldview of Southeast Asian peoples. The magico-religious medicine of Southeast Asian countries is derived from magico-animistic beliefs that suffuse their cultures. In this cultural orientation, healers are shamans and mediums, and healing is effected through sorcery, exorcism, and spirit possession, assisted when necessary by herbal concoctions and massage.

Spirit possession is believed to be a channel by which deities or spirits of a high order (e.g., spirits of monks or saints) use their divine power to heal the sick. Healing includes a diagnosis of illness and the performance of corresponding magical rites. These magical activities are usually conducted within the religious framework of the healer. Thai Buddhist shamans, for example, do not practice on *wan phra*, a Buddhist Sabbath observed at the four phases of the moon, and they make use of recitations from the Pali Buddhist texts. The Malay Muslim shamans add verses from the Qur'an to their healing, while the Taoist shamans in Singapore recite Tao incantations in their practice.

Herbalists, folk medicine doctors, and monks

While the magico-religious medicine of Southeast Asia is tied to its culture, its naturalistic medicine is heir to the Indian ayurvedic medical system and traditional Chinese medicine. In these medical traditions disease is understood as a disturbance of inner equilibrium that can be corrected through the administration of herbal solutions. Thus this form of medicine is designated as naturalistic or herbal, and its practitioners are known as herbalists, ayurvedics, or folk medicine doctors. In Thailand many of these healers are Buddhist monks, who usually combine herbal treatment with religious rituals (e.g., the taking of religious vows and the sprinkling of lustral water) and meditation. Some of these monks have been credited with successful rehabilitation of drug addicts. The use of meditation differentiates traditional Thai medicine from the medicines of other Southeast Asian countries.

Medical ethics in traditional medicine

The preoccupation of traditional medicine with magic, religion, and herbal concoctions is due to its holistic approach to health and health care. The practitioners work on their patients at both the physical level and the psychological/spiritual level. While herbal concoctions are mainly used to cure patients' physical illness, magico-religious rites have a therapeutic effect on their minds. The rites reassure patients of divine blessing and protection, and strengthen their self-confidence.

This traditional method of healing may be especially suitable today for Southeast Asians, who, living in societies with increased urbanization and industrialization, need physical, psychological, and spiritual care to enable them to cope with such change and the strains and stresses of modern life. Modern Western medicine with its advanced knowledge and technology has more effective means of healing, but it divides the patient into organ systems and treats only those parts of the person that are afflicted by a specific disease, rather than the whole person. Southeast Asians, who do not divide the person in such a way but need treatment with scientific medicine, will often seek traditional medicine as a supplement to scientific medicine. For example, a patient with a brain tumor might request magico-religious rites from a Buddhist shaman in order to ensure the success of an operation to be performed by a neurosurgeon. It was reported in the Thai press that the patient who uses this approach experiences such an operation with great calm and recovers more quickly.

Medical ethics in Southeast Asian traditional medicine is not codified but is inherent in the values and practices of its practitioners. Some of these healers are Buddhist monks whose ethic of conduct approximates the Buddhist ideal of showing compassion and loving kindness. For example, they do not charge fees and solicit no gifts for their healing. Other healers may demand fees for their service, but their code of ethics requires that they be under some self-imposed moral restraints, for example, that they not practice for monetary gain; that they serve their patients impartially, with only their benefit in mind; and that they not take cases that they cannot treat successfully. Having no common standard of practice to follow, the healers' success depends on their own virtues and healing powers. Their services are sought as long as they can instill belief and faith. They sink into anonymity when they are seen as charlatans or when doubt about their powers arises.

Modern medicine and health-care allocation

Modern medicine came to Southeast Asia during the colonial period, starting in the eighteenth century. Since then it has made tremendous progress. It has greatly benefited people in Southeast Asia, but beneath the surface of these benefits there is a multitude of attendant ethical problems.

The most important concerns the macroallocation of limited health care resources, specifically, grave inadequacies and inequalities in their distribution. Nearly 80 percent of the population of Southeast Asia lives in rural areas. Most of these people are poor and need more medical services than affluent people. Their health depends mostly on medical services provided by the government through hospitals and public health centers. Yet many of these services are inaccessible to them. In Thailand, for example, 62 percent of doctors and nurses are in Bangkok, where most of the country's hospitals are, while there are too few doctors and nurses in the provinces, where most of the people are. There are also too many hospitals in Bangkok and too few neighborhood clinics and public health centers in rural areas.

Southeast Asian countries, eager to bring the benefits of modern medicine to their people, have modeled patterns of health care and education of health personnel in their countries on those in more affluent and developed nations in the West, particularly Britain and the United States, without regard to social, economic, and cultural differences. As a result, limited health-care resources are allocated to catastrophic or hospital-oriented medicine, despite the fact that most of the diseases afflicting the majority of people in these countries are preventable. Even though it has become increasingly clear that these patterns are irrelevant to the health needs of developing Southeast Asian countries, Western-trained health policymakers are very reluctant to deviate from these models, which are being questioned even in the developed nations where they originated.

Politically pressured to show more concern for the poor, governments in some Southeast Asian countries are now acting to correct some of the imbalance of resource allocation. The present Thai government, for example, though still following Western models, has increased funding for preventive health measures and public health services. More provincial hospitals and health clinics are being built, and paramedics and auxiliaries trained to staff them. Thai medical schools now require medical graduates to spend at least three years in the provinces and rural areas, and a plan is being devised to provide incentive subsidies to doctors and nurses working in poor rural areas. Many more corrective measures are needed to create a just and reasonable allocation of the country's overall health-care resources such that the general standard of health and health care can be raised nationwide.

Shortages of health personnel in Southeast Asia have been aggravated by the fact that so many doctors and nurses are lured from their homelands, where they are in desperately short supply, to serve the less critical health needs of affluent nations. The Filipino Department of Health, for example, reported in 1990 that two hundred towns in the Philippines had no resident doctors and that seven out of ten persons died without even being seen by a physician. Only an estimated 32 percent of all qualified Filipino doctors and nurses practice their profession in their own country. This shortage of doctors and nurses, typical of developing Southeast Asian countries, makes it much more difficult for governments to provide adequate health care to many of their people.

Human experimentation

Another important ethical issue in Southeast Asia concerns human experimentation. Since the adoption of modern medicine in the nineteenth century, medical schools in Southeast Asian countries have become more research oriented and are increasingly moving into the area of human experimentation. In violation of international agreements, Western researchers who have been restricted in the kind of human experiments they may do in their own countries are turning to Southeast Asia to conduct their research where there is less public awareness of the issue and less government regulation. These researchers are usually assisted by Southeast Asian colleagues, who engage in all kinds of human experimentation no longer permitted in the West, including forms of psychosurgery and genetic experiments. Drug testing and tests of new contraceptives have been carried out in Southeast Asian countries on a massive scale. Nearly all of these experiments use poor people as subjects, without their informed consent. Abuse of poor patients and the violation of their human rights in public hospitals often occur.

The governments and the medical communities in Thailand and the Philippines have taken some measures to prevent the exploitation of the poor by researchers. In 1985 the National Research Council of Thailand formulated guidelines for research involving human subjects; these guidelines were later revised and made more elaborate. In 1987 the Philippine Council for Health Research and Development published *National Guidelines for Biomedical Research Involving Human Subjects,* similar to those delineated by the World Medical Association at Helsinki in 1964 and revised at Tokyo in 1975. These guidelines on human experimentation laid special emphasis on voluntary informed consent of research subjects. Unfortunately, both in Thailand and in the Philippines there is as yet little compliance with these guidelines or accountability for their violation.

The creation of national ethics committees and institutional review committees in Thailand and the Philippines is another Southeast Asian response to the issue of human experimentation. These institutional committees are concerned primarily with the evaluation of the scientific value of research proposals; the national ethics committees are expected to deal with the ethical aspects of experiment proposals and their protocols. Both the proper role and the composition of national ethics committees are still being debated. At present such committees are far from being instruments for effective control of experimentation in Southeast Asian countries. The Thai committee, for example, does not scrupulously supervise procedures for gaining the needed informed consent. Nor does the committee intervene when it believes an experiment is being conducted without proper ethical consideration. A 1988 study in Thailand indicated that often the procedures followed in many hospitals made it unlikely that the patients were fully informed or gave genuinely voluntary consent. Though many questions are being raised about it, this national committee could become an effective means to prevent morally questionable experiments on human subjects from being performed.

Traditional morality and new ethical issues

The traditional morality of Southeast Asia is permeated by the ethical traditions of Hinduism, Buddhism, Christianity, and Islam. The emergence of modern medicine has produced many new ethical issues that challenge traditional morality. For example, within this morality is the cardinal Buddhist principle of *adhimsa*, which directs that life not be taken and harm not be done. Modern medicine with its advanced technologies has produced ethical dilemmas concerning how to abide by these precepts. For example, does removal of a life-support system constitute violation of these precepts? Is allowing a seriously defective infant to die untreated a form of "harming" or "killing"? Is it morally acceptable for patients to take their own lives in cases of lingering terminal illness or chronic severe pain or disability? Is it morally acceptable that doctors or nurses act upon the expressed desire of patients and assist them in committing suicide when they are unable to act for themselves or to find the means to do so? Is removal of a kidney from a live donor a morally justified form of harming?

Traditional morality also dictates that we not deceive others. One of the five precepts of Buddhist morality prohibits falsehood. Does this include failing to tell a terminally ill patient the truth about his or her prognosis? Is administering placebos a morally justified exception to the moral rule against deception? Can the patient be deceived about a treatment if the doctor or nurse thinks it is in the patient's best interest? Must all the truth about a double-blind trial in human research be told in order to obtain the "informed consent" that the new medical ethics calls for? These are examples of new questions raised as a result of the encounter between modern medicine and traditional morality in Southeast Asia. Traditional morality is no more prepared to deal with these new moral issues than are the Southeast Asian scientists and physicians caught in the middle of them.

The development of modern medicine has raised questions about the adequacy of traditional morality. For example, the traditional Buddhist concept of death as the cessation of all vital functions cannot accommodate the recent development in modern medicine, in which some cells or organs may be sustained by artificial means after the cessation of all vital functions. Nor does it facilitate early retrieval of organs for transplantation. Southeast Asians must rethink and reinterpret the applications of their traditional morality to cope with the advanced knowledge and technologies of modern medicine. For example, as technologies for behavior control and modification are available through drugs, electrostimulation, electroshock treatments, psychological manipulation, psychosurgery, and genetic engineering, the traditional precept of "do no harm" to an existent being may be stretched to cover the question of whether we have the right to "create" a being of our own design.

Teaching and other bioethical activities

Southeast Asian medical students usually learn about medical ethics in classes, and from time to time through lectures outside of regular classes. They are also encouraged to follow the example of morally respected elder doctors. In the past the teaching of medical ethics at medical schools in Southeast Asian countries was integrated into other courses and was primarily concerned with professional etiquette as developed in the West or culled from the teachings of Buddhism, Hinduism, or Islam.

The new medical ethics, or bioethics, was initiated in Southeast Asian countries as a response of scholars and medical professionals to the impact of modern medicine on the life and well-being of people in their countries. Through the combined efforts of Christian clergy and doctors, the Center for Biomedical Ethics Development was established in Indonesia in 1983, primarily to enhance the development of bioethics and Christian values in medicine. Its present activities include the formulation of hospital ethical codes for Indonesian doctors and nurses, and the promotion of bioethics education at hospitals and universities through lectures, seminars, and regular meetings.

Also in 1983, the Bioethics Study Group, consisting principally of Western-trained philosophers and doctors, was established at Mahidol University, a major education and research university in Thailand, to initiate the teaching of bioethics at the university and to bring the awareness of bioethical issues to the public and concerned authorities. By 1988 three full-credit, separate courses were being taught. Through these courses students are exposed to bioethical issues and the way these issues are being addressed and resolved in the United States and other Western countries. They are also encouraged to engage in ethical reflection on those issues as they arise in Thailand, and to find solutions that reflect Thai cultural values. The group has planned to initiate a graduate program in bioethics in 1993 and has created small teams at six other medical schools to stimulate and promote bioethical activities there.

The Southeast Asian Center of Bioethics was established in the Philippines in 1987 by a group of Catholic priests and doctors as a result of the visit of the International Federation of Catholic Universities in the same year. Since its inception the Center has focused its activities on the promotion of interest in and concern with bioethics through teaching, research, seminars, and monthly meetings to discuss bioethical issues confronted by the scientific and medical community in the Philippines. Thus the value of bioethics is appreciated in Thailand, Indonesia, and the Philippines, but it is less recognized in other countries.

All the work done in bioethics has been based on Western models of health and health-care delivery systems, and on principles derived from the Western moral tradition and specific ethical issues that are relevant to the particularities of Western culture. It is urgent that Southeast Asian academics and medical professionals begin the task of defining and clarifying bioethical issues as they affect their own countries' health and health-care systems, and that they find resolutions in keeping with the moral principles, values, priorities, and social needs of their countries.

PINIT RATANAKUL

While all the articles in this entry are relevant, see especially the GENERAL SURVEY *and other articles in this section, which discuss* INDIA, CHINA, *and* JAPAN. *Directly related to this article are the entries* ISLAM; BUDDHISM; TAOISM; *and* HINDUISM. *For a further discussion of topics mentioned in this article, see the entries* ALTERNATIVE THERAPIES; BIOETHICS EDUCATION; DEATH, *article on* EASTERN THOUGHT; DEATH, ATTITUDES TOWARD; ENVIRONMENT AND RELIGION; ETHICS, *article on* RELIGION AND MORALITY; HEALTH AND DISEASE; HEALTH-CARE RESOURCES, ALLOCATION OF, *article on* MACROALLOCATION; INFORMATION DISCLOSURE; INFORMED CONSENT; MEDICINE, ANTHROPOLOGY OF; MEDICINE, SOCIOLOGY OF; MULTINATIONAL RESEARCH; RESEARCH, HUMAN: HISTORICAL ASPECTS; RESEARCH ETHICS COMMITTEES; RESEARCH POLICY; SOCIAL MEDICINE; *and* WOMEN, *article on* HISTORICAL AND CROSS-CULTURAL PERSPECTIVES. *Other relevant material may be found under the entries* AUTHORITY; AUTONOMY; COMPASSION; HEAL-ING; JUSTICE; PATERNALISM; RIGHTS; TECHNOLOGY; *and* VALUE AND VALUATION.

Bibliography

BRYANT, JOHN. 1969. *Health and the Developing World.* Ithaca, N.Y.: Cornell University Press.

DE CASTRO, LEONARDO D. 1990. "The Philippines: A Public Awakening." *Hastings Center Report* 20, no. 2 (March–April):27–28.

HEINZE, RUTH-INGE. 1988. *Trance and Healing in Southeast Asia Today.* Bangkok: White Lotus.

KLEINMAN, ARTHUR. 1980. *Patients and Healers in the Context of Culture: An Exploration of the Borderland Between Anthropology, Medicine and Psychiatry.* Berkeley: University of California Press.

LESLIE, CHARLES, ed. 1976. *Asian Medical Systems: A Comparative Study.* Berkeley: University of California Press.

MITCHELL, DAVID, ed. 1982. *Indonesian Medical Traditions: Bringing Together the Old and the New.* Clayton, Victoria: Monash University.

PHILIPPINE COUNCIL FOR HEALTH RESEARCH AND DEVELOPMENT. 1985. *National Guidelines for Biomedical Research Involving Human Subjects.* Manila: Author.

RATANAKUL, PINIT. 1988. "Bioethics in Thailand: The Struggle for Buddhist Solutions." *Journal of Medicine and Philosophy* 13, no. 3:301–312.

———. 1990. "Thailand: Refining Cultural Values." *Hastings Center Report* 20, no. 2:25–27.

TUMBIAH, S. J. 1973. "Form and Meaning of Magical Acts: A Point of View." In *Modes of Thought: Essays on Thinking in Western and Non-Western Societies,* pp. 199–229. Edited by Robin Horton and Ruth Finnegan. London: Faber and Faber.

IV. EUROPE

A. ANCIENT AND MEDIEVAL

1. GREECE AND ROME

Ancient Greece and Rome are often treated together by scholars who seek to describe in a limited space any aspect of those two civilizations. Greek history is typically divided into the Mycenaean period (2000–1200 B.C.E.), the "dark age" (1200–750 B.C.E.), the archaic period (750–500 B.C.E.), the classical age (500–323 B.C.E.), and the Hellenistic period (323–30 B.C.E.); and Roman history into three phases: monarchy (753–509 B.C.E.), Republic (509–31 B.C.E.), and Empire (31 B.C.E.–476 C.E.). During the archaic period the Greeks engaged in considerable colonization in the Near East and throughout the Mediterranean basin, including southern Italy. The Hellenistic period, which was immediately preceded by Alexander the Great's conquest of much of the Near East, was marked by a fusion of Greek and various Near Eastern civilizations. Roman culture was influenced by the Greeks of southern Italy and, to a much greater degree, by the various Hellenized peoples whom the Romans conquered during the last two centuries of the Republic. The culture of the first three centuries of the Empire is appropriately labeled Graeco-Roman. During the last two centuries of the Empire, a gradual division between the Latin West and the Greek East culminated in the emergence of the European Middle Ages in the former and the Byzantine era in the latter.

The ancient medical profession

Although some herbal medicine and primitive surgery were employed by Greeks as early as the time represented in the Homeric epics (before 750 B.C.E.), the understanding and treatment of disease were predominantly magico-religious. It was not until the late sixth or early fifth century B.C.E. that Greek philosophy provided a rational/speculative theoretical framework for understanding health and disease, and hence for the emergence of what may be called a medical profession. The development of such a framework for the practice of medicine marks the origin of the expectation that physicians are above all products of a scientific training and orientation; that is, that they deal with disease and other physical ailments both empirically and rationally, not magically, mystically, or superstitiously (Amundsen and Ferngren, 1983). Desacralized medicine was an important aspect of Greek culture that spread throughout the Mediterranean world during the Hellenistic period and was adopted and adapted by the Romans during the late Republic.

There were no institutions that granted medical degrees or certification, nor was there a licensure requirement at any time or place. All who wished could call themselves physicians and practice medicine. Nevertheless, from the fifth century B.C.E. until the end of the period under consideration, the prevailing picture is of a population that typically distinguished between physicians (*iatroi* in Greek, *medici* in Latin) and those who practiced a magico-religious healing.

The Hippocratic oath. Professional standards enforceable by sanctions against physicians did not exist. Those who chose to call themselves physicians and undertake the practice of medicine were not required to swear any oath or to accept and abide by any formal or informal code of ethics. Several medical oaths, however, are known from classical antiquity. The most famous is the Hippocratic oath, though no scholar today believes it was written by the historically elusive "father of medicine." Even the date of the oath's composition is unknown; some scholars place it as early as the sixth century B.C.E. and others as late as the first century C.E. Apparently it did not evoke much attention before the Christian era; the first known reference to it was made by the physician Scribonius Largus in the first century C.E.

Some of the stipulations in the oath are not consonant either with ethical precepts prevalent elsewhere in the Hippocratic Corpus and other classical literature or with medical practice as revealed in the sources. Attempts have been made either to explain away these inconsistencies or to attribute the oath to an author or school whose views were, in other respects as well, discordant with those characteristic of classical society. Most influential has been Ludwig Edelstein's theory (1967) that the oath was a product of the Pythagorean school, whose tenets included belief in reincarnation, the practice of vegetarianism and sexual purity, and a condemnation of abortion, suicide, and the shedding of blood. Although his thesis has appealed to many scholars, few now accept it (Deichgräber, 1955; Kudlien, 1970; Lichtenthaeler, 1984; Nutton, 1993). Parallels for even the most esoteric injunctions in the oath can be found outside Pythagoreanism. Furthermore, the Greek text offers many variant readings, some of which can be translated in significantly different ways.

The ideal physician. One constant emerges from the variegated history of ancient medical ethics. When a Greek spoke of *iatroi* or a Roman of *medici*, each was using a word charged with meaning. Unless modified by a pejorative adjective, both meant compassionate, objective, unselfish persons, dedicated to their responsibilities. By the fifth century B.C.E. *iatros* was thus employed in a simile and metaphor; the good ruler, legislator, or statesman was frequently referred to as the physician of the state, and philosophers often described themselves as physicians of the soul. Such usage was carried over to the Latin *medicus*. The popular ideal of the physician was a dedicated, unselfish, and compassionate preserver or restorer of health—and, sometimes, inflicter of health-giving pain—always committed to the good of the patient, regardless of how far short of this ideal many physicians undoubtedly fell.

Beginning in the fifth century B.C.E., a body of medical literature developed that describes the ethics of Greek physicians. These books dealt with eminently practical concerns suggested by medical practitioners for their own benefit, such as issues of the physician–patient relationship, and obligations to the arts, to humanity, and to life itself.

General etiquette and deportment

Greek physicians' formulation of a standard of general etiquette and deportment provided the basis for a social expectation that has remained since that time: physicians are guided by certain basic standards of deportment or professional etiquette in dealing with patients (Amundsen and Ferngren, 1983). The physician should look healthy and be of suitable weight, "for the common crowd considers those who are not of excellent bodily condition to be unable to take care of others" (*The Physician* 1; in the Hippocratic Corpus). This is of particular significance, especially for classical Greek culture, in which health was considered by many both a virtue and an indicator of virtue. Health, the highest good, was set above beauty, wealth, and inner nobility. Health was a goal in itself, for without health, nothing else had value.

Especially in dealings with their patients, physicians should be cheerful and serene, but neither harsh nor silly. They should be reserved, speak decisively and briefly, exercise self-control, and not be excitable. Ostentation was regarded with particular distaste. Further, "It is disgraceful in any art and especially in medicine, to make a parade of much trouble, display, and talk, and then to do no good" (*On Joints* 44; in the Hippocratic Corpus). Physicians were urged to refrain from holding lectures for the purpose of drawing a crowd. Conducting one's practice with much fuss, although it might appeal to the vulgar crowd, smacked of charlatanism. Charlatans avoided consultations; good physicians, recognizing their own limitations and respecting their colleagues' knowledge, turned to other competent physicians for advice. Since consultations could lead to disputes, "Physicians who meet in consultation must never quarrel or jeer at one another" (*Precepts* 8; in the Hippocratic Corpus).

The physician–patient relationship

Physicians' relationships with their patients usually commenced with an examination followed by a prognosis. Then the physician was faced with two or three ethical decisions: (1) whether to take the case if it appeared to be dangerous or hopeless; (2) what to tell the patient; and (3) what treatment to pursue.

Informing the patient. When determining what to tell their patients, two considerations impinged upon physicians: (1) the effect of their statement on the patient and (2) the effect of these cases on their own reputation. There was considerable reluctance to take hopeless or doubtful cases. Some physicians, if they considered their cases hopeless, merely informed the patients that they were going to die, and left them. A treatise in the Hippocratic Corpus, probably written in the second century B.C.E., advises physicians to "conceal most things from the patient while you are attending to him . . . revealing nothing of the patient's future or present condition. For many patients through this cause have taken a turn for the worse" (*Decorum* 16). If the case was dangerous and the outcome uncertain but not hopeless, it was sometimes suggested that the patient's relatives or some other third party be informed,

or that the patient should be told and advised to make a will. Sextus Empiricus, a physician and philosopher of the second century C.E., argued that "The physician who says something false regarding the cure of his patient, and promises to give him something but does not give it, is not lying though he says something false," since in saying it he has regard to the cure of the person he is treating (*Against the Logicians* 1, 43). The great diversity of advice and examples in both medical and other literature shows that opinions on this delicate question varied considerably then, just as they do now.

Choice of treatment. The question of what treatment to pursue posed an ethical problem for some ancient physicians. Therapeutics were placed in three categories: the mildest, dietetics; next, drug therapy; and the most drastic, cutting or cauterizing. Those who abided by the Hippocratic oath swore not to "cut for stone," which some scholars interpret as a rejection of all operative surgery. Especially in the last century B.C.E. and the first century C.E., different medical sects vigorously debated whether drug therapy was unethical and whether milder therapeutics were preferable. But some, like Scribonius Largus, argued that it was even more unethical to refuse to employ drugs responsibly when their benefit to patients was so obvious (Hamilton, 1986).

The patient's cooperation. The cooperation of patients was, of course, recognized as important (*Aphorisms*; in the Hippocratic Corpus), for if they did not obey their physicians' instructions, their condition might worsen or they might die, in which case their physicians would be blamed (*The Art*; *Decorum*; both in the Hippocratic Corpus). A brilliant prognosis, including a description of what course their illnesses had already taken, might so impress the patients that they would be inclined to obey their physicians (*Prognostics*; in the Hippocratic Corpus). Persuasion might be used; a passage in the *Laws* of Plato advances the idea that good physicians will reason with their patients and persuade them to follow the treatments prescribed (cf. *The Statesman*). Galen remarks on the importance of convincing patients that remarkable benefit will ensue if their physicians' orders are obeyed. But it is the patients' respect and admiration for their physicians that are most desirable. Since faith in one's physician could render treatment more efficacious, Galen, for example, maintained that patients should admire their physician like a god.

Confidentiality. Should physicians treat as confidential any information they acquired in their contact with patients? In the Hippocratic oath, the following injunction appears: "What I may see or hear in the course of the treatment or even outside of the treatment in regard to the life of men, which on no account one must spread abroad, I will keep to myself, holding such things shameful to be spoken about." Edelstein sees in this stipulation a clear indication of Pythagorean purity, an insistence on secrecy "not as a precaution but as a duty" (1967, p. 37). Those things that one ought not spread abroad, whether encountered within or outside of practice, are categorized as "shameful to be spoken about," or in another translation, "holy secrets." Elsewhere in the Hippocratic Corpus the physician is advised to "say only what is necessary. For . . . gossip may cause criticism of his treatment" (*Decorum* 7). In another treatise in the Hippocratic Corpus, the physician is urged "not only to be silent but also of a great regularity of life, since thereby his reputation will be greatly enhanced" (*The Physician* 1). While the stipulation to refrain from speaking too much may be motivated by a sense of duty to keep inviolable especially those private things physicians encounter in practice, the other two quotations belong in the context of a self-interested regard for reputation rather than a concern for the supposed "rights" of patients.

Sexual propriety. A very practical stipulation in the Hippocratic oath reads, "Whatever house I may visit, I will come for the benefit of the sick, remaining free of all intentional injustice, of all mischief, and in particular of sexual relations with both female and male persons, be they free or slaves." Edelstein (1967) stresses again the Pythagorean tone of this injunction, especially the emphasis on justice, and sees in the prohibition of sexual relations with members of the patient's household evidence of Pythagorean severity in sexual morality. Whether this advice was motivated by ideals of purity or by merely pragmatic concerns, physicians who used their close contact with patients or their households to satisfy their sexual passions would earn not only disrespect and contempt but also distrust. Having a reputation as a seducer of patients and their family members simply did nothing to enhance one's medical career (see also *The Physician*).

Duty to the art, society, and life

Love of humanity. Sometimes ancient medical literature addresses very fundamental questions of motivations for practicing medicine, physicians' role in society, and the obligations incumbent upon them in that role. One statement in the Hippocratic Corpus—"Where there is love of humanity [*philanthropia*] there is also love of the art [*philotechnia*]" (*Precepts* 6)—has often been taken to demonstrate that for Greek physicians, love of humanity and love of the art were the foundational motivations for their practicing medicine. Sir William Osler saw in it the Greek physician's "love of humanity associated with the love of his craft—*philanthropia* and *philotechnia*—the joy of working joined in each one to a true love of his brother" (Edelstein, 1967,

pp. 319f.). The precept in question, however, may not be so lofty. Vivian Nutton, for example, sees it as simply a pragmatic assertion that physicians' showing love for humanity will foster in their patients a love for the medical art (Nutton, 1993). In any event, it is evident that for many physicians, love of one's honor, glory, and reputation provided a greater motivation than *philanthropia* (Amundsen and Ferngren, 1982).

The statement quoted from the *Precepts* in the preceding paragraph occurs in the context of a discussion about fees that is introduced by the admonition "I urge you not to be too unkind." The noun *apanthropia*, the antonym of *philanthropia*, is here translated by the adjective "unkind." In the Hippocratic Corpus *philanthropia* generally is little more than kindness and compassion. Owsei Temkin, however, emphasizes that one must take care not to trivialize their philanthropy (1991), which one may easily do by contrasting it with the nearly religious flavor that philanthropy took on during subsequent eras. A profound change occurred in late Hellenistic and Roman thought, which, affected by the influence of humanitarian and cosmopolitan ideas on both philosophical and popular ethics, began to see *philanthropia* (Latin, *humanitas*) as humane and civilized feeling toward humanity in general; that is, the principle of the common humanity of all people as expressed by the Stoic philosopher Sarapion around 100 C.E. in a poem titled "On the Ethical Duties of the Physician": "Like a savior god, let [the physician] make himself the equal of slaves and of paupers, of the rich and of rulers of men, and to all let him minister like a brother; for we are all children of the same blood" (Oliver, 1949, p. 246).

This sentiment is strongly present in Galen (second century C.E.), for whom the best physician was also a philosopher, motivated by *philanthropia* (Brain, 1977). Galen, however, conceded that many physicians were motivated not by *philanthropia* but by the pursuit of money or love of glory (Temkin, 1973). Although a few sources, such as Scribonius Largus, held that to be truly a physician, one must be motivated by *philanthropia* (Hamilton, 1986), a majority of our sources concur with Plato that the motivation to practice any art, including medicine, has little or nothing to do with the integrity of the art itself: the practitioner must only be competent (*Republic*). Nevertheless, while few physicians or laymen may have regarded *philanthropia* as essential for the physician, most people probably regarded lack of kindness and compassion as distinctly undesirable for a physician. Ample evidence suggests that the "presence of compassion among doctors was taken for granted by authors of the first century" and that, even much earlier, physicians "could think of compassion as rooted in medical ethics" (Temkin, 1991, pp. 33, 34).

Fees.   Ancient medical writers expressed much concern about fees. Physicians were acutely aware that the appearance of greed could have a detrimental effect on their reputations. Hence, in the Hippocratic Corpus physicians are urged to be more concerned with their reputation than with financial reward, sometimes to give their "services for nothing, calling to mind a previous kindness or [their] present reputation," and to avoid beginning a case by discussing fees, since it could adversely affect patients, particularly those whose condition was acute (*Precepts* 6). Physicians were admonished to consider their patients' economic situation in setting fees and to provide less expensive remedies for the poor than for the rich (*On Diet*). In spite of such sentiments, physicians do not appear to have engaged in much charitable activity from a sense of duty to humanity, to the community, or to the poor (Hands, 1968). Furthermore, the subject of medical fees in antiquity is complicated because some physicians objected to being considered "hirelings" and, especially during the Empire, some insisted that medicine was a liberal art, which entangled their remuneration with the complexities of Roman laws governing honoraria (Kudlien, 1976; Temkin, 1979).

Experimentation.   Ancient physicians strove to improve their proficiency and the efficacy of their art. The most extreme example of medical experimentation was vivisection of human subjects, a very controversial subject (Ferngren, 1982). Celsus states that Herophilus and Erasistratus in Ptolemaic Alexandria performed vivisections on condemned criminals supplied by the crown. Whether or not Celsus's statement is accurate is debated (Von Staden, 1989; Scarborough, 1976), but he presents the arguments for and against the value of vivisection, concluding that "to lay open the bodies of men while still alive is as cruel as it is superfluous . . . [since] actual practice will demonstrate [what can only be learned from the living] in the course of treating the wounded in a somewhat slower yet much gentler way" (pr. 74f.). There is ample evidence for the vivisection of animals either to gain new knowledge or to test new theories (Galen, *On Anatomical Procedures*).

Some physicians recognized that without attempting new procedures and remedies, medical knowledge and techniques would not advance (Michler, 1968). The author of *On Joints* in the Hippocratic Corpus, after describing the failure of a novel attempt at reducing a dislocation, writes, "I relate this for a purpose: Those things which after a trial show themselves to have failed and which show why they failed, also provide good instruction" (*On Joints* 47). The author of the same treatise urges physicians to study incurable cases. Commenting on the Hippocratic maxim "Experiment is perilous" (which can also be translated "Experience is unreliable"), Galen cautions that "In the human body,

to try out what has not been tested is not without peril in case a bad experiment leads to the destruction of the whole organism" (Temkin, 1991, p. 60). Further, he asserts that in several instances he had refrained from testing some remedies when he had others whose effects he knew better, and he points out that rash experimentation presents a danger to the life of the patient (Ferngren, 1985).

Some physicians may have been deterred from experimenting on patients by a fear of being brought to court. Complaints can be found in classical sources that only the physician can commit homicide with complete impunity, but there were some very limited means for seeking redress against the negligent or incompetent physician, at least in Athenian and Roman law (Amundsen, 1973; 1977). But most physicians were probably deterred from any compelling desire to experiment primarily by concern for their reputations rather than by fear of litigation. Classical literature provides numerous examples of the worry expressed by laymen that physicians experiment at their patients' risk (Ferngren, 1982; 1985).

Sharing new techniques.   When new knowledge and techniques were discovered or developed, physicians were faced with the question of whether they should share this information with their colleagues—their competitors—and with the public at large. The Hippocratic oath appears to have been composed for an exclusive sect. In it physicians swear not to impart their knowledge to those outside their sect. Similar sentiments are expressed elsewhere in the Hippocratic Corpus: "Things . . . that are holy are revealed only to men who are holy. The profane may not learn them until they have been initiated into the mysteries of the science" (*The Law* 5).

Apart from a few such statements, a desire to share new techniques or knowledge with other physicians pervades the medical literature. Those who published their medical knowledge and experience obviously did not desire to keep them secret. Galen was motivated in part by the wish to help physicians after him. But many physicians undoubtedly guarded their special techniques with jealousy. Galen shows no surprise at a surgeon's intentionally concealing his operative procedures from view, but expresses disappointment that even some of his own pupils would not share their anatomical knowledge with others (*On Anatomical Procedures*). His "philanthropy is not only that of the physician, but more comprehensively that of a philosopher who subjectively delights in study and objectively labors for the good of mankind. He thinks of his work as belonging to posterity . . ." (Temkin, 1973, p. 50). Some physicians wrote to instruct other physicians and also to edify laymen. In their desire to share medical knowledge with contemporaries and with posterity, at least a few Greek and Roman physicians achieved the most enduring manifestation of their *philanthropia* and *philotechnia* (Temkin, 1949).

Respect for life

How did physicians view their responsibility to nature and, more specifically, to life? Or, to put it differently, how might they have interpreted and applied the maxim frequently quoted in the Hippocratic Corpus, "to help or at least to do no harm" (*Epidemics* 1.11)? Did the Greek or Roman physician feel bound by any sense of "respect for life"?

Abortion.   The Hippocratic oath enjoins that the physician "will not give a pessary to a woman to cause abortion" (Jones's translation [1924]; Edelstein's [1967] "I will not give to a woman an abortive remedy" appears broader in scope than the Greek). Here again we encounter a situation in the oath that runs counter to the realities of ancient medical practice. Many physicians did perform abortions, and various techniques are described in the medical literature (Carrick, 1985). Both Plato (*Republic*) and Aristotle (*Politics*) encouraged abortion as a means of population control and for eugenics. Objections to abortion were relatively rare before the beginning of the Christian era; in both Greek and Roman law, abortion was a criminal offense only if performed without the consent of the woman's husband (or father, if she was not married). By the first century c.e., some pagan physicians such as Scribonius Largus (Hamilton, 1986), influenced as much by an increasing humanitarianism as by the Hippocratic oath per se, refused to perform abortions under any circumstances. The physician Soranus of Ephesus (late first/early second century c.e.) gives three reasons for which a woman seeks an abortion: to rid herself of the consequence of adultery, to maintain her beauty, and to preserve her health. Only for the last would he perform an abortion (*Gynaecia*). Soranus was highly critical of physicians who so strictly adhered to the injunction in the oath that they refused to perform an abortion even to save the life of the mother. It appears, then, that some physicians would perform abortions on request, some refused to do so for any reason, and others assumed a position on therapeutic abortion consonant with that of Soranus. The decision to perform or not to perform an abortion ultimately rested on the convictions of the individual physician. The opposition to abortion of the author of the Hippocratic oath and such physicians as Scribonius Largus and Soranus was based less upon an idea of the inherent value or sanctity of life than on an abhorrence of physicians' using their art in actively terminating even fetal life.

Defective newborns.   While some voices were raised against exposure of healthy newborns, the morality of killing weak, sickly, or deformed newborns appears not to have been questioned by either nonmedical or medical authors (Amundsen, 1987). Soranus, who condemned any but therapeutic abortion, not only raised no objection to rejecting a defective newborn; he also provided criteria to be used by midwives in determining which newborns were worth rearing (*Gynaecia*).

Prolonging life and passive euthanasia.   *The Art*, a treatise in the Hippocratic Corpus, defines medicine as having three roles: doing away with the sufferings of the sick, lessening the violence of their diseases, and refusing to treat those overwhelmed by their diseases, realizing that in such cases medicine was powerless. The decision whether to take on a possibly incurable case was entirely the individual physician's. Some cases in the therapeutic treatises in the Hippocratic Corpus are introduced with the advice that certain procedures should be followed *if* the physician chooses to attempt treatment (Amundsen, 1978). Ancient medical literature is divided on the question of whether physicians should withdraw from cases once it becomes clear that they will not be able to help. Some urged that physicians ought not to withdraw, even if by so doing they might avoid blame. Others felt that they should withdraw if they had a respectable excuse, particularly if continuing treatment might hasten the patient's death.

Physicians did, however, sometimes attend cases considered incurable. In the Hippocratic Corpus many diseases that then generally ended in death are described with no mention of prognosis and with no recommendation to the physician that such cases be undertaken or rejected. For most of them, medications to be employed are named. It was recognized that it was necessary to deal with incurable conditions in order to learn how to prevent curable states from advancing to incurability, particularly in the case of wounds (Michler, 1968). Opinions varied on the physician's responsibility to undertake treatment of hopeless or dangerous cases. In recent times it has become almost dogma to assert that the Hippocratic physician would not take on hopeless cases, but this is demonstrably false (Von Staden, 1990). Nevertheless, some laymen in antiquity held that, as Cicero wrote to his friend Atticus, "Hippocrates too forbids employing medicine in hopeless [cases]" (Temkin, 1991, p. 139).

Celsus, a medical compiler of the first century c.e., appears to represent the mainstream of medical thought: "For it is the part of a prudent man first not to touch a case he cannot save, and not to risk the appearance of having killed one whose lot is but to die; next when there is grave fear without, however, absolute despair, to point out to the patient's relatives that hope is surrounded by difficulty, for then if the art is overcome by the malady, he may not seem to have been ignorant or mistaken" (*De Medicina* 5.26.1.c). Available evidence suggests that physicians who prolonged or attempted to prolong the life of patients who could not ultimately recover their health were generally viewed as acting unethically (Amundsen, 1978).

Assisted suicide or active euthanasia. Would the ancient physician have thought it helping or harming to agree to assist those who for any reason wished to end their lives? To this question a majority of ancient physicians would probably have replied, "Helping, or at least not harming." The right of a free person to control his or her life as each saw fit—if not always in its living, at least in its termination—was a generally accepted view (Cooper, 1989). Suicide was, under most circumstances, outside the moral interest of the law; the exception was whether the suicide of one accused of a crime should be construed as an admission of guilt (Hooff, 1990). If a person who wished to commit suicide enlisted the aid of a second party, the latter was not legally culpable for rendering such assistance. Extralegal sources contain few objections to suicide in general, fewer still to the suicide of the hopelessly ill (Gourevitch, 1969; Hooff, 1990). Assisting in suicide was a relatively common practice for Greek and Roman physicians, and condemnations of the practice were infrequent.

One such condemnation appears in the Hippocratic oath: "I will neither give a deadly drug to anybody, not even if asked for it, nor will I make a suggestion to this effect" (following Kudlien's translation, 1970, p. 118, n.47). This statement immediately precedes the prohibition of abortion. Both prohibitions have at least this much in common: They are inconsistent with the values expressed by the majority of sources and atypical of the realities of ancient medical practice as revealed in most medical and lay literature. Some physicians, however, may have preferred not to assist a suicide, for it could prove to be a messy business, at least from a legal point of view. Under Greek and Roman law, physicians could be charged with poisoning their patients. Indeed, physicians were sometimes charged with, or at least frequently suspected of, doing so (Kudlien, 1970; Nutton, 1985). Some physicians refused to aid anyonoe in committing suicide; perhaps they condemned assisting suicide under all circumstances for philosophical or religious reasons, or on the grounds that such action was inconsistent with the role of medicine (e.g., the first-century physicians Scribonius Largus [Hamilton, 1986] and Aretaeus [Amundsen, 1978]).

At the most, a limited "respect for life." In light of the Hippocratic oath and several later sources that also condemn abortion and active euthanasia, Temkin asserts that "Sufficient material has now been gathered to prove the existence of a tradition which, in its uncompromising form, did not sanction any limit to the respect for life, not even therapeutic abortion . . ." (1976, p. 5). This tradition appears to have been entirely negative in its emphasis: The physician would not actively terminate life by abortion or euthanasia. But it laid no stress on the positive correlate that would require the physician actively to attempt to prolong life. This negative tradition did, indeed, become stronger with the rise of Christianity and its introduction of the principle of sanctity of life: Abortion, infanticide, suicide, and euthanasia became sins. In addition, philanthropy became a virtue—the highest virtue, in fact—and the love of humanity and Christian compassion became central to the Western ideal of medical practice.

DARREL W. AMUNDSEN

While all the articles in this section and the other sections of this entry are relevant, see especially the other articles in this subsection: EARLY CHRISTIANITY, *and* MEDIEVAL CHRISTIAN EUROPE. *For a further discussion of topics mentioned in this article, see the entries* ABORTION; BENEFICENCE; COMPASSION; CONFIDENTIALITY; CONSCIENCE; DEATH AND DYING: EUTHANASIA AND SUSTAINING LIFE; FIDELITY AND LOYALTY; HEALTH AND DISEASE; INFANTS, *article on* HISTORY OF INFANTICIDE; INFORMATION DISCLOSURE; MEDICAL CODES AND OATHS; MEDICINE, ANTHROPOLOGY OF; MEDICINE, ART OF; MEDICINE, PHILOSOPHY OF; MEDICINE, SOCIOLOGY OF; MEDICINE AS A PROFESSION; PATIENTS' RESPONSIBILITIES; PROFESSIONAL–PATIENT RELATIONSHIP; PROFESSION AND PROFESSIONAL ETHICS; RESEARCH, HUMAN: HISTORICAL ASPECTS; RESPONSIBILITY; SEXUAL ETHICS AND PROFESSIONAL STANDARDS; TRUST; *and* VIRTUE AND CHARACTER. *Other relevant material may be found under the entries* AUTONOMY; CARE; JUSTICE; LOVE; *and* VALUE AND VALUATION. *See also the* APPENDIX (CODES, OATHS, AND DIRECTIVES RELATED TO BIOETHICS), SECTION II: ETHICAL DIRECTIVES FOR THE PRACTICE OF MEDICINE.

Bibliography

AMUNDSEN, DARREL W. 1973. "The Liability of the Physician in Roman Law." In *International Symposium on Society, Medicine and Law, Jerusalem, March 1972*, pp. 17–31. Edited by Heinrich Karplus. New York: Elsevier Scientific Publishing.

———. 1977. "The Liability of the Physician in Classical Greek Legal Theory and Practice." *Journal of the History of Medicine and Allied Sciences* 32, no. 2:172–203.

———. 1978. "The Physician's Obligation to Prolong Life: A Medical Duty Without Classical Roots." *Hastings Center Report* 8, no. 4:23–30.

———. 1987. "Medicine and the Birth of Defective Children: Approaches of the Ancient World." In *Euthanasia and the Newborn: Conflicts Regarding Saving Lives*, pp. 3–22. Edited by Richard C. McMillan, H. Tristram Engelhardt,

Jr., and Stuart F. Spicker. Dordrecht, Netherlands: D. Reidel.

AMUNDSEN, DARREL W., and FERNGREN, GARY B. 1982. "Philanthropy in Medicine: Some Historical Perspectives." In *Beneficence and Health Care*, pp. 1–31. Edited by Earl E. Shelp. Dordrecht, Netherlands: D. Reidel.

———. 1983. "Evolution of the Patient–Physician Relationship: Antiquity Through the Renaissance." In *The Clinical Encounter: The Moral Fabric of the Patient–Physician Relationship*, pp. 1–46. Edited by Earl E. Shelp. Dordrecht, Netherlands: D. Reidel.

BRAIN, PETER. 1977. "History of Medicine: Galen on the Ideal of the Physician." *South African Medical Journal* 52, no. 23:936–938.

CARRICK, PAUL. 1985. *Medical Ethics in Antiquity: Philosophical Perspectives on Abortion and Euthanasia*. Dordrecht, Netherlands: D. Reidel.

COOPER, JOHN M. 1989. "Greek Philosophers on Euthanasia and Suicide." In *Suicide and Euthanasia: Historical and Contemporary Themes*, pp. 9–38. Edited by Baruch A. Brody. Dordrecht, Netherlands: Kluwer.

DEICHGRÄBER, KARL. 1955. *Der hippokratische Eid*. Stuttgart: Hippokrates-Verlag.

EDELSTEIN, LUDWIG. 1967. *Ancient Medicine: Selected Papers of Ludwig Edelstein*. Edited by Owsei Temkin and C. Lilian Temkin. Baltimore, Md.: Johns Hopkins University Press.

FERNGREN, GARY B. 1982. "A Roman Declamation on Vivisection." *Transactions and Studies of the College of Physicians of Philadelphia* 4, no. 4:272–290.

———. 1985. "Roman Lay Attitudes Toward Medical Experimentation." *Bulletin of the History of Medicine* 59, no. 4:495–505.

FERNGREN, GARY B., and AMUNDSEN, DARREL W. 1985. "Virtue and Health/Medicine in Pre-Christian Antiquity." In *Virtue and Medicine: Explorations in the Character of Medicine*, pp. 3–22. Edited by Earl E. Shelp. Dordrecht, Netherlands: D. Reidel.

GOUREVITCH, DANIELLE. 1969. "Suicide Among the Sick in Classical Antiquity." *Bulletin of the History of Medicine* 43, no. 6:501–518.

HAMILTON, J. S. 1986. "Scribonius Largus on the Medical Profession." *Bulletin of the History of Medicine* 60, no. 2:209–216.

HAMMOND, NICHOLAS G. L., and SCULLARD, HOWARD HAYES, eds. 1970. *The Oxford Classical Dictionary*. 2d ed. Oxford: At the Clarendon Press. This work should be consulted for references to available texts and English translations of primary sources cited in this article but not listed in the bibliography.

HANDS, ARTHUR ROBINSON. 1968. *Charities and Social Aid in Greece and Rome*. Ithaca, N.Y.: Cornell University Press.

HOOFF, ANTON J. L. VAN. 1990. *From Autothanasia to Suicide: Self-Killing in Classical Antiquity*. London: Routledge.

JONES, WILLIAM HENRY SAMUEL. 1924. *The Doctor's Oath: An Essay in the History of Medicine*. Cambridge: At the University Press.

KUDLIEN, FRIDOLF. 1970. "Medical Ethics and Popular Ethics in Greece and Rome." *Clio Medica* 5, no. 2:91–121.

———. 1976. "Medicine as a 'Liberal Art' and the Question of the Physician's Income." *Journal of the History of Medicine and Allied Sciences* 31, no. 4:448–459.

LICHTENTHAELER, CHARLES. 1984. *Der Eid des Hippokrates: Ursprung und Bedeutung*. Cologne: Deutscher Ärzte-Verlag.

MICHLER, MARKWART. 1968. "Medical Ethics in Hippocratic Bone Surgery." *Bulletin of the History of Medicine* 42, no. 4:297–311.

NUTTON, VIVIAN. 1985. "Murders and Miracles: Lay Attitudes Towards Medicine in Classical Antiquity." In *Patients and Practitioners: Lay Perceptions of Medicine in Pre-Industrial Society*, pp. 23–53. Edited by Roy Porter. Cambridge: At the University Press.

———. 1993. "Beyond the Hippocratic Oath." In *Doctors and Ethics: The Earlier Historical Setting of Professional Ethics*, pp. 10–37. Edited by Roger K. French, Andrew Wear, and Johanna Geyer-Kordesch. Amsterdam: Rodopi.

OLIVER, JAMES H. 1949. "Two Athenian Poets." *Hesperia* suppl. 8:243–258.

SCARBOROUGH, JOHN. 1976. "Celsus on Human Vivisection at Ptolemaic Alexandria." *Clio Medica* 11, no. 1:25–38.

TEMKIN, OWSEI. 1949. "Changing Concepts of the Relation of Medicine to Society: In Early History." In *Social Medicine: Its Derivations and Objectives*, pp. 3–12. Edited by Iago Galdston. New York: Commonwealth Fund.

———. 1973. *Galenism: The Rise and Decline of a Medical Philosophy*. Ithaca, N.Y.: Cornell University Press.

———. 1976. "The Idea of Respect for Life in the History of Medicine." In *Respect for Life in Medicine, Philosophy, and the Law*, pp. 1–23. By Owsei Temkin, William K. Frankena, and Sanford H. Kadish. Baltimore, Md.: Johns Hopkins University Press.

———. 1979. "Medical Ethics and Honoraria in Late Antiquity." In *Healing and History: Essays for George Rosen*, pp. 6–26. Edited by Charles E. Rosenberg. New York: Science History Publications.

———. 1991. *Hippocrates in a World of Pagans and Christians*. Baltimore, Md.: Johns Hopkins University Press.

VON STADEN, HEINRICH. 1989. *Herophilus: The Art of Medicine in Early Alexandria: Edition, Translation, and Essays*. Cambridge: At the University Press.

———. 1990. "Incurability and Hopelessness: The *Hippocratic Corpus*." In *La maladie et les maladies dans la collection Hippocratique. Actes du VIe colloque international Hippocratique*, pp. 75–112. Edited by Paul Potter, Gilles Maloney, and Jacques Desautels. Quebec: Éditions du Sphinx.

2. EARLY CHRISTIANITY

Christianity arose in Palestine during the first half of the first century C.E. among the followers of Jesus of Nazareth, called the Christ, who believed him to be the Messiah and the Son of God. Although the first followers were almost exclusively Jews, this new faith spread quickly through the Mediterranean basin and soon attracted many non-Jewish converts. For its first three centuries it remained a religion of a small but steadily growing minority. Officially declared a forbidden religion by the Roman imperial government, its adherents endured spasmodic persecutions that culminated in the Great Persecution (303–311). Emperor Constantine, a convert to Christianity, pronounced it a legal religion in 313; Emperor Theodosius I (379–395) declared it the official religion of the state and abolished the public practice of pagan religious rites.

This article covers the Christian religion from its origins to the fifth century. The sources for early Christianity are primarily literary: the New Testament, composed by followers of Jesus during the first century; and the patristic literature (the writings of early church leaders and theologians until the end of the fifth century). During this era, the beliefs and practices of the new faith were articulated and refined amid many controversies, particularly about the divinity of Christ and the nature of redemption. Gradually, a core of beliefs and a canon of literature predominated as orthodox and a church organization emerged that promoted these beliefs. By the late fifth century, orthodoxy had achieved its enduring form in doctrine and hierarchy, both of which differed in some respects between western Europe and the Byzantine culture of the East. At the same time, certain heterodox or heretical Christian groups existed peripherally. One of these, Arianism, became a powerful political and religious force.

Medical theories and practice in the varied milieu of Greek and Roman paganism were so religiously neutral that a discussion of classical medical ethics need pay relatively little attention to the subject of religion. Christianity, however, is fundamentally different in its most basic tenets and principles from the salient features of the religious pluralism in which it took root. Issues of health, sickness, healing, life, and death are so integral to Christian theology that two questions need to be addressed before anything meaningful can be said about early Christian medical ethics: (1) What was Christianity's theological understanding of illness? (2) Were the use and practice of medicine regarded as appropriate for Christians?

What was the theological understanding of illness? Patristic theology viewed physical health as a good but not an absolute good, and much less the supreme good. Physical health could even be an obstacle to the supreme good, which was spiritual health. The church fathers emphasized that the soul is infinitely more valuable than the body, and that care for the latter is not to conflict with care for the former. Yet the majority of the sources maintained that the body is to be reasonably cared for, since God has provided the means for its care. The church fathers saw health as a blessing from God, but since it was only a relative good, it could be an evil if given a higher priority than it deserved. Conversely, sickness could be a good thing. A survey of the writings of the church fathers reveals the firm conviction that

Christians should rejoice in sickness as well as in health. Sickness can correct or restrain one from sin, refine, admonish, increase patience, reduce pride, cause one to be less self-reliant and more dependent upon God, and make one more mindful of eternity and one's own mortality, thus helping to wean one from the material to the spiritual, from the temporal to the eternal (Amundsen, 1982).

Sin lurked in the background of all conditions of suffering. Without sin there would be no suffering, because the fall of the first humans created by God, Adam and Eve, was the ultimate explanation for the miseries of the present. Sin, in this sense, was generic in the human race. When the church fathers identified personal sin as the cause of sickness, it was usually in the context of pastoral exhortations intended to comfort and correct rather than to foster guilt.

In the literature of the first several centuries of Christianity, three sources of disease or illness were identified: God, demons, and nature. They were not mutually exclusive. While there appears to have been a hesitancy to attribute disease directly to God, the more his sovereignty was stressed, the more he was viewed as either sending or permitting illness through demonic or natural instrumentality. The subject of disease causality in the early Christian literature is rife with confusion and interpretive problems, especially considering the perceived role of demons.

What was thought to cause disease in any given case greatly affected the choice of means of healing: spiritual/miraculous (e.g., prayer, the sacraments, exorcism, and, beginning in late antiquity, the cult of saints and relics); medical (drugs, dietetics, and surgery—typically administered by a physician); or magical (demonic or occult practices). The first two of these approaches were often combined, and sometimes magic was employed, although its use was consistently condemned in Christian literature. A Christian was to depend upon God. Sometimes the line of dependence was direct; at other times it included one or several intermediaries. The church itself (i.e., its clergy and sacraments) and the saints became variable parts of a chain of dependence to which a spiritual/miraculous healing model was essentially integral. A magical model offered an inherently incompatible, conflicting, and competing structure of dependence. A medical model was not necessarily either harmonious and compatible with the church's structure of dependence, or incompatible, conflicting, and competing with it.

Did the potential for tension between Christianity and medicine ever lead to a rejection of medicine? Some scholars have maintained that several church fathers were diametrically opposed to medicine in any form for Christians (e.g., Harnack, 1892; Frings, 1959; Schadewaldt, 1965). Most sources that have been thus interpreted have lately been shown not to be hostile to medicine per se (Amundsen, 1982; Temkin, 1991). Although more scholarly work remains to be done, it is unlikely that any patristic source will ultimately prove to have made a blanket condemnation of medicine. Nevertheless, some church fathers maintained that only those who lacked spirituality sufficient for them to be able to rely exclusively on divine healing should use medicine (e.g., Origen [ca. 184–ca. 253], *Contra Celsum*). Others practiced an asceticism that so glorified suffering and disease that they would not avail themselves of help from any source, although they did not deny the propriety of medicine for other Christians (Harvey, 1985; Amundsen, 1982).

Even if no patristic sources totally condemned medicine, the existence of those passages that have been thus interpreted, together with numerous cautionary statements about medicine made by other church fathers, demonstrates an uneasiness and a real potential for tension. Scholars like Adolf Harnack (1892), Hermann-Josef Frings (1959), Hans Schadewaldt (1965), and Vivian Nutton (1985), have advanced two possibly complementary theories to account for the supposedly unequivocal condemnation of medicine by some church fathers and the general uneasiness about Christians' using medicine expressed by others: (1) An early, conservative hostility against medicine was gradually ameliorated by a Hellenistic, liberalizing influence; (2) Christianity's supposed emphasis on, and ostensible promise of, miraculous physical healing was a constant, major obstacle to compatibility. Both views betray a misunderstanding of the nature of the inherent, and hence enduring, tensions and compatibilities between Christianity and medicine (Amundsen, 1982), and the second compounds the error by exaggerating the importance of miraculous healing in the propagation of the Gospel and in the Christian community, especially during the second and third centuries (Ferngren, 1992). Generally the patristic sources see medicine and physicians as God's gifts. Christianity inherited from Hellenistic Judaism an appreciation of Greek medicine that defined disease naturalistically while denying neither God's sovereignty nor his prerogative to intervene in mundane affairs. Nevertheless, the church fathers regarded as both sinful and foolish the use of physicians and medicine apart from faith in God and the failure to recognize that all healing, other than magical (demonic or occult), comes from God (Amundsen, 1982; Temkin, 1991).

The ideal physician of early Christianity

The tension between Christianity and medicine was overshadowed by their compatibility in one important sense: Jesus Christ was described as the great physician, the true physician, both the physician and the medication (Pease, 1914; Arbesmann, 1854; Schipperges, 1965; Temkin, 1991). Early Christian authors thus adopted and adapted a long-established tradition in classical literature that employed, in simile or metaphor, the idea of physicians as dedicated, unselfish, and compassionate preservers or restorers of health and, sometimes, inflicters of health-giving pain, always committed to the good of their patients. It was not uncommon for the term "Hippocratic art" to be used metonymously for the medical art, and Christian authors occasionally mention Hippocrates as an ethical ideal for the medical practitioner. Indeed, Christ was himself spoken of as being, "as it were, a spiritual Hippocrates" (Pease, 1914, p. 75), and it is to Hippocrates as the type of physician that Jerome (ca. 345–ca. 419), compares the Christian healer (*In Ioanem Commentarii*; cf. *Epistle* 125).

Early Christians found the "Hippocratic ideal" of decorum very appealing. Jerome wrote to a priest that it

> is part of your duty to visit the sick, to be acquainted with people's households, with matrons, and with their children, and to be entrusted with the secrets of the great. Let it therefore be your duty to keep your tongue chaste as well as your eyes. Never discuss a woman's looks, nor let one house know what is going on in another. Hippocrates, before he will instruct his pupils, makes them take an oath and compels them to swear obedience to him. That oath exacts from them silence, and prescribes for them their language, gait, dress, and manners. How much greater an obligation is laid on us who have been entrusted with the healing of souls! (*Epistle* 52.15; see Temkin, 1991, p. 182)

In a collection of letters incorrectly attributed to Clement of Alexandria (ca. 150–ca. 220), there is a passage that reads, "We are to visit the sick . . . without guile or covetousness or noise or talkativeness or pride or any behavior alien to piety. . . . [I]nstead of using elegant phrases, neatly arranged and ordered . . . act frankly like men who have received the gift of healing from God, to God's glory" (*De virginitate* 1, 112). This advice, which sounds as if it had been written for physicians, was intended for exorcists dealing with the demon-possessed. Every detail enunciated here, save for reference to piety and to God, is mentioned in the classical literature on medical etiquette, but one need not assume that the anonymous author of this letter was intentionally adopting principles of medical etiquette. Rather, the guidelines for conduct in both instances seem to be little more than practical etiquette for clergy as well as for physicians.

Compassion or philanthropy was the one feature of the "Hippocratic ideal" that the church fathers regarded as especially Christian. Origen writes that he followed "the method of a philanthropic physician who seeks the sick so that he may bring relief to them and strengthen them" (*Contra Celsum* 3.74). In demonstrating the superiority of Christianity to pagan philosophy, he says that "Plato and the other wise men of Greece, with their fine sayings, are like the physicians who confine their attention to the better classes and despise the common man while the disciples of Jesus carefully study to make provision for the great mass of men" (ibid., 7.60). It was in caring for common people, especially for the destitute and the poor, that physicians evinced a Christlike compassion. Augustine (354–430) regarded his friend, the physician Gennadius, as "a man of devout mind, kind and generous heart, and untiring compassion, as shown by his care of the poor" (*Epistle* 159). He frequently mentions physicians who, motivated by charity, asked no remuneration for their services but undertook the most desperate cases among the poor with no thought of receiving any recompense (e.g., *Sermon* 175).

Eusebius of Caesarea (ca. 265–ca. 339) writes that Christ, "like some excellent physician, in order to cure the [spiritually] sick, examines what is repulsive, handles sores, and reaps pain himself for the sufferings of others" (*Ecclesiastical History* 10.4.11). And Origen paraphrases a well-known Hippocratic aphorism that a physician "who sees terrible things and touches unpleasant wounds in order to heal the sick . . . does not wholly avoid the possibility that he may fall into the same plight" (*Contra Celsum* 4.15; see Temkin, 1991, pp. 141ff.). Physicians, according to Augustine, should always have their patients' cure at heart (*Sermon* 9), for the practice of medicine would be cruelty if physicians were only concerned about engaging in their art (*In Psalmos*). Gregory of Nyssa (ca. 335–394) began a letter to the physician Eustathius with the statement that, "Philanthropy is the way of life [*epitedeuma*, "one's business"] for all of you who practice the medical art" (although almost certainly written by Gregory of Nyssa, it is usually printed as *Epistle* 189 of his elder brother, Basil). While philanthropy was a highly desirable attribute for many pagan physicians, it is no exaggeration to say that Christianity made it an ethical obligation for Christian physicians (Temkin, 1991). Indeed, for some it became the chief motivating factor for the practice of medicine.

Hence it is not surprising that Christians adopted and adapted the so-called Hippocratic oath at some time before the end of the period under consideration. Several manuscripts of an "Oath of Hippocrates insofar as a Christian may swear it" are extant (Jones, 1924, pp. 54f.). The Christian oath omits the enigmatic prohibition of cutting for stone and makes more specific and definite the antiabortion statement. Where the pagan oath reads "Into whatsoever houses I enter, I shall do so to help the sick, keeping myself free from all intentional wrongdoing and harm," The Christian oath has "Into whatsoever houses I enter, I will do so to help the sick,

keeping myself free from all wrongdoing, both intentional and unintentional, tending to death or to injury." While one should not make too much of the addition of the promise to keep oneself free from even unintentional harm, it is reasonable to suggest that this concern, although not inconsistent with pagan medical ethics, is even more consonant with an early Christian ethics of respect for life that manifested itself not only in a condemnation of such practices as infanticide and suicide (including active euthanasia) but also in a philanthropy that was regarded as owed to the destitute and the ill.

Philanthropy

There is an enormous gap between pagan and Christian concepts of philanthropy. Christian philanthropy was an outgrowth of the Jewish insistence that love, mercy, and justice were attributes of God and were essential for true worship of God (e.g., Mic. 6:6–8). Christian philanthropy was the expression of agape, an unlimited, freely given, sacrificial love that was not dependent on the worthiness of its object, since it was the manifestation of the very nature of God, who himself is agape (1 John 4:8). It was incumbent upon all Christians to extend care to the needy, especially to the sick. By late antiquity the care of the sick had become a highly organized activity under the supervision of the local bishop (Ferngren, 1988). Institutions that with some qualification may be called hospitals, were established and maintained beginning in the fourth century. The most famous of these was the *nosokomeia* or *ptocheion* of Basil, who was the bishop of Caesarea from 370 to 379 (Miller, 1985; Temkin, 1991). These institutions, as well as orphanages and homes for the care of the elderly and destitute, first arose after the legalization of Christianity, were distinctly Christian, and were a direct outgrowth of Christian philanthropy.

During various outbreaks of plague, Christians responded with spectacular daring in their attempts to succor the ill, both Christian and pagan. One particular group, on whom we have only scant information, were known as the *parabalani* ("reckless ones") because of the risks they faced by caring for plague victims (Philipsborn, 1950). Their zeal in the face of imminent danger was motivated in part by the belief that death thus incurred ranked with martyrdom (Eusebius, *Ecclesiastical History*). Christians were so well known for their care of the destitute that Julian the Apostate (r. 361–363), the only pagan emperor after the legalization of Christianity, complained that the "impious Galileans support not only their own poor but ours as well" (*Epistle* 22). Henry Sigerist did not overstate the case when he said that Christianity introduced "the most revolutionary and decisive change in the attitude of society toward the sick. . . . It became the duty of the Christian to attend to the sick and the poor of the community. . . . The social position of the sick man thus became fundamentally different from what it had been before. He assumed a preferential position which has been his ever since" (1943, pp. 69f.).

The sanctity of human life

The Christian imperative to a practical philanthropy that extended to the poor and the sick was not solely a manifestation of Christian love but was ultimately articulated as a theology of respect for life, a principle of the sanctity of human life predicated on the concept of the *imago Dei*, the belief that every human being was formed in the image of God (Ferngren, 1987). By virtue of sharing the *imago Dei*, all human life was of value, and therefore was owed compassion and care. Specific condemnations of contraception, abortion, and infanticide, however, are not found in the New Testament. And when they first appear in Christian literature during the second century, they seem not to be predicated upon a developed concept of the *imago Dei* as the basis of human value. Rather, such condemnations appear in the context of broad and fervent denunciations of the most offensive sins to which Christians felt pagans were especially prone, such as gladiatorial shows and other exhibitions of extreme cruelty, and sexual immorality of an extravagantly imaginative variety.

The history of the treatment of contraception and abortion in the early church is rife with difficulties. First, the distinction between contraception and abortion, at least in the early stages of pregnancy, was blurred in both medical and popular perceptions (Noonan, 1966). The question of when human life begins was, and still is, hotly debated. Ancient embryology, although scientifically inaccurate, was more helpful than modern science in answering this question. Aristotle's theory of fetal succession of souls—nutritive, sensitive, rational—had a profound impact on patristic discussions of abortion. A fetus that is "fully formed" (a very imprecise concept) is "ensouled," that is, possesses a sensitive soul and is "animate" (an equally imprecise concept). One that is not "fully formed" is not "animate," in that it is not yet "ensouled" with a sensitive rather than a nutritive soul. The transition from a nutritive to a sensitive soul—that is, animation—is marked by "quickening," the first movement of the fetus, which ostensibly happens about the fortieth day with males and the ninetieth day with females.

Furthermore, Christian condemnations of contraception and abortion were based on two quite different principles. One is that contraception and abortion before "ensoulment" are essentially sexual sins but not the destruction of human life. The other is that contraception and abortion at any stage are indeed the destruction of human life. Both, of course, regarded abortion after "ensoulment" as homicide (Noonan, 1970; Connery, 1977; Gorman, 1982; Dombrowski, 1988). Some recent revisionist historians advance the argument that the early Christian community did not condemn abortion at any stage of fetal development until two factors conduced to condemning it: the desire to rely not only on evangelism to increase the Christian community but also on internal growth, and the developing contempt for women within the church that relegated them to the role of childbearers (e.g., Hoffmann, 1990). Such special pleading has little to commend it.

The Christian condemnation of infanticide, including exposure, however, was unequivocal and inclusive, counting the active or passive killing of any newborn, whether healthy, sickly, defective, or even grossly deformed, as the murder of one made in the image of God (Amundsen, 1987).

Active euthanasia, except as it was condemned in the "Hippocratic oath insofar as a Christian may swear it," is not discussed in the sources, but must have been regarded as murder, especially given the early Christian community's attitude toward suicide. Although suicide was not included in the broad spectrum of sins of pagans that aroused the moral indignation of early Christians, it was condemned by numerous church fathers, beginning with Justin Martyr, who in the second century replied to the hypothetical question why Christians do not just kill themselves and save pagans the trouble, "If we do so, we shall be opposing the will of God" (2 *Apology* 4). At about the same time the anonymous *Epistle to Diognetus* states that Christians do not kill themselves because God has assigned them for an important purpose to a post that they must not abandon. Clement of Alexandria flatly states that suicide is not permitted for Christians (*Stromateis*). The anonymous *Clementine Homilies*, which reached their present form in the mid-fourth century, but were based on an original composed in the late second or early third century, assign to suicides a severe future punishment (*Homily* 12). Lactantius (ca. 240–320) condemns suicides as worse than homicides, since they not only commit violence against nature but are impious as well. Nothing, in his opinion, can be more wicked than suicide (*Divine Institutes; Epitome* 39). John Chrysostom (ca. 349–407) writes that all Christians justly regard suicide with horror, "for if it is base to destroy others, much more is it to destroy one's self" (*Commentary on Galatians* 1:4). His contemporaries Ambrose and Jerome also categorically condemn suicide, the former flatly stating that "Scripture forbids a Christian to lay hands on himself" (*Concerning Virgins* 3.7.32), and the latter that Christ will not receive the soul of a suicide (*Letter* 39). Both Ambrose and Jerome make one exception to their condemnation of suicide: when it is committed to preserve one's chastity.

Augustine's rejection of this one exception led him to engage in a thorough analysis of suicide in books I and XIX of his *City of God.* His argument against the permissibility of suicide is fivefold. First, Scripture neither commands it nor expressly permits it, either as a means of attaining immortality or as a way to avoid or escape any evil. Second, the Sixth Commandment of the Mosaic law, "Thou shalt not kill," must be understood to forbid it. Third, since individuals have no right on their own authority to kill even a person who justly deserves to die, those who kill themselves are homicides. Fourth, the act of suicide allows no opportunity for repentance. And fifth, suicide violates the foundational Christian principle of patient endurance of all that the sovereign Creator permits to befall humanity (Amundsen, 1989).

While the church fathers firmly held that death was not to be sought, they proclaimed that Christians should not fear physical death, since it would furnish them entry into the ineffable delights of heaven. Hence numerous patristic sources marveled at Christians who were afraid of dying, and especially at those who desperately clung to any hope of sustaining their lives when afflicted with seemingly hopeless illness. They viewed such conduct as tantamount to blasphemy, or at least as a sad contradiction of Christian values (Amundsen, 1989).

It was bad enough to stake one's futile hope of a temporary reprieve on physicians; but to resort to magic was even more reprehensible (Amundsen and Ferngren, 1986). For example, in the late fourth or early fifth century, John Chrysostom praised a mother who chose to allow her sick child to die rather than use amulets, although her ostensibly Christian friends had urged her to do so and she herself was confident that it could save her daughter's life (*Homily 8 on Colossians*). About 150 years later, the physician Alexander of Tralles employed quite different reasoning when he argued that it was sinful not to apply any remedy that might possibly save a patient's life, even amulets and incantations (Temkin, 1991). Alexander's attitude is interesting for three reasons. First, it demonstrates that magical remedies had already obtruded themselves into medicine. Second, it graphically illustrates a conflict of priorities between the physician and the theologian. And third, it is a very early, perhaps the earliest, hint of a physician's expressing a moral, indeed a religious, obligation to prolong life, in this case based on the reasoning that the supposedly greater sin of not doing all in one's power to save a patient was justifiably avoided by the lesser sin of using magical remedies.

Christianity developed a theological basis for the sanctity of human life, condemning contraception, abortion, infanticide (even of the sickly and deformed), suicide, and (by implication) active euthanasia. Although it did not embrace any sense of obligation to attempt to prolong life (nor did it until several centuries more had elapsed), its theology of sanctity of life did conduce to the reasoning of Alexander of Tralles that is described above, an attitude that grew even stronger during the Middle Ages.

Conclusion

In early Christian literature a reasonably clear, if not exhaustive, picture emerges of ideal physicians who were "Hippocratic" in their decorum and motivated by Christian philanthropy, and who so cherished the sanctity of human life that they would neither perform abortions nor assist in suicide, yet regarded desperate attempts to forestall death as inconsistent with ultimate Christian values. Nevertheless, such a description tells us nothing directly about the ethics of early Christian physicians except insofar as individual physicians may have agreed with and attempted to conform to such an ideal.

The ideal physician had been posited in classical antiquity, and that ideal included compassion as a desirable characteristic. However, agape—Christian love, which was the basis of philanthropy—was so central a tenet of Christian theology that it was applied to the physician as not merely a desirable but as an essential characteristic. The philanthropic basis of medical practice and the principle of the sanctity of human life became the hallmarks of Western medical ethics until modern times.

DARREL W. AMUNDSEN

While all the articles in this section and the other sections of this entry are relevant, see especially the other articles in this subsection: GREECE AND ROME, *and* MEDIEVAL CHRISTIAN EUROPE. *Directly related to this article are the entries* ROMAN CATHOLICISM; JUDAISM; *and* COMPASSION. *For a further discussion of topics mentioned in this article, see the entries* ABORTION, *section on* RELIGIOUS TRADITIONS, *articles on* JEWISH PERSPECTIVES, *and* ROMAN CATHOLIC PERSPECTIVES; BENEFICENCE; FERTILITY CONTROL; HEALTH AND DISEASE; PASTORAL CARE; *and* SUICIDE. *Other relevant material may be found under the entries* DEATH: ART OF DYING, *article on* ARS MORIENDI; LIFE; LITERATURE; *and* OBLIGATION AND SUPEREROGATION. *See also the* APPENDIX (CODES, OATHS, AND DIRECTIVES RELATED TO BIOETHICS), SECTION II: ETHICAL DIRECTIVES FOR THE PRACTICE OF MEDICINE, OATH OF HIPPOCRATES.

Bibliography

AMUNDSEN, DARREL W. 1982. "Medicine and Faith in Early Christianity." *Bulletin of the History of Medicine* 56, no. 3:326–350.

————. 1987. "Medicine and the Birth of Defective Children: Approaches of the Ancient World." In *Euthanasia and the Newborn: Conflicts Regarding Saving Lives*, pp. 3–22. Edited by Richard C. McMillan, H. Tristram Engelhardt, Jr., and Stuart F. Spicker. Dordrecht, Netherlands: D. Reidel.

————. 1989. "Suicide and Early Christian Values." In *Suicide and Euthanasia: Historical and Contemporary Themes*, pp. 77–153. Edited by Baruch A. Brody. Dordrecht, Netherlands: Kluwer.

AMUNDSEN, DARREL W., and FERNGREN, GARY B. 1982. "Philanthropy in Medicine: Some Historical Perspectives." In *Beneficence and Health Care*, pp. 1–31. Edited by Earl E. Shelp. Dordrecht, Netherlands: D. Reidel.

————. 1986. "The Early Christian Tradition." In *Caring and Curing: Health and Medicine in the Western Religious Traditions*, pp. 40–64. Edited by Ronald L. Numbers and Darrel W. Amundsen. New York: Macmillan.

ARBESMANN, RUDOLPH. 1954. "The Concept of 'Christus Medicus' in St. Augustine." *Traditio* 10:1–28.

CONNERY, JOHN R. 1977. *Abortion: The Development of the Roman Catholic Perspective*. Chicago: Loyola University Press.

D'IRSAY, STEPHEN. 1927. "Patristic Medicine." *Annals of Medical History* 9, no. 4:364–378.

DOMBROWSKI, DANIEL A. 1988. "St. Augustine, Abortion, and *Libido Crudelis*." *Journal of the History of Ideas* 49, no. 1:151–156.

FERNGREN, GARY B. 1987. "The Imago Dei and the Sanctity of Life: The Origins of an Idea." In *Euthanasia and the Newborn: Conflicts Regarding Saving Lives*, pp. 23–45. Edited by Richard C. McMillan, H. Tristram Engelhardt, Jr., and Stuart F. Spicker. Dordrecht, Netherlands: D. Reidel.

————. 1988. "The Organisation of the Care of the Sick in Early Christianity." In *Actes: Proceedings of the XXX International Congress of the History of Medicine*, pp. 192–198. Leverkusen, Germany: Vicom KG.

————. 1992. "Early Christianity as a Religion of Healing." *Bulletin of the History of Medicine* 66, no. 1:1–15.

FRINGS, HERMANN JOSEF. 1959. "Medizin und Arzt bei den griechischen Kirchenvätern bis Chrysostomos." Ph.D. diss., University of Bonn.

GORMAN, MICHAEL. 1982. *Abortion and the Early Church: Christian, Jewish, and Pagan Attitudes in the Greco-Roman World*. Downers Grove, Ill.: Intervarsity.

HARNACK, ADOLF. 1982. *Die griechische Übersetzung des Apologeticus Tertullians Medizinisches aus der ältersten Kirchengeschichte*. Texte und Untersuchungen zur Geschichte der altchristlichen Literatur, vol. 8, no. 4. Leipzig: J. C. Heinrichs.

HARVEY, SUSAN ASHBROOK. 1985. "Physicians and Ascetics in John of Ephesus: An Expedient Alliance." In *Symposium on Byzantine Medicine*, pp. 87–93. Edited by John Scarborough. Dumbarton Oaks Papers, no. 38. Washington, D.C.: Dumbarton Oaks Library and Collection.

HOFFMANN, R. JOSEPH. 1990. "Faith and Foeticide." *Conscience: A Newsjournal of Prochoice Catholic Opinion* 11, no. 6:1, 3–6.

JONES, WILLIAM HENRY SAMUEL. 1924. *The Doctor's Oath: An Essay in the History of Medicine*. Cambridge: At the University Press.

MILLER, TIMOTHY S. 1985. *The Birth of the Hospital in the Byzantine Empire*. Baltimore: Johns Hopkins University Press.

NOONAN, JOHN T., JR. 1966. *Contraception: A History of Its Treatment by the Catholic Theologians and Canonists*. Cambridge, Mass.: Harvard University Press.

————. 1970. "An Almost Absolute Value in History." In *The Morality of Abortion: Legal and Historical Perspectives*, pp. 1–59. Edited by John T. Noonan, Jr. Cambridge, Mass.: Harvard University Press.

NUTTON, VIVIAN. 1985. "From Galen to Alexander, Aspects of Medicine and Medical Practice in Late Antiquity." In *Symposium on Byzantine Medicine*, pp. 1–14. Edited by John Scarborough. Dumbarton Oaks Papers, no. 38. Washington, D.C.: Dumbarton Oaks Library and Collection.

PEASE, ARTHUR STANLEY. 1914. "Medical Allusions in the Works of St. Jerome." *Harvard Studies in Classical Philology* 25:73–86.

PHILIPSBORN, ALEXANDRE. 1950. "La compagnie d'ambulanciers 'parabalani' d'Alexandrie." *Byzantion* 20:185–190.

QUASTEN, JOHANNES. 1950–1986. *Patrology*. 4 vols. Westminster, Md.: Newman Press. Should be consulted for references to available texts and English translations.

RENGSTORF, KARL HEINRICH. 1953. *Die Anfänge der Auseinandersetzung zwischen Christusglaube und Asklepiosfrömmigkeit*. Münster: Aschendorff.

SCHADEWALDT, HANS. 1965. "Die Apologie der Heilkunst bei den Kirchenvätern." *Veröffentlichungen der Internationalen Gesellschaft für Geschichte der Pharmazie* 26:115–130.

SCHIPPERGES, HEINRICH. 1965. "Zur Tradition des 'Christus Medicus' in frühen Christentum und in der älteren Heilkunde." *Arzt und Christ* 11:12–20.

————. 1990. "Krankheit IV. Alte Kirche." In vol. 19 of *Theologische Realenzyklopädie*, pp. 686–689. Edited by Frank Schumann and Michael Wolter. Berlin: Walter de Gruyter.

SIGERIST, HENRY E. 1943. *Civilization and Disease*. Ithaca, N.Y.: Cornell University Press.

TEMKIN, OWSEI. 1991. *Hippocrates in a World of Pagans and Christians*. Baltimore: Johns Hopkins University Press.

3. MEDIEVAL CHRISTIAN EUROPE

The Middle Ages are typically divided into early (500–1050) and high and late (1050–1545). This survey of the history of medical ethics in medieval Europe will first examine the sparse evidence from the early Middle Ages, and then deal thematically with significant developments during the high and late Middle Ages. The Middle Ages was a period of monumental changes. There was, however, one constant—the nearly complete identification of society with the Catholic church, which became the most thoroughly integrated involuntary religious system in human history. The Catholic church, of course, evolved throughout the Middle Ages. Nevertheless, the indirect influence of the church on most—perhaps all—aspects of life, as well as the effects of its efforts to define, direct, and regulate the details of secular and religious life, provide a backdrop for much of the discussion that follows.

The early Middle Ages

We know of the existence of a variety of medical practitioners from the early Middle Ages. Here and there in the sources are physicians who had been trained in Alexandria or in Constantinople, Jewish or Islamic physicians, and public or civic physicians in some of the surviving Roman cities of Italy and southern France. But primarily there are those who seem to have been little more than craftsmen who had learned their techniques as apprentices. The sources, nevertheless, call all these varied types *medici*, and often contrast them with *incantatores* (enchanters, magicians, witch doctors). *Medici*, although sometimes depicted negatively in the predominantly religious literature of the early Middle Ages, are presented favorably as practitioners of an art not inherently inconsistent with the teachings of the church. The *incantatores*, however, are invariably condemned in the literature, including secular and canon law, as diabolical practitioners of illicit arts inherently opposed to the church (Flint, 1989, 1991). In this sense the physicians of the early Middle Ages—indeed, throughout the Middle Ages—were regarded by those who spoke for the church as providing a theologically neutral alternative to the spiritually pernicious ministrations of the nearly ubiquitous practitioners of those healing arts that the church condemned (Amundsen, 1986).

Not only are these physicians, of whose ethics we have little or no direct evidence, contrasted with the *incantatores*; they also are distinguished from monks or other clergy who practiced medicine as part of their religious calling. Surveys of medical history typically describe the early Middle Ages as a time when medicine was practiced predominantly by monks who treated the ills not only of their fellow monks but also of the laity of the surrounding community, as an act of Christian charity. The rule of Saint Benedict, founder of the Benedictine order (early sixth century), is often cited in this regard. Chapter 36 of the rule is addressed to those who tend ill monks. Since, however, this chapter says nothing about medical care of the laity, scholars have emphasized that the rule may not be used as evidence for a policy of monastic medical care of the ill by the Benedictines (e.g., Park, 1992). But the steward, who, according to chapter 36, is largely responsible for the logistics of the care of sick monks, is admonished elsewhere in the rule to "take the greatest care of the sick, of children, of guests, and of the poor, knowing without

doubt that he will have to render an account for all these on the Day of Judgment" (ch. 31). The "children, guests, and poor" in this context certainly would not be monks, nor should the "sick" here be limited to them. Still, this is far from a concise articulation of a monastic obligation to succor the ill of the lay community at large.

In the mid-sixth century, Cassiodorus wrote a rule for the members of a monastery he had founded. The section governing monk-physicians begins with praise for their performing "the functions of blessed piety for those who flee to the shrines of holy men" (*Institutiones* 1.31), which suggests his expectation that the ill would come to the monastery for medical care. The availability and quality of medical care at monasteries varied enormously during those early centuries. Only from the ninth century on can we speak with any certainty about monasteries' playing a key role in providing medical care for the sick poor (Park, 1992). Various church councils during the early Middle Ages enjoined bishops to provide accommodations for the destitute. These, originally called *xenodochia*, but soon more commonly known as *hospitia* or *hospitalia*, were attached to cathedrals or other churches (Ullmann, 1971). These *hospitalia* were not hospitals in the modern sense of that term (Miller, 1978). Often they provided only food, shelter, and some amenities; only occasionally were they staffed with medical attendants, who would then not have been monks but other clergy who devoted part of their energies to practicing medicine.

Cassiodorus wrote two documents that describe the duties of physicians. One, already cited as evidence for monastic medical care of the laity, gives inspirational guidance to those of his monks who were also physicians (*Institutiones*). The other, which he wrote as an official in the service of King Theodoric, regulated the activities of the civic physicians of Ostrogothic Rome and of the royal household (*Variae*). While in both documents Cassiodorus lauds the medical art, there is little other similarity between them. He urges the secular physicians to place their confidence in their art, while the monk-physicians are to place their hope in the Lord and not in the medical art itself. Although Cassiodorus stresses that the secular physicians are to be dedicated to their learned art and mindful of the oath by which they were consecrated, swearing "to hate iniquity and to love purity," his major concern is nevertheless with correcting negative aspects of medical practice: professional jealousies, envy, an unwillingness to share techniques with colleagues, and bedside bickering. While this secular document places a minor emphasis on the calling, motivation, or qualities of the secular physicians, the monk-physicians are to be deeply compassionate, distressed with personal sorrow at the misfortunes of others, and grieved by their suffering and peril. Motivated by compassion, they will "perform the functions of blessed piety," and their reward will be received from the Lord. Similarly, Cassiodorus' contemporary, Benedict, had charged his monk-physicians, "Before all things and above all things care must be taken of the sick, so that they may be served in very deed as Christ himself" (*Rule*, ch. 36). Their reward would come from the Lord.

While Cassiodorus' guidance to the secular physicians has no distinctly Christian flavor, the peculiar qualities of the monk-physicians are those of the ideal physicians of earlier Christian thought and of a variety of clergy who were to devote their lives to the charitable care of the sick, especially the poor, during the high and late Middle Ages. The best-known example is the Knights Hospitallers of Saint John of Jerusalem (late eleventh to the mid-sixteenth century), an order founded to provide shelter and care for pilgrims. These Hospitallers vowed to "serve our lords, the sick" (Hume, 1940). This phrase not only is an inversion of the lord/vassal relationship but also conveys the same ideal as the injunction in the Rule of Saint Benedict that the monk-physicians should serve the sick as if the latter were "Christ himself." These highly spiritual ideals of monastic medicine merged with the secular tradition of medical ethics and etiquette in the medicoethical literature of the seventh through the tenth century.

Numerous medical manuscripts survive from the early Middle Ages, including several that deal with medical ethics and etiquette (MacKinney, 1952). Unfortunately the authorship, intended audience, and purpose of these medicoethical treatises remain uncertain. They may have been composed by monks or other clergy as purely literary efforts. They may have been used as part of clerical education in the liberal arts, of which medicine was typically a subdivision (Amundsen, 1979). It is most unlikely that they were intended for, or used in, the training of physicians. These treatises present a fusion of the classical tradition of medical etiquette with Christian principles of compassion and charity. The bulk of each treatise was apparently drawn from, and sometimes directly attributed to, Hippocratic writings on etiquette: the physician's aptitude and ideal character, conscientiousness and diligence in practice, bedside manner, confidentiality, sexual propriety, proper relations with colleagues, and the preservation of one's reputation, that is, decorum in the broadest sense of the word. There is nothing distinctly Christian about any of this. But intermingled with such commonsensical precepts are distinctly Christian emphases: the physician should serve the rich and the poor alike, looking for eternal rather than material rewards, making "the cases of others his own sorrow." MacKinney correctly observes that "the monastic spirit dominated . . . medical hand-

books of the period." They were "classical as well as pious, and secular as well as ascetic" (1952, p. 5).

We know little about the ethics of early medieval physicians except for some monks and other clergy who practiced medicine as an act of Christian charity, without thought of remuneration. We do not even know by whom, for whom, and for what purposes treatises devoted to medical ethics and etiquette were composed. Anyone could claim to be a physician and practice medicine. There were no licensure requirements and no professional organizations. Only rarely do we encounter evidence of legal efforts to regulate physicians' activities, for example, by the Visigoths (Amundsen, 1971). Nor did the church make any concerted effort, during these early centuries, to define the responsibilities and regulate the conduct of secular or monastic/clerical physicians, other than to wage vigorous warfare against the use of illicit means of healing that typically were employed not by *medici* but by *incantatores*. Much of the time, the lines blur between secular physicians and those practitioners of medicine who were monks or clergy but practiced medicine for financial gain; many physicians who appear to have been secular were in fact clergy. Nor do we have any evidence about the behavior of physicians during epidemics that affected the villages and countryside during the early Middle Ages. But all these matters were to change during the high and late Middle Ages.

The high and late Middle Ages

Medical and surgical practice by the clergy. At the beginning of the high Middle Ages most monasteries could provide medical care for their members without resorting to the services of secular physicians. Nunneries typically engaged secular physicians for serious illnesses, although nuns attended to the minor health needs of members of their communities. There were some nuns, however, who were as medically sophisticated as any monastic/clerical or secular physician. The outstanding example is Hildegard of Bingen (1098–1179). Well known to her contemporaries as a visionary and mystic, she was also famous for her scientific and medical writings. While the propriety of monks treating monks and nuns treating nuns appears not to have been questioned, the role of the clergy generally as physicians and surgeons was beginning to be subjected to close scrutiny.

In the early twelfth century, the Cistercian abbot Bernard of Clairvaux received a demand from another abbot to send back to his former monastery a monk who had fled to Clairvaux. This monk had left because his abbot "used him not as a monk but as a doctor," and compelled him "to serve not God but the world; that in order to curry favour with the princes of this world he was made to attend tyrants, robbers, and excommunicated persons" (Amundsen, 1986, p. 84), which had brought considerable financial reward to his monastery. The monk was troubled about the spiritual propriety of this. Bernard permitted him to remain. The Cistercians shortly thereafter forbade their monk-physicians to practice outside their monasteries or to treat the laity (Miller, 1978).

A general church council, Lateran II, in 1139 promulgated a regulation having the rubric "Monks and canons regular are not to study jurisprudence and medicine for the sake of temporal gain," which condemned the avarice that motivated some clergy to pursue such studies: "[T]he care of souls being neglected . . . they promise health in return for detestable money and thus make themselves physicians of human bodies" (Schroeder, 1937, pp. 201–202). This law also expresses concern that clergy who practiced medicine would see "inappropriate things." But the major focus was that if financial gain were the motive for the study and practice of medicine and secular law, such pursuits were not appropriate for those who had dedicated themselves to a religious life. We should note, first, that this stipulation did not apply to most clergy but only to monks and canons regular ("regular" means living under a "rule," which did not include most clergy) and, second—and worth noting—that it was never incorporated into canon law. A regional council at Tours in 1163 enacted a law much narrower than the one of Lateran II. It simply prohibited monks and other regular clergy from leaving their religious institutions to study medicine or secular law (Amundsen, 1978). This regulation, which did not forbid the practice of medicine by clergy, became part of canon law.

In 1219 Pope Honorius III issued a rescript, also included in canon law, that extended the prohibition of the study of medicine and secular law to virtually all clergy whose major responsibility was the performance of spiritual duties. Many clergy, however, were not affected by this stipulation, whose prohibitions were significantly lessened by subsequent enactments (Amundsen, 1978). By the end of the Middle Ages, canon law still had not prohibited the clergy from practicing medicine. Surgery, however, was a somewhat different matter, since it involved much greater risk to the patient and increased the danger that a clerical practitioner might be held responsible for a patient's death and hence excluded from exercising his clerical office. In 1215, Lateran IV forbade clergy in major (holy) orders (subdeacons, deacons, and priests) to practice the part of surgery that involved cautery and cutting, in which clergy in minor orders (porters, acolytes, exorcists, and lectors) could still engage (Amundsen, 1978).

Although the practice of medicine by the clergy was permitted, the church was obviously uneasy about their motivation and the possible effects that it might have on their spiritual obligations. Many of the clergy who continued to practice medicine and surgery, at least with the tacit blessing of the church, did so predominantly for charity. For example, some clergy composed medical treatises so that their fellow clerics could treat the poor gratis. Many clergy also wrote medical handbooks to help the poor help themselves. The outstanding example is Petrus Hispanus, "who publicly taught, wrote on, and practised medicine during the early stages of a highly successful ecclesiastical career that culminated with his election as Pope John XXI in 1276" (Siraisi, 1990, p. 25). He is the probable author of the *Treasury for the Poor*, which describes herbs the poor could gather to treat themselves.

During the high Middle Ages rapid urbanization brought about widespread suffering and disease in the growing towns and cities. In the late eleventh century, Augustinian canons (who were regular clergy like monks, but unlike them in that they did not live apart from society) and various lay brotherhoods established charitable institutions that included facilities for the destitute ill (Miller, 1978). A variety of such institutions were founded by bishops, kings, feudal lords, wealthy merchants, guilds, and municipalities as endowed charitable institutions. Members of various orders, like the Knights Hospitallers of St. John of Jerusalem, sometimes staffed these hospitals. Nursing orders also arose, committed to caring for the destitute ill in such institutions. The Knights Hospitallers' phrase "to serve our lords, the sick," perfectly captures both the idealism and spiritual motivation of these orders and the very essence of their ethics. But such practitioners constituted only a small proportion of physicians and surgeons of the high and late Middle Ages. By the mid-fourteenth century, most monasteries were paying secular physicians to treat their ill monks (Park, 1992). The church's desire to decrease clerical involvement in medical practice, especially for financial gain, combined with rapidly changing social conditions that, beginning around 1050, significantly altered the practice of medicine and the nature of medical ethics.

Licensure, guilds, universities, and a reciprocity of obligations. Stimulated by a dynamic revival of a commercial economy, dormant since the collapse of Roman civilization, a gradual transformation of European society began around 1050, an urban revolution that created a starkly altered context for nearly all aspects of life. One of its most salient features was the corporate nature of late medieval urban society, as manifested in increasing institutional sophistication and formalized specialization of labor, regulated either internally by guilds or corporations or externally by secular or ecclesiastical authority. Both regulatory features changed the basis for the practice of most trades and professions, including medicine and surgery. No longer would the practice of medicine be a right that anyone could claim, a free enterprise constrained only by individual conscience and criminal law. The practice of medicine would now be a privilege granted, enforced, and protected by the state or the church, at the state's or church's initiative or at the request of guilds or corporations of physicians or surgeons.

The earliest datable law instituting medical licensure is from the Kingdom of Sicily. In 1140, Roger II issued a statute specifying that those who wished to practice medicine were to appear before his officers and judges and be examined by their court. Those who practiced in defiance of this statute were to be imprisoned and their property confiscated. ". . . this has been arranged so that subjects in our kingdom may not be experimented on by inexperienced physicians" (Powell, 1971, p. 130; Hartung, 1934). A considerable advance over this legislation was made by Roger's grandson, Emperor Frederick II, who in his capacity as king of Sicily, in 1231 promulgated the *Liber Augustalis.* Thereafter the examination for licensure was to be conducted by the masters of the medical school at Salerno, and the license to practice would be issued by the emperor or his representative. Before the examination, the aspirant was to study logic for three years and medicine (to include surgery) for five years, and to practice for one year under the direction of an experienced physician. These revisions are introduced by the following justification: "We see a special usefulness when we provide for the common safety of our [faithful subjects]. Therefore, since we are aware of the serious expense and irrecoverable loss that can occur because of the inexperience of physicians . . ." (Powell, 1971, p. 131). Physicians must visit their patients twice a day and, at the request of the patient, once during the night. Fees were to be determined in part by the distance involved. The physician was required to swear to abide by the regulations fixed by the government, treat the poor gratuitously, and inform the authorities of any apothecary who prepared drugs at less than the required strength. Physicians were forbidden to make any contracts with apothecaries or to own apothecary shops (Powell, 1971; Hartung, 1934).

On the Iberian Peninsula, the first medical licensure regulation, in 1289, imposed no requirement for a course of study in a medical school; forty years later a new law established a university medical degree as a prerequisite for practice (García-Ballester et al., 1989). The law of 1329 and subsequent legislation provided very specific regulations governing physicians' conduct and responsibilities. These regulations, which benefited both the general public and the qualified and responsible phy-

sician, evince a reciprocity of obligations between the profession and the state. Elsewhere in Europe, by contrast, artisans, merchants, surgeons, physicians, and professors were organizing into guilds, gaining charters from municipal, royal, or ecclesiastical authorities, and guaranteeing standards of quality of goods or services in exchange for the privilege of holding a monopoly in their service or commodity.

One of the most striking features of late medieval urban life was its corporative aspect, particularly its guild organization. Perhaps originally formed simply as social organizations under the auspices of a patron saint, guilds had three major interests: (1) social, manifested in both internal and external charitable efforts, and social life within the guild (banquets, etc.); (2) political, especially guilds involved in the production of economically vital commodities; and (3) commercial, involving the protection of financial and vocational interests. In respect to the last, the guilds, by obtaining charters, secured the right to exercise a monopoly on their product or service in a particular geographical area. Such a monopoly entailed the right to make and enforce standards of quality in their products or services, to control hours and working conditions, to limit competition among members, to limit entry into the craft or profession, and to ensure the proper treatment of customers. Part of the monopoly was the right to train and license new members, thus eliminating competition from outside the guild. Although one of the major aims of such measures was economic, the guilds frequently claimed that such restrictions were necessary to maintain a high level of competence and ethics in the trade or profession. Distinct from the merchant and craft guilds, the medieval universities were essentially educational guilds. Beginning in the late twelfth century, some universities gained charters and thus became corporate bodies designed to further educational interests and to protect their members. The *collegium* of teachers who examined the candidates for a degree was, at some universities, vested with the authority to grant a license or, at others, to recommend to secular or ecclesiastical authorities that a license be awarded.

Conditions were so diverse that generalities are often misleading. But usually surgeons were organized in craft guilds; physicians, at least in cities having a university, were not members of a craft guild but were part of, affiliated with, or under the supervision of the medical faculty of the university. In university cities, medical licensure requirements were generally instituted earlier than in those without a university but, from the early fourteenth century on, many cities and towns required those who wished to practice medicine within their jurisdiction to have a degree and license from an acceptable university. Physicians practicing in such places often organized themselves into *collegia* or guilds, and in some instances obtained the authority to examine and license physicians who wanted to practice within the community, regardless of the degrees held by the applicants (Siraisi, 1990).

Practitioners brought to trial for practicing without a license often accused medical and surgical guilds and faculties of self-interest (Kibre, 1953; Cosman, 1973). However, restrictions on medical and surgical practice, whether imposed by authorities or requested by medical faculties or medical or surgical guilds, were justified in terms of the common good, especially the grave dangers to the people if charlatans and quacks were permitted to undertake medical or surgical care. For example, the medical faculty of the University of Paris initiated medical licensure provisions and, in seeking ecclesiastical and royal support to enforce these regulations, continually appealed to the "public interest." The same appeal was made in the medical faculty's attempts to establish a right to oversee the activities of surgeons, apothecaries, barbers, and herbalists, and to prosecute unlicensed practitioners in ecclesiastical or secular courts. The unlicensed practitioners often were women who were frequently "caught in the crossfire" (to use Green's phrase, 1989, p. 447) of the legal battles between licensed groups like physicians and surgeons (see also Park, 1992, for analysis; Kibre, 1953, for narrative examples). As in the early Middle Ages, there was also a concerted effort to exclude the illicit supernatural from healing procedures. Often suspected of being "witches and exorcisoresses of the devil," unlicensed women practitioners were in double jeopardy (Amundsen, 1986, pp. 93–94).

Although guilds were organized to serve their members' self-interest, guild ethics generally were beneficial to the public. In 1423, the physicians and surgeons of London petitioned the mayor and aldermen to authorize the creation of a joint *collegium* of the two crafts. George Unwin, a historian of English guilds, remarks that their petition illustrates "the best spirit of professionalism at this period of London history." He summarizes its contents as follows:

> Their rules were meant to ensure that all practitioners in both branches should be duly qualified, if possible, by a university training, and they sought to provide a hall where reading and disputation in philosophy and medicine could be regularly carried on. No physician was to receive upon himself any cure [i.e., case], "desperate or deadly," without showing it within two or three days to the Rector or one of the Surveyors in order that a professional consultation might be held, and no surgeon was to make any cutting or cauterization which might result in death or maiming without similar notice. Any sick man in need of professional help but too poor to pay for it, might have it by applying to the Rector. In other cases the physician was not to charge excessive fees, but to fix them in accordance with the power of

the sick man, and "measurably after the deserving of his labour." A body composed of two physicians, two surgeons, and two apothecaries, was to search all shops for "false or sophisticated medicines," and to pour all quack remedies into the gutter. (1963, p. 173)

The foundational principles of medieval medicosurgical guild ethics were that each guild member must (1) be ready to help the other; (2) protect the well-being and honor of the guild; and (3) help the sick. The order of these principles is very important. The guilds were functional, inherently selfish organizations designed to promote and protect members' special interests. They were brotherhoods, companies of people united more often than not by a common economic activity. The well-being and honor of the craft depended upon the mutual cooperation of its members. If these conditions were met, then the third—the service rendered or the commodity produced—could be effectively delivered. All these, in late medieval urban life, hinged upon the freedom of the artisans, merchants, professors, physicians, or surgeons to perform their functions unmolested by those who would illicitly meddle in their affairs. Hence they sought an exclusive right to fill a particular role; in exchange, a guild would guarantee a level of expertise in the production of its commodity or in the rendering of its service, and would assume the responsibility to police and to supervise its own members, both in respect to their qualifications, that is, training (leading to licensure), and to their performance. Regulations governing the minutiae of conduct, both within the guild and in relationships with customers or the community, varied considerably from guild to guild and from city to city. But the obligation to ensure competence and quality seems to have been a constant feature.

The highest guarantee of competence to practice medicine, recognized throughout Europe in the late Middle Ages, was a degree granted by a university medical faculty. A university curriculum in medicine, a set body of literature, and the presence of instructors qualified to teach and to test demonstrate that a standard of competence existed. The reality of such a standard has important ethical implications. Luis García-Ballester goes so far as to assert that "Everything connected with the conduct of the physician—from strictly technical matters . . . to the question of fees or the problems of etiquette . . .—was derived from this strictly technical organizational scheme . . . what later became known as medical ethics had this technical, intellectual origin. The specific morality of the practitioner derived, therefore, from his being a healer technically trained, and was essential for his status as an expert in medicine" (1993, pp. 44–45).

An underlying and sometimes articulated principle of medical and surgical guilds was that the guild would ensure that the ill of the community, including the poor and the hopelessly ill, would not be abandoned at the whim of individual physicians or surgeons. This was based at least in part on the conviction, which was very strong in the late Middle Ages, that one had an *officium*, that is, an office or calling, that carried with it certain duties and obligations. In a work devoted to the responsibilities attached to kingship, Thomas Aquinas wrote, "Nor has [the king] the right to question whether or not he will so promote the peace of the community, any more than a physician has the right to question whether he will cure the sick committed to him. For no one ought to deliberate about the ends for which he must act, but only about the means to those ends" (*De regimine principum* 2). In late medieval urban (i.e., corporate) life, physicians and surgeons, by virtue of their privilege of engaging in a legitimate *officium* within the corporate structure of society, had responsibilities both to their *officium* itself, as represented by the guild, company, craft, or *collegium*, and to the community that granted them their privileges.

The church's efforts to define the responsibilities of physicians.

In 1215, a general church council, Lateran IV, promulgated a decree that required annual confession by all Catholics, on pain of excommunication. This decree was widely publicized and strictly enforced. In response, lengthy treatises on moral theology and numerous manuals to aid priests in interrogating penitents during confession were written by moral theologians in an effort to subject the broadest spectrum of human activities to Christian moral principles, including a wide variety of occupations. The discussion that follows is a very condensed summary of the sections of ten primary sources from the early fourteenth through the early sixteenth century that provided priests with a range of questions and moral guidance to be addressed to physicians and surgeons during their mandatory annual confession (Amundsen, 1981). Where the word "physician" appears, it should be understood to include "surgeon."

Competence and diligence. Physicians who are not competent according to accepted standards within the profession sin by practicing medicine. Simply possessing a degree in medicine does not in itself guarantee competence. Competent physicians sin if they do not conscientiously exercise diligence. Rashness, which may result from incompetence or negligence, is a sin in medical practice, especially if patients are harmed. Hence physicians should be cautious and not administer medicines about whose effects they are in doubt; patients should be left in God's hands rather than be exposed to additional danger. Generally, physicians sin if they engage in any experimentation at the patient's risk, especially if they experiment on the poor whom they treat without charge. Physicians also sin if they are so cautious

that they fail to give the appropriate medicines, and especially if they do so in order to prolong the illness and thereby increase their fees.

Fees and charity. Beginning with the assumption that it is licit to receive remuneration for what one is not bound to do gratuitously, but bypassing consideration of how the scholastic principle of "just price" for services could be applied to medical practice, the moral theologians discuss a wide variety of moral aspects of medical fees. The most basic principle is that physicians should ensure that they accept only a "reasonable" fee, as determined by the quality of care; the physician's labor, diligence, and conscientiousness; the custom of the place; and the patient's means. A patient who is rich must not be exploited by exorbitant rates. More problematic is the sick pauper. Is the physician obligated to give free medical care to the poor? This, as we shall see when discussing the medicoethical literature of the high and late Middle Ages, was a source of great frustration for physicians. Thomas Aquinas, beginning with the premise that "no man is sufficient to bestow a work of mercy on all those who need it," suggests that kindness ought first to be shown to those with whom one is united in any way. As for others, if one "stands in such a need that it is not easy to see how he can be succored otherwise, then one is bound to bestow the work of mercy on him." Hence a lawyer is not always obligated to defend the destitute, "or else he would have to put aside all other business and occupy himself entirely in defending the poor. The same holds with physicians in respect to attending the sick" (*Summa theologiae* 2–2, 71, 1). The authors of the confessional literature generally follow Aquinas and specify that physicians must treat the poor gratuitously if the patient would die without treatment.

An obligation to care (especially for hopeless cases). With the advent of medical licensure requirements and medicosurgical guild monopolies, the physicians' option of refusing to treat or of deserting hopelessly ill patients became more circumscribed. Social and religious pressures also changed. Typically the moral theologians maintain that "Desperate cases that, according to the judgments of men, are held to be fatal, sometimes the diligent physician is able to cure, but rarely . . . therefore, clear to the end the physician ought to do what he can to cure the patient" and should not entirely withdraw from the patient "as long as nature does not succumb." If a rich miser is unwilling to employ the services of a physician, the physician is obligated to treat him or her gratis, even to provide medicines without charge; otherwise the physician is killing such a person indirectly. If the rich miser recovers, the physician may sue for fees and expenses; if the miser dies, the heirs are obligated to pay (Amundsen, 1981).

Spiritual obligations of physicians to patients. While the theologians were quite concerned to protect the patient from physical harm and financial exploitation, they were even more determined to guard the well-being of the patient's soul. At Lateran IV in 1215, the following decree was enacted:

> Since bodily infirmity is sometimes caused by sin, the Lord saying to the sick man whom he had healed: "Go and sin no more, lest some worse thing happen to thee" [John 5:14], we declare in the present decree and strictly command that when physicians of the body are called to the bedside of the sick, before all else they admonish them to call for the physician of souls, so that after spiritual health has been restored to them, the application of bodily medicine may be of greater benefit, for the cause being removed the effect will pass away. We publish this decree for the reason that some, when they are sick and are advised by the physician in the course of the sickness to attend to the salvation of their soul, give up all hope and yield more easily to the danger of death. If any physician shall transgress this decree after it has been published by the bishops, let him be cut off from the church till he has made suitable satisfaction for his transgression. And since the soul is far more precious than the body, we forbid under penalty of anathema that a physician advise a patient to have recourse to sinful means for the recovery of bodily health. (Schroeder, 1937, p. 236)

The stipulation that physicians must advise and persuade patients, before all else, to call a priest concerns the curative effect of confession rather than the opportunity to confess before dying. The moral theologians' discussions of this stipulation vary enormously in length, detail, and sensitivity to the problems that it posed. Several maintain that this requirement applied only to cases of extremely dangerous or mortal illnesses. Some go so far as to provide lists of applicable diseases, symptoms, or injuries, especially those demanding immediate attention. This interpretation of the decree is surprising, since it flies in the face of the specific intent that patients be made aware that the requirement to call a confessor is not to be taken as an indication that their condition is hopeless. And some of the authors of the confessional literature interpret it strictly along such lines, making no exceptions. They wrestle with the question of whether a physician is obliged to withdraw from a case if the patient refuses to call a confessor, and reach a variety of answers ranging from a strict "yes" to an unequivocal "no," some of the latter maintaining that if the physician were required to abandon the stubborn patient, "the precept of the church [would] seem against the precept of God." At the end of the Middle Ages, there was no uniformity either of practice or of interpretation of this piece of canonical legislation.

In the context of discussions of the requirement that physicians have their patients summon a confessor, some moral theologians raise the question of whether physi-

cians are obliged to inform terminally ill patients of their condition. There is some disagreement among the moral theologians who address this issue, particularly since physicians (and here Galen is cited) typically tell patients that they will recover, even if there is little hope, since predicting a fatal outcome will likely remove all hope of recovery and hasten death. Generally the authors of the confessional literature insist, however, that unless physicians are certain that their terminally ill patients have set both their spiritual and their temporal affairs in order, they must inform them of their imminent demise, since otherwise harm may ensue to patients' souls and estates.

The second requirement of the legislation in question is for physicians to refrain from advising sinful means for the recovery of health. Several of the moral theologians simply quote that stipulation without elaboration. Others condemn specific matters, such as advising fornication, masturbation, incantations, consumption of intoxicating beverages, breaking the church's fasts, and eating meat on forbidden days.

Abortion and euthanasia. The authors of the confessional literature almost entirely ignore the subject of abortion when discussing the responsibilities and sins of physicians. While all include thorough discussions of abortion under the rubric "homicide" or "abortion" or both, only two include it in their extensive considerations of medical ethics. Apparently the rest did not think that physicians or surgeons were confronted with requests for abortions. Women who sought abortions would probably not have turned to physicians or surgeons, the overwhelming majority of whom were men during the high and late Middle Ages, but to another woman, such as a midwife or an unlicensed female practitioner.

Abortion, regarded both as a sexual sin and, under some circumstances, as homicide, was an issue fraught with interpretive problems during the Middle Ages (Noonan, 1970; Connery, 1977). The opinion of Jerome and Augustine (fourth century) that abortion is not homicide unless the fetus is "formed," that is, vivified or ensouled, was incorporated into medieval canon law, which also included a conflicting decree that applied the penalty for homicide to the induced abortion of a fetus at any stage of development. Theologians, canon lawyers, and the authors of the confessional literature were split between these two positions. The stricter interpretation generally forbade abortion at all times and under all circumstances. The more liberal interpretation, which was influenced by Aristotelian embryology, did not classify induced abortion as a mortal sin within the first forty days of pregnancy in the case of a male fetus, and eighty (or, according to some, ninety) days in the case of a female, and permitted abortion during these periods under a variety of extenuating circumstances. The conflict between the interpretations of these two camps was not resolved until long after the Middle Ages. Both, however, clearly condemned abortion as reprehensible if performed simply to destroy the unwanted consequence of sexual intercourse.

What we call active euthanasia is a subject that the moral theologians thus far surveyed never raised when discussing the sins of physicians; it was probably regarded throughout the Middle Ages simply as homicide on the physician's part and suicide on the patient's, assuming willing involvement by the latter. Martin Azpilcueta, better known as Navarrus, a leading canon lawyer and moral theologian of the sixteenth century, wrote in 1568 that the physician sins who gives any medicine that he knows is harmful, "even if he administers it out of pity or in order to please the patient." Navarrus's statement seems clear and unambiguous: active euthanasia, whether motivated by pity or by the wish of the patient, is sinful. This must be one of the earliest articulations regarding active euthanasia in such precise terms. Navarrus gives as his authority the canon lawyer Panormitanus (early fifteenth century), who had simply given the opinion that those having custody or serving a sick person sin greatly if, motivated by "a sort of pity," they obey or indulge the "corrupted desire" of the ill. Before active euthanasia was seen as a separate moral category, the closest the authors of the confessional literature could have come to including relevant comments in their sections on physicians' sins would have been to have stated that it was a sin for physicians to kill or poison their patients intentionally.

The effects of the moral theologians' efforts.   Medieval European society was, with the exception of a small number of Jews and heretics (e.g., Albigensians and Waldensians), exclusively Catholic. Guaranteed the allegiance of virtually the entire population of western Europe and the prestige of ecclesiastical institutions, the church could exercise jurisdiction over areas of life that now would be the concern of either secular authority or the individual conscience. The church promulgated laws and expected obedience. Ecclesiastical courts imposed penalties ranging from penance to imprisonment to excommunication. The extent to which the confessional influenced ethics and conduct cannot be gauged with certainty. The authors of the confessional literature strove both to educate the laity so that they might be able to identify previously unknown sins, both of commission and of omission, and to correct sinful practices. The best confession was one that led to a changed life, and a changed life should be one in as close conformity to the expectations and standards of the church as possible. The priest's authority "to loose and to bind," although ultimately of eternal consequence, applied also to this life in that it included the authority—indeed, the responsibility—to grant forgiveness and restoration only

to those who satisfied the requirements of the confessional, and to impose sanctions upon those who refused. The ultimate sanction, excommunication, when imposed upon those who exercised their vocation by license, would deprive them of their livelihood. Whether such steps were ever taken against physicians during the high and late Middle Ages remains unclear. Nevertheless, the morally educating (or possibly alienating) effects of this annual interrogation, which employed the detailed scrutiny available to every priest in his confessional manual, must have been profound.

Physicians' and surgeons' advice on ethics and etiquette.   In the extensive medical and surgical literature that has survived from the high and late Middle Ages, one occasionally encounters comments made directly on matters of medical ethics or etiquette. Surgical manuals, for example, often begin with a discussion of the moral and educational qualifications of a practitioner, bedside manner, fees, and a variety of related matters. Medical and surgical literature also contains comments that indirectly reveal aspects of the ethical standards of the author, especially in the tractates written by physicians who attempted to understand and deal with the outbreaks of plague that struck Europe during the late Middle Ages.

Loren MacKinney perceived that, by the twelfth century, a change in spirit had occurred in medical literature from monastic to secular, a "shift of emphasis from ideals to practical considerations," a "despiritualization of the medical physician," particularly in the introduction of various "tricks of the trade" and a predominant concern with fees (1952, pp. 23ff.). He credits this change to such factors as rapid urbanization, and he is probably right to a degree. But it is important to note the different walks of life from which the authors of the sources came. While the literature from the early Middle Ages was likely composed by monks, that of the high and late Middle Ages was written mainly by secular physicians. So it is not surprising that its tone is less otherworldly than that of the earlier treatises. The later literature was written with the clear intention of providing practitioners with two types of information: (1) the ideal physician's character, preparation, and practice; and (2) very practical and sometimes questionable advice on how best to survive in the profession. Both were at least moderately informed by the teachings of the medieval Catholic church.

The first category consists of the same range of commonsensical advice as appears in Hippocratic treatises and in the medicoethical literature of the early Middle Ages. The second appeared especially in discussions of fees. As early as the tenth century, the physician is advised: "At the outset, accept at least half of the remuneration without hesitation, for he who wishes to buy [your services] is disposed to pay and to beg [for treatment]. Get it while he is suffering, for when the pain ceases, your services also cease" (MacKinney, 1952, p. 24). Somewhat more enlightened is the suggestion by William of Saliceto (thirteenth century) that "a high salary, if demanded, imparts to the physician an air of authority, which strengthens the confidence of the patient in him . . . so that the sick man imagines from this that he is more skillful than others and ought therefore to be successful in curing him" (Mirfeld, 1936, p. 132).

Some of the advice that follows, written by physicians or surgeons, may appear particularly crass. It is, however, important to realize that the medical literature of the time stressed, in Luis García-Ballester's words,

> the mutual confidence that should exist between doctor and patient. Without such confidence the efficacy of the curative action would be greatly undermined. . . . the physician's or surgeon's confidence in his patient was demonstrated by two conditions of equal significance: the first was that the patient should carry out what had been prescribed by the healer; the second that the patient should pay the remuneration agreed upon. The fee would be for the doctor the objective and tangible expression of his relationship with the patient and that of the patient with the doctor, while, at the same time, it would be a guarantee of continuity in treatment. (1993, p. 51)

Henry de Mondeville (fourteenth century) laments that "The chief object of the patient, and the one idea which dominates all his actions, is to get cured, and when once he is cured, he forgets his own obligations and omits to pay; the object of the surgeon, on the other hand, is to obtain his money, and he should never be satisfied with a promise or a pledge, but he should either have the money in advance or take a bond for it" (Hammond, 1960, p. 159; Welborn, 1938, p. 356). Mondeville's attitude was probably the fruit of bitter experience. Official documents from the late Middle Ages record many cases of physicians suing patients in order to collect their fees. In most cases in which the treatment had been unsuccessful, the suit went in favor of the patient. Quite unreasonable demands by patients for extensive credit, the necessity that physicians sometimes demand securities before undertaking treatment, and lucrative contractual arrangements all contribute to the complex and ethically ambiguous way in which late medieval medical and surgical practitioners made a living (Rawcliffe, 1988, for late medieval England).

One area in which physicians seemed to act against their more mercenary interests was in providing advice that would keep potential patients from needing their services. Mondeville wrestled with the problem presented by surgeons' advising their patients how to stay healthy, "because the treatment which stops the onset of a new disease is more useful to a patient than all other treatments. But this is, as one can see, useless and harmful to the surgeon because he thus stops the appearance of a disease whose treatment would be advantageous to himself" (Hammond, 1960, p. 155; Welborn, 1938, p. 355).

Neither Mondeville nor his contemporary, John Arderne, seem to have felt any embarrassment over pressing for as high a fee as possible. The former recommends that "The surgeon should pretend that he has no living nor capital except his profession, and that everything is as dear as possible, especially drugs and ointments; that the fee is nothing as compared with his services; and the wages of all other artisans, masons, for example, have doubled of late" (Hammond, 1960, p. 156). He considered it essential that the fee not be reduced too much. It would be better, then, to charge nothing.

In determining how much to charge, Mondeville recommends that the surgeon consider three things: "First, his own standing in the profession, then the [financial] condition of the patient, and, third, the seriousness of the illness" (Hammond, 1960, p. 156; Welborn, 1938, p. 356). It was the second of these that was probably the most trying. Mondeville advises the doctor not "to have too much faith in appearances. Rich people have a bad habit of appearing before him in old clothes, or if they do happen to be well dressed, they make up all sorts of excuses for demanding lower fees" (Welborn, 1938, p. 356). So strong, though, is the sense of obligation to succor the poor gratis, or at least to give the appearance of doing so, that physicians and surgeons probably were quite frequently faced with very difficult judgments.

The motivation of physicians and surgeons to extend charity to the poor was more than the advantages that might accrue to their reputation and to the honor of the profession; it was a product of enlightened self-interest, with eternal consequences, fully compatible with the theology of the time, as is succinctly expressed by Mondeville: "You, then, surgeons, if you operate conscientiously upon the rich for a sufficient fee and upon the poor for charity, you ought not to fear the ravages of fire, nor of rain nor of wind; you need not take holy orders or make pilgrimages nor undertake any work of that kind, because by your science you can save your souls alive, live without poverty, and die in your house" (Hammond, 1960, p. 156).

While some effect of the church's teaching is manifest in even Mondeville's fee policies, in other areas spiritual concerns are more evident. An anonymous twelfth-century Salernitan treatise advises: "When you reach [a patient's] house and before you see him, ask if he has seen his confessor. If he has not done so, have him either do it or promise to do it. For if he hears mention of this after you have examined him and have considered the signs of the disease, he will begin to despair of recovery, because he will think that you despair of it too" (De Renzi, 1852–1857, vol. 2, p. 74). This work was composed some time before Lateran IV of 1215, and thus before physicians were required "before all else to advise and persuade" their patients to call a confessor. The anonymous author of this treatise does not appear unusually devout. Indeed, were one to attach an adjective to the work, "eminently practical" would describe it better than any other. The author, of course, was a member of a society in which the belief in the necessity of confession before death was deeply ingrained. While he may not have considered it especially his own spiritual duty to look after his patients' spiritual as well as physical health, he must have considered the alternative of advising patients to confess only when in dire straits to be potentially dangerous to them.

The advice on confession, as it appears in a treatise attributed to Arnald of Villanova (late thirteenth century), is significantly different in emphasis from that in the anonymous Salernitan piece: "[W]hen you come to a house, inquire before you go to the sick whether he has confessed, and if he has not, he should immediately or promise you that he will confess immediately, and this must not be neglected because many illnesses originate on account of sin and are cured by the Supreme Physician after having been purified from squalor by the tears of contrition, according to what is said in the Gospel: 'Go, and sin no more, lest something worse happens to you'" (Sigerist, 1946, p. 141). This version, written after Lateran IV, quoting the same Scripture as the canon law, demonstrates the direct influence of a constitution of canon law on a strictly secular piece of medical literature, as does even more strongly the following passage in an anonymous plague tractate composed in 1411: "If it is certain from the symptoms that it is actually pestilence that has afflicted the patient, the physician first must advise the patient to set himself right with God by making a will and by making a confession of his sins, as is set forth according to the Decretals; since a corporal illness comes not only from a fault of the body but also from a spiritual failing as the Lord declares in the gospel and the priests also tell us" (Amundsen, 1977, p. 416). About a century earlier, similar advice had been given by Mondeville: "Do not let the patient be concerned about any business except spiritual matters only, such as confession and his will and arranging similar affairs in accordance with the rules of the Catholic faith" (Amundsen, 1986, p. 90). Whether these writings composed after Lateran IV are simply examples of lip service to ecclesiastical authority or reflect genuine approval of the underlying principle upon which the legislation was based must remain an open question.

An eleventh-century treatise advises that the physician should "never become involved knowingly with any who are about to die or who are incurable" (Mac-

Kinney, 1952, p. 23). Although from the earliest times such counsel was common, in the late Middle Ages it was becoming increasingly less so. The previously quoted anonymous Salernitan treatise from the twelfth century advises the physician, just before leaving, to "promise the patient that with the help of God you will cure him. As you go away, however, you should tell his servants that he is seriously ill, because if he recovers you will receive greater credit and praise, and if he dies, they will testify that even from the beginning you despaired of his health" (De Renzi, 1852–1857, vol. 2, p. 75). Although this treatise may be described as eminently practical, it is not clear that this particular bit of advice is ethical.

A parallel passage in a treatise attributed to Arnald of Villanova (late thirteenth century) is nearly identical, with the significant difference that instead of promising the patient "that with the help of God you will cure him," which still leaves the matter in doubt and at least partially in God's hands, it advises more crassly that "you promise health to the patient who is hanging on your lips" (Sigerist, 1946, p. 142). This treatise appears to have been hastily thrown together from various sources, since elsewhere it flatly contradicts the advice that the physician should promise health to the patient. Later it suggests that the physician "must be . . . circumspect and cautious in answering questions, ambiguous in making a prognosis, just in making promises; and he should not promise health because in doing so he would assume a divine function and insult God. He should rather promise faithfulness and attentiveness . . ." (Sigerist, 1946, p. 141). For two such opposing pieces of advice to be found in the same treatise is unusual. Such conflicting opinions, however, are typical of medical ethics in the late Middle Ages. For example, Bernard de Gordon (thirteenth/fourteenth centuries) advised that if there was little likelihood of a patient's recovering, "One should try to escape from such cases, provided one can do so honorably" (Demaitre, 1980, p. 153). Nevertheless, he also expresses a concern to do everything possible to postpone the death of terminally ill patients.

William of Saliceto (thirteenth century) recommends that the physician should "comfort his patient, and on every occasion should promise him restoration to health, even if the physician himself shall regard the case as desperate." He justifies this on the grounds that this will greatly encourage the patient, increasing his chances of recovering. He further suggests that the physician "acquaint the friends of his patient with the truth, and discuss the case fully with them as he shall deem best, lest he incur scandal or loss of reputation from inability to offer a satisfactory statement of the case, and lest the friends of the patient regard him with distrust: nor will he then be held responsible for having caused the death of a patient who shall die; but he will be given credit for having cured the man who lives and is restored to health" (Mirfeld, 1936, p. 122). William's reason for giving a favorable prognosis to the critically ill patient is strictly for the latter's benefit. He recommends that the physician tell the patient's friends the truth for the physician's own protection, a far different piece of advice from that in the two treatises previously discussed, which recommend that the physician, regardless of the patient's actual condition, advise those close to him or her that the case is dangerous and that the patient is not faring well.

Mondeville wrote that the surgeon "ought to promise a cure to every sick person, but he should refuse as far as possible all dangerous cases, and he should never accept desperately sick ones" (Welborn, 1938, p. 350). Physicians and surgeons were sometimes charged with the deaths of patients in the late Middle Ages, and the fear of facing blame for a patient's death still motivated some to recommend, as Mondeville did, that dangerous cases not be taken on. Mondeville, incidentally, writes at some length about how to ensure that a patient's friends or relatives can be compelled to exonerate the surgeon if a case should end in the patient's death (Welborn, 1938). Nevertheless, advice not to take on dangerous cases occurs much less often in late medieval sources than in the medical literature of ancient Greece and Rome. Instead, physicians are advised to protect themselves either by telling the relatives or friends of the patient that the situation is critical, regardless of the patient's condition, or to tell the truth in cases that actually are critical.

Plague and medical ethics in the late Middle Ages. The devastating plague epidemics that periodically swept through Europe, beginning in 1348 and continuing well beyond the Middle Ages, tried and tested the ethics of medieval physicians far beyond conditions encountered in ordinary practice. Contemporary sources almost uniformly express the conviction that plague was extremely contagious. Merely being in the vicinity of the sick, many supposed, doomed one to become infected and die. Numerous sources describe parents deserting their dying children, children their parents, wives fleeing from their sick husbands, and husbands from their wives. All who could, fled the cities and towns to take refuge in the countryside. Not only were the sick deserted by their families; physicians would not come near them, and even priests would not meet the final spiritual needs of the dying. Such accounts are plentiful. But they must be set against abundant accounts of responsible actions by family members, magistrates, physicians, and clergy.

Some physicians undoubtedly did flee. In 1382 Venice stipulated that physicians who fled during epidemics would lose their citizenship. Barcelona and Cologne took similar action during the sixteenth century. While

it is impossible to determine the extent to which physicians actually did flee from plague-ridden communities, the percentage was probably relatively small. A study of nearly three hundred plague tractates written by physicians between 1348 and the early sixteenth century found not even one allusion to physicians who fled from areas afflicted with plague (Amundsen, 1977). Medieval physicians were not at all timid in castigating their colleagues in writing. Vitriolic criticism, particularly of fellow physicians' theories and medical techniques, is found throughout the medical literature. If the flight of physicians had been extensive, then one should encounter among the plague tractates such statements as "Although many other physicians fled, I remained."

Many physicians did advise people to flee from plague-infected areas as the best form of prevention. This advice, however, was typically followed by the concession that since flight "rarely is possible for most people, I advise that, while remaining, you. . . ." Prevention is the primary concern of most of the plague tractates. Even if they are unanimous in urging flight, it does not follow that the physicians who wrote them intended by doing so to justify flight for themselves and their colleagues. The authors of the tractates appear simply to have assumed that their readers would be able to avail themselves of the services of physicians during plague epidemics.

Did physicians who fled, or who refused to visit and diagnose those perhaps afflicted with pestilence, or who abandoned patients actually suffering from plague, violate their responsibilities as conceived at that time? Contemporary sources make it abundantly clear that both the public at large and physicians themselves viewed those physicians who fled from plague as having acted disgracefully. In the mid-fourteenth century, Guy de Chauliac, at one time personal physician to the pope, wrote concerning his own activities during the Black Death, the earliest and most devastating of a long series of plague epidemics: "It was so contagious . . . that even by looking at one another people caught it. . . . And I, to avoid infamy, dared not absent myself but with continual fear preserved myself as best I could" (Campbell, 1931, p. 3). Faced with both extreme peril to themselves and with the knowledge of the extremely high mortality rate of plague victims, physicians found themselves in an ethical quandary. Chauliac wrote, "It was useless and shameful for the doctors, the more so as they dared not visit the sick, for fear of being infected. And when they did visit them, they did hardly anything for them, and were paid nothing" (Campbell, 1931, p. 3).

One tractate maintains that physicians "must treat the ill," and another that "they must treat or visit the ill" (Amundsen, 1977, p. 414). The difference between these two is very important. While the first holds that physicians must treat plague victims, the second asserts that physicians must treat *or* visit the afflicted. Physicians who fled from a plague-infected area or hid in fear obviously failed even to attempt to diagnose the condition. But if the sick were indeed afflicted with the plague (since not all who became ill during a time of plague were necessarily afflicted with the plague), did physicians have an ethical obligation to attempt treatment?

A basic feature of medieval medical and surgical guild ethics was an obligation to be available to treat the ill or injured of the community and not to abandon hopeless cases. To the moral theologians who wrote the confessional literature, the duty to treat and to stay with the patient was unequivocal, although they were considering normal conditions rather than the exigencies of plague epidemics. Physicians were ambivalent about whether to take on hopeless cases; so were authors of the plague tractates. During outbreaks of plague, some physicians viewed the disease as treatable and others as at least potentially curable. Many physicians felt compelled to investigate the various strains of plague and to seek ways both to prevent and to treat them. Many of the plague tractates discuss treatment, distinguishing among different varieties of plague and stressing their faith in the efficacy of their curative methods. Some physicians, however, considered all forms of plague to be incurable. Of course physicians had to visit the ill to determine whether they were suffering from pestilence. If the condition was diagnosed as plague, some physicians then sought to determine whether the patient was possibly curable.

A plague tractate composed in 1411 advises: "If the patient is curable, the physician will undertake treatment in God's name. If he is incurable, the physician should leave him to die, in accord with the commentary on the second of the aphorisms [probably a medieval commentary on *Aphorisms* II in the Hippocratic Corpus]. Those who are going to die must be distinguished by prognostic signs and then you should flee from them. He labors in vain who attempts to treat such as these" (Amundsen, 1977, pp. 416–417). A plague tractate written in 1406 suggests that physicians not immediately inform patients if their condition is diagnosed as hopeless. Nevertheless, the physician "should refrain from administering anything to the patient that will cause him to die quickly, for then he would be a murderer" (Amundsen, 1977, p. 417, n. 64).

Various contemporary lay accounts from the time of the Black Death accuse some physicians of hiding in their houses and refusing to visit the sick for fear of infection. The authors of many plague tractates, while advising the general public to avoid contact with those afflicted with plague, do not direct such advice to their colleagues. They recommend varied and imaginative prophylactic techniques for use when visiting plague vic-

tims. The variety and abundance of such recommended precautions show the extent to which many physicians thought they were effective; moreover, there are numerous artistic representations of physicians who employed prophylactic measures while visiting plague victims. Many tractates deal exclusively with prophylaxis because their authors feel that treatment must be left to the discretion of the physician handling the case. Those that do include a discussion of treatment generally express great confidence in the curative methods prescribed. Many introduce new methods claimed effective by physicians who say they have employed them.

Some people did recover from the plague, from some strains of the disease more than from others; and although such cases of recovery were often in spite of the treatments to which the patients had been subjected, the attending physicians would have thought that their techniques had indeed been effective. The success rate in medieval medicine was, of course, much lower than in modern medicine; hence the expectations of both physicians and the public were not nearly as high as those of the present. The efforts of physicians to combat and cure various strains of plague, as well as their attempts to educate people in prevention and treatment by writing plague tractates, graphically demonstrate a high level of ethical and professional responsibility.

Summary and conclusions

The medicoethical treatises of the early Middle Ages blend Hippocratic etiquette with Christian morality, particularly emphasizing compassion and charity. The high and late medieval treatises, while loyal to the traditional concerns of the genre, suggest a new pragmatism born of the realities of medical practice by secular Catholic practitioners in a society starkly different from that of the monastic ethos of the early medieval medical literature. Although no mention of guilds or universities appears in this later literature, its tone and emphasis demonstrate that its authors regarded the practice of the art of medicine as a privilege that required training and skill, and carried consequent responsibilities. While there is no direct articulation of physicians' obligations to their immediate community in this literature, the obligation to the Christian community at large—an obligation to extend medical charity to the poor and destitute—is implicit and sometimes explicit.

Treating dangerous and even desperate cases is not discouraged in the later literature nearly as often as it had been before. Warnings against it are so infrequent, compared with advice on what to tell critically ill patients and their relatives or friends, that one may conclude there was a growing tendency to take on dangerous or even hopeless cases. But were physicians who in the late Middle Ages declined to treat patients for whom they foresaw little or no hope of recovery, still acting within the strictures of accepted ethics? This was a time during which popular attitudes toward physicians' responsibilities to the terminally ill were changing. Physicians who refused to treat patients were accused of deserting them because they thought they would not be paid for their services, while physicians who continued to treat such patients were suspected of greed for ministering to patients they know would not recover.

We see these two extremes illustrated by two sermons preached in fourteenth-century England. Lanfranc of Milan exclaimed, "O wretched physician, who for the money that you may not hope to get, desert the human body travailing in peril of death; and allow him, whom, according to the law of God, you should love and have most concern for, of all creatures under heaven, to be in jeopardy of life and limb, when you can and know how to apply a suitable remedy" (Owst, 1966, p. 351). John Bromyard, by contrast, asserted, "All craftsmen would at once refuse a job for which unsuitable materials were provided. If a carpenter were offered wages for the building of a house with planks that were too short or otherwise unsuitable, he would at once say: 'I will not take the wage or have anything to do with it, because the timber is of no use.' Similarly the physician who can see no hope of saving his patient" (Owst, 1966, p. 351).

Bromyard's sentiments were deeply rooted in tradition, but attitudes were changing. This change is very significant for the history of medical ethics. It seems to have been the product of two complementary and possibly related catalysts. The first is that the practice of medicine and surgery had been changed from a right to a privilege. A specific authority, whether royal, ecclesiastical, or municipal, granted to a select few the privilege of practicing in a specified, limited region. The authorities who granted what was essentially a monopoly also were ostensibly responsible for protecting that monopoly, and the privilege of holding a monopoly carried certain responsibilities, among them to service the sick of the community indiscriminately.

The second source of the growing tendency to take on dangerous or hopeless cases is the increasing theological insistence that physicians should do all they could to cure until the end, or nearly the end, and the church's support for their right to receive fees under such circumstances. One sees in the confessional literature the seeds of what was later to blossom into a medical duty to prolong life. The view is strongly articulated that physicians are religiously obligated to extend care to a rich miser even if he or she both resists treatment and refuses to pay. Some moral theologians also maintain that even if patients refuse to call a confessor, physicians must not desert them, since help must be given to those who are

in danger, regardless of how stubborn they are. While this is still far from an imperative to prolong life, it is a significant change from earlier medical attitudes and practice.

This fundamental change in perceived responsibilities of physicians to their patients is illustrated by the acts of a late-twelfth-century and a mid-eighteenth-century pope, both of whom address the request of physicians to enter the priesthood. Clement III, in the late twelfth century, ruled that the physician in question should search his memory to ensure that he had never, even inadvertently, harmed a patient by any treatment that he had administered. In the mid-eighteenth century, Benedict XIV's ruling centered on the problem that physicians can never be entirely positive that they have consistently used every available means for patients who died under their care (Amundsen and Ferngren, 1983). The concern in the twelfth century was with harm perhaps inflicted actively on patients: "Did you ever harm patients by the treatment you gave them?" But by the eighteenth century, attention focused on harm that may have resulted from oversight: "Did you ever harm patients by failing to give them the treatment you should have given?" These two papal rulings highlight a fundamental change both in physicians' sense of responsibility to their patients and in social and religious expectations, a change that occurred primarily in the late Middle Ages.

We look nearly in vain in the medicoethical literature of the late Middle Ages for statements on two topics of medical ethics: abortion and euthanasia. We cannot conclude from this that both theologians and physicians considered abortion and euthanasia ethical for physicians to perform. Indeed, the presumption is quite the opposite. Theologians and physicians alike took it for granted that both were sinful, so much so that their sinfulness need not be mentioned explicitly. Rather, it would seem that abortion was a procedure for which women would turn to someone other than a male physician or surgeon. Facilitating the death of a patient was undoubtedly so repugnant to medieval moral principles that to mention it as unethical for a physician to do would have been gratuitous, at least in a general treatise on medical ethics.

When the contents of the late medieval medicoethical treatises are supplemented by guild ethics and the moral pronouncements of the theologians, as well as by the evidence of physicians' conscientious response to the outbreaks of plague, the picture that emerges is of relatively high ethical standards. Although "Hippocratic ideals" persisted throughout the Middle Ages and provided the basis for medical etiquette, the role and responsibilities of physicians and surgeons were variously affected by Christian morality. This is particularly evident in concern for the gratuitous treatment of the poor, both by individual physicians and by professional associations. The discipline of moral theology provided distinct criteria for medical ethics from a late medieval Catholic perspective. Secular law and medicosurgical organizations, including university faculties, established regulations and standards of competence for medical licensure, and guilds and university faculties set precise codes of conduct. Essentially, the creation of medical licensure, medical faculties, and professional organizations helped to formulate medical professionalism and ethics in a sense that is still very much present today.

DARREL W. AMUNDSEN

While all the articles in this section and the other sections of this entry are relevant, see especially the other articles in this subsection: GREECE AND ROME, *and* EARLY CHRISTIANITY. *Directly related to this article are the entries* HOSPITAL, *article on* MEDIEVAL AND RENAISSANCE HISTORY; ROMAN CATHOLICISM; MEDICINE AS A PROFESSION; *and* NATURAL LAW. *For a further discussion of topics mentioned in this article, see the entries* ABORTION, *section on* RELIGIOUS TRADITIONS, *article on* ROMAN CATHOLIC PERSPECTIVES; DEATH: ART OF DYING, *article on* ARS MORIENDI; DEATH AND DYING: EUTHANASIA AND SUSTAINING LIFE; *and* INFORMATION DISCLOSURE. *Other relevant material may be found under the entries* BENEFICENCE; CASUISTRY; DEATH, *articles on* WESTERN RELIGIOUS THOUGHT, *and* DEATH IN THE WESTERN WORLD (*with its* POSTSCRIPT); EASTERN ORTHODOX CHRISTIANITY; ETHICS, *article on* RELIGION AND MORALITY; EUGENICS AND RELIGIOUS LAW, *article on* CHRISTIANITY; HEALTH AND DISEASE, *article on* HISTORY OF THE CONCEPTS; *and* MEDICAL CODES AND OATHS, *article on* HISTORY.

Bibliography

AMUNDSEN, DARREL W. 1971. "Visigothic Medical Legislation." *Bulletin of the History of Medicine* 45, no. 6: 553–569.

———. 1977. "Medical Deontology and Pestilential Disease in the Late Middle Ages." *Journal of the History of Medicine and Allied Sciences* 32, no. 4:403–421.

———. 1978. "Medieval Canon Law on Medical and Surgical Practice by the Clergy." *Bulletin of the History of Medicine* 52, no. 1:22–44.

———. 1979. "Medicine and Surgery as Art or Craft: The Role of Schematic Literature in the Separation of Medicine and Surgery in the Late Middle Ages." *Transactions and Studies of the College of Physicians of Philadelphia*, n.s. 1, no. 1:43–57.

———. 1981. "Casuistry and Professional Obligations: The Regulation of Physicians by the Court of Conscience in the Late Middle Ages." *Transactions and Studies of the College of Physicians of Philadelphia* 3, no. 1:22–39, and 3, no. 2:93–112.

———. 1986. "The Medieval Catholic Tradition." In *Caring and Curing: Health and Medicine in the Western Religious Traditions*, pp. 65–107. Edited by Ronald L. Numbers and Darrel W. Amundsen. New York: Macmillan.

AMUNDSEN, DARREL W., and FERNGREN, GARY B. 1983. "Evolution of the Patient–Physician Relationship: Antiquity Through the Renaissance." In *The Clinical Encounter: The Moral Fabric of the Patient–Physician Relationship*, pp. 1–46. Edited by Earl E. Shelp. Dordrecht, Netherlands: D. Reidel.

CAMPBELL, ANNA MONTGOMERY. 1931. *The Black Death and Men of Learning.* New York: Columbia University Press.

CONNERY, JOHN R. 1977. *Abortion: The Development of the Roman Catholic Perspective.* Chicago: Loyola University Press.

COSMAN, MADELEINE PELNER. 1973. "Medieval Medical Malpractice: The Dicta and the Dockets." *Bulletin of the New York Academy of Medicine* 49, no. 1:22–47.

DEMAITRE, LUKE E. 1980. *Doctor Bernard de Gordon: Professor and Practitioner.* Toronto: Pontifical Institute of Medieval Studies.

DE RENZI, SALVATORE, ed. 1852–1857. *Collectio salernitana.* 5 vols. Naples: Filiatre-Sebezio.

FLINT, VALERIE J. 1989. "The Early 'Medicus,' the Saint—and the Enchanter." *Social History of Medicine* 2, no. 2: 127–145.

———. 1991. *The Rise of Magic in Early Medieval Europe.* Princeton, N.J.: Princeton University Press.

GARCÍA-BALLESTER, LUIS. 1993. "Medical Ethics in Transition in the Latin Medicine of the Thirteenth and Fourteenth Centuries: New Prospects on the Physician–Patient Relationship and the Doctor's Fee." In *Doctors and Ethics: The Earlier Historical Setting of Professional Ethics*, pp. 38–71. Edited by Andrew Wear, Johanna Geyer-Kordesch, and Roger K. French. Amsterdam: Rodopi.

GARCÍA-BALLESTER, LUIS; MCVAUGH, MICHAEL R.; and RUBIO-VELA, AGUSTÍN. 1989. *Medical Licensing and Learning in Fourteenth-Century Valencia.* Transactions of the American Philosophical Society, vol. 79, pt. 6. Philadelphia: American Philosophical Society.

GREEN, MONICA. 1989. "Women's Medical Practice and Health Care in Medieval Europe." *Signs* 14, no. 2:434–473.

HAMMOND, E. A. 1960. "Incomes of Medieval English Doctors." *Journal of the History of Medicine and Allied Sciences* 15:154–169.

HARTUNG, EDWARD F. 1934. "Medical Regulations of Frederick the Second of Hohenstaufen." *Medical Life* 41: 587–601.

HUME, EDGAR E. 1940. *The Medical Work of the Knights Hospitallers of Saint John of Jerusalem.* Baltimore: Johns Hopkins University Press.

KIBRE, PEARL. 1953. "The Faculty of Medicine at Paris, Charlatanism and Unlicensed Medical Practices in the Later Middle Ages." *Bulletin of the History of Medicine* 27, no. 1:1–20.

MACKINNEY, LOREN C. 1952. "Medical Ethics and Etiquette in the Early Middle Ages: The Persistence of Hippocratic Ideals." *Bulletin of the History of Medicine* 26, no. 1:1–31.

MILLER, TIMOTHY S. 1978. "The Knights of Saint John

and the Hospitals of the Latin West." *Speculum* 53, no. 4: 709–733.

MIRFELD, JOHN. 1936. *Johannes de Mirfeld of St. Bartholemew's, Smithfield: His Life and Works.* Edited by Percival Horton-Smith Hartley and Harold Richard Aldridge. Cambridge: At the University Press.

NOONAN, JOHN T., JR. 1970. "An Almost Absolute Value in History." In *The Morality of Abortion: Legal and Historical Perspectives*, pp. 1–59. Edited by John T. Noonan, Jr. Cambridge, Mass.: Harvard University Press.

OWST, GERALD R. 1966. *Literature and Pulpit in Medieval England: A Neglected Chapter in the History of English Letters and of the English People.* Oxford: Basil Blackwell.

PARK, KATHARINE. 1992. "Medicine and Society in Medieval Europe, 500–1500." In *Medicine in Society: Historical Essays*, pp. 59–90. Edited by Andrew Wear. Cambridge: At the University Press.

POWELL, JAMES M., trans. 1971. *The Liber Augustalis or Constitutions of Melfi, Promulgated by the Emperor Frederick II for the Kingdom of Sicily in 1231.* Syracuse, N.Y.: Syracuse University Press.

RAWCLIFFE, CAROLE. 1988. "The Profits of Practice: The Wealth and Status of Medical Men in Later Medieval England." *Social History of Medicine* 1, no. 1:61–78.

SCHROEDER, HENRY JOSEPH, ed. 1937. *Disciplinary Decrees of the General Councils.* St. Louis, Mo.: Herder.

SIGERIST, HENRY ERNEST. 1946. "Bedside Manners in the Middle Ages: The Treatise *De Cautelis Medicorum* Attributed to Arnald of Villanova." *Quarterly Bulletin of the Northwestern University Medical School* 20:136–143.

SIRAISI, NANCY G. 1990. *Medieval and Early Renaissance Medicine: An Introduction to Knowledge and Practice.* Chicago: University of Chicago Press.

ULLMANN, WALTER. 1971. "Public Welfare and Social Legislation in the Early Medieval Councils." In *Councils and Assemblies: Papers Read at the Eighth Summer Meeting and the Ninth Winter Meeting of the Ecclesiastical History Society*, pp. 1–39. Edited by G. J. Cuming and Derek Baker. Studies in Church History, vol. 7. Cambridge: At the University Press.

UNWIN, GEORGE. 1963. *The Guilds and Companies of London.* 4th ed. London: Frank Cass.

WELBORN, MARY CATHERINE. 1938. "The Long Tradition: A Study in Fourteenth-Century Medical Deontology." In *Medieval and Historiographical Essays in Honor of James Westfall Thompson*, pp. 344–357. Edited by James Lea Cate and Eugene N. Anderson. Chicago: University of Chicago Press.

B. RENAISSANCE AND ENLIGHTENMENT

Medicine in early modern Europe (from the later fifteenth century to the end of the eighteenth century) is best characterized by its diversity of practitioners, practices, and conceptual foundations. Even by the end of the eighteenth century, few places in Europe had effective regulations to restrict medical practice to people with certain kinds of certification, or to regulate their practices. University-educated practitioners differed sharply with one another about the true conceptual foundations of good and effective medical practice, while among the merely literate, or even the illiterate, practitioners, views about the constitution of good medicine varied even more.

Many medical changes occurred during the period: The number of university-educated physicians rose considerably, as did the number of other formally trained (usually apprenticed) practitioners. With the proliferation of schooling, the educational level of many ordinary practitioners rose. And while the beginning of the period was marked by the proliferation of various philosophical and medical systems, by the end of the eighteenth century most of those systems had been set aside by the educated elite in favor of varieties of a more unified "science."

Throughout the period, no formal systems of medical ethics existed per se. Yet medical practitioners took varying degrees of interest in ethical issues, issues that commonly focused on the personal character of the practitioner. The discussion of the period that follows is therefore divided into two parts: a description of the general structures of the period and the organization of medical practice; and the debates among the literate, and especially among the learned, over the foundations of good medical practice and behavior.

Social structures of medical practice

European society underwent a major transformation from the fifteenth to the eighteenth century. Throughout the period, Europe remained an overwhelmingly rural region, and at times the population grew rapidly. And, because of demographic, economic, political, and intellectual changes, city life came to typify refinement. As a result, most of the great changes in medical practices and mores took place in the cities, although most of the people needing care continued to live in the countryside.

The vast majority of the people in Europe—nine in ten, or more, depending on when and where—lived in a rural environment: in small towns or villages, in hamlets, or on rural manors; a few even resided in the forests and fields. In the fifteenth century, many rural laboring people lived relatively well, since after the fourteenth-century plague (the Black Death), there was land enough for most. But during the sixteenth century, the European population increased rapidly (perhaps about 1 percent per year); it generally leveled off during the seventeenth and early eighteenth centuries; and late in the eighteenth century again began to increase rapidly. While at first, people could generally grow enough food for themselves and their landlords and a little extra, with the increasing population of the sixteenth century, the number of rural itinerant laborers and destitute began to rise rapidly (Flinn, 1981).

Ordinarily, rural people bartered with neighbors and used money only occasionally, relying on mental accounts of who owed what to whom. At local markets, though, they might purchase a few goods manufactured locally or imported from afar, and sell their own goods or labor. When they needed medical care, most ill people and those caring for them relied on practices long used: self-help; recipes for home remedies (or "kitchen physic") passed down through kin or neighbors; and other traditional practices that could be gathered from local people, which might include ritual and invocation (or what the educated sometimes called "superstitious" practices). Beyond the resources of neighbors and kin, the sick often had available to them the services of people with special knowledge or powers: clergymen, herb wives, sorcerers or witches, and people who healed by special powers of touch. In return for medical help, payment might be in coin, but probably more commonly added a debt to the mental balance of favors, or earned the practitioner goods or services such as chickens or eggs, pasturing an animal on the patient's land, or the patient's help in doing certain chores.

In a few regions, however—mainly from northern Italy along the Mediterranean coast to southern Spain, in the Low Countries and northern France, a thin strip along the south edge of the Baltic, and in southeastern England—urban life was more common. In the fifteenth and early sixteenth centuries, people in towns and cities raised animals for slaughter, and sometimes kept a plot of ground nearby on which they grew food. But by the later sixteenth century, many towns were becoming too large and too densely settled for such practices. Much of the increasing population was drawn from the countryside into the cities or, later, pushed to the overseas colonies. Many people spent a part of their lives in a city working as laborers or servants, returning to their towns or villages after accumulating enough money to establish a family. Others migrated to the towns and cities permanently, causing a huge expansion of wealthy, middling, and poor neighborhoods. The largest city in Europe, Naples, soon had rivals in Paris and London. Just how brutal were the conditions of urban life has been vigorously debated; what is clear is that urban mortality and morbidity rates in the age before plumbing and sewerage were very high indeed.

The cities wrought important economic changes, especially a greater use of money. The demand for food among the urban populations also transformed nearby regions into centers of market agriculture where individuals or landlords produced cash crops. In some areas, such as southeastern England and the Netherlands, this agricultural revolution brought into being a free yeomanry; in other regions, such as Prussia and Russia, it brought about a reenserfment of the peasantry by great landlords. Whatever the local consequences, throughout Europe people increasingly grew used to buying and selling labor and goods, and to handling money; even rural laborers often had a few copper pennies at their disposal.

With the increasing importance of money as a means of exchanging value, more and more people supplemented their incomes by engaging in medical practice for money, or relied upon it entirely for their living. Many, undoubtedly most, such people offered their services to ordinary people, doing so in their neighborhoods or traveling to offer their services among strangers. If itinerant, they found their customers wherever gatherings occurred: markets, crossroads, taverns, inns, alehouses, coffeehouses, and even street fights. They might also gather a crowd by saying something interesting from a platform or from horseback, or by presenting an entertainment from a table, wagon, or stage: These people soon acquired the name of "quacksalver" or "quack" (a term of obscure origin), or "mountebank" (probably from climbing on benches).

With the spread of the printing press and the growth of literacy in the later sixteenth century, medical advertising could be used to heighten the practitioner's reputation or to attract more people to the shows. Medical advertising could also publicize the practice of someone who did not travel but practiced out of a shop, inn, or house. By the later seventeenth century, as the postal systems of many regions of Europe developed, advertisements could be sent to agents for posting throughout a region, and medical customers could order remedies through the mail. The medical practitioners who relied on such methods for their incomes might offer special services (like cutting for cataracts or bladder stones, or setting bones), or sell special remedies (what became known by the eighteenth century as "patent remedies") (Cook, 1986; Porter, 1989; Porter and Porter, 1989).

In the cities and a few large towns, craft guilds of medical practitioners came into being or expanded from their late medieval roots. Guilds had municipal charters allowing their members the rights and privileges of citizenship, and the group the right to act as a corporation: to stand as one person before the local courts, to own property, to pass internal rules regulating their members and organizing them by rank, and often to restrict certain practices to their own members. Throughout early modern Europe, guilds of barber-surgeons and surgeons, or groups of barber-surgeons and surgeons in other guilds, could be found. In general, guilds of barber-surgeons and surgeons restricted the use of instruments on the body to their members.

The barber-surgeons undertook barbering and minor operations, such as opening a vein to let blood, and were ordinarily among the lower-ranking members of the guild (Pelling, 1986). The surgeons, far fewer in number and generally among the higher-ranking liverymen, undertook major operations, such as amputating limbs, setting bones, repairing hernias and fistulas, extracting teeth, and tending to wounds, sores, and ulcers. Among the armies and navies of Europe, surgeons performed most of the general medical tasks, and the kinds of operations that could be successfully performed gradually increased. Consequently, the status and income of surgeons grew during the period, and they began to be increasingly trusted by monarchs to develop certain kinds of medical policies for their kingdoms or principalities (Temkin, 1951; Gelfand, 1980).

Another kind of medical craftsmen were the apothecaries, or pharmacists. Originally wholesale importers of spices, by the early modern period many sold medicines from retail shops; some of the medicines they sold could be dangerous unless used under careful supervision. Many cities therefore had guilds of apothecaries, who were subject to rigorous municipal regulations. In the Scandinavian and Germanic lands, cities often restricted the selling of medicines to a very few official apothecaries, sometimes to just one. As their numbers increased, so did the tendency of apothecaries to give medical advice. It was from the surgeon-apothecaries that the general practitioners eventually arose (Loudon, 1986).

One other kind of medical corporation proliferated in the early modern period: that of the university-educated physicians, usually called a "college" (collegium) of physicians. Ordinarily, colleges of physicians had formal standing from a municipal or royal charter that gave members of the group sole right to practice "physic"— the giving of medical advice—in their city and the surrounding area. Regular members had to possess a university degree in medicine (by the sixteenth century, ordinarily Medicinae Doctor). The colleges of physicians ordinarily were not authorized to grant degrees (an important exception to this rule was the Faculty of Medicine in Paris, which had its roots in the medieval university; the professors of medicine of the university were elected from the Faculty). Independent colleges of medicine first came into being in several northern Italian cities, and by the early sixteenth century had spread to Spain, France, and England. By the seventeenth century, physicians in northern European cities like Amsterdam had established their own colleges. These colleges not only governed the physicians of a city but also, sometimes, took on other regulatory powers, such as inspecting the apothecaries' shops, examining apprentices in surgery and pharmacy, and even looking into the behavior of all local medical practitioners.

In the view of the learned physicians, a medical hierarchy should exist: the physicians at the top, governing the practices of the apothecaries and surgeons, and

most other practitioners being outlawed. While this ideal could seldom be thoroughly enforced, physicians often worked to obtain its legal foundations from municipal or national governments. As an important part of their argument, they fostered the idea that physicians ought to be trusted more than other practitioners because of their learning, which not only gave them knowledge but also inculcated good character. Physicians spoke often of defending the "dignity" of their profession, and concerned themselves with cultivating the outward manners that would best exhibit their inward virtues.

A final medical institution must be mentioned, that of the city physician and, eventually, the physician or surgeon officer of state. In the later Middle Ages, on the Continent, some large cities began to revive the ancient tradition of employing a physician to see to the needs of the municipality. In return for an annual salary, the city physician treated poor citizens, advised on medical regulations (including plague orders), and often served in one or more of the municipal hospitals for the sick poor (if the city had any) (Russell, 1981). By the later sixteenth century, city physicians had become important officers of local government in many places. Moreover, as unified territorial states came into being in the seventeenth century, and sovereigns tried to impose more uniform codes of law and government, they, too, began to use medical advisers to help them govern. Given contemporary international competition, princes deeply felt the need to try to increase the general wealth and power of their countries. Part of their domestic policy therefore was concerned with bettering the health of the public and increasing the population. To do so, sovereign rulers frequently tried to co-opt existing medical corporations or to establish new ones.

In central Europe, by the later eighteenth century, medical advice had become important enough to government that the phrase "medical police" (meaning medical policy promoted and enforced through government agents) had become a common topic in discussions about the structure of state institutions (Rosen, 1974; Hannaway, 1981; Jordanova, 1981; Fischer-Homberger, 1983). But associating themselves with magistrates and government might give physicians and surgeons more authority among those who supported the government; it also might make them more subject to criticism during periods of public unease. The revolutionaries in France, for example, demolished most formal medical institutions during the mid-1790s.

With a rising population, increased urbanization, the spread of the market economy, greater literacy and formal education, and the development of nations, the significance of medical help outside networks of kin and neighbors increased. These changes had many implications for those who practiced medicine. With regard to the gender of the practitioner, for example, women seem to have dominated the practice of traditional medicine, while it was predominantly men who flourished in the commercial medical market (although not to the total exclusion of women). When it came to medical guilds, outside of Italy, memberships were generally limited to men or to the widows of members. Since virtually all European universities excluded women from receiving degrees, nearly all medical doctors were men. In the eyes of the governments, if not always in the eyes of the public, a group who recognized themselves as professional men sat at the top of the medical hierarchy: the physicians, and gradually the surgeons. They obtained many new mechanisms of medical regulation from the state (for example, the French crown established a new College of Surgery in Paris in 1750, and a Royal Society of Medicine in 1776), and increasingly tried to regulate all other practitioners. They could not always succeed in imposing medical order on society, but their professional ideals were influential.

Debates about medical practice and practitioners

Because the increasingly literate and monied public of the towns and cities had a host of medical practitioners from whom to choose, the medical professionals could not impose their ideals on others. While noble and wealthy patients often consulted physicians, they often also consulted surgeons, apothecaries, "quacks," and traditional healers. Without a single, inclusive medical profession and firm regulation to govern practitioners or establish uniform requirements for their training, patients could pick and choose the kind of medicine they preferred, as long as they could pay for it or obtain it through charity. Consequently, medical practitioners cajoled and persuaded their paying patients to do what they considered right (Jewson, 1974; Porter, 1985). (Those they helped through charity could take what was offered or go without.) As a result, the various medical groups, even the physicians, had few clear ethical codes on how to treat patients that were distinct from general sentiments. Notions of virtue and good behavior existed everywhere; concepts of "medical ethics" per se were few (Waddington, 1975).

The humanist movement of the Renaissance brought to light a plethora of ancient philosophies of nature, each with its own ethical foundations. Renewed Aristotelianism, Platonism, Stoicism, Epicureanism, Hermeticism, and Hippocratism: Among the learned, each had its medical adherents. When modern natural philosophers began to take precedence over the old, physicians of a Baconian, Cartesian, or Newtonian stripe often adopted moral notions consistent with their philosophical system. For instance, with a renewed interest in Hippocratism came a renewed interest in the Hippocratic Oath (Smith, 1979); with the spreading of Cartesianism came a hard-hearted attitude toward the use of living automata (animals) in bloody experiments (Guerrini, 1989). But none of these philosophical positions was solely medical, and so none of the ethical implications were strictly medical. The physician took no more and no less interest in the ethical implications of the natural philosophy he adopted than did any other learned person.

Moreover, it is possible to discern some of the general public's ideas of ethical medicine. One can see such general notions at work in the plague. During the first outbreaks (from the mid-fourteenth century), the best advice on avoiding the pestilence that a practitioner could give or take was to "flee fast and far." But as magistrates worked to prevent or ameliorate epidemics, in part by working with city physicians, a sense that the legally privileged physicians ought to help in times of crisis grew up alongside older notions of charity and self-sacrifice (Amundsen, 1977). By the seventeenth century, colleges of physicians suffered public embarrassment when many of their members (even those who held no public office) left town during an epidemic. In the London plague of 1665, for instance, many of the physicians' rivals, especially the chemical physicians, gained the respect of the public by staying and treating victims of the plague, showing by this disinterested public service that they ought to take precedence over the cowardly physicians. For whatever reason, the public was beginning to expect higher standards of behavior from medical practitioners than from all but a few others.

Another place where public notions of ethics in medicine can be found is in the general sense that physicians should not be overly commercial. Journals of literate sentiment, like *The Spectator* or *Gentleman's Magazine* (both of London), made fun of medical commercialism. For their part, physicians generally tried to avoid becoming personally involved in public medical disputes, frowned on advertising their practices or medicines as beneath the dignity of their calling, considered fee splitting and the taking of part of a fee in advance as "quackish," and even began to accept "honoraria" instead of fees. They also continued to treat without charge some of the poor who sought their help and, when they took up hospital posts (where they saw the sick poor inmates), received no fees for their once-a-week (or so) visits. Such general notions of good and charitable behavior, ordinarily shared between patient and practitioner, underlay the more detailed treatment of medical etiquette in the statutes of the various medical corporations.

The topics of more specific debate about moral medical behavior in the early modern period included what constituted the best medical learning; what kind of person made a good practitioner; what kinds of people ought to be prohibited from practice; and what medical practices should be encouraged and which discouraged. Debates about each of these topics could hardly be separated from the others, however, since they all surrounded what might be called the early modern equivalent of "virtue" ethics.

The two most numerous kinds of documents regarding early modern medical practice illustrate how interconnected were ideas about good practice and good character. One kind is the internal regulations of medical guilds and colleges of physicians. The statutes of the London College of Physicians, Society of Apothecaries, and Surgeons' Company, for instance, governed the behavior of the members closely but had almost nothing to say about medical practice per se. (One of the few explicit prohibitions in the College statutes is against making prognoses from the inspection of urine alone; the practices of "urine-casters" came in for much scathing comment from physicians in the early seventeenth century.) In drafting the statutes of the College of Physicians, the officers devoted much attention to whether and in what kinds of cases members might consult non-members, how members should behave during consultations, what the order of precedence would be during meetings and on ceremonial occasions, how they should write prescriptions, and so on, all trying to maintain the dignity, gravity, and exclusivity of the group. The same is true of the College of Physicians in Amsterdam, and colleges elsewhere in Europe; and it is equally true for guilds. One sees the same concern with character in the record of whom the London College of Physicians tried for medical misbehavior: They rarely distinguished between illicit practice and malpractice, insisting that in their examinations for membership, applicants had to show that they were the right sort of people in character as well as in knowledge, anyone else being de facto and de jure incapable of practice.

The second major class of historical documentation discussing the foundations of good or ill medical practice is the antiquackery tracts that proliferated during the early modern period. In them, physicians and others discussed practitioners' behavior far more than their medical practices. In England, perhaps the best-known early piece of antiquackery literature is by John Cotta, who passionately condemned the multitude of nonphysicians: empirics, women practitioners, fugitives, jugglers, quacksalvers, practicing surgeons and apothecaries, practicers of spells, witches, wizards, the servants of physicians, "the methodian learned deceiver or hereticke Physition," beneficed practitioners, astrologers, urine-casters, and itinerants (Cotta, 1612).

Cotta not only condemned the ignorance and bad practices of such people, he condemned above all their undisciplined characters. He explained how even good remedies cause harm when recommended by those who do not possess the learning, and hence the virtue, of physicians (Cotta, 1612, pp. 2–8). As one of his contemporaries noted, because learning and character were so closely associated, ignorance in medical practitioners could be recognized by bad behavior: "loquaciousness," "haste" in judging diseases and promising cures before the cause had been ascertained, "forwardness" in condemning and slandering proper physicians, and "boastfulness" about their own skills (Dunk, 1606, pp. 20–21). These behaviors exhibited by empirics were not tests of their knowledge but demonstrations of their indiscipline: outward signs of an inward character. Character had so foundational a role in medical practice because, as Cotta explained, "the dignitie and worth of Physicks skill consisteth *not (as is imagined commonly) in the excellence and preheminence of remedies, but in their wise and prudent use*" (1612, p. 7; emphasis added). Wisdom and prudence could be built only on the coupling of solid learning with good character. Similar works on how the good physician alone could exhibit proper medical behavior can be noted throughout early modern Europe: Gabriele de Zerbi's *De cautelis medicorum* (1495); Laurent Joubert's *Erreurs populaires* (1578); Govanni Condronchi's *De Christiana ac tuta medendi ratione* (A Christian and Careful Manner of Healing, 1591); Rodericus à Castro's *Medicus-politicus* (The Responsible Physician, 1614); Paolo Zacchia's *Questiones medicolegales* (1621); and Friedrich Hoffman's *Medicus politicus* (1738).

In countering the links made by physicians between learning and virtue, other practitioners discussed their own notions of the sources of good character, frequently arguing that it came not from academic discipline but from an inner light. Since all knowledge ultimately stemmed from God and God's creation, they argued, their direct apprehension of things through experience and a properly prepared intuition made them the possessors of a more immediate wisdom than that of the pagan- and Islamic-influenced university physicians (as they often put it). Such arguments had been put forward forcefully by the influential chemical physician Paracelsus in the early sixteenth century; by the seventeenth century, these views had spread widely among medical chemistry's advocates (Debus, 1977; Webster, 1982).

Not only chemists but also many nonphysicians took the same view about godly practice. For instance, the Swiss Protestant surgeon Gulielmus Hildanus Fabricius wrote:

> Though godlinesse be needfull for all sorts of men, yet it is most requisite in such as practise Physick, for God Almighty doth often abate the power of the Medicines, when he which administers them, is an ungodly and

blasphemous man: and contrariwise, doth give wonderfull power to things despicable and vile, when they are administered by good and godly Physitians. (Fabricius, 1640, pp. 53–54)

Given the deep and bloody struggles over religion in the early modern period, comments about character and godliness divided people. Fabricius's ideas about the personal godliness of the practitioner affecting the efficacy of his medicines is quite different from the learned physician Cotta's view that even good medicines used by the unlearned could cause harm. Different kinds of medical practitioners had very different views about the inner qualities necessary for good practice, and how those qualities could be acquired. For a good Anglican like Cotta, or for his professional colleagues in all orthodox churches, sentiments about intuition and inner light such as Fabricius's smacked of dangerous religious "enthusiasm" (the sense of being inspired directly by God); for practitioners like Fabricius, linking virtue with higher education could only reinforce the position of the "dogmatists" (those who privileged reason over intuition and experience).

By the later seventeenth century, however, many physicians, too, had come to accept the importance of learning from experience, although they continued to believe that it had to be coupled with a disciplined and knowledgeable mind rather than based on intuitions. The scientific revolution had introduced notions that associated virtue with knowledge as much as (or even more than) dignity, and associated knowledge with experience (or, in English, "experiment") rather than learned debate (Shapin and Schaffer, 1985). The "virtuosi" of Europe launched detailed investigations into things, finding the best evidences of God not in human testimony and argument but in creation itself. Consequently, by the eighteenth century, many physicians, as well as surgeons, apothecaries, and empirics, placed great weight on furthering curative and preventive medicine through scientific trials.

The foundation for experiments such as James Lind's work on scurvy, or William Withering's on digitalis, or Lady Wortley Montague's on smallpox inoculation and Edward Jenner's on vaccination, or Antoine Mesmer's on "animal magnetism," had been "folk" custom. Ignoring what they considered the superstitious explanations of what happened, and concentrating instead on the material causes and consequences of various practices, such medical investigators throughout Europe explored new medicaments and treatments. In this enterprise, surgeons and apothecaries, and even unlicensed ordinary practitioners, could make contributions equal to those of physicians. Debates among medical practitioners still implied notions of who might be the best sort of person; but as the nineteenth century loomed, medical debates focused increasingly on what might be the best treatment rather than who might be the best treater.

Conclusion

Throughout Europe in the early modern period, one finds implicit and explicit notions about what constituted a good medical practitioner. Given prevailing public ideas about morality being linked first to character and only second to behavior, the question of *who* ought to practice *what* dominated medical debates. Oral codes and written rules governing medical etiquette proliferated, while people devoted relatively little attention to what we might consider medical ethics per se in the rules of good practice. Without a united and powerful profession, no group of medical practitioners could hope to universalize their own rules, although they often tried. Instead, they had to abide by the ordinary notions of virtue and morality held by their peers and the public. Notions of public and private virtue could be vigorously contested and undoubtedly affected the behavior of practitioners, but they were seldom strictly medical.

HAROLD J. COOK

While all the articles in this entry are relevant, see especially the articles in the other subsections in this section: ANCIENT AND MEDIEVAL, NINETEENTH CENTURY, *and* CONTEMPORARY PERIOD. *For a further discussion of topics mentioned in this article, see the entries* ADVERTISING; ANIMAL RESEARCH; HEALTH-CARE FINANCING, *article on* PROFIT AND COMMERCIALISM; LICENSING, DISCIPLINE, AND REGULATION IN THE HEALTH PROFESSIONS; MEDICAL CODES AND OATHS; MEDICAL EDUCATION; MEDICAL MALPRACTICE; OBLIGATION AND SUPEREROGATION; PROFESSION AND PROFESSIONAL ETHICS; UNORTHODOXY IN MEDICINE; *and* VIRTUE AND CHARACTER. *For a discussion of related ideas, see the entries* ALTERNATIVE THERAPIES; CASUISTRY; DEATH: ART OF DYING, *article on* ARS MORIENDI; EPIDEMICS; HOSPITAL, *article on* MEDIEVAL AND RENAISSANCE HISTORY; MEDICINE, ANTHROPOLOGY OF; MEDICINE, SOCIOLOGY OF; PHARMACY; PROFESSIONAL–PATIENT RELATIONSHIP; PUBLIC HEALTH; SOCIAL MEDICINE; TRUST; *and* WOMEN, *article on* HISTORICAL AND CROSS-CULTURAL PERSPECTIVES.

Bibliography

AMUNDSEN, DARREL W. 1977. "Medical Deontology and Pestilential Disease in the Late Middle Ages." *Journal of the History of Medicine and Allied Sciences* 32, no. 4:403–421.

COOK, HAROLD J. 1986. *The Decline of the Old Medical Regime in Stuart London.* Ithaca, N.Y.: Cornell University Press.

COTTA, JOHN. 1612. *A Short Discoverie of the Unobserved Dan-*

gers of Severall Sorts of Ignorant and Unconsiderate Practisers of Physicke in England. London: William Jones and Richard Boyle.

DEBUS, ALLEN G. 1977. *The Chemical Philosophy: Paracelsian Science and Medicine in the Sixteenth and Seventeenth Centuries*. New York: Science History Publications.

DUNK, ELEAZAR. 1606. *The Copy of a Letter Written by E. D. Doctour of Physicke to a Gentleman, by Whom It Was Published*. London: M. Bradwood.

FABRICIUS, HILDANUS GULIELMUS. 1640. *Lithotomia vesicae: That Is, an Accurate Description of the Stone in the Bladder*. London: John Norton.

FISCHER-HOMBERGER, ESTHER. 1983. *Medizin vor Gericht: Gerichtsmedizin von der Renaissance bis zur Aufklärung*. Bern, Switzerland: Hans Huber.

FLINN, MICHAEL W. 1981. *The European Demographic System 1500–1820*. Baltimore: Johns Hopkins University Press.

GELFAND, TOBI. 1980. *Professionalizing Modern Medicine: Paris Surgeons and Medical Science and Institutions in the Eighteenth Century*. Westport, Conn.: Greenwood Press.

GUERRINI, ANITA. 1989. "The Ethics of Animal Experimentation in Seventeenth-Century England." *Journal of the History of Ideas* 50:391–406.

HANNAWAY, CAROLINE. 1981. "From Private Hygiene to Public Health: A Transformation in Western Medicine in the Eighteenth and Nineteenth Centuries." In *Public Health: Proceedings of the Fifth International Symposium on the Comparative History of Medicine—East and West*, pp. 108–128. Edited by Teizo Ogawa. Tokyo: Saikon.

JEWSON, NORMAN D. 1974. "Medical Knowledge and the Patronage System in Eighteenth Century England." *Sociology* 8:369–385.

JORDANOVA, LUDMILLA J. 1980. "Policing Public Health in France 1780–1815." In *Public Health: Proceedings of the Fifth International Symposium on the Comparative History of Medicine—East and West*, pp. 12–32. Edited by Teizo Ogawa. Tokyo: Saikon.

LOUDON, IRVINE. 1986. *Medical Care and the General Practitioner, 1750–1850*. Oxford: Oxford University Press.

PELLING, MARGARET. 1986. "Appearance and Reality: Barber-Surgeons, the Body and Disease." In *London 1500–1700: The Making of the Metropolis*, pp. 82–112. Edited by Augustus L. Beier and Roger Finlay. London: Longman.

PORTER, DOROTHY, and PORTER, ROY. 1989. *Patient's Progress: Doctors and Doctoring in Eighteenth-Century England*. Stanford, Calif.: Stanford University Press.

PORTER, ROY. 1989. *Health for Sale: Quackery in England 1650–1850*. Manchester, U.K.: Manchester University Press.

———, ed. 1985. *Patients and Practitioners: Lay Perceptions of Medicine in Pre-Industrial Society*. Cambridge: At the University Press.

ROSEN, GEORGE. 1974. *From Medical Police to Social Medicine: Essays on the History of Health Care*. New York: Science History Publications.

RUSSELL, ANDREW W., ed. 1981. *The Town and State Physician in Europe from the Middle Ages to the Enlightenment*. Wolfenbüttel: Herzog August Bibliothek.

SHAPIN, STEVEN, and SCHAFFER, SIMON. 1985. *Leviathan and the Air-Pump: Hobbes, Boyle, and the Experimental Life*. Princeton, N.J.: Princeton University Press.

SMITH, WESLEY D. 1979. *The Hippocratic Tradition*. Ithaca, N.Y.: Cornell University Press.

TEMKIN, OWSEI. 1951. "The Role of Surgery in the Rise of Modern Medical Thought." *Bulletin of the History of Medicine* 25, no. 3:248–259.

WADDINGTON, IVAN. 1975. "The Development of Medical Ethics: A Sociological Analysis." *Medical History* 19, no. 1:36–51.

WEBSTER, CHARLES. 1982. *From Paracelsus to Newton: Magic and the Making of Modern Science*. Cambridge: At the University Press.

C. NINETEENTH CENTURY

1. EUROPE

In the course of the nineteenth century, medical ethics was profoundly transformed in European countries. Social, political, economic, professional, and scientific developments influenced the relationship of physicians to their patients, to their colleagues, and to the state. Focusing on continental Europe, this article first briefly characterizes medical ethics in the eighteenth century and then discusses its transformation after 1800, in connection with the evolution of the medical profession, public health and social medicine, and medical science. Most examples are drawn from Germany and France, where debates on ethical issues in medicine became particularly intense. The codification of medical morality was based on different models in these two countries. While in the German states (and to some extent also in Spain) medical ethics was clearly influenced by the early Anglo-American professional codes, in France national traditions of codes of honor in nineteenth-century bourgeois society appear to have shaped doctors' rules of conduct.

The gentleman doctor

Medical ethics in the eighteenth century was determined by the personal integrity and gentlemanly manners of the physician. His moral decisions were generally based, not on written rules of conduct of a college of physicians, nor directly on the Hippocratic code, but mainly on his medical knowledge, reasoning, and an internal code of honor. Enlightenment natural law theory, as developed by Samuel Pufendorf and Christian Thomasius, may have contributed to this approach. It encouraged a morality based upon rational reflection and individual conscience, rather than upon religious and ecclesiastical precepts (Geyer-Kordesch, 1993b). Eighteenth-century doctors usually treated only a small number of wealthy patients, leaving the majority of the population to the care of barber-surgeons (trained by apprenticeship), midwives, and diverse lay healers. Physicians, like their patients, felt bound to the traditional Platonic and Christian virtues of wisdom, moderation, courage, justice, and faith, hope, charity, as well as to bourgeois Enlightenment virtues like order, cleanliness, and industry (von Engelhardt, 1985).

In the German-speaking world of the eighteenth century, particularly in Prussia, modern professional ethics began to take shape within the academic discipline of medical jurisprudence. Physicians who were called on to give expert testimony on legal cases (e.g., consummation of marriage, paternity, infanticide, murder, poisoning, assault) were exhorted to build their statements truthfully on empirical findings, to admit uncertainty in medical evidence, and to behave with dignity (Geyer-Kordesch, 1993a, 1993b). At some universities, such as Halle and Göttingen, graduating physicians had to take vows of faithfulness to and respect for the academic institutions, careful and rational treatment of poor as well as rich patients, and medical confidentiality (Helm, 1992). Ethical demands like these helped physicians distinguish their conduct from that of quacks.

Social and professional change

The industrial revolution, urbanization, and pauperization shaped new forms of medical care during the late eighteenth and the first half of the nineteenth century. The migration of working people to the industrial regions led to an expansion of hospital medicine. Towns created publicly funded posts for physicians to treat the registered poor (i.e., those who were officially entitled to financial support from the municipal poor-relief fund). Accordingly, doctors were now confronted with a much broader range of patients, especially from the lower classes. At the same time, medical education began to require the acquisition of practical skills in surgery and obstetrics. Surgery was integrated as an academic discipline, and eventually the occupation of barber-surgeons was abolished.

Doctors became involved in public health through campaigns of smallpox vaccination, which was made compulsory in several European states as early as the first third of the nineteenth century, for example, in Bavaria (1807), Sweden (1816), and Württemberg (1818). Other states (e.g., France and Prussia) tried to support their national vaccination programs with a combination of encouragement (bonus paid to parents per vaccinated child, cash prizes and medals for vaccinators), constraint (refusal of welfare benefits to parents of unvaccinated children), and education (La Berge, 1992).

In France a public-health movement coalesced in the 1820s, in which "hygienists" of various professional backgrounds (physicians, pharmacist-chemists, engi-

neers, veterinarians, and administrators) made efforts to solve common health problems by undertaking scientific investigations into their causes. Pioneering studies in occupational and industrial hygiene were carried out by the leaders of this movement, the physicians Alexandre Parent-Duchâtelet and Louis-René Villermé. Differential mortality studies by Villermé and the statistician Louis-François Benoiston de Châtauneuf further demonstrated a strong correlation between standard of living, and health and longevity. Following the model of the Paris health council (founded in 1802), conseils de salubrité were soon formed in other French cities and departments to advise prefects and mayors in regulating public health. Some hygienists, especially Villermé, saw themselves as moral reformers who would enable workers through better material and environmental conditions to emulate the values of the middle class (La Berge, 1992).

As the connection between bad living conditions and disease became more and more obvious—particularly after the onset of cholera epidemics in Europe beginning in the 1830s, and through the experience of the typhus epidemic in parts of Silesia in 1848—liberal physicians such as Rudolf Virchow argued for the social character of medicine and recognition of the doctor as an "advocate for the poor" (Ackerknecht, 1953).

In this period of social and professional change, physicians' concern about medical competition and secure incomes deepened. The breakdown of the so-called patronage system, in which a doctor's services were remunerated by the patient with a voluntary lump sum at the end of the year, raised debates about new models of payment that could maintain the dignity and independence of the physician and defuse competition. The concept that all practitioners should become medical officials (employees of the state)—an idea originating from reform proposals of the French Revolution—was discussed in France and Germany, and was temporarily implemented in the German duchy of Nassau (Brand, 1977). An 1823 proposal to found societies of physicians that would collect and redistribute fees, suggested by the Bonn clinician Christian Friedrich Nasse in a monograph *Von der Stellung der Ärzte im Staate* (On the Position of Physicians in the State), was apparently not realized (Nasse, 1823). Instead, Russia, Prussia, Hanover, and Bavaria instituted a policy of limiting the number of licensed physicians during the first decades of the nineteenth century. Some medical ordinances, for instance, those of Baden (1807) and of the canton of Zurich (1821), made licensing as a physician contingent on a number of ethical obligations, such as helping patients at any time irrespective of their social status, being discreet, and continuing one's medical education (Anner, 1979; Brand, 1977).

Duties and rights

Increasingly, doctors wrote about the duties entailed by their profession, often using the expression "deontology" (science of duty), a title that is still sometimes found in European literature about medical ethics. In 1831 the Spanish physician Félix Janer published a book *Elementos de moral médica,* which dealt with the "dignity and importance" of the medical profession and examined the doctor's relations to the patient, within the profession and to other healers, and to the state and law (Janer, 1831). Being strongly influenced by the *Lectures on the Duties and Qualifications of a Physician* (1772) of the Edinburgh professor of medicine John Gregory (Gregory, 1772), Janer adopted the Scotsman's demand that medical men show temperance, sobriety, firmness of character, humanity, and candor. Interestingly, he also extended these moral requirements to surgeons. These developments in Spain occurred in the context of arising competition and disputes over competence between traditional university-trained physicians (*médicos puros*) and new *médicos colegiales,* who from 1827 on began to graduate from colleges for medicine and surgery. These institutions granted the title *médico-cirujano,* which gave access to hospital positions. Janer himself was involved in teaching these future "medico-surgeons," eventually becoming director of the Barcelona College. Not surprisingly therefore, he defended the unity of medicine and surgery and pleaded for harmonious relations between the two types of medical practitioners (Ortiz Gómez et al., 1991).

Other important examples of literature on medical deontology from the first half of the nineteenth century are Christoph Wilhelm Hufeland's "*Die Verhältnisse des Arztes*" ("The Relationships of the Physician," the last chapter of his authoritative manual of medical practice, *Enchiridion medicum,* 1836; ten editions until 1857; English, 1842) and Maximilien Armand Simon's *Déontologie médicale* (1845; Spanish, 1852). Like Janer, both these authors dealt with the relationships and ethical duties of the doctor to colleagues, to patients, and to society. Simon added a part on the moral rights of physicians, including a right to political activity, especially in the reform of laws pertaining to public health. Here Simon differed from Hufeland, who wanted to keep physicians out of any involvement in politics, permitting them only to educate the public on rational behavior in matters of health and disease. Both Hufeland and Simon described altruism as the central moral principle of the medical profession. For Simon, Christian faith formed the undisputable basis of this altruism and of all specific duties of the physician.

Both physicians' renewed admonition to care equally for the rich and the poor reflects the larger social spectrum of patients, as compared to the eighteenth century. Simon welcomed the "now multiplied" number of hospitals and dispensaries for the sick poor, yet warned his colleagues, as did Hufeland, not to abuse this group of patients for harmful scientific experiments. On the question of euthanasia, both physicians stressed that the sufferings of the dying should be alleviated, if necessary by a liberal use of opium, but that any life-shortening measures were strictly forbidden, even if the patient demanded them. Hufeland feared dire consequences for society if the physician once transgressed the line by judging the necessity of a human being's existence; Simon advanced the religious argument that man is not the master of his life. These statements were in keeping with those of the Göttingen professor of medicine Carl Friedrich Heinrich Marx, who had discussed the topic in detail in his inaugural lecture *De euthanasia medica* (1826). They expressed a general point of view within the medical profession that remained undisputed until the end of the nineteenth century.

Contemporary problems involving competition among doctors are reflected in Hufeland's strong plea for cooperative conduct—"Disparaging a colleague means disparaging the art and oneself!" (Hufeland, 1836, p. 906)—and in his discussion of proper behavior during joint consultations, a topic treated in 1798 by the Hanoverian court physician Johann Stieglitz in a monograph *Über das Zusammenseyn der Ärzte am Krankenbett* (On the Meeting of Doctors at the Bedside). In cases of malpractice, however, Hufeland exhorted his profession to set greater store by the "saving" of the patient than by consideration for the colleague. Difficulties with the transition of medical practice from a gentlemanly calling to a modern, economically oriented profession are evident in Simon's energetic defense against the reproach that doctors were guided by commercial interests.

Codification and control

For physicians in the states of the North German Confederation, and soon for those of the whole German Empire, the trade ordinance of 1869 became an important step in that transition. It defined medical practice as a trade that anyone could exercise (*Kurierfreiheit*), yet granted legal protection of the title *Arzt* (physician). It abolished the doctor's duty to help any patient in case of "urgent danger," which had been included in the Prussian penal code in 1851 and was regarded by many physicians as a coercion to provide treatment. The trade ordinance intensified the resolve of academic, state-certified physicians to distinguish themselves from lay healers by establishing professional societies.

In 1873, two years after the foundation of the German Empire, an association of German societies of physicians (*Deutscher Ärztevereinsbund*) was formed. Its main activities consisted of representing professional and economic interests. Many societies of physicians had codes of appropriate conduct, some of which were modeled directly on the code of ethics of the American Medical Association of 1847, and thus basically on Thomas Percival's *Medical Ethics* of 1803 (Percival, 1803). The disciplinary powers of those societies were limited to their own members, however.

In contrast to this, the so-called chambers of physicians (*Ärztekammern*), founded in German states beginning in the mid-1860s, formed state-controlled medical courts of honor, which were given authority to punish professional misconduct by all physicians in the respective district (except army doctors and medical officials, who were under the direct control of the state). Once created, the medical courts of honor seem to have been very active. It has been estimated that they engaged in more than 3,000 proceedings between 1904 and 1909 in Prussia, which at this time had about 15,000 physicians who were not employed by the state or the army. Most proceedings dealt with charges of misconduct in medical competition, such as unlawful advertising, underbidding other doctors, disparaging colleagues in the presence of laypeople, and unauthorized use of specialist titles (Huerkamp, 1985).

This German path toward well-organized intraprofessional self-control, authorized by the state, contrasted with developments in France. Here, the formation of medical professional organizations was hindered by post-revolutionary legislation that followed the principle of liberal individualism. The Le Chapelier law of 1791 prohibited members of the same occupation from forming organizations that would promote their common interests, and in 1810 associations of more than twenty people formed without approval of the government were forbidden. Physicians were subject to legal responsibility for malpractice: Harm to a patient was a tort, as defined by the civil code of 1803, and was also punishable as a criminal offense under some articles of the penal code of 1810 (Ramsey, 1988).

The "medical marketplace" of early–nineteenth-century France, however, led to proposals for additional disciplinary provisions. Legislation in 1803 had established the first uniform licensing system for medical practitioners in the whole of France, distinguishing "doctors of medicine" and "doctors of surgery," *officiers de santé* (health officers), and certified midwives. While the doctors were required to have studied at least four years at a medical school, health officers could qualify after three years' study but also by serving six years under a doctor or five years in a hospital. Unlike doctors, the *officiers*, destined to provide constant medical care for the rural population, were permitted to work only within the *département* that had given them license to

practice. On the one hand, these legal requirements drew a sharp line between regular, licensed practitioners and irregular healers, such as itinerant quacks, sedentary empirics (vendors of special remedies), and folk healers, who could now be prosecuted for illegal medical practice. On the other hand, the institution of health officers, who represented a class of less-well-trained physicians, created fears of a lapse in standards and professional decline among doctors. Moreover, economic need caused many regular practitioners to collaborate with unqualified empirics, to promote their own proprietary medicines, or to offer special cures. In these circumstances, medical reform commissions from 1812 onward repeatedly suggested the establishment of "chambers of discipline" or "medical councils," whose jurisdiction would include both illegal practice and professional misconduct. None of these proposals was put into action, however, partly because they were linked to the controversial question of reforming the institution of health officers, and partly because many doctors did not wish any further intervention by the state. In 1892 legislation abolished the title of *officier de santé*, as well as that of "doctor of surgery" (Ramsey, 1988).

Beginning in the 1850s, the number of physicians relative to the population grew steadily in France, leading to still fiercer competition and precarious incomes. In addition, legislation between 1874 and 1905 imposed new duties on French doctors, such as treating poor patients in return for a moderate state remuneration, testifying as experts in courts, and surveying the standards of public health (e.g., quality of water supply, housing conditions). In the 1880s, in response to these developments, doctors began to form medical unions (*syndicats*) to promote their professional interests. Initially illegal but tolerated, the *syndicats* were legally recognized in 1892. The ultimate aim of their most radical members was to create an obligatory *Ordre des Médecins*, analogous to the *Ordre des Avocats* for lawyers (founded in 1810). Such an order did not emerge; Both the government and a majority within the medical profession opposed it. But in an attempt to set ethical standards for doctors, to regulate intraprofessional relationships, and to form a unified front toward the public, the medical syndicates adopted deontological statutes that were binding on their membership.

These syndical deontologies were modeled upon the male honor codes of bourgeois social and recreational societies (*cercles* or *sociétés à plaisance*), which flourished in mid-nineteenth-century France (Nye, 1993b). Like these societies, the syndicates regarded the personal honorability (*honnêteté*) of their members as essential and had a policy of solving internal conflicts *intra muros* (i.e., without recourse to the courts). Members were obliged to report cases of malpractice to the *syndicat*, which had the right to withdraw membership. In this context, the old idea of "chambers of discipline" was taken up again, for example, by the medical syndicate of the *arrondissement* of Avesnes, which prescribed the formation of such a "tribunal of honor" in its statutes of 1910 (Nye, 1993a). Generally, however, the disciplinary powers of French professional organizations remained relatively weak throughout the nineteenth century, compared to those of their counterparts in Germany, Britain, and the United States (Ramsey, 1988).

In 1900 the Paris medical syndicate organized an international congress on "professional medicine and medical deontology," at which key speakers proposed that the problems created by overcrowding and competition should be solved through "confraternity" and "the force of moral law." Many French treatises on medical deontology, published around the time of the congress, reflected the same demands. They furthermore insisted on medical confidentiality to protect not only the privacy of the patient but also the reputation of the profession. Accordingly, the medical syndicates in the 1890s resisted requirements of the public-health legislation to divulge the names of patients with contagious diseases, whereas doctors in the first half of the nineteenth century had done so freely during smallpox and cholera epidemics (Nye, 1993a).

Controversial issues

In the second half of the nineteenth century, ethical issues arising from developments in preventive medicine, medical science, and hospital medicine became topics of intraprofessional as well as public debate in several European countries. Following the introduction of compulsory smallpox vaccination in the German Empire in 1874, the many newly established antivaccination societies agitated intensely until World War I. Refusal to have one's children vaccinated was based mainly on reasons of conscience resulting from individual weighing of benefits and risks. In part, the reasons also reflected a protest against the restriction of personal freedom in matters of health (Maehle, 1991). This aspect had surfaced as a problem already around 1800, when Johann Peter Frank, then director general of public health of Lombardy (Cisalpine Republic), proposed universal state-controlled health care in his *System einer vollständigen medicinischen Polizey* (Haun, 1993). Antivaccinationism was basically a medical lay movement. Societies against vaccination were guided by academics and few physicians, who were influenced by ideas of natural healing (through water cures, diet, exercise, sun, and fresh air) and social hygiene. The same was true for the organized antivivisection movement (Maehle, 1993), which emerged as a result of the increasing scientific use of animals associated with the rise of experimental physiology (Claude Bernard, Carl Ludwig), pathology (Vir-

chow), and bacteriology (Louis Pasteur, Robert Koch). Antivivisectionist activities, imported from Britain in the 1860s, were particularly strong in Tuscany, Germany, Switzerland, and Sweden (Rupke, 1990). A general antiscientific and antimaterialistic attitude was often behind the overt argument that animal experiments were useless cruelties (Maehle, 1993).

The growing importance of hospital medicine, reflected in the large clinics of Vienna and Paris in the first half of the nineteenth century, combined with the progress in medical science, brought the ethical problems of human experimentation into the foreground. In 1880 the courts of Bergen, Norway, sentenced Gerhard Armauer Hansen, the discoverer of the leprosy bacillus, for inoculating a female hospital patient suffering from a particular type of leprosy with leprous material from another patient (with a different type of the disease) without prior information or consent (Vogelsang, 1963). Albert Neisser, professor of dermatology in Breslau, was fined in 1900; hoping to induce immunity against syphilis, he had injected syphilitic blood serum into eight uninformed female hospital patients (three children and five prostitutes) in 1892. These and other cases stimulated intensive public debate, which—like the vivisection controversy—often had antiscientific and antisemitic undercurrents. Prevented from careers in the German civil service, Jews were strongly represented in the so-called free professions, such as medicine or law. In medical university careers, doctors of Jewish origin tended to concentrate in the experimental disciplines (physiology, pharmacology, immunology) and the new specialty of dermatology and venereology, because they could hardly find entry to the prestigious "classic" professorships in internal medicine and surgery. Anti-Semites advanced propaganda arguments that animal and human experimentation was an expression of "Jewish materialism" (Elkeles, 1991).

A concrete consequence of the debate on human experiments was a decree by the Prussian Ministry of Education in 1900 that required informed consent of the research subjects and prohibited scientific experimentation on minors and other persons who were not fully competent (Grodin, 1992).

New ethical challenges also emerged with the passage in the German Empire of the Health (1883), Accident (1884), and Retirement and Disability (1889) Insurance Acts; the scheme was soon copied by Austria (1888), Hungary (1891), Luxembourg (1901), and Switzerland (1911). The task of certifying sickness and disability placed physicians between the often conflicting interests of patients and insurance companies. Medical insurance tended to strengthen the patient's position; doctors began to complain that patients behaved as if they were their employers (Brand, 1977). On the other hand, insurance companies owned by factories could serve as a means for the social control of working-class patients (Frevert, 1984). For physicians the insurance scheme created hopes of economic improvement. In the long run, however, it heightened medical competition by drawing an increasing number of individuals into the profession.

Teaching medical ethics

Against this background, the proposal to include medical ethics in the curriculum for medical students was debated in Germany during the 1890s. At an 1898 conference on internal medicine at Wiesbaden, those who argued that an ethical attitude must be inculcated by the family, not at the university, and that ethics could not be subdivided according to the different professions, won the day. Yet the debate generated a spate of books that advocated the teaching of medical ethics. The Berlin medical historian Julius Pagel published a *Medicinische Deontologie* for prospective medical practitioners in 1897 (Pagel, 1897), the Wiesbaden physician Oswald Ziemssen, cousin of the renowned clinician Hugo von Ziemssen, a monograph *Die Ethik des Arztes als medicinischer Lehrgegenstand* (The Doctor's Ethics as a Medical Teaching Subject) in 1899. Pagel gave a great deal of space to cooperative behavior among medical colleagues, demanded solidarity in cases of professional error, and advised doctors to act with self-confidence when seeing patients. Furthermore, the doctor should take care not to speak familiarly with members of the lower classes. Ziemssen built his book on codes of German societies of physicians and above all on Jukes de Styrap's *A Code of Medical Ethics* of 1878 (de Styrap, 1878). To some extent, he also drew on German philosophical traditions, arguing that the ethics of the physician were based on a combination of Immanuel Kant's categorical imperative, Arthur Schopenhauer's voice of feeling, and Johann Friedrich Herbart's practical judgment.

Contemporary philosophers, such as Friedrich Paulsen and Max Dessoir, also acknowledged the importance of teaching medical ethics with books and lectures. Paulsen pointed to the growing importance of medicine for modern society (von Engelhardt, 1989). Dessoir wanted the profession to compensate for a loss of ethical values in depersonalized doctor–patient relationships that resulted from specialization and the influence of medical science. Accordingly, he suggested a teaching program that would cover not only the "profession and character of the physician" and his "relationship to colleague and to the public" but also "vivisection and human experimentation" and "ethical principles in general" (Dessoir, 1894, p. 382).

Dessoir also served as an adviser to the Berlin neurologist Albert Moll, who provided the most significant contribution of this period with his 650-page *Ärztliche Ethik* (Moll, 1902). Moll argued that concern for medical ethics had concentrated on the physician's duties to colleagues and the profession (i.e., on medical etiquette), rather than on duties to the patient. He therefore put particular emphasis on ethical problems of medical practice, such as the doctor's refusing and breaking off treatment, euthanasia, deceiving the patient, advising extramarital sexual intercourse (e.g., in neurasthenia due to sexual abstinence, or in impotence), cosmetic surgery, and abortion. Moll devoted much attention to the issue of human experimentation, quoting numerous examples from the scientific literature. He oriented medical ethics to the well-being of the individual patient, not to the general welfare. Explicitly renouncing any basis in theological or philosophical systems of morality, he defined the doctor–patient relationship in legal terms, as a contract. This implied the physician's duty to fulfill the contract and the patient's obligation to respond by paying the fee. With this positivist approach, Moll reflected a general intellectual tendency of his time. In its comprehensiveness, his book provides a good overview of ethical issues in late-nineteenth-century European medicine.

Summary

In the nineteenth century there was a significant shift from reliance on largely implicit and nonsystematic notions concerning the gentleman doctor to written codes of professional etiquette and to a growing body of literature and theoretical perspectives concerning specific issues in medical ethics. In this century many of the concerns and methods now employed in medical ethics were first articulated.

ANDREAS-HOLGER MAEHLE

While all the articles in this section and the other sections of this entry are relevant, see especially the companion article in this subsection: GREAT BRITAIN. *For a further discussion of topics mentioned in this article, see the entries* ANIMAL RESEARCH, *articles on* HISTORICAL ASPECTS, *and* PHILOSOPHICAL ISSUES; AUTONOMY; BIOETHICS EDUCATION; CONFLICT OF INTEREST; DEATH AND DYING: EUTHANASIA AND SUSTAINING LIFE, *articles on* HISTORICAL ASPECTS, *and* ETHICAL ISSUES; EPIDEMICS; ETHICS; HEALTH-CARE RESOURCES, ALLOCATION OF, *article on* MACROALLOCATION; HEALTH AND DISEASE; HOSPITAL, *articles on* MEDIEVAL AND RENAISSANCE HISTORY, *and* MODERN HISTORY; INFORMED CONSENT; LICENSING, DISCIPLINE, AND REGULATION IN THE HEALTH PROFESSIONS; MEDICAL CODES AND OATHS; MEDICAL MALPRACTICE; MEDICINE, ANTHROPOLOGY OF; MEDICINE, SOCIOLOGY OF; MEDICINE AS A PROFESSION; NATURAL LAW; PROFESSIONAL–PATIENT RELATIONSHIP; PROFESSION AND PROFESSIONAL ETHICS; PUBLIC HEALTH; RESEARCH,

HUMAN: HISTORICAL ASPECTS; RIGHTS; SURGERY; VIRTUE AND CHARACTER; *and* WOMEN, *article on* HISTORICAL AND CROSS-CULTURAL PERSPECTIVES. *Other relevant material may be found under the entries* ADVERTISING; CONFIDENTIALITY; DEATH; FREEDOM AND COERCION; HARM; HEALTH-CARE FINANCING, *article on* PROFIT AND COMMERCIALISM; JUSTICE; LIFE; PROTESTANTISM; RACE AND RACISM; RESPONSIBILITY; *and* ROMAN CATHOLICISM. *See also the* APPENDIX (CODES, OATHS, AND DIRECTIVES RELATED TO BIOETHICS), SECTION II: ETHICAL DIRECTIVES FOR THE PRACTICE OF MEDICINE, OATH OF HIPPOCRATES.

Bibliography

ACKERKNECHT, ERWIN HEINZ. 1953. *Rudolf Virchow: Doctor, Statesman, Anthropologist.* Madison: University of Wisconsin Press.

ANNER, ERNST. 1979. *Gelöbnisse der Medizinalpersonen im Kanton Zürich seit 1798.* Zurich: Juris.

BRAND, ULRICH. 1977. *Ärztliche Ethik im 19. Jahrhundert: Der Wandel ethischer Inhalte im medizinischen Schrifttum—ein Beitrag zum Verständnis der Arzt–Patient-Beziehung.* Freiburg im Breisgau: H. F. Schulz Verlag.

DESSOIR, MAX. 1894. "Der Beruf des Arztes." *Westermanns Illustrierte Deutsche Monatshefte* 77:375–382.

DE STYRAP, JUKES. 1878. *A Code of Medical Ethics.* London: Churchill.

ELKELES, BARBARA. 1991. "Der moralische Diskurs über das medizinische Menschenexperiment zwischen 1835 und dem Ersten Weltkrieg." Hannover: Habilitationsschrift Medizinische Hochschule Hannover.

FREVERT, UTE. 1984. *Krankheit als politisches Problem, 1770–1880: Soziale Unterschichten in Preußen zwischen medizinischer Polizei und staatlicher Sozialversicherung.* Göttingen: Vandenhoeck & Ruprecht.

GEYER-KORDESCH, JOHANNA. 1993a. "Infanticide and Medicolegal Ethics in Eighteenth Century Prussia." In *Doctors and Ethics: The Earlier Historical Setting of Professional Ethics,* pp. 181–202. Edited by Andrew Wear, Johanna Geyer-Kordesch, and Roger French. Amsterdam: Rodopi.

———. 1993b. "Natural Law and Medical Ethics in the Eighteenth Century." In *The Codification of Medical Morality: Historical and Philosophical Studies of the Formalization of Western Medical Morality in the Eighteenth and Nineteenth Centuries,* vol. 1, pp. 123–139. Edited by Robert Baker, Dorothy Porter, and Roy Porter. Dordrecht, Netherlands: Kluwer.

GREGORY, JOHN. 1772. *Lectures on the Duties and Qualifications of a Physician.* Corrected and enlarged ed. London: W. Strahan.

GRODIN, MICHAEL A. 1992. "Historical Origins of the Nuremberg Code." In *The Nazi Doctors and the Nuremberg Code,* pp. 121–144. Edited by George J. Annas and Michael A. Grodin. New York: Oxford University Press.

HAUN, IRENE. 1993. "Ethische Gesichtspunkte der Präventivmedizin in Johann Peter Franks (1745–1821) 'System einer vollständigen medicinischen Polizey.'" Göttingen: M.D. thesis, Georg-August-Universität.

HELM, JÜRGEN. 1992. "Tradition und Wandel der ärztlichen Selbstverpflichtung: Der Göttinger Promotionseid 1737–1889." Göttingen: M.D. thesis, Georg-August-Universität.

HUERKAMP, CLAUDIA. 1985. *Der Aufstieg der Ärzte im 19. Jahrhundert: Vom gelehrten Stand zum professionellen Experten: Das Beispiel Preussens.* Göttingen: Vandenhoeck & Ruprecht.

HUFELAND, CHRISTOPH WILHELM. 1836. *Enchiridion medicum, oder Anleitung zur medizinischen Praxis: Vermächtnis einer fünfzigjährigen Erfahrung.* 2d enlarged ed. Berlin: Jonas Verlagsbuchhandlung.

JANER, FÉLIX. 1831. *Elementos de moral médica.* Barcelona: Verdaguer.

LA BERGE, ANN ELIZABETH FOWLER. 1992. *Mission and Method: The Early Nineteenth-Century French Public Health Movement.* Cambridge: At the University Press.

MAEHLE, ANDREAS-HOLGER. 1991. "Präventivmedizin als wissenschaftliches und gesellschaftliches Problem: Der Streit über das Reichsimpfgesetz von 1874." In *Medizin, Gesellschaft und Geschichte,* vol. 9, pp. 127–148. Edited by Robert Jütte. Stuttgart: Franz Steiner Verlag.

———. 1993. "The Ethical Discourse on Animal Experimentation, 1650–1900." In *Doctors and Ethics: The Earlier Historical Setting of Professional Ethics.* Edited by Andrew Wear, Johanna Geyer-Kordesch, and Roger French. Amsterdam: Rodopi.

MOLL, ALBERT. 1902. *Ärztliche Ethik: Die Pflichten des Arztes in allen Beziehungen seiner Thätigkeit.* Stuttgart: F. Enke.

NASSE, CHRISTIAN FRIEDRICH. 1823. *Von der Stellung der Ärzte im Staate.* Leipzig: Cnobloch.

NYE, ROBERT A. 1993a. "Honor Codes and Medical Ethics in Modern France." Norman: Department of History, University of Oklahoma.

———. 1993b. *Masculinity and Male Codes of Honor in Modern France.* New York: Oxford University Press.

ORTIZ GÓMEZ, TERESA; VALENZUELA, JOSÉ; and RODRÍGUEZ OCAÑA, ESTEBAN. 1991. "Ética y profesion en la medicina española del siglo XIX: Los 'Elementos de moral médica' (1831) de Félix Janer (1781–1865)." In *Actas del IX Congreso Nacional de Historia de la Medicina,* vol. 1, pp. 291–302. Edited by Francesc Bujosa i Homar et al. Zaragoza: Secretariado de Publicaciones Prensas Universitarias de Zaragoza.

PAGEL, JULIUS. 1897. *Medizinische Deontologie: Ein Kleiner Katechismus für angehende Praktiker.* Berlin: O. Coblentz.

PERCIVAL, THOMAS. 1803. *Medical Ethics: A Code of Institutes and Precepts, Adapted to the Professional Conduct of Physicians and Surgeons.* Manchester: S. Russell.

RAMSEY, MATTHEW. 1988. *Professional and Popular Medicine in France, 1770–1830: The Social World of Medical Practice.* Cambridge: At the University Press.

RUPKE, NICOLAAS A., ed. 1990. *Vivisection in Historical Perspective.* Rev. ed. London: Routledge.

SIMON, MAXIMILIEN ISIDORE ARMAND. 1845. *Déontologie médicale; ou, des devoirs et des droits des médecins dans l'état actuel de la civilisation.* Paris: J. B. Bailliere.

VOGELSANG, T. M. 1963. "A Serious Sentence Passed Against

the Discoverer of the Leprosy Bacillus (Gerhard Armauer Hansen), in 1880." *Medical History* 7:182–186.

VON ENGELHARDT, DIETRICH. 1985. "Virtue and Medicine During the Enlightenment in Germany." In *Virtue and Medicine: Explorations in the Character of Medicine*, pp. 63–79. Edited by Earl E. Shelp. Dordrecht, Netherlands: D. Reidel.

———. 1989. "Entwicklung der ärztlichen Ethik im 19. Jahrhundert—medizinische Motivation und gesellschaftliche Legitimation." In *Medizinische Deutungsmacht im sozialen Wandel des 19. und 20. Jahrhunderts*, pp. 75–88. Edited by Alfons Labisch and Reinhard Spree. Bonn: Psychiatrie-Verlag.

2. GREAT BRITAIN

Questions of medical ethics acquired heightened significance in nineteenth-century Great Britain. The reform of the medical profession and the growing prominence of medicine within public policy brought ethical and medicolegal issues into sharper focus. For the first time, medical ethics assumed codified form.

The period from the early sixteenth century to the close of the eighteenth saw the founding of medical colleges and societies in Britain, among them the Royal College of Physicians. But such bodies played only a minor part in imposing ethical codes upon the profession as a whole—or even suggesting them. The Royal College of Physicians and the Royal College of Surgeons possessed jurisdiction over one city, London. There was no centralized medical regulation over most of the nation. With few exceptions, it was only in the nineteenth century that medical ethics were written down, the watershed being the publication in 1803 of Thomas Percival's *Medical Ethics; or, A Code of Institutes and Precepts Adapted to the Professional Conduct of Physicians and Surgeons*. Two circumstances provided impetus for codification, one intellectual, the other socioeconomic. Intellectually, the moral philosophy of the Scottish Enlightenment and the reawakening of religious conscience associated with Evangelicalism concentrated attention on man's (concern was almost wholly with males) duties to society. John Gregory, professor of medicine at Edinburgh, had published his *Observations on the Duties of a Physician* in 1770, and Rev. Thomas Gisborne, a friend of Percival, had included a section on obligations attending the calling of a physician in his *An Enquiry into the Duties of Men in the Higher and Middle Classes of Society in Great Britain, Resulting from their Respective Stations, Professions and Employments* (1794). Percival certainly drew on both in shaping his *Medical Ethics*, though it would be a mistake to assume that Percival was significantly concerned with academic philosophy. His handbook was first and foremost practical. It contained no discussion of any philosopher by name and did not refer to particular formal philosophical schools.

At the same time, the tremendous social transformations precipitated by the industrial revolution were posing exacting problems for medical practitioners. Newly emergent urban communities had severe medical needs but no deep-rooted traditions of professional service. In Britain's laissez-faire, free-market economy, doctors were tempted to adopt entrepreneurial attitudes, operating according to the law of "let the buyer beware." Moreover, new medical institutions were springing up, above all charity hospitals and dispensaries for the poor. Codes of practice governing the duties of doctors attached to these distinctive establishments needed to be formulated.

Thomas Percival (born in 1740) had studied medicine at Edinburgh. He became a senior and well-respected Manchester practitioner, and a leading light in the town's Literary and Philosophical Society. When a virulent intraprofessional feud flared up at the Manchester Infirmary in 1792—a sordid fracas concerning nepotistic appointments—he had been called in as a kind of peacemaker. His *Medical Ethics* arose from his musing on that unseemly rumpus. It was thus a work that spoke directly to the needs of its times. Percival set out some precepts, of a somewhat platitudinous nature, about the general duties and responsibilities of the physician to his patients, to society, and to his calling. Above all, he addressed himself in a direct manner to the tangible difficulties facing doctors in a commercial society.

High on Percival's list of priorities was the desire to secure harmony among practitioners and between the different grades of the profession. He addressed such questions as seniority and precedence, spelling out in detail the protocols of joint consultations. Though little interested in formal professional bodies, he was adamant that "medical men" should not compete against each other; instead they should cultivate, and be seen to cultivate, a comradely esprit de corps. Professional rivalries, naked jealousies, and controversies in public conducted through the medium of pamphlets would poison intraprofessional relations and ultimately work to the disadvantage of patients. Charging lower than normal fees, for instance, would deny a living to poorer brethren, and discourage the young from investing in a thorough medical education and training. A liberal profession could not be supported, Percival insisted, except as a "lucrative one."

Sentiments such as these give support to those, like Chauncey Leake and Ivan Waddington, who argue that Percival's *Medical Ethics* was misnamed, being in truth a work of "medical etiquette," primarily designed to bolster the collective status, dignity, and monopolistic power of the profession vis-à-vis the public. Percival certainly aimed to regulate "the official conduct and mutual intercourse of the faculty"; but it should not be forgotten that he added that this was to be accomplished "by precise and acknowledged principles of urbanity and rec-titude"—that is, the unwritten but generally acknowledged code of gentlemanly behavior. In other words, he was concerned not with self-serving expediency but with humanitarianism, prudence, and honorable standards of virtuous conduct as understood by a gentleman.

Some American philosophers of medical ethics are inclined to see Percival as having written a work with strong foundations in academic ethical philosophies. It has, for example, been suggested that Percival and his successors may have drawn upon utilitarianism. There is little warrant for this reading in Percival himself. The great bulk of his text was concerned with resolving practical problems among medical men.

Percival upheld the ideal of the professional pyramid. Where wealth and density of population permitted a professional division of labor, the traditional hierarchical separation between physicians, surgeons, and apothecaries was to be maintained because it stimulated specialist skills. Yet physicians were not to lord it over the lesser "gentlemen of the faculty": in small communities, the humble apothecary was often the best expert on the circumstances of patients, and so his advice should be heeded.

Percival thus required courtesy among practitioners. A compassionate man, he insisted that the fears and feelings of the sick should be respected. Ever the realist, he acquiesced in the authority deriving from social status that the gentry were accustomed to wield. Wealthy patients would exercise the right to a second or third opinion: It was up to the doctors involved to manage such delicate circumstances with tact, preventing the dangers of "divide and rule." Likewise, though nostrums were an abomination, Percival judged that the astute physician would sometimes comply when a patient insisted on a worthless, but safe, favorite proprietary remedy.

With affluent patients, the one who paid the piper would evidently call the tune. But different rules must apply, Percival observed, when practitioners gave their services without charge. Charity patients in infirmaries could not expect to pick and choose among the physicians or to negotiate over treatments. Disobedient hospital patients must face dismissal. Likewise, it was permissible to experiment with new remedies or surgical procedures upon charity patients, so long as such innovations were attempted with due caution and humanity.

Prizing the close clinical relationship between practitioner and patient, Percival believed this depended primarily upon the character of the physician. The ideal practitioner was an academically educated, liberal gentleman who would combine "tenderness with steadiness," and "condescension with authority," displaying proper composure, dignity, tact, and courtesy. He must govern himself: be temperate, avoid intoxication, and take care to retire from practice before age eroded his powers and judgment. He must be civil to colleagues, benevolent toward patients. It was a paternalist ideal, entailing a gentlemanly noblesse oblige.

Percival's book became immensely influential in the United States, serving as the basis for the American Medical Association's code of 1847. Though reprinted in 1849, it achieved less celebrity in Britain. This was not because it was superseded by any other more illustrious tome or rival ethical scheme. For subsequent works, like William Ogilvie Porter's *Medical Science and Ethicks: An Introductory Lecture* (1837) and Abraham Banks's *Medical Etiquette* (1839), largely echoed Percival's platitudes; and as late as 1878, Jukes de Styrap was still lifting phrases out of Percival in *A Code of Medical Ethics*. Rather, in contrast to that in the United States, the medical profession in nineteenth-century Britain seems to have felt little need for explicit ethical codifications.

The contrast is readily explained. In early-nineteenth-century America, no standard, universal, and accredited licensing procedures unambiguously demarcated orthodox practitioners from quacks and irregulars. Hence, when regulars banded together into state medical societies to enhance their prestige, the adoption of a code of ethics was of immense significance as a conspicuous shibboleth. In Britain, by contrast, licensing was already well entrenched; since 1815, the Apothecaries Act had stipulated nationwide minimum qualifications for practice as an apothecary or general practitioner. Thus, in Britain, regular doctors did not need written codes of ethics to prove their standing in relation to irregulars. In Britain regulars were already adequately defined in contrast with quacks.

Nor did regulars need codes of medical ethics to affirm their personal bona fides. British practitioners were confident that they were, first and foremost, *gentlemen*. Gentility came from birth and breeding, education, wealth, contacts, manners, mien, and so forth—or at least from the capacity to create a show of such attributes. (Needless to say, most medical practitioners were not, in the literal sense, the sons of gentlemen; rather, they aspired to genteel status.) Gentlemanly behavior depended heavily upon notions of personal honor rather than upon formal ethical or religious principles. A written ethical code might have seemed to impugn a gentleman's honor, rather as the British prided themselves politically upon not having a formal written constitution. It is thus no surprise that the British medical profession was indifferent to collections of medical ethics. Neither the Royal College of Physicians nor the Royal College of Surgeons drew up an ethical code for its members.

From professors of forensic medicine, students learned a little about the rules governing evidence to be given in court. The Manchester Medical Ethical Association was formed in 1847, aiming to bind its members to a slate of regulations outlawing the marketing of nostrums and the giving of testimonials for patent medicines. And the British Medical Association—the newly formed society of general practitioners and family doctors—set up its own medical ethics committee in 1853. Over the next fifteen years, however, it signally failed actually to draw up a corpus of medical ethics. Despite such token activities, no comprehensive manifesto of ethical principles was codified in Britain that was binding upon the profession as a whole.

Yet this is not to say that the profession was indifferent to ethics. As was vehemently argued in Thomas Beddoes's *A Letter to the Right Honourable Sir Joseph Banks . . . on the Causes and Removal of the Prevailing Discontents, Imperfections, and Abuses, in Medicine* (1808) and in countless subsequent works, it was at bottom ethical commitments that distinguished honorable practice from quackery (although, Beddoes implied, all too often eminent regulars disgraced their vocation by unprincipled practices). And, of course, ethical dilemmas often arose that urgently needed resolution. A formal mechanism for upholding ethical standards was constituted in 1858 as a consequence of the establishment of the Medical Register, a public roll of all duly licensed practitioners. The body appointed to act as guardian of the register was the General Council of Medical Education and Registration of the United Kingdom, commonly known as the General Medical Council (GMC). The GMC was to admit properly qualified practitioners to the register, and to delete those whose conduct was professionally inadmissible—for example, those who had been convicted of a crime or who had been judged guilty of infamous professional conduct (such as adultery with a patient or vilification of colleagues). Sitting in camera, the GMC thus served as a sort of moral inquisition for the profession.

But what constituted "unprofessional conduct"? For most of the Victorian age, practitioners were held to less taxing standards than have generally been enforced in twentieth-century Britain. Considerable leeway was still permitted to engage in commercial and entrepreneurial activities. It was not unknown for eminent Victorian physicians to puff proprietary preparations with impunity, or to lend their names to extravagant publicity for spas, clinics, and balneological establishments. Such respectable medical organs as the *British Medical Journal* and *Lancet* published advertisements every week for nostrums, health foods, and medical institutions of doubtful probity (for example, so-called nursing homes that probably served as abortion clinics).

Nevertheless, the profession grew increasingly mindful of the fact that, in an age priding itself upon public probity, respectability, and heightened moral sensibilities, doctors had to be seen as above scandal. Trying situations easily occurred. For example, from the 1840s,

thanks in part to the development of anesthetics, the scope for surgical intervention rapidly grew. Enterprising gynecologists and surgeons newly claimed to be able to treat a wide range of women's ailments, physical and psychosexual, through hysterectomy, ovariotomy, and similar operations upon the reproductive system. In the first flush of enthusiasm, some practitioners leapt in before the ethical implications had been adequately debated and resolved: Was proper informed consent being obtained for such operations? In the case of the removal of a womb, was it desirable to obtain the consent of the husband as well as of the patient? In the absence of diseased organs, was it permissible to perform operations for purely preventive or psychological reasons? Anxiety that the good name of the profession was being jeopardized by overenthusiastic intervention led to the expulsion, in the 1860s, of Isaac Baker Brown, a prominent advocate of clitoridectomy and similar surgery, from the Obstetrical Society (though he was disciplined not for the operations he performed but for the self-seeking manner in which he publicized them). Greater caution was subsequently exercised.

Whenever possible, the medical profession aimed to police its operations discreetly, retaining in its own hands the right to set moral standards. Thus, in ethically sensitive areas such as abortion, it was contended that termination of pregnancy was essentially a matter of clinical judgment in the individual case; in the last resort, only the personal physician was in a position to decide. Likewise, when legislation was proposed to control the sale of dangerous drugs, the profession was successful in safeguarding the right to supply narcotics on prescription.

In other medical spheres, however, ethical controversies arose that could not be kept within the circuit of professional discretion. This was because the Victorian age witnessed an unprecedented expansion of doctors' involvement in implementing state policy. For example, by 1900 new lunacy laws resulted in the compulsory confinement of nearly 100,000 mental patients. All had to be certified by due medical authorization. This created ethical predicaments for doctors that could not be resolved within Percival's notion of a tacit contract between physician and patient. Certain doctors, like the distinguished early Victorian psychiatrist John Conolly, warned of what a later generation was to call "psychiatric abuse": Some patients, Conolly feared, were being stripped of their rights and liberty not because they were sick but because they were nuisances or were merely eccentric.

It was in public health that the greatest ethical dilemmas arose. Before 1800, Great Britain had lacked the apparatus of medical police controls already in place on the Continent. This changed. The success of Jenner's variolation techniques (giving a dose of cowpox to create immunity against smallpox) led Parliament to make smallpox vaccination compulsory in 1853. Poor Law doctors—doctors appointed under the New Poor Law (1834) to tend to the parish poor, particularly those confined to workhouses—were to act as state agents in enforcing the legislation. Resistance and protests grew common during the next half-century, condemning compulsory vaccination as an iniquitous annulment of natural liberties and condemning doctors for serving as the lackeys of a coercive state.

A similar crisis arose in 1864 with the Contagious Diseases Acts. These sanctioned, under certain circumstances, medical inspection for signs of venereal disease of women detained by the police under suspicion of prostitution. Once again, opponents accused medical men of prostituting their art in the service of a corrupt state, and feminists argued that the acts were designed to provide disease-free vice for men. Around the same time, antivivisection agitators began accusing medical experimenters and scientists of inflicting cruelty upon dumb and defenseless experimental animals. The widening circle of medicine began to raise medical-ethical issues never dreamed of in the innocent days of Percival's *Medical Ethics*. Just before World War I these dilemmas came to a head when convicted suffragettes (militant feminists) went on a hunger strike, and prison doctors were instructed to administer forced feeding. Did their duty lie to society or to the prisoner (hardly a patient in the normal sense of the term, one who voluntarily seeks medical aid)?

In a characteristically British manner, professional bodies judged that the decision must be left to the doctor's scruples. The ingrained habits of individuality, specific to English liberal politics, and the cult of the gentleman that formed the unspoken code of male elites in all contemporary European societies meant that in professional eyes and, to a large degree, equally in the public mind the ethical dilemmas raised by medicine were best handled not by the law courts, jurists, academic philosophers, or Parliament but by the integrity of private practitioners following clinical judgment and their own consciences. These precepts, for better or worse, left a potent legacy to twentieth-century Britain. They certainly offered great latitude to the medical profession while placing heavy burdens upon its shoulders. Radical critics of the professions and their ideologies have contended, surely correctly, that the formulation of medical ethics enhanced the status and exalted the independence of the nineteenth-century doctors. How far this process helped to protect the public is more difficult to judge.

ROY PORTER

While the other articles in this section and the other sections of this entry are relevant, see especially the companion article in this subsection: EUROPE. *For a further discussion of* topics mentioned in this article, see the entries CIRCUMCISION; CLINICAL ETHICS; HEALTH-CARE FINANCING, *article on* PROFIT AND COMMERCIALISM; HEALTH OFFICIALS AND THEIR RESPONSIBILITIES; HEALTH SCREENING AND TESTING IN THE PUBLIC-HEALTH CONTEXT; HOSPITAL, *articles on* MEDIEVAL AND RENAISSANCE HISTORY, *and* MODERN HISTORY; INFORMED CONSENT; LICENSING, DISCIPLINE, AND REGULATION IN THE HEALTH PROFESSIONS; MEDICAL CODES AND OATHS, *article on* HISTORY; MEDICAL MALPRACTICE; MEDICINE, ANTHROPOLOGY OF; MEDICINE, SOCIOLOGY OF; MEDICINE AS A PROFESSION; PATIENTS' RESPONSIBILITIES; PHARMACEUTICS; PROFESSIONAL–PATIENT RELATIONSHIP; PROFESSION AND PROFESSIONAL ETHICS; PROSTITUTION; PROTESTANTISM; PSYCHIATRY, ABUSES OF; PSYCHOSURGERY; PUBLIC HEALTH; PUBLIC HEALTH AND THE LAW; PUBLIC POLICY AND BIOETHICS; RESEARCH, HUMAN: HISTORICAL ASPECTS; SEXISM; SURGERY; VIRTUE AND CHARACTER; *and* WOMEN. *Other relevant material may be found under the entries* BENEFICENCE; CONSCIENCE; FEMINISM; JUSTICE; OBLIGATION AND SUPEREROGATION; PATERNALISM; *and* RESPONSIBILITY. *See also the* APPENDIX (CODES, OATHS, AND DIRECTIVES RELATED TO BIOETHICS), SECTION II: ETHICAL DIRECTIVES FOR THE PRACTICE OF MEDICINE, CODE OF ETHICS [1847] *of the* AMERICAN MEDICAL ASSOCIATION.

Bibliography

BARTRIP, PETER. 1994. "Secret Remedies, Medical Ethics and the Finances of the *British Medical Journal*." In vol. 2 of *The Codification of Medical Morality: Historical and Philosophical Studies of the Formalization of Medical Morality in the Eighteenth and Nineteenth Centuries*. Edited by Robert Baker, Dorothy Porter, and Roy Porter. Dordrecht, Netherlands: Kluwer.

BEDDOES, THOMAS. 1808. *A Letter to the Right Honourable Sir Joseph Banks . . . on the Causes and Removal of the Prevailing Discontents, Imperfections, and Abuses in Medicine.* London: Richard Phillips.

BURNS, CHESTER. 1974. "Reciprocity in the Development of Anglo-American Medical Ethics, 1765–1865." In vol. 1 of the *Proceedings of the XXIII International Congress of the History of Medicine*, pp. 813–819. London: Wellcome Institute for the History of Medicine.

CRAWFORD, CATHERINE. 1987. "The Emergence of Forensic Medicine: Medical Evidence in Common Law Courts, 1730–1830." D. Phil. diss., Oxford University.

CROWTHER, M. ANN. 1994. "Forensic Medicine and Medical Ethics in Nineteenth-Century Britain." In vol. 2 of *The Codification of Medical Morality: Historical and Philosophical Studies of the Formalization of Medical Morality in the Eighteenth and Nineteenth Centuries*. Edited by Robert Baker, Dorothy Porter, and Roy Porter. Dordrecht, Netherlands: Kluwer.

GAY, PETER. 1984. *Education of the Senses.* Vol. 1 of *The Bourgeois Experience, Victoria to Freud.* New York: Oxford University Press

———. 1986. *The Tender Passion.* Vol. 2 of *The Bourgeois Experience, Victoria to Freud.* New York: Oxford University Press.

LEAKE, CHAUNCEY D. 1971. "Percival's *Medical Ethics*: Promise and Problems." *California Medicine* 114, no. 4:68–70.

MOSCUCCI, ORNELLA. 1990. *The Science of Woman: Gynaecology and Gender in England, 1800–1929.* Cambridge: At the University Press.

PELLEGRINO, EDMUND. 1986. "Percival's *Medical Ethics*: The Moral Philosophy of an 18th–Century English Gentleman." *Archives of Internal Medicine* 146, no. 114:2265–2269.

PERCIVAL, THOMAS. 1803. *Medical Ethics; or, A Code of Institutes and Precepts Adapted to the Professional Conduct of Physicians and Surgeons.* Manchester: J. Johnson and R. Bickerstaff.

PETERSON, M. JEANNE. 1978. *The Medical Profession in Mid-Victorian London.* Berkeley: University of California Press.

PICKSTONE, JOHN V. 1993. "Thomas Percival and the Production of Medical Ethics." In *Medical Ethics and Etiquette in the Eighteenth Century,* pp. 161–178. Vol. 1 of *The Codification of Medical Morality: Historical and Philosophical Studies of the Formalization of Western Medical Morality in the Eighteenth and Nineteenth Centuries.* Edited by Robert Baker, Dorothy Porter, and Roy Porter. Dordrecht, Netherlands: Kluwer.

PORTER, DOROTHY, and PORTER, ROY. 1988a. "The Enforcement of Health: The British Debate." In *AIDS: The Burdens of History,* pp. 97–120. Edited by Elizabeth Fee and Daniel M. Fox. Berkeley: University of California Press.

———. 1988b. "The Politics of Prevention: Anti-Vaccinationism and Public Health in Nineteenth-Century England." *Medical History* 32, no. 3:231–252.

PORTER, ROY. 1989. *Health for Sale: Quackery in England 1650–1850.* Manchester, U.K.: Manchester University Press.

SMITH, RUSSELL. 1994. "Legal Precedent and Medical Ethics: Some Problems Encountered by the General Medical Council in Relying upon Precedent When Declaring Acceptable Standards of Professional Conduct." In vol. 2 of *The Codification of Medical Morality: Historical and Philosophical Studies of the Formalization of Medical Morality in the Eighteenth and Nineteenth Centuries.* Edited by Robert Baker, Dorothy Porter, and Roy Porter. Dordrecht, Netherlands: Kluwer.

WADDINGTON, IVAN. 1975. "The Development of Medical Ethics—A Sociological Analysis." *Medical History* 19, no. 1:36–51.

———. 1984. *The Medical Profession in the Industrial Revolution.* Dublin: Gill and Macmillan.

D. CONTEMPORARY PERIOD

1. INTRODUCTION

Bioethics is flourishing in most of the countries of late-twentieth-century Europe. However, as a field of ethical reflection and an instrument of public policy, bioethics is hardly uniform across the continent. The development of medical science and technology, as in many countries throughout the world, has stimulated an interest in the attendant ethical issues. Yet the ways various countries have experienced that development differ, as has their ethical response. Although influenced by social and political events, and by philosophical, literary, religious, and cultural ideas common to the European milieu, various countries and cultures have contributed in unique ways to the formulation of bioethical ideas. There is now a European Association of Bioethics, and in its deliberations, the commonalities of European bioethics can be found, as well as the distinct accents of the various national participants. This introduction will state some of the common themes; the articles that follow will emphasize national and regional distinctions.

Role of medical science and technology

An important prerequisite to twentieth-century discussions and positions was the establishment in the nineteenth century of a natural scientific basis of medicine. Impressive progress in diagnosis and treatment, coupled with this development, led to new ethical problems. Concurrent with this process was an anthropological reduction—a loss of humanistic dimensions in the natural sciences and medicine leading to various attempts at balance and correction in the early twentieth century.

Philosophical influences

Anthropological medicine and philosophical or existential psychiatry are important twentieth-century reactions to the one-sided natural scientific orientation of medicine. Various philosophical directions, associated with the names of Edmund Husserl, Martin Heidegger, Karl Jaspers, Jean-Paul Sartre, Maurice Merleau-Ponty, Gabriel Marcel, and José Xavier Zubiri, have influenced medicine. Theology has also made important contributions. An independent, intramedical discussion of methods and theory, beginning in the late nineteenth century, and the integration of psychology and sociology into medicine in the last decades, have also affected contemporary European bioethics.

The situation of medical history in the medical faculties of the universities of Europe presents a different picture. The grand tradition of the presentation of history and theory, including the study of medical ethics, as part of the formal education required of medical students during the preclinical and clinical years, was abandoned in the empirical, scientific nineteenth century. Only in Germany was it possible to establish a chair for medical history in almost every medical faculty.

These impulses and initiatives sought to bridge the separation between the natural sciences and humanities. The history of the patient was considered to be as important as the history of the illness. The ethical dimension was recognized anew in the understanding of disease, the concept of treatment, and the physician–patient relationship.

After 1900, discussions of the concept of cause led to a new appreciation of the anthropological dimensions of medicine. The concept of monocausality has been countered by that of multiconditionalism; disease cannot be explained by one cause but by several causes. Constitution and disposition (i.e. the physical conditions of the individual) supplement the principle of exogenous infection; cause (= causa efficiens) and aim (= causa finalis) should not mutually exclude one another. Physical as well as mental illness can fulfill a purpose or meaning, can represent freedom in unfreedom, in the type of coping with these damages.

Literary influence

The arts—in particular literary texts—also proffer important influences and models. Medical ethics has profited and will continue to profit from a unification with medical humanities. Novels and stories describe the attitudes and behavior of the patient as well as the physician in detail, drawing the reader into the context of the hospital as well as the wider social environment. Such literary depictions and interpretations, in providing examples, can play an important role in medical training. The scientific pleas for euthanasia at the beginning of the twentieth century find their supplementation or preparation in the literature of the nineteenth century. The texts of Guy de Maupassant, Henrik Ibsen, Theodor Storm, Anton Chekhov, and Hjalmar Söderberg describe conflicts in which the killing of a suffering and dying person is suggested; at the same time, there are warnings against active euthanasia. Normative opinions that equate health with the positive and illness with the negative are relativized or even reversed in the works of Marcel Proust, Thomas Mann, Robert Musil, Virginia Woolf, and many other writers. Health should also be understood as the ability to live with illnesses and disabilities, which may harbor opportunity and challenge. The patient has rights and duties, as does the physician; both can exhibit virtues. Their relationship manifests both asymmetry and symmetry such as differences in medical knowledge and experiences of pain and disease.

Political influences

Ethical discussions of medical issues took place in all European countries even before World War II. Numerous essays and monographs were published on the ethics of the physician, ethics in research, and the ethics of patients, as well as the ethics of the family and of society. In 1901, the first Congrès International de Médecine Professionelle et de Déontologie Médicale took place in Paris. Many conventions on the subject of forensic medicine had already taken place. Bioethics in Europe is not uniform. Different accents can be found in theory and practice. The differences are based on each country's respective artistic traditions as well as on the respective political and economic situations and legal regulations.

Undoubtedly, World War II and, after its end, the Nuremberg Code were turning points in bioethics. On the one hand, an increased tendency toward international uniformity in bioethics was reflected in such international declarations as, for example, Helsinki (1964) and Tokyo (1975), and in the introduction of ethics committees. On the other hand, the multitude of differing orientations retains its validity, even gaining a new weight through the presence of foreign labor and long-term migration in the European countries. Radical political changes in Eastern Europe and Germany through the collapse of communism has made manifest the continuity of ethical opinions and social conditions that had been thought to be relics of the past; these hold new meaning for bioethics in the future.

Problems in bioethics must be solved on many levels, particularly in the Eastern European countries. At the center stands the task of finding a convincing ethical or humanistic solution for the vacuum of ideals left by the collapse of communism and the pressure of technical–scientific progress. Here, as is generally the case in the realization of ethical principles, the applicable legal regulations are of decisive importance. When moral principles are weak, laws can offer protection.

Medical ethics and bioethics

Because of the plurality of traditions that make up contemporary European bioethics, it is not possible to isolate a single path of development. The word "bioethics" itself denotes many things. "Bioethics" has been used to propose norms in the practices of modern biomedicine, norms of a religious-ethical nature, and norms of legal or philosophical ethics. Sometimes, under the new label "bioethics," the method and arguments of already consolidated disciplines (moral theology, law, ethical guidelines for health professionals, moral philosophy) are easily recognizable, enriched only by the content of new problems.

In the different European cultural contexts, bioethics has had to confront a strong tradition of medical ethics that was developed and defended by physicians as their exclusive property. The proprietary claims of health professionals on medical ethics have produced ambivalent results. The independence of medical ethics has sometimes been able to protect the profession from the pressures that totalitarian ideology exerts on physicians to conform their behavior to the values imposed by the regime. Under the fascist and Nazi regimes (Italy and Germany) and in countries ruled by communism, medical ethics was denied an independent status in order to subordinate it to particular ideological visions (including racism, eugenics, the class struggle, and the dictatorship of the proletariat). In such situations, medical ethics' independence from the values that regulate the society created space for an ethics tied to philanthropic and universalistic ideals.

Nevertheless, the medical ethics elaborated by professional physicians can also obstruct the rise of formulations better adapted to the changing cultural situation. This is evident in many European countries by the many physicians who turn to traditional medical ethics, inspired by the ideals of Hippocratic medicine and strongly anchored in a paternalistic attitude toward the sick person, in order to oppose the medical models centered on the value of individual autonomy and the practice of informed consent.

The thrust toward bioethics is characterized, if compared with the strong tradition of an ethics developed by the medical profession itself, by the need for a civil ethics or an ethic of ordinary life elaborated in many voices. Bioethics is differentiated from medical ethics in being a consensual reformulation of rights and obligations in the context of medical practice and health care. This includes the professional obligations of physicians, but does not derive only from these. A further characteristic trait of bioethics in regard to civil or general ethics is the minimal ethical consensus, which obliges all citizens, in contrast to the maximal ethical consensus, which focuses on individual preferences.

A second issue that bioethics in Europe must face is its relationship with religious ethics. The weight of religious ethics relative to the moral problems posed by the corporality of man (sexuality, procreation, disease, health, death) and health care varies according to cultural context and type of religious communities in the society. In societies in which a single religion dominates, especially of the Catholic tradition (Ireland, Poland, Italy, Spain), religious ethics tends to superimpose itself onto bioethics, shaping it to its own norms. In countries in which a tradition of pluralism prevails, the two normative contexts—religious ethical and bioethical—are more clearly distinct.

Where religious ethics is seen as antithetical to secular ethics, a clear polarization can appear in the society; possible examples are Ireland, Poland, or Portugal, with their Catholic tradition. Justification of ethical judgment then consists of making reference exclusively to one set of values instead of another. This happens, for example, when clinical decisions are evaluated exclusively in terms of values considered to be absolute: sacredness of life versus quality of life, benefit of the medical act versus self-determination of the patient, and so on.

A third issue in the contemporary development of bioethics in Europe relates to the challenge of universalism. Developments in the ethics of medicine and biological sciences reveal two opposing challenges for bioethics: the need to be rooted in the particular, with respect to the cultures, traditions, and local communities of belonging, and the need to refer itself to universal values. Universalism is an intrinsic dimension of ethical rationalism. At the same time, universalism is necessary to ensure normative rules and moral obligations. The directives, for example, of "Good Clinical Practice for Trials on Medical Products in European Community" (1991) have had the aim of producing one practice of experimentation in this field. In Europe, in fact, the crowded national frontiers would easily create "enclaves" where biomedical practices prohibited beyond these frontiers would be legitimate. An international consensus has to be created to prevent a "tourism" in medical research.

The various bioethics developing in Europe face the challenge of particularism as much as that of universalism. The best forms of European bioethics are clearly those that are trying to respond to both these challenges.

DIETRICH VON ENGELHARDT
SANDRO SPINSANTI

While the other articles in this section and the other sections of this entry are relevant, see especially the other articles in this subsection: SOUTHERN EUROPE, THE BENELUX COUNTRIES, UNITED KINGDOM, REPUBLIC OF IRELAND, GERMAN-SPEAKING COUNTRIES AND SWITZERLAND, NORDIC COUNTRIES, CENTRAL AND EASTERN EUROPE, *and* RUSSIA. *For a further discussion of topics mentioned in this article, see the entries* AUTONOMY; BIOETHICS EDUCATION; HEALTH AND DISEASE; INFORMED CONSENT; LITERATURE; MEDICINE, ANTHROPOLOGY OF; MEDICINE, SOCIOLOGY OF; PATERNALISM; PROFESSION AND PROFESSIONAL ETHICS; PROTESTANTISM; ROMAN CATHOLICISM; SOCIAL MEDICINE; *and* VALUE AND VALUATION.

2. SOUTHERN EUROPE

The term "southern European countries" includes all the occidental European countries in the Mediterranean area (Spain, France, Italy, Greece, Malta, and Cyprus), plus an Atlantic country closely related to them (Portugal). In addition to geographical and climatological affinities, these seven countries have for many centuries shared a common history centered on the Mediterranean Sea. Although they maintain local peculiarities and differences, the nations of southern Europe can be said to have a common identity.

This common identity is particularly evident in ethical issues (Gracia, 1993). Occidental ethics had its origin in the Mediterranean Greco-Latin culture, and since the days of the Greek philosophers, this ethics has centered on the concepts of virtue and vice. Only with the Enlightenment did a new ethical tradition, with right and duty as its main concepts, begin to take shape in central Europe. Since then the two approaches have widely been considered opposites, although they are in fact complementary. The ethics of virtue has persisted in those countries in which the Enlightenment had less influence, such as the Catholic or Orthodox southern European nations, while the ethics of duty has prevailed in the Protestant central European and Anglo-Saxon countries (MacIntyre, 1984).

Today the Occidental world harbors three palpably different ethical traditions, each with its own characteristics: the Anglo-Saxon, the central European, and the Mediterranean. Because modern bioethics is a product of the Anglo-American culture, Mediterranean countries have not attempted simply to import or "translate" bioethics but, rather, to "re-create" or "remake" the discipline according to their own cultural and ethical traditions (Gracia, 1990).

A "Latin model" of bioethics

If traditional Anglo-American philosophy is generally classified as empiricist, European philosophy has been more influenced by rationalism. Anglo-American ethics is generally more teleological and consequentialist, and European ethics more deontological. This explains why, for instance, the term "autonomy" has acquired a different meaning in the United States than in Europe. According to North American ethics, autonomy is the capacity to act intentionally, with understanding, and without controlling influences. On the other hand, European ethicists often interpret the principle of autonomy in a Kantian sense, as the capacity of human reason to impose absolute moral laws upon itself. The latter is a metaphysical assumption, while the former is only the lack of constraints. In the European, acting autonomously means that the human reason is capable of freely establishing absolute and compulsory moral laws (freedom to). In the Anglo-American, on the contrary, freedom is understood only negatively, as the capacity to act without constraints (freedom from). The first is a maximal concept of autonomy, and the second a minimal one. These two meanings are so disparate that an autonomous person, according to the European point of view, may not act autonomously from the Anglo-American perspective because of constraints such as ignorance or coercion. Moreover, it is also possible to deny the capacity of reason to impose on itself absolute moral laws, and to accept the concept of autonomous choice as the absence of external constraints.

The rational foundation of ethics is closely linked to the discussion of whether the principle of autonomy is relative or absolute. In Europe, the Anglo-American propensity to base ethical analysis on several theories, such as utilitarianism and contractualism, and on a few principles, such as autonomy and beneficence, is usually considered insufficient or less adequate. Europeans generally search for more "universal" or "transcendental" ethical foundations. The meaning of the concept of "transcendental" differs in central and southern Europe. Central European ethics often attempts to reach the transcendental dimension through an intersubjective procedure, such as the universalization of personal interests. According to many Mediterranean ethicists, the transcendental universality of ethical norms is reached in a more objective way, based on metaphysical concepts like "reality," "human nature," or "personhood" (Russo, 1992). The latter is, of course, the most "classical" position in Occidental philosophy. It is no coincidence that this classical concept of metaphysics was born on the Mediterranean coast.

Modern northern European ethics, based on the concepts of "right" and "duty," has been the matrix of ethical minimalism (or the ethics of duty), while the traditional Mediterranean ethics, based on "virtue," has tended more toward ethical maximalism (or the ethics of happiness). While minimalistic ethics looks for the basic rights and duties of every human being and society, maximalistic ethics is concerned with life projects and ideals of perfection and happiness (in Greek, *eudaimonia*). During the sixteenth century, Mediterranean countries adopted anti-Protestant, and therefore anti-modern, attitudes; they considered certain aspects of modernity to be fundamentally hostile to their cultural traditions: their medieval political, ethical, and religious ideals. These attitudes may explain why many Mediterranean nations belatedly and with difficulty adopted the doctrines of human rights and parliamentary democracy, the greatest achievements of the Anglo-American world. This may also explain the relative weakness of democratic practices in these countries in comparison with other areas. This antimodern stance enables us to understand the history of southern Europe since the nineteenth century, particularly the potency of anti-democratic movements and authoritarianism during the first half of the twentieth century. And while western European countries definitively adopted democracy and liberal systems following World War II, some of the Mediterranean countries maintained a markedly different identity.

All these elements help clarify why southern European countries have tried to elaborate a "Latin" model of bioethics (Leone, 1990). While the Anglo-American model is structured around the four classical principles of autonomy, nonmaleficence, beneficence, and justice, Salvino Leone, following Elio Sgreccia, bases the so-called Latin model on the four principles of the fundamental value of life; liberty and responsibility; totality (or therapeutic wholeness); and social subsidiarity (the idea that smaller units are always preferred to larger ones when it comes to addressing social problems) (Sgreccia, 1988; Palazzani, 1993).

This search for distinctiveness also led Mediterranean ethicists to seek to establish their own terminology. The French expression *éthique biomédicale*, "meaning the desire to promote a new style of questioning in the field of biomedical sciences, both theoretical and educational" (Moulin, 1988, p. 280), has been adopted as an alternative term to the Anglo-American bioethics not only in French but also in other Mediterranean languages, such as Italian (Spinsanti, 1987) and Spanish. The reason for this terminological change is that for many authors, the word "bioethics" seems overly biologistic and suggests that ethical behavior is biologically determined. The alternative expression "biomedical ethics" was coined to avoid this danger. It situates the term "ethics" as the noun, with "biology" and "medicine" in secondary adjectival position. Of course, the term "bioethics" is also frequently used in Mediterranean countries, just as North American literature occasionally uses the expression "biomedical ethics" (Beauchamp and Childress, 1983).

The ethics of virtue and the doctor-patient relationship

Mediterranean countries have created a "realistic" and "personalist" model of biomedical ethics, based on the classical Aristotelian-Scholastic philosophy and complemented with more modern European philosophical traditions such as phenomenology, axiology, and hermeneutics (Viafora, 1990). In it, the idea of virtue acquires much more significance than in any other Occidental tradition, a fact that has important consequences in the medical field. For example, trustworthiness is considered more crucial than the right to information (Dalla-Vorgia et al., 1992). Patients in southern European nations are generally less concerned with receiving detailed information or having their autonomy respected than with finding a doctor in whom they can place their full confidence (Gordon, 1990; Spinsanti, 1992; Fletcher, 1992; Loewy, 1992).

One virtue is particularly important in establishing a satisfactory doctor-patient relationship: friendship. The Spanish physician and humanist Pedro Laín En-

tralgo has written extensively on this topic, especially in his book *The Doctor-Patient Relationship* (Laín Entralgo, 1969, 1983). This relationship must be based on what Laín Entralgo calls "medical friendship," composed of benevolence, beneficence, and confidence. His studies have had a substantial but not exclusive impact in Mediterranean and Latin American medicine; as a result, the idea of friendship as the cornerstone of the relationship between doctor and patient has gradually acquired importance in bioethics. The influence of his studies is also visible in North American bioethical literature (Siegler, 1979, 1981; Pellegrino and Thomasma, 1981; U.S. President's Commission, 1982; Cassell, 1984; Drane, 1988).

Friendship includes trust and confidence, which is why we talk about "intimate" friends; friendship is the ambit of trust. The three theological virtues (faith, hope, and love) are common between friends. The core of this relation is hope, understood as trust: we trust friends, we have faith in them, and we trust them because we love them. Friendship is more than ethics; it is almost a religion. Charity, or agape, is considered the most important virtue in the Judeo-Christian tradition. But, according to Laín Entralgo, the agape can be considered perfect only when benevolence and beneficence, its main components, join friendship's trust and confidence (Laín Entralgo, 1985). The result is, as Edmund Pellegrino (Pellegrino, 1986, 1988, 1989) and Warren T. Reich (Reich, 1989, 1991), two U.S. authors influenced by Laín Entralgo, have written, "com-passion," the act of putting oneself in the place of another in order to understand his or her experiences. Compassion is not pity but, rather, the human relationship based on devotion, constancy, personal respect, and responsibility. As Reich says, it is the relation with the other, based on love, benevolence, comprehension, and friendship. Mediterranean bioethics has emphasized the study of the friendship aspect of the physician–patient relation, and the Spanish contribution has been important (Gracia, 1989).

Ethics and law

The relationship between ethics and law is peculiar in the Mediterranean. In its origins, Roman law was substantially influenced by Stoicism, a school of thought that assimilated law and morality. Stoics considered nature the source of both law and morality; natural law could be known rationally, and thus formulated deontologically and axiomatically into a legal code. Because law expresses what is morally correct, ethics and law converged. Ethical "goodness," the intention with which an act is performed, only added to the legal "rightness" of the act and to the "virtue" of the person involved.

Christian thinkers adopted this relationship between ethics and law without substantial changes, and it has been a latent presence both in canon law and in the moral theology of the Roman Catholic church. Thus, in Catholic nations such as those of southern Europe, law and morality are difficult to distinguish conceptually.

One of the problematic outgrowths of this tradition is legalism, the tendency to believe that every human act can be legally prefigured, that laws precede facts, making it possible to regulate beforehand every real or possible situation. Thus, in these countries court rulings are considered nothing more than the concrete application of statutory law. This law is prior to individual rulings, quite the opposite of the Anglo-Saxon common-law system. The traditions also diverge in that the Roman model is largely centralized and state-oriented and places less importance on social dynamics. The prevalence of state over society explains why Mediterranean countries have fostered more authoritarian and less democratic political practices than Anglo-Saxon ones.

Health systems

That the state must, in southern European countries, take responsibility for what in other countries is considered the realm of private enterprise, illuminates another distinctive characteristic of Mediterranean bioethics: its overwhelming concern with health-care justice. In fact, the health systems of these countries are mainly state-run. Justice plays the decisive role in European biomedical ethics that autonomy plays in North American bioethics (Thomasma, 1985).

France, Italy, Greece, Portugal, and Spain have similar national health insurance systems. Their common origins date back to the German *Krankenkassen* (patients' fund) system, designed by Otto von Bismarck in the final decades of the nineteenth century as a means of assuring medical assistance for workers. In distinction to the socialist European countries, where all the population was covered by an insurance system financed by public funds, Mediterranean countries, following the German model, began insuring only workers, and financing the system with the economic support of both workers and employers. Coverage was later extended by public funding, and today nearly the entire population of each country is protected. This process of generalization of the health insurance system took place during the zenith years of the welfare state, between the end of World War II and the economic crisis of 1973. In the mid-1970s, health insurance as well as the entire social security system, and perhaps the welfare state itself, experienced a crisis, mainly because of the "costs explosion," which made it impossible to satisfy the population's health expectations. To find solutions for this complex problem, most countries set up reform commissions aimed at proposing measures to make health insurance viable in the future.

In Spain, compulsory health insurance for all workers was enacted in 1942 and implemented in 1943. Over the next three decades, coverage was gradually extended. In 1986 it became a national health system very similar to those in Britain and Italy, covering the health care of most of the country's population (Gracia, 1987). This satisfied one of the people's greatest wishes but at the same time gave birth to a new problem, which became more and more acute as time went by: the scarcity of economic resources and the subsequent need to limit free health services. In order to analyze and evaluate the needs of the national health system, the Spanish parliament in 1990 set up a commission, known as the Comisión Abril Martorell. The commission's main report, published in July 1991, asserted the importance of the national health system in maintaining the level of health and well-being in Spain, and proposed certain amendments to increase efficiency without altering the basic system. One such modification would require every user of health-care services to pay a percentage of the total cost, in an attempt to make everyone shoulder the burden of the constant increases in health expenses.

Patients' rights

The way patients' rights were established marks another differentiating factor of Mediterranean countries. In the United States these rights, particularly the right to informed consent, took shape in the field of common law, while in Mediterranean countries their entry was directly through statutory laws and codes (Council of Europe, 1976; Gracia, 1989). In these countries, protecting patients' rights is a duty of the state more than the duty of individuals. In Spain, patients' rights were first established legally (Article 10 of the Health Law of 1986) and then socially.

In all Mediterranean countries the respect for patients' autonomy and their right to make decisions about their own bodies has grown remarkably in the last decades (Cattorini and Reichlin, 1992). This has produced profound changes in the role of health-care professionals, as well as more litigation against physicians and other health-care workers. The old juridical terms "professional incompetence" and "negligence," which referred to faulty medical procedures, are today overshadowed by new complaints about health workers' lack of skill or their negligence in giving information, or about battery, for handling the patient's body without consent.

The patients' rights movement of the 1970s provoked wide-ranging legislative changes (Council of Europe, 1976). For example, the large antipsychiatry movement in 1978, led in the Mediterranean area by Italy, prompted some countries to modify laws on the compulsory restraint of the mentally ill by passing new legislation more respectful of these patients' human rights and providing greater protection against possible abuse by family members or health professionals.

Additional consequences of this new respect for patients' rights are the strict regulation of biomedical experimentation and the creation of institutional review boards to monitor every clinical trial and research project protocol, analyzing not only technical and methodological but also ethical aspects. The Council of the European Community on November 24, 1986, approved a directive on the protection of the animals used in research and other scientific projects. Every country of the European Community adopted its own legislation in the following years, and today research with animals is strictly controlled (Illera, 1989).

In an attempt to promote organ transplants while avoiding any kind of commerce and abuse in the donation process, all Mediterranean countries have introduced legislative criteria for brain death and have elaborated laws regulating transplants. The legal regulation of medical care to the dying has encountered greater obstacles, and has provoked heated debates over euthanasia (Gracia, 1987; Gracia, 1988; Lefevre, 1988; Dracopolou and Doxiadis, 1988; Bompiani, 1992).

Issues related to the origin of life, especially abortion and new techniques for human reproduction, have been the subject of the most intense debates. Mediterranean countries have adopted conservative positions in these debates. In these nations the U.S. Supreme Court decision *Roe* v. *Wade* (1973), based on the right to privacy, restricting the right of states to legislate on abortion in terms of viability and trimesters, is not easily understood. In Mediterranean countries, abortion is held to be a public rather than a private issue and therefore a matter of justice and not of autonomy, since the life of a human being is believed to be at stake. Hence, in these countries, laws governing the interruption of pregnancy are based on exceptional circumstances or "indications" rather than on periods of time or "terms." These laws allow abortion in three exceptional indications: great danger to the mother's health or life; important defects of the fetus; and rape. Only a few countries, such as Italy and Cyprus, have included a fourth indication: socioeconomic incapacity, valid during the first trimester of gestation. The Veil Law (1975) in France established that any pregnant woman can undergo an abortion during the first ten weeks if gestation is a source of anguish (*détresse*) for her, an indication that, in practice, is analogous to a law of terms (a period of time in which abortion is permitted without any indication). Since 1986 Greece has had a law of terms: abortion is permitted in the first twelve weeks of pregnancy. After

this period, gestation can be interrupted only with an ethical (nineteen weeks), eugenic (twenty-four weeks), or therapeutic indication (Glendon, 1987).

The problems presented by new techniques of human reproduction are so various and complex that every southern European country has established a specific commission for their study. The Comisión Palacios of Spain and the Commissione Santosuosso of Italy are examples. Both bodies have elaborated reports for legislative enactment, which has been achieved in Spain but not in Italy (Gracia, 1988; Fagot-Largeault, 1987; Mori, 1987; Walters, 1987; Bompiani, 1992). But more important, these commissions became aware of the need for national committees of bioethics, which today are firmly established in the Mediterranean area. This same process has taken place in Europe as a whole, where the Council of Europe in 1983 established the Ad Hoc Committee on Ethical and Legal Problems Related to Genetic Engineering, which a few years later became the Ad Hoc Committee of Experts on Bioethics and is now called the Steering Committee of Bioethics.

National committees of bioethics

National committees of bioethics have been set up because of the increasing complexity of biomedical research and to avoid dangerous research like that which made possible the construction of nuclear weapons during the 1940s and 1950s, and the experiments carried out in Nazi concentration camps. The main aim of these committees is to help those involved in biomedical research by offering prudent criteria for conduct.

On February 23, 1983, French President François Mitterrand created the first national bioethics commission in a European country, the Comité Consultatif National d'Éthique pour les Sciences de la Vie et de la Santé (CCNE). Its purpose is mainly to elaborate recommendations on ethical problems stemming from scientific research in biology, medicine, and other health professions (Isambert, 1989). It deals not with healthcare problems but with ethical questions raised by biomedical research. The CCNE is composed of thirty-six members plus a chairman who is appointed by the president of the republic. The departments of Education, Research, Industry, Health, Justice, Family, and Communication appoint sixteen members with proven competence and interest in ethical issues. Fifteen posts are filled by researchers and representatives of universities and the National Institutes of Health and Research. Five members, named by the president of the republic, are drawn from the "spiritual and philosophical" fields. Committee members are divided into working teams to prepare reports and recommendations (*avis*). The documents so far produced have dealt with the use of fetal and embryonic tissues for diagnostic, therapeutic, or research purposes; techniques of artificial procreation; prenatal and perinatal diagnosis; the use of the abortion-causing drug RU-486; and the noncommercialization of the human body, among other topics. Every year, the committee organizes meetings of study and debate called the *Journées Annuelles d'Éthique*, in order to release the year's work to the public.

The French commission's work has stimulated bioethics studies in the Mediterranean area, much as the National and President's Commissions have done in the United States. Of the two possible methodologies identified by the Belgian philosopher of medicine François Malherbe—that of the lowest common denominator (the search for a formula everybody agrees with, even if it is ambiguous and makes room for very different interpretations) and that of the highest common denominator (requiring much more work, reflection, and dialogue)—the Comité Consultatif National opted for the second. This decision had an evident impact on the text of a report the committee issued, "Biomedical Research and Respect for the Human Being" (CCNE, 1988). French bioethics is coming to be, as Malherbe says, "an active center of public morality in the life of people" (Malherbe, 1990, p. 227). The French ethics of the highest common denominator is similar to some of the most creative ideas from Jürgen Habermas and Karl O. Apels's "ethics of communication," which is based on the idea that in the context of a pluralistic society, ethics will flourish only if it takes into account the interests of every person actually or virtually involved in the conflict. The French committee has integrated German dialogic ethics with French personalism, widespread among French philosophers of the last century, and firmly established in certain Catholic (Maurice Nédoncelle), Protestant (Paul Ricoeur), and Jewish (Emmanuel Lévinas) phenomenological thinkers. According to Lucien Séve, these ideas have proved fundamental for the elaboration of a working procedure based on "rational consensus" and not on a merely strategic consensus (Séve, 1988).

The French committee has had great success, and hence this model has spread throughout Europe, including the Mediterranean countries. Malta instituted its Health Ethics Consultative Committee in 1989 (Le Bris, 1992). In March 1990 the Italian government approved the creation of the Comitato Nazionale per la Bioetica, directly responsible to the prime minister. The body is composed of forty members and, like the French group, is aimed at controlling research involving human beings. It has published documents on gene therapy, definition of human death, ethics of the use of seminal fluid for diagnostic purposes, biotechnological security, bioethical learning in the clinical setting, health care and terminally ill patients, organ donation, and ethics committees.

Portugal, following the French pattern, in June 1990 established the National Ethical Council for Life Sciences (Martinho da Silva, 1990). The body started functioning January 1, 1991, and in its three first years published three reports: on organ donation and transplantation (1991), on the use of human corpses in research and teaching (1991), and on new reproductive technologies (1993).

In 1984 Spain created a special committee known as the Comité Palacios to study problems related to new techniques of assisted reproduction (artificial insemination, in vitro fertilization, and so forth). In addition, in September 1990 the Department of Health elaborated a legal project outlining the objectives and functions of the National Committee of Bioethics, but it was not approved. In July 1992 the Department of Health published a legal order creating a health advisory committee whose main goal was assessing and informing the secretary of the department on scientific, ethical, professional, and social questions. This committee deals not only with problems of biomedical research but also with those raised by health care. This innovative feature distinguishes it from others in the region.

In southern Europe, institutional ethics committees are rare, in part due to the prevalence of socialized medicine and in part because Mediterraneans are not completely conscious of patients' rights. In Spain, for instance, such committees have only recently begun to appear in hospitals, following the General Health Law of 1986 that specifically mandates the protection of patients' rights.

New goals for the 1990s

In recent years new problems have appeared. They will probably be the most important in the last decade of the twentieth century. Two of them are population ethics and ecology. Ecology is acquiring increasing importance in all Mediterranean countries, and is beginning to be not only an ethical and intellectual issue but also a political force (Gafo, 1991; Poli and Timmerman, 1991). Latin European countries are neighbors of the underdeveloped nations situated on the southern Mediterranean coast, and they therefore understand very well that only a sustainable development can correct the unsustainable development of the First World and the underdevelopment of the Third World. Ecology in these countries will be not only an ethical compromise but also a political project, prompted by the left-wing parties. With the death of the Marxist ideology, ecology assumes the place once held by economic theory.

Due to the increasing importance of bioethics in the life of these countries, research and teaching are growing quickly. The teaching of bioethics is being introduced not only in schools directly related to health care, such as medicine, pharmacy, and biology, but also in theology, philosophy, and humanities (Comitato Nazionale per la Bioetica, 1991; Gracia, 1992). Literature is being published, and universities are supporting new research centers (Viafora, 1993). All of the research centers have been integrated into the European Association of Centers of Medical Ethics. Since 1990 the Milazzo Group has published *International Journal of Bioethics*.

Bioethics has acquired a very important place in the culture of Mediterranean countries, where, as in most developed countries, it is coming to be the ethics of the end of the twentieth century and the beginning of the third millenium.

DIEGO GRACIA
TERESA GRACIA

While all the articles in this section and the other sections of this entry are relevant, see especially the INTRODUCTION *and other articles in this subsection:* THE BENELUX COUNTRIES, UNITED KINGDOM, REPUBLIC OF IRELAND, GERMAN-SPEAKING COUNTRIES AND SWITZERLAND, NORDIC COUNTRIES, CENTRAL AND EASTERN EUROPE, *and* RUSSIA. *See also the section on* EUROPE, *subsection on* NINETEENTH CENTURY, *article on* EUROPE. *Directly related to this article are the entries* ROMAN CATHOLICISM; *and* EASTERN ORTHODOX CHRISTIANITY. *For a further discussion of topics mentioned in this article, see the entries* ABORTION; ANIMAL RESEARCH; AUTONOMY; BENEFICENCE; BIOETHICS EDUCATION; CLINICAL ETHICS, *article on* INSTITUTIONAL ETHICS COMMITTEES; COMPASSION; DEATH, DEFINITION AND DETERMINATION OF; DEATH AND DYING: EUTHANASIA AND SUSTAINING LIFE; ETHICS; FRIENDSHIP; HEALTH-CARE DELIVERY; HEALTH-CARE RESOURCES, ALLOCATION OF, *article on* MACRO-ALLOCATION; INFORMATION DISCLOSURE; INFORMED CONSENT; JUSTICE; LAW AND MORALITY; LOVE; MEDICAL MALPRACTICE; PATIENTS' RIGHTS; PROFESSIONAL–PATIENT RELATIONSHIP; REPRODUCTIVE TECHNOLOGIES; RESEARCH ETHICS COMMITTEES; RIGHTS; SUSTAINABLE DEVELOPMENT; TRUST; *and* VIRTUE AND CHARACTER. *Other relevant material may be found under the entries* ENVIRONMENTAL ETHICS; LIFE; PERSON; *and* RESPONSIBILITY.

Bibliography

BEAUCHAMP, TOM L., and CHILDRESS, JAMES F. 1983. *Principles of Biomedical Ethics.* 2d ed. New York: Oxford University Press.

BOMPIANI, ADRIANO. 1992. *Bioetica in Italia: Lineamenti e tendenze.* Bologna: Edizioni Dehoniane.

BONDOLFI, ALBERTO. 1990. "Orientamenti e tendenze della bioetica nell'area linguistica tedesca." In *Vent'anni di bioetica: Idee, protagonisti, istituzioni,* pp. 317–359. Edited by Corrado Viafora and Alberto Bondolfi. Padua: Fondazione Lanza/Gregoriana Libreria Editrice.

BRODY, BARUCH A. 1989. "The President's Commission: The Need to Be More Philosophical." *Journal of Medicine and Philosophy* 14, no. 4:369–383.

CASSELL, ERIC J. 1984. *The Place of the Humanities in Medicine.* Hastings-on-Hudson, N.Y.: Hastings Center.

CATTORINI, PAOLO, and REICHLIN, MASSIMO. 1992. "The Physician, the Family, and the Truth." *Journal of Clinical Ethics* 3, no. 3: 219–220.

COMITATO NAZIONALE PER LA BIOETICA. 1991. *Bioetica e formazione nel sistema sanitario.* Rome: Presidenza del Consiglio dei Ministri, Dipartimento per l'Informazione e l'Editoria.

COMITÉ CONSULTATIF NATIONAL D'ÉTHIQUE POUR LES SCIENCES DE LA VIE ET DE LA SANTÉ (CCNE). 1988. *Recherche biomédicale et respect de la personne humaine.* Paris: Documentation Française.

COUNCIL OF EUROPE. 1976. *Recommendation 779, on the Rights of the Sick and Dying.* Strasbourg: Author.

DALLA-VORGIA, PANAGIOTA; KATSOUYANNI, KLEA; GARANIS, TINA N.; TOULOUMI, GIOTA; DROGARI, POTITSA; and KOUTSELINIS, ANTONIOS. 1992. "Attitudes of a Mediterranean Population to the Truth-telling Issue." *Journal of Medical Ethics* 18, no. 2:67–74.

DRACOPOULOU, SOUZY, and DOXIADIS, SPYROS. 1988. "In Greece, Lament for the Dead, Denial for the Dying." *Hastings Center Report* 18 (spec. suppl., August-September):15–16.

DRANE, JAMES F. 1988. *Becoming a Good Doctor: The Place of Virtue and Character in Medical Ethics.* Kansas City, Mo.: Sheed & Ward.

FAGOT-LARGEAULT, ANNE. 1987. "In France, Debate and Indecision." *Hastings Center Report* 17 (spec. suppl., June): 10–12.

FLETCHER, JOHN C. 1992. "On Grinding Axes and Examining Practices." *Journal of Clinical Ethics* 3, no. 3:221–224.

GAFO, JAVIER, ed. 1991. "Ética y ecología." Part 5 of *Dilemmas éticos de la medicina actual.* Madrid: Publicaciones de la Universidad Pontificia Comillas.

GLENDON, MARY ANN. 1987. *Abortion and Divorce in Western Law.* Cambridge, Mass.: Harvard University Press.

GORDON, DEBORAH. 1990. "Embodying Illness, Embodying Cancer." *Culture, Medicine, and Psychiatry* 14, no. 2:275–297. Issue title is *Traversing Boundaries Between Inside/Outside, Individual/Society, and European/North American Anthropology.*

GRACIA, DIEGO. 1987. "Spain: From the Decree to the Proposal." *Hastings Center Report* 17 (spec. suppl., June): 29–31.

———. 1988. "Spain: New Problems, New Books." *Hastings Center Report* 18 (spec. suppl., August-September): 29–30.

———. 1989. *Fundamentos de bioética.* Madrid: EUDEMA.

———. 1990. "Orientamenti e tendenze della bioetica nell'area linguistica spagnola." In *Vent'anni di bioetica: Idee, protagonisti, istituzioni,* pp. 269–299. Edited by Corrado Viafora and Alberto Bondolfi. Padua: Fondazione Lanza/Gregoriana Libreria Editrice.

———. 1992. "Enseñanza postgraduada y formación continuada en ética médica," *Organización médica colegial* 21: 25–28.

———. 1993. "The Intellectual Basis of Bioethics in Southern European Countries." *Bioethics* 7, nos. 2–3:97–107.

ILLERA, MARIANO. 1989. *Trabajar en experimentación animal.* Madrid: Fundación Universidad-Empresa.

ISAMBERT, FRANÇOIS-ANDRÉ. 1989. "Ethics Committees in France." *Journal of Medicine and Philosophy* 14, no. 4: 445–456.

LAÍN ENTRALGO, PEDRO. 1969. *Doctor and Patient.* Translated by Frances Partridge. New York: McGraw-Hill.

———. 1983. [1964]. *La relación médico-enfermo: Historia y teoría.* Madrid: Alianza.

———. 1985. [1972]. *Sobre la amistad.* Madrid: Espasa-Calpe.

LE BRIS, SONIA. 1992. *National Ethics Bodies.* Strasbourg: Council of Europe.

LEFEVRE, CHARLES. 1988. "In France, Terminal Stage Medicine Is Not Hopelessly Ill." *Hastings Center Report* 18 (spec. suppl., August-September):19–20.

LEONE, SALVINO. 1990. "Il problema dei 'valori comuni' nelle deliberazioni dei comitati." In *I comitati di bioetica: Storia, analisi, proposte,* pp. 143–158. Rome: Edizioni Orizzonte Medico.

LOEWY, ERICH H. 1992. "Consent, Ethics, and Community." *Journal of Clinical Ethics* 3, no. 3:224–228.

MACINTYRE, ALASDAIR. 1984. *After Virtue. A Study in Moral Theory.* 2d ed. Notre Dame, Ind.: University of Notre Dame Press.

MALHERBE, JEAN-FRANÇOIS. 1990. "Orientamenti e tendenze della bioetica nell'area linguistica francese." In *Vent'anni di bioetica: Idee, protagonisti, instituzioni,* pp. 199–235. Edited by Corrado Viafora and Alberto Bondolfi. Padua: Fondazione Lanza/Gregoriana Libreria Editrice.

MARTINHO DA SILVA, PAULA. 1990. "A bioética, o direito e um breve resumo sobre o quadro legislativo português." *Revista do Ministério público* 11, no. 43:163–167.

MORI, MAURIZIO. 1987. "Italy: Pluralism Takes Root." *Hastings Center Report* 17 (spec. suppl., June):34–36.

MOULIN, ANNE MARIE. 1988. "Medical Ethics in France: The Latest Great Political Debate." *Theoretical Medicine* 9, no. 3:271–285.

PALAZZANI, LAURA. 1993. "Modello argomentativo. Per una valutazione bioetica nella prospettiva personalistica." In *Centri di bioetica in Italia,* pp. 36–54. Edited by Corrado Viafora. Padua: Fondazione Lanza/Gregoriana Libreria Editrice.

PELLEGRINO, EDMUND D. 1986. "Health Care: A Vocation to Justice and Love." In *The Professions in Ethical Context: Vocations to Love and Justice,* pp. 97–126. Edited by Francis A. Eigo. Villanova, Pa.: Villanova University Press.

———. 1988. "Every Sick Person Is My Brother or Sister." *Dolentium Hominum* 3, no. 1:65–70.

———. 1989. "Agape and Ethics: Some Reflections on Medical Morals from a Catholic Perspective." In *Catholic Perspectives on Medical Morals: Foundational Issues,* pp. 277–300. Edited by Edmund D. Pellegrino, John P. Langan, and John C. Harvey. Dordrecht, Netherlands: Kluwer.

PELLEGRINO, EDMUND D., and THOMASMA, DAVID C. 1981. *A Philosophical Basis of Medical Practice: Toward a Philosophy and Ethic of the Healing Professions.* New York: Oxford University Press.

POLI, CORRADO, and TIMMERMAN, PETER, eds. 1991. *L'etica nelle politiche ambientali.* Padua: Fondazione Lanza/Gregoriana Libreria Editrice.

REICH, WARREN THOMAS. 1989. "Speaking of Suffering: A Moral Account of Compassion." *Soundings* 72:83–108.

———. 1991. "The Case: Denny's Story, and Commentary: Caring as Extraordinary Means." *Second Opinion* 17: 41–56.

RUSSO, GIOVANNI. 1992. *Sessualità ed embriopoiesi nella genesi della bioetica in Italia.* Messina, Sicily: Istituto Teologico S. Tommaso.

SÉVE, LUCIEN. 1988. *Recherche biomédicale et respect de la personne humaine.* Paris: Documentation Française.

SGRECCIA, ELIO. 1988. *Bioetica: Manuale per medici e biologi.* Milan: Vita e Pensiero.

SIEGLER, MARK. 1979. "The Nature and Limits of Clinical Medicine." In *Changing Values in Medicine,* pp. 19–41. Edited by Eric J. Cassell and Mark Siegler. Frederick, Md.: University Publications of America.

———. 1981. "Searching for Moral Certainty in Medicine: A Proposal for a New Model of the Doctor-Patient Encounter." *Bulletin of the New York Academy of Medicine* 57, no. 1:56–69.

SPINSANTI, SANDRO. 1987. *Etica bio-medica.* Milano: Paoline.

———. 1992. "Obtaining Consent from the Family: A Horizon for Clinical Ethics." *Journal of Clinical Ethics* 3, no. 3:188–192.

SYMPOSIUM OF THE COUNCIL OF EUROPE ON BIOETHICS. 1990. *Europe and Bioethics: Proceedings of the 1st Symposium of the Council of Europe on Bioethics.* Strasbourg: Council of Europe.

THOMASMA, DAVID C. 1985. "The Philosophy of Medicine in Europe: Challenges for the Future." *Theoretical Medicine* 6, no. 1:115–123.

U.S. PRESIDENT'S COMMISSION FOR THE STUDY OF ETHICAL PROBLEMS IN MEDICINE AND BIOMEDICAL AND BEHAVIORAL RESEARCH. 1982. *Making Health Care Decisions.* Vol. 1. Washington, D.C.: U.S. Government Printing Office.

VIAFORA, CORRADO. 1990. "Bioetica oggi: Un quadro storico e sistematico." In *Vent'anni di bioetica: Idee, protagonisti, instituzioni,* pp. 19–76. Edited by Corrado Viafora and Alberto Bondolfi. Padua: Fondazione Lanza/Gregoriana Libreria Editrice.

———. 1993. *Centri di bioetica in Italia: Orientamenti a confronto.* Padua: Fondazione Lanza/Gregoriana Libreria Editrice.

WALTERS, LEROY. 1987. "Ethics and New Reproductive Technologies: An International Review of Committee Statements." *Hastings Center Report* 17 (spec. suppl., June): 3–9.

3. THE BENELUX COUNTRIES

The Benelux countries—Belgium (population 10 million), the Netherlands (population 15 million), and Luxembourg (population 385,000)—with a total of just over 25 million inhabitants, three languages (Dutch, spoken by 20 million; French, by 5 million; and German, by 500,000), and two Christian religions (Roman

Catholicism and Protestantism)—have been leaders in European bioethics. Here the first institutes for bioethics were founded in the early 1980s, here the European universities first developed a full curriculum for medical ethics, and here the initiatives for European associations of both organizations and individuals working in the field were established.

During the first half of the twentieth century, in the Benelux, very much as in other countries, medical ethics was covered from three different perspectives: the deontological approach by medical associations (*ordres des médecins*), highlighting duties and professional etiquette of doctors; the forensic approach by lawyers who deal with health law; and the philosophical and (pastoral) theological approach by various denominational and religious groups. The third approach has produced, particularly since the 1960s, a considerable amount of literature in both religious and lay ethics. Early forms of interdisciplinary bioethics are found in nations where medical ethics was largely a branch of traditional Catholic moral theology. Thus, "moralists" wrote, or co-authored with medical doctors, "manuals" (Salsmans, 1919), comprehensive tracts on ethics for the daily use of physicians. Their content was consistently the following: (1) general moral concepts of responsibility, charity, and justice; (2) general duties of physicians—knowledge and diligence, professional secrecy, and fairness in charging and sharing fees; (3) specific duties of physicians regarding chastity and marriage, procreation and childbirth, and the religious duties of the Catholic physician.

Rarely did any single issue attract universal interest. What was then called "neo-Malthusian contraceptive practices" constituted perhaps the only exception to the rule. Even in the 1930s they revealed the profound opposition between religious and lay ethics in Belgium; in the Netherlands they also illustrated a conflict between Roman Catholics and Protestants. A well-known example is the firm opposition of Catholic moralists to contraceptive practices acceptable in the more liberal view of Protestant and lay ethics.

As in most other Western countries, the Benelux saw a sudden rise in interest in medical ethics soon after World War II. Medical experiments on prisoners during the war, as well as increased development of medical technologies during the same period, had sharpened people's awareness and perception of possible ethical problems in medicine. With the standard of living rising steadily within the first five postwar years, new technologies were adding promising greater future quality of life. Health and health care came within reach for the many. In the Netherlands, through an early form of resource allocation, health care was available for all (Wachter, 1988).

During the 1960s, early warning signals were issued by physicians and philosophers. Prominent among them was Jan H. van den Berg (1961; 1969), who warned against inevitable medical failures once patients become objects of medical science instead of persons and subjects of care.

The real boom in bioethics, however, did not come until the mid-1970s and 1980s, when bioethics, more or less imitating developments in the United States, gained institutional status. From then on, not only doctors and a few ethicists but also ordinary people, among them patients and politicians, were interested. In 1974 a famous case of active euthanasia in the Netherlands, in which a physician terminated the life of her terminally ill mother, at the latter's request, marked the beginning of a debate that would last several decades. Bioethics now plays a role in the democratic decision-making process about health care.

The institutionalization of bioethics is apparent in the existence of three centers for bioethics in Belgium (two in Brussels, one in Leuven [Louvain]) and five centers in the Netherlands (Amsterdam, Ede, Maastricht, Nijmegen, Utrecht), as well as in a number of interfaculty working groups. In Luxembourg a national consultative ethics commission for the life sciences and health has existed since 1988 by government decree.

Belgium

Geographically and culturally, Belgium belongs to two regions, north and south, as well as to two cultures, Roman and Germanic. Religiously speaking the country was (and nominally still is) almost entirely Roman Catholic, though in matters of medical ethics—for example, contraception—a group of postwar Catholic doctors and moral theologians of the personalist tradition has taken a rather liberal stance. Today the Roman Catholic church still plays an influential role in Belgian bioethics. Academically, its bioethical message is carried by the universities of Leuven-Louvain. During the last decades strong lay trends have entered bioethics. The universities of Brussels, Ghent, and Liège established centers or study groups for bioethics. The Center of Interdisciplinary Research in Bioethics, founded in 1987 and run by Gilbert Hottois at the Free University of Brussels, promotes medical ethics from a strictly secular view. In 1973 the Belgian Society for Ethics and Medical Ethics was founded by Jacques Achslogh. Since 1990, this association has had a Flemish-language section. Another important society is the Belgian Academy of Medicine, whose president, Armand André, is a well-known hematologist at the University of Liège as well as an expert on legal and ethical matters of international repute.

Medical ethics at universities was usually taught by faculty from either theology or philosophy departments. Rare exceptions where physicians taught medical ethics, such as Dr. Marcel Renaer at Leuven, proved the rule.

In 1980 Leuven University created a chair of medical ethics that is currently held by Paul Schotsmans. The Leuven (Flemish-language) center and the Louvain (French-language) center, under the direction of Jean-François Malherbe, belong to the Catholic University and have developed teaching programs for medical ethics at the graduate level. All other universities are still in the process of setting up a full curriculum.

At the national level, few concrete projects have been undertaken. In the mid-1980s, the Ministry of Health organized a national convention, "Bioethics in the 1990s" (Demeester, 1987). Internationally, an important role was played by the conventions on health law at Ghent University (Dierkens). Started in the 1960s, these yearly conventions bring together health lawyers and bioethicists from around the world.

Bioethics in the 1990s.   In 1987 a national convention explored the key bioethical issues of the future: medically assisted procreation, technologies of reproduction and the status of the embryo, genetics and the beginning of life, the end of life, and medical experiments on human subjects. Organized by the Ministry of Health, the congress was expected to generate significant policy recommendations. In fact, only a general proposal resulted: that vehicles for ongoing debate should be created and that medical practice ought to be protected against wild growth and carelessness in the above-mentioned fields.

Ethics committees.   As a self-regulating body, the Belgian medical establishment has controlled biomedical science and research not only from a scientific but also from an ethical viewpoint. The National Foundation for Medical Research installed an ethics committee during 1976. Its prime task was to review research at university centers. The National Council of the Order of Physicians had already developed a set of ethical rules and guidelines in what was called a "code of deontology" (1975), to be respected by all physicians. In the 1980s, an important initiative was taken by several academic institutions to ensure that medical research be done under proper conditions. University hospitals and major centers quickly established institutional review boards (Delfosse, 1990). In 1984 the National Council ruled that research ethics committees had to give their approval before research could be initiated in any hospital. By the end of 1990, about one hundred ethics committees were in place.

Gradually many of these ethics committees have expanded their mandate: the original research ethics committees (or institutional review boards) became hospital ethics committees, thus involving themselves in the ethics of clinical cases and health-care policy. In principle these committees are advisory. At the end of the 1980s in Belgium, as in many other European countries—for example, the Netherlands (Bergkamp, 1988)—there was a lack of uniformity in rules and regulations among these committees, and diversity in method and application of moral principles. It is fair to say that during the 1990s efforts will be made to create greater consistency, if not uniformity, in the normative as well as the procedural working methods of ethics committees.

Belgium is still in the process of creating its national ethics committee. In February 1991 a bill for the creation of a national committee that would have an advisory role on biomedical and health care research was tabled. Comparable with the French *comité national*, it would also be responsible for documentation and public education programs.

The Netherlands

Medical ethics in the Netherlands has an increasingly solid basis and infrastructure. More than half of the universities have medical faculties where medical ethics is taught. Research and training institutes provide medical ethics information for health-care institutions and for policymakers, and, joined by professional organizations, they offer systematic ethical training for health-care workers. In the world of health care, numerous ethics committees are in place, and at the public level, the media and politics play an important role.

In the Netherlands, medical ethics is rooted in both religious and secular traditions. However, during the 1960s Christian traditions lost their grip on social life, leaving a gap that was gradually filled by, among other things, the new (medical) ethics. The debate on contraception, for instance, was carried out partly on religious and partly on strictly ethical grounds. This debate, as well as all other debates on bioethics, was characterized by lively public participation, including patients and their organizations, as well as the movements for autonomy and self-determination. Examples of a similar public debate are the abortion issue during the 1970s and the euthanasia issue during the 1970s and 1980s, and well into the 1990s.

In the immediate post-World War II period, a number of theologians as well as physicians were active in the field: Johannes H. van den Berg, Jaap de Graaf, Herman Heering, Gerrit A. Lindeboom, Bernard Metz, Cees van der Meer, and Paul Sporken. In the late 1960s and early 1970s, others joined the chorus of medical ethicists: Theo Beemer, Heleen Dupuis, Harry Kuitert, and Maurice de Wachter. Many bioethicists, even during the 1980s and 1990s, still have a religious if not a theological background, although a profound change has occurred in their interaction with society. Having gone through secularization, many of them have acknowledged the "humanum" as a basic norm that carries common agreement in this pluralistic society. Thus, the gradual secularization of religious ethics, the occasional substitution of secular ethics for religious ethics, and the contributions of critical philosophers have reinforced the significance of strictly humanistic (nontheological) traditions.

Institutionalized bioethics.   A major instance of institutionalization of bioethics in the Netherlands lies in the area of ethics committees for both research and hospital ethics. The number of independent review boards (IRBs), which began to be established in the early 1970s, grew rapidly after 1984; hospital ethics committees (HECs) seem to have grown more slowly, principally since the second half of the 1980s. The Netherlands has also played an international role, developing a system of insurance for researchers and subjects of research.

A number of professional organizations (physicians, nurses, hospitals) have their own study services for ethics that help them to research and develop policies in health care. Moreover, the Netherlands counted, as of 1992, five established centers for bioethics, two of which are independent institutes (Maastricht and Lindeboom-Ede); the others are university based (Amsterdam, Nijmegen, Utrecht). Several medical schools offer, in addition to academic teaching programs for ethics, services to clinics and physicians as well as research projects in bioethics.

Dutch society, particularly Dutch politicians, has at its disposal five major advisory organs to assist in making health-care decisions: the Health Council, the National Council for Public Health, the Sickness Fund Council, the Central Organism for Fees, and the College of Hospital Provisions. All these organizations may offer advice without being asked. The Netherlands Organization for Technology Assessment (NOTA), created at the request of the Dutch Parliament, monitors the ethical aspects of applied medical technology. All of the above organizations have sections or subsections for medical ethics. Obviously, applied medical ethics is the major contribution of all of these institutions.

Dutch universities played an important role in the development of medical ethics. In the 1970s the universities of Maastricht (Paul Sporken), Nijmegen (Theo Beemer, Maurice de Wachter), and Leiden (Heleen Dupuis) were leaders in curriculum development. During the 1980s several other teaching units were established throughout the country. Most medical schools offer some form of medical ethical training to their students.

Major topics.   During the 1960s the Netherlands focused on contraception and abortion; the new reproductive technologies have attracted increasing interest in recent years. Euthanasia has been a key issue since the 1970s, and scarce resources and distributive justice, during the 1980s. A few issues that otherwise might not have been considered of importance have become so due to their link with scarcity of resources, for example, reproductive technologies, organ transplantation, and the issue of insurance in the context of clinical genetics. What follows is a description of these major topics.

Decisions concerning the end of life.   Euthanasia, in principle still punishable under criminal law although legal under certain conditions, has played a prominent role since 1974. Under the influence of an increased acceptance of the patient's absolute right to self-determination and of lenient jurisprudence, the medical practice of euthanasia and assisted suicide has emerged. Despite the publication of a well-documented national survey made for the government (van der Maas et al., 1992), stating that only 2,300 cases of requested euthanasia and 400 cases of assisted suicide occur, as well as 1,000 cases of active termination of the patient's life without request, some estimates still range between 2,000 and 20,000 cases per year. The then governing coalition of Christian Democrats and Socialists made a two-pronged proposal that was approved by a large majority in the Lower House and Senate in February 1993. The proposal retains Article 293 of the Penal Code, which states that "He who takes another person's life, even at his explicit and serious request, will be punished by imprisonment of approximately twelve years or a fine of the fifth category"; on the other hand, it is proposed to change the law on the burial of the dead by adding a clause that makes it obligatory for any physician who terminates the life of a patient, at the latter's request or without it, to report to legal authorities. The implementation of conditions such as the patient's explicit request, a situation of utter distress, and collegial consultation warrant the physician's recourse to "emergency" (force majeure) assistance in the death of a patient. There is a quasi certainty that no prosecution will follow. A reporting procedure is to be developed. It is fair to describe the Dutch euthanasia development over two decades as a transition from a moral debate, carried out on a large public scale during the 1970s and early 1980s, to discussions about careful implementation of policies, procedures, and guidelines, bringing about a clearer perception of the real practice.

Health-care system and reallocation issues.   The Dutch health-care system is based on principles of egalitarianism and solidarity. The latter principle is characteristic of the financial organization of health care in the Netherlands. Solidarity used to mean that individuals felt responsible for others in need. In the religious context of the past, solidarity stood for mercy and charity. In today's welfare state the moral principle is not primarily to feel individually responsible for others in need but to be held communally responsible for helping those in need. In a sense society imposes the duty to contribute financially in order to succor the needy in society. Individuals agree with this principle out of well-understood self-interest (Government Committee, 1992). At the same time, in the actual system of health-care distribution, regulatory and marketing strategies are not necessarily contradictory (Wachter, 1988). While the population does not like cuts in health care or increased premiums for health-care insurance, there is general agreement that health care is for all, and that the cost of individual preferences of patients beyond the basic package should be paid by the individual. The government has legislated on hospital provisions (1973), on fees (1980), and on budgeting in hospitals (1983). Recently, a reform system based on the following principles was introduced: (1) private initiative is possible, and government controls only quality of care, access, and cost (for example, the government controls the drug compensation system); (2) hospitals may plan according to local needs; and (3) insurers are free to market care.

Reproductive technologies. During the 1980s the emphasis on reproductive technologies was prominent. Contraception had become less problematic. In 1981 abortion was legalized, offering women in distress the possibility to be treated in officially licensed clinics. A conscience clause warrants the right of health-care workers to refuse to participate. Meanwhile, artificial procreation had become the issue of the day. This can be seen from the following points in the agreement between Christian Democrats and Socialists when forming a government in 1989; commercial surrogacy will be prohibited; artificial insemination by donor ought to be available in all kinds of relationships; a follow-up study will be made on consequences for children who have no access to the identity of their biological/genetic parents; a legal regulation on embryo experimentation will be made.

In vitro fertilization was an issue from the viewpoint of medical insurance coverage. In 1989 the Health Insurance Fund decided to continue a financial subvention for the practice.

Organ transplantation. A bill on organ transplantation intends to increase donations, to have a just distribution of organs, and to fight commercialization. The future law would follow an opting-in system: people decide to donate. Donation by the living would be permitted only if no permanent damage to health occurs.

Clinical genetics. Several commissions have studied issues of clinical genetics: counseling, registration, access, screening and testing, as well as therapy. During 1990 the government took a position on various issues. For instance, the government agrees with the intention of the private insurers to exempt applicants from the obligation to disclose data resulting from a previous genetic diagnosis. In the case of life insurance, for example, the exemption applies to a limit of 200,000 florins, meaning that for insurance below that amount the insurer will not ask for genetic information. The insurers have shown readiness to try this policy for five years. They also will not ask for additional genetic investigation. Based on principles of privacy, confidentiality, and solidarity, this position finds broad support among ethicists. Some, however, do not agree (Luijk, 1991) with this policy and suggest retaining the applicants' obliga-

tion to communicate the knowledge already available but, at the same time, compensating them for possible financial disadvantages. These positions rest on arguments of justice as well as solidarity.

Also in the context of clinical genetics, the government asked in early 1993 that the research community end all embryo research of its own volition. Moreover, the government intends to prohibit by law numerous types of embryo research, such as research on embryos older than fourteen days and the creation of embryos for the sole purpose of research. Should the research community not stop of its own free will, the government would then by Order of Council impose a moratorium for two years that would be renewable once. It would also prohibit research on embryos less than fourteen days old. The government intends to prohibit germ-cell line therapy but has no objections to somatic-cell gene therapy.

Luxembourg

The smallness of the territory of Luxembourg and the closeness of contacts intensify mutual knowledge and exchange of information. Within medical circles this has produced a remarkable amount of self-regulation. Having no medical school of its own, Luxembourg sends its medical students to neighboring countries, where they study in Belgian, French, or German universities. The "medical college" equivalent of a medical association published a code of medical deontology in 1991.

In 1988 the government established the National Consultative Committee on Ethics in the life sciences and health care. As an advisory group it is supposed to study problems in a pluralistic perspective and to suggest solutions. The commission is also expected to develop programs of public information in bioethics. Reports thus far have covered patenting genetically modified organisms, reproductive technologies, youth protection, genetic research, and anonymity.

Ethics committees in hospitals and research centers are currently being developed.

MAURICE A. M. de WACHTER

While all the articles in this section and the other sections of this entry are relevant, see especially the INTRODUCTION *and other articles in this subsection:* SOUTHERN EUROPE, UNITED KINGDOM, REPUBLIC OF IRELAND, GERMAN-SPEAKING COUNTRIES AND SWITZERLAND, NORDIC COUNTRIES, CENTRAL AND EASTERN EUROPE, *and* RUSSIA. *For a further discussion of topics discussed in this article, see the entries* ABORTION; BIOETHICS EDUCATION; CLINICAL ETHICS, *article on* INSTITUTIONAL ETHICS COMMITTEES; DEATH AND DYING: EUTHANASIA AND SUSTAINING LIFE; FERTILITY CONTROL; FETUS, *article on* FETAL RESEARCH; GENETIC TESTING AND SCREENING; HEALTH-CARE RESOURCES, ALLOCATION OF,

article on MACROALLOCATION; ORGAN AND TISSUE PRO-
CUREMENT; PROTESTANTISM; RESEARCH ETHICS COM-
MITTEES; *and* ROMAN CATHOLICISM. *Other relevant
material may be found under the entries* COMPASSION; JUS-
TICE; *and* RESPONSIBILITY.

Bibliography

BERG, JAN H. VAN DEN. 1961. *Het menselijk lichaam: Een me-
tabletish onderzoek.* 2 vols. Nijkerk, Netherlands: G. F.
Callenbach.
————. 1969. *Medische macht en medische ethiek.* Nijkerk,
Netherlands: G. F. Callenbach.
BERGKAMP, LUCAS. 1988. *Het proefdier mens: De normering en
regulering van medische experimenten met mensen.* Alphen
aan de Rijn, Netherlands: Samson.
BLOMQUIST, CLARENCE. 1978. "Medical Ethics, History of:
Western Europe in the Twentieth Century." In vol. 1 of
Encyclopedia of Bioethics, pp. 982–987. Edited by Warren
T. Reich. New York: Macmillan.
DELFOSSE, MARIE-LOUISE. 1990. "Les comités d'éthique en
Belgique." In *Contrôler la science? La question des comités
d'éthique,* pp. 81–102. Edited by Madeleine Moulin. Brus-
sels: De Boeck–Wesmael.
DEMEESTER–DE MEYER, WIVINA. 1987. *Bioéthique dans les an-
nées '90.* Ghent: Omega Editions.
DUPUIS, HELEEN M., and THUNG, PAUL. 1988. *Voordelen van
de twijfel.* Alphen aan de Rijn, Netherlands: Samsom Sta-
fleu.
GOVERNMENT COMMITTEE ON CHOICES IN HEALTH CARE.
1992. *Choices in Health Care.* Zoetermeer, Netherlands:
Ministry of Welfare, Health, and Cultural Affairs.
JANSSENS, LOUIS. 1963. "Morale conjugale et progestogènes."
Ephemerides theologicae lovanienses 39:287–307.
————. 1980–1981. "Artificial Insemination: Ethical Consid-
erations." *Louvain Studies* 8:3–29.
KUITERT, HARRY M. 1989. *Mag alles wat kan? Ethiek en medisch
handelen.* 2d ed. Baarn, Netherlands: Ten Have.
LUIJK, HENK J. VAN. 1991. "Genetica en levensverzekeringen:
Ethische aspecten." In *Genetica en levensverzekeringen:
Ethische en juridische aspecten.* Edited by Maurice A. M.
de Wachter. Maastricht, Netherlands: Institute for Bio-
ethics.
MAAS, PAUL J. VAN DER; DELDEN, JOHANNES J. M. VAN; and
PIJNENBORG, LUCAS. 1992. *Euthanasia and Other Medical
Decisions Concerning the End of Life.* Amsterdam: Elsevier.
SALSMANS, JOSEPH. 1919. *Geneeskundige plichtenleer.* Leuven:
Deontologia Medica.
SPORKEN, PAUL. 1969. *Ethiek en gezondheidszorg.* 3d ed. Baarn,
Netherlands: Ambo.
WACHTER, MAURICE A. M. DE. 1988. "Ethics and Health Pol-
icy in the Netherlands." In *Health Care Systems: Moral
Conflicts in European and American Public Policy,* pp. 97–
116. Edited by Hans M. Sass and Robert U. Massey. Dor-
drecht, Netherlands: Kluwer.
WACHTER, MAURICE A. M. DE; WERT, GUIDO M. W. R.;
MEULEN, RUUD H. J. TER; BERGHAMANS, RON L. P.;
RAVENSCHLAG, INGRID; and SIMONS-COMBECHER, A. K.
1992. "Bioethics in the Netherlands: 1989–1991." In *Regional Developments in Bioethics: 1989–1991,* pp. 191–210.
Edited by B. Andrew Lustig, Baruch A. Brody, H. Tristram Engelhardt, Jr., and Laurence B. McCullough. Dordrecht, Netherlands: Kluwer.

4. UNITED KINGDOM

This article surveys the development of medical ethics
in Britain in the twentieth century and some substantive
medical ethical issues arising in that period. It describes
the involvement of important organizations concerned
with medical ethics, the development of academic
courses in the subject, and the establishment of a privately sponsored national bioethics committee and of
national forums for teachers and students of bioethics.
It suggests that a typically British antitheoretical, commonsense, and situational approach to medical ethics is
gradually modifying so as to include at least some theoretical issues in the teaching and study of medical ethics.

Medical ethics at the beginning of the twentieth century

Respect for the professions and for the established Anglican church were well-entrenched characteristics of
British society at the beginning of the twentieth century, and medical ethics conformed to these cultural
realities. Thus the normative standards of medical ethics
were left almost entirely to the profession itself to establish and maintain. It did so largely in conformity with
Hippocratic medical tradition and the ethical norms
(e.g., prohibition of active euthanasia and of abortion
except to save the life of the pregnant woman) of the
Church of England. (The latter, as the established
church of the nation, was the dominant religious influence on official medicine, even as practiced in the other
constituent nations: Scotland, Wales, and Ireland.) The
Medical Act of 1858 had, at the instigation of the newly
established British Medical Association, established the
General Medical Council to protect the public by controlling admission to the medical register on the basis of
explicit medical educational standards, including ethical standards, both to exclude "quacks" (unqualified
practitioners claiming to be doctors) from practicing
medicine and to ensure that only those orthodox
practitioners who had attained the prescribed standards
were admitted to the register of medical practitioners.

Moreover, qualified medical practitioners who fell
below the prescribed standards were liable to disciplinary
action, including removal from the register (and thus
loss of their professional livelihood) if they were found
guilty of "infamous conduct in a professional respect."
Among the infamous activities that could result in removal were the carrying out of abortion or active euthanasia, and sexual relationship with a patient. Other

matters of considerable ethical concern to the General Medical Council included abuse of alcohol and drugs, fee splitting, "covering" for medical practice carried out by unregistered persons, convictions in the courts that would bring dishonor on the medical profession, abuse of the financial opportunities afforded by medical practice, improper denigration of professional colleagues, advertising for the doctor's own financial advantage, and canvassing for patients. Thus, at the beginning of the century, British medical ethics was almost entirely the prerogative of the medical profession and concerned itself with a paternalistic concern to protect the public and to maintain its own honor and dignity.

Social justice and health care: 1911, 1946, and beyond

If concerns about more equitable distribution of health care were not part of the medical profession's medical ethics agenda at the beginning of the twentieth century, they undoubtedly were a concern for the reforming liberal government elected with a large parliamentary majority in 1906. By 1911 David Lloyd George, then chancellor of the Exchequer and later prime minister, achieved passage of his National Insurance Act; this provided working people (not their families) with medical and unemployment insurance, and was funded by compulsory contributions from workers, employers, and government (Braithwaite, 1957; Fox, 1986). The medical profession, though not opposed to the principle of such general provision of health care, fought the government on grounds of inadequate fees and inadequate protection for patients' choice of doctor; more than twenty-seven thousand doctors threatened to withhold their services. However, by 1913 Lloyd George, after compromising with the doctors, had won the day (Lloyd, 1968).

The extension of medical care to the general population remained a popular political objective in Britain, and the wartime report by Sir William Beveridge (1942) led, via the 1946 National Health Service Act, to the Labour government's establishment of the National Health Service (NHS) in 1948. This offered preventive as well as curative medical care to every member of the British public; it was provided in response to need, free at the time of that need, and financed by taxes (Bruce, 1971). While the objectives and provisions of the NHS remain widely accepted, Beveridge's (in retrospect somewhat naive) expectations of producing a healthy nation—leading to reduced requirements for health care, with the poor and socially disadvantaged as healthy as the rest of society—have never been achieved. On the contrary, concerns about increasing, yet inadequate, health expenditure multiplied, especially from the 1970s (Maxwell, 1975); a government committee chaired by Sir Douglas Black showed vast in-

equalities of health status in the population correlating with economic and other social disadvantages. However, the committee's recommendations for government expenditure to remedy these inequalities were rejected by the secretary of state for health in his foreword, in which he categorically declined to endorse the report's recommendations (Black, 1980).

Instead, the Conservative government of Margaret Thatcher responded to the escalating costs of health care by initiating radical reforms in the late 1980s and early 1990s, setting up internal markets within the NHS with clear distinctions between "purchasers" and "providers," and establishing competition (at least in theory) between the providers of health care, in order to encourage the efficient and discourage or even eliminate the inefficient. Supporters see these reforms as ways to improve the efficiency and accountability of the NHS; opponents view them as a step toward its dismantling in favor of a two-tier system of health care: a basic and limited state provision for those who cannot afford to insure themselves privately, alongside unlimited private provision of medical services for those who can afford to pay.

Voluntary euthanasia: 1936 and beyond

A quite different issue of health-care ethics—voluntary euthanasia—has been of public concern in Britain for almost as long as the issue of justice in the provision of health care. Medical proposals for its legislation had appeared early in the twentieth century; and in 1936, following the creation of the Voluntary Euthanasia Society, the House of Lords debated and rejected a proposal to legalize voluntary euthanasia, which would have provided the legal right to request and be given medical assistance to die when suffering from incurable and fatal illness. Despite the admission by Lord Dawson, an eminent doctor, that euthanasia was carried out by many doctors (*Parliamentary Debates,* House of Lords 5th series, vol. 103 [1936], cols. 488–489), he and another medical peer, Lord Horder, opposed the bill on the grounds that its proposals involved too many legal formalities and that, in any case, euthanasia was a matter best left to the discretion of doctors. (Many years later state archives were opened and revealed that Lord Dawson had deliberately accelerated the death of the dying King George VI, partly in order to enable the quality morning newspapers to report it first rather than risk the death being announced by a less suitable evening newspaper (*Times of London,* November 27 and 28, 1986).

Euthanasia remains an intermittently burning public issue. Further proposals to legalize it were rejected by the British Parliament in 1969 and in 1990; and in 1988 the British Medical Association (BMA) declared that, while allowing patients to die was properly a matter of medical discretion, active killing, even if requested by the patient in circumstances of severe and incurable suffering and disease, was always unacceptable and should remain illegal (British Medical Association, 1988a). In 1992 a British doctor was convicted of attempted murder for administering undiluted potassium chloride to a long-standing patient of his who, in intractable pain, had repeatedly requested him to end her life (Brahams, 1992). However, his sentence of one year's imprisonment was suspended and the General Medical Council, while admonishing him, permitted him to continue practicing (*Lancet*, 1992a). After the verdict a *British Medical Journal* editorial called for a royal commission to study active and passive euthanasia—its subtitle was "The Tide Seems to Be Running for Euthanasia" (R. Smith, 1992); a *Lancet* editorial criticized the BMA's "unsympathetic public line" on euthanasia (*Lancet*, 1992b).

Experimentation on human subjects: 1947 and beyond

Medical ethics in Britain—as in all parts of the civilized world—was given a shocking impetus after World War II by the revelations at the Nuremberg trials of Nazi medical war crimes, and the 1947 Nuremberg Code on Human Experimentation was as readily accepted within Britain as elsewhere. In the early 1960s, however, an English physician claimed that many orthodox medical research investigations were unethical, and in a book first published in 1967 he enraged the British medical establishment by likening examples of British medical research to the research of the notorious Nazi doctors (Pappworth, 1967). Whether cause and effect or coincidence, in the same year the Royal College of Physicians (RCP) published a recommendation that all clinical research proposals should be subject to ethical review; this advice was widely circulated by the British government's Department of Health and Social Security. Over the next few years "ethical committees," or research ethics committees, were established in the majority of hospitals and other institutions conducting medical research.

Nonetheless, development and practice of these committees was recognized to be variable and in 1984 the RCP published guidelines for research ethics committees (RECs), updated in 1990 (Royal College of Physicians, 1990a), as well as reports titled *Research Involving Patients* (1990b) and *Research on Healthy Volunteers* (1986). In 1991 the Department of Health published its own guidelines for RECs (Department of Health, 1991). In both sets of guidelines the advice is detailed; it is designed, in the words of the RCP document, "to facilitate medical research in the interest of society, to protect subjects of research from possible harm, to preserve their rights, and to provide reassur-

ance to the public that this is being done. Committees also protect research workers from unjustified attack." While the RCP guidelines are widely accepted in Britain as the national standard for ethics committees, and while research on human subjects must be submitted to RECs, there is considerable doubt about what proportion of British ethics committees actually implement them (Nicholson, 1986; Gilbert et al., 1989; Neuberger, 1992). Continuing development and standardization of REC activities can be predicted.

Abortion: 1938 and beyond

Another major medicomoral issue of British concern in the second half of the century has been abortion. Under the Offences Against the Person Act of 1861, procuring an abortion was a felony punishable by life imprisonment. In 1938 an English obstetrician-gynecologist, Alec Bourne, challenged the law by reporting himself to the police after carrying out a therapeutic abortion on a girl who had been the victim of multiple rape. He was found not guilty on the grounds that the patient's life, in the sense of her mental well-being, was at risk if the pregnancy continued; just as "child destruction" (as the Act calls it) to preserve the life of the mother was legally permissible under the Infant Life Preservation Act of 1929, so abortion for the mother's well-being might be lawful (See Mason and McCall Smith, 1987). In 1967 the law was liberalized to permit abortion in cases where two doctors certify that the continuation of the pregnancy would be a greater risk to the life or health of the pregnant woman, or her existing children, than a termination; or that termination would prevent grave permanent injury to the physical or mental health of the pregnant woman; or that there is a substantial risk that the child would suffer serious physical or mental handicap.

In practice many British doctors, accepting that during the first three months of any pregnancy the risk of continuing to normal birth is greater than the risk of therapeutic abortion, agree to abortion for any woman who after deliberation continues to request it. The upper limit of gestation at which abortion is permitted was reduced by the Human Fertilisation and Embryology Act (1990) from twenty-eight weeks to twenty-four weeks. No upper limit applies in cases where the mother's life is seriously threatened and in cases where the child, if born, would probably be seriously handicapped. Significant, though minority, opposition to abortion persists both within the medical profession and among the public. In Northern Ireland, a part of the United Kingdom, opposition to abortion among the Protestant as well as the Roman Catholic population is sufficiently widespread for the Abortion Act not to apply there.

"Official" British medical ethics, as represented in this context by the General Medical Council, the British Medical Association, and the Royal College of Obstetricians and Gynaecologists, accepts abortion when carried out according to the law while recognizing any doctor's or nurse's right of conscientious objection. Such practitioners are expected to inform their patients of their moral objections to abortion and advise them that they may seek assistance elsewhere, and give information about sources of such assistance if requested (BMA, 1988b).

Reproductive technology: 1978 and beyond

In July 1978 the pioneering work of Patrick Steptoe and Robert Edwards led to the birth of the world's first "test-tube baby"—and to a paradigm shift in bioethical thinking about human reproduction and genetics. From 1982, when the British government appointed a Committee of Inquiry into Human Fertilisation and Embryology (Warnock, 1984), until the passing of the Human Fertilisation and Embryology Act in 1990, the British public and the British medical profession were gripped by a vigorous debate about the moral issues associated with in vitro fertilization (Snowden and Mitchell, 1983; Council for Science and Society, 1984; Bock and O'Connor, 1986; Bromham et al., 1990). As with abortion, the central moral issue was seen by many to be the moral status of the embryo/fetus, though other issues included possible adverse physical and psychological effects on children conceived artificially, and also on the women involved with such techniques, especially in the case of surrogacy. Feminist concerns included the continuing debate about access by single heterosexual women and lesbian women to reproductive technology (Hanscombe and Forster, 1982; Chadwick, 1987). The issues were resolved in an extensive government bill that, unusually, offered alternative clauses on the most contentious issue of all: research on, followed by destruction of, the human embryo. Members of Parliament (MPs) were given a free vote (i.e., without any party pressure to vote in one way rather than another) and asked to choose between allowing such research up to fourteen days of embryo development, as recommended by the Warnock Committee majority report, or forbidding all such research on human embryos except where it was done therapeutically—that is, to facilitate transfer of the embryo into the uterus of a woman. (The latter is the position of the Roman Catholic church, though it is worth noting that the eminent Jesuit theologian Professor John Mahoney had argued that the early embryo is "unlikely to be possessed of a soul and personhood in its existence at the simple cell-multiplication stage prior to diversification" [Mahoney, 1984, p. 85]). After cliff-hanging public, professional, and parliamentary debate, the MPs ac-

cepted research up to fourteen days of embryonic development and established the national Human Fertilisation and Embryology Authority to monitor and control all such activities.

Informed consent: 1985 and beyond

Of the many other medicomoral issues that have exercised both the public and health-care professionals in Britain, two legal cases are particularly notable: the Sidaway case on informed consent to treatment and the Gillick case on treatment of minors without parental consent. In the Sidaway case, finally determined by the House of Lords in 1985, the plaintiff complained that her surgeon had been negligent in not warning her of the small risk of spinal nerve root damage, which had occurred. Their lordships decided by a majority (Lord Scarman dissenting) to uphold the existing English legal doctrine according to which a doctor is not negligent if acting in a way supported by a body of reasonable medical opinion (the "Bolam test"). However, by indicating what reasonable doctors could be expected to do in certain circumstances (for example, answer their patients' questions and warn them of any substantial risks!) the judges brought English law "edging toward" the American "reasonable patient standard" whereby the requirements of a reasonable person in the patient's situation would determine what information was required (Kennedy and Grubb, 1989)—though not all legal commentators agree that even this modest degree of change was achieved in the case (Brazier, 1992).

In the Gillick case a mother asked the court to rule that doctors should not be allowed to give medication (birth-control pills) to her children under the age of sixteen without obtaining parental consent. Once again the case went to the House of Lords, which in 1986 rejected Mrs. Gillick's claim; it ruled that a doctor ought to try to persuade the minor to involve the parents in the consultation, but if the patient refused—provided the doctor had good reason to assess the minor as having sufficient maturity and understanding—treatment could be prescribed without involving the parents (Kennedy and Grubb, 1989).

The organization of medical ethics in Britain

At the beginning of the twentieth century, medical ethics was entirely determined by the General Medical Council (GMC). Toward the end of the century the GMC's role remains pivotal, though far more influenced by others than it had been. In 1991 the GMC was composed of 103 members, of whom 54 were directly elected by the medical profession; 36 appointed by the medical faculties of universities, by medical royal colleges or by other academic medical organizations; and 13 appointed by the government, of whom 12 were not physicians (the thirteenth was the government's chief medical officer). Among the medical ethics functions of the GMC are the promotion of high standards of medical education, including education in medical ethics, quasi-judicial assessment of complaints against doctors, and provision of advice on ethical standards and professional conduct in its "little blue book" (GMC, 1992b) and in its annual reports (GMC, 1992a).

The British Medical Association, which is the doctors' professional association and trade union, though it has no official authority in matters of medical ethics, in fact provides considerable guidance on these issues to its members, to the government, and to the public. It has a Central Ethical Committee and provides individual advice to members as requested; it publishes booklets relevant to medical ethics (e.g., BMA, 1988b, 1988c). The BMA even produced what may have been one of the world's first computer programs offering doctors medicomoral advice (Sieghart and Dawson, 1987).

Other professional influences on medical ethics are exerted during medical education by individual teachers, themselves influenced not only by the GMC and (often) the BMA but also by the Medical Research Council (MRC) and specialty organizations; the latter include the Royal Colleges of Physicians, Surgeons, Obstetricians and Gynaecologists, General Practitioners, Psychiatrists, and so on, all of which offer advice and guidance on medical ethics relevant to their specialties. So, too, do the medical malpractice organizations, such as the Medical Defence Union and the Medical Protection Society. In addition the employment contracts of most doctors in Britain exert some legally binding ethical pressure on their behavior. For example, general practitioners, though they are independent contractors, are required by their contracts with the NHS to provide emergency care in their vicinity whether or not those needing such care are registered with them; and they are also required by their contracts to accept "difficult to place patients" for a minimum of three months, when required by the NHS to do so. And in NHS hospitals a surgeon does not meet the requirements of his or her contract of service if, in normal circumstances, he or she does not obtain written consent from the patient prior to operating. In addition there is a strong tradition in British medicine of consultation, especially with more experienced colleagues, about any difficult medical problem, including difficult medicomoral problems.

Nonmedical influences on British medical ethics include the range of forces typical of a modern Western democracy. The most important is undoubtedly the law, which, as noted above, has a major role in defining the arenas within which the medical profession may make its own choices about medicomoral issues. Nurses have undergone a metamorphosis from doctors' handmaidens to independent health professionals, and have become increasingly influential in British health-care ethics, especially through the activities and pronouncements of their disciplinary body, the United Kingdom Central Council for Nursing, Midwifery and Health Visiting, or UKCC (1992a, 1992b), and of their professional association and trade union, the Royal College of Nursing (1991).

Many public pressure groups, patient groups, and special medical interest groups exist to try to influence the profession, the media, Parliament, and the public on such matters as health-care ethics issues. Among many others, the Patients Association, the College of Health, the Consumers Association, MIND (which promotes the interests of the mentally ill), MENCAP (which promotes the interests of the mentally handicapped or impaired), CERES (Consumers for Ethics in Research), and the local community-health councils are important examples. The media constantly, even daily, publish and broadcast on medical ethics issues.

From a plethora of possible examples, one media event is particularly worth noting: the prestigious BBC Radio Reith Lectures, given in 1980 by Ian Kennedy, then a lecturer in academic law (later a professor of medical law and ethics). Later published under the profession-provoking title *The Unmasking of Medicine* (Kennedy, 1981), the lectures brought into the arena of intelligent public discussion many of the standard themes of medical ethics, and argued forcefully that while doctors had special training and expertise in technical medical matters, they had no such training and expertise in moral matters. Even if they had had such training (which Kennedy advocated), they had no right to assume that moral decisions in medical practice were solely for doctors to make, in the way technical decisions in medical practice might be. The resulting public and professional debate did much to achieve Kennedy's objective of bringing medical ethics "out of the hushed halls of Academe into the noisy market place of ideas" (Kennedy, 1981, p. xi).

The study and development of medical ethics in Britain has also been promoted by the Institute of Medical Ethics (IME). Originally named the Society for the Study of Medical Ethics, it was founded in the early 1960s by a Church of England priest, Dean Edward Shotter, who at the time had pastoral responsibility for medical students in London. Shotter soon recruited two other clerics, both from Scotland, who were to become influential in British medical ethics: Dr. Kenneth Boyd (Boyd, 1979, 1987, 1990, 1992; Boyd et al., 1986; Smith and Boyd, 1991; Gallagher and Boyd, 1991) and Professor Alastair Campbell, founding editor of the IME's *Journal of Medical Ethics* (Campbell, 1972, 1978, 1984; Campbell and Higgs, 1982). Among the IME's activities have been the establishment of multidisciplinary ethics study groups within most of the British medical schools, the establishment of multidisciplinary working groups to study and report on specific issues of medical ethics, and the founding of two publications, the *Journal of Medical Ethics* (1975) and the *Bulletin of Medical Ethics* (1985; now independent of the IME).

Other organizations stimulating the early development of health-care ethics in Britain include the Centre for Medical Law and Ethics at King's College, London; the Centre for the Study of Philosophy and Health Care at the University of Wales at Swansea; the Centre for Social Ethics and Policy at the University of Manchester; the Social Values Research Centre at the University of Hull; various centers at the University of Oxford, including Rewley House, the Ramsey Centre, the Department of Philosophy and the Oxford Practice Skills Project; the Centre for Philosophy and Public Affairs at the University of St. Andrews; the Centre for Business and Professional Ethics at Leeds University; and the Centre for Applied Ethics, University of Wales at Cardiff.

In addition, the Society for Applied Philosophy is concerned with philosophical illumination of "areas of practical concern" that often include issues of health-care ethics; it publishes the *Journal of Applied Philosophy*. Of various influential academic disciplines with a secondary interest in medical ethics that has stimulated their development, health economics deserves mention, in the context of its particular concern with resource allocation. Alan J. Williams (1985, 1991), Alan Maynard (1986), and Anthony J. Culyer (1992), from the Centre of Health Economics at York University, and Gavin Mooney and Alistair McGuire (1988) are influential in this area of health economics—especially Williams, with his advocacy of the maximization of quality-adjusted life years as the centrally relevant criterion for health-service resource allocation.

Academic courses

The first British academic course in medical ethics seems to have been started by the ancient City of London guild, the Worshipful Society of Apothecaries (still a medical licensing body), when it instituted a diploma course in the philosophy of medicine in 1978. An annual one-week "intensive course in medical ethics for medical and nursing teachers" was started in 1983 at Imperial College, London, and in 1984 the Centre of Medical Law and Ethics at King's College, London, initiated a one-year postgraduate diploma in medical law and ethics, upgraded in 1987 to a master's degree. In 1985 the University of Wales introduced a highly popular part-time M.A. in health-care ethics, and in 1987 the University of Manchester offered a multidisciplinary M.A. in health-care ethics, administered by its Centre for Social Ethics and Policy. Since then various other British

universities and colleges have developed a wide variety of courses in health-care ethics.

British medical schools were slow to introduce the formal study of medical ethics, the Scots leading the way at Edinburgh University and Glasgow University. King's College Hospital led the way in London. Full-time philosophers were appointed to teach the subject at medical schools at Liverpool and at the London Hospital; and a London University medical school, St. Mary's Hospital Medical School, was the first to appoint a (part-time) visiting professor of medical ethics. Medical schools were stimulated into activity by the report of an Institute of Medical Ethics working group (Boyd, 1987) urging that they introduce the critical study of medical ethics.

In 1991 two national groups concerned with medical ethics were established. The first, the UK Forum for Health Care Ethics and Law, was designed to bring together the increasingly numerous and various academic and other organizations, teachers, and students in Britain concerned with health-care ethics. The second was the Nuffield Council on Bioethics, a national multidisciplinary committee established by the private philanthropic Nuffield Foundation, to review the ethical issues raised by medical research, starting with those raised by genetic manipulation; the committee is anticipated to provide the antecedents of a national committee on bioethics. In 1992 a further national organization, the Association for Healthcare and Medical Ethics Teachers, was founded for medical ethics teachers in British medical and nursing schools.

Two continental European influences on the British approach to medical ethics are also important to note, though at the time of writing the likely extent of their influence is difficult to assess. The Council of Europe is in the process of drafting a European Convention on Bioethics (analogous to and derived from its European Convention on Human Rights), and the European Community has begun to distribute significant funding for bioethics research projects requiring cooperation between member nations.

Religious influences on medical ethics

Religious organizations are influential in medical ethics in Britain, both at a personal level, affecting the decisions of patients, health-care workers and others concerning medicomoral issues, and as a result of institutional activities. Relevant institutions include the Church of England Board for Social Responsibility (an account of its activities is provided by one of the doyens of British medical ethics, the Rev. Prof. Gordon Dunstan; see Dunstan, 1987; Dunstan and Seller, 1983); the (Roman) Catholic Bishops' Joint Committee on Bioethical Issues (see, e.g., Catholic Bishops' Joint Committee on Bioethical Issues, 1987); the (Roman Catholic) Linacre Centre (see, e.g., Linacre Centre, 1982); the (evangelical Protestant) Christian Medical Fellowship (which holds regular meetings and publishes the *Journal of the Christian Medical Fellowship*); and the Jewish Chief Rabbinate (one of whose members, Lord Immanuel Jakobovits, obtained the first doctorate devoted to Jewish medical ethics; see Jakobovits, 1959).

The national "flavor" of medical ethics in Britain

While it is always risky to generalize, a pragmatic, situationist, commonsense, antitheoretical, and antiregulatory approach tends to characterize the British approach to medical ethics (as to many other aspects of British life). However, despite this national reluctance to theorize, it is increasingly acknowledged that some theoretical underpinning is needed even for commonsense ethical decisions. In the context of medical ethics, a distinction is increasingly recognized between two medical ethical concepts (*Journal of Medical Ethics*, 1985b). The first is traditional medical ethics, in the sense of promulgating and enforcing within the medical profession certain medicomoral norms—what Dunstan calls "the obligations of a moral nature which govern the practice of medicine" (Dunstan, 1981, xxviii–xxxi). This sort of medical ethics has characterized medical education and practice since Hippocratic times. The second, more recent sort—philosophical or critical medical ethics—sets out rigorously and in the light of argument, justification, and counterargument, to examine the issues of medical ethics, including the claims of traditional medical ethics.

Prompted from without as well as from within, the British medical profession has, since the mid-1970s, begun cautiously and gradually to accept the latter medical ethical concept as a proper part of medical thinking and education. Evidence for this includes the General Medical Council's increased interest in medical ethics since it held a conference on medical ethics teaching in 1984 (General Medical Council, 1985); publication in 1985/1986 by the *British Medical Journal* of a series of twenty-six articles under the title "Philosophical Medical Ethics" (Gillon, 1985–1986); publication of *The Pond Report* on medical ethics teaching (Boyd, 1987), recommending such teaching in medical schools; and the increasing teaching of critical or philosophical medical ethics in medical schools. But virtually all involved in the British medical ethics scene agree on one issue: the central importance of real cases, manifesting real medicomoral problems, for any adequate critical study, teaching, or understanding of this constantly developing subject.

RAANAN GILLON

While all the articles in this section and the other sections of this entry are relevant, see especially the INTRODUCTION *and other articles in this subsection:* SOUTHERN EUROPE, THE BENELUX COUNTRIES, REPUBLIC OF IRELAND, GERMAN-SPEAKING COUNTRIES AND SWITZERLAND, NORDIC COUNTRIES, CENTRAL AND EASTERN EUROPE, *and* RUSSIA. *See also the section on* EUROPE, *subsection on* NINETEENTH CENTURY, *article on* GREAT BRITAIN. *For a further discussion of topics mentioned in this article, see the entries* ABORTION; BIOETHICS EDUCATION; CHILDREN, *article on* HEALTH-CARE AND RESEARCH ISSUES; CLINICAL ETHICS; DEATH AND DYING: EUTHANASIA AND SUSTAINING LIFE; HEALTH-CARE DELIVERY; HEALTH-CARE RESOURCES, ALLOCATION OF, *article on* MACROALLOCATION; INFORMATION DISCLOSURE; INFORMED CONSENT; LICENSING, DISCIPLINE, AND REGULATION IN THE HEALTH PROFESSIONS; MATERNAL–FETAL RELATIONSHIP, *article on* MEDICAL ASPECTS; PROFESSION AND PROFESSIONAL ETHICS; REPRODUCTIVE TECHNOLOGIES; RESEARCH, UNETHICAL; RESEARCH ETHICS COMMITTEES; *and* WOMEN, *article on* HEALTH-CARE ISSUES. *Other relevant material may be found under the entries* ETHICS; FEMINISM; JUSTICE; *and* UTILITY.

Bibliography

ALMOND, BRENDA, ed. 1990. *AIDS: A Moral Issue—The Ethical, Legal and Social Aspects.* London: Macmillan Press.

BEVERIDGE, SIR WILLIAM. 1942. *Social Insurance and Allied Services.* Cmd 6404. London: His Majesty's Stationery Office.

BLACK, SIR DOUGLAS. 1980. *Inequalities in Health: Report of a Research Working Group (the Black Report).* London: Department of Health and Social Security. Also published as *Inequalities in Health: The Black Report*, by Sir Douglas Black, Jeremy Morris, Cyril Smith, and Peter Townsend. Harmondsworth, U.K.: Penguin, 1982.

BOCK, GREGORY, and O'CONNOR, MAEVE, eds. 1986. *Human Embryo Research: Yes or No?* London: Tavistock.

BOYD, KENNETH. 1979. *The Ethics of Resource Allocation.* Edinburgh: Edinburgh University Press.

———, ed. 1987. *The Pond Report: The Teaching of Medical Ethics.* Report of a Working Party of the Institute of Medical Ethics. London: Institute of Medical Ethics.

———, ed. 1990. "Assisted Death: Institute of Medical Ethics Working Party on the Ethics of Prolonging Life and Assisting Death." *Lancet* 336:610–613.

———. 1992. "HIV Infection and AIDS: The Ethics of Medical Confidentiality—Report of an Institute of Medical Ethics Working Party." *Journal of Medical Ethics* 18:173–179.

BOYD, KENNETH; CALLAGHAN, BRENDAN; and SHOTTER, EDWARD. 1986. *Life Before Birth: Consensus in Medical Ethics.* London: SPCK.

BRAHAMS, DIANA. 1992. "Medicine and the Law: Euthanasia Doctor Convicted of Attempted Murder." *Lancet* 340: 782–783.

BRAITHWAITE, WILLIAM J. 1957. *Lloyd George's Ambulance Wagon: Papers Edited by Sir Henry N. Bunbury.* London: Methuen and Cox.

BRAZIER, MARGARET. 1992. *Medicine, Patients and the Law.* 2d ed. Harmondsworth, U.K.: Penguin.

BRAZIER, MARGARET, and LOBJOIT, MARY, eds. 1991. *Protecting the Vulnerable: Autonomy and Consent in Health Care.* London: Routledge.

BRITISH MEDICAL ASSOCIATION. 1988a. *The Euthanasia Report: Report of a Working Party to Review the British Medical Association's Guidance on Euthanasia.* London: Author.

————. 1988b. *Philosophy and Practice of Medical Ethics.* London: Author.

————. 1988c. *Rights and Responsibilities of Doctors.* London: Author.

BROMHAM, DAVID; DALTON, MAUREEN; and JACKSON, JENNIFER, eds. 1990. *Philosophical Ethics in Reproductive Medicine: Proceedings of an International Conference Held in 1988.* Manchester, England: Manchester University Press.

BRUCE, M. 1972. *The Coming of the Welfare State.* London: Batsford.

CAMPBELL, ALASTAIR. 1972. *Moral Dilemmas in Medicine.* Edinburgh: Churchill Livingstone.

————. 1978. *Medicine, Health and Justice: The Problem of Priorities.* Edinburgh: Churchill Livingstone.

————. 1984. *Moderated Love: A Theology of Professional Care.* London: SPCK.

CAMPBELL, ALASTAIR, and HIGGS, ROGER. 1982. *In That Case: Medical Ethics in Everyday Practice.* London: Darton, Longman and Todd.

CATHOLIC BISHOPS' JOINT COMMITTEE ON BIOETHICAL ISSUES (U.K.). 1987. *On Human Infertility Services and Embryo Research: Response to the Department of Health and Social Security's Consultation.* Abingdon, England: Author.

CHADWICK, RUTH F. 1987. "Having Children" and "The Perfect Baby." In *Ethics, Reproduction, and Genetic Control,* pp. 3–43, 93–135. Edited by Ruth F. Chadwick. London: Routledge.

CLOTHIER, SIR CECIL. 1988. *The Patient's Dilemma.* London: Nuffield Provincial Hospitals Trust.

COUNCIL FOR SCIENCE AND SOCIETY. 1984. *Human Procreation: Ethical Aspects of the New Techniques.* Oxford: Oxford University Press.

CULYER, ANTHONY J. 1992. "The Morality of Efficiency in Health Care: Some Uncomfortable Implications." *Health Economics* 1:7–18.

DEPARTMENT OF HEALTH (U.K.). 1991. *Local Research Ethics Committees: Health Service Guidelines.* Ref.: HSG (91) S-19/8/91. London: Author.

DOWNIE, ROBIN, and CALMAN, KENNETH. 1987. *Healthy Respect.* London: Faber. 2d ed. Oxford: Oxford University Press, 1993.

DOYAL, LEN, and GOUGH, IAN. 1991. *A Theory of Human Need.* London: Macmillan.

DUNSTAN, GORDON R. 1981. "Medical Ethics." In *Dictionary of Medical Ethics.* Rev. ed. Edited by Archibald S. Duncan, Gordon R. Dunstan, and Richard B. Welbourn. London: Darton, Longman and Todd.

————. 1987. "The Authority of a Moral Claim." *Journal of Medical Ethics* 13:189–194.

DUNSTAN, GORDON, and SELLER, MARY, eds. 1983. *Consent in Medicine: Convergence and Divergence in Tradition.* Oxford: Oxford University Press.

DUNSTAN, GORDON, and SHINEBOURNE, ELLIOT, eds. 1989. *Doctors Decide: Ethical Conflicts in Medical Practice.* Oxford: Oxford University Press.

EVANS, DON, ed. 1990. *Professional Studies in Health Care Ethics: Why Should We Care?* London: Macmillan.

FAIRBAIRN, GAVIN. 1991. "Complexity and Value of Lives: Some Philosophical Dangers for Mentally Handicapped People." *Journal of Applied Philosophy* 8:211–217.

FOX, DANIEL M. 1986. *Health Policies, Health Politics: The British and American Experience, 1911–1965.* Princeton, N.J.: Princeton University Press.

FULFORD, K. WILLIAM M. 1990. *Moral Theory and Medical Practice.* Cambridge: At the University Press.

GALLAGHER, URSULA, and BOYD, KENNETH. 1991. *Teaching and Learning Nursing Ethics.* London: Scutari.

GENERAL MEDICAL COUNCIL (U.K.). 1992a. *Annual Report of the General Medical Council for 1991.* London: Author.

————. 1992b. *Professional Conduct and Discipline: Fitness to Practise.* London: Author.

GILBERT, CLAIRE; FULFORD, K. WILLIAM; and PARKER, C. 1989. "Diversity in the Practice of District Ethics Committees." *British Medical Journal* 299:1437–1439.

GILLON, RAANAN. 1985. "Philosophical Medical Ethics." A twenty-six-part series first published in *British Medical Journal* and subsequently published as *Philosophical Medical Ethics.* Chichester: Wiley, 1986.

————, ed. 1993. *Principles of Health Care Ethics.* Chichester: Wiley.

GLOVER, JONATHAN. 1977. *Causing Death and Saving Lives.* Harmondsworth, U.K.: Penguin.

HANSCOMBE, GILLIAN E., and FORSTER, JACKIE. 1982. *Rocking the Cradle: Lesbian Mothers—A Challenge in Family Living.* London: Sheba Feminist Publishers.

HARRIS, JOHN. 1985. *The Value of Life: An Introduction to Medical Ethics.* London: Routledge & Kegan Paul.

HIGGS, ROGER. 1985. "On Telling Patients the Truth." In *Moral Dilemmas in Modern Medicine,* pp. 187–202. Edited by Michael Lockwood. Oxford: Oxford University Press.

HOFFENBERG, SIR RAYMOND. 1987. *Clinical Freedom.* London: Nuffield Provincial Hospitals Trust.

HOLMES, JEREMY, and LINDLEY, RICHARD. 1989. *The Values of Psychotherapy.* Oxford: Oxford University Press.

HOPE, ANTHONY; SPRIGINGS, DAVID; and CRISP, ROGER. 1993. "Not Clinically Indicated: Patients's Interest or Resource Allocation?" *British Medical Journal* 306:379–381.

JACKSON, JENNIFER. 1991. "Telling the Truth." *Journal of Medical Ethics* 17:5–9.

JAKOBOVITS, LORD IMMANUEL. 1959. *Jewish Medical Ethics.* New York: Bloch. Reprinted 1975.

JENNETT, BRYAN. 1984. *High Technology Medicine—Benefits and Burdens.* London: Nuffield Provincial Hospitals Trust.

Journal of Medical Ethics. 1985a. "Fourteen Papers from the General Medical Council's Symposium on Medical Ethics." 11:5–41.

———. 1985b. "Two Concepts of Medical Ethics." 11:3. Editorial.

KENNEDY, IAN. 1981. *The Unmasking of Medicine.* London: George Allen and Unwin.

———. 1991. *Treat Me Right: Essays in Medical Law and Ethics.* Oxford: At the Clarendon Press.

KENNEDY, IAN, and GRUBB, ANDREW. 1989. *Medical Law: Texts and Materials.* London: Butterworth.

LAMB, DAVID. 1985. *Death, Brain Death and Ethics.* Beckenham, U.K.: Croom Helm.

Lancet. 1992a. "Decision on Dr. Cox." 340:1283. Unsigned article.

———. 1992b. "The Final Autonomy." 340:757–758. Editorial.

LINACRE CENTRE. 1982. *Euthanasia and Clinical Practice: Trends, Principles and Alternatives—the Report of a Working Party.* London: Author.

LLOYD, WYNDHAM E. B. 1968. *A Hundred Years of Medicine.* 2d ed. London: Duckworth.

LOCKWOOD, MICHAEL, ed. 1985. *Moral Dilemmas in Modern Medicine.* Oxford: Oxford University Press.

MAHONEY, JOHN. 1984. *Bioethics and Belief.* London: Sheed and Ward.

MASON, J. KENNETH, and McCALL SMITH, R. ALEXANDER. 1987. *Law and Medical Ethics.* 2d ed. London: Butterworths.

MAXWELL, ROBERT. 1975. *Health Care: The Growing Dilemma.* New York: McKinsey.

MAYNARD, ALAN. 1986. "National Health Service: Reflections on Enthoven." *Lancet* 1 (January 11):108.

MEDICAL RESEARCH COUNCIL (U.K.). 1991. *The Ethical Conduct of AIDS Vaccine Trials; The Ethical Conduct of Research on Children; The Ethical Conduct of Research on the Mentally Handicapped.* London: Author.

MOONEY, GAVIN, and McGUIRE, ALISTAIR, eds. 1988. *Medical Ethics and Health Care.* Oxford: Oxford University Press.

NEUBERGER, JULIA. 1992. *Ethics and Health Care: The Role of Research Ethics Committees in the United Kingdom.* London: King's Fund Institute.

NICHOLSON, RICHARD, ed. 1986. *Medical Research with Children: Ethics, Law, and Practice.* Report of an Institute of Medical Ethics Working Group on the Ethics of Clinical Research Investigations on Children. Oxford: Oxford University Press.

PAPPWORTH, MAURICE H. 1967. *Human Guinea Pigs.* London: Routledge & Kegan Paul. 2d ed. Harmondsworth, U.K.: Penguin, 1969.

PHILLIPS, MELANIE, and DAWSON, JOHN. 1985. *Doctors' Dilemmas: Medical Ethics and Contemporary Science.* Brighton, U.K.: Harvester Press.

POLKINGHORNE, JOHN. 1989. *Review of the Guidance on the Research Use of Fetuses and Fetal Material* (the Polkinghorne Report). Cmd. 762. London: Her Majesty's Stationery Office.

ROWSON, RICHARD. 1990. *An Introduction to Ethics for Nurses.* London: Scutari.

ROYAL COLLEGE OF NURSING. 1991. "Issues in Nursing and Health." London: Author. Guidance notes on the nature and scope of professional practice; patient records and research (requiring anonymization of notes before use in audit and patient consent before use in research); research trials; living wills; the case for good nursing care; responding to sexual assault; fetal cell transplantation; and guidelines on commercial sponsorship.

ROYAL COLLEGE OF PHYSICIANS. 1986. *Research on Healthy Volunteers.* London: Author.

———. 1990a. *Guidelines on the Practice of Ethics Committees in Medical Research Involving Human Subjects.* London: Author.

———. 1990b. *Research Involving Patients.* London: Author.

SEEDHOUSE, DAVID. 1986. *Health: The Foundations for Achievement.* Chichester: Wiley.

SIEGHART, PAUL, and DAWSON, JOHN. 1987. "Computer-Aided Medical Ethics." *Journal of Medical Ethics* 13: 185–188.

SMITH, JANE, and BOYD, KENNETH. 1991. *Lives in the Balance: The Ethics of Using Animals in Biomedical Research.* Report of a Working Party of the Institute of Medical Ethics. Oxford: Oxford University Press.

SMITH, RICHARD. 1992. "Euthanasia: Time for a Royal Commission: The Tide Seems to Be Running for Euthanasia." *British Medical Journal* 305:728–729.

UNITED KINGDOM CENTRAL COUNCIL FOR NURSING, MIDWIFERY AND HEALTH VISITING (UKCC). 1992a. *Code of Professional Conduct.* London: Author.

———. 1992b. *The Scope of Professional Practice.* London: Author.

WARNOCK, LADY MARY. 1984. *Report of the Committee of Inquiry into Human Fertilisation and Embryology.* Cmd. 9314. London: Her Majesty's Stationery Office.

WILLIAMS, ALAN J. 1985. "The Value of QALYs." *Health and Social Services Journal* 94:3–5.

———. 1991. "Is the QALY a Technical Solution to a Political Problem? Of Course Not." *International Journal of Health Services* 21:365–369.

WILSON-BARNETT, JENIFER. 1986. "Ethical Dilemmas in Nursing." *Journal of Medical Ethics* 12:123–126, 135.

5. REPUBLIC OF IRELAND

"Ireland" here refers to that part of the island of Ireland (twenty-six of the thirty-two counties) that achieved independence from British rule in 1921 and was declared a republic in 1949.

Ireland's moral traditions and its history in ethics are inextricably linked with centuries of religious history that is primarily rooted in the Roman Catholic church. After experiencing religious suppression and persecution under British rule, the government of the new Irish state reinforced the traditional religious ethos in its laws and institutions, particularly education and health care. The Irish Constitution of 1937 recognized the "special position" of the Holy Roman church as guardian of the faith of the great majority of Irish people. This recognition was deleted in 1972, when Ireland was preparing for membership in the European Economic Community.

In what follows, medical ethics in the Republic of Ireland will be discussed by looking at two time periods:

1922–1972 and 1973 forward. Three areas of significant development are then taken as a focus: ethics of reproduction; clinical trials legislation and the role of ethics committees; and changing expectations for doctor–patient relationships.

Between 1922 and 1972 a religious homogeneity of tradition and practice prevailed. On January 1, 1973, Ireland became a member of the European Economic Community and increasingly interacted with other countries whose philosophies of life were based on secular viewpoints. Moral questioning in the society, in politics, and in medical practice became more open and more tolerated.

Ethics of reproduction

In the early 1970s, women's groups actively began to protest a prevailing legal ban on contraceptives and the complete ban on elective abortion even in cases where women were victims of rape or incest. Women who could afford private health care could get contraceptives and abortion advice. The justice of a two-tier health system came under moral and political scrutiny. A private citizen, Mrs. McGee, challenged the Irish government's long-standing prohibition of the sale and importation of contraceptives. Her efforts led to the Health (Family Planning) Act of 1979, in which the Irish state allowed restricted access to contraceptives. Outsiders may be incredulous at Ireland's preoccupation with reproductive ethics. However, this area of morality is central in Irish traditional religious teachings, which have consistently reaffirmed the primacy of women's procreative capacity and fetal life.

Until the 1980s, the topic of abortion was largely a closed moral and legal issue. Ireland had never rescinded the complete ban on abortion specified under the British Offences Against the Person Act of 1861. In practice, termination was permitted under the principle of double effect in exceptional cases, such as ectopic pregnancy. Yet Irish women did procure abortions. On average, four thousand Irish women a year went to England to have abortions under the provisions of the 1969 British abortion legislation. Irish women gradually became more politicized and organized public demonstrations, claiming their rights to control fertility. Serious polarization of views developed as other groups in society feared that elective abortion might be legalized in Ireland. A national campaign began to guarantee protection of embryonic life by means of constitutional amendment.

In 1983, the eighth amendment to the Irish Constitution gave "the unborn" the same rights to life as other citizens. Since then, this amendment has generated a complex series of political, legal, and moral challenges, issuing in a Supreme Court judgment of 1992, *Attorney General* v. X *and Others,* which argues that

abortions may lawfully be carried out in Ireland where continuance of the pregnancy constitutes a real and substantial risk to the life of the pregnant woman. A threat of suicide was specified as such a risk. The Irish government now must provide legislation to specify the conditions under which it is lawful to have abortions in Ireland.

Moral concerns to protect fetal life also influenced the development of guidelines for in vitro fertilization (IVF). Issued by the Institute of Obstetricians and Gynaecologists, the guidelines specify that IVF should be offered to married couples who have been appropriately counseled and have given informed consent. Only sperm and ova from the consenting couple may be used, and all resulting fertilized ova should be placed in the potential mother's uterus.

Research legislation and ethics committees

For years, medical research and clinical trials in Ireland were assessed by institutional review boards whose composition and procedures lacked any nationally agreed guidelines. The ethical norms from the Declaration of Helsinki were applied. The death of a male participant in a nontherapeutic drug trial in Ireland resulted in the government's issuing of the Control of Clinical Trials Act of 1987 (amended in 1990). The principal features of this legislation are that, with certain exceptions, all proposed clinical medical trials must be authorized by the minister for health and have the approval of an ethics committee approved by the minister. Ethics committees are charged with the responsibility for ensuring that participants in any trial give their informed consent personally or by proxy. The latter provisions allow for clinical trials with psychiatric patients who might not be considered competent to consent. Proxy consent must not be given by any investigators involved in the clinical trial.

Ethics committees in Irish public hospitals have frequently been given the job of adjudicating requests from doctors for female sterilizations. Women's groups and gynecologists are now rejecting this role for ethics committees, and criticize what is judged to be unwarranted religious influence on decisions of ethics committees in public hospitals. Doctors are increasingly trying to minimize intrusions into the privacy of the doctor–patient relationship. No case is being made in Ireland for expanding the functions of ethics committees beyond that legally required by the Clinical Trials Act.

Changing expectations for doctor–patient relationships

With the rapid increase of diagnosed AIDS patients and escalating reports of child sexual abuse, incest, and domestic violence, doctors continue their efforts to clarify exceptions to confidentiality. Ethical guidelines on third-party disclosure are available from the Medical Council of Ireland, which officially registers doctors to practice in Ireland and is responsible for taking professional disciplinary action against doctors accused of unethical conduct, proceedings that could issue in deregistration.

In 1989, a law reform commission studying the problem of child sexual abuse recommended a mandatory reporting law that requires cooperation among social workers, community health nurses, and family doctors. Cultural silence about sexual abuse and domestic violence has, in the past, made reform of confidentiality obligations in these areas a complex and onerous challenge. The task of reassessing obligations on third-party disclosures will try to adjudicate the combined moral values of respect for patient autonomy, the need for a competent patient's consent, and the genuine probability of third-party harm.

Since the 1980s, doctors in Ireland have experienced increasing lawsuits for alleged malpractice or negligence. Further analysis is required to determine the multiple causes for such an increase, but the Medical Defence Union, an indemnity insurer for doctors, continues to urge doctors to reflect on the quality of their relationships with patients and to work consistently to improve communication. Litigation is a concern for psychiatric professionals, who recognize the need for clearer procedures for involuntary admissions and for reviewing long-term hospital detention of patients.

Irish patients are now requiring more communication about diagnoses and prognoses, and also expect increased participation in medical decision making. Women who wish to have amniocentesis or chorionic villus sampling for determining fetal health find that they must go to England, since these tests are rarely available in Irish hospitals. Many doctors agree that fetal testing should be provided, but institutions are slow to comply, on the grounds that such tests might contribute to an abortion decision.

The previously dominant model of strong paternalism characterizing the doctor–patient relationship is now under challenge due to changing educational experiences of doctors and a more questioning Irish population. Courses in ethics are taught in Irish medical schools, where almost 20 percent of students are now non-Irish. Nurses and medical students are now encouraged to reflect on reasons for their moral views and to consider the possible validity of diverse ethical positions. Religious orthodoxy is no longer taken for granted. Such courses are usually required of medical students and nurses, and vary in length from several weeks to a full year.

Awareness is growing among an increasingly educated population that living wills are available in other countries, and that decisions about withholding life-support systems for the terminally ill are areas of medical decision making where patients and family members ought to have more voice. In trying to determine moral boundaries in the prolongation of life, the Roman Catholic tradition distinguishing obligatory and nonobligatory treatment (ordinary and extraordinary) may be justly recognized as a well-argued basis for granting patients considerable voice in their treatment decisions.

As Ireland continues to be more actively integrated into the European Community, ethical pluralism is being acknowledged as a reality requiring open debate. The hope is that such efforts at public discussion will yield a stronger, because more consensual, public morality that will signal respect for the now undeniable differences of ethical viewpoints among Irish people. In the years ahead, the scope of Irish medical ethics can be expected to broaden in order to encompass issues such as genetic research and testing, biotechnology, environmental ethics, and distributive justice in determining health-care priorities.

DOLORES DOOLEY

While all the articles in this section and the other sections of this entry are relevant, see especially the INTRODUCTION *and other articles in this subsection:* SOUTHERN EUROPE, THE BENELUX COUNTRIES, UNITED KINGDOM, GERMAN-SPEAKING COUNTRIES AND SWITZERLAND, NORDIC COUNTRIES, CENTRAL AND EASTERN EUROPE, *and* RUSSIA. *Directly related to this article is the entry* ROMAN CATHOLICISM. *For a further discussion of topics mentioned in this article, see the entries* ABORTION, *section on* CONTEMPORARY ETHICAL AND LEGAL ASPECTS, *and section on* RELIGIOUS PERSPECTIVES, *article on* ROMAN CATHOLICISM; AUTONOMY; CLINICAL ETHICS, *article on* INSTITUTIONAL ETHICS COMMITTEES; CONFIDENTIALITY; DOUBLE EFFECT; ETHICS, *article on* RELIGION AND MORALITY; FERTILITY CONTROL; HEALTH-CARE DELIVERY, *article on* HEALTH-CARE SYSTEMS; INFORMED CONSENT; JUSTICE; LAW AND MORALITY; LICENSING, DISCIPLINE, AND REGULATION IN THE HEALTH PROFESSIONS; MEDICAL MALPRACTICE; MENTALLY DISABLED AND MENTALLY ILL PERSONS, *article on* RESEARCH ISSUES; OBLIGATION AND SUPEREROGATION; PATERNALISM; PATIENTS' RIGHTS; POPULATION ETHICS, *section on* RELIGIOUS TRADITIONS, *article on* ROMAN CATHOLIC PERSPECTIVES; PRIVACY IN HEALTH CARE; PROFESSIONAL-PATIENT RELATIONSHIP; REPRODUCTIVE TECHNOLOGIES, *article on* IN VITRO FERTILIZATION AND EMBRYO TRANSFER; RESEARCH ETHICS COMMITTEES; RESEARCH POLICY; *and* WOMEN, *articles on* HISTORICAL AND CROSS-CULTURAL PERSPECTIVES; *and* HEALTH-CARE ISSUES.

Bibliography

CLARKE, DESMOND M. 1984. *Church and State: Essays in Political Philosophy.* Cork, Ireland: Cork University Press.

Consultation Paper on Child Sexual Abuse. 1989. Dublin: Law Reform Commission.

Control of Clinical Trials Act. 1987. Annotated by Robert A. Pearce. London: Sweet and Maxwell. Reprinted from *Irish Current Law Statutes Annotated.*

DOOLEY, DOLORES. 1991. "Medical Ethics in Ireland: A Decade of Change." *Hastings Center Report* 21, no. 1:18–21.

EDMONDSON, RICCA. 1992. "Moral Debate and Social Change." *Doctrine and Life* 42, no. 5:233–243. This entire issue is a collection of articles titled "Abortion, Law and Conscience."

FOGARTY, MICHAEL P.; RYAN, LIAM; and LEE, JOSEPH. 1984. *Irish Values and Attitudes: The Irish Report of the European Value Systems Study.* Dublin: Dominican Publications.

HANNON, PATRICK. 1989. "In Vitro Fertilisation." *Irish Theological Quarterly* 55, no. 1:7–17.

HENSEY, BRENDAN. 1988. *The Health Services of Ireland.* 4th rev. ed. Dublin: Institute of Public Administration.

IRELAND. STUDY GROUP ON THE DEVELOPMENT OF THE PSYCHIATRIC SERVICES. 1984. *The Psychiatric Services: Planning for the Future.* Dublin: Stationery Office.

MACCURTAIN, MARGARET, and Ó CORRÁIN, DONNCHADH, eds. 1978. *Women in Irish Society: The Historical Dimension.* Dublin: Arlen House Women's Press.

McMAHON, BRYAN M. E. 1982. "The Law Relating to Contraception in Ireland." In *Morality and the Law,* pp. 20–30. Edited by Desmond Clarke. Cork, Ireland: Mercier Press.

MEDICAL COUNCIL OF IRELAND. 1989. *A Guide to Ethical Conduct and Behaviour and to Fitness to Practise.* 3d ed. Dublin: Author.

O'ROURKE, KEVIN. 1989. "On Prolonging Life." *Doctrine and Life* 39, no. 7:352–366.

REIDY, MAURICE, ed. 1982. *Ethical Issues in Reproductive Medicine.* Dublin: Gill and Macmillan.

RYNNE, ANDREW. 1982. *Abortion: The Irish Question.* Dublin: Ward River.

SMYTH, AILBHE, ed. 1992. *The Abortion Papers, Ireland.* Dublin: Attic Press.

WHYTE, JOHN H. 1980. *Church and State in Modern Ireland, 1923–1979.* 2d ed. Dublin: Gill and Macmillan.

6. GERMAN-SPEAKING COUNTRIES AND SWITZERLAND

This article discusses the origin and current status of bioethics in German-speaking countries, specifically, Germany, Austria, and Switzerland. Topics covered in this article include bioethics institutions and teaching, the role and function of ethics committees, euthanasia and assisted suicide, abortion, new reproductive technologies, genetics, organ transplantation, and resource allocation.

General remarks

As elsewhere, interest in bioethics in the German-speaking countries originated with medical-ethics questions related to both modern biotechnological potential and societies' growing ethical pluralism. Also as elsewhere, this not only induced physicians to debate these issues, but was part of the reason for a "rehabilitation of practical philosophy" among a number of German academic philosophers and theologians—a renewed interest and focus on moral, social, and political problems.

Several factors make bioethics in Germany, Switzerland, and Austria different than that in the United States or other European countries. First, as a major and collective effort, it developed relatively late, that is, in the mid-1980s. Some explanations for this are the lack of civil rights movements that would have endorsed issues of patients' rights; a widespread and deeply rooted (patient-voluntary) medical paternalism; general access to medical care, and thus little need for allocation debates; a different philosophical tradition (discussed later); and, in Germany, a severely disturbed moral self-assurance due to the recent experiences of Nazi Germany's undescribable immoralities. Second, there are many theological voices in German bioethics. In the German world theology is given a legitimate academic presence within universities, where it enjoys the same juridical status as all other disciplines. It also possesses relative independence from the churches. Third, German law is solely statutory in nature and is not linked to case law as in the American judicial system. Hence, going to court is a far less common way to trigger public discussion on difficult bioethics cases. For Switzerland it is important to mention its plebiscites (direct voting by the population on an issue) as an instrument of legislative decision making, and the fact that legal authority resides partly with the Bund (federation) and partly with the 26 different cantons (states), which show remarkable legal differences in handling some bioethics problems. Fourth, Germans place great importance on the study of the history of medicine and medical anthropology, the philosophical clarification of fundamental medical categories. And finally, Germany labors under the historical weight of the Nazi regime's deadly medical experimentation, eugenics, and so-called "euthanasia," and of the concomitant moral degradation of many physicians.

Not only does the Nazi specter affect the discussion of bioethics in Germany even more profoundly than in the rest of the world, but it is seen by many in Germany to have a direct connection to a number of issues discussed in contemporary bioethics. Concern is heightened by the fact that Nazi experimentation occurred despite the existence of guidelines for therapeutic and scientific research on human subjects that prohibited such treatment. These guidelines, thought to be the first of their kind, were published originally as a Circular of the Reich Minister of the Interior dated February 28, 1931, and remained in force until 1945 (Sass, 1993). Thus, several groups and movements take permissive positions on selective abortion, euthanasia, or gene therapy to be not only deeply immoral but Nazi-like, and also (falsely) to be definitive of "bioethics" as such, which they therefore attack harshly.

Philosophical bioethics in Germany

The philosophical clarification of medicine's role, and of its fundamental categories such as pathology, illness, and healing, in Germany still has an influential intramedical tradition as medical anthropology (e.g., *Weizsäcker*, 1951). Also, as already mentioned, German medicine has long cultivated historical study, and the many institutes devoted to medical history increasingly view part of their work as preparatory to or incorporating moral reflection on medicine. Whereas medical ethics has traditionally focused primarily on aspects of the physician–patient relationship (e.g., truth-telling, confidentiality, humaneness), its spectrum has by now been broadened to cover all issues addressed by Anglo-American "bioethics." However, the latter is sharply opposed by many—be it merely as a label, as the writing of those who call themselves bioethicists, or as a discipline in general. Thus, in sharp contrast to (welcome) medical ethics, "bioethics" is frequently understood as an ideological and uncritical defense of any biotechnology and of the resulting cultural and lifestyle changes, or on a par with a dangerous pro-euthanasia movement (see below), or at least with a suspected (i.e., "analytical") style of philosophy.

It is in part for this last reason that professional German philosophers have by and large been late to join the contemporary Anglo-American debate on any issue in applied ethics. Analytical philosophers had to leave the country under the Nazi regime; moreover, continental philosophy had rarely been attracted by either utilitarianism or pragmatism, which are among the dominant theories in contemporary Anglo-Saxon ethics debates. Kant, with his rejection of material ethical values and his predominant interest in a metaphysico-rational justification of ethics, has certainly been the major influence to the contrary.

Institutions and teaching

Paralleling the belated onset of bioethical debates in German-speaking countries, the development of institutions focused on the study of bioethics has also been comparatively slow. A few such institutions have, however, developed recently, most of them university-based. Many of them offer optional courses, and some receive support for research from resources outside the university. The *Institut für Geschichte der Medizin* (Institute for History of Medicine) at the University of Freiburg in Breisgau is among these initiatives. The first university program established in Germany specifically for bioethics research is at the University of Tübingen. Its bioethics projects began in 1985 in the context of an ongoing colloquium involving professors from all faculties; in 1986 this became a research unit (*Forschungsstelle*); and in 1990 the University converted this to a multidisciplinary Center for Ethics in the Sciences and Humanities (*Zentrum für Ethik in den Wissenschaften*). The center draws fellows and postgraduate students from different disciplines into collaboration and common discourse on ethical aspects of medicine, science, and the law. Although sometimes directed by moral theologians, the center does not espouse any particular religious or theological point of view. It publishes a series, "*Ethik in den Wissenschaften.*" In 1986 Hans-Martin Sass and Herbert Viefhues created an influential center at the University of Bochum: the *Zentrum für Medizinische Ethik Bochum* (the Bochum Institute for Medical Ethics). This center is involved in teaching, consultation, and research and publishes a series of short papers ("*Medizinethische Materialien*") on specific issues in bioethics, including translations from the international literature.

The *Forschungsinstitut für Philosophie* (Research Institute for Philosophy) in Hannover was founded with financing from and under the auspices of the Roman Catholic church. Since its inception in 1988, it has focused on issues at the intersection of religion and philosophy in the Catholic tradition of philosophical thought. The most recently founded (1993) German bioethics institution is the *Institut für Wissenschaft und Ethik* at the University of Bonn; it brings together a large number of scholars from different backgrounds to explore and debate science–ethics problems in interdisciplinary projects, conferences, and teaching.

In Switzerland, two institutes are active in the study of bioethics at the University of Zurich: the *Institut für Sozialethik* and the *Arbeits- und Forschungsstelle für Ethik*. The latter was founded in 1989 and performs research activities on practically the whole spectrum of applied ethics. Other Swiss institutes operate within the theological faculties at Freiburg and Lucerne.

The first German-language journal for medical ethics, *Arzt und Christ* ("Physician and Christian"), was founded in Austria in 1955 by Dr. Wolfgang Mueller-Hartburg, a Viennese clinician. Since 1993 the journal has been called *Zeitschrift für medizinische Ethik* ("Journal of Medical Ethics"), and is published in Bonn, Germany. Also in Austria, a pioneer institute, *Senatsinstitut für Ethik in der Medizin* ("Senate Institute for Ethics in Medicine"), was founded at the University of Vienna in 1992 to pursue research and teaching activities in bioethics. Also, the *Wissenschaftliche Landesakademie für Niederösterreich* (Scientific State's Academy for Lower Austria) has established an institute for the research, teaching, and study of bioethics.

Teaching of bioethics in Switzerland is part of the curriculum of theological ethics at Lausanne and Geneva, as well as the curriculum of philosophical ethics at Basel and Freiburg. The Austrian and German worlds have just begun to take the first steps necessary to include the teaching of ethics as part of the regular and required curriculum of medical students. Although such teaching has so far mainly been a matter of personal initiative by interested professors, it has been attempted by numerous medical faculties. Traditional obstacles to incorporating such teaching are evident; these include resistance to introducing a new discipline into an already burdensome curriculum; the difficulty physicians have in according ethics the status of a discipline that is epistemologically and materially independent of the study of medicine; and concern about the trend of entrusting the teaching of ethics to physicians who may, from a professional bias, be blinded to difficulties of the medical profession. But increasing efforts are being made to promote a coherent teaching program within the medical curriculum. Of note is the German students' association for medical ethics (*Studentenverband Ethik in der Medizin*, Freiburg), founded in 1989. These and other efforts and activities (see below) have led to planned revisions of the federal regulations of the German medical curriculum which require medical ethics to be a subject of both teaching and exams for future medical students. At present, however, no medical ethicist has ever been appointed to a permanent position in Germany.

Professional bodies/"Akademien"/ government-appointed bodies

Common to all German-speaking countries is the existence of a governing body that holds normative power over health-care professionals. Characteristically these institutions focus on determining professional ethics and have recognized authority in judging new medical practices.

In Switzerland, the *Schweizerische Akademie der medizinischen Wissenschaften* (Swiss Academy of Medical Sciences) is a foundation comprised of all the medical schools and the Swiss physicians' associations. Its Central Ethics Commission prepares guidelines on specific issues of medical or research practice that are considered ethically problematic, such as policies for new reproductive technologies and withdrawing life-supporting treatment. These published guidelines regulate the practices of health-care professionals. Internally imposed sanctions are administered by the profession to those who do not respect the directives. In addition, the fourteen-

member commission serves as a permanent ethics counseling body for physicians and the public.

Similarly, in Germany, the Federal Chamber of Physicians (*Bundesärztekammer,* membership in which is obligatory for German physicians) has established an Ethics Advisory Board to its Scientific Council to issue ethics guidelines for intraprofessional self-regulation and to serve as a counseling body. Particularly in areas of conduct that lack legal regulation, this type of binding professional self-legislation functions somewhat as a legal substitute. Other important bodies are "societies of experts" (*Gesellschaften* or *Akademien*). They aim at promoting scientific debates and research among their members and the public. For medical ethics, there exists in Germany the *Akademie für Ethik in der Medizin* (Academy for Medical Ethics). Founded in 1986, it has an interdisciplinary membership of approximately 200 members, most of whom are German. The Akademie receives a mix of public and private funding and provides a forum for research (working groups on specific topics), for expert and public debate, and for teaching medical ethics. Since 1989 it has published the second German language journal on medical ethics, *Ethik in der Medizin,* and in 1993 it established the first German bioethics literature data base. Another professional body (of both law and medicine) worth mentioning is the *Deutsche Gesellschaft für Medizinrecht* (German Society for Medical Law), which formulated recommendations on the treatment of severely disabled newborns (the Einbecker Recommendations, see below). In Switzerland, the most important professional body is the *Schweizerische Gesellschaft für biomedizinische Ethik* (Swiss Society for Biomedical Ethics).

Finally, governments in these countries have sometimes appointed political working groups or expert commissions to issue advisory reports on a variety of bioethico-legal issues. The first to be published in Germany (*Bundesminister für Forschung und Technologie,* 1985) was the Report of the Benda Commission on assisted fertilization, genome analysis, and gene therapy. This commission, appointed by the Federal Ministers of Law and of Research and Technology, and chaired by the former president of the Constitutional Court, Ernst Benda, was composed of nineteen members, most of them scholars from different backgrounds. The Swiss issued the Amstad Report dealing with the same subjects (*Expertenkommission Humangenetik und Reproduktionsmedizin,* 1988). Another ongoing German expert commission works on cost-saving strategies in public-health care and issues yearly reports. The ethical analyses contained in such reports are certainly less in-depth and also less balanced than, for example, the Reports of the President's Commission. Participants with a background in philosophy served on these bodies only in rare instances. The German Parliament also established an Office for

Technology Assessment (*Büro für Technologiefolgen-Ab-schätzung beim Bundestag*; under Herbert Paschen), which issued a 1993 report on genome analysis.

In Austria, the Parliament and its commissions (membership may include experts) remain the major participants in drafting laws or new regulations on issues such as patient treatment, research, and health-care financing.

"Ethics committees" for human experimentation

So-called *Ethikkommissionen* exist in Austria, Germany, and Switzerland—functioning, however, almost exclusively as review boards for medical experiments on human subjects. Only in the early 1990s have scattered committees been established upon personal initiative in a very few hospitals to consider questions such as treatment decisions for individual patients or the development of institutional ethics guidelines. As in other Western countries, the institutionalization of review boards for medical research on humans occurred in response to the Nuremberg Trials of Nazi physicians, and is in accord with the 1964 Declaration of Helsinki and its subsequent revisions.

In Switzerland, the pioneering 1970 (revised in 1989) guidelines on research involving human subjects issued by the Swiss Academy of Medical Sciences (*Schweizerische Akademie der Wissenschaften*, or SAMW) required the establishment of ethics committees at hospitals and research institutes to make certain that proposed projects were important, well designed, and of acceptable risk, and that subjects were insured and had given informed consent. Participation of nurses on these committees was required, leaving other details to institutional discretion. No federal law exists covering experimentation on human subjects, and only half of Switzerland's cantons have established legal guidelines to oversee research or protect patients. The 1989 revision of the SAMW guidelines did much to increase uniformity in approach and method among committees, but many differences still exist in method and scope of review (*Schweizerische Akademie der Wissenschaften*, 1989). On average, membership consists of seven members (mostly physicians and predominantly male), one nurse, and one lay member. Concerns exist about the lack of oversight of protocols conducted in private practice. In 1992 the SAMW established an Overregional Ethics Committee for Clinical Research, which approves of multicenter research protocols and offers consultation to local committees.

In Germany, the introduction of *Ethikkommissionen* was not recommended until 1979, with endorsement

from both the German Federal Chamber of Physicians (*Bundesärztekammer*) for the chambers on state and federal levels, and the Federal Association of Medical Schools for each medical school. The purpose of such ethics committees (approval by which is required for projects funded by governmental agencies such as the national German Research Foundation, *Deutsche Forschungsgemeinschaft*) is to give advice to researchers in the assessment of the ethical and legal aspects of proposed clinical research on humans. In 1983 the Workgroup of Medical Ethics Committees (*Arbeitskreis Medizinischer Ethik-Kommissionen*) was founded, comprised of all ethics committees at the state physicians chambers or the medical faculties. The workgroup meets annually to share experiences, promote standardization, and revise/update its procedural principles. In 1985 the *Bundesärztekammer* turned the requests for ethics committee review into an obligatory standard of professional practice. The German Drug Law (*Arzneimittelgesetz*, AMG) requires approval by an Ethics Committee for Controlled Clinical Trials; the State Chambers of Physicians (*Landesärztekammern*) and university-based Departments of Medicine request approval of all protocols prior to the initiation of research. In accordance with the *Arbeitskreis* recommendations, committees have at least five (and up to eleven) members, that is, four physicians plus one expert in medical law. In addition, theologians often serve, but only few committees include a philosopher or laypeople. Critics of the present state of ethics committees thus question the autonomy and independence from institutional pressure of such "peer groups." In addition they express regret at the absence of legal standing for the committees and of standardized criteria to determine their and their individual members' ethical competence. Other issues raised include whether committee notification of research results should be mandatory; oversight of commercial or "free" (not institution-affiliated) committees; and a lack of clarity as to whether research conducted on human cells and tissues should be subject to review and whether review should then extend to the use or disposal of human cells or tissues collected for diagnostic or other nonresearch purposes. In addition, they claim that inadequate attention is given to coordinating the review of different ethics committees in multicenter research.

In Austria research ethics committees are legally required since 1988 for the medical faculties as well as for every research hospital. These prescriptions have been revised in detail in 1993, requiring that the states issue legal regulations according to which members of every ethics committee have to include women; at least one independent and one physician with particular expertise in the research at stake; at least one representative of the hospital's chaplain or somebody else with ethical expertise of patients, staff and legal service; and a pharmacist.

Specific ethical issues

Allowing to die/euthanasia.

The *Guidelines on Assistance in Dying* of the Swiss Academy of Medical Sciences (initially issued in 1976) emphasize a patient's right to turn down any treatment. They further permit withholding treatment for irreversibly dying patients as well as for patients with a loss of consciousness considered irreversible. Treatment in such cases explicitly includes respiration and artificial nutrition. Decisions must include substituted judgments made with the help of the patient's next of kin and must consider the patient's best interests. As of 1988, valid and relevant living wills must be followed. Active voluntary euthanasia, however, is ruled out; it is illegal under the Swiss Penal Code.

The German Federal Chamber of Physicians modeled its 1979 guidelines on "assistance in dying" almost verbatim after the Swiss guidelines (Baumann, 1986). Remarkably, however, two points were left out without further discussion: the explicit permission to withhold or withdraw respiration and artificial nutrition in the irreversibly dying patient, and the explicit permission to forgo treatment in patients with an irreversible loss of consciousness. Moreover, the German guidelines. (here again copying the former Swiss ones) consider living wills merely as a nonbinding piece of evidence among others. In a 1993 update of these guidelines, this last point is explicitly reaffirmed.

Another noteworthy aspect of these German guidelines is that they give moral backing to restricted truthtelling to terminally ill patients "so as to save him or her from anxiety." And finally, they reaffirm—against a climate of decreasing unanimity in this respect—the impermissibility of active voluntary euthanasia. Both in Switzerland and Germany the latter is illegal under the Penal Code. The German Roman Catholic Conference of Bishops and the Protestant church have repeatedly and strongly argued against active euthanasia while emphasizing the need and Christian obligation to care in a humane and Christian way for the suffering and dying. A hospice movement that provides palliative care for the dying is seen by many as an appropriate way both to fulfill the obligation to care for the terminally ill and to eliminate the very reasons patients ask for voluntary euthanasia. In addition, any use of the term "euthanasia" in Germany conjures up vivid images of the use of the term by the Nazis as they carried out their goal of exterminating millions of fellow human beings who were of "inferior" quality. The killing began with individuals institutionalized because of physical or mental impair-

ments and spread to those deemed racially or genetically inferior. The deeply emotional nature of this historical association explains current objections by many Germans even to open discussions of euthanasia. The media and public culture are so aware of Nazi cruelties that lectures by Peter Singer and Helga Kuhse—Australian bioethicists who support both voluntary euthanasia and the permissibility of passive as well as active euthanasia (withholding treatment as well as directly killing) for severely disabled neonates on parental request—in Germany or Austria have been prohibited or protested (Schöne-Seifert, 1993). In the aftermath of this so-called "Singer affair" (starting in 1989), organizations of disabled people and other political and interest groups have vehemently argued that those in favor of euthanasia for severely disabled newborns make an indirect judgment about the worth of a life and are on a slippery slope toward a climate where elimination of the unfit or discrimination toward the sick, feeble, and disabled will again be accepted. These objections have often been paralleled in debates about selective abortion and have been the beginning of a rather widespread antibioethics climate in both Germany and Austria.

Withdrawing treatment for most severely disabled newborns is considered morally permissible and is narrowly specified as such by the above-mentioned Swiss guidelines. Again, the corresponding German guidelines have eliminated this passage. However, the German Society for Medical Law had issued rather similar recommendations (so-called *Einbecker Empfehlungen*) in 1986. The society considered it morally permissible to let newborns die who either suffer from most severe mental disabilities or can only be kept alive by permanent intensive care. After the Singer affair, these recommendations were revised (1992) such that forgoing treatment is restricted to newborns with irreversible medical problems that will lead to death within a short period of time.

Legalized active euthanasia on request of terminally ill patients has been advocated by some German voices, too. One such voice has been raised by the *Deutsche Gesellschaft für Humanes Sterben* (the German Society for Humanely Dying, or DGHS), founded in 1980, which argues for respect for the dying patient's autonomy. This lay organization, which does not enjoy much support in the medical or legal communities, also provides its members with forms for living wills and, in the past, has provided assistance in suicide. Because suicide is not a criminal offense, assisting it is not illegal either. However, physicians are seen by law to stand under specific professional obligations (*garantenpflichten*), which some courts—in contrast to the view dominant in legal literature—have interpreted to include suicide intervention. Hence, there is an unresolved legal tension that makes jurisdiction on physicians' assistance (and consequent nonintervention) in suicide unpredictable. The credibility of DGHS, moreover, was shaken in early 1993 when its founder and president, H. H. Atrott, was arrested for selling cyanide capsules at inflated prices (Tufts, 1993).

In 1986, an Alternative Draft of a Law for Assistance in Dying (*Alternativentwurf eines Gesetzes über Sterbehilfe*) was published by a number of reputable experts in medicine and law (Baumann, 1986). Among its suggestions was one to waive prosecution of (nevertheless still "illegal") euthanasia on persistent request, if the euthanized patient was competent and suffering from terminal illness. However, the draft never succeeded, due to lack of sympathy by the Federal Chamber of Physicians and by the German Legal Association.

Advance directives, be they in the form of living wills or of durable powers of attorney, are rarely used by patients and hence play a minor role in medical decision making in all three German-speaking countries. Although the 1992 Care Law (*Betreuungsgesetz*) in Germany in principle provides for both instruments, and although various forms for living wills are publicly available, the legal status of advance directives is disputed, has not yet been tested in the courts, and is widely considered uncertain. This situation further discourages its already low acceptance by the medical profession and wider use by patients.

In Austria, the overall situation is very similar to that in Switzerland and Germany: Active euthanasia is illegal under the national Penal Code; withdrawing treatment is not, by either law or policies, regulated in any detail; and advance directives as yet have little practical impact.

Abortion. With the 1990 reunification of the German nation, divided since the end of World War II, most laws and regulations of the former Federal Republic of Germany (West Germany) were applied to the citizens of the former German Democratic Republic (East Germany). However, the abortion paragraph of the Penal Code resulted in heated debate because there were very different models of legal abortion in the former two Germanys. In the West, a 1974 law permitted pregnant women to choose abortion until the end of the first trimester. Based on a charge of nonprotection of the rights of the unborn, the constitutionality of this law was challenged in 1975; the resulting interpretation of the constitution (*Grundgesetz*) by the German Constitutional Court (*Bundesverfassungsgericht*) held that human dignity (*Menschenwürde*)—a conceptually loose term that is used by both sides of the abortion debate to support their position—is constitutionally protected from the moment of conception. It enforced an "indication model," permitting legal abortion until the end

of the first trimester only if a physician certified that certain social or medical indications were present. Under this model, the physician was the ultimate moral agent and an acknowledged right to life of the unborn was to be balanced against medical or social hardship. Generous interpretation of these criteria often lead to a de facto policy of abortion on demand in the first trimester, but with different standards and variability in enforcement in the various states of the Federal Republic. In the German Democratic Republic, a "term model" for legal abortions operated since 1972, wherein abortion was allowed until the end of the first trimester and was cost-free.

In the new Germany a heated public debate—involving, however, little philosophical analysis—took place on the underlying theological, moral, and political positions motivating the clashing views on abortion. In 1992 the Federal Parliament approved a compromise law under which abortion would be legal in the first trimester (and paid for by health insurance) as long as the woman had a consultation session prior to abortion. Mandatory counseling and education were intended as an additional step to strengthen fetal protection (a goal that had been emphasized almost unanimously) and include informing pregnant women about existing supportive social, welfare, and employment programs, as well as kindergarten settings for the child, that would enable her to choose to continue her pregnancy. However, conservative parliamentarians and the Roman Catholic church petitioned the *Bundesverfassungsgericht* to declare the law unconstitutional. The German Supreme Court did so in May 1993, stating that the counseling sessions did not go far enough in protecting fetal human life as required by the (formerly West) German constitution. The Court argued that the constitutional rights of a woman (to physical integrity, human dignity, right of personality) do not go so far as to allow her to claim a fundamentally protected legal right to kill an unborn child by means of abortion; that abortions at any point during a pregnancy are fundamentally wrong and thus illegal; and that the state's duty to protect the unborn also includes maintaining and raising the public's consciousness of the unborn child's legal right of protection. However, the Court held that a future abortion law would be considered constitutional even if it abstained from prosecution of those (nevertheless "illegal") first-trimester abortions that were performed at the pregnant woman's request, so long as they followed mandatory and explicit pro-life counseling. Abortion other than for pregnancy resulting from rape or for medical reasons should, moreover, not be paid for by health insurance. Among the many voices that strongly objected to this decision, some admitted that it was at least more consistent than the former compromise of both acknowledging a fetal right to life and legalizing abortion on demand. A future abortion law is planned to respond to these Supreme Court requirements.

In Switzerland (where women first began to acquire the political right to vote only in 1971), abortions are permitted only for serious medical indications or in case of grave emergency (commonly interpreted to include rape and embryopathy). In the 1970s, opinion polls suggested that a majority of the Swiss people would opt for a liberalization of abortion law. However, a plebiscite in 1977 resulted in a vote narrowly against abortion on demand in the first trimester of pregnancy (with a majority of French-speaking and dominantly Protestant cantons [states] in favor of liberalization, and German-speaking and dominantly Catholic cantons against). Various initiatives aiming at a revision of the Swiss Penal Code such that first-trimester abortions will no longer be prosecutable offenses have so far been unsuccessful.

In predominantly (85%) Roman Catholic Austria, first-trimester abortion on demand has been legally permitted since 1975. Costs of medically indicated abortions are covered by insurance, while those resulting from abortions performed for nonmedical reasons must be paid for by the women themselves. A pro-life referendum initiated the year before the introduction of this law won only 18% of Austrian voters, and none of the three major political parties supported the initiative.

New reproductive technologies and embryo research. A great deal of the public debate in German, Austrian, and Swiss bioethics continues to focus on reproductive issues. Germany criminalizes all forms of sperm, egg, and embryo donation and embryo testing, manipulation, or research, while Austria and Switzerland are less restrictive and do not use their penal law to sanction these positions as does Germany.

In Germany, the Benda Report of 1985 recommended that a future reproduction law ban all forms of surrogate motherhood; heterologous in vitro fertilization (IVF) and assisted insemination by donor (AID), at least for single women; research on other than embryos that are purposefully left over from IVF; and any genetic manipulation of germ-line cells. These measures were considered necessary to prevent violations of "human dignity." The first regulations, issued in 1985 by the Federal Chamber of Physicians had the status of intraprofessional self-regulation. They were revised in 1988 and in January 1994 and now permit only homologous (using only the spouses' egg and sperm) IVF and GIFT (gamete-intra-fallopian-tube transfer) and only in married couples. Only somatic infertility is explicitly accepted as an indication for IVF, for example, and in a detailed commentary, the aforementioned restriction to homology and marriage are justified by the well-being of the child-to-be. In accordance with the 1991 Embryo Protection

Law (see below), embryo donation and all forms of surrogate motherhood are prohibited. Theoretically, in rare cases, (unpaid-for) donor sperm may be used, and in those instances, the mature child-to-be has the right to know on request the donor's identity. Moreover, it is conceivable that either the child-to-be or its social father may legally contest the latter's paternity, with the effect that the biological father might have to fulfill paternal duties. However, no cases of AID have occurred since 1985 and these issues of access to (heterologous) IVF and its ramifications for family law still await a long-planned Reproductive Medicine Law.

In a second set of guidelines issued in 1985, the chamber prohibited the production of embryos for research and restricted embryo research to important questions of infertility treatment or embryo development and to spare embryos before day 14, after approval of the central commission. After heated public debates on the implications of human dignity, reproductive autonomy, and the permissibility of research even on spare embryos, the German Embryo Protection Law (*Embryonenschutzgesetz*) was introduced in 1991. Because this law is so restrictive, it is still controversial. In summary, the law prohibits: (1) artificial insemination of an oocyte for any purpose other than a nonsurrogate pregnancy of the "possessing" woman, and (2) any kind of nontherapeutic manipulation or research on the embryo, even in case of spare embryos (whose occurrence is made unlikely by the first prohibition). In addition, (3), any single totipotent cell (an early embryonic cell from which a whole organism could still develop) is given the same legal status as the embryo. Further restrictions rule out (4) egg donation and any form of surrogate motherhood, as well as (5) cloning or the creation of chimeras (organisms with a combination of human and animal genes). Violating these regulations can result in lengthy prison terms and monetary fines, but punishment applies only to third parties (i.e., physicians, researchers, and agencies), not to biological, gestational, or social mothers-to-be.

This Embryo Protection Law has been criticized heavily for setting up an ethical double standard because it forbids preimplantation diagnosis—by (2) plus (3) above—even for those with a family history of severe hereditary disease, while at the same time other laws allow elective abortion for medical or other reasons in later stages of pregnancy. The law also has been accused of interfering with self-determination, responsible parenthood, and reproductive choice, and for putting an end to all research even on spare embryos (except on oocytes excluded from use for fertilization or fetal cells that will not be cloned or transferred).

The law does not specifically address the use of fetal tissue; guidance is provided by recommendations issued by the Federal Chamber of Physicians. It determined that researchers may use tissue from a dead fetus only if an ethics committee determines that the research protocol is well designed and cannot be done without the fetal tissue. The woman's consent must be obtained in all instances, but a woman may not consent to research use of fetal tissue prior to aborting the fetus. Tissue from a living fetus may be used only if the research is restricted to the direct benefit of the particular fetus.

Austria's Law on Reproductive Medicine (*Fortpflanzungsmedizingesetz*) regulates both the use of new reproductive technologies and embryo protection. It was introduced in 1992 after long and heated debates and represents a political compromise between the Roman Catholic opposition to reproductive technologies on theological grounds and more liberal approaches that emphasize the benefits of new reproductive technologies to support individual reproductive freedom and choice. With regard to embryo protection, both germ-line manipulation and any form of nontherapeutic research are prohibited. Preimplantation diagnostics, though not expressly permitted, might be acceptable if avoidance of severe hereditary disease was at issue.

In reproductive medicine, homologous as well as heterologous IVF or GIFT are permitted as infertility treatments for married couples or those in stable relationships. Embryo donation and all forms of surrogate motherhood are forbidden. Only freely donated sperm from living donors may be used, and—based on the concept of human dignity—a child conceived from donor sperm is permitted to know the identity of the biological father once he or she reaches maturity; records must be kept thirty years. Issues of inheritance and other matters affecting IVF offspring are regulated elsewhere in the law.

In Switzerland, the Swiss Academy for Medical Sciences (SAMW) issued guidelines on the use of new reproductive technologies in 1990. Homologous IVF in married or quasi-married couples, as well as IVF using anonymously donated sperm or egg in married couples, are permitted as either infertility treatment or as a means to prevent transmission of a genetic disease. Embryo donation, all forms of surrogate motherhood, preimplantative sex selection, germ-line manipulation, and any research on embryos are prohibited.

In 1992, the Swiss accepted a new constitutional Article 24, which requires federal regulation of embryo protection and of reproductive technologies according to the following restrictions: The manipulation of germ-line cells and embryos, the creation of chimeras, and the production of spare embryos are illegal. Homologous and heterologous IVF are legal as an infertility treatment (allowing—like German and Austrian law, and in contrast to the SAMW guidelines—for later access to informa-

tion about one's biological parent) or as a means to prevent transmission of a genetic disease; embryo donation and all forms of surrogate motherhood are illegal; research on spare embryos (which ought, however, not to be produced) is not explicitly ruled out.

Human genetics. Use of genetic testing techniques in Germany, Switzerland, and Austria is regulated quite strictly. Each of these countries has regulations regarding the use of genetic testing, the need for informed consent of the individuals involved, and the need to integrate genetic testing into a larger process of genetic counseling. The memory of eugenic experiments during the Third Reich inevitably generates negative emotions, especially in Germany, toward any medical intervention concerned with the prevention of hereditary disease. German reflection seems much concerned with the question of how far society and parents should go to accept disabilities that can be easily discovered using prenatal diagnosis while at the same time protecting the woman's right to decide whether or not to use prenatal diagnosis. Another main issue discussed in all three countries is the appropriate balance between people's autonomy (to know about a carrier status or genetic disease in themselves or their embryo and to draw consequences they consider appropriate) and the protection of the same people from unwelcome or unbearable information, from unreasonable risk assessment, or from external sanctions upon their genetic status. There seems to be a strong public consensus for a ban on germ-line manipulation, whereas somatic gene therapy, although met with a lot of public suspicion, was applied for the first time in 1994, on cells other than eggs and sperm. The Federal Chamber of Physicians is currently at work on guidelines on somatic gene therapy.

The German Gene Technology Law of 1990 (revised in 1993) does not address questions of genetic testing or engineering in humans. Three commissions, one at the level of the Federal Parliament and two composed of executives from state and federal governments (*Bund/Länder-Arbeitsgruppen*), have already (in 1987, 1988, and 1990, respectively) issued recommendations for a law that would specifically regulate issues of genetic counseling and testing in embryos, neonates, carriers, high-risk persons, or at the workplace. For the time being these issues are partly regulated intraprofessionally. In 1992 guidelines of the German Federal Chamber of Physicians urged that genetic testing must always be integrated with genetic counseling, that such counseling may be provided by nonmedical personnel under medical supervision, and that consent is required for testing. The Commission of the German Society for Human Genetics also supports genetic testing only within nondirective genetic counseling and confirms its earlier 1990 position that screening for nonmedical information such as the sex of the fetus should be prohibited and that information obtained by genetic testing is to be held strictly confidential.

In Switzerland the Federation of Swiss Physicians asserted in 1991 that genetic analysis for occupational health or insurance issues always must be rejected even if consent is given and the information is to be confidential. The Swiss Academy of Medical Sciences guidelines of 1993 asserted that genetic testing must be part of a larger counseling relationship. The academy supports voluntary testing for (1) diagnosis of hereditary diseases; (2) carrier testing and genetic counseling for family or career planning; and (3) presymptomatic testing whenever medical intervention or changes in lifestyle may reduce or postpone disease. Counseling and education prior to testing are obligatory. The mentioned Article 24 of the Swiss constitution, amended in 1992, states that "the genetic endowment of a person cannot be analyzed, registered or revealed without that person's consent or a legal prescription."

In Austria a Gene Law was introduced in July 1994, regulating genetic counseling, diagnostics, and manipulation both inside and outside human beings. It prohibits any release of genetic information to third parties, notably insurance companies and employers.

Organ transplantation. In Germany the current policy of posthumous organ retrieval presupposes explicit prior consent by the donor or substitute consent by his or her proxy. Various drafts for a transplantation law have been debated over several years. The most likely legal regulation so far has been a policy requiring that donation be requested of the deceased potential donor's proxy, consent of the patient being presumed if he or she had not objected to organ donation. However, much protest has been raised against these suggestions on the grounds that they disregard the right to self-determination due to an uncritical pro-transplantation ideology. Among the protestors are a number of Protestant theologians, despite the fact that both the Protestant and the Catholic churches had officially praised organ donation as a means of love of neighbor (Council of Protestant Churches in Germany, German Roman Catholic Bishops' Conference, 1989). A proposed German transplantation law, moreover, confirms current policy by restricting live donation, ruling out any commercialization, and legalizing the whole-brain-death definition of death. This last point is also at the center of much current debate and protest. German physicians officially adopted the whole-brain-death definition of death in 1982, but this position has been a matter of intraprofessional policy (issued by the Federal Chamber of Physicians, with the most recent revision of test criteria in 1991) rather than legal statute. Rising concerns about the definition's underlying, allegedly reductionist con-

cept of human life (spurred by recent cases involving attempted continuation of pregnancy in brain-dead women by maintaining them for weeks on life support, and rumors that authorities of the former East Germany sold organs, sometimes prior to fulfillment of death criteria) have fueled public suspicion and professional objections, and have even raised the possibility of revision of the 1991 brain-death formula.

In Austria, the 1982 *Krankenanstaltengesetz* presumes consent to organ procurement if the donor or his or her proxy do not oppose it—without, however, explicitly requiring that the proxy be informed about his or her right to oppose. The same policy is recommended by guidelines of the Swiss Academy of the Medical Sciences issued in 1981 (under revision in 1994). The legal situation, however, is different in Switzerland. Among the cantons (states), fifteen have a presumed consent policy, while four have an explicit consent policy. Furthermore, the above Academy issued the intraprofessional acceptance of the whole-brain-death definition and specified its test criteria (guidelines of 1969, revised in 1983). A committee of the Swiss Society for Transplantation is developing guidelines for improved education regarding the benefits of and the need for more organ donation in Switzerland and the dangers of seeking transplants in Third World countries. Efforts to regulate organ procurement on a European level have not yet been implemented by the European Parliament in Strasbourg.

Germany is a member of the Netherlands-based Eurotransplant Center, which computerizes distribution of available organs, primarily according to tissue compatibility, among a network of European transplantation units. Organ information and distribution centers in Switzerland and Austria are more loosely affiliated with Eurotransplant.

Resource allocation. Social welfare systems in each of these countries provide almost universal coverage for health-related costs, as well as allowances for certain conditions (e.g., maternity, disability, old age, work-related injuries, and dependent children). Overall health conditions, health care, and access to physicians are great in each of these countries.

However, steadily increasing costs of modern medical care have begun to endanger the unlimited approval of the underlying "solidarity principle" by which the rich and healthy pay for health care of the sick and needy. Moreover, various cost containment policies that claim to increase cost effectiveness without decreasing the quality of care have slowly increased public awareness of the underlying ethical questions of distributive justice and permissible rationing criteria. The debates on a decent maximum of generally accessible health care have only started. Again, public concern about a renaissance of Nazi spirit is raised by the prospect of rationing treatment, which might discriminate against the disabled and elderly.

Animal experimentation. Strong concern exists throughout Europe for the ethical use and protection of animals in research. Swiss guidelines, inspired by animal rights activists, have served as the basis for regulations in other countries. Germany's special 1986 Animal Protection Law (*Tierschutzgesetz*) was implemented by specific regulations approved by the Federal Ministry of Agriculture and Forestry in 1988. These requirements detail the type of experiments permissible, selection criteria for animals, supervision by qualified veterinarians, and standards for the treatment of animals in agriculture and as pets. In addition, notice must be given to qualified animal welfare commissioners. Animal welfare committees exist in all states; membership is based on nomination by animal welfare groups and by academic training and professional experience. This legislation is supplemented by public education and information campaigns designed to bring about more humane treatment of animals in all spheres. Austria passed an Animal Research Law (*Tierversuchsgesetz*) in 1989 that provides for criminal penalties if research is not reviewed or performed ethically or responsibly and according to current scientific standards. The law also calls for a reduction in the number of experiments performed and the number of animals affected.

Conclusion

Despite strong disagreement on many bioethical topics and some tendencies to avoid debate on certain issues regarding human life because of past atrocities, a long history of interest in philosophical and theological ethics in the German tradition make it likely that the new questions of bioethics will find a lasting place in a respected intellectual tradition. What shape this will take is not yet known.

BETTINA SCHÖNE-SEIFERT
HANS-MARTIN SASS
LAURA JANE BISHOP
ALBERTO BONDOLFI

While all the articles in this section and the other sections of this entry are relevant, see especially the INTRODUCTION *and other articles in this subsection:* SOUTHERN EUROPE, THE BENELUX COUNTRIES, UNITED KINGDOM, REPUBLIC OF IRELAND, NORDIC COUNTRIES, CENTRAL AND EASTERN EUROPE, *and* RUSSIA. *Directly related to this article are the entries* EUGENICS, *article on* HISTORICAL ASPECTS; HOSPITAL, *article on* MODERN HISTORY; MEDICINE AS A PROFESSION; NATIONAL SOCIALISM; *and* PROFESSIONAL–PATIENT RELATIONSHIP, *article on* HISTORICAL PERSPECTIVES. *Other relevant material may be found under the en-*

tries BENEFICENCE; CARE, *article on* HISTORY OF THE NOTION OF CARE; CASUISTRY; DEATH, *articles on* WESTERN RELIGIOUS THOUGHT, *and* DEATH IN THE WESTERN WORLD (with its POSTSCRIPT); EASTERN ORTHODOX CHRISTIANITY; HEALTH AND DISEASE, *article on* HISTORY OF THE CONCEPTS; MEDICAL CODES AND OATHS, *article on* HISTORY; PROTESTANTISM; *and* ROMAN CATHOLICISM.

Bibliography

ACH, JOHANN S., and GAIDT, ANDREAS, eds. 1993. *Herausforderung der Bioethik.* Stuttgart: Frommann-Holzboog.

BAUMANN, JÜRGEN; BOCHNIK, HANS-JOACHIM; BRAUNECK, ANNE-EVA; et al., eds. 1986. *Alternativentwurf eines Gesetzes über Sterbehilfe (AE-Sterbehilfe): Entwurf eines Arbeitskreises von Professoren des Strafrechts und der Medizin sowie ihrer Mitarbeiter.* Stuttgart: Thieme Verlag.

BAYERTZ, KURT, ed. 1991. *Praktische Philosophie: Grundorientierungen angewandter Ethik,* pp. 278–321. Reinbek bei Hamburg: Rowohlt.

BENNETT, CHARLES L.; SCHWARTZ, BERNHARD; and MARBERGER, MICHAEL. 1993. "Health Care in Austria: Universal Access, National Health Insurance, and Private Health Care." *Journal of the American Medical Association* 269, no. 21:2789–2794.

BERNAT, E. 1992. "Regulating the 'Artificial Family': An Austrian Compromise." *International Journal of Bioethics* 3, no. 2:103–108.

BIRNBACHER, DIETER. 1991. "Mensch und Natur: Grundzüge der ökologischen Ethik." In *Praktische Philosophie: Grundorientierungen angewandter Ethik.* Edited by Kurt Bayertz. Reinbek bei Hamburg: Rowohlt Verlag.

BUNDESMINISTER FÜR FORSCHUNG UND TECHNOLOGIE, BONN. 1985. *In-vitro-Fertilisation, Genomanalyse und Gentherapie: Bericht der gemeinsamen Arbeitsgruppe.* [Benda Report.] München: J. Schweitzer Verlag.

BUNDESMINISTERIUM FÜR LANDWIRTSCHAFT. 1993. *Tierschutzbericht.* Bonn: Author.

CHRISTOPH, FRANZ, and ILLIGER, HORST, eds. 1992. *Notwehr gegen die neue Euthanasiebedrohung.* Neumünster: Brücke-Neumünster.

DAELE, W. VAN DEN, and MÜLLER-SALMON, H. 1990. *Die Kontrolle der Forschung am Menschen durch Ethikkommissionen.* Stuttgart: Enke Verlag.

DOERNER, KLAUS. 1988. *Tödliches Mitleid: Zur Frage der Unerträglichkeit des Lebens, oder, die soziale Frage, Entstehung, Medizinisierung, NS-Endlösung heute, morgen.* Gütersloh: Verlag Jakob van Hoddis.

ESER, ALBIN, and KOCH, HANS-GEORG. 1988. *Schwangerschaftsabbruch im internationalen Vergleich: Rechtliche Regelungen, soziale Rahmenbedingungen, empirische Grunddaten. Band 1. Europa.* Baden-Baden: Nomos Verlag.

Ethik in der Medizin. 1989–. Heidelberg: Springer Verlag (by the Akademie für Ethik in der Medizin). 4 issues per year.

EXPERTENKOMMISSION HUMANGENETIK UND REPRODUKTIONSMEDIZIN. 1988. *Amstad Bericht.* Bern: Author.

HEERKLOTZ, BRIGITTE. 1989. *Biomedizinische Ethik: Europäische*

Richtlinien und Empfehlungen. Medizinethische Materialien, 52. Bochum: Zentrum für medizinische Ethik.

HEGSELMANN, RAINER, and MERKEL, REINHARD, eds. 1991. *Zur Debatte über Euthanasie: Beiträge und Stellungnahmen.* Frankfurt: Suhrkamp Verlag.

HEISTER, ELISABETH. 1989. "Ethik in der ärztlichen Ausbildung an den Hochschulen der Bundesrepublik Deutschland." *Ethik in der Medizin* 1, no. 1:13–23.

HOERSTER, NORBERT. 1991. *Abtreibung im säkularen Staat: Argumente gegen den §218.* Frankfurt: Suhrkamp Verlag.

ILLHARDT, FRANZ-JOSEF. 1985. *Medizinische Ethik: Ein Arbeitsbuch.* Berlin: Springer Verlag.

KELLER, ROLF; GÜNTHER, HANS-LUDWIG; and KAISER, PETER. 1992. *Embryonenschutzgesetz: Kommentar.* Stuttgart: W. Kohlhammer.

KOCH, HANS-GEORG; MERAN, JOHANNES GOBERTUS; and SASS, HANS-MARTIN. 1994. *Patientenverfügung und stellvertretende Entscheidung in rechtlicher, medizinischer und ethischer Sicht.* Medizinethische Materialien, no. 93: Bochum: Zentrum für medizinische Ethik.

LEIST, ANTON. 1990. *Eine Frage des Lebens: Ethik der Abtreibung und künstlichen Befruchtung.* Frankfurt: Campus Verlag.

———. 1993. "Bioethics in a Low Key: A Report from Germany." *Bioethics* 7, no. 2/3:271–279.

LORZ, ALBERT. 1992. *Tierschutzgesetz mit Rechtsverordnungen und europäischen Übereinkommen: Kommentar.* 4th ed. Munich: C. H. Beck Verlag.

MCGREGOR, ALAN. 1992. "Switzerland: Limits on Genetic Research and Artificial Insemination." *Lancet* 339, no. 8805:1345.

MedR-Medizinrecht. 1983–. Heidelberg: Springer Verlag. 12 issues per year.

MEGGLE, GEORG; RIPPE, KLAUS PETER; and WESSELS, ULLA, eds. 1992. *Almanach der praktischen Ethik.* Opladen, Germany: Westdeutscher Verlag.

PATZIG, GÜNTHER. 1993. *Angewandte Ethik.* Göttingen: Wallstein Verlag.

RAT DER EVANGELISCHEN KIRCHE IN DEUTSCHLAND UND SEKRETARIAT DER DEUTSCHEN BISCHOFSKONFERENZ. 1989. *Gott ist ein Freund des Lebens: Herausforderungen und Aufgaben beim Schutz des Lebens.* Gütersloh: Gütersloher Verlagshaus Gerd Mohn.

SASS, HANS-MARTIN. 1983. "Reichsrundschreiben 1931: Pre-Nuremberg Regulations Concerning New Therapy and Human Experimentation." *Journal of Medicine and Philosophy* 8, no. 2:99–111.

———, ed. 1988. *Ethik und öffentliches Gesundheitswesen: Ordnungsethische und ordnungspolitische Einflussfaktoren im öffentlichen Gesundheitswesen.* Berlin: Springer Verlag.

———, ed. 1991. *Genomanalyse und Gentherapie: Ethische Herausforderungen in der Humanmedizin.* Berlin: Springer Verlag.

———. 1992. "Bioethics in German-Speaking Western European Countries: Austria, Germany, and Switzerland." In *Bioethics Yearbook Vol. 2: Regional Development in Bioethics—1989–1991*, pp. 211–231. Edited by B. Andrew Lustig, Baruch A. Brody, H. Tristram Engelhardt, Jr., and Laurence B. McCullough. Dordrecht, Netherlands: Kluwer Academic.

———. 1994. "Bioethics in German-Speaking Western European Countries: Austria, Germany, and Switzerland." In *Bioethics Yearbook Vol. 4: Regional Developments—1992–1993*, pp. 247–268. Edited by B. Andrew Lustig, Baruch A. Brody, and H. Tristram Engelhardt, Jr. Dordrecht, Netherlands: Kluwer Academic.

SASS, HANS-MARTIN, and VIEFHUES, HERBERT, eds. 1991. *Güterabwägung in der Medizin: Ethische und ärtzliche Probleme.* Heidelberg: Springer Verlag.

SCHÖNE-SEIFERT, BETTINA, and KRÜGER, LORENZ, eds. 1993. *Humangenetik: Ethische Probleme der Beratung, Diagnostik und Forschung.* Stuttgart: Gustav Fischer Verlag.

SCHÖNE-SEIFERT, BETTINA, and RIPPE, KLAUS-PETER. 1991. "Silencing the Singer: Antibioethics in Germany." *Hastings Center Report* 21, no. 6:20–27.

SCHWEIZERISCHE AKADEMIE DER WISSENSCHAFTEN (SAMW). 1989. *Medizinisch-ethische Richtlinien der Schweizerischen Akademie der Wissenschaften.* Basel: Author.

SPAEMANN, ROBERT. 1992. "Wir dürfen das Tabu nicht aufgeben." *Die Zeit* 25:14.

THÉVOZ, JEAN-MARIE. 1992. "Research and Hospital Ethics Committees in Switzerland." *HEC (HealthCare Ethics Committee) Forum* 4, no. 1:41–47.

TOELLNER, RICHARD, ed. 1990a. *Die Ethik-Kommission in der Medizin, Problemgeschichte, Aufgabenstellung, Arbeitsweise, Rechtsstellung und Organisationsformen Medizinischer Ethick-Kommissionen.* Stuttgart: Gustav Fischer Verlag.

———, ed. 1990b. *Organtransplantation—Beiträge zu ethischen und juristichen Fragen.* Stuttgart: Gustav Fischer Verlag.

WEIZSÄCKER, VIKTOR VON. 1951. *Fälle und Probleme: Anthropologische Vorlesungen in der medizinischen Klinik.* 2d ed. Stuttgart: F. Enke.

WESSELS, URSULA. 1991. *Genetic Engineering and Ethics in Germany.* Diskussionsbeiträge zur Ethik, Nr. 5. Saarbrücken: Projekt Praktische Ethik, Universität Saarbrücken.

WIESING, URBAN. 1993. "In Vitro Fertilization: Regulations in Germany." *Cambridge Quarterly of Healthcare Ethics* 2, no. 3:321–326.

WIKLER, DANIEL, and BARONDESS, JEREMIAH. 1993. "Bioethics and Anti-Bioethics in Light of Nazi Medicine: What Must We Remember?" *Kennedy Institute of Ethics Journal* 3, no. 1:39–55.

WOLF, JEAN-CLAUDE. 1992. *Tierethik: Neue Perspektiven für Menschen und Tiere.* Freiburg, Switzerland: Paulusverlag.

Zeitschrift für medizinische Ethik (successor of *Arzt und Christ,* 1955–1992). 1992–. Ostfildern, Austria: Schwabenverlag. 4 issues per year.

Zeitschrift für Medizinrecht. 1985–. Heidelberg: Springer Verlag. 12 issues per year.

7. NORDIC COUNTRIES

This article gives a brief overview of the modern development of medical ethics in the Nordic countries: Denmark, Finland, Iceland, Norway, and Sweden. With a few exceptions, the focus is on the period since the beginning of the 1960s. First, an account is given of the establishment of ethics review committees and other medical ethics bodies and organizations. Then, changes in the educational and research situation are treated, as well as the establishment of special institutions for medical ethics. Finally, attention is given to some essential features of the debate on a few principal issues.

Codes, ethics bodies, and organizations

The attempt formally to regulate physicians' duties toward both patients and colleagues goes far back in the history of medicine. Ethics codes in the Nordic countries can be traced to the early practice of physicians taking an oath of office and allegiance. For example, in seventeenth-century Sweden, when physicians still received their doctoral degrees abroad (usually in Holland), permission to practice medicine required taking an examination given by the association of physicians, the Collegium Medicorum (founded 1663). Upon passing the examination, the physician had to take a special oath. The taking of an oath was an obligatory part of the examination of physicians in Sweden until the late nineteenth century, and is still required in Denmark, Finland, and Iceland.

It was only after World War II, however, that the codification in the Nordic countries came to encompass areas outside clinical practice and to include professional categories other than physicians. The current ethical guidelines for physicians' clinical work were adopted in their original forms by the Danish Medical Association in 1976; by the Finnish in 1956; by the Icelandic in 1918; by the Norwegian in 1961; and by the Swedish in 1951. During the 1950s and 1960s, other health professional groups—for example, nurses and physical therapists—began to develop their current ethical codes. The 1964 adoption of the Helsinki Declaration by the World Medical Association extended the codification to explicit inclusion of ethics in research. To facilitate its implementation, the Nordic countries created a system of ethics review committees.

These committees are organized somewhat differently in the different countries. Denmark and Norway have regional committees, whereas Finland and Iceland have local hospital committees, and Sweden has both regional and local committees. The Danish system, established in 1978, consists of seven regional committees and a central scientific-ethical committee. The committees in Norway are organized in a similar way. In 1985, regional committees were set up in each of Norway's five national service regions. In order to establish a coordinating and advisory body for these regional committees, the existing Norwegian Medical Research Council's Committee for Medical Research Ethics, formed in 1978, became the National Committee for Medical Re-

search Ethics in 1990. In Finland the first ethics committee was set up at Helsinki University in 1972; since 1977, all medical faculties have had ethics committees. In Iceland the two national university hospitals have had ethics committees since 1976. In Sweden, an advisory council was formed at the Karolinska Hospital in Stockholm in 1965. This council was superseded the following year by the first medical-faculty ethics committee, established at the Karolinska Institute. By 1967 similar committees were in place at all medical faculties in the country.

Since these committees were established, the call for assessment of the ethical implications of new technologies and other advances in medicine has increased. To respond to growing pressures on political decision makers, an additional and new type of national ethics body was created. Its principal task is twofold: to provide expert knowledge to government, Parliament, and the health-service authorities, and to contribute generally to a continuous exchange of information and opinions on medical ethics issues among researchers, politicians, and the public. To this end, the Danish Council of Ethics was established by the Parliament in 1987; the National Research Ethics Committee, by the Finnish Parliament in 1991; the National Biotechnology Advisory Board, by the Norwegian government in 1991; and the National Council of Medical Ethics, by the Swedish government in 1985. Iceland still lacks a national body of this kind. (For further information about the origin, composition, and activities of these national bodies and of the review committees, see Council of Europe, 1992; Solbakk, 1991.) In 1988 the Nordic Committee for Ethics in Biotechnology was created by the Nordic Council of Ministers. Like some of the national bodies, this committee deals with bioethical issues in a broad sense of the term. Besides issues in medicine, the Nordic Committee addresses ethical questions in, for example, stockbreeding and agriculture.

Several other bodies and organizations play an important role in the analysis and debate of medical-ethics issues. For example, ethics committees were set up within the medical associations of Denmark (1969), Finland (1975), Norway (1962), and Sweden (1979), as well as within the National Finnish Board of Health (1988), the National Swedish Board of Health and Welfare (1984), and the Ministry of Health and Social Affairs in Norway (1988). In 1989, the Council of Ethics was established at the Office of the Director General of Health in Iceland. A number of medical societies should also be mentioned: the Delegation for Medical Ethics, established in 1969 within the Swedish Society of Medicine (earlier called the Swedish Society of Medical Sciences); the Society for Medical Law and Ethics founded in Finland in 1980; the Danish Society for Medical Philosophy, Ethics, and Methodology in 1988; and the

Swedish Society for Medical Ethics in 1989. In 1988, a section for medical ethics in the Nordic countries was established within the European Society for Philosophy of Medicine and Health Care.

Education and research

Since the beginning of the 1970s, medical ethics has been taught at the medical faculties and nursing schools in all of the Nordic countries. However, there are no uniform requirements regarding the scope and content of this teaching in any of the countries. At a meeting in Reykjavik, Iceland, in 1991, the medical associations of the Nordic countries agreed to work toward making medical ethics a compulsory subject at all medical faculties in the Nordic countries and toward creating teaching positions in the subject (Oldinger, 1991). Textbooks have been written in most of the countries. For a long time *Medicinsk etik* (1971), a doctoral dissertation by Clarence Blomquist, a pioneer in Swedish medical ethics, was the only general introduction; it deals with both metaethics and normative ethics and covers most of the principal medical-ethics issues at that time. Subsequently, a number of textbooks have appeared, including some broad general introductions (Fagerberg, 1984; Andersen et al., 1987; Tranøy, 1991; Wretmark et al., 1983); some more philosophically oriented (Malmgren, 1990; Tännsjö, 1990); and some dealing not only with ethics but also with other philosophical issues in medicine (Bjarnason, 1991; Tranøy, 1978; Wulff et al., 1986).

The philosophical rather than the medical faculties have been responsible for most postgraduate education in medical ethics. Blomquist's *Medicinsk etik*, the first doctoral dissertation, was defended at the Department of Philosophy at Uppsala University in 1973. Philosophy departments since then have produced dissertations on specific medical ethics issues, like suicide (Anderberg, 1989), paternalism (H. Häyry, 1990), and abortion (Munthe, 1992), as well as on the nature and scope of philosophical medical ethics in general (M. Häyry, 1990). Partly empirical doctoral dissertations, focusing primarily on medical-ethics issues, have been written within sociology; for example, on conflicts between ideal and operative norms in treatment research (Johansson, 1986); and within nursing research, for example, on ethical reasoning in feeding severely demented patients (Åkerlund, 1990); as well as within medicine, for example, on decision making in dialysis and renal transplantation (Kjellstrand, 1988).

The establishment of two special institutions for medical ethics, one in Norway and the other in Sweden, as well as the foundation of a unit for the philosophy of medicine in a broader sense in Denmark, have improved the opportunities at medical faculties for both graduate and postgraduate education in medical ethics. The Center for Medical Ethics at the University of Oslo was founded in 1989. A chair in medical ethics was created at the University of Oslo Medical Faculty in 1992. In Sweden, Lund University established the Department of Medical Ethics in 1991. The department came into existence through the creation of a chair in medical ethics at the Swedish Medical Research Council in 1990. In 1988 the University of Copenhagen established the Unit of Medical Philosophy and Clinical Theory at the Panum Institute.

These institutions have strengthened the position of medical ethics as an independent research field at medical faculties. Research in medical ethics is otherwise normally carried on only in the form of time-limited projects, and mainly outside medical faculties, in philosophy departments and departments of theology. Some institutions focus on medical ethics as one of their principal areas of research. For example, the Department of Health and Society at Linköping University in Sweden has had a chair of philosophy of medicine since 1987. Two institutes have been established, one in Iceland in 1989 (the Ethics Institute at the University of Iceland) and the other in Sweden in 1988 (the Ersta Institute for Health Care Ethics, Stockholm). In Finland, the Center for Bioethics was founded in 1991 at the University of Turku.

Principal issues

Artificial insemination and in vitro fertilization. Of the Nordic countries, only Norway and Sweden have laws specifically regulating the use of noncoital reproductive technologies for achieving pregnancy. The use of human sperm, ova, zygotes, and early embryonic forms (blastemas) for research purposes also is restricted in the Nordic countries. (For an overview of the development of the legislation in the Nordic countries, see U.S. Congress, 1988.)

The ethical and legal debate in the Nordic countries over the use of noncoital reproductive technologies has focused mainly on artificial insemination by donor semen (AID), in vitro fertilization (IVF), and ovum donation. The closely related issues of artificial insemination by husband's semen (AIH) and gestational surrogacy (surrogate motherhood) have attracted less attention. Except among certain religious minorities, the use of AIH has been generally accepted.

To a large extent, the 1987 Norwegian legislation on artificial insemination and IVF corresponds to the 1985 Swedish legislation. One point on which the Norwegian and Swedish laws differ is of particular ethical interest: the issue of whether it should be possible for the child to obtain information about the identity of his or her natural father. Sweden legislated in favor of the child's right to this information, but Norway legislated against it.

According to the Swedish legislation, (1) only women married or cohabiting with a man under circumstances of marital character should be allowed insemination treatment; (2) insemination requires written consent by the husband or cohabitant, who will, by this act, be regarded as the legal father of a child born as a result of the treatment; (3) AID should be undertaken only in general hospitals under the supervision of a physician who specializes in obstetrics and gynecology, and the sperm donor should be chosen by the physician; (4) information about the sperm donor should be kept in a special hospital record for at least seventy years; (5) when a child conceived by donor insemination is mature enough, he or she has a right to obtain information about the identity of the natural father; and (6) when requested, the public welfare committee is duty bound to assist the child in retrieving this information. (For literature on the debate and official reports preceding this law, see Lindahl, 1985, 1988; U.S. Congress, 1988.)

The most controversial issue has been (5). The main point of departure of the Swedish legislation was the needs and interests of the child. In this respect, the legislators decided to follow the general direction of modern legislation toward a gradual strengthening of children's judicial standing and the movement in society toward a greater openness in family relations, rather than the traditional patient-oriented perspective of clinical medical ethics. These two contrasting perspectives have dominated much of the debate.

Prenatal diagnostics and abortion.   The laws on abortion vary among the Nordic countries. In Denmark, women have a legal right to abortion, regardless of the reasons, before the twelfth week (law of 1973, in force the same year); in Norway, until the end of the twelfth week (law of 1975, in force from 1979); and in Sweden, before the end of the twelfth week or, after special consultation with a social worker, up to the end of the eighteenth week (law of 1974, in force from 1975). In Finland (law of 1970, in force the same year) and Iceland (law of 1975, in force the same year) abortion is permissible before the twelfth week, but only on certain indications (see below).

The development in Sweden clearly illustrates how the legal status of the fetus, and the understanding of its relationship to the mother, have changed during the twentieth century. Until the abortion act of 1974, the fetus was viewed as a separate individual, even during the first three months, and as such was legally protected. According to the earliest legislation, in the eighteenth century, abortion carried a penalty of death because it was equated with infanticide. As late as the 1920s, the penalty for abortion was one to six years' imprisonment

at hard labor. However, exceptions were made if abortion was necessary to preserve the health or life of the woman. This practice was ratified by law in 1938. As of 1939, abortion was permissible up to the end of the twentieth week on any of the following three indications: medical (i.e., when, due to disease, physical defect, or weakness, childbirth would cause serious danger to the life or health of the woman); humanitarian (e.g., pregnancy following rape or incest, or in minors); and eugenic (i.e., when there was reason to believe that the expected child would inherit mental disease, mental deficiency, or serious physical disease). After the twentieth week, abortion was permissible only on medical grounds. Two additional indications were introduced before the abortion act of 1974: in 1946, sociomedical (i.e., when, considering the living conditions and other circumstances, it might be assumed that childbirth or care of the child would seriously reduce the woman's physical or emotional strength); and, in 1963, teratogenetic (i.e., when there was reason to believe that the expected child, due to injury during the fetal stage, would suffer from a serious disease or serious defect). All these indications, somewhat differently formulated, are still used in Finland and Iceland.

In the debate surrounding the 1974 law on abortion, the fetus often was no longer viewed as a separate individual but as a part of the woman's body. Abortion therefore became, according to this view, not a matter of weighing the value of one individual's life against another's but a question of the woman's right to make decisions regarding her own body. The only legal limit to this right is the point in time at which the fetus has become viable, that is, able to survive outside the uterus. In Sweden the operation may then still be performed, but only if the woman suffers from a disease or physical defect and continued pregnancy therefore constitutes a serious threat to her life or health. Unless the operation cannot be postponed without danger to the woman, permission from the National Board of Health and Welfare is always required after the eighteenth week of pregnancy.

This exception has been questioned in an official Swedish investigation of the abortion law (Justitiedepartementet, 1989). The investigation points out that since abortion, according to the common medical definition, amounts to the expulsion of a nonviable fetus, this exception must mean that the operation is performed in such a way that the fetus is dead at delivery. The investigation found this unacceptable and required that instead, efforts should be made to save the life of both the woman and the fetus at this stage of pregnancy.

The investigation calls attention to the revaluation of the legal status of the fetus undertaken since the abortion law was instituted. During the 1980s, recurrent demands were made that the unborn child be protected from the risk of injury because of the mother's abuse of alcohol or narcotics. This request led to the conclusion that the woman and the prospective child can no longer be viewed as a single individual.

Euthanasia and the concept of death. Until the 1990s, the dominant view on euthanasia in the medical profession of the Nordic countries was virtually that expressed in the mid-1800s by the Finnish physician Immanuel Ilmoni in his book on medical ethics, *Om läkarens yrke och pligter* (1847). Ilmoni called euthanasia one of the most important special disciplines of the art of medicine. At the same time, he made it clear that the physician may not, under any circumstances, deliberately contribute to shortening the patient's life—not even in cases where the patient is "incurably ill, tormented beyond description, [and] fervently desires and demands death" (Ilmoni, 1847, pp. 45–46).

In the late 1960s and during the 1970s, when the debate on euthanasia was most intensive in the Nordic countries, it would have been hard to imagine the medical profession supporting legislation that allowed physicians to comply with a terminally ill patient's wish to die. Among the earliest and most thorough contributions to this debate was Clarence Blomquist's book on euthanasia, *Livet, döden och läkaren* (1964). In this book Blomquist discusses the five principal definitions of euthanasia used in the debate: (1) the original meaning: medical care in the terminal phase of life, for example, the mitigation or relief of pain and discomfort of the dying; (2) causing death as a predicted but not intended side effect of treatment; (3) the acceleration of death; (4) passive euthanasia: discontinuing treatment or refraining from initiating treatment; and (5) active euthanasia: intentional killing in accordance with the patient's explicit or implicit wish to die or irrespective of the patient's will. Obviously these different forms of euthanasia may overlap.

A fundamental issue in the debate has been, of course, where to draw the line between life and death. Brain-related criteria of death were introduced by law in Finland in 1971, in Norway in 1977, in Sweden in 1988, in Denmark in 1990, and in Iceland in 1991. The introduction of these criteria eliminated a minor but important part of the problem.

Throughout the 1970s, even euthanasia as medical care in the terminal phase of life was disputed. The administration of painkillers was restricted, in order to prevent terminally ill patients from becoming addicted to the drugs used. In Sweden, for example, this restriction was not lifted until 1979. There was also a concern that a more liberal administration of painkillers and tranquilizers might shorten the patient's life. Blomquist was among those who found this unintentional form of euthanasia, and the passive form, morally justifiable but did not support active euthanasia. Others, like the Swedish professor of practical philosophy Ingemar Hedenius, advocated active euthanasia.

In 1992 Denmark was the first Nordic country to break with the traditional legal view on medical care in the terminal phase of life, passing a law according to which—unless there is particularly good authority for acting differently—the physician may not initiate or continue life-sustaining treatment of a terminally ill patient against wishes expressed in his or her "living will." The law further provides that the physician may, in the absence of a "living will," discontinue or refrain from initiating treatment that may prolong the life of a terminally ill patient. The physician also may administer painkillers, tranquilizers, and similar substances necessary for easing the terminally ill patient's suffering, even when this may shorten the patient's life.

Three organizations for terminal care have been formed: in Sweden in 1973, the national organization Right to Our Death; in Norway in 1977, the national association My Living Will—the Right to a Death in Dignity; and in Finland in 1993, EXITUS. In 1985 a special organization for active euthanasia, EXIT, was founded in Sweden.

Concluding remarks

Among other areas that have attracted special attention in the Nordic countries are ethical problems in medical research, for example, questions of integrity and the difficulties of meeting the requirements of informed consent in epidemiological and health-care research. The frequent use of personal numbers in computerized official registers provides unique potential opportunities for population studies. At the same time, it creates special ethical problems (see, e.g., Hermerén, 1988). Another field of increasing importance is the ethical consequences of the technological and scientific developments in human genetics (for an overview, see Berg and Tranøy, 1989; Bischofberger et al., 1989; Therkelsen et al., 1989; Nordisk Ministerråd, 1992, 1994). Finally, the ethical questions of health economics and setting priorities in health care should be mentioned. In 1987 in Norway, a government-appointed commission produced a report on guidelines for priorities in public health care (Sosialdepartementet, 1987).

To sum up, from the early 1960s to the 1990s, medical ethics has undergone a sweeping transformation in the Nordic countries. From being viewed primarily as a concern between the patient and the physician, and between colleagues, medical ethics has evolved into a field of systematic studies and extensive interdisciplinary and public debate. The scope has broadened from discussions of normative ethical issues to include metaethical analyses of the norms, values, and basic concepts of medicine. The general awareness of the conflicts of interest and the incompatibility of goals inherent in medical decision making and research has increased considerably, a development we all benefit from, both as patients and as medical professionals.

B. I. B. LINDAHL

While all the articles in this section and the other sections of this entry are relevant, see especially the INTRODUCTION *and other articles in this subsection:* SOUTHERN EUROPE, THE BENELUX COUNTRIES, UNITED KINGDOM, REPUBLIC OF IRELAND, GERMAN-SPEAKING COUNTRIES AND SWITZERLAND, CENTRAL AND EASTERN EUROPE, *and* RUSSIA. *For a further discussion of topics mentioned in this article, see the entries* ABORTION; BIOETHICS EDUCATION; DEATH AND DYING: EUTHANASIA AND SUSTAINING LIFE; LICENSING, DISCIPLINE, AND REGULATION IN THE HEALTH PROFESSIONS; MATERNAL–FETAL RELATIONSHIP; MEDICAL CODES AND OATHS; REPRODUCTIVE TECHNOLOGIES; *and* RESEARCH ETHICS COMMITTEES. *Other relevant material may be found under the entry* INFORMED CONSENT.

Bibliography

AIRAKSINEN, TIMO, and VUORIO, MANU J. 1988. "Medical Ethics in Finland: Some Recent Trends." *Theoretical Medicine* 9, no. 3:299–307.

ÅKERLUND, BRITT MARI. 1990. *Dementia Care in an Ethical Perspective: An Exploratory Study of Caregivers' Experiences of Ethical Conflicts When Feeding Severely Demented Patients.* Medical Dissertations, n.s., no. 299. Umea, Sweden: Umeå University.

ANDERBERG, THOMAS. 1989. *Suicide: Definitions, Causes, and Values.* Lund, Sweden: Lund University Press.

ANDERSEN, DANIEL; MABECK, CARL ERIK; and RIIS, POVL. 1983. *Medicinsk etik.* Arhus, Denmark: FADL.

BERG, KARE, and TRANØY, KNUT ERIK. 1989. "Ethics and Medical Genetics in Norway." In *Ethics and Human Genetics: A Cross-Cultural Perspective,* pp. 317–338. Edited by Dorothy C. Wertz and John C. Fletcher. Berlin: Springer-Verlag.

BISCHOFBERGER, ERWIN; LINDSTEN, JAN; and ROSENQVIST, URBAN. 1989. "Ethics and Medical Genetics in Sweden." In *Ethics and Human Genetics: A Cross-Cultural Perspective,* pp. 339–352. Edited by Dorothy C. Wertz and John C. Fletcher. Berlin: Springer-Verlag.

BJARNASON, ÖRN. 1991. *Siðfræði og siðamá lækna.* Reykjavik: Idunn.

BLOMQUIST, CLARENCE. 1964. *Livet, döden och läkaren: Om medicinsk dödshjälp.* Göteborg, Sweden: Zinderman Förlag.

———. 1971. *Medicinsk etik.* Stockholm: Natur och Kultur.

COUNCIL OF EUROPE. AD HOC COMMITTEE OF EXPERTS ON BIOETHICS. 1992. *National Ethics Bodies.* Strasbourg, France: Council of Europe.

FAGERBERG, HOLSTEN, ed. 1984. *Medicinsk etik och människosyn.* Malmö, Sweden: Liber Förlag.

FINLANDS LÄKARFÖRBUND. 1991. *Läkarens etik.* Helsinki: Author.

GIERTZ, GUSTAV. 1984. *Etik i läkarens vardag.* Stockholm: Svenska Läkaresällskapets Förlag.

HÄYRY, HETA. 1990. *Freedom, Autonomy, and the Limits of Medical Paternalism.* Helsinki: Department of Philosophy, University of Helsinki.

———. 1991. *The Limits of Medical Paternalism.* London: Routledge.

HÄYRY, MATTI. 1990. *Critical Studies in Philosophical Medical Ethics.* Helsinki: Department of Philosophy, University of Helsinki.

HERMERÉN, GÖRAN. 1988. "Ethical Problems in Register Based Medical Research." *Theoretical Medicine* 9, no. 2:105–116.

HJELT, OTTO E. A. 1891–1893. *Svenska och finska medicinalverkets historia 1663–1812.* Helsinki: Helsingfors Central-Tryckeri.

ILMONI, IMMANUEL. 1847. *Om läkarens yrke och pligter.* Helsinki: Simelii.

JOHANSSON, STINA. 1986. *Forskare—behandlare—patient: En studie i praktisk forskningsetik.* Stockholm: S. Academise Ubsaliensis.

JUSTITIEDEPARTEMENTED. 1989. *Den gravida kvinnan och fostret—två individer. Om fosterdiagnostik. Om sena aborter.* Stockholm: Allmänna Förlaget.

KJELLSTRAND, CARL M. 1988. "Giving Life—Giving Death: Ethical Problems of High-Technology Medicine." *Acta Medica Scandinavica,* suppl. 725.

KJØNSTAD, ASBJØRN. 1987. *Helserett.* Oslo: TANO.

LINDAHL, B. INGEMAR B. 1985. "Philosophy of Medicine in Scandinavia." *Theoretical Medicine* 6, no. 1:65–84.

———. 1988. "Medical Ethics in Sweden." *Theoretical Medicine* 9, no. 3:309–335.

———. 1989. "Sweden: Growing Interest in Ethics." *Hastings Center Report* 19, no. 4 (spec. suppl.):S30–S31.

MALMGREN, HELGE. 1990. *Medicinsk etik: En socialfilosofisk analys.* Stockholm: Almqvist and Wiksell.

MUNTHE, CHRISTIAN. 1992. *Livets slut i livets början: En studie i abortetik.* Stockholm: Thales. English summary, pp. 405–417.

NORDISK MINISTERRAD. NORDISKT UTSKOTT FÖR ETIK INOM BIOTEKNOLOGI. 1992. *Risk, bioteknologi och etik.* Copenhagen: Author.

———. 1994. *Bioetisk debatt i Norden 1993.* Copenhagen: Author.

OLDINGER, EVA. 1991. "Undervisning i medicinsk etik bör vara obligatorisk vid alla medicinska fakulteter i Norden." *Nordisk medicin* 106, no. 11:308–309.

SOLBAKK, JAN HELGE. 1991. "Ethics Review Committees [in Biomedical Research] in the Nordic Countries: History, Organization, and Assignments." *Health Care Ethics Committee Forum* 3, no. 4:215–220.

SOSIALDEPARTEMENTET. 1987. *Retningslinjer for prioriteringer innen norsk helsetjenste.* Oslo: Universitetsforlaget.

SWEDISH MINISTRY OF HEALTH AND SOCIAL AFFAIRS. 1984. *The Concept of Death.* Stockholm: Swedish Committee on Defining Death.

SYSE, ASLAK. 1993. *Abortloven: Juss og verdier.* Oslo: Ad No-tam Gyldendal.

TÄNNSJÖ, TORBJÖRN. 1990. *Vårdetik.* Stockholm: Raben and Sjögren.

———. 1991. *Välja barn: Om forsterdiagnostik och selektiv abort.* Stockholm: SESAM.

———. 1993. "Should We Change the Human Genome?" *Theoretical Medicine* 14, no. 3:231–247.

THERKELSEN, AAGE J.; BOHLUND, LARS; and MORTENSEN, VIGGO. 1989. "Ethics and Medical Genetics in Denmark." In *Ethics and Human Genetics: A Cross-Cultural Perspective,* pp. 141–155. Edited by Dorothy C. Wertz and John C. Fletcher. Berlin: Springer-Verlag.

TRANØY, KNUT ERIK. 1978. *Fra filosofi til fysiologi.* Bergen, Norway: Universitetsforlaget.

———. 1988. "Medical Ethics in Norway: Modern Medicine—Traditional Morality." *Theoretical Medicine* 9, no. 3:337–350.

———. 1991. *Medisinsk etikk i vår tid.* Søreidgrend, Norway: Sigma Forlag.

U.S. CONGRESS. OFFICE OF TECHNOLOGY ASSESSMENT. 1988. *Infertility: Medical and Social Choices.* OTA-BA-358. Washington, D.C.: U.S. Government Printing Office.

WRETMARK, GERDT; ANDERSSON WRETMARK, ASTRID; and LUNDVIGSSON, JOHNNY. 1983. *Etik i vården—teori, praktik, forskning.* Lund, Sweden: Studentlitteratur.

WULFF, HENRIK R.; PEDERSEN, STIG ANDUR; and ROSENBERG, RABEN. 1986. *Philosophy of Medicine: An Introduction.* Oxford: Blackwell Scientific Publications.

8. CENTRAL AND EASTERN EUROPE

This article covers Poland, the Baltic states, Hungary, Romania, the Czech and Slovak republics, the former Yugoslavia, Bulgaria, Albania, and Cyprus. In these nations, to the east and southeast of the Elbe River, the doctor–patient relationship and biomedicine itself have been characterized by the paternalism and dominance of a powerful elite within the medical establishment. Furthermore, a number of factors have profoundly influenced the status of health care as well as bioethics in this region. Among the most important are (a) a relatively small percentage (no more than 4 percent) of the gross national product spent on health care, biomedical research, and environmental protection; (b) Prussian-like feudalistic attitudes (e.g., a rigid hierarchical system with a small and arrogant elite at the top and a large number of disempowered people below) preserved within universities and medical colleges. For physicians the idea of being the "captain of the ship" is still self-evident, and many believe that the behavior of older doctors provides the right ethical model for future ones.

In Hungary, Poland, Romania, the former Yugoslavia and Czechoslovakia, the Baltic republics, Bulgaria, and Albania another determining factor that shaped medicine, health care, and bioethics was the form of Marxism that became the official ideology after the end of World War II. The hard ideology of Stalinist Marxism prevailed in Albania much longer than anywhere in eastern and central Europe. These ideologies constructed morals and morality, so that only behaviors that brought people closer to communism were considered morally correct. Only infallible and omniscient party leaders knew exactly what acts and behaviors these were.

Before World War II

In central and eastern Europe a feudal-capitalistic system existed prior to World War II. Agriculture was so dominant that in most of these countries the peasantry, unskilled agricultural toilers employed by owners of huge tracts of land, made up more than half of the population. These peasant workers were not able to rise from serfdom to free citizenry. This situation existed in large part because there had never been any genuine democracy in this region. The high degree of illiteracy, and the struggle for survival within the context of wars and ethnic strife, had a great impact on the people's health as well as on medical ethics.

A significant majority of people (normally peasants and poor urban dwellers) had no health insurance, and thus no access to professional care. Infant mortality, tuberculosis, and high overall death rates due to lack of treatment were very common. It was quite natural, for example, to view patients, usually those who were unable to pay, as teaching objects in university clinics and teaching hospitals. Health care was basically private, a profit-oriented endeavor that brought high earnings and social prestige to physicians—who carefully controlled their own numbers, especially the number of specialists. There existed a unified medical profession and a system of professional and ethical control. Within the profession certain basic norms concerning referrals, regulation of payments (neither overcharging nor undercharging), and advertisements were generally honored and violators were punished.

Some dedicated individuals in these countries, usually physicians, kept the Hippocratic ethics alive by writing books and articles that, for generations, exerted a strong influence over the practice of doctors: for example, in Hungary, Jozsef Imre's *Orvosi Ethika* (*Physicians' Ethics*), 1925; in Poland, Wiadislav Bieganski's *Mysli i aforyzmy o etyce lekarskiej* (*Thoughts and Aphorisms on Medical Ethics*), 1899. These authors concentrated almost as much on the duties of the patient as on those of the physician. In addition to the Hippocratic works as a source of ethical standards, Polish physicians relied heavily on Catholic moral theology in the development of bioethics, especially concerning such issues as abortion, birth control, genetics, and euthanasia.

After World War II

As a result of the Yalta agreement dividing Europe into spheres of interest, a large part of central and eastern Europe came under the dominance of the Soviet Union. The communist leaders launched a massive industrialization program in most countries of the region. Among other things, this resulted in an unprecedented mobilization of people that contributed to significant changes in class structures, (e.g., millions of peasants became industrial workers), disintegration of large family units, and increased migration to urban areas. All these changes occurred just after World War II.

These countries became monolithic states soon after the war. Moral pluralism existed only underground. Marxism shaped by Soviet communism or distorted forms of materialistic socialism provided the basis for the dominant philosophy and ethics. Moral rules were dictated by party leaders who claimed infallibility and ruled coercively. This resulted in a monopolistic moral climate. Behind these rules there stood an irrefutable state power and an excessive bureaucratization of power, with extreme centralization of decision making. Political theoreticians presented a future-oriented ethics in which every desirable human goal was placed in the future state of communism. At the same time they denied the right of existence to any autonomous professional ethics, believing that their form of Marxist ethics was adequate to answer all questions raised in any area of human endeavor. Ironically, the principal slogan in all these states was "The highest value in socialism is the human being."

However, as soon as a little freedom of speech appeared in the 1980s, it became obvious that the morals of socialism were in ruins, as was the socialist economy. Despite claims that the socialist health-care system was of high quality, free, and accessible to everyone, it became evident that this was not so. Sociological surveys in these countries showed a very poor general state of health in the populations, high mortality rates, and severely reduced life expectancies. For example, Hungary has (as of 1994) the highest cardiovascular mortality rate in Europe for people below age sixty-five, and for all ages it places fourth, after Romania, Bulgaria, and the former Soviet Union. The percent of women in Hungary dying from cervical cancer is twice as high as the regional average; the suicide rate is the highest in Europe and about three times the regional average; the mortality rate from malignant neoplasm is also the highest in Europe, accounting for 21 percent of all deaths. Hungary and the former Czechoslovakia have the highest mortality rates for ischemic heart disease among countries in the region. In life expectancy the difference is almost five years between central/eastern and western Europe.

In addition, the crime, divorce, and suicide rates in Hungary rank highest in the world. A low priority has been given to the prevention of accidents and illnesses and to occupational diseases in these countries. Their notorious environmental pollution and destruction was justified through the repeated use of slogans regarding the need to subdue nature for the sake of human progress.

The Soviet type of health-care system was introduced in all these central and eastern European countries. Some of the features of the Soviet system, besides those already mentioned, were little if any freedom for patients to choose their doctors; bribes and corruption, manifested mainly in the practice of patients' tipping physicians for services; injustices in distributing limited resources; prejudice against the elderly; mechanistic patient care; and a clash between heavy demand and very limited resources. There was also, incidentally, a predominance of women in the medical profession.

For decades the problems could be hidden because fact-finding studies were regarded as "top secret" and revealing them was a serious political offense. Writers on the sociology or ethics of medicine were mostly either Communist party hacks or individuals afraid of writing the truth lest they lose their jobs. Consequently, it is little wonder that people in Western countries did not understand the decay and injustice that characterized the socialist health-care systems of the region. Only after the political and economic collapse of these once-praised systems did they come under fierce criticism. In the health laws of these countries very little was mentioned about patient rights, and nothing at all about such principles as patient autonomy. In practice, physicians and health-care institutions had no freedom in choosing patients, nor had patients in choosing doctors. Nevertheless, people could have access to health care that was theoretically free and "officially" had a high quality level. There is no doubt that many millions of people who, before World War II, might have died due to an inability to pay for medical care, could get essential treatments under the socialist system. This, in itself, was a great achievement.

Since no professional ethics beyond an exclusive Marxist version was accepted by the state and party officials, teaching ethics meant teaching Marxist ethics. Its main features were the unrelenting struggle against the enemies of the working class and the constant urging of people to work and produce more. Ethics was taught in colleges and universities only by the departments (or institutes) of Marxism-Leninism. These institutes occasionally smuggled into medical universities issues pertaining to medical ethics alongside the allowed themes of the Hippocratic oath and the moral ills of private medical practice. Noticing the great interest of students in ethical issues in medicine, some teachers began to deal with euthanasia, transplantation, and confidentiality. But nowhere in these countries was the teaching of medical ethics/bioethics formally established or officially supported during the Marxist-Leninist era.

The pioneers who introduced a more contemporary medical ethics in health colleges and medical universities were quite often physicians. In Hungary, the first textbook was written by a psychiatrist (Szilard, 1972); the second comprehensive textbook, written by a medical ethicist with a background in law and philosophy, appeared eighteen years later (Blasszauer, 1990). In Poland, a popular collection of essays written by doctors was recommended for teaching medical ethics at medical universities (Kielanowski, 1985). These broadly based works on bioethics contained a number of previously undiscussed issues, including patient rights, informed consent, reproductive medicine, and refusal of treatment.

In Poland and Hungary, more than six thousand hours are devoted to the six-year medical curriculum, and only thirty of these are assigned to the teaching of medical ethics. In Poland, these hours consist of surveying standard medical codes and existing laws (Szawarski, 1987). In Hungary, almost all the issues of bioethics are in the curriculum, especially such topics as informed consent, euthanasia, human experimentation, and patient rights.

Only now, some years after the radical political changes throughout central and eastern Europe, is the teaching of bioethics encouraged and is bioethics beginning to achieve a prominent place in the medical school curriculum. Whereas all Hungarian medical universities and health colleges teach thirty hours of bioethics, usually in the third year, in the Czech and Slovak republics bioethics is taught in ten medical schools; in Slovenia thirty hours of bioethics are given to medical students and fifteen hours to dental students. In Romania bioethics is on the medical school curriculum in Bucharest and Temesvar, and in Estonia, one priority is to train bioethicists and to begin teaching in this area.

Medical ethics in Croatia was given an impetus for development by the war in the territory of what had been Yugoslavia. Until that event, medical ethics was not taught as a separate subject in medical faculties but was a part of the history of medicine, social medicine, or forensic medicine. Since 1982, Zagreb, the capital of Croatia, has been the seat of the Yugoslav Center for Medical Ethics and Quality of Life. In 1992, the medical faculty of Rijeka introduced medical ethics as an independent subject. It is the ambition of the Department of Social Studies at Rijeka to establish an international center of medical ethics for the neighboring countries. Since Croatia is still at the beginning of a more general development of medical ethics, there are no ethics committees at the state level. There are, however, ethics commissions that formerly belonged to various institutions; they have no real programs that could form a nucleus of future ethics committees.

Main areas of ethical concern

Tipping. Sometimes referred to as *parasolventia,* gratuity, or even bribery, tipping was one of the most hotly debated medical ethics issues in Hungary (Adam, 1986), Czechoslovakia (Page, 1976), Poland (Szawarski, 1987), and Romania (Bologa, 1963). Outside of the health-care system, tipping has long been a common practice in many of these societies. Where there is a real or artificially created scarcity, and a tradition of some occupations with obligatory tips (e.g., waiters, barbers, concierges), the spreading of the practice to medicine may not be so surprising. The practice of slipping envelopes containing money into physicians' pockets for the treatment that was provided was not only unlawful but a violation of the basic idea of free health care, an idea that was supposed to make socialism superior to capitalism. In Hungary, from the 1950s until the 1980s, a campaign was waged by the Communist party and the government against tipping.

Still, in the few articles on medical ethics or medical deontology that did appear in these countries, only the most courageous or the most trusted authors dared to write about tipping. Generally, they would have been prosecuted for damaging the reputation of the socialist health-care system. Moreover, though it was (and is) a well-known phenomenon, nobody could ever prove who took such money, how much, when, and why. In Poland, since tipping makes health care unregulated and uncontrolled, the new Code of Medical Ethics forbids accepting tips (Polish Code of Medical Ethics, 1991).

In undergraduate medical education, ethics classes were devoted to this phenomenon. Ethics teachers were expected to educate future doctors to uphold socialist morality, which condemns taking money or any other form of bribe or gift from patients. Tipping has penetrated the whole system of medical care and has been hindering radical reforms in the system. Whether the cause is low professional salary, lack of public resources, the patient's feeling of gratitude, or simply a general moral decay, widespread tipping has morally eroded the system of health care. Experts believe that the system would collapse without this extra income, which, in some cases, is many times greater than the state-paid salary.

To a much smaller degree other health professionals supplement their wages with occasional tips. A common feature of central and eastern European state health-care systems is the very low salaries of doctors and other health workers. Still, some of these professions remain attractive because financial rewards can be hoped for as long as the system of gratuities persists. One can expect that debates will continue to probe the causes of this practice, which has been causing major problems in the physician–patient relationship and also greatly distorts the relationship between physicians and nurses, as well as nurses and patients.

Euthanasia of adults and infants.   Although discussion of euthanasia was long tabu in central and eastern Europe, it surfaced from time to time and aroused tremendous public interest. While laws in these countries forbid both active and passive euthanasia—by obliging physicians to do the utmost, regardless of the status and prognosis of the patient (thus making no distinction between the active and the passive forms)—the latter is widely accepted and practiced. In Poland, euthanasia debates have been rare because the Auschwitz, Birkenau, Stuthof, Gross-Rosen, Treblinka, and Majdanek concentration camps were the sites of Nazi doctors' criminal practices and experiments. The memories of crimes against humanity and the moral teachings of the Catholic church made the Polish people very hostile to any argument favoring either form of euthanasia (Szawarski, 1987, 1988). In Romania, even under the communist dictatorship of Nicolae Ceausescu, there were scholars who openly advocated passive euthanasia (Kiraly, 1982). Erno Kiraly and Karoly Daniel (Daniel, 1981) have introduced and endorsed the use of the living will in that country. In Romania it was not even possible to talk about bioethics until 1989. Now there are hospital ethics committees for special care issues. In Czechoslovakia a physician, Pavel Lukl, has advanced the idea of passive euthanasia (Lukl, 1970). In Slovenia the practice of passive euthanasia is openly accepted while active euthanasia, as everywhere else, is rejected (Straziscar and Milcinski, 1979).

The Hungarian euthanasia debate dates back to the early 1920s, when a crusade to legalize active euthanasia, led by Karl Binding and Alfred Hoche (a German lawyer and physician, respectively), was rejected. In the 1970s the debate was renewed, and several articles and a book appeared (Boldizsar, 1970; Blasszauer, 1984; Czeizel, 1982). Those sympathetic to euthanasia were accused of deviating from the socialist norms and advocating discrimination among people on the basis of social worth (Horvath, 1973; Monory, 1982). The Hungarian Health Act of 1972 states, without mentioning the word "euthanasia," that the physician's duty is to do the utmost until the very end for all patients, even those who suffer from incurable conditions. There is no mention of consulting the patient about his or her wishes. Nor is there discussion of what is to be done when legally mandated heroic efforts require respirators, dialysis machines, or other lifesaving devices that are in short supply.

In the case of seriously ill newborns, those who argued for the need to select infants to receive life-sustaining treatment were harshly condemned and even accused of behaving like the notorious Nazi doctor of Auschwitz, Joseph Mengele (Mestyan, 1985). Because of Hungary's low birthrate, obstetricians were rewarded with promotions or premiums for infants who survived at least to the age of one. Therefore, up to the age of one the statistics are closely monitored, while beyond that age there is no incentive to provide high-quality health care. The decision to extend treatment to seriously ill infants belongs exclusively to physicians; no infant-care ethics committee exists, and in most cases the parents are not consulted.

Only now, after the radical political changes, can such topics be discussed openly without accusations and reprisal. In Hungary a survey asked physicians, "Do you believe, in all circumstances, every possible effort should be made to sustain life?" Seventy-nine percent of responding physicians who worked in neonatal intensive-care units answered no (Schultz, 1993).

Informed consent and truth-telling.   In harmony with the existing paternalism, patients in central and eastern Europe usually receive little, if any, information about their conditions. Physicians' unwillingness to discuss diagnosis, prognosis, and intended therapy with the patient is due to their training, their limited knowledge of contemporary bioethics, and their characteristically negative judgment regarding their patients' medical knowledge and ability to make rational medical decisions. Since the physician is the "captain of the ship," it is taken for granted that the patient's duty is to follow his or her orders. Hungarian sociologist Agnes Losonczi described the situation well when she stated that a sick person does not have as many rights as someone who seeks to have a washing machine repaired (Losonczi, 1986).

Generally, the relatives of the patient are given medical information and left to decide whether to reveal that knowledge to the patient. Disclosure is very rare in cases of incurable disease; silence is believed justified by fear of patient suicide. The claim is simplistic and unsupported by fact, but despite arguments against deceiving patients, the dominant principle remains: "One must never tell a hopeless prognosis, instead one must always give hope" (Magyar, 1978). As long as a high court judge writes that an incurably ill patient must not be informed that a planned surgical intervention will bring only temporary relief, there is little hope that lawyers will fight for patients' autonomy (Toro, 1986).

Considering the prevalence of this practice of silence in central and eastern Europe, little can be said about the principle of informed consent. Although the law requires it, in reality the principle is seldom honored. The Hungarian Health Act of 1972 requires physicians to give information to patients but also extends to them the therapeutic privilege of withholding medical information in the interest of the patient. However, doctors considered therapeutic privilege as the main law, and the legislation had to be revised in 1991. The mention of therapeutic privilege was deleted, and there is no longer any legal excuse for withholding information from the patient about his or her illness (Sandor, 1991). Nevertheless, throughout the region people are infamous for paying little attention to what laws dictate.

Human experimentation, reproductive medicine, and genetic screening.   Because high technology is rare in these countries, research is primarily related to pharmaceuticals. The Helsinki Declaration (1975) is accepted everywhere as a guideline for ethical research using human subjects, and in some of these countries (e.g., Hungary and Romania) the guidelines have been incorporated into laws regulating biomedical research. Prisoners are excluded from any experimental or research protocol, and nontherapeutic research uses volunteers, usually students. The Polish Code of Medical Ethics (1991) makes no distinction between therapeutic and scientific research.

The policy of presumed consent for the donation of organs, tissues, or other biological material is universal in these countries and provides an almost unlimited possibility for procurement of such materials for research, transplantation, and drug production. Lawmakers influenced by prominent members of the medical establishment were instrumental in enacting presumed-consent legislation that made organ procurement quite easy and opened the way to organ transplantation. There is little or no control because, in most cases, research ethics committees are just being established. To the extent that such groups exist, they are rather ineffectual, since they cannot enforce the rules.

In a few clinics and hospitals, artificial insemination, in vitro fertilization, and GIFT programs proceed under vague and inadequate legal and ethical norms. In some countries (e.g., Romania and the Baltic states) in vitro fertilization and surrogate motherhood are virtually unknown or quite new concepts. In none of these countries is there legislation concerning human artificial procreation.

Genetic screening is done in most central and eastern European countries, but in some of them (e.g., Hungary and Poland) it meets with opposition from the Catholic church. In Cyprus, President Archbishop Makarios introduced compulsory screening for thalassemia, a hereditary blood disease. The screening has considerably decreased the occurrence of this disease.

Confidentiality.   Throughout this region confidentiality is highly valued. Cases of its violation hardly ever come before the courts because the laws in these lands allow many exceptions (the interest of the state, divorce cases, etc.). In practice, however, the violation of medical confidence is very common and goes hand in hand with the frequent violation of privacy. Moreover, the state has exclusive access to all patient records—patients are not allowed to see them. In certain countries, like Hungary, the laws overregulate confidentiality; thus everything is viewed as a secret, which leads to the fact that nothing is.

Abortion.   In most of the former communist countries abortion was considered a hard-won right for women. Laws were lenient, allowing abortion for simple social reasons. In Hungary, for example, 4.5 million abortions were performed between 1956 and 1990. Some view it as a national tragedy. Only after the Communist party's demise has the pro-life voice been heard. Abortion was (and is) a major method of birth control. In the former Czechoslovakia there were ninety-four abortions for each 100 live births. In Romania, however, abortion was forbidden; as a result of illegal abortions at least ten thousand women died from complications. In Poland, a heated debate accompanies the attempt, strongly urged by the Catholic church, to reverse liberal abortion laws. The 1991 Polish Code of Medical Ethics allows abortion under two special circumstances: if the mother's life and health are at risk or if conception was the result of rape. In Lithuania, opposition to abortion is increasing, and the law that allows abortion on demand in the first trimester is considered by the pro-life group to be a crime against humanity. The debate is especially intense and interesting in what was East Germany, where abortion laws were far more liberal than in West Germany (Beese, 1990).

Transplantation.   In these countries, transplantation has so far been largely limited to kidneys. In spite of the policy of presumed consent for donation, organs are scarce and demand is high. Thus, the problem of organ procurement cannot be blamed on individuals' lack of willingness to donate their organs, but on the indifference of many health professionals. Their lack of motivation leaves many available kidneys unreported: It is estimated that only 10 percent of potential donors in Hungary are made available to transplant centers. Age is one of the main criteria for transplant recipients, and no "new" kidney is available for persons over the age of fifty. Heart and liver transplants have also taken place (e.g., in Hungary) and have received tremendous media coverage. Consequently, the problem of obtaining organs has drawn great public interest and has become an important ethical issue for discussion. In these countries, where the medical establishments are strong and have significant political influence, it is doubtful that consent by the spouse or relatives of the dead person to use organs will ever be necessary or that their refusal will be honored.

Malpractice.   Charges of malpractice are very rare in central and eastern Europe, and successful lawsuits are even rarer. The most likely reason is not the superior professional skills of physicians working in these countries but the lack of patient rights, and the very powerful medical establishment that displays a high level of solidarity at critical times. The laws are worded in such a way that carelessness, negligence, or incompetence is difficult to prove as causally connected with the patient's state of health. Slowly, however, with the process of democratization and the planned reform of health care, and especially with the introduction of market conditions, malpractice is finding its way into the patient–physician encounter. Insurance against malpractice has already appeared in several of these countries.

Western help: Promising changes

In central and eastern Europe the transition from a one-party system to political pluralism has opened the way to democracy with free elections, public control, and constitutional guarantees. The reform of health care has begun: free choice of doctors; health insurance; mechanisms to finance health provision; separation of health care and social services; extension of private practice; reimbursement in accordance with the type of disease and number of patients.

The changes have already brought to the surface a divergence of opinions on bioethical issues. Help in many forms is coming from such world organizations as WHO, UNESCO, and the Council of Europe. These organizations hold meetings, work out guidelines, keep data banks on bioethical activities, and encourage such endeavors. The Hastings Center in the United States has played a key role in helping to bring together the central and eastern European bioethicists and their western counterparts. It has provided books, journals, forums, and scholarships to a number of bioethicists in this region. The Centre for the Study of Philosophy and Health Care of Swansea, Wales, joined the Hastings Center's Eastern European Program. It obtained support from the Nuffield Foundation, which has been quite generous in giving scholarships, libraries, and journals to many of these countries. The European Society for Philosophy of Medicine and Health Care, the European Association of Centers of Medical Ethics, Jefferson Medical College of Philadelphia, the Inter-University Centre of Dubrovnik, the Center of Medical Ethics of Oslo, and the International Association of Bioethics have done their share in helping to move bioethics out

of the underground. Without such international help, bioethics in the region would be still back in Hippocratic times and would be poorer both intellectually and materially.

BELA BLASSZAUER

While all the articles in this section and the other sections of this entry are relevant, see especially the INTRODUCTION *and other articles in this subsection:* SOUTHERN EUROPE, THE BENELUX COUNTRIES, UNITED KINGDOM, REPUBLIC OF IRELAND, GERMAN-SPEAKING COUNTRIES AND SWITZERLAND, NORDIC COUNTRIES, *and* RUSSIA. *For a further discussion of topics mentioned in this article, see the entries* ABORTION, *section on* CONTEMPORARY ETHICAL AND LEGAL ASPECTS, *article on* CONTEMPORARY ETHICAL PERSPECTIVES, *and section on* RELIGIOUS TRADITIONS, *article on* ROMAN CATHOLIC PERSPECTIVES; BIOETHICS EDUCATION; CONFIDENTIALITY; DEATH AND DYING: EUTHANASIA AND SUSTAINING LIFE; ETHICS, *article on* SOCIAL AND POLITICAL THEORIES; HEALTH CARE, QUALITY OF; HEALTH-CARE DELIVERY, *article on* HEALTH-CARE SYSTEMS; HEALTH-CARE FINANCING, *article on* PROFIT AND COMMERCIALISM; HEALTH-CARE RESOURCES, ALLOCATION OF; HEALTH POLICY, *article on* POLITICS AND HEALTH CARE; INFORMATION DISCLOSURE; INFORMED CONSENT; MEDICAL CODES AND OATHS; MEDICAL MALPRACTICE; MEDICINE, ANTHROPOLOGY OF; MEDICINE, SOCIOLOGY OF; PATERNALISM; PATIENTS' RESPONSIBILITIES, *article on* DUTIES OF PATIENTS; PROFESSIONAL–PATIENT RELATIONSHIP; PROFESSION AND PROFESSIONAL ETHICS; PUBLIC POLICY AND BIOETHICS; *and* ROMAN CATHOLICISM. *Other relevant material may be found under the entries* AUTHORITY; AUTONOMY; FREEDOM AND COERCION; JUSTICE; *and* OBLIGATION AND SUPEREROGATION. *See also the* APPENDIX (CODES, OATHS, AND DIRECTIVES RELATED TO BIOETHICS), SECTION II: ETHICAL DIRECTIVES FOR THE PRACTICE OF MEDICINE, OATH OF HIPPOCRATES; *and* SECTION IV: ETHICAL DIRECTIVES FOR HUMAN RESEARCH, DECLARATION OF HELSINKI *of the* WORLD MEDICAL ASSOCIATION.

Bibliography

ADAM, GYORGY. 1986. *Az orvosi halapenz Magyarorszagon.* Budapest: Magveto Kiado.

———. 1989. "Gratuity for Doctors and Medical Ethics." *Journal of Medicine and Philosophy* 14, no. 3:315–322.

BIEGANSKI, WLADISLAV. 1899. *Mysli i aforyzmy o etyce lekarskiej.* Czestochowa, Poland: Logika Medycyny.

BLASSZAUER, BELA. 1984. *A jo halal.* Budapest: Gondolat Konyvkiado.

———. 1990. *Orvosi egeszsegugyi etika.* Budapest: Tankonyvkiado.

BOLDIZSAR, FERENC. 1970. "Eutanazia—Igen? Nem?" *Valosag* 13, no. 10:34–41.

BOLOGA, VALERIU L. 1963. "Jegyzetek az orvosi etikarol." *Korunk* 22, no. 6:746–750.

BRAHAMS, DIANA. 1989. "Kidney for Sale by Live Donor." *Lancet* 1, no. 8632:285–286.

BREESE, WOLFGANG. 1990. "Twist in My Sobriety: Abortion in Germany." *Bulletin of Medical Ethics,* no. 61 (September):13–16.

CZEIZEL, ENDRE. 1982. "A teratanazia." *Valosag* 25, no. 6: 56–67.

——. 1988. *The Right to Be Born Healthy. The Ethical Problems of Human Genetics in Hungary.* Budapest: Kiado.

DANIEL, KAROLY. 1981. "Az eutanazia es a rakos betegseg utolso szakasza." *Korunk* 40, no. 6:16–24.

DOROSZEWSKI, J. 1988. "Medical Ethics in Poland." *Theoretical Medicine* 9, no. 3:351–370.

Health Law and Act of its Execution: Egeszsegugyi torveny es vegrehajtasi rendelet. 1972. Budapest: Egeszsegugyi Miniszterium Kiadvanya.

HORVATH, TIBOR. 1973. "Eutanazia—az orvosetika es a bunteto-jog dilemmaja." *Magyar tudomany,* no. 10:644–652.

IMRE, JOZSEF. 1925. *Orvosi ethica.* Budapest: "Studium" Kiadasa.

KIELANOWSKI, T., ed. 1985. *Etyka i deontologia lekarska.* Warsaw: PZWL. Essays written by doctors and recommended for teaching of medical ethics at medical universities.

KIRALY, ERNO. 1982. "Eutanazia es buntetojog." *Korunk* 2: 123–127.

KOVACS, JOZSEF. 1991. "Bribery and Medical Ethics in Hungary." *Bulletin of Medical Ethics,* no. 66 (March):13–18.

LANG, SLOBODAN; WOOLHANDLER, STEFFIE; BANTIC, ZELJKO; and HIMMELSTEIN, D. 1984. "Yugoslavia: Equity and Imported Ethical Dilemmas." *Hastings Center Report* 14, no. 6:26–27.

"London Kidney Exchange in Trouble." 1989. *Nature* 337, no. 6026 (February):393.

LOSONCZI, AGNES. 1986. *A kiszolgaltatottsag anatomiaja az egeszegugyben.* Budapest: Magveto Kiado.

LUKL, PAVEL. 1970. "Medizinisch-ethische Probleme der Reanimation." *Zeitschrift für innerliche Medizin* 25, no. 21:8–13.

MAGYAR, IMRE. 1970. "Az orvos es a halal." *Orvosi hetilap* 111, no. 51:3011–3041.

——. 1978. "Remenyt kell nyujtani." *Egeszsegugyi dolgozo,* no. 2:8.

MESTYAN, GYULA. 1985. "Eletet—de milyet?" *Orvosi hetilap* 126, no. 41:2563–2565.

MONORY, BULCS. 1982. "Az eutanazia modern ertelmezese." *Magyar jog* 29, no. 4:307–312.

PAGE, BENJAMIN B. 1976. "A Letter from Czechoslovakia: Socialism, Health Care, and Medical Ethics." *Hastings Center Report* 6, no. 5:20–23.

Polish Code of Medical Ethics. 1991. Resolution of the Extraordinary Congress of Physicians, December 14.

SANDOR, JUDIT. 1991. "A Missing Sentence." *Bulletin of Medical Ethics,* no. 66 (March):19.

SCHULTZ, KAROLY. 1993. "A Report from Hungary: Hungarian Pediatricians' Attitudes Regarding the Treatment and Non-Treatment of Defective Newborns. A Comparative Study." *Bioethics* 7, no. 1:41–56.

STRAZISCAR, STEFAN, and MILCINSKIJ, JANEZ. 1979. *Some Attitudes Toward Euthanasia in Slovenia.* Ghent, Belgium: World Congress of Health Law.

SZAWARSKI, ZBIGNIEW. 1987. "Poland: Biomedical Ethics in a Socialist State." *Hastings Center Report* 17 (spec. suppl., June):27–29.

——. 1988. "Treatment of Defective Newborns—a Survey of Pediatricians in Poland." *Journal of Medical Ethics* 14, no. 1:27–29.

——. 1990. "Poland Moves Against Abortion." *Bulletin of Medical Ethics,* no. 62 (October):3–4.

SZILARD, JANOS. 1972. *Az orvosi etika kerdesei.* Budapest: Semmelweis Orvostudomanyi Egyetem.

TORO, KAROLY. 1986. *Az orvosi jogviszony.* Budapest: Kozgazdasagi es Jogi Konyvkiado.

9. RUSSIA

The history and state of medical ethics in Russia in the twentieth century has been defined by the influence of the communist regime. Communism, its evolution, and its deterioration, exercised, and will exercise for a long time to come, a pervasive influence on the most diverse spheres of social life, including the area of medicine and health care.

Prerevolutionary period

The ascendancy of the Bolsheviks in 1917 sharply interrupted the stormy development of Russian health care, whose beginnings coincided with the great reforms of 1861, which eliminated serfdom for a peasant population that comprised the overwhelming majority of the country. Prior to those reforms, peasants could turn only to the village folk doctor (practitioner of popular medicine) or, in certain cases, healers from among the Russian Orthodox monks. For the most part, the health care of serfs had been the responsibility of their owners.

One of the most important of the mid-nineteenth-century reforms was the creation of elected local self-governments: the *zemstvos,* which received some autonomy from the central authority. The organs of local self-government levied taxes that were used for general needs, including building and equipping hospitals, ambulances, homes for orphans and for the elderly, and other needs. *Zemstvos* also hired and paid doctors, doctors' assistants, nurses, and other medical personnel.

In 1864, 530 medical centers were opened in Russia. Each center served an average area of 4,860 square *versts* (one *versta* equals two-thirds of a mile) and a population of about 100,000 people. After fifty years, in 1914, there were 2,800 such centers, each of which served an area of 880 square *versts* and 27,000 people. Expenditures for *zemstvos* health care grew from 2.5 million rubles in 1870 to 57.7 million rubles in 1912. Before 1861, the country had 519 hospitals; by 1914, it had 1,715 (Solov'ev, 1970).

The local doctor's ideals formed the ethos of Russian medicine. The ordinary zemsky (hired and paid by the zemstvos) physician had a modest social standing and a very modest income. He earned about as much as a factory worker. Zemsky physicians represented one of the largest groups within the Russian intelligentsia, along with zemsky teachers. Service to the people (i.e., the peasants) was a defining characteristic of the intelligentsia. The ignorance and poverty of the peasants, whose work fed the whole country, evoked among the intelligentsia that considered itself dependent on the peasant class not only sympathy, but a guilt that moved them to active work on behalf of the peasants. Many of the intelligentsia, neglecting their own material well-being, saw as the highest meaning of their lives the unselfish service to the people. Thus was born the movement called the narodniki, that is, representatives of the intelligentsia who saw that their responsibility was to "go to the people," to work selflessly in the most faraway places in Russia. "Every comfort of life I have," wrote one of the most committed leaders of the narodniki movement, the philosopher and sociologist Petr Lavrov, ". . . is purchased with the blood, sufferings, and work of the millions. . . . I will discharge my responsibility for the cost in blood of my development, if I use my development to lessen evil now and in the future" (Solov'ev, 1970, p. 43).

Along with the more radically disposed social-democratic intelligentsia, the mass of zemsky physicians were very dissatisfied with the actual state of affairs, but they preferred the path of reform and the laborious work of education to the revolutionary path of violence. The first obstacles of the path of reform were the deep prejudices and lack of confidence of the peasants, their resistance to change from traditional lifestyles, including acceptance of medical aid or elementary hygienic recommendations.

The zemstvos system permitted physicians to achieve an unprecedented degree of professional autonomy; the government, however, constantly strove to curtail this autonomy. During these years, periodic meetings of local physicians were held to discuss current problems within the profession. In the zemstvos, physicians, together with representatives of the administration, participated in the formulation of local policies for health care. In 1883, the newly formed Society of Russian Doctors to the Memory of N. E. Pirogov assembled physicians of all specialties. The society, named in honor of the outstanding Russian surgeon Nikolai Pirogov (1810–1881), was the first independent organization of physicians. The Pirogov Society significantly influenced the formulation of ideas and policies about health care. It fought actively for improvements in the working conditions of peasants and factory workers, and mostly because of its efforts, in 1903 a law was adopted regarding the liability of owners for accidents in the workplace. The society strove to improve the health education of the people and battled for increases in budgets for medicine and health care. In 1910, the society blocked efforts of the authorities to unify the health-care system and impose upon it strict government control. The society monitored physicians with regard to the norms of medical ethics, and fostered discussions about medical practice that touched on moral and ethical problems.

Medical ethics in Russia evolved, for the most part, in the light of European traditions, even though the specifics of Russian medicine left a noticeable mark. General practitioner and hygienist Matvei Mudrov (1776–1831), one of the first in Russia to concern himself with problems of medical ethics, believed that the Hippocratic oath could be the foundation of a code of conduct for Russian physicians. Nikolai Pirogov, whose ideas attracted particular attention to the problem of medical mistakes, and Vjacheslav Manassein (1841–1901), general practitioner and organizer of state and local medicine as well as editor of the journal Vrach (Physician; 1880–1901), which devoted significant attention to discussions of medical ethics, developed their ideas along the same lines. Among the characteristics of Russian medical ethics of the prerevolutionary period, the marked paternalism connected with the long-standing tradition of subjugation of the personality to the state or to the peasant community stands out. Typical patients were illiterate and ignorant peasants who were considered unable to make reasonable decisions in their own best interests and, therefore, required direction from others.

The other significant characteristic was the peculiar understanding of social justice, which generated a feeling of eternal indebtedness to the most impoverished and unfortunate people in society. Not by accident, a physician of German origin, Fyodor Gaaz (1780–1853), who settled in Moscow and devoted himself to the medical care of prisoners in jails and their children, enjoyed great moral authority both during and after his life. Unselfish and self-sacrificing service was demanded of physicians who understood their duty, including the willingness to work at any time of the day or night, to venture into any weather at the first call to reach the bedside of a sick person as quickly as possible, and to spend as much time at his or her bedside as necessary. To appreciate this high idealism, one should bear in mind the vast expanses of Russia, which were (and are) far from being fully connected by roads.

These ideals were also reflected in the literary works of doctors who became famous writers: Anton Chekhov (1860–1904), Vikentii Veresa'ev (1867–1945), and Mikhail Bulgakov (1891–1940). Writers in Russia were traditionally leaders of public opinion and exerted great moral influence, so the works of Chekhov and Veresa'ev that were dedicated to *zemsky* physicians deeply influenced the education of the intelligentsia. In his *Physician's Notes* (first published in 1901), Veresa'ev sharply criticized violations of ethics in medical practice and research. For many years this book was at the center of significant discussions in Russian as well as western European literature. The ideal of the *zemsky* doctor was so deeply ingrained that it even survived the Bolshevik regime.

Communist period

The communist regime came to power on the crest of a world war that was especially terrible and destructive for Russia. Immediately, the new government had to confront serious problems inherited from previous governments. Social collapse, hunger, and poor sanitary conditions caused huge epidemics of cholera, typhoid, and smallpox, so that the new government mounted a fierce fight against contagion (mass vaccinations, disinfections, isolation of infected, sanitary measures, and so on). Measures were taken to coordinate health-care activities, resulting in extreme centralization. In July 1918, the Peoples' Commissariat for Health Care in the Russian Republic was founded.

This commissariat was the first national ministry for health care in the world, created a year before the British Ministry (Kazer, 1976). Under the leadership of the first Soviet People's Health Care Commissar, Nicholas Semashko (1874–1949), a doctor close to Lenin, all the departments of the government having anything to do with medical services were united under one ministry (Knaus, 1981). In subsequent years, however, organizations that were autonomous from this commissariat gradually appeared, though health-care services for the railroads, the army, and other kinds of special services remained centralized. Health-care services were supported financially by the state and were free to the people.

These measures of the new authorities provoked severe criticism from members of the Pirogov Society who complained that the introduction by Soviet authorities of free health care would deprive physicians of their independence and initiative, both of which had been fought for during the earlier reforms. The regime, however, was not inclined to compromise with critics, especially with any type of organized opposition. The all-Russian Federation of Medical Workers (*Medsantrud*) was created in opposition to the Pirogov Society. The Pirogov Society was liquidated by 1922.

Medsantrud attempted to conserve the remains of democratic self-management of the ranks of medical

workers, and this brought upon it the wrath of the authorities. For example, one of the principal organizers of Soviet health care, the People's Deputy Commissar for Health Care, Zinovii Solov'ev (1876–1928), wrote in 1923: "What is this 'public' and what in general can 'public' mean in the conditions of the Soviet government? Two different answers to these questions are not possible. Our public is to work on all aspects of Soviet life on the basis of the independent revolutionary class, the bearer of the proletarian dictatorship, the proletariat and its ally, the impoverished and the middle peasant class" (Solov'ev, 1970, p. 54).

In this way the regime essentially redefined the social role of the physician. The physician was now considered a representative of the hostile bourgeois class, tolerated only as a specialist and permitted to work only under the strict control of the proletariat. In essence, however, that control was exercised by government and Party bureaucrats.

Meanwhile, the 1917 revolution and the ensuing civil war led to a serious decrease in the number of physicians in the country. In the first years after the revolution, about eight thousand physicians left Russia. Many doctors died from hunger and disease. Between November 1917 and August 1920, 46 percent of all physicians in Petrograd died (Knaus, 1981). In response, the authorities attempted the rapid training of new physicians. People were admitted into medical schools without even a secondary education and, at times, without even being able to read or write; final exams were eliminated. A system of "brigade education" was introduced whereby the knowledge of the group of students was evaluated on the basis of an oral exam of one of the students, on the grounds that the better prepared students would help the unprepared students in their training. There was, then, a rapid increase in the number of physicians, although, of course, at the cost of serious decline in professional standards.

Such reliance on collectivism was anything but accidental. Medicine, like everything else, was viewed from the class perspective. Individualistic bourgeois medicine was countered by collectivist proletarian medicine. The aim of the new medicine became the following: "The conservation of the life forces of the proletariat and the building of socialism in and of itself, of course, must be for us the main compass with respect to which a question regarding the tasks of our contemporary medical practice will be posed" (Solov'ev, 1970, p. 187). Consequently, the entire area of medical practice had to be reconsidered: "Characteristic of today's clinics is the fact that they were formed and exist today as the products of a discipline that is strictly individualistic. Contemporary capitalist society leaves its mark on medicine in the area of theory as well as particularly in the area of practice. The individualistic demand for care of a single person and not of a human collective creates corresponding methods of thought and practice" (p. 175). Key to the problem of shaping the approach and content of medical practice, according to Solov'ev, was the answer to the question of how "it is possible to strengthen the health of the human collective and restore [its] health once it has been destroyed" (p. 171).

These words affirmed the traditional approach of Russia regarding the importance of prevention in health care. This approach was implemented by making the work conditions and living conditions of people healthier, as well as by considering the social and ecological causes of many illnesses. At the same time, these comments by one of the leaders of Soviet medicine in its formative stages show clearly Bolshevism's negation of the self-worth of the individual, the reduction of human individuals to the role of cogs in a system of production, and the subjection of the individual to social expediency.

In the view of the Bolsheviks, considerations of class expediency defined the areas of morals and ethics. For example,

> The much celebrated theoretician of petty bourgeois morals, Immanuel Kant, advanced in his time a moral demand: "Never look on another person as a means to an end but always as an end in itself. . . ." Can you imagine how far the proletariat would have advanced in its revolution if it had allowed itself to be guided by such a demand and not by the completely contrary demand of class interests. . . . The highest wisdom of the proletarian struggle consists not in that everyone claims his own rights, but in that everyone must selflessly, almost spontaneously, without phrases of superfluous gestures, without demanding anything for himself, pour all of his energy and enthusiasm into the common stream, and work for the goal, with the entire class, perhaps be the first to fall on the road. (Preobrazhenskii, 1923, pp. 72–73)

A systematic elaboration of medical ethics that could have corresponded to the ideological purposes of the new regime and the new system of health care was, with rare exceptions, not attempted. To the extent that the physician was considered as only an auxiliary, rather than as an independent professional, the idea of posing questions of specific medical ethics was deemed superfluous. Even though some problems had a distinctly moral/ethical content and as such were quite controversial (for example, abortion, confidentiality, and medical mistakes), they were not viewed as problems specific to medical ethics. In general, medical ethics or, as it was usually referred to, "physicians' ethics" was understood as the affirmation of a corporate morality opposed to the class interest of the proletariat. The viewpoint was rather widespread that Soviet people, regardless of their sex and profession, should be guided solely by the norms of communist morality, and that any specific norms of professional morality would only limit the scope of and adherence to the general norms.

With respect to medical education, systematic courses in medical ethics did not exist in prerevolutionary Russia nor were they created by the new regime. After the revolution, in fact, the initiation of new physicians by means of a professional oath, a revision of the Hippocratic oath, was eliminated, even though that practice had been obligatory since the beginning of the twentieth century. The social humanitarian preparation of medical students was limited to a course in Marxism-Leninism.

Against this background of ethical relativism and nihilism characteristic of the Bolshevik scorn for traditional moral values and principles, the earlier traditions of medical ethics could still be found. Among those who received medical education, many were inspired by the ideals of disinterested and self-sacrificing service that had characterized the ethos of *zemstvos* health care. The medical profession attracted intellectuals drawn to that sphere because it was not under the sway of particularly severe ideological control. The norms and values of medical ethics were transmitted under these conditions by means of informal communication and daily contact between professors and students and between experienced physicians and new colleagues.

Stabilization of the regime. From the end of the 1920s to the beginning of the 1930s, the communist regime consolidated itself; its radical revolutionary policies were gradually transformed into pragmatism. This pragmatism, of course, was specifically Soviet, oriented to the resolution of problems of building a communist state. All aspects of civil life began to be affected by organs of administrative and bureaucratic planning and management. Health care also fell under the planning system: The number of physicians in various specialties and the number of hospital beds, hospitals, and polyclinics in cities and villages, the direction and topics of medical research, the development of facilities in sanitoriums and health resorts—all were centrally planned.

Planning presupposes qualitative evaluations and measurements, and from this perspective Soviet medicine obtained impressive results. The number of doctors had long since passed one million (about 1.2 million in 1983), and a single doctor had about half as many patients as his or her counterpart in the United States. Many infectious diseases were practically eliminated, the frequency of infant mortality was significantly lowered, and the average life expectancy was increased. By these and certain other indicators the country approached the level of more developed countries or became equal to them. The results of the Soviet organization of health care attracted much attention outside the Soviet Union, particularly among Third World countries.

Policy in the area of health care, however, was always viewed as subordinate to policy in the economic sphere. Thus, when the Communist Party began to emphasize the industrialization of the country in 1929, the central task of the health-care system was designated as the improvement of medical services to workers in the industrial centers, especially in the mining and metallurgic centers.

The system of health care that developed and remained relatively stable for many years was quite original in several respects. The physician became a civil servant, a kind of clerk, whose activities, regulated by numerous bureaucratic rules, consisted largely of writing reports that reflected his or her implementation of these rules. Any appearance of personal initiative was dangerous, especially because the physician's mistake could easily be interpreted as intentional, the act of a class enemy.

In relations with patients, the physician was a representative of state authority rather than an autonomous actor. Lack of autonomy, in its turn, made less urgent the problems of personal choice and responsibility. Low salaries of ordinary physicians as well as their low social prestige were among the reasons for the large number of female physicians in the country (about 80 percent). It was thought that physician's work was not so difficult, did not demand essential physical force, and therefore was well suited for women.

The social interaction of the physician and the patient was paradoxically characterized by two mutually exclusive elements. On the one hand, the long-reigning paternalism became even more entrenched, to the point where the individual regarded his or her health as a kind of state property—and therefore no one's—which could be squandered. On the other hand, health was viewed as the highest and ideal value, so high in fact that it was simply indecent to measure it by any sort of material equivalent, such as money. So, it was presupposed that self-sacrifice and unselfishness on the part of a physician was a kind of moral norm. The combination of these alternative, conflicting attitudes permitted the rather modest financing of medicine and health care, at a level that would ensure only the replacement of the labor force. Another characteristic of Soviet medicine was that patients were not permitted to choose their physicians.

Medical deontology

In 1939, the famous surgeon and oncologist Nikolai Petrov (1876–1964) published an article, "Questions of Surgical Deontology," in the *Bulletin of Surgery*. In 1945, he published a small book by the same title. These publications were the first steps in the rehabilitation of medical ethics. Petrov justified the use of the term "medical deontology" by arguing that the concept of "physicians'

ethics" had a narrower meaning. The latter, Petrov maintained, referred only to a corporate morality, reflecting the scientific and professional career interests of doctors (Petrov, 1956). This may have been a subterfuge designed to circumvent the ideological taboo on the problems of medical ethics. It is noteworthy that such an attempt was made by a doctor who received his training and education before the 1917 revolution.

Wide discussion of the problems of deontology did not begin until the middle and at the end of the 1960s when writings on this topic by medical practitioners and philosophers began to appear. The 1969 First All-Union Conference on the Problems of Medical Deontology in Moscow played an important role in this development. In 1971, state authorities approved the text of a document called "The Oath of the Physician of the Soviet Union." The oath was required for all graduates of medical institutes who intended to enter into professional activities. The text of the oath demanded that physicians be governed by the norms of communist morals and spoke more of their responsibility to the people and to the Soviet government than to the patient.

At the same time, medical deontology was introduced into the curricula of the medical institutes. However, notwithstanding reports to the contrary in a number of Western sources, courses on deontology and medical ethics appeared only in the beginning of the 1990s. In most medical schools the subject of deontology appeared to be spread out in separate courses in medical specialties, and philosophers had not been drawn into its teaching.

After 1971, the stream of literature in the area of deontology increased sharply. The contents of these publications, however, were often one-dimensional, moralizing reflections: criticism of the anti-humanist Western medical system coupled with a confirmation of the indisputable moral superiority of Soviet free medicine and the disinterested Soviet doctor. Attention to concrete cases, mainly from the personal practices of the authors, was frequent. Authors, however, avoided discussion of truly difficult cases that presented moral or ethical conflicts. Apart from the fact that this literature signaled the presence of ethical problems in medicine, its real interest lay in its increasing references to the moral authority of prerevolutionary Russian medicine and its attempt to present Soviet medicine as a direct and uninterrupted continuation of the best traditions of the past.

Crisis and breakdown of state medicine

The government-supported awakening of interest in medical deontology coincided with the first signs of crisis in Soviet medicine. Starting in the 1970s, but primarily in the 1980s, the authorities and a small circle of specialists, and then finally the public at large, became aware of the high rates of infant mortality and the consequent reduction of life expectancy. The press began to write more often about failures in the medical field and about the callousness, greed, and low level of competence of physicians and other medical personnel. Notwithstanding the state's propaganda efforts, the people, who were losing confidence in physicians and in official medicine, turned more often to practitioners of alternative medicine.

These failures, as well as many others, revealed that the centrally planned and managed free medical system had used up all its own resources, among them the moral resource that had enabled the authorities to make do with "cheap" medicine for so long. It was clear that the communist modernization was accompanied by an erosion of traditional values, which was particularly noticeable as the medical profession became so large and more and more specialized. The turn to deontology was in some sense dictated by the efforts to mobilize the neglected moral factor in the face of growing medical crises. This attempt, to the extent that it appealed to values from the past, however glorious it might have been, could not succeed.

The attempt made during perestroika in 1987 to reform the system of health care without changing anything essential turned out to be unproductive. In 1991 the Russian parliament adopted a law providing for medical insurance for Russian citizens: This was an admission of the failure of state medicine. The stability during the last decades of the state system of health care was assured, even though the principles of free medicine and equal access to health care for all, in practice, deteriorated. The bribes that had to be given to physicians by patients and their families to some extent compensated for the pitiful financial circumstances surrounding health care. The availability of a special medical-care system for party members and other members of the nomenklatura, people given leading positions in various fields by the Communist party, made them less inclined to pursue radical reforms.

Previous stability itself made the process of thoroughgoing reform particularly painful for the people. The deeply rooted tradition of paternalism hindered the acceptance of personal responsibility for one's own health. In addition, social justice often was viewed as a pure leveling of differences. Finally, most people could not accept the idea that health care could be paid for, even though "free medicine" proved very inefficient.

Acute economic, ecological, sociopsychological problems during the period of reforms led to serious worsening of health of the population. For the first time since the beginning of the nineteenth century, mortality in Russia exceeded birth rate; morbidity, including infectious diseases, grew rapidly. These factors along with barely controlled commercialization of health care, limitation in access to medical services for most people, expense, and shortage of many crucial drugs generated on the part of many Russians a nostalgia about the free health-care system of the past.

Specific areas of ethical debate and decisions

This section provides an overview of only those problems of medical ethics that have been treated in Russia in a rather original fashion.

Abortion.   Abortions in prerevolutionary Russia were considered criminal acts. In 1920, the Soviet government became the first in the world to legalize the artificial termination of a pregnancy at the request of the woman. Then, in 1936, in seeking means to improve the demographics, abortions were once again criminalized; in 1955, with some liberalization of the regime, they were again legalized to lessen the negative social consequences of widespread illegal abortions. The passage of legislation in 1993 permitted abortion at the request of the woman up to twelve weeks of pregnancy for any reason, and up to twenty-two weeks with consent of the woman for medical reasons. Abortion became a common means of birth control. The use of abortion for birth control may have resulted from a lack of contraceptive alternatives, as well as inadequate public knowledge and education about these matters.

Although abortions have been considered morally reprehensible, the attitude of people in concrete situations has been rather liberal. For many years the Russian Orthodox church, the most influential confession in Russia, was prohibited from taking positions on any question of social significance. Even after the persecution of religion ceased, the church had not shown itself ready to express an opinion on most matters of biomedical ethics. One exception was the stance the church took on abortion. In 1990, the Patriarch of the Russian Orthodox church confirmed the church's unequivocal censure of abortion; yet on a practical level priests tended to be more tolerant because of the hard economic situations of many women. In 1992, the Right to Life Society was formed to oppose abortions and was supported by the Russian Orthodox church.

Confidentiality.   Controversial discussions occurred in the 1920s concerning the problem of physicians' secrets. The People's Commissar for Health Care, N. Semashko, announced "the abolition of physicians' secrets," which were understood as holdovers of bourgeois medicine. This position was based on the notion that an illness was not a disgrace but, rather, a misfortune. Full abolition of physicians' secrets would occur, it was thought, when that concept was accepted by the population. Until that time the necessity of maintaining physicians' secrets was linked to the fear that eliminating them would create an obstacle for people seeking doctors' advice and help.

Even though Semashko himself, no longer a people's commissar but a practitioner, spoke out in favor of physicians' secrets in 1945, his earlier viewpoint turned out to be more influential, for many health-care workers did not understand the need for confidentiality. The requirement of confidentiality gained a legal basis only in 1970. Up to 1993, however, a patient who returned to work after illness was obliged to bring a sick-leave certificate from a physician. This certificate containing the patient's diagnosis was available to many people. New legislation changed this norm: A diagnosis would be filled in only with the consent of a patient; without consent only general reasons (disease, trauma, etc.) could be indicated.

Disclosure to patients.   The subject of disclosure to patients has been marked by strong paternalistic tendencies. The overwhelming majority of those writing on the subject considered it unacceptable to inform a terminally ill patient of his or her diagnosis and prognosis. The practice of informing patients was not generally regulated, so concrete decisions were left to the discretion of the treating physician.

However, Russian laws on psychiatric treatment and on transplantation of human organs and tissues, which were adopted in 1992, contained norms of informed consent for patients and donors. Included in the legislation were norms governing the protection of the health of citizens, granting the patient the right to know his or her diagnosis and prognosis as well as the right to refuse this information.

The law also established specific rules regarding receipt and documentation of informed consent of patients undergoing biomedical experiments. The advent of *glasnost* (openness) in 1985 permitted public disclosure of the terrifying information about fatal biomedical experiments (such as testing of nuclear or chemical weapons, new drugs, etc.) carried out on soldiers of the Soviet Army and on prisoners under Joseph Stalin (1879–1953) and Lavrenti Pavlovich Beria (1899–1953) and even later. Some steps were undertaken for ethical control of biomedical experiments, but as of 1994 most researchers were not aware of internationally accepted norms of experimentation.

Euthanasia.   As early as prerevolutionary times the well-known Russian jurist Anatoly Koni (1844–1927), opposing the dominant view, defended the admissibility of euthanasia under certain exceptional circumstances: (1) conscious and insistent requests of the patient; (2) the impossibility of lessening the suffering with known methods; (3) agreement by a commission of doctors on the impossibility of saving the life; and (4) preliminary notice of the decision to the prosecutors. A law permitting mercy killing of a patient was adopted

in the criminal code of 1922, but in subsequent legislation it vanished. It was practically inoperative and little is known about its utilization.

Sociological studies conducted among physicians in Moscow indicated that about 40 percent of them viewed euthanasia as permissible if the patient wishes it or in exceptional cases. However, many respondents did not seem to know what the word "euthanasia" meant (Bykova et al., 1994). The public's attitude toward euthanasia appeared more tolerant: According to the findings of one public opinion poll, 55 percent of the respondents approved and 19 percent opposed the mercy killing by a physician of a terminally ill patient who wishes to die.

The majority of specialists in medical ethics, including physicians, jurists, and philosophers, have with rare exceptions adopted a sharply negative opinion of active euthanasia. The prohibition of active euthanasia, understood as acceding to a patient's request to hasten his or her death by medical means, was included in a law for "the protection of the health of citizens of the Russian Federation." Nonetheless, such forms of passive euthanasia as the refusal by the patient of treatment or the withdrawal of life-sustaining treatment from a hopeless patient were considered acceptable. The public's attitude toward euthanasia remained rather tolerant.

Eugenics and medical genetics.   In the first decades of the twentieth century, Russia was among the world's leaders in the development of genetics. This interest in genetics generated a rather strong eugenics movement, which flowered in the 1920s. To some extent this interest may be explained by the consonance of eugenics with the central communist ideology of the creation of a "new man" who would be free of the "birthmarks" of capitalism. One of the leaders of Russian genetics, Nikolai Kol'tsov (1892–1940), following Francis Galton, spoke of eugenics as the religion of the future that still awaited its prophets. It was the powerful ruler of nature and the creator of life that would permit the creation of a perfect type of human being (Adams, 1990). In the 1920s, when ideological control was not yet particularly strong, the possibilities for forming a new human being were suggested by psychoanalysts as well as by those in other areas of scientific research.

The paths of communist ideology and eugenics diverged rather quickly, however. The principal criticism of eugenics was that the new human being should be formed by social, and not by biological, methods. Eugenic projects in Russia, because of such criticism, were interrupted long before they had achieved any practical realization. Inasmuch as Russian eugenics at that time was a form of medical genetics, the blow to eugenics also impeded research in human genetics. This setback was only the first of many caused in the Soviet Union by the reigning ideology associated with Trofim Lysenko, who taught the thesis of inheritance of acquired characteristics, which lasted until Khrushchev fell from power in 1964. Even afterward the development of medical genetics ran up against ideological obstacles, since many associated it with the eugenics that served as a basis for the murderous racism of the German Nazis. Since the beginning of *glasnost* and the end of ideological censorship, some far-reaching proposals with possible eugenic interventions in the Russian population have been published, among them, killing newborns with serious defects and forced sterilization of alcoholics and drug abusers. Genetecists, however, have been rather passive in relation to public discussions of these topics. Despite the growing public concern about the genetic effects of radiation and environmental pollution and despite rather intensive research in the field of medical genetics, Russia now has only limited capacity for genetic screening and counseling except in a few large cities. In 1994, the Russian human genome project started to study possible ethical implications of recent developments in human genetics.

Repressive psychiatry. The practice of using psychiatry as a weapon in the struggle against political dissidents began under the regime of Nikita Khrushchev. The first victim was Zhores Medvedev, who was punished for wanting to publish a book on the crushing of genetics in 1948. Medvedev was diagnosed by state psychiatrists as mentally deranged and was committed for treatment. The widespread use of psychiatry in this manner did not occur until later, during the regime of Leonid Brezhnev. Hundreds of victims, without any judicial proceedings and often without even being physically present, were sentenced for indeterminate lengths of time to special psychiatric hospitals under the jurisdiction not of the Ministry of Health but of the Ministry of Internal Affairs. "Treatment" ranged from "wall therapy"—merely keeping patients inside four walls—to forcible psychotropic injections. The practice came to be used even against ordinary citizens who had conflicts with local authorities. The Soviet psychiatrist Andrei Snezhnevsky (1904–1987) worked out the basis for this method of repression, using the concept of "creeping schizophrenia" with symptoms such as the "spreading of slander," "exaggerated religiosity," and "excessive appreciation for the West." The center for expert studies and diagnoses of such afflictions was the V. Serbsky Institute for Forensic Psychiatry in Moscow.

Many cases of psychiatric repression became well known in the West. This caused the breach in 1983 in relations between the World Psychiatric Association (WPA) and the Soviet All-Union Society of Psychiatrists and Narcologists. The membership of the society in the association was renewed only in 1989. That same year, the Independent Psychiatric Association, founded in the Soviet Union in 1988 and actively involved in exposing psychiatric abuses, gained unconditional membership in the WPA.

A 1989 fact-finding mission of U.S. psychiatrists to Soviet psychiatric hospitals discovered that the malice of psychiatrists or of repressive state bodies was not the only cause of the abuse of psychiatry. Other factors included the poor training of medical personnel, the absence of adequate judicial mechanisms for the protection of the rights of patients, and the low level of ethical standards for hospital personnel. The aim of a 1992 law was the improvement of psychiatric treatment. According to this law, involuntary hospitalization in a psychiatric hospital was permissible only on the basis of a court's decision. The position of supervisor, to protect the rights of patients, was to be established in every psychiatric hospital. In 1993 the Russian Society of Psychiatrists—the most influential psychiatric association—adopted the Code of Professional Ethics of the Psychiatrist.

Transplantation. The adoption in 1992 of a "law on the transplantation of human organs and tissues" provided an example of the direction of the reforms in Russian health care. Before adoption of this law, questions such as the determination of brain death, the rights of donors and recipients, and the permission for the removal of organs and tissues from cadavers were decided on by internal instructions of the Ministry of Health, instructions that were unknown to the population. On the one hand, this situation impeded the practice of organ and tissue transplants and, on the other hand, facilitated abuses, such as commercial use of human organs or the too-hasty declaration of brain death. The law on transplantation at last provided a legal basis for this area of medicine, and more important, became one of the first laws relating to health care using principles and practices accepted in the world community.

Perspectives for Russian bioethics

Interest in the problems of bioethics grew as Russia emerged from isolation. Such interest evolved mainly through the efforts of a small group of enthusiasts. Neither the leadership of the health-care system nor the government bureaucracy nor the public itself grasped the critical importance of problems in bioethics. Democratic reforms, to the extent that they will continue, will change this situation. As reforms develop, health care will become one of the most important priorities of social legislation and public interest. The reform of medicine and health care will make both physicians and patients much more independent and, consequently, responsible parties in social interactions.

Foundations of Legislation of Russian Federation on the Protection of the Health of Citizens, adopted in 1993, as well as other laws filled in many gaps in health-care and legal regulations. The law opened the door for the creation of ethical committees (commissions) at federal (similar to France), regional, and local levels as well as in hospitals and biomedical research institutes to defend human rights in health-care areas.

In 1992 the Russian National Committee on Bioethics (RNCB) was established under the aegis of the Russian Academy of Sciences. The main activities of the RNCB include the development of ethical guidelines for scientific research, proposal of legislation in health care and biomedicine, promotion of bioethical training and education, preparation of textbooks and methodical materials, stimulation of discussions on bioethical issues in the mass media, and encouragement of bioethics in Russian regions as well as in countries of the Commonwealth of Independent States. The RNCB prepared documents on such acute problems as mass vaccination and protection of human rights, ethical aspects of transplantation of organs, ethical regulation of new reproductive technologies, ethical control of biomedical experiments, and so forth.

"Free medicine" has not been a social priority, and whoever leads the government can find more critical need for expenditures than health care. But the failure of free medicine, however painful for the population, will provide the basis to hope for a better future. Already the harsh reality has caused people to realize that the government or the Ministry of Health is not alone responsible, nor will either pay for the people's health; people themselves must do so. People are also beginning to realize that medicine and health care are areas in which the fundamental rights and vital interests of people are realized (or not realized) and, consequently, this area requires moral and ethical consideration as well as legal regulation.

BORIS YUDIN
TRANSLATED BY RICHARD SCHNEIDER

While all the articles in this section and the other sections of this entry are relevant, see especially the INTRODUCTION *and other articles in this subsection:* SOUTHERN EUROPE, THE BENELUX COUNTRIES, UNITED KINGDOM, REPUBLIC OF IRELAND, GERMAN-SPEAKING COUNTRIES AND SWITZERLAND, NORDIC COUNTRIES, *and* CENTRAL AND EASTERN EUROPE. *Directly related to this article are the entries* EASTERN ORTHODOX CHRISTIANITY; *and* SOCIAL MEDICINE. *For a further discussion of topics mentioned in this article, see the entries* ABORTION; CONFIDENTIALITY; DEATH AND DYING: EUTHANASIA AND SUSTAINING LIFE; DIVIDED LOYALTIES IN MENTAL-HEALTH CARE; EUGENICS; INFORMATION DISCLOSURE; ORGAN AND TISSUE PROCUREMENT; PRIVILEGED COMMUNICATIONS; *and* PSYCHIATRY, ABUSES OF. *Other relevent material may be found under the entries* HEALTH POLICY, *article on*

HEALTH POLICY IN INTERNATIONAL PERSPECTIVE; INTERNATIONAL HEALTH; MEDICINE AS A PROFESSION; PRISONERS; *and* PUBLIC POLICY AND BIOETHICS.

Bibliography

ADAMS, MARK B. 1990. "Eugenics in Russia, 1900–1940." In his *The Wellborn Science: Eugenics in Germany, France, Brazil, and Russia,* pp. 153–216. New York: Oxford University Press.

AMNESTY INTERNATIONAL. 1975. *Prisoners of Conscience in the USSR: Their Treatment and Conditions.* London: Author.

BYKOVE, SVETLANA Y.; YUDIN, BORIS G.; and YASNAYA, LJUDMILA V. 1994. "Is Euthanasia Permissible? Opinions of Physicians." *Chelovek* 2:87–92. In Russian.

CRAWSHAW, RALPH. 1974. "Medical Deontology in the Soviet Union." *Archives of Internal Medicine* 134, no. 3:592–594.

DE GEORGE, RICHARD T. 1990. "Biomedical Ethics." In *Science and the Soviet Social Order,* pp. 195–224. Edited by Loren R. Graham. Cambridge, Mass.: Harvard University Press.

HYDE, GORDON. 1974. *The Soviet Health Service: A Historical and Comparative Study.* London: Lawrence and Wishart.

IVANYUSHKIN, ALEKSANDR J. 1990. *Professional Ethics in Medicine.* Moscow: Medicine Publishers. In Russian.

KAZER, MICHAEL CHARLES. 1976. *Health Care in the Soviet Union and Eastern Europe.* Boulder, Colo.: Westview Press.

KNAUS, WILLIAM A. 1981. *Inside Russian Medicine: An American Doctor's First-Hand Report.* New York: Everest House.

KOTEL'NIKOV, VALENTIN PROKHOROVICH. 1987. *Ot Gippokrata do hashikh dnei.* Moscow: Znanie.

MALKOV, SERGEI M., and OGYRTZOV, ALEKSANDR P., eds. 1992. *Bioethics: Problems and Prospects.* Moscow: Institute of Philosophy of Russian Academy of Sciences. In Russian.

PAGE, BENJAMIN B. 1978. "Medical Ethics, History of: Eastern Europe in the Twentieth Century." *Encyclopedia of Bioethics,* vol. 3, pp. 977–982. Edited by Warren T. Reich. New York: Macmillan.

PETROV, NIKOLAI NIKOLAEVICH. 1956. *Voprosy khirurgicheskoi deontologii.* Leningrad: Medgiz Publishers.

PETROVSKII, BORIS VASIL'EVICH. 1988. *Deontologiia v meditsine.* 2 vols. Moscow: Medicine Publishers.

PREOBRAZHENSKII, EVEGENII ALEKSEEVICH. 1923. *O morali i klassovykh normakh.* Moscow: Gos. izd–vo.

RYAN, MICHAEL. 1979. "USSR Letter: Aspects of Ethics (2)." *British Medical Journal* 2, no. 6191:648–649.

SOLOV'EV, ZINOVII PETROVICH. 1970. *Voprosy sotsial'noi gigieny i zdravookhraheniia.* Moscow: Meditsina.

TICHTCHENKO, PAVEL D., and YUDIN, BORIS G. 1992. "Toward a Bioethics in Post-Communist Russia." *Cambridge Quarterly of Healthcare Ethics* 1, no. 4:295–303.

"A Topical Interview Given by the Holy Patriarch Pimen." 1990. *Journal of the Moscow Patriarchate,* no. 7, pp. 12–21.

VEATCH, ROBERT M. 1989. "Medical Ethics in the Soviet Union." *Hastings Center Report* 19, no. 2:11–14.

VERESA'EV, VIKENTII VIKENTEVICH. 1904. "Physician's Notes."

In *The Confessions of a Physician*. Translated by Simeon Linden. London: Grant Richards.

YUDIN, BORIS G. 1992. "Bioethics for the New Russia." *Hastings Center Report* 22, no. 2:5–6.

V. THE AMERICAS

A. COLONIAL NORTH AMERICA AND NINETEENTH-CENTURY UNITED STATES

North American physicians fashioned their ethics as professionals from the dominant cultural ideals of their era, from norms hallowed through centuries of professional tradition, from rules and regulations of newly established medical institutions, and from laws and legal institutions operative in the communities in which they practiced.

Christian practitioners

The soil of religious values grounded the quest for professional ethics. For the majority of British and French physicians who settled North America in the seventeenth and eighteenth centuries, Jesus was as real and significant as Asclepius, Hygeia, and Panaceia had been to the author of the Hippocratic Oath. An intimate causal connection existed between character and professional righteousness. The beliefs and rituals of Christian institutions formed character. The ethically acceptable physician displayed the characteristics of a Christian.

Cotton Mather, a Puritan cleric who wielded considerable power throughout New England during the early eighteenth century, was a major figure in the evolution of North American medical ethics. He believed that Christian physicians who abided by the secrecy clause of the Hippocratic Oath became special confessors who had extraordinary opportunities for offering "admonitions of piety" to their trusting and needful patients (Mather, 1966). Because sin was the ultimate cause of all diseases—spiritual, mental, and physical—Mather expected physicians to prescribe Christian beliefs as well as drugs (Mather, 1972). Though he acknowledged confusion about the variety of remedies proposed as cures for any single disease, he would not dishonor "skillful and faithful" physicians (Beall and Shryock, 1954).

Though many Bostonians objected, Mather advocated inoculation during smallpox epidemics. He believed that the ultimate success of smallpox inoculation depended on God's mercy, but the validity of inoculation required trial-and-error testing and statistical comparisons between those naturally infected and those artificially inoculated. If deaths were prevented or suffering mitigated, as had occurred in Africa and Turkey, then inoculation was a good practice for doctors in North America. Its goodness as praxis was determined by the scientific demonstrations of practical trials involving mathematical standards and utilitarian outcomes that would be the basis for the reform of medical therapeutics during the nineteenth and twentieth centuries.

Gentlemen practitioners

North American physicians repeatedly urged students and colleagues to be both Christians and gentlemen in their interactions with each other and with patients. The principal characteristics of a gentleman included proper birth, sufficient wealth, unblemished character, adequate learning, and civic service. While the importance of birth and wealth faded in the more egalitarian atmosphere of the New World, that of character, learning, and civic virtue grew stronger. Was a physician good because he cured many sick patients, or because he was a Christian and a gentleman? Doctors who prepared the earliest biographical dictionaries of deceased physicians in the United States and Canada judged their worth by Christian and gentleman standards, not by curative or preventive statistics (Thacher, 1967). Hallmarks of professional goodness depended on allegiance to the dominant cultural ideals.

Educated doctors

Those who promoted higher standards for judging physicians frequently decried the immoralities of uneducated practitioners. In 1765, two years after the British assumed rule of New France (Canada) and ten years before the battles of Lexington and Concord, John Morgan proclaimed that most North American practitioners were ignorant, unsteady, irresolute, idle, negligent, and merciless. After six years as an apprentice to John Redman in Philadelphia, four years as a military surgeon, three years of medical studies in London and Edinburgh, and the luster of a European "grand tour," it was easy for Morgan to feel superior.

Wanting to improve this deplorable situation, Morgan and others established the first colonial medical school at the College of Philadelphia (1765). Samuel Bard, another Edinburgh graduate, delivered the first commencement address at King's College Medical School in New York City in 1769. Bard's judgment, no less harsh than Morgan's, was a fusion of Christian ethics, gentlemanly values, and academic ideals: "As those who have neither emulation nor honesty, who neither have abilities, or will give themselves the trouble of acquiring them, I would recommend it to such, seriously to consider the sixth commandment, 'Thou Shalt Do No Murder'" (Bard, 1769, p. 6). Morgan, Bard, and others fervently advocated formal education to produce morally acceptable doctors.

Because of the influx of practitioners from the United States and Great Britain, and because of British restrictions on degree-granting institutions in the colonies, enduring medical schools were not established in Canada until the third decade of the nineteenth century. In 1830, when the medical school at McGill University was one year old, twenty regular medical schools functioned in the United States. Graduates of these schools usually championed academic norms as measures of professional goodness: collegiate studies before medical ones, a systematic formal education in a medical school, improving medical science by careful clinical observations, development of effective teacher–pupil relationships, and continuing studies after formal education. Physicians were professionally good if they were Christians, gentlemen, and scholars.

Legal proprieties

North American physicians were not considered wholly ethical unless they were law-abiding citizens. Throughout Canada's early history, its doctors associated professional propriety with approval by licensing authorities, established as early as 1788 when the British Parliament passed a licensure act governing the Canadian settlements (Heagerty, 1928). Two Canadian groups assumed licensing responsibilities: the College of Physicians and Surgeons of Lower Canada in 1847 and the College of Physicians and Surgeons of Ontario in 1869. The voluntary medical societies organized in Canada before 1850 were not concerned with licensing.

The situation was quite different in the United States. Legislators granted exclusive licensing rights to medical societies in some states and to separate boards of physicians in other states. Such licensing bodies had been established in most states by 1832. During the subsequent forty years, however, existing states repealed or ignored their medical licensing laws, and new states adopted none. Since possession of a medical degree was sufficient for licensing in many states, there seemed to be little need for sustaining separate powers for societies or boards. No group enforced these laws uniformly or effectively. Nor had the laws prevented the growth and development of medical quackery and sectarianism.

Legislators believed that free Americans could be trusted to discover the good physician and to sue the bad one. Even if a physician in the United States could be judged a good professional without being licensed, as was the situation between 1835 and 1875, he did not want to be accused of malpractice, much less convicted in court.

During the first half of the nineteenth century, the American culture, unlike the Canadian, experienced an outburst of religious pluralism, the populist effects of expansion to the West, an economic atmosphere of laissez-faire, and widespread opposition to centralized regulation by governmental authorities. These conditions fostered the lack of interest in licensure laws and the willingness of legislators to charter schools for homeopaths, hydropaths, and other sectarian practitioners.

These social and cultural conditions caused many practitioners to believe that standards of professional propriety were disappearing in a sea of populist relativism. If models of personal morality, such as Christian or gentleman, were so varied and even conflicting (Could Jewish doctors be good?), and if standards of knowing were so pluralistic that legislators relinquished efforts to distinguish among them, what could be done by practitioners who still believed in the integrity and dignity of a medical profession?

Codes of ethics

To cope with the pluralism and relativism of the modern era, physicians created codes of professional ethics. During the last decade of the eighteenth century, Thomas Percival, a general practitioner in Manchester, England, had developed a systematic view of medical ethics based on the premise that it was possible to comprehend a moral order suitable for all medical practitioners. Universal truths about good professional behavior could be learned and applied by all conscientious and respectable doctors. Percival delineated these truths within a fourfold categorization of physicians as persons, caregivers, livelihood competitors, and civil servants.

The following admonitions exemplify Percival's approach. Physicians should be Christian gentlemen: considerate, reasonable, self-critical, temperate, educated. Doctors ought to interrogate patients privately and have special regard for their feelings and prejudices. Practitioners should consult openly and respectfully with each other, searching for proper remedies and sharing responsibilities in the care of the sick. Doctors ought to honor the trust of their communities by providing medical services free to public institutions and by providing medical knowledge needed by courts and governing officials. Percival included these and numerous other exhortations in a book on medical ethics published in 1803.

This book, together with John Gregory's lectures on medical education and medical ethics published in 1772, became a handy guide for North American practitioners who wanted practical criteria for judging propriety but had little interest in theoretical formulations of moral philosophy that might bring them too close to the Catholic traditions of the medieval universities. Most of these doctors were Protestants, and many were stalwart Puritans who, like Cotton Mather, deliberately rejected the "new moral philosophy" of the seventeenth and eighteenth centuries. In their view, these modern philosophies contained too much ancient paganism and too little Christianity, and placed more reliance on observation and reason than on faith and ritual.

Despite such theoretical objections, American physicians became exemplars of the "new moral philosophy" as they created codes of professional ethics during the first half of the nineteenth century. In 1808 an association of Boston physicians adopted a code of medical ethics composed of nine sections that addressed consultations between physicians, interfering with another doctor's practice, arbitration of differences between doctors, discouraging the use of quack medicines, promoting professional respectability, fees and exemptions from fees, practicing for a sick or absent doctor, and seniority among practitioners. All of these precepts could be found in the second chapter of Percival's *Medical Ethics*. Titled "Boston Medical Police," this code became the model for codes adopted by at least thirteen medical societies in eleven states during the ensuing thirty-four years.

In 1823 the New York State Medical Society adopted a code that resurrected the broader scope of Percival's original view. The New York doctors presented ethical claims about the personal character of physicians, quackery, consultations, patient care, and public obligations. In 1832 an original code was adopted by the Medico-Chirurgical Society of Baltimore. Norms were offered about the obligations of physicians to each other, quackery, consultations, and fees. This code also included a separate section about duties of patients toward physicians, an approach that had been taken by Benjamin Rush in a lecture to students. Rush thought that citizens should employ only serious-minded, educated doctors. Patients should not burden doctors with too many details of their illnesses, and they should strictly follow their doctors' orders and pay their fees promptly.

These examples of distinctive codes from Boston, New York City, Baltimore, and Philadelphia demonstrate the extraordinary interest in codifying professional ethics among American doctors, an interest that culminated in the adoption of a national code in 1847 by the newly established American Medical Association (AMA).

The AMA doctors accepted Percival's fourfold pattern of categorizing professional ethics and many of the specific claims cherished by the British practitioner. They advocated excellence of moral character, though Christian norms were no longer identified as the exclusive grounds for this character, probably because Isaac Hays, a prominent Jewish physician in Philadelphia, was a member of the committee that drafted the code. Though the AMA doctors valued proper education, they insisted that loyalty to professional colleagues was more important than scientific attainments. Article IV explicitly forbade association or consultation with irregular

practitioners, that is, physicians whose "practice is based on an exclusive dogma, to the rejection of the accumulated experience of the profession," an injunction directed primarily against homeopaths. Standards of patient care included careful attention to professional secrecy, a proper number of visits to the sick, absence of gloomy prognoses, and refusal to abandon patients who have incurable diseases.

Physicians also had excellent opportunities for influencing the personal character of patients. Section 7 of Article I of Chapter 1 of the code is quite specific: "The opportunity which a physician not unfrequently enjoys of promoting and strengthening the good resolutions of his patients, suffering under the consequences of vicious conduct, ought never to be neglected." Sustaining Cotton Mather's view of the sickroom as a stage for confession and redemption, the AMA doctors accepted professional roles as moral therapists. Since "moral" then included what would be called psychotherapy today, the AMA code also sanctioned the devotion of those physicians who had chosen careers as superintendents of institutions caring for the mentally ill.

The AMA doctors emphasized the ideal of shared obligations between physicians and patients, between the profession and the public. Copying Rush, the AMA committee codified the rights of American physicians in a long list of obligations of patients toward their physicians. In the last chapter of the code these duties of patients were expressed more generally as the obligations of the public to the profession, for example, in supporting medical schools and allowing them to acquire cadavers for anatomical dissection. In return, the profession acknowledged a relatively new dimension of professional ethics by its willingness to provide medical knowledge to the governing groups of their communities. This knowledge was needed, for example, in adjudicating civil and criminal proceedings as well as in deliberations about the proper kinds of laws and institutions needed for sanitation, quarantine, and other public health measures.

Worthington Hooker, a general practitioner who later became a professor at Yale, focused on the ideal of reciprocal obligations in *Physician and Patient* (1849), the only comprehensive view of professional ethics published in book form by a North American practitioner before 1900. Hooker's religious beliefs were almost as conservative as those of Cotton Mather, but Hooker believed that moral philosophizing was acceptable for a Christian apologist. He became a moral philosopher of medicine. Like other conscientious midcentury doctors, he knew that religious, educational, and legal institutions had failed to provide a fully acceptable set of moral standards for judging physicians. Hooker believed that doctors were obliged to discover acceptable standards of professional behavior, to publicly proclaim these standards in a format that would be comprehensible to both professionals and the public, and to determine whether such standards had been honored by individual doctors. A code of medical ethics adopted and enforced by a national organization could become the cultural and social instrument for shaping a uniform and universal moral order for American doctors. Hooker viewed his book as an extensive commentary on the AMA code.

Thus, Hooker and many others touted the advantages of the AMA code. Professional righteousness in the United States could be measured by the extent of adherence to this code. Professionally virtuous doctors maintained professional secrecy, made the proper number of visits to the sick, did not offer gloomy prognoses, cared for the incurably sick, requested consultations as needed, and abided by the numerous other precepts in this code that was adopted voluntarily by many societies. In 1855, the AMA decided that all state and local societies wishing to send delegates to its meetings had to adopt its code of ethics.

Not a few chided the AMA's officers about the absence of enforcement procedures. Some state and local societies reprimanded members for consulting with irregular practitioners and occasionally expelled members for criminal offenses, gross immorality, or the sale of secret medicines. The AMA established a judicial council in 1873, but there is no evidence that the council enforced the code regularly or extensively. Similar difficulties affected Canadian practitioners.

One year after its establishment in 1867, the Canadian Medical Association adopted a code of ethics that was almost identical with the AMA code. Minor changes had been made in wording. One clause in the article about obligations of the public to physicians had been omitted, and a new paragraph in Section 3 of Article I permitted beginning practitioners to announce the existence of their offices in the public press. Although some doctors lauded its rules and enforcement was attempted, this code was hardly the final word in matters of medical ethics for most Canadian practitioners.

The attitudes of Canadians contrasted sharply with the sentiments of many practitioners in the United States who believed that the AMA code was as important as the Bible and the Constitution. If the American government could create a bill of rights suitable for all citizens, then the American medical profession could prepare a bill of rights suitable for all reputable medical practitioners. The AMA code of 1847 was that document. In filling a moral vacuum caused by religious pluralism, unacceptable educational standards, loss of confidence in traditional remedies, and ineffective licensure laws, the AMA code became the set of sacred

values voluntarily created and professed by respectable and honorable doctors. Sick patients could place their trust in practitioners who gave their allegiance to this code.

In 1880, when one editor doubted that the majority of Canadian medical practitioners had ever read the code adopted by the Canadian Medical Association ("Code of Medical Ethics," 1880a), journal editors in the United States were about to receive an onslaught of articles for and against the AMA code. The problem involved the prohibition against consultation with any practitioners other than those exhibiting allegiance to the code. In 1882 the New York State Medical Society revised its code of ethics so that its members could consult with legally qualified practitioners regardless of their scientific or sectarian status. Seventeen state societies condemned this action, and the AMA refused to admit the New York delegates to its annual meeting. In the following year, the AMA expected all delegates to sign a pledge to obey its original code of ethics. Articles for and against the code and supporting or opposing the renegade New York physicians appeared in nearly all state medical journals. The code-loving conservatives withdrew from the New York State Medical Society and started a new organization that became larger than the original society. Conservatism was the order of the day; the code of 1847 withstood revision until 1903.

Exemplifying a practical application of the moral philosophy taught as a senior year course in most American colleges of the nineteenth century, the AMA code and its predecessors had nurtured professional unity and social respectability during the heyday of Jacksonian egalitarianism in the United States. These codified norms sustained important traditions in Western medicine, reminded all practitioners of essential duties to their patients and colleagues, and encouraged doctors to participate in those public institutions designed for the health and welfare of all.

Science versus codes

Those members of the New York State Medical Society who revised their code of ethics in 1882 exemplified a new breed of medical practitioner emerging in North America during the last three decades of the nineteenth century. These individuals could not accept the AMA code's claim that intraprofessional loyalty was more important than scientific truth. When Francis Delafield announced in 1886 that he and his colleagues wanted an association in which there would be no medical politics and no medical ethics, he heralded a fundamental change in the approach of North American practitioners to the perennial challenge of fashioning an acceptable set of professional ethics. Delafield and his colleagues wanted to associate with those practitioners who were able "to contribute something real to the common stock of knowledge" in medical practice (Konold, 1962, p. 39). They could no longer tolerate those practitioners who rested secure with a fundamentalist allegiance to the code of one organization whose precepts were rooted in eighteenth-century British experiences. The iconoclastic doctors of the late nineteenth and early twentieth centuries advocated a professional morality that would judge physicians in terms of their skillful application of specialized scientific knowledge in caring for the sick and the healthy. This new moral philosophy of medicine gradually became institutionalized in some medical schools and societies between 1870 and 1900.

The more progressive schools established teaching and research laboratories, and hundreds of North American practitioners journeyed to the laboratories and clinics of Europe for instruction in the basic sciences, especially microbiology and pathology, and in the clinical specialties, especially the surgical ones. Between 1864 and 1894, American physicians organized more than a dozen national societies for medical specialists (e.g., pediatrics, obstetrics, urology).

These groups did not adopt written codes of ethics. Instead they proclaimed—by word and deed—the values of a liberal premedical education and a thorough education in the medical sciences, allegiance to the experimental method as the proper approach to truths about health and disease, and a strong belief in research and continuing education.

These doctors espoused the rightness of their values as dogmatically as those who believed in the AMA code. Physicians and patients knew of numerous practitioners who did not accept the code but were reputable as persons and successful as healers. The same could not be said for doctors who ignored the bacteriological discoveries, the vaccines, the antiseptic principles, the improvements in diagnostic technology, the pharmacological therapeutics—all based on the methods of experimental science and clinical trials. Good doctors were those who competently and humanely applied this medical science.

These values led to numerous reforms in North American medical education, facilitated and sanctioned by the reestablishment of licensure policies in all of the United States by 1898. In 1902 the Medical Council of Canada became the central licensing agency for the provinces. These new licensure approaches not only sanctioned the reform measures adopted by the progressive American and Canadian medical schools but also upheld obedience to law as an important measure of professional virtuosity.

The physicians who supported these laws and schools recognized that the AMA code said nothing about the more technically proficient environments of the modern hospitals emerging after 1870. To provide competent surgical care, doctors needed instruments and assistants. By the late 1890s, scientific practitioners needed X-ray equipment and laboratory machines that could not be carried in black bags. Technically imprecise care was immoral to these doctors.

Technically adequate care, especially surgical care, required the services of trained nurses. As hospitals became cathedrals of applied science, doctors supported the training schools for nurses initiated by London's Florence Nightingale in 1860. At least fifteen of these schools existed in North America by 1880 (Rosenberg, 1987, p. 219). The ethical values espoused by these professional nurses encompassed certain cultural ideals about women, as well as specific norms about knowledge and obedience. Women were believed to be the moral standard-bearers of Victorian society. Those who chose to become nurses were special women who sacrificed much for the glory of God and the needs of the sick. Soldiers in the fight against disease, these nurses organized militaristic training schools that prepared women, attired in starched and pressed white uniforms, to assist physicians obediently in applying scientifically derived medical knowledge.

The AMA code had said nothing about nurses or women or blacks. Physicians and patients welcomed trained nurses who were social products of a new moral philosophy of medicine that assigned special values to some women. Overcoming objections by most males, other women became doctors. Nearly 400 women physicians practiced in 21 states by 1881 (Burns, 1988). Excluded from the AMA, black physicians adapted to the segregationist culture of their era by organizing the National Medical Association in 1895. The AMA codifiers made no revisions to accommodate these scientific, professional, and social changes.

The most significant change involved the transformation of the hospital into a powerful institution that incorporated the moral values of religious charity, scientific excellence, specialized patient care, and social justice. The number of hospitals in North America grew from about 300 in the 1870s to more than 4,000 by 1910. These hospitals became arenas for moral confrontations between medical practitioners and nonprofessional administrators and other laypersons. They fostered the emergence of new health-care workers and professionals, including laboratory technicians, nurses, occupational and physical therapists, social workers, and hospital chaplains. Each group forged its particular ethical agenda. Hospitals also supported the rapidly expanding urge for specialty differentiation among physicians. At the turn of the twentieth century, hospitals became the interpersonal crucibles that sustained and transformed the legacies of North American medical ethics.

Conclusion

Before 1900, North American physicians were morally acceptable if they cherished dominant religious ideals, behaved as gentlepersons, learned the fundamentals of medical science, revered a code of professional ethics, and abided by the laws of their communities. Professional virtuousness was measured by the extent of allegiance to the cultural and professional traditions of the West, as those traditions had been adapted to North American conditions. During the last quarter of the nineteenth century, a small group of doctors began to challenge some of the value claims for professional orthodoxy. They believed that favorable results in curing and preventing specific diseases in particular humans made possible by the technically proficient behaviors of skilled professionals applying scientifically derived knowledge were more important than the status-seeking rituals of AMA codifiers or the religious beliefs of the professionals. Yet, the conservative tendencies were so tenacious that the majority of practitioners, at the opening of the twentieth century, still believed in codification as the primary method for establishing professional ethics and still displayed loyalty to the values of one association's code even though major changes in the cultural, scientific, technological, and institutional legacies had changed the nature of the quest for professional ethics.

CHESTER R. BURNS

While all the articles in this entry are relevant, see especially the companion articles in this section: THE UNITED STATES IN THE TWENTIETH CENTURY, CANADA, *and* LATIN AMERICA. *For a further discussion of topics mentioned in this article, see the entries* BIOETHICS EDUCATION; EPIDEMICS; ETHICS; HOSPITAL, *article on* MODERN HISTORY; LICENSING, DISCIPLINE, AND REGULATION IN THE HEALTH PROFESSIONS; MEDICAL CODES AND OATHS; MEDICAL EDUCATION; MEDICAL MALPRACTICE; MEDICINE AS A PROFESSION; NURSING ETHICS; NURSING AS A PROFESSION; PATIENTS' RESPONSIBILITIES; PROFESSIONAL–PATIENT RELATIONSHIP; PROFESSION AND PROFESSIONAL ETHICS; RACE AND RACISM; SEXISM; UTILITY; *and* WOMEN. *Other relevant material may be found under the entries* FREEDOM AND COERCION; NURSING, THEORIES AND PHILOSOPHY OF; RIGHTS; *and* VIRTUE AND CHARACTER. *See also the* APPENDIX (CODES, OATHS, AND DIRECTIVES RELATED TO BIOETHICS), SECTION II: ETHICAL DIRECTIVES FOR THE PRACTICE OF MEDICINE.

Bibliography

BARD, SAMUEL. 1769. *A Discourse upon the Duties of a Physician with Some Sentiments on the Usefulness and Necessity of a Public Hospital: Delivered Before the President and Governors of King's College, at the Commencement Held on the 16th of May, 1769, as Advice to Those Gentlemen Who Then Received the First Medical Degrees Conferred by That University.* New York: A. & J. Robertson.

BEALL, OTHO T., JR., and SHRYOCK, RICHARD H. 1954. *Cotton Mather: First Significant Figure in American Medicine.* Baltimore: Johns Hopkins University Press.

BLAKE, JOHN B. 1952. "The Inoculation Controversy in Boston: 1721–1722." *New England Quarterly* 25:489–506.

BURNS, CHESTER R. 1969. "Malpractice Suits in American Medicine Before the Civil War." *Bulletin of the History of Medicine* 43, no. 1:41–56.

———. 1977a. "American Medical Ethics: Some Historical Roots." In *Philosophical Medical Ethics: Its Nature and Significance,* pp. 21–26. Edited by Stuart F. Spicker and H. Tristram Engelhardt, Jr. Dordrecht, Netherlands: D. Reidel.

———. 1977b. "Richard Clarke Cabot (1868–1939) and Reformation in American Medical Ethics." *Bulletin of the History of Medicine* 51, no. 31:353–368.

———. 1977c. "Thomas Percival: Medical Ethics or Medical Jurisprudence?" In *Legacies in Ethics and Medicine,* pp. 284–299. Edited by Chester R. Burns. New York: Science History Publications.

———. 1988. "Fictional Doctors and the Evolution of Medical Ethics in the United States, 1875–1900." *Literature and Medicine* 7:39–55.

"Code of Medical Ethics." 1880a. *Canada Lancet* 12:286. Editorial.

"Code of Medical Ethics: Of the Duties of Physicians to Their Patients, and of the Obligations of Patients to Their Physicians." 1880b. *Canada Lancet* 12:257–264. Editorial.

FIERING, NORMAN. 1981. *Moral Philosophy at Seventeenth-Century Harvard: A Discipline in Transition.* Chapel Hill: University of North Carolina Press.

GREGORY, JOHN. 1772. *Lectures on the Duties and Qualifications of a Physician.* London: W. Strahan.

GROB, GERALD. 1973. *Mental Institutions in America: Social Policy to 1875.* New York: Free Press.

HAMPTON, ISABEL, et al. 1893. *Nursing of the Sick.* New York: McGraw-Hill.

HEAGERTY, JOHN JOSEPH. 1928. *Four Centuries of Medical History in Canada and a Sketch of the Medical History of Newfoundland.* 2 vols. Toronto: Macmillan.

HOOKER, WORTHINGTON. 1972. [1849]. *Physician and Patient; or, A Practical View of the Mutual Duties, Relations and Interests of the Medical Profession and the Community.* New York: Arno Press.

KETT, JOSEPH F. 1967. "American and Canadian Medical Institutions, 1800–1870." *Journal of the History of Medicine and Allied Sciences* 22, no. 4:343–356.

KONOLD, DONALD E. 1962. *A History of American Medical Ethics, 1847–1912.* Madison: State Historical Society of Wisconsin for the University of Wisconsin.

LUDMERER, KENNETH. 1985. *Learning to Heal: The Development of American Medical Education.* New York: Basic Books.

MATHER, COTTON. 1966. [1710]. *Bonifacius: An Essay upon the Good.* Edited by David Levin. Cambridge, Mass.: Harvard University Press.

————. 1972. [1724]. *The Angel of Bethesda: An Essay upon the Common Maladies of Mankind*. Edited by Gordon W. Jones. Barre, Mass.: American Antiquarian Society.

PERCIVAL, THOMAS. 1975. [1803]. *Medical Ethics; or, A Code of Institutes and Precepts, Adapted to the Professional Conduct of Physicians and Surgeons*. Huntington, N.Y.: Krieger.

ROLAND, CHARLES G. 1984. *Health, Disease and Medicine: Essays in Canadian History*. Toronto: Hannah Institute for the History of Medicine.

ROSENBERG, CHARLES. 1987. *The Care of Strangers: The Rise of America's Hospital System*. New York: Basic Books.

SLOAN, DOUGLAS. 1971. *The Scottish Enlightenment and the American College Ideal*. New York: Teachers College Press, Columbia University.

SMITH, WILSON. 1956. *Professors and Public Ethics: Studies of Northern Moral Philosophers Before the Civil War*. Ithaca, N.Y.: Cornell University Press.

STEVENS, ROSEMARY. 1971. *American Medicine and the Public Interest*. New Haven, Conn.: Yale University Press.

THACHER, JAMES. 1967. [1828]. *American Medical Biography; or, Memoirs of Eminent Physicians Who Have Flourished in America. . . .* New York: DaCapo. Reprint of 1828 edition and 1845 supplement by Stephen Williams.

B. THE UNITED STATES IN THE TWENTIETH CENTURY

The field now called bioethics originated in the 1960s in the United States. It has its roots in the traditional medical ethics of Anglo-American medicine, in the cultural setting of American health care, and in certain social, religious, and moral perceptions that had emerged in the American ethos. This article will first delineate the background for the development of bioethics and then relate the events, issues, and concepts that have stimulated its growth during the latter half of the twentieth century.

The culture of U.S. health care

Bioethics, in the broad sense of the study of ethical problems encountered as humans interact with the biological within themselves and in their environment, comprehends much more than medicine and medical science. However, the development of bioethics can best be understood against the background of the development of medicine in the United States from 1900. The twentieth century has seen enormous growth in American medicine—in the amount of money devoted to medical care, the number of persons with access to care, the number of personnel and specialities, the complexity of institutional systems, and the extent of scientific technology. Three principal lines of development that contribute to the interest in ethical questions are the changing role of the hospital, the predominance of science and technology, and the development of specialization.

Beginning in the late nineteenth century, hospitals were founded at an increasing rate and eventually became the principal sources of medical care in the United States. As medical diagnosis and treatment increasingly involved elaborate techniques and devices, it was seen as more efficient and economical to centralize care in hospitals. Physicians could allocate their time more conveniently; nurses, technicians, and medical specialists could coordinate their work more effectively. Communities desired hospitals as a matter of pride; cities needed hospitals for indigent patients. The passage of the Hill-Burton Act, which provided federal support for local hospital construction (1946), and the tendency of the newly popular health insurance to reimburse hospital care rather than office or home care accelerated the evolution of the hospital in the United States (Rosenberg, 1987; Stevens, 1989).

With seminal discoveries in bacteriology, pathology, and physiology during the nineteenth century, scientific medicine came into its own. However, it became an integral part of medical practice in the United States only after the extensive reorganization of medical schools in the decades around 1900—a period marked by the vigorous efforts of the American Medical Association to reform medical education and to improve the standards of medical practice. Medical school reform was greatly stimulated by the Flexner Report, *Medical Education in the United States and Canada*, sponsored by the Carnegie Foundation (Flexner, 1910). Scientific investigation, increasingly supported by the federal government, especially during and after World War II, brought research physicians into medical education and patient care. Experimentation involving human subjects, both patients and health volunteers, became more widespread as the National Institutes of Health opened and sponsored clinical research centers in the 1950s. The twentieth century brought a "new" medicine, one profoundly shaped by the biological sciences. Diagnosis and treatment took on forms dictated by the scientific knowledge generated in the laboratory, tested in clinics, and assessed by statistical methods.

The fascination of scientific knowledge and techniques drew many physicians into narrower fields of concentration. The vastly increased body of knowledge became too much for individual physicians to master. Moreover, it became possible for physicians to build careers by performing procedures focused on limited aspects of patient care. Thus, scientific medicine fostered the growth of specialties. Specialty boards, organized to test and certify competence in the particular fields of medicine, were established in a variety of specialties and subspecialties, beginning in the United States with the

Board of Ophthalmology in 1917 (Stevens, 1971). The social and economic status of physicians improved significantly during the first half of the twentieth century and American physicians gradually moved from middle- to upper-class status, which distinguished them in attitudes, lifestyle, and place of residence from many of their patients (Starr, 1982).

In general, the three developments described above set the scene for the ethical concerns that began to surface in the United States in the 1960s. The concentration of specialized medical care in hospitals encouraged an impersonal, organizational approach to medical care. While social, behavioral, environmental, and personal aspects of illness were not totally neglected, scientific medicine focused on the biological and physical aspects; complaints that physicians had lost the ability to care for "the whole patient" were increasingly heard. As scientific knowledge increased, teaching in the sciences tended to crowd other concerns from the basic medical curriculum. Specialization narrowed attention to particular organ systems and diseases, and patients were shuttled between a variety of specialists rather than cared for by the family doctor. Leading medical educators felt obliged continually to stress the more comprehensive view of medicine, but educational, economic, and professional pressures constantly obscured these calls. By the 1960s, physicians, formerly close and familiar to their patients, had become "strangers at the bedside." This alienation was an important impetus toward the emergence of bioethics (Rothman, 1991).

Social and cultural trends

In addition to these directions within medicine, cultural and social movements involved the public in the ethics of medical care to an unprecedented extent. The mass media stimulated public interest in medicine. By emphasizing new discoveries, dramatic incidents, and "human interest" stories, the media underlined growing tensions between complex medical technology and its humane use. Growing urbanization and the consequent uneven distribution of population heightened existing obstacles to health care. A higher standard of living and increased educational achievement for many increased the sophistication of patients. Growing support of biomedical research by the federal government during the 1950s and 1960s thrust research into the realm of public policy. The ability of persons to purchase health care, dramatically improved by the introduction of employment-based insurance in the 1930s and augmented for the poor and the elderly by the passage of Medicare and Medicaid in 1965, gradually began to erode. Health care in the United States, while technically superb, became extremely costly and, due to its cost and organi-

zation, excluded large numbers of Americans from adequate care. This had become a social and political crisis by the late 1980s.

The slow but incessant influence of consumerism, from the concern about adulteration of food in the early decades of the century to the militant demands for consumers' rights in the 1970s, began to influence the health-care system. The patients'-rights movement in the 1970s was a segment of a larger movement for civil rights. The women's movement brought attention to the care of women patients and the distribution of women professionals in health care. These movements heightened sensitivity to the unmet health-care needs of women and people of color. The issues of birth control and abortion divided the public on the role of health professionals in family and population policies. Medicine began to draw practitioners from a culturally broader population, and many new allied health professions and technical specialties were added to the health-care team, enriching and intensifying debates over values among health-care providers. The peace movements of the 1960s and 1970s and growing ecological movements drew attention to burgeoning international health problems arising from war, environmental hazards, and pollution (McCally and Cassel, 1990; Leaf, 1989). These concerns challenged the role of medicine in maintaining the overall health and well-being of Earth's population. Physicians for Social Responsibility was founded in 1971, on the premise that the health risks of nuclear armaments fell within the social responsibilities of physicians. Although threats to the global biological environment emerged as major research and political concerns in the 1970s, the study of ethical issues in these areas remained rather separate from the study of ethical issues in medicine and health sciences (Geiger, 1971; Jonsen and Jameton, 1977; Cassel and Jameton, 1982).

These social and cultural trends, together with the direction of the biological and medical sciences, were the background for the bioethics movement that began in the 1960s. Bioethics as we know it today had its roots in general public concerns over issues of individual rights, social justice, and environmental quality that marked American culture in that era. Before examining the bioethics movement itself, it is advisable to examine the ideas, activities, and interests that were its precursors.

Traditional medical ethics

The effort to establish a unified medical profession during the nineteenth century and the accompanying internecine strife among physicians of various doctrinal allegiances profoundly influenced the nature and content of medical ethics at the opening of the twentieth century. Although strains of the Hippocratic, medieval, and Enlightenment tradition were invoked, the dominant themes stressed the respectability and collegiality of the profession and detailed the etiquette of professional relationships that promoted those themes. At the beginning of the twentieth century, this goal of a unified profession was within reach. The American Medical Association (AMA), through the strenuous efforts of its chief spokesman, Joseph McCormack, represented the profession as dedicated to orthodox scientific medicine, the advancement of medical education, the elimination of quackery, and the promotion of public health, particularly through support of pure food and drug legislation (Burrow, 1977).

One crucial mandate of professional ethics—that ethical physicians did not consult with or refer patients to unorthodox practitioners—was firmly in place in the early twentieth century. Decades before the turn of the century and for several decades afterward, many ill-trained or untrained persons practiced "medicine." A vast number of substances and devices were promoted as cures for various or all disorders. A strong public voice favored freedom of choice of practitioner, claiming that the "scientific" practitioners and drugs offered nothing better than their untutored and untested competitors. Others, particularly the more educated practitioners, set out to discredit quacks, nostrums, and patent medicines.

This concern stimulated the debate among physicians over cooperation between physicians and "irregular" practitioners. Many regular physicians refused to treat patients who had received prior treatment from irregulars; medical society codes of ethics barred irregular practitioners from society membership, hospital admitting privileges, and joint practice with regular practitioners (Gewitz, 1988). During the years before World War I, the AMA led a fight that finally persuaded state legislatures and Congress to pass legislation controlling the practice of medicine and the sale of drugs. Midwives were among the targets of the campaign against quackery, and despite better health outcomes by many midwives at the turn of the century, the campaign for "scientific" practice won public support and midwives have been largely displaced by obstetricians (Leavitt, 1986). During that era, medical ethics appeared to some as exclusively concerned with the criteria that restricted practice to "orthodox" physicians. While self-interested motives can be imputed to organized medicine, many repudiated the "freedom of choice" argument out of the sincere concern that medicine "at least do no harm" (Burrow, 1977). Still, as many commentators have noted, medical ethics, in this matter, served the ends of medical monopoly (Berlant, 1975).

A second important question about consultation and referral was vigorously debated: whether referring

physicians were entitled to a fee or "kickback" for having sent a patient to a specialist or consultant. This practice was particularly common in surgery. Some surgeons solicited patients through general practitioners who, in turn, found it lucrative to refer patients who sometimes did not require surgery. The abuses of fee splitting scandalized the public and many professionals. The American College of Surgeons, founded in 1915, required its fellows to take an oath that explicitly repudiated fee splitting. The problem, although branded by all professional organizations as unethical, continued in a covert way for many years (Davis, 1960).

Perhaps the most agitated debate in traditional medical ethics during the first half of the twentieth century was over the integrity of the patient–physician relationship. Fee-for-service practice by solo practitioners who sought to develop their own followings of patients was the predominant model. However, some "contract practice," in which a physician undertook to provide unlimited service to a designated population for an agreed amount had long existed. Plantations in the American South had utilized this method for the medical care of slaves. Fraternal organizations formed by immigrant populations had insured their members in this way, and in the West, the railroad and lumber industries contracted with physicians to care for their workers. However, many in the organized profession objected to contract practice, condemning it as "cut-rate medicine," as inferior to private practice in the quality of care and personal relationship, and as allowing a "third party" to dictate conditions of care, to the possible detriment of the patient. The same objections met the forms of group practice that evolved from contract practice in the first half of the twentieth century. Bitter battles raged over these issues; many medical societies excluded physicians who were involved in these "schemes." A series of antitrust decisions by the U.S. Supreme Court, beginning in the 1940s and continuing into the 1970s, gradually cleared the way for the development of a variety of corporate practice forms, such as health maintenance organizations, that a few decades before would have been considered unethical forms of medical practice.

Another ethical issue was closely related: the debate over payment for medical care. The traditional ethics had required physicians to charge their patients fairly and to provide free or discounted services to those who could not pay. The emergence of free public clinics and hospitals in the late nineteenth century threatened that ethic. Many physicians claimed that even patients who could pay sought free care, draining their practices and making it impossible for them to provide charitable services, which depended on a steady income from paying patients. Thus, at the turn of the century, extensive public use of free clinics was debated as an ethical question. Some argued that it was conducive to continued pauperization; others claimed that forcing poor people to pay for needed medical care was immoral. Some practitioners opposed free clinics because they viewed them as unfair competition by medical schools, which they saw as using free clinics to obtain patients for medical education. At the same time, the organized profession realized that the costs of care were beyond many persons and that physicians' incomes were low. Initial support was given to proposals emanating from organized labor for government-supported compulsory health insurance. By 1916, a broad coalition of organized medicine, labor, and social reformers had almost achieved the passage of national health insurance. World War I intervened, and the coalition was weakened: National health insurance seemed a "Germanic" proposal (Germany had long had such a program) to many and "socialistic" to others. Organized medicine, from then on, firmly opposed almost all forms of government health insurance. Again, it was proclaimed that since this would interpose government between doctor and patient, such programs would be unethical. This opposition persisted down to the passage of Medicaid and Medicare in 1965 (Marmor, 1970; Fein, 1986).

The AMA revised its 1847 Code of Ethics in 1903, 1912, 1947, 1957, and 1980. The revisions, successively more succinct, reflected an increased sense of professionalism and ideals about the scientific excellence of the practitioner. At the same time, the professional ethics expressed in official codes and in the positions taken by organized medicine on social questions reflected an interest in maintaining the status quo of the profession and the practice of medicine as it had been evolving in the late nineteenth and early twentieth centuries. With few exceptions, such as increased tolerance for group practice, the 1957 revision of the AMA Code, which consists of a condensation into ten "principles of medical ethics," bears little evidence of the major social changes that had begun to affect medical care in the United States. In 1985, the AMA Judicial Council changed its name to the Council on Ethical and Judicial Affairs; it now issues regular statements on issues of current ethical import, such as euthanasia, the obligation to care for patients with AIDS, and financial conflict of interest. Many major medical organizations, such as the American College of Physicians and the American Academy of Pediatrics, have formed ethics committees with a similar purpose. Although commentaries and informal codes on the conduct of nurses can be found as far back as the inception of the profession by Florence Nightingale, the American Nurses' Association did not adopt an official code of ethics for nurses until 1950.

Thus, during the first half of the twentieth century, medical ethics consisted of professionally devised propositions to enhance the unity and monopoly of the profession. Professional self-interest sometimes hid behind ethical claims that were often to the detriment of the public. At the same time, the profession, in encouraging improved medical education and advocating public-health and safety measures, lived up to its more noble traditions (Jonsen, 1990).

The influence of theological and philosophical ethics

The medical profession in the United States imbibed an ethic from the Judaeo-Christian culture of the nation. The ethical physician was expected to be respectful of religion and to be a "good Christian gentleman" (Burns, 1977). The dominant Protestant culture offered some admonitions about health and medicine. For example, the enactment of strict laws against abortion in the nineteenth century was urged by physicians with strong Protestant faith (Mohr, 1978). However, theological ethics was relatively silent on particular issues concerning medicine and health.

Roman Catholic moral theology, however, had a long tradition of concern with moral questions in medicine. Since the seventeenth century principles of Scholastic philosophy and theology had been applied to such issues as abortion, sterilization, and the duties of physician and patient. Acute analyses had been made of the duty to sustain life and the circumstances under which the death of a patient could be permitted. This tradition was conveyed to students in the Catholic medical schools that were founded in the nineteenth century. Father Charles Coppens, S.J., lectured in the Medical Department of Creighton University at the turn of the century. His book, *Moral Principles and Medical Practice: The Basis of Medical Jurisprudence,* treated abortion, sexual behavior, and the duties of physicians in light of philosophical and theological principles (Coppens, 1905). His work represented "the emergence of medical ethics as a medical school subject, especially at religiously affiliated schools" (Burns, 1980, p. 282). During the 1940s and 1950s, this tradition was carried on in the extensive writings of theologians Edwin Healy, Gerald Kelly, Charles McFadden, Francis Connell, and Patrick Finney. In 1949, the Catholic Hospital Association issued *Ethical and Religious Directives for Catholic Health Facilities* (revised in 1954 and 1971), which obliged all physicians and health professionals working in Catholic institutions to follow Catholic moral tenets with regard to a number of specific medical procedures (U.S. Catholic Conference, 1971).

Catholic reflection on medical moral issues continues in the *Linacre Quarterly,* published by the National Federation of Catholic Physicians' Guilds since 1932. Theologians Charles Curran, Richard McCormick, Kevin O'Rourke, Margaret Farley, and Lisa Sowle Cahill are now the principal voices of this tradition. The Catholic tradition, in its doctrine of natural law, has affirmed that moral questions can be analyzed from a philosophical viewpoint, without explicit reference to revealed theological truths. Thus, common ground can be found with those who do not share the Catholic faith. This somewhat nonsectarian approach has allowed Catholic analysis of problems to have a significant influence on the intellectual development of secular bioethics.

The Protestant denominations, while not producing a detailed analysis of medical-moral problems, had taken positions on such questions as suicide, euthanasia, abortion, and contraception. In 1950, Willard Sperry, Dean of Harvard Divinity School, published lectures given at Massachusetts General Hospital and the University of Michigan Medical School, entitled *The Ethical Basis of Medical Practice* (Sperry, 1950). He offered reflective, humane, literary, but unsystematic commentary on such problems as truth telling, prolongation of life, and euthanasia as the era of medical technology was opening. Four years later, Episcopal theologian Joseph Fletcher published the ground-breaking and prescient study *Morals and Medicine*. Fletcher's work was the first to emphasize the patient's rights as the center of an ethics of medicine and to argue "the ethical case for our human rights . . . to use contraceptives, to seek insemination anonymously from a donor, to be sterilized and to receive a merciful death from a medically competent euthanasist." He strongly asserted the patient's right to be told the truth about his or her diagnosis and prognosis (Fletcher, 1954, p. 25). Fletcher's book is the pioneering work of the new medical ethics.

Sixteen years later, Methodist theologian Paul Ramsey produced the foundational work of bioethics, *Patient as Person*. Ramsey, professor of religion at Princeton University, took the unusual step of spending a year in intense dialogue with physicians, scientists, and students at Georgetown University and immersing himself in the clinical activities of the Georgetown University Hospital. *Patient as Person*, first delivered as the Beecher Lectures at Yale in 1969, examined questions, such as organ transplantation, experimentation with human subjects, and the use of life-supporting technologies, that had not been on the agenda of previous commentators on the moral aspects of medicine. Although he spoke from a very different theological ground than did Fletcher, Ramsey also placed the freedom and rights of the patient at the center of his ethic but subsumed patient and physicians within the scope of a theologically defined covenant. Despite the theological tone and language of Ramsey's work, its cogent analyses of issues such as consent were widely influential. At about the same time, James Gustafson of Yale Divinity School produced thoughtful essays on the implications of medical and scientific advances (Gustafson, 1970). Many Prot-

estant theologians followed the paths laid down by these pioneers, among them Kenneth Vaux, William May, Harmon Smith, James Childress, and Stanley Hauerwas. In 1987, the Park Ridge Center for the Study of Health, Faith and Ethics was founded under the auspices of the Lutheran Hospital Association to foster religious reflection on the issues of bioethics. The center has published a fine series of volumes describing the teachings about medicine and morality of major Christian denominations and other world religions (Marty, 1983; Vaux, 1984). The distinctive features of modern bioethics begin to appear in Fletcher and Ramsey: attention to the effects of new technologies, affirmation of the centrality of the patient as free and responsible agent, and the invocation of the concepts and method of moral analysis from the classical disciplines of theology and philosophy.

The Jewish faith has an ancient tradition of reflection upon questions of life, death, health, and medical care. Issues in medical ethics, such as allocation of scarce resources, risk–benefit evaluation, quality of life, indications of death, abortion, and contraception are discussed in great detail in Talmudic literature. The doctoral thesis of Immanuel Jakobovits, published in 1959 as *Jewish Medical Ethics*, drew these teachings together and brought them into contact with modern scientific advances. In so doing, Jakobovits gave a distinct identity to a field of study that had not been previously singled out in Jewish scholarship (Jakobovits, 1959). This effort has been continued by Talmudic scholars such as Moses Tendler, David Bleich, David Feldman, and the physician Fred Rosner. The first course in Jewish medical ethics was taught by Rabbi Tendler at Yeshiva University in 1956, and the Institute for Jewish Medical Ethics was established in San Francisco in the early 1980s.

The influence of moral philosophy came rather late to the analysis of medical-moral questions. Although the first AMA code of ethics was strongly influenced by the English physician Thomas Percival, who was affected to some extent by the philosophers of the Scottish Enlightenment, American philosophers paid scant attention to these questions. In 1927, Chauncey Leake noted in his edition of *Percival's Medical Ethics* that all of the classic codes represented "medical etiquette" or the tenets of professional courtesy rather than medical ethics. "It is interesting," he wrote, "that writers on medical ethics have seldom availed themselves of the philosophical analyses of the principles of ethical theory made by recognized ethical scholars." In words that predict the bioethics movement of the 1960s, he called for a medical ethics that would bring the systems of moral philosophy to bear on the problems of medical practice (Percival, 1927, p. 3). Leake undertook to do this in a dialogue with philosopher Patrick Romanell (Leake and

Romanell, 1950). Three decades later, moral philosophers were important figures in the elaboration of ethics of health care.

Secular academic philosophy did not find it easy to approach the practical problems posed by evolving science and medicine. In the 1950s, philosophical ethics was struggling with the diverse theoretical challenges of naturalism, relativism, utilitarianism, Marxism, linguistic analysis, and positivism; hardly any attention was paid to the analysis of actual moral problems. This began to change in the 1960s as questions about the moral legitimacy of the Southeast Asian war and racial discrimination were vociferously put to professors of moral philosophy by their students. Interest in practical philosophy slowly appeared within academic philosophy. The questions of life and death raised by new technologies began to intrigue some philosophers. Nicholas Rescher wrote an early article on the allocation of "exotic medical lifesaving therapy," such as dialysis and transplantation (Rescher, 1969). Medical ethics began to be taught as an undergraduate philosophy course for which textbooks were produced (Gorovitz et al., 1973; Gorovitz, et al., 1976). Daniel Callahan, trained in the analytic philosophy tradition at Harvard, realized the ethical dimensions of the new medicine and in 1979 founded, with psychiatrist Willard Gaylin, the Institute for Society, Ethics and the Life Sciences, later renamed the Hastings Center. Although slower to enter the field of practical ethics than the theologians, philosophers such as Baruch Brody, K. Danner Clauser, Tom Beauchamp, and Stephen Toulmin made significant contributions to the methods and substantive analysis of biomedical problems. Indeed, as Toulmin has claimed, "Medical ethics saved the life of philosophy," imparting an intellectual vitality and moral urgency to a field that had turned from the moral concerns of personal and social life to arid speculation (Toulmin, 1982).

Legal scholars were also prominent in the early years of bioethics. William Curran and Paul Freund of Harvard and Jay Katz of Yale contributed to the important symposium on experimentation with human subjects sponsored by the American Academy of Arts and Sciences in 1966; Katz subsequently published major work in this area (Freund, 1970; Katz et al., 1972). John Noonan wrote perceptively on abortion and contraception. As the issues surrounding death and dying became prominent, particularly with the Karen Ann Quinlan case in 1975, lawyers became deeply involved, since law has always taken a serious interest in the determination of the causes of human death. Similarly, the evolution of the doctrine of informed consent has been strongly influenced by jurisprudence and judicial opinion. It is difficult to distinguish between the lawyer and the bioethicist in such figures as George Annas, John Robert-

son, Alexander Capron, and William Winslade. Indeed, one of these scholars has asserted, "American law, not philosophy or medicine, is primarily responsible for the agenda, development and current state of American bioethics" (Annas, 1993, p. 2).

Many physicians and scientists have become interested and adept in bioethics. However, as the field developed, the majority of its practitioners came from theology and philosophy; relatively few physicians have devoted themselves to scholarly productivity. Notable exceptions are Edmund Pellegrino, Mark Siegler, Howard Brody, Eric Cassell, and Christine Cassel. They bring to their contributions the sense and sensitivity of the practicing physician.

Although ethics was once taught in American colleges as the summit of the curriculum (often by the president of the college), as the twentieth century opened, ethics had retreated from that academic prominence to a refined and remote subspecialty of philosophy. Many believed that ethics was "caught" rather than taught. Medical ethics, it was said, was best conveyed to medical students by the example of prominent physicians, such as William Osler, as well as by the role models of the leading teachers in individual medical schools. Their lives and writings were common touchstones of discussion. Moreover, resolution of ethical issues tended to emphasize the need for the excellent overall character and reputation of the physician, that is, an ethics of virtue. This emphasis on the good intentions of the physician was congruent with the model of practice then supported by the AMA—the independent practitioner in contract with the individual patient.

Although medical jurisprudence, the study of the relationship between medical practice and the law, had been taught in American medical schools with some regularity during the nineteenth century, no course on medical ethics as such is known to have been offered until the late 1920s, except in the Catholic medical schools. The curriculum of the first known course in a secular medical school, offered by Park White at Washington University School of Medicine, St. Louis, in 1924, included discussion of group practice, consultations, relations with other practitioners, quackery, eugenics, euthanasia, and birth control (Burns, 1980). In 1926, the AMA recommended that medical ethics be made part of the medical curriculum. By 1931, it was reported that 43 percent of the sixty-seven American medical schools offered a course in medical ethics, most of these courses in the required curriculum. Approximately the same level was maintained through the 1950s, although course time was stretched to cover other subjects, such as medical sociology and economics, and it is unclear what topics were covered as medical ethics. During this era, Richard Cabot, who was both professor of medicine and professor of social ethics at Harvard, was a dominant figure. He stressed the importance of personal integrity and honesty in the physician, as had the earlier professional ethics, but placed this within the evolving framework of scientific medicine: Integrity must be manifested in clinical competence, the primary ethical obligation of the practitioner (Burns, 1977).

As the century progressed and the social and psychological sciences spread in collegiate education, discussion of the art of character development became increasingly overlaid with psychological and psychiatric analysis of the physician's character. Indeed, in the 1940s and 1950s, the Freudian model of psychological dynamics and of the doctor–patient relationship became prominent in the analyses of the virtues of physicians (Binger, 1945). Meanwhile, the increasing midcentury confidence in the social science tended to displace ethics terminology with concepts of "professional development," "human engineering," and so forth, sometimes even denigrating the admonitions of traditional morality as no more than "taboos." Ethics was often seen as so colored by religion that its teaching was bound to be covert indoctrination. In the secular climate of that time, any formal acknowledgment of ethics was suspect: Even the National Endowment for the Humanities, which eventually became a strong supporter of bioethics, originally excluded ethics from the list of the humanities whose study it would fund. Thus, ethics was rarely taught in higher education and even more rarely in medical education. This hiatus in the teaching of medical ethics during the 1950s may be seen as a prelude to the bioethics movement, in which neglected ethical questions forced their way back into the consciousness of the profession and the public alike.

The first national conference on the teaching of medical ethics was held under the sponsorship of the Institute for Society, Ethics and the Life Sciences and the Columbia University College of Physicians and Surgeons in 1972. By this time, out of 114 medical schools, only three required an ethics course and only thirty-three offered ethics as an elective (Veatch et al., 1973). The Society for Health and Human Values, formed in 1969, and its attendant Institute on Human Values in Medicine, encouraged medical ethics teaching. In the decade that followed, the number of schools providing organized teaching of ethics increased, and faculty members, often philosophers and theologians, were appointed. The content of the course shifted from the traditional topics, such as truth telling, confidentiality, care of the poor, care of the dying, and relations among practitioners, to the newer problems raised by technology and the social setting of modern medical care. In 1987, ninety-five American medical schools reported

that they required a course in medical ethics, and the Association of American Medical Colleges strongly urged the inclusion of ethics in the curriculum (Bickel, 1987).

Nursing ethics

Although medical students received little formal instruction in ethics, nursing schools developed a strong tradition of ethics teaching. Several major works on ethics were published by nurses at the turn of the century, notably *Nursing Ethics* by Isabel Hampton Robb (Robb, 1901). Although her text is marked by a stern and self-sacrificing message to nurses, it includes sensitive discussion of many aspects of nurse–patient and nurse–physician relations. Textbooks on nursing ethics published in the first two decades of the century went through many editions before fading from popularity in the 1940s and 1950s. Notable among the authors were Charlotte Aikens and Thomas Verner Moore, whose books made extensive use of case studies (Aikens, 1916; Moore, 1935). In 1931, religious educator Paul Limbert published a defense of nursing ethics courses: They were needed, he argued, to make ethical concerns explicit and to assist student nurses in interpreting their clinical experiences in such a way as to foster good professional character (Limbert, 1931). As in the medical ethics of that era, the emphasis was on the character development of the nurse rather than on principle-centered or patient-centered ethics. An important theme for nursing ethics has always been the impact of the feelings and character—the "humanness" of the practitioner—on the care and cure of the patient. As new technologies developed with increasing efficacy, practitioners felt the need to redefine the role of their personality in relationship to those technologies.

At the beginning of the twentieth century, nursing was predominantly a home-based practice; by the end of the century, it had become predominantly institutionally based. This redefinition of the nursing role provided a stimulus for some of the recurring issues in the nursing literature of the early part of the century. For instance, whether a nurse should do housework, such as washing diapers or tending the fire in the grate, was a significant issue until the 1950s. How the nurse should react to the errors of quacks and regular physicians continued to be a prominent issue. In all such cases, texts resolve the questions in terms of dedication to the welfare of patients. Indeed, nursing ethics took an early stand against permitting patients to be injured by other practitioners, including physicians, and nurses have taken an increasing role in institutional quality control.

Like physicians, nurses struggled with the problem of "irregular" practitioners. In the earliest part of the century, the "untrained nurse" was represented in the nursing ethics literature as ethically, as well as technically, incompetent. The emergence of the licensed practical nurse in the 1930s and the increasing number of nursing aides during the century have challenged professional nursing, and the ethics of relationships with these occupations has been delicate. In the 1970s, the ANA took a stand that a bachelor's-level education was necessary for professional nursing, calling into question the standing of nurses trained in hospitals and community colleges. In the 1980s, nursing was again challenged by a recommendation from the AMA, calling for the creation of a "registered care technician" to perform some of the technical functions of nurses. The ethics of the relationship of nurse to physician is still being debated in the nursing ethics literature. It is commonly asserted that power and gender relationships are central to the ethics of nursing. Original presentations of the ethics of nursing have appeared: The works of Mila Aroskar, Martin Benjamin, Joy Curtis, Anne Davis, Marsha Fowler, Sara T. Fry, Sally Gadow, Amy Haddad, Andrew Jameton, Christine Mitchell, James Myskens, and Michael Yeo are notable. Their work carries the themes of nursing ethics into the broader stream of bioethics. The bioethics movement has also touched the many other professions involved in the care of patients: dentists, occupational therapists, pharmacists, physical therapists, physician assistants, medical technicians, and social workers.

Ethical issues in the emerging biomedical technologies

In the years after World War II, the rapid advances of biomedical science were translated into clinical interventions that could save and sustain life in ways never before possible. These technological advances brought not only the benefits of improved health and prolonged life but also a range of puzzling moral questions. One of the first of these technologies to raise explicit ethical concerns was the 1961 invention by Belding Scribner at the University of Washington of a technique for chronic hemodialysis of persons with end-stage renal disease. Because the first artificial kidney center in Seattle, Washington, had limited machines and trained personnel, it could serve only a tiny portion of the 15,000 or so persons in need of such lifesaving care. A committee consisting of seven lay members and two physician-advisers was chosen to select patients who would be admitted. Those who were not admitted would die. The committee employed social criteria, such as productive livelihood and respectable citizenship, for selecting candidates from among the many medically eligible patients. There was a strong public reaction and much se-

vere criticism of using social values in life-and-death decisions (Fox and Swazey, 1974).

Philosophers and theologians noticed the issue and engaged in debate over it (Rescher, 1969; Childress, 1970; Ramsey, 1970b). The issue of rationing the scarce resource of dialysis was resolved in 1972 by an amendment to the Social Security Act providing payment for about 90 percent of the high cost of dialysis. This led to further discussion comparing the plight of other persons in high-cost disease categories, such as hemophilia, with that of kidney patients. In justice, the argument ran, various other groups ought to receive similar public aid. This early example of the ethical dilemmas posed by the new technology exemplified some of the themes that would become central to bioethics: the acceptance of lay opinion into decisions formerly reserved to physicians, the appearance of philosophical and theological analyses of the issue, the recognition of questions of fairness in application of medical resources, and the profound implications of life-and-death decisions. Indeed, the questions "Who Should Live? Who Should Die? Who Should Decide?" became almost thematic of bioethics.

The first heart transplantations were done in South Africa in 1968; similar operations were attempted shortly thereafter in the United States. Optimistic claims by medical innovators fostered public enthusiasm, which turned to disillusionment when, after three years, the very poor survival rate resulted in a virtual moratorium on heart transplants (Fox and Swazey, 1974). As heart and kidney transplantation became more-effective, ethical issues surrounding organ donorship arose. To encourage cadaver donorship, the Uniform Anatomical Gift Act was proposed by the U.S. National Conference of Commissioners on Uniform Laws in 1968 and subsequently adopted by all states (Katz et al., 1972). Because of high costs and the scarcity of organs, transplantation forcefully raised questions of whether the gains of new technology could justify the costs. At the same time, the determination of death, traditionally done by noting the cessation of cardiorespiratory functions, began to be questioned: These criteria seemed obsolete under conditions of artificial respiratory support and did not allow for removal of organs for transplantation. A vigorous debate ensued about the ethical and legal implications of shifting to clinical criteria that would focus on cessation of brain activity. In 1968, a committee at Harvard Medical School formulated a statement defining "brain death" as a criterion for declaring death (Harvard Medical School, 1968). "Brain death" criteria were accepted and legalized slowly, beginning in Kansas in 1970. Still, considerable confusion required further refinement of the concept, leading eventually to the recommendation of a Uniform Statute for the Determination of Death, which has now been adopted in most jurisdictions (U.S. President's Commission for the Study of Ethical Problems in Medicine, 1981).

During this same period, artificial implants to assist or replace the heart were being developed. Denton Cooley in Houston, Texas, unsuccessfully attempted to implant an artificial heart in 1969. In anticipation of the time when such a device might be ready for use in humans, the National Heart and Lung Institute in 1971 established a panel to study the possible ethical, social, economic, legal, medical, and psychiatric consequences of its development. This was the first effort by the federal government to explore the ethical implications of new medical technologies (National Heart and Lung Institute, 1973; Jonsen, 1973). The first actual implantation of an artificial heart—in Barney Clark, at Salt Lake City in 1982—aroused considerable debate about the appropriateness of this device (Shaw, 1984).

By the mid-1960s, issues of research ethics had begun to ferment among scientists (Ladimer and Newman, 1963). The Nuremberg trials in 1947 revealed the horrors of the Nazi concentration camps, where cruel and lethal medical experiments were performed on prisoners. Several articles on the ethics of human experimentation had appeared in the American medical literature, but the ethical issues of biomedical experimentation with human beings were not widely discussed, perhaps because many believed that nothing so horrible could happen here (Alexander, 1949; Annas and Grodin, 1992). However, during World War II, the intense efforts to improve the capabilities of military medicine spurred researchers occasionally to design experiments in which persons were treated dangerously and without their consent. In the years after the war, biomedical research was fueled by large infusions of funds from the newly expanded National Institutes of Health, and research projects were sponsored in hospitals throughout the country. As the volume and intensity of research increased, questionable practices appeared and were tolerated as the price to be paid in the war against disease. Informed consent of research subjects was rarely obtained, and oversight by anyone other than the researcher was unusual. In 1962, a number of children were born with serious congenital defects due to their mothers' ingestion of thalidomide, an unapproved drug. This tragedy stimulated congressional hearings at which the ethics of human experimentation, then largely uncontrolled, was aired. Subsequently, amendments to the Federal Food, Drug and Cosmetic Act in 1964 required full and free consent of all subjects of drug trials.

In 1966, Henry Beecher, professor of anesthesia at Harvard, brought problems in the ethics of experimentation to the attention of the medical community. He detailed twenty-two medical experiments carried on by respected investigators that he branded as unethical due to lack of consent or inappropriate assessment of risks in relation to benefits (Beecher, 1966; Rothman, 1991). In 1966 (with revisions in 1968) the U.S. Public Health Service formulated guidelines for protection of rights and welfare of human subjects in all federally supported research. In 1971, these guidelines became regulations of the Department of Health, Education, and Welfare, requiring research institutions to set up medical and lay panels to review all federally funded experimentation in order to ensure that subjects are informed and freely consent to the research procedure, and to determine that the scientific benefits justify the risks of the research (Levine, 1986).

A number of scandals in research ethics brought public attention to the need for regulation. At Willowbrook State Hospital in New York, from 1965 to 1971 a series of studies on hepatitis involved inoculating mentally retarded children with hepatitis virus. At the Jewish Chronic Disease Hospital in Brooklyn in 1963, live cancer cells were injected into senile patients without their knowledge or consent. In 1971 a study begun in the 1930s at Tuskegee, Alabama, came to public attention: A number of rural black men suffering from syphilis had been left untreated in order to ascertain the "natural history" of the untreated disease (Jones, 1981). In response to these and several other scandals, the U.S. Congress established the National Commission for the Protection of Human Subjects in Biomedical and Behavioral Research (1974–1977) to make recommendations for federal policy on the broad problems of human subjects in research as well as the special problems posed by research with fetuses, children, prisoners, and other dependent or vulnerable persons. These recommendations were codified in federal regulations and are now widely enforced in research institutions. The field of bioethics was significantly advanced by the work of this commission. Several scholars in ethics sat on the commission, and many philosophers, theologians, lawyers, and sociologists were asked to contribute to its deliberations, thereby stimulating thought about the issues and making public careful analyses of the problems and principles. Its *Belmont Report,* stating the principles of research with human subjects, first enunciated the triad of bioethical principles: autonomy, beneficence, and justice (National Commission for the Protection of Human Subjects, 1978).

It has become increasingly common during the twentieth century for people to die in a hospital, often under conditions of dehumanizing technology. This reawakened age-old discussions of death, dying, and euthanasia, now in light of the new technical potential of modern medicine. Although there had been several unsuccessful attempts to sanction euthanasia legally in the early years of the century, death and dying had become a taboo subject in medicine. Elisabeth Kübler-Ross's sensitive interviews with dying patients did much to awaken interest in the psychology of dying (Kübler-Ross, 1969).

In 1976, the state of California passed novel legislation about termination of life support. The Natural Death Act authorized patients to sign a legal document directing physicians to remove or to withhold life-support devices under carefully defined circumstances. Many states have followed California by enacting legal forms of "advance directives" to guide physicians in following the wishes of their dying, incompetent patients. In 1976 a New Jersey Supreme Court decision allowed the parents of Karen Ann Quinlan—a young woman quite dead by the Harvard brain death criteria, but who could be maintained indefinitely on a respirator with no hope of recovery—to have their daughter removed from the respirator after a much-publicized debate over the right to die and active and passive euthanasia (*In the Matter of Karen Ann Quinlan,* 1976). Subsequent judicial decisions in many states and one U.S. Supreme Court decision—*Cruzan v. Missouri Health Department* (1990)—have elucidated the conditions under which life support might be forgone. Many of these decisions have been influenced by the bioethical literature. In the 1990s, the debate over legalization of active euthanasia was renewed, spurred by the Hemlock Society, which advocated legislation that would authorize physicians to provide "aid in dying" at the request of terminal patients. These questions about the nature of appropriate care for the terminally ill, as well as many other ethical questions, are made more urgent by the increase in the numbers of elderly people in the United States: Since the turn of the century, the number of Americans over the age of sixty-five has tripled in proportion to the general population (Jecker, 1991).

In 1978, the U.S. Congress reestablished the National Commission for the Protection of Human Subjects of Biomedical Research as the U.S. President's Commission for the Study of Ethical Problems in Medicine and in Biomedical and Behavioral Research. Among the new commission's mandates were studies of brain death, genetic screening, access to health care, and use of life-sustaining technologies (U.S. President's Commission, 1981, 1983a, 1983b, 1983c). Like its predecessor, it called on scholars from many disciplines to contribute to its deliberations. Its reports make up a veritable canon of bioethics.

The ascendancy of technological medicine inspired critical study of the nature of the health-care professions and institutions. Popular and academic works investigated the conceptions of health employed in medicine and the efficacy of medical services offered (Illich, 1976). They explored the nature and authority of the health professions and raised questions about ethical responsibilities of health professionals whose attitudes are shaped by economic and social forces (Freidson, 1970). The proper role of health professionals has been questioned in many contexts, including the right of health professionals to strike and the extent to which they bear responsibility for patients' lives, for behavioral factors affecting health, and for social and political factors causing disease. The helplessness of individuals in the face of a massive medical establishment led to a patients' rights movement. As evidence of this concern, the American Hospital Association published *A Patient's Bill of Rights* in 1973, with the suggestion that it be adopted by all hospitals.

Reproduction and reproductive technology also fostered debate. During the first part of the century, birth control was an important issue in the feminist movement. Not until the late 1960s were restrictions on the use and teaching of birth control removed in most states. The feminist movement, especially through Margaret Sanger, also sponsored and encouraged research on new birth-control methods (Gordon, 1976). In the 1960s abortion became a center of debate. The discussion began with the American Law Institute's model statute permitting abortion for medical and psychological conditions as well as after rape and for fetal defect. The "responsibility for pregnancy" issue for the most part dropped from the debate as it became an issue of women's right to control their bodies, on one side, and the claim of the fetus's right to life, on the other, a claim largely, although not exclusively, urged by Catholics. The U.S. Supreme Court in *Roe v. Wade* (1973) chose a position protecting the mother's decision in the first trimester of the pregnancy, with increasing possibility for legal restrictions during the second and third trimesters. Abortion, because of its intriguing questions about personhood, stimulated considerable professional, philosophical, and theological reflection (Callahan, 1970; Grisez, 1970). That reflection has, in the 1990s, ceded to vigorous, even violent political activism. Whether the reflection or the activism will prevail in policy remains to be seen.

In the 1960s, advances in genetics and reproductive technology caused much speculation about social consequences of such possible innovations as cloning, in vitro fertilization, and extrauterine gestation (Ramsey, 1970a). Interest in the potential and the dangers of genetic manipulation was heightened by the development of recombinant DNA technology in the mid-1970s. Amniocentesis (a test to diagnose certain fetal disorders during early pregnancy) and improvements in genetic history-taking made possible the development of genetic counseling as a profession in the late 1960s, with attendant ethical questions (Hilton et al., 1973). Many questions considered speculative in the 1980s have come close to realization today. The federally sponsored project to map the entire human genome has become a focus for the study of the ethical questions involved in genetic diagnosis, treatment, and social policy (Juengst and Watson, 1991). In 1992, the National Advisory Board on Ethics and Reproduction was established as a private entity to examine and advise on these questions.

Questions about the biological basis of personality, achievement, and social behavior continued to arise. In the early part of the century the eugenics movement fostered many state laws requiring or allowing sterilization of persons with mental retardation or illness. Debate over sterilization arose again around 1970, when protection of women and minority groups against pressure for sterilization became an issue. The role of genetics in behavior continued to be debated with the development of sociobiology and studies on IQ and heredity. There was disagreement over the goals of genetic counseling, as well as over whether genetic factors in behavior could or should be identified. Screening of populations for genetically determined conditions was much debated (U.S. President's Commission, 1983c; Holzman, 1989).

Biology and behavior was also an issue in treatment of mental disorders by surgical methods. Prefrontal lobotomy was widely used but much debated after its introduction in 1935. With improvements in surgical techniques in the 1960s, new types of brain surgery were attempted for treatment of violence and other indications. The use of psychosurgery on prisoners became a public issue (Valenstein, 1974). The National Commission for Protection of Human Subjects issued a report on this practice that recommended only its strictly controlled experimental application. A related but quite different form of brain surgery involves the implantation of tissue from aborted fetuses into those suffering from certain neurological and endocrine disorders. This practice, initiated in the late 1980s, aroused great debate. Several advisory committees convened by the National Institutes of Health approved this form of research as acceptable public policy, yet the federal government refused for almost six years to fund studies (Vawter et al., 1990). This research was finally approved by the Clinton administration in 1993.

Although psychosurgery is the most physically invasive mode of treatment for behavioral problems, all levels of psychiatric treatment were subject to ethical inquiry. The warrant and nature of involuntary commitment to mental hospitals had been a source of contention for many years (Rothman, 1980). Commitment laws in many of the United States were modified in the 1960s to increase protection of individuals from arbitrary commitment, although at the same time, the policy of deinstitutionalization thrust many mental patients into a world for which they were unprepared. The right of hospitalized mental patients to receive treatment was established in the United States initially by the Supreme Court decision in *Wyatt v. Stickney* (1972). The use of

drugs in treating psychiatric disorders became an issue after chlorpromazine and related major tranquilizers became widely available in the 1950s, reducing the need for hospitalization. The use of medicines and medical language in treatment of behavioral problems came under attack from radical psychiatrists such as Thomas Szasz (Szasz, 1961). Goals and values in psychotherapy came to the fore in discussions about treating patients who manifested "antisocial" behavior. The growth of behaviorism and behavior modification seemed also to challenge traditional libertarian values.

In 1981, a previously unknown disorder of the immune system appeared, at first in men known to engage in homosexual activities. This disorder, named acquired immunodeficiency syndrome (AIDS), was quickly traced to a bloodborne retroviral infection. The resulting disease was relatively slow to appear but was, given the therapeutic possibilities available, inevitably fatal. It spread in epidemic fashion among gay men and among those who shared needles while taking drugs intravenously. Fear of the disease and widespread homophobia led to discriminatory actions against those infected. Old ethical questions about restricting freedom of persons suspected of having a communicable disease were revived. Public-health needs appeared to conflict with personal rights. The duty of health-care professionals to treat infected persons was vigorously debated, as was the right of infected care providers to practice. Bioethics, by now adept at the discussion of practical ethics, made a major contribution to these debates (Bayer, 1989).

The problem of just allocation of health care had been noticed in the earliest days of bioethics. However, at that time it was largely defined in terms of selection of patients for rare and expensive technologies, such as dialysis. In the early 1980s, it was recognized that some thirty-five million Americans were not covered by any health-care insurance (U.S. President's Commission, 1983b; Dougherty, 1988; Churchill, 1987). Ethical questions about the justice of such a system were raised just as health-policy experts began to note the rapid inflation in health-care costs. Lack of access to care competed with cost containment in public debate and political maneuvering. These problems became central to the concerns of many bioethicists, who began to produce acute analyses of the issues of justice in the health-care system and its financial base. These ethicists raised and examined the politically unpalatable issue of rationing of health-care resources (Daniels, 1985; Callahan, 1988; Menzel, 1990).

Academic bioethics

As the 1970s opened, a number of scholars were beginning to attempt to analyze these issues within the perspectives and methodologies of the disciplines traditionally concerned with ethics: philosophy and theology. As these scholars began to publish and communicate, a distinct field of study called bioethics came into being. The word "bioethics" was first applied to the ethics of population and environment (Potter, 1971), and soon became the rubric for a diverse collection of considerations about the ethical issues inherent in health care and the biological sciences (Callahan, 1973). The term, although considered unsatisfactory even by some of those who employed it, was canonized by the inauguration of the *Encyclopedia of Bioethics* project in 1972 and by the publication of that work in 1978 (Reich, 1978). The scholars in this new field now come from many disciplines, such as theology, philosophy, social sciences, and law. It concentrates on a specific set of issues, such as those mentioned above, and employs a range of analytic methodologies, explained in texts such as *Principles of Biomedical Ethics* (Beauchamp and Childress, 1989) for the more theoretical questions and in *Clinical Ethics* (Jonsen et al., 1992) for the more practical questions. It has professors, students, texts, journals, learned societies, and research centers. In 1993, a dozen graduate programs offered higher degrees to students trained in the topics and methods of the field.

Bioethicists show considerable interest in the theoretical definition of the field and its methodologies. Albert Jonsen and André Hellegers published an assay in the early era of the field's existence in which they saw it as a mélange of traditional professional ethics, philosophical ethics, and theological ethics (Jonsen and Hellegers, 1974). Robert Veatch, however, was the first to attempt a full exposition of the theoretical underpinnings of bioethics. His *Theory of Medical Ethics* set the field firmly on the ethical considerations relative to autonomy of the patient (Veatch, 1981). H. Tristram Engelhardt, Jr., followed with *The Foundations of Bioethics*, an even more strongly stated thesis about autonomy as the basis of the discipline (Engelhardt, 1986). However, some have asserted that bioethics, while it had its origins in the strong affirmation of autonomy for patients, may have moved too far in this direction and thereby neglected other aspects of health care, such as benevolence, community, and social justice.

The study of bioethics, together with other fields in applied ethics, has inspired much debate about the methods appropriate to studying practical ethics in general. Many of these nascent methods have lent a richer, more detailed texture to ethical discussion than is permitted by principle- and theory-based ethics. The long-abandoned casuistry that employs rhetorical and analogical reasoning to examine cases is now being viewed with renewed and critical interest (Jonsen and Toulmin, 1988; Arras, 1991). Mathematical decision analysis has been used to study values through systematically related cases (Smith and Wigton, 1987).

Stories, real and fictional, are used as texts open to moral interpretation according to the methods of hermeneutics (Brody, 1987; Hunter, 1991), and phenomenology seeks to capture the ethical subtleties of clinical encounters (Zaner, 1988; Carson, 1990). Echoing the language of ethics from the nineteenth century, but with much greater attention to depth and detail, interest in virtue- and character-based ethics is vigorous (Drane, 1988; Shelp, 1985).

Although the early development of bioethics was dominated by male scholars, women such as Elizabeth Fee, Renée Fox, Loretta Kopelman, Karen Lebacqz, Ruth Macklin, Ruth Purtilo, and Judith Swazey have made significant contributions to theoretical and practical bioethics, and feminist ethics has begun to attract much attention. Feminist bioethics offers social criticism of the treatment of women as patients and physicians, discusses the interrelationship between gender and power, provides fresh analyses of issues of traditional concern to women (such as pregnancy, birth, and reproductive choices), and emphasizes important theoretical concepts—such as caring, community, and responsibility—neglected by male scholars (Holmes and Purdy, 1992; Sherwin, 1992).

Other authors note the ethnocentricity of U.S. bioethics; it has been charged with a failure to reflect the concerns of people of color, and new work is beginning to appear that increasingly reflects diverse viewpoints. Collections of narratives of the black experience with disease and health care have begun to appear (Secundy and Nixon, 1992; White, 1990). Authors discuss the tensions between expressed philosophical ideals and systematic patterns of discrimination, such as abuses of birth control, sterilization, and selection of subjects for research (Dula, 1991; Flack and Pellegrino, 1992). Moreover, U.S. bioethics is becoming more international and less ethnocentric in its concerns: American bioethicists visit many nations and bioethicists from around the world spend time in American programs, stimulating cross-cultural comparisons and analyses (Fox and Swazey, 1984; Harding, 1987; Sagoff, 1991).

The tendency of ethics researchers to study clinical questions cooperatively with clinicians has inspired empirical study of ethics in health care. This in turn has fostered cooperation between the social sciences and normative philosophical ethics. Termed the "contextual approach" by some authors, it has begun to call attention to significant social and cultural features of life that affect ethical expression and debate (Weisz, 1990; Thomasma, 1984). Some researchers have used in-depth ethnographic techniques, such as participant observation and interviews, to study the microcontext of clinical settings; others are employing epidemiological methods to ascertain frequency of behaviors, such as resuscitation. The empirical social sciences and philosophy are beginning to converse with each other on the common ground of bioethics (Guellemin and Holmstrom, 1986; Bosk, 1979).

In the 1970s, as faculty members were appointed to teach ethics in medical schools, it became common for the ethicist to accompany physicians on teaching rounds. This led to the participation of ethicists in consultations about cases that presented particularly difficult ethical decisions. This practice came to be called clinical ethics. In 1977, ethicist John Fletcher was appointed assistant for bioethics to the director, Clinical Center, National Institutes of Heath, with responsibility for ethics consultation. Since philosophy itself provides little guidance about how to assist in actual decision making, various methods were devised to apply principles to practice. Clinical ethics spread from university hospitals to community hospitals; many individuals, physicians and philosophers alike, now act as clinical ethics consultants. The *Journal of Clinical Ethics* was initiated in 1991, and the Society for Bioethics Consultation enrolls some 300 persons who engage in clinical consultation. As might be expected, some dispute surrounds the idea and practice of ethics consultation, since it seems to imply that some persons are "ethical experts," a notion rather foreign to a morally pluralistic culture (Fletcher et al., 1989).

As the field of bioethics was beginning to form and as yet lacked institutional support for regular teaching and discussion, conferences and symposia were an important source for developing literature, teaching, and publicity. Some of the more important early conferences were the Joseph P. Kennedy, Jr., Foundation's International Conference on Abortion, held in 1967 in Washington, D.C.; a New York Academy of Sciences' Conference, New Dimensions in Legal and Ethical Concepts for Human Research (Ladimer and Newman, 1963); the U.S. National Academy of Sciences Institute of Medicine's conference Health Care and Changing Values in 1973; a series of transdisciplinary symposia on philosophy and medicine, the first of which was held in Galveston, Texas, in 1974 (Engelhardt and Spicker, 1975); and the 1975 conference Experiments and Research with Humans: Values in Conflict, sponsored by the National Academy of Sciences (National Academy of Sciences, 1975). In the 1990s, such conferences, on a wide variety of topics, are announced at a dizzying pace.

Several privately funded institutes are devoted primarily to the study of bioethics. The Institute of Religion, established in 1954 at the Texas Medical Center, Houston, began to devote attention to bioethical issues in the late 1960s. The Society for Health and Human Values evolved in 1969 from a smaller interdisciplinary group that had formed the Committee on Health and Human Values in 1963 with support from the ecumeni-

cal United Ministries in Higher Education. The society, with some 700 members, provides a meeting place for a variety of individuals from all disciplines who are interested in the medical humanities; in its early years, it sponsored the Institute on Human Values in Medicine. The Institute of Society, Ethics and the Life Sciences, now officially named the Hastings Center, founded in 1969 by Daniel Callahan and Willard Gaylin, investigates social, legal, and ethical aspects of the health sciences. In conducts a program for visiting fellows and associates; publishes the most widely read of the ethics journals, *Hastings Center Report*, and *IRB: A Review of Human Subjects Research*; organizes study groups on special topics; and conducts courses for health professionals and others. In 1993, the Hastings Center had ninety-seven fellows and almost 12,000 members.

For several years in the 1970s, the Joseph P. Kennedy, Jr., Foundation funded the Interfaculty Program in Medical Ethics, which joined Harvard University's Medical School, School of Public Health, and Divinity School to train scholars in this new field. In 1971 André Hellegers founded the Joseph and Rose Kennedy Institute for the Study of Human Reproduction and Bioethics, now known as the Kennedy Institute of Ethics, at Georgetown University. This program, initially financed by the Kennedy Foundation, has supported research by permanent and visiting scholars, courses and workshops in bioethics, and cooperative and consulting programs with private and governmental institutions. The Kennedy Institute has specialized in the creation of fundamental research tools in the field of bioethics. Starting in 1972, the institute sponsored Warren Reich's project for the preparation of the *Encyclopedia of Bioethics,* a landmark in U.S. bioethical studies (Reich, 1978). Its National Resource Center prepares the computer-based bibliography of bioethical literature called Bioethicsline, a part of the National Library of Medicine's Medlars network, which is also published in book form as *Bibliography of Bioethics* (Walters, 1975–). The Kennedy Institute originated the important *Journal of Philosophy and Medicine,* which is now published independently, and currently produces the *Kennedy Institute of Ethics Journal.* In 1993, the American Association of Bioethics came into existence to promote the exchange of ideas among bioethics scholars, encourage the development of new scholars, and maintain contact with international societies in bioethics.

As bioethics flowered, many ethical issues were being debated as matters of public policy. Some bioethicists found themselves working as public employees to aid in policy formation, and others served as members of and consultants to advisory bodies such as the National Commission for the Protection of Human Subjects, the U.S. President's Commission, the now defunct Ethics Advisory Board of the Department of

Health and Human Services, and state bodies such as New York's Task Force on Life and the Law and New Jersey's Bioethics Commission. Ten of the eighty-two "special government employees" working with the 1993 Clinton Task Force on Reform of Health Care were persons identifiable as bioethicists. Beyond these official bodies, several thousand physicians, nurses, clergy, and laypersons sit, often with bioethicists, on the hospital ethics committees that have, since the 1980s, become part of most medical centers in the United States. Grassroots bioethics activities, such as the Oregon Health Decisions Project, strive to involve laypersons in making decisions about the ethics of health-care allocation policy. Bioethics has become, to some extent, a philosophy for the people.

The bioethics movement has demonstrated extraordinary vitality in the United States since the 1970s. Its work effected significant changes in the practices of health care. Its first historian, David Rothman, wrote, "The record since 1966, I believe, makes a convincing case for a fundamental transformation in the substance as well as the style of medical decision making" (Rothman, 1991, p. 251). That transformation consists largely in the flow of lay opinion and judgment into the formerly closed world of medical decision and policy, in both clinical and research settings.

By the 1990s, bioethics was firmly established as a field of study within academic settings. This gives it a prestige and institutional base that it had previously lacked, but that may also imperil its vitality and independence. Although initially seen by some as a fad, bioethics is linked with social and personal issues deeply rooted in the culture of the United States during the twentieth century. The impact of technology on human life, the distribution of increasingly scarce health resources in an otherwise affluent society, the role of government in the pursuit of health by individuals and populations, and the voice of the consumer-patient in decisions about medical care—all these issues are central to the concerns of bioethics. Inevitably, ethical issues in the life sciences also embrace the larger social problems of environment and population. It is likely that the diffuse field of bioethics will take shape as it increasingly finds its place in the education of future health professionals, as it becomes part of the attempt by schools and consumer organizations to increase personal responsibility for health and environment, and as it attends to the formulation of public policy about social life in the biosphere.

ALBERT R. JONSEN
ANDREW JAMETON

While all the articles in the other sections of this entry are relevant, see the companion articles in this section, espe-

cially COLONIAL NORTH AMERICA AND NINETEENTH-CENTURY UNITED STATES. *Directly related to this article are the entries* BIOETHICS; HEALTH-CARE DELIVERY; HEALTH-CARE FINANCING; MEDICINE AS A PROFESSION; NURSING AS A PROFESSION; PATIENTS' RIGHTS, *article on* ORIGIN AND NATURE OF PATIENTS' RIGHTS; PROFESSIONAL–PATIENT RELATIONSHIP; *and* PROFESSION AND PROFESSIONAL ETHICS. *For a further discussion of topics mentioned in this article, see the entries* ACADEMIC HEALTH CENTERS; ALTERNATIVE THERAPIES, *article on* SOCIAL HISTORY; BIOETHICS EDUCATION; CLINICAL ETHICS, *article on* ELEMENTS AND METHODOLOGIES; DEATH, DEFINITION AND DETERMINATION OF; DEATH AND DYING: EUTHANASIA AND SUSTAINING LIFE; ETHICS, *article on* TASK OF ETHICS; MEDICAL EDUCATION; PUBLIC POLICY AND BIOETHICS; *and* TECHNOLOGY, *article on* HISTORY OF MEDICAL TECHNOLOGY. *For a discussion of related ideas, see the entries* AUTONOMY; BENEFICENCE; COMPETENCE; INFORMATION DISCLOSURE; *and* INFORMED CONSENT, *article on* HISTORY OF INFORMED CONSENT. *See also the* APPENDIX (CODES, OATHS, AND DIRECTIVES RELATED TO BIOETHICS), SECTION II: ETHICAL DIRECTIVES FOR THE PRACTICE OF MEDICINE, *and* SECTION III: ETHICAL DIRECTIVES FOR OTHER HEALTH-CARE PROFESSIONS.

Bibliography

AIKENS, CHARLOTTE. 1916. *Studies in Ethics for Nurses.* Philadelphia: W. B. Saunders.

ALEXANDER, LEO. 1949. "Medical Science Under Dictatorship." *New England Journal of Medicine* 241, no. 2:39–47.

AMERICAN HOSPITAL ASSOCIATION. 1973. *A Patient's Bill of Rights.* Chicago: Author.

ANNAS, GEORGE J. 1993. *Standard of Care: The Law of American Bioethics.* New York: Oxford University Press.

ANNAS, GEORGE J., and GRODIN, MICHAEL A. 1992. *The Nazi Doctors and the Nuremberg Code: Human Rights in Human Experimentation.* New York: Oxford University Press.

ARRAS, JOHN D. 1991. "Getting Down to Cases: The Revival of Casuistry in Bioethics." *Journal of Medicine and Philosophy* 16, no. 1:29–51.

BAYER, RONALD. 1989. *Private Acts and Social Consequences: AIDS and the Politics of Public Health.* New York: Free Press.

BEAUCHAMP, TOM L., and CHILDRESS, JAMES F. 1989. *Principles of Biomedical Ethics.* 3d ed. New York: Oxford University Press.

BEECHER, HENRY K. 1966. "Ethics and Clinical Research." *New England Journal of Medicine* 274, no. 24:1354–1360.

BERLANT, JEFFREY L. 1975. *Profession and Monopoly: A Study of Medicine in the United States and Great Britain.* Berkeley: University of California Press.

BICKEL, JANET. 1987. "Human Values Teaching Programs in the Clinical Education of Medical Students." *Journal of Medical Education* 62, no. 5:369–378.

BINGER, CARL A. L. 1945. *The Doctor's Job.* New York: W. W. Norton.

BOSK, CHARLES L. 1979. *Forgive and Remember: Managing Medical Failure.* Chicago: University of Chicago Press.

BRODY, HOWARD. 1987. *Stories of Sickness.* New Haven, Conn.: Yale University Press.

BURNS, CHESTER R. 1977. "Richard Clark Cabot (1868–1939) and Reformation in American Medical Ethics." *Bulletin of the History of Medicine* 51, no. 3:353–368.

———. 1980. "Medical Ethics and Jurisprudence." In *The Education of American Physicians: Historical Essays,* pp. 273–289. Edited by Ronald L. Numbers. Berkeley: University of California Press.

BURROW, JAMES G. 1963. *AMA: Voice of American Medicine.* Baltimore: Johns Hopkins University Press.

———. 1977. *Organized Medicine in the Progressive Era: The Move Toward Monopoly.* Baltimore: Johns Hopkins University Press.

CALLAHAN, DANIEL. 1970. *Abortion: Law, Choice, and Morality.* New York: Macmillan.

———. 1973. "Bioethics as a Discipline." *Hastings Center Studies* 1, no. 1:66–73.

———. 1988. *Setting Limits: Medical Goals in an Aging Society.* New York: Simon and Schuster.

CARSON, RONALD A. 1990. "Interpretive Bioethics: The Way of Discernment." *Theoretical Medicine* 11, no. 1:51–59.

CASSEL, CHRISTINE K., and JAMETON, ANDREW. 1982. "Medical Responsibility and Thermonuclear War." *Annals of Internal Medicine* 97, no. 3:426–432.

CHILDRESS, JAMES F. 1970. "Who Shall Live When Not All Can Live?" *Soundings* 53:339–355.

CHURCHILL, LARRY R. 1987. *Rationing Health Care in America: Perceptions and Principles of Justice.* Notre Dame, Ind.: University of Notre Dame Press.

COPPENS, CHARLES. 1905. *Moral Principles and Medical Practice: The Basis of Medical Jurisprudence.* 4th rev. ed. New York: Benziger Brothers.

DANIELS, NORMAN. 1985. *Just Health Care.* Cambridge: At the University Press.

DAVIS, LOYAL EDWARD. 1960. *Fellowship of Surgeons: A History of the American College of Surgeons.* Springfield, Ill.: Charles Thomas.

DOUGHERTY, CHARLES J. 1988. *American Health Care: Realities, Rights, and Reforms.* New York: Oxford University Press.

DRANE, JAMES F. 1988. *Becoming a Good Doctor: The Place of Virtue and Character in Medical Ethics.* Kansas City, Mo.: Sheed and Ward.

DULA, ANNETTE. 1991. "Toward an African-American Perspective on Bioethics." *Journal of Health Care for the Poor and Underserved* 2, no. 2:259–269.

ENGELHARDT, H. TRISTRAM, JR. 1986. *The Foundations of Bioethics.* New York: Oxford University Press.

ENGELHARDT, H. TRISTRAM, JR., and SPICKER, STUART F., eds. 1975. *Evaluation and Explanation in the Biomedical Sciences: Proceedings of the First Trans-Disciplinary Symposium on Philosophy and Medicine, Held at Galveston, May 9–11, 1974.* Dordrecht, Netherlands: D. Reidel.

FEIN, RASHI. 1986. *Medical Care, Medical Costs: The Search for a Health Insurance Policy.* Cambridge, Mass.: Harvard University Press.

FLACK, HARLEY E., and PELLEGRINO, EDMUND D., eds. 1992. *African-American Perspectives in Biomedical Ethics.* Washington, D.C.: Georgetown University Press.

FLETCHER, JOHN C.; QUIST, NORMAN; and JONSEN, ALBERT, R., eds. 1989. *Ethics Consultation in Health Care.* Ann Arbor, Mich.: Health Administration Press.

FLETCHER, JOSEPH F. 1954. *Morals and Medicine: The Moral Problems of the Patient's Right to Know the Truth, Contraception, Artificial Insemination, Sterilization, Euthanasia.* Princeton, N.J.: Princeton University Press.

FLEXNER, ABRAHAM. 1910. *Medical Education in the United States and Canada.* Carnegie Foundation for the Advancement of Teaching, Bulletin no. 4. New York: Carnegie Foundation.

FOX, RENÉE C., and SWAZEY, JUDITH F. 1974. *The Courage to Fail: A Social View of Organ Transplants and Dialysis.* Chicago: University of Chicago Press.

———. 1984. "Medical Morality Is Not Bioethics: Medical Ethics in China and the United States." *Perspectives in Biology and Medicine* 27, no. 3:336–360.

FREIDSON, ELIOTT. 1970. *The Profession of Medicine: A Study of the Sociology of Applied Knowledge.* New York: Harper & Row.

FREUND, PAUL A., ed. 1970. *Experimentation with Human Subjects.* New York: George Braziller.

GEIGER, H. JACK. 1971. "Hidden Professional Roles: The Physician as Reactionary, Reformer, Revolutionary." *Social Policy* 1, no. 6:24–33.

GEWITZ, NORMAN, ed. 1988. *Other Healers: Unorthodox Medicine in America.* Baltimore: Johns Hopkins University Press.

GILLIGAN, CAROL. 1982. *In a Different Voice: Psychological Theory and Women's Development.* Cambridge, Mass.: Harvard University Press.

GORDON, LINDA W. 1976. *Woman's Body, Woman's Rights: A Social History of Birth Control in America.* New York: Grossman.

GOROVITZ, SAMUEL; JAMETON, ANDREW L.; MACKLIN, RUTH; O'CONNOR, JOHN M.; PERRIN, EUGENE V.; ST. CLAIR, BEVERLY PAGE; and SHERWIN, SUSAN, eds. 1976. *Moral Problems in Medicine.* Englewood Cliffs, N.J.: Prentice-Hall.

GOROVITZ, SAMUEL; MACKLIN, RUTH; JAMETON, ANDREW; SHERWIN, SUSAN; PERRIN, EUGENE V.; and O'CONNOR, JOHN. 1973. *Teaching Medical Ethics: A Report on One Approach.* Cleveland: Case Western Reserve University, Department of Philosophy and School of Medicine.

GRISEZ, GERMAIN G. 1970. *Abortion: The Myths, the Realities, and the Arguments.* New York: Corpus.

GUELLEMIN, JEANNE HARLEY, and HOLMSTROM, LYNDA LYTLE. 1986. *Mixed Blessings: Intensive Care for Newborns.* New York: Oxford University Press.

GUSTAFSON, JAMES. 1970. "Basic Ethical Issues in the Bio-Medical Field." *Soundings* 53:430–455.

HARDING, SANDRA. 1987. "The Curious Coincidence of Feminine and African Moralities: Challenges for Feminist Theory." In *Women and Moral Theory,* pp. 296–315. Edited by Eva Feder Kittay and Diana T. Meyers. Totowa, N.J.: Rowman and Littlefield.

HARVARD MEDICAL SCHOOL. AD HOC COMMITTEE OF THE HARVARD MEDICAL SCHOOL TO EXAMINE THE DEFINITION

OF BRAIN DEATH. 1968. "A Definition of Irreversible Coma." *Journal of the American Medical Association* 205, no. 6:337–340.

HILTON, BRUCE; CALLAHAN, DANIEL; HARRIS, MAUREEN; CONDLIFFE, PETER; and BERKELEY, BURTON, eds. 1973. *Ethical Issues in Human Genetics: Genetic Counseling and the Use of Genetic Knowledge.* Fogarty International Proceedings, no. 13. New York: Plenum.

HOLMES, HELEN BEQUAERT, and PURDY, LAURA MARTHA, eds. 1992. *Feminist Perspectives in Medical Ethics.* Bloomington: Indiana University Press.

HOLTZMAN, NEIL A. 1989. *Proceed with Caution: Predicting Genetic Risks in the Recombinant DNA Era.* Baltimore: Johns Hopkins University Press.

HUNTER, KATHRYN MONTGOMERY. 1991. *Doctors' Stories: The Narrative Structure of Medical Knowledge.* Princeton, N.J.: Princeton University Press.

ILLICH, IVAN. 1976. *Medical Nemesis: The Expropriation of Health.* New York: Pantheon.

In the Matter of Karen Ann Quinlan. 1976. 2 vols. Arlington, Va.: University Publications of America.

JAKOBOVITS, IMMANUEL. 1959. *Jewish Medical Ethics: A Comparative and Historical Study of the Jewish Religious Attitude to Medicine and Its Practice.* New York: Bloch.

JECKER, NANCY, ed. 1991. *Aging and Ethics: Philosophical Problems in Gerontology.* Clifton, N.Y.: Humana.

JONES, JAMES H. 1981. *Bad Blood: The Tuskegee Syphilis Experiment.* New York: Free Press.

JONSEN, ALBERT R. 1973. "The Totally Implantable Artificial Heart." *Hastings Center Report* 3, no. 6:1–4.

———. 1990. *The New Medicine and the Old Ethics.* Cambridge, Mass.: Harvard University Press.

JONSEN, ALBERT R., and HELLEGERS, ANDRÉ E. 1974. "Conceptual Foundations for an Ethics of Medical Care." In *Ethics of Health Care: Papers of the Conference on Health Care and Changing Values, November 27–29, 1973,* pp. 3–20. Edited by Laurence R. Tancredi. Washington, D.C.: National Academy of Sciences.

JONSEN, ALBERT R., and JAMETON, ANDREW. 1977. "Social and Political Responsibilities of Physicians." *Journal of Medicine and Philosophy* 2, no. 4:376–400.

JONSEN, ALBERT R.; SIEGLER, MARK; and WINSLADE, WILLIAM J. 1992. *Clinical Ethics: A Practical Approach to Ethical Decisions in Clinical Medicine.* 3d ed. New York: Macmillan.

JONSEN, ALBERT R., and TOULMIN, STEPHEN E. 1988. *The Abuse of Casuistry: A History of Moral Reasoning.* Berkeley: University of California Press.

JUENGST, ERIC, and WATSON, JAMES. 1991. "Human Genome Research and the Responsible Use of New Genetic Knowledge." *International Journal of Bioethics* 2:99–102.

KATZ, JAY; CAPRON, ALEXANDER M.; and GLASS, ELEANOR SWIFT, eds. 1972. *Experimentation with Human Beings: The Authority of the Investigator, Subject, Professions, and State in the Human Experimentation Process.* New York: Russell Sage Foundation.

KÜBLER-ROSS, ELISABETH. 1969. *On Death and Dying.* New York: Macmillan.

LADIMER, IRVING, and NEWMAN, ROGER W., eds. 1963. *Clinical Investigation in Medicine: Legal, Ethical, and Moral Aspects.* Boston: Law-Medicine Research Institute, Boston University.

LEAF, ALEXANDER. 1989. "Potential Health Effects of Global Climatic and Environmental Changes." *New England Journal of Medicine* 321, no. 23:1577–1583.

LEAKE, CHAUNCEY D., and ROMANELL, PATRICK. 1950. *Can We Agree? A Scientist and a Philosopher Argue About Ethics.* Austin: University of Texas Press.

LEAVITT, JUDITH W. 1986. *Brought to Bed: Childbearing in America, 1750–1950.* New York: Oxford University Press.

LEVINE, ROBERT. 1986. *Ethics and Regulation of Clinical Research.* 2d ed. Baltimore: Urban and Schwarzenberg.

LIMBERT, PAUL M. 1931. "Are Courses in the Ethics of Nursing Worthwhile?" *Trained Nurse and Hospital Review* 87, no. 4:472–476.

MARMOR, THEODORE R. 1970. *The Politics of Medicare.* London: Routledge & Kegan Paul.

MARTY, MARTIN E. 1983. *Health and Medicine in the Lutheran Tradition: Being Well.* New York: Crossroad.

McCALLY, MICHAEL, and CASSEL, CHRISTINE K. 1990. "Medical Responsibility and Global Environmental Change." *Annals of Internal Medicine* 113, no. 6:467–473.

MENZEL, PAUL T. 1990. *Strong Medicine: The Ethical Rationing of Health Care.* New York: Oxford University Press.

MOHR, JAMES C. 1978. *Abortion in America: The Origins and Evolution of National Policy, 1800–1900.* New York: Oxford University Press.

MOORE, THOMAS VERNER. 1935. *Principles of Ethics.* Philadelphia: J. B. Lippincott.

NATIONAL ACADEMY OF SCIENCES. 1975. *Experiments and Research with Humans: Values in Conflict.* Washington, D.C.: Author.

NATIONAL HEART AND LUNG INSTITUTE. ARTIFICIAL HEART ASSESSMENT PANEL. 1973. *The Totally Implantable Artificial Heart: Economic, Ethical, Legal, Medical, Psychiatric, and Social Implications.* Bethesda, Md.: National Institutes of Health.

PERCIVAL, THOMAS. 1927. *Percival's Medical Ethics.* Edited by Chauncey D. Leake. Baltimore: Williams and Wilkins.

POTTER, VAN RENSSELAER. 1971. *Bioethics: Bridge to the Future.* Englewood Cliffs, N.J.: Prentice-Hall.

RAMSEY, PAUL. 1970a. *Fabricated Man: The Ethics of Genetic Control.* New Haven, Conn.: Yale University Press.

———. 1970b. *Patient as Person: Explorations in Medical Ethics.* New Haven, Conn.: Yale University Press.

REICH, WARREN T., ed. 1978. *The Encyclopedia of Bioethics.* 4 vols. New York: Free Press.

RESCHER, NICHOLAS. 1969. "The Allocation of Exotic Medical Lifesaving Therapy." *Ethics* 79, no. 3:173–186.

ROBB, ISABEL HAMPTON. 1901. *Nursing Ethics: For Hospital and Private Use.* Cleveland: J. B. Savage.

ROSENBERG, CHARLES E. 1987. *The Care of Strangers: The Rise of America's Hospital System.* New York: Basic Books.

ROTHMAN, DAVID J. 1980. *Conscience and Convenience: The Asylum and Its Alternatives in Progressive America.* Boston: Little, Brown.

———. 1991. *Strangers at the Bedside: A History of How Law and Bioethics Transformed Medical Decision Making.* New York: Basic Books.

SAGOFF, MARK. 1991. "Zuckerman's Dilemma: A Plea for Environmental Ethics." *Hastings Center Report* 21, no. 5: 32–40.

SECUNDY, MARIAN GRAY, and NIXON, LOIS LACAVITA, eds.

1992. *Trials, Tribulations, and Celebrations: African-American Perspectives on Health, Illness, Aging, and Loss.* Yarmouth, Me.: Intercultural Press.

SHAW, MARGERY W., ed. 1984. *After Barney Clark: Reflections on the Utah Artificial Heart Program.* Austin: University of Texas Press.

SHELP, EARL E., ed. 1985. *Virtue and Medicine: Explorations in the Character of Medicine.* Dordrecht: D. Reidel.

SHERWIN, SUSAN. 1992. *No Longer Patient: Feminist Ethics and Health Care.* Philadelphia: Temple University Press.

SMITH, DAVID G., and WIGTON, ROBERT S. 1987. "Modeling Decisions to Use Tube Feeding in Seriously Ill Patients." *Archives of Internal Medicine* 147, no. 7:1242–1245.

SPERRY, WILLARD. 1950. *The Ethical Basis of Medical Practice.* New York: P. B. Hoeber.

STARR, PAUL. 1982. *The Social Transformation of American Medicine.* New York: Basic Books.

STEVENS, ROSEMARY. 1971. *American Medicine and the Public.* New Haven, Conn.: Yale University Press.

———. 1989. *In Sickness and in Wealth: American Hospitals in the Twentieth Century.* New York: Basic Books.

SZASZ, THOMAS S. 1961. *The Myth of Mental Illness: Foundations of a Theory of Personal Conduct.* New York: Harper & Row.

THOMASMA, DAVID C. 1984. "The Context as a Moral Rule in Medical Ethics." *Journal of Bioethics* 5, no. 1:63–79.

TOULMIN, STEPHEN. 1982. "How Medicine Saved the Life of Ethics." *Perspectives in Biology and Medicine* 25, no. 4: 736–750.

U.S. CATHOLIC CONFERENCE. DEPARTMENT OF HEALTH AFFAIRS. 1971. *Ethical and Religious Directives for Catholic Health Facilities.* Washington, D.C.: Author.

U.S. NATIONAL COMMISSION FOR THE PROTECTION OF HUMAN SUBJECTS OF BIOMEDICAL AND BEHAVIORAL RESEARCH. 1978. *The Belmont Report: Ethical Principles and Guidelines for the Protection of Human Subjects of Research.* Washington, D.C.: U.S. Government Printing Office.

U.S. PRESIDENT'S COMMISSION FOR THE STUDY OF ETHICAL PROBLEMS IN MEDICINE AND BIOMEDICAL AND BEHAVIORAL RESEARCH. 1981. *Defining Death: A Report on the Medical, Legal and Ethical Issues in the Determination of Death.* Washington, D.C.: U.S. Government Printing Office.

———. 1983a. *Deciding to Forego Life-Sustaining Treatment: A Report on the Ethical, Medical, and Legal Issues in Treatment Decisions.* Washington, D.C.: U.S. Government Printing Office.

———. 1983b. *Screening and Counseling for Genetic Conditions. A Report on the Ethical, Social and Legal Implications of Genetic Screening, Counseling & Education Programs.* Washington, D.C.: U.S. Government Printing Office.

———. 1983c. *Securing Access to Health Care: A Report on the Ethical Implications of Differences in the Availability of Health Services.* Washington, D.C.: U.S. Government Printing Office.

VALENSTEIN, ELLIOT S. 1974. *Brain Control: Critical Examination of Brain Stimulation and Psychosurgery.* New York: Wiley.

VAUX, KENNETH L. 1984. *Health and Medicine in the Reformed Tradition: Promise, Providence, and Care.* New York: Crossroad.

VAWTER, DOROTHY E.; KEARNEY, WARREN; GERVAIS, KAREN G.; CAPLAN, ARTHUR L.; GARRY, DANIEL; and TANER, CAROL. 1990. *The Use of Human Fetal Tissue: Scientific, Ethical, and Policy Concerns.* Minneapolis: Center for Biomedical Ethics, University of Minnesota.

VEATCH, ROBERT M. 1981. *A Theory of Medical Ethics.* New York: Basic Books.

VEATCH, ROBERT M.; GAYLIN, WILLARD; and MORGAN, COUNCILMAN. 1973. *The Teaching of Medical Ethics: Proceedings of a Conference Sponsored by the Institute of Society, Ethics and the Life Sciences and Columbia University College of Physicians and Surgeons, June 1–3, 1972.* Hastings-on-Hudson, N.Y.: Institute of Society, Ethics and the Life Sciences.

WALTERS, LEROY, ed. 1975–. *Bibliography of Bioethics.* Washington, D.C.: Kennedy Institute of Ethics.

WEISZ, GEORGE, ed. 1990. *Social Science Perspectives on Medical Ethics.* Philadelphia: University of Pennsylvania Press.

WHITE, EVELYN C., ed. 1990. *The Black Women's Health Book: Speaking for Ourselves.* Seattle: Seal Press.

ZANER, RICHARD M. 1988. *Ethics and the Clinical Encounter.* Englewood Cliffs, N.J.: Prentice-Hall.

C. CANADA

This article presents the most important and distinctive features of bioethics in Canada. It begins by sketching the development of medical ethics in the nineteenth and twentieth centuries; the main focus, however, is on the emergence and flowering of modern bioethics from the 1960s to the present. Two aspects of Canadian society are described as particularly determinative of the Canadian approach to bioethics: the country's health-care system and the role of law. A few of the multitude of bioethical issues that have occupied Canadians since the 1960s are analyzed to illustrate the three major areas of bioethical activity—namely, clinical ethics, research ethics, and ethics in public policy.

From medical ethics to bioethics

The period under consideration can be divided into two phases: 1800 to the 1960s, and the 1960s to the present. During the first phase medical ethics predominated, although theological ethics and the ethics of nursing were also important. In the second phase, medical ethics has been incorporated into the broader field of bioethics.

Phase I: 1800–1960s. The history of medical ethics in Canada during the nineteenth and early twentieth centuries is still to be written. The following sketch focuses on certain association activities and some publications in the field.

In 1829, the Quebec Medical Society adopted a code of ethics entitled *Laws of the Quebec Medical Society.* The code's influence was minimal, since the society became inactive in 1832. In 1867, the year of Canada's formation as a nation, a more permanent medical organization, the Canadian Medical Association (CMA), came into being. At its first annual meeting in 1868, the CMA adopted a Code of Ethics, closely modeled on the Code of the American Medical Association. The three major divisions of the CMA Code have been retained to the present: the duties of physicians to their patients, to each other and the profession at large, and to the public. The CMA Code underwent a major revision in 1936–1937 and another in 1956–1957.

In 1878 the Quebec College of Physicians and Surgeons (established in 1847) formed a committee to prepare a code of medical etiquette. The committee recommended adoption of the CMA code of ethics. In August of that year the governing body of the college, the Bureau provincial de médecine, adopted this code. However, it did not receive the power to enforce the code until 1898. The college was reorganized as the Corporation professionnelle des médecins du Québec in the 1970s; its code of ethics has been revised and incorporated into the provincial Medical Act.

The Canadian Nurses Association was established in 1908. However, the association did not have a code of ethics until 1954, when it adopted the one that had been prepared the previous year by the International Council of Nurses.

The Roman Catholic church has played an important role in health care in Canada since colonial times. The Catholic Hospital Association of the United States and Canada (CHAUSC), founded in 1915, adopted a code of ethics in 1921, which dealt primarily with surgical issues in obstetrics and gynecology. This document was updated in 1935, and the following year a version was adopted by the Catholic hospitals of Montreal as binding on all their medical personnel. The code was revised and expanded in 1949 and published as *Ethical and Religious Directives for Catholic Hospitals*. A French edition was published in Montreal in 1950. In 1954 the Catholic Hospital Council of Canada, established in 1942, declared its independence from CHAUSC, and renamed itself the Catholic Hospital Association of Canada. It adopted its own moral code in 1955.

Canadian contributions to the medical ethics literature were few and far between until the 1940s. The most renowned Canadian physician of this period, Sir William Osler (1849–1919), made few references to "medical ethics" in his 1500 publications. He did, however, have a great deal to say about the practice of medicine and physician behavior. The chief virtue of the individual physician is variously referred to in his writings as equanimity (*aequanimitas*), imperturbability, and detachment. His stated ideal for the medical profession was "noblesse oblige" (Osler, 1985).

Not until the 1940s did a significant number of Canadian publications in medical ethics begin to appear, most of them written by Catholic theologians (e.g., LaRochelle and Fink, 1940). Some Catholic schools of

medicine (for example, the University of Ottawa) and nursing (for instance, the Université de Montréal) made faculty appointments in medical ethics; these professors contributed to the growing body of Catholic literature in this field (e.g., Paquin, 1954). Comparable work by philosophers and health professionals was noticeable by its absence.

Phase II: 1960s–1990s. Beginning in the mid-1960s, the field of medical ethics underwent a radical transformation and by the end of the 1970s displayed all the features of what has become known as bioethics. In Canada the major actors in the development of bioethics have been professional associations, public commissions, and academic institutions.

The major health-professional associations expanded their ethics activities during this period. In the early 1980s, the Canadian Medical Association remandated its Committee on Ethics to deal with the whole range of bioethical issues rather than those affecting only physicians. In 1989 the CMA established a Department of Ethics and Legal Affairs with three full-time professional staff members. The Royal College of Physicians and Surgeons of Canada created a Biomedical Ethics Committee in 1977, and the College of Family Physicians followed suit in 1991. Although the Canadian Nurses Association does not have a standing committee on ethics, it has involved ethicists in three revisions of its code of ethics since 1970. The Catholic Health (formerly Hospital) Association of Canada updated its moral code in 1971 and again in 1991 and has been heavily involved in educational programs on bioethical issues for its members. Many other health associations have developed mechanisms for dealing with bioethics.

A favored Canadian way of dealing with contentious social issues is to establish a public commission. Since 1970 there have been more than thirty commission inquiries into bioethical issues (Williams, 1989). Some of these were created with a time-limited mandate to study certain problems, such as the nonmedical use of drugs or the new reproductive technologies. Others were given a semipermanent status, such as the federal and provincial law reform commissions. The federal Law Reform Commission was established in 1971 to review on a continuing basis the federal laws of Canada and to make recommendations for their improvement, modernization, and reform. Bioethical issues were dealt with in the Protection of Life Project, one of four commission projects. Between 1979 and 1992, a dozen or so study papers, working papers, and reports to Parliament were published on topics such as euthanasia and assisted suicide, experimentation on human subjects, and medically assisted procreation. None of the commission's recommendations has been implemented by the federal government, and in 1992 the commission was terminated by the government for budgetary reasons. The commission's recommendations, however, have influenced important court decisions dealing with life-prolonging treatment, as will be discussed below.

Academic institutions have experienced tremendous growth in the area of bioethics since the 1960s. Courses in this field have proliferated in philosophy and religious-studies departments, where they are often the most heavily subscribed offerings. Bioethics instruction is now offered in every Canadian medical school at the basic degree level and is rapidly expanding into residency training programs. The Université de Montréal, for example, has an annual case-method course in clinical ethics for surgery residents. Nursing, health administration, and dentistry programs have also formalized ethics teaching; and in many universities, instruction in the ethical aspects of animal experimentation is required for zoology and psychology students.

Research in bioethics has been fostered by the creation of centers, institutes, and professional associations for practitioners in this field. The Center for Bioethics of the Clinical Research Institute of Montreal, Quebec, established in 1976, was the first such organization in Canada. It was followed three years later by the Westminster Institute for Ethics and Human Values in London, Ontario. By 1993 there were at least sixteen research centers and groups in Canada, most of them university based. A national association, the Canadian Bioethics Society, was formed in 1988 through a fusion of two previously established associations.

Institutional matrix of bioethics

The Canadian health-care system and Canadian law have been two of the most important forces shaping the context within which bioethics has developed in Canada. The health-care system has also been, and will continue to be, the source of some of the most difficult bioethical issues Canadians have faced since 1971, when the country's national health-insurance program was fully in place (Taylor, 1987). Although Canadian legislation and jurisprudence have largely guided and supported work in bioethics, there have also been points on which they have clashed.

The Canadian health-care system.   The Canadian health-care system is in reality not a single system but rather a network of ten distinct provincial and two territorial health-care systems. The coherence of this network derives from a series of accords between the federal and provincial governments. The federal government provides a considerable part of the funds to the provinces and territories for health care; the latter governments, in return, agree to incorporate the essential features of the national health-insurance program into their health-care systems.

The principal features of Canada's national health-insurance program (comprehensiveness; universality; accessibility; portability—that is, coverage across Canada

and, in part, in other countries also; public administration) derive from Canadians' commitment to the principle of equality. The Canadian national health-insurance system, as defined in the Hospital Insurance Act (1957) and as reaffirmed in the Canada Health Act (1984), is founded on a principle of public ethics to which the Canadian people fiercely adhere. Equality before the health-care system, as Robert Evans has phrased it, is as strong a principle in Canada as equality before the law (Evans, 1988). The governing idea of this principle is that all Canadians should have access to a similar level of care, regardless of their ability to pay for it.

There have been challenges to the Canadian health-care system's principle of universal, equal access to hospital and medical services. The practice of extra billing by doctors represented one such challenge. Extra billing would allow doctors to bill patients for charges exceeding what the national health-insurance plan paid doctors for a medical service. The practice of extra billing by doctors was prohibited by the Canada Health Act in 1984.

The way a country organizes its health-care system as a whole is not just an issue of economics and administration. It is also an issue of public ethics rooted deeply in a clash between powerful interest groups and the requirements of justice, as interpreted in the light of a society's governing ethos. The Canadian ethos of universal access with equal terms and conditions for all is being challenged by new questions of fairness. For example, a debate has arisen over whether more expensive but safer radiological contrast agents (injected chemicals that make it possible to visualize anatomic structures by X ray) should be used, at great cost to the health budget: Is it fair to use these agents only for persons judged at higher risk of adverse reactions to the older agents?

Bioethics and law in Canada.   Since a comprehensive discussion of the interactions between bioethics and law on biomedical issues in Canada would require at least a book-length discussion (Roy et al., 1994), we limit our attention here to selected illustrations of the impact each has exerted on the other.

In Canada, the Constitution Act (1867), originally known as the British North American Act, was amended in 1982 by introduction of the Canadian Charter of Rights and Freedoms. The charter obliges government agencies not to violate rights considered fundamental. Such rights include life, liberty, and security of the person; freedom of conscience, thought, belief, and expression; and freedom from discrimination. Democratic support for legislation that violates the charter does not compel the courts to uphold the legislation, since the charter protects fundamental freedoms and legal rights against even democratically composed majorities. This is illustrated in the 1988 decision of the Supreme Court of Canada regarding abortion (discussed more extensively below).

A central ethical principle of palliative care and palliative medicine is that physicians should have wide discretion in using every proportionate means available to relieve the dying of their pain and symptom-related distress so that they can die in tranquillity rather than in agony. Canada has played a leading role in the development of palliative medicine; yet, given the ambiguity of Canada's criminal code, some physicians believe they have to be courageous and daring to go far enough with their use of drugs to relieve suffering effectively (Roy and Rapin, 1992). For this reason, the Law Reform Commission of Canada has strongly reinforced the ethical foundations of palliative medicine in Canada in proposing to amend the criminal code so that it cannot be interpreted as obliging doctors to curtail the use of pain-killing drugs because of a fear that pain relief will shorten an incurably ill patient's life. The commission holds that any possible effect of analgesics on a dying person's length of life is no basis whatsoever for holding physicians criminally liable when they administer palliative medicine proportionate to the need for relief.

A leading instance of bioethics influencing case law occurred in the 1991 Ontario Court of Appeal decision in *Malette v. Shulman*. A Jehovah's Witness was taken to the hospital unconscious and bleeding after a vehicle accident. The physician attending her was informed that she was carrying a signed card refusing blood products, but he undertook transfusion in order to prevent her death from heavy loss of blood. The patient, Georgette Malette, sued him for the civil wrong of battery, meaning unauthorized touching, and was awarded a favorable judgment, which the Ontario Court of Appeal upheld. The trial judge observed that transfusion may have saved her life, but he and the unanimous appeal judges agreed that, in this case, the bioethical principle of respect for autonomous persons prevailed over principles of beneficence and nonmaleficence. Society may not share her priority of interests but, in a pluralistic country, can tolerate her freedom of preference.

From the mid-1970s to the mid-1980s, numerous symposia, workshops, and position papers reflecting the thinking of a cross-section of Canadians supported the conclusion that contraceptive sterilization, in some circumstances, would be truly beneficial for some mentally disabled persons, because it would allow them to enjoy sexual fulfillment without the burden of bearing and rearing children. Controversy centered on the decision-making process: Who should be involved, and what conditions had to be fulfilled, to protect mentally disabled persons from being sterilized for someone else's benefit.

The ethical consensus that resulted came from the grass-roots initiative of many people to solve a pressing problem in the absence of legal guidelines. However, a 1986 decision of the Supreme Court of Canada in the *Eve* case clarified the law in this matter (*Eve v. Mrs. E.*,

1986). The Court declared categorically that sterilization should never be authorized for nontherapeutic purposes. In the absence of the affected person's consent, the Court believed that it can never be safely determined that such sterilization is for the benefit of that person. This decision has proved to be difficult for clinicians, parents, those carrying institutional responsibility for the care of mentally retarded persons—and, perhaps, for the latter themselves, whose social lives and privacy in relations with members of the other sex may be restricted for fear of pregnancy. Of course, mentally disabled persons may never fully comprehend why they are being restrained from being with the persons to whom they are attracted and whom they would want to love. The decision also serves as a focus for continuing discussions in Canada about what should be done when what is judged by many to be ethically justifiable has been declared illegal.

Key issues

Although Canadians have been preoccupied with most bioethics issues, the following discussion is limited to selected issues that have most intensively mobilized the thought and action of Canadians in the fields of clinical ethics, research ethics, and ethics in public policy.

Clinical ethics. Several court cases in Canada illustrate the interplay between clinical ethics and jurisprudence when decisions have to be made regarding cessation of treatment.

In the 1983 case of Stephen Dawson, Justice Lloyd McKenzie of the Supreme Court of British Columbia overturned an earlier ruling of the Provincial Court and ordered that corrective surgery be performed to replace the shunt, now blocked, that had been implanted in Dawson's brain to draw off excess cerebrospinal fluid (*Superintendent, In re*, 1983). That decision emphasized how ethically crucial it is to be very careful about verifying descriptions of persons that serve as a basis for life-and-death decisions. The second ethical point supported by that decision is that it would be just as wrong to conclude that all disabled persons have to be given life-prolonging treatment to the end as it would be to refuse such treatment on the bias that life with a disability is not worth living.

In 1986, the Quebec Court of Appeal upheld the right of family members to refuse life-prolonging chemotherapy for their terminally ill children. The judgment in the case of Carole Couture-Jacquet, a three-year-old girl afflicted with a rare and progressive pelvic cancer, was noteworthy for its sensitive use of proportionality reasoning (*Couture-Jacquet v. Montreal Children's Hospital*, 1986). Liberating Carole from the chemotherapy's continuing and increasingly distressful side effects was seen by the judge to be more important than taking the treatment's estimated 10 to 20 percent chance of arresting the progression of the tumor for an admittedly limited time.

An ethical consensus has grown in Canada since the late 1970s in support of the view that physicians are quite justified in withholding or discontinuing treatments that do little more than prolong a patient's dying and suffering (Baudouin and Blondeau, 1993). However, physicians, nurses, hospital administrators, and others have demonstrated a reluctance to disconnect a respirator from intelligent, conscious, and lucid patients, particularly when the prognosis is for continued life for a considerable period of time.

In an important judicial decision, the Superior Court of Quebec affirmed that the request of a competent patient to discontinue life-supporting treatment should be honored by the authorities at the Hôtel-Dieu Hospital in Quebec City (*Nancy B. v. Hôtel-Dieu de Québec*, 1992). Nancy B., a twenty-five-year-old woman, was permanently dependent on a respirator due to Guillain-Barré syndrome; after two years, while lucid and without clinical depression, she asked that the respirator be stopped, knowing that this would lead to her death. The court's decision to allow this stated that doing so would not constitute criminal negligence or homicide. In so ruling, it cited the Canadian Law Reform Commission's recommendation that ambiguous sections of the criminal code should be changed so that the criminal law of Canada could not be interpreted as obliging physicians either to treat patients against their informed and free refusal, or to initiate or continue treatments that are therapeutically useless and not in patients' best interests (Law Reform Commission, 1983).

This decision also confirms and reflects the direction of numerous day-to-day practical judgments of clinical ethics in Canada on issues involving life-prolongation decisions. This trend is toward an ethic based primarily upon the dignity and quality of life rather than on the duration of life taken as an absolute value.

Research ethics. Canadians have been quite intensively occupied with elaborating the conditions for the ethically acceptable conduct of research with human subjects.

In August 1961, Walter Halushka volunteered to be a research subject in a project to test a new anesthetic drug. Halushka suffered a cardiac arrest during the experiment, and though successfully resuscitated, he was left with some brain damage and could no longer continue his university studies. The Court of Appeal found that the physician-researchers had failed to inform Halushka that the test was of a new drug, that they had little previous knowledge about this drug, that the drug was an anesthetic, and that there was accordingly risk involved in its use. The physician-investigators also failed to tell the subject that the test would involve passage of a catheter up a vein in his arm into his heart.

The Court of Appeal clarified the requirements for consent in the research setting:

> There can be no exceptions to the ordinary requirements of disclosure in the case of research as there may well be in ordinary medical practice. . . . The subject of medical experimentation is entitled to a full and frank disclosure of all the facts, probabilities and opinions which a reasonable man might be expected to consider before giving his consent. (Halushka, 1965)

Though patients are rarely harmed seriously in clinical research, such harm, even death, can occur. It is particularly tragic when a research-related death occurs that could have been avoided if consent negotiations had been adequate.

On October 13, 1981, Julius Weiss, sixty-two years old, died in a Montreal hospital while participating in a research project conducted to test the efficacy of a drug (indomethacin, administered by eyedrops) to reduce swelling in the eye after cataract surgery. This project also required that Weiss undergo a series of radiological examinations called fluorescein angiograms to gauge the effects of the indomethacin eyedrops. Weiss had a history of heart problems and went into convulsions following a drop in blood pressure after the first injection of dye. His heart stopped, resuscitation attempts failed, and he died. Weiss's widow and children sued the two physicians involved in the clinical study and the hospital where the study was conducted. In his judgment on this case, rendered on February 23, 1989, Judge Louis De Blois of Quebec Superior Court found that the patient would not have agreed to be in this project had he known it carried even a small risk of cardiac arrest and death (*Weiss v. Solomon*, 1989). It also seems that the key physician-investigator in the project was not aware of Weiss's heart condition. Although this tragic case raises many complex issues beyond the scope of this article (Freedman and Glass, 1990), it clearly emphasizes that informed consent is a two-way transaction (Dickens, 1982). Physician-investigators need information about patients as much as patients need information about the trial.

The basic assumption in Canada is that controlled clinical trials are as necessary ethically as they are scientifically. A physician's professional and ethical obligation to offer each patient the best available treatment cannot be separated from the twin clinical and ethical imperatives of basing the choice of treatment on the most reliable available or obtainable evidence. However, controlled clinical trials can be an ethical imperative only if it is possible to conduct them in an ethically justifiable manner.

In 1987, the Medical Research Council of Canada (MRC) published *Guidelines on Research Involving Human Subjects*. The guidelines emphasize items that are particularly important in controlled clinical trials of therapies. Patients whose enlistment in such trials is sought need to know about their prognosis if treatment of their disease is undertaken; about the availability of treatments other than those to be studied in the clinical trial; and about treatments that will not be available to them if they decide to participate in the trial (Medical Research Council, 1987). In view of the concerns voiced by members of the pediatric-research community about the adequacy of the MRC guidelines for research undertaken with children, the National Council on Bioethics in Human Research (NCBHR), with the support of the Canadian Paediatric Society, published its *Report on Research Involving Children* (1992).

The Canadian HIV Trials Network, established in 1990, has formed two committees—the Safety and Efficacy Review Committee (SERC) and the National Ethics Review Committee (NERC)—to supervise and update the conditions for the ethical conduct of trials of new treatments for HIV disease. NERC's specific function is to serve as a research ethics committee for clinical researchers in the community who have no access to an institutional review board.

Ethics in public policy.   Between the 1960s and the 1990s, the issue of abortion dominated the public-policy debate in bioethics. The debate was ignited in the late 1960s, when the federal government proposed changes to the criminal code that would relax restrictions on divorce, homosexual acts between consenting adults, the distribution of contraceptives, and abortion. The last issue was the most contentious and engendered widespread public discussion and lobbying of members of Parliament. In 1969 a new abortion law (section 251 of the Criminal Code) was adopted that retained criminal sanctions against both the woman seeking abortion and anyone who would perform the act unless certain conditions were met: (1) the abortion had to be performed by a qualified medical practitioner in an accredited or approved hospital; (2) it had to be approved by a therapeutic abortion committee of the hospital; and (3) the continuation of the pregnancy would or would be likely to endanger the life or health of the woman seeking abortion.

The number of legal abortions in Canada increased rapidly during the 1970s, from 11,152 in 1970 to 75,071 in 1982. It then leveled off and even declined slightly, to 72,693 in 1988. Throughout this period, there were many complaints of unequal access to abortion services, as well as accusations from antiabortion groups that the law was being applied too loosely. Since the federal government refused to revise the law, both proponents and opponents of abortion decided to challenge the law in the courts. In Montreal Dr. Henry Morgentaler had established in 1970 a clinic solely for performing abortions, in clear opposition to the law. After his third jury

acquittal in 1976 on charges of performing an illegal abortion, the Quebec government allowed his clinic to operate, despite vigorous protests from antiabortion forces.

In 1983 Dr. Morgentaler set up an abortion clinic in Toronto and was promptly arrested and charged, along with two colleagues. He was once again acquitted by a jury. This decision was appealed, and the Ontario Court of Appeal in 1985 overturned the decision of the jury and ordered a new trial. Dr. Morgentaler appealed this ruling to the Supreme Court of Canada. On January 28, 1988, the Supreme Court, in a 5 to 2 decision, overturned the Court of Appeal decision and restored the original jury acquittal. The Court also declared the 1969 abortion law unconstitutional and no longer in effect.

The Supreme Court heard another abortion-related case in 1988, this one initiated by an opponent of abortion. In 1981, Joe Borowski, a former Manitoba politician and antiabortion activist, challenged the 1969 abortion law on behalf of the unborn child. A Saskatchewan court heard the case in 1983 and in its judgment rejected Mr. Borowski's claim that the fetus is a person with legal rights. The Supreme Court upheld this judgment.

Between 1988 and 1991, the federal government made several attempts to pass a new abortion law, but none was successful. A bill introduced in 1989 would have recriminalized abortion except when performed by a doctor "of the opinion that, if the abortion were not induced, the health or life of the female person would be likely to be threatened." Health was defined as including physical, mental, and psychological aspects. The bill was approved by the House of Commons in May 1990 and was then sent to the Senate, where it received detailed examination. In January 1991, a vote was taken and the result was a tie. Under Canada's Senate rules, a tie is considered a defeat. As a result, Canada is one of the few countries where abortion is not mentioned in the criminal law.

The new reproductive technologies have generated considerable public-policy activity in Canada and have been the subject of several public inquiries, including a federal Royal Commission that reported in November 1993. The commission received many submissions focusing on the ethical aspects of reproductive technology. Feminist concerns (e.g., regarding commercialization in surrogate mothering) have figured prominently in the Canadian discussion of these issues (Overall, 1989; Sherwin, 1992).

Increasing attention is being given to ethical issues related to the use of Human Genome Project–derived technology for the diagnosis, treatment, and prevention of disease. The Privacy Commissioner of Canada has emphasized that people must have meaningful control over the communication of genetic information in the private sector and in governments (Privacy Commissioner, 1992). Protecting the privacy and confidentiality of genomic information is central to the protection of human dignity (Knoppers, 1991). The Medical Research Council of Canada has issued guidelines regarding gene therapy (Medical Research Council, 1990).

Conclusion

Canada is a nation of immigrants, and its multicultural character is becoming more evident with each passing year. During its developmental phase, bioethics has been clearly monocultural, reflecting the values of the white, largely Anglo-Saxon professional class that has dominated Canadian society, including its science and medicine. This approach is inadequate. If bioethics is to be relevant to Canadian society in the future, it must develop a multicultural sensitivity. This must include a growing recognition of, and respect for, aboriginal culture and health-care practices. More specifically, bioethics in Canada will have to take account of the role and status of aboriginal herbal and psychiatric medical practices and of the prioritization in traditional cultures of community entitlements over individual or autonomous rights.

DAVID J. ROY
JOHN R. WILLIAMS

While all the articles in this entry are relevant, see especially the section on EUROPE, *subsections on* RENAISSANCE AND ENLIGHTENMENT, *and* NINETEENTH CENTURY, *and the companion articles in this section:* COLONIAL NORTH AMERICA AND NINETEENTH-CENTURY UNITED STATES, THE UNITED STATES IN THE TWENTIETH CENTURY, *and* LATIN AMERICA. *For a further discussion of topics mentioned in this article, see the entries* ABORTION; BIOETHICS EDUCATION; CLINICAL ETHICS; DEATH AND DYING: EUTHANASIA AND SUSTAINING LIFE; GENOME MAPPING AND SEQUENCING; HEALTH-CARE DELIVERY, *article on* HEALTH-CARE SYSTEMS; LAW AND BIOETHICS; MEDICAL CODES AND OATHS; RESEARCH, UNETHICAL; *and* RESEARCH ETHICS COMMITTEES. *Other relevant material may be found under the entries* HEALTH-CARE FINANCING; HEALTH POLICY, *article on* POLITICS AND HEALTH CARE; NURSING ETHICS; *and* PUBLIC POLICY AND BIOETHICS. *See also the* APPENDIX (CODES, OATHS, AND DIRECTIVES RELATED TO BIOETHICS), SECTION II: ETHICAL DIRECTIVES FOR THE PRACTICE OF MEDICINE, CODE OF ETHICS AND GUIDE TO THE ETHICAL BEHAVIOUR OF PHYSICIANS *of the* CANADIAN MEDICAL ASSOCIATION, *and selections from the* HEALTH-CARE ETHICS GUIDE *of the* CATHOLIC HEALTH ASSOCIATION OF CANADA; SECTION III: ETHICAL DIRECTIVES FOR OTHER HEALTH-CARE PROFESSIONS, CODE OF ETHICS FOR NURSING *of the* CANA- DIAN NURSES ASSOCIATION; *and* SECTION V: ETHICAL DIRECTIVES PERTAINING TO THE WELFARE AND USE OF ANIMALS, ETHICS OF ANIMAL INVESTIGATION *of the* CANADIAN COUNCIL ON ANIMAL CARE.

Bibliography

BAUDOUIN, JEAN-LOUIS, and BLONDEAU, DANIELLE. 1993. *Éthique de la mort et droit à la mort.* Paris: Presses universitaires de France.

Borowski v. Attorney General of Canada. 1987. 39 D.L.R. (4th) 731; 33 C.C.C. (3d) 402; 2 W.C.B. (2d) 96.

Couture-Jacquet v. Montreal Children's Hospital. 1986. 28 D.L.R. (4th) 22.

DICKENS, BERNARD M. 1982. "The Modern Law on Informed Consent." *Modern Medicine of Canada* 37:706–710.

EVANS, ROBERT G. 1988. "'We'll Take Care of It for You': Health Care in the Canadian Community." *Daedalus* 117, no. 4:155–189.

Eve v. Mrs. E., In re. 1986. 31 D.L.R. (4th) 1.

FREEDMAN, BENJAMIN, and GLASS, KATHLEEN C. 1990. "*Weiss v. Solomon:* A Study in Institutional Responsibility for Clinical Research." *Law, Medicine & Health Care* 18, no. 4:395–403.

Halushka v. The University of Saskatchewan et al. 1965. 53 Dominion Law Reports (2d) 436.

KNOPPERS, BARTHA M. 1991. *Human Dignity and Genetic Heritage: A Study Paper.* Ottawa: Law Reform Commission of Canada.

LAROCHELLE, S. A., and FINK, C. T. 1940. *Précis de morale médicale pour infirmières, médecins et prêtres.* Quebec: L'Action catholique. English translation by M. E. Poupore of the 4th edition: *Handbook of Medical Ethics for Nurses, Physicians and Priests.* Montreal: Catholic Truth Society, 1943.

LAW REFORM COMMISSION OF CANADA. 1983. *Euthanasia, Aiding Suicide and Cessation of Treatment.* Report no. 20. Ottawa: Minister of Supply and Services Canada.

Malette v. Shulman. 1990. 67 D.L.R. (4th) 321; 71 O.R. (2d) 417; 20 A.C.W.S. (3d) 301.

MEDICAL RESEARCH COUNCIL OF CANADA. 1987. *Guidelines on Research Involving Human Subjects.* Ottawa: Author.

———. 1990. *Guidelines for Research on Somatic-Cell Gene Therapy in Humans.* Ottawa: Minister of Supply and Services Canada.

Morgentaler, Smoling and Scott v. The Queen. 1988. 44 D.L.R. (4th) 385; 37 C.C.C. (3d) 449; 3 W.C.B. (2d) 332.

Nancy B. v. Hôtel-Dieu de Québec. 1992. 86 D.L.R. (4th) 385; 69 C.C.C. (3d) 450; 31 A.C.W.S. (3d) 160.

OSLER, SIR WILLIAM. 1985. [1904–1928]. *The Collected Essays of Sir William Osler.* Vol. 1, *The Philosophical Essays.* Edited by John P. McGovern and Charles G. Roland. Birmingham, Ala.: Classics of Medicine Library.

OVERALL, CHRISTINE, ed. 1989. *The Future of Human Reproduction.* Toronto: Women's Press.

PAQUIN, JULES. 1954. *Morale et médecine.* Montreal: Comité des Hôpitaux du Québec.

PRIVACY COMMISSIONER OF CANADA. 1992. *Genetic Testing and Privacy.* Ottawa: Minister of Supply and Services Canada.

ROY, DAVID J., and RAPIN, CHARLES-HENRI, eds. 1992. *Les annales de soins palliatifs.* Vol. 1, *Les défis.* Montreal: Centre de bioéthique—IRCM.

ROY, DAVID J.; WILLIAMS, JOHN R.; and DICKENS, BERNARD M. 1994. *Bioethics in Canada.* Scarborough, Ont.: Prentice-Hall Canada.

ROYAL COMMISSION ON NEW REPRODUCTIVE TECHNOLOGIES. 1993. *Proceed with Care.* Final Report. Ottawa: Canada Communication Group.

SHERWIN, SUSAN. 1992. *No Longer Patient: Feminist Ethics and Health Care.* Philadelphia: Temple University Press.

Superintendent of Family and Child Service and Dawson et al., In re. Russell et al. and Superintendent of Family and Child Service et al., In re. 1983. 145 D.L.R. (3d) 610.

TAYLOR, MALCOLM G. 1987. *Health Insurance and Canadian Public Policy: The Seven Decisions That Created the Canadian Health Insurance System.* Montreal: McGill-Queen's University Press.

Weiss v. Solomon. 1989. R.J.Q. 731.

WILLIAMS, JOHN R. 1989. "Commissions and Biomedical Ethics: The Canadian Experience." *Journal of Medicine and Philosophy* 14, no. 4:425–444.

D. LATIN AMERICA

This article presents a historical panorama of biomedical ethics in Latin America, the name given to a linguistic and cultural community encompassing South America, Central America, Mexico, and part of the Caribbean. From political, economic, and social points of view, the Latin American nations are quite different, although at present they have underdevelopment in common.

Since bioethics as a discipline flourished first in the United States, it is useful to compare medical ethics in North America, with its predominantly Anglo and northern European culture, and in Latin America, pointing out the differences between the two traditions within the Western culture.

First, the Latin American tradition of medical ethics is described; next, the incipient bioethics movement in Latin America is considered; then the major bioethical problems of the region are noted; and finally, the challenge to Latin American bioethics is discussed.

The Latin American tradition of medical ethics

When Spain and Portugal established colonies in the Americas, they brought with them the profound influence of the Roman Catholic Church, heir to that Western culture whose roots are Greek philosophy, Judaism, and Roman law. The Catholic tradition has in fact defined Latin American ethics and the Latin American ethos. First, Catholic moral theology built a system of medical ethics based on (1) natural-law theory as the basis of morality; (2) the principle of the sanctity of human life as a moral criterion; and (3) the commandment of love, or the virtue of charity, as the golden rule. Second, through their pastoral role and religious authority, priests reinforced the paternalistic medical ethos of the Hippocratic tradition. The paternalistic model of medical responsibility centered on the principle of beneficence (that benefit must be produced and harm avoided); the principle of autonomy is not taken into account. Beneficent paternalism has dominated the relationships between doctor and patient, and between medicine and society, in Latin America up to the present day.

As the cultures of northern and southern Europe evolved in the Americas, the differences between the two were accentuated. Modernity did not have the same secular, liberal, and pluralistic cast in Latin America as it did in North America. In Latin America, morality was not detached from metaphysics and religion; it did not establish a new basis in scientific and political rationalism, nor did it set itself up as critical and autonomous over against the natural and supernatural order of the medieval epoch.

Beginning in the eighteenth century, it is possible to contrast two ethics: the classical tradition of virtue, represented by the Mediterranean peoples (particularly the Italians and Spaniards), and the tradition in which principles are central, dominant in the English- and German-speaking countries (McIntyre, 1984). In Latin America, the political paternalism of the ancien régime and the medical paternalism of the Hippocratic tradition go together; the result is a paternalistic model on both the individual-clinical and the social policy levels.

The ethics and ethos of Latin American medicine are expressed in professional codes of ethics and in health policy and legislation. The forebear of all these normative institutions was the *protomedicato.* Originating in the Roman Empire, the *protomedicato* was a tribunal of royal physicians (*protomédicos*) that granted professional licenses and acted as a judicial and legislative body in health matters. In the thirteenth century, Castile was one of the first kingdoms to establish legal regulations for medical practice and public health; examples of this were found in the School of Salerno, and the laws of Frederick II in Sicily (Mainetti, 1989). The *protomedicato* was transplanted from Spain to the Americas, where it endured until the period of independence (early nineteenth century), at which point medical instruction, practice, and policy began to be modernized.

In the twentieth century, professional associations or medical colleges in various countries began to formulate their own codes of ethics, in accordance with the deontological tradition that regulates the relationships of doctors among themselves, with the public, and with the state. One of the first such codes was drawn up in 1918 by Luis Razetti (Razetti, 1963), a leading Venezuelan physician who specialized in medical deontology, under the influence of the French, an influence that was at that time very perceptible in Latin American society in general and in the medical culture in particular. This same code was later adopted in Colombia (1919) and in Peru (1920); it provided a basic model for other Latin American codes, which are essentially traditional guides for professional courtesy or etiquette, the relationships of physicians among themselves, with the patient, and with the state (León, 1978).

The medical codes promulgated in many Latin American countries are influenced by a variety of factors, among them biomedical progress, malpractice legislation, and the political changes throughout the region after decades of military rule. Brazil's Federal Code of Medical Ethics (1988), for example, incorporates concern about new problems like AIDS, and reformulates the rule of medical confidentiality. The Medical College of Chile has been very active since 1984, demonstrating its sensitivity to—among other issues—the participation of Chilean physicians in torture during the years of authoritarian rule that ended in 1984 (Mainetti, 1990a).

The state's responsibility for health care has constitutional status in Latin American countries (Pan American Health Organization, 1989). The right to health care is included among social and economic rights. The first nation to incorporate the right to health care in its constitution was Chile, in 1925, followed by Bolivia, Cuba, Guatemala, Guyana, Haiti, Honduras, Mexico, Nicaragua, Paraguay, Peru, Uruguay, and Venezuela. The responsibility of the state for health planning is legislated by many Latin American countries, which provide for universal access to essential medical services and a national health-care system that is either free or based on copayments, but with limited coverage. In Latin America government health policy generally demonstrates a significant gap between principle and practice: between justice, which theoretically endorses the equal right to health care, and actual practice in societies that, owing to their social and economic development, are not able to guarantee that this and other rights will be respected.

Codes of ethics and health legislation are based on a moral view that is both dogmatic (codified and legalistic, in contrast with philosophic, analytic, and critical) and authoritarian (based on professional authority, which is partly religious and partly governmental, rather than civic or democratic). The Latin American tradition of medical ethics can be defined as naturalistic, paternalistic, dogmatic, and authoritarian. The new Latin American medical ethics, represented by bioethics, has developed in contrast with this older tradition.

The bioethics movement in Latin America

The bioethics revolution that has occurred in the industrialized nations has arisen both from the scientific and technological progress of biomedicine and from the liberal and pluralistic character of those nations. By contrast, in the developing Latin American countries bioethical interests correspond more to those of a low-technology society and a tradition of confessional morality (Mainetti, 1988a). Bioethics, based on the principles of beneficence, autonomy, and justice, may be seen as civic morality to which the parties to an increasingly conflictual relationship—physician, patient, and society—appeal. Or bioethics may be seen as medical culture, expressed in the "introduction of the moral subject into medicine," the promotion of the rational, free agent in the therapeutic relationship. It is fair to say, however, that bioethics has barely arrived in Latin America in either guise.

Public and academic interest in bioethical topics did appear in the 1980s, with the proliferation of new medical technologies, such as those used in intensive care units, transplants, and assisted reproduction, and with the appearance of democratic governments in the region. On the one hand, legal intervention in medical cases increased, due perhaps to the distances created between the professional and the patient by specialization. Malpractice and a patient's rights movement in Latin America imitated the early history of U.S. bioethics. On the other hand, there was an academic rehabilitation of practical, moral, and political philosophy as they could be applied to medicine. This development was in keeping with the kind of ideological pluralism and consensus formation that has characterized bioethics as a discipline in the United States.

The academic and professional development of bioethics in Latin America has been a process of incorporating the U.S. model in stages. As the twentieth century nears its end, the institutionalization of the discipline as expressed in the creation of research centers, professorships at universities, ethics committees at hospitals, and national commissions on bioethics cannot be said to be significant. Nor have the three main functions of bioethical studies been carried out. These are the educational function (deontology and legal medicine still stand for ethics at medical schools); the consultative function (clinical and health-care ethics are not practiced in hospitals and other health-care facilities); and the political function (groups of experts have not formed to advise public institutions on biomedical norms).

Bioethics is also just beginning to capture the attention of the public and the media.

Among the groups active on the Latin American bioethics scene, several deserve mention: the Instituto de Humanidades Médicas y Centro de Bioética of the Fundación Mainetti (Institute for the Medical Humanities and Center for Bioethics of the Mainetti Foundation) in La Plata, Argentina, and the Instituto Colombiano de Estudios Bioéticos (Colombian Institute for Bioethical Studies) in Bogotá, Colombia. The former, established in 1972, combines the European and Anglo-American traditions of medical humanism, serving as a model and resource center for other countries in the region, particularly through its Escuela Latinoamericana de Bioética (Latin American School of Bioethics, ELABE), directed by Juan Carlos Tealdi. The latter, founded in 1985 by Fernando Sánchez Torres, former dean of the National University of Colombia, together with the ASCOFAME (Colombian Association of Medical Faculties) with its Center for Medical Ethics, directed by Alfonso Llano Escobar, S.J., and the Colombian School of Medicine and its Health Care Ethics Committee, also lead in the process of renovating medical ethics in the region.

Other academic and professional associations have emerged in Latin American countries in recent years for the purpose of developing programs of bioethical studies: The Department of Bioethics of the Catholic University of Uruguay; the Sindicato Médico of Uruguay (a very important professional organization), which appointed a bioethics commission; the Department of Bioethics of the Chilean Catholic University; and the Chilean Medical College, mentioned above, work actively on deontological questions, and the Brazilian Association of Medical Ethics Teachers emphasizes bioethical issues.

The bioethics enterprise also can be evaluated by the number of people interested in the discipline; by courses, conferences, and other scientific activities; and by the publication of books and articles. The classic 1973 Latin American text on medical ethics, by Augusto León, was followed by several bioethics texts (Mainetti, 1988a; Varga, 1988; Vélez Correa, 1989). According to a 1990 report issued by the Pan American Health Organization, conditions in Latin America should encourage the development of programs to integrate medical ethics into the health system. This integration could occur along a broad spectrum ranging from legislation and public policies to academic curricula, and should include the revision of the ethics codes of established medical associations. To this end the Latin American School of Bioethics has been coordinating a regional program of hospital ethics committees since 1989 (Tealdi and Mainetti, 1990). The growth of interest in bioethics justifies a Latin American bioethics association to unite isolated efforts, and thus to offer a concerted response to the needs of the region. Meeting in La Plata, Argentina, in December 1991, representatives from several Latin American nations founded the Federación Latinoamericana de Instituciones Bioéticas (Latin American Federation of Bioethics Institutions, FELAIBE).

Major topics in Latin American bioethics

Latin American countries share a concern about a number of problems with implications for both law and policy. A common sociocultural and public-health situation defines the Latin American biomedical ethos. Ethnomedical ethics ought to be an essential topic, because the health and disease conceptions, practices, and values, as well as the needs, of the native (precolonial) Latin American peoples, are not properly understood by academic medicine and the health policy of the dominant culture. These peoples still await the fulfillment of the World Health Organization's proclamation calling for the integration of their healing arts into modern medicine. Among the most pressing bioethical issues facing Latin America are the following.

Reproductive ethics.   Both the prevention of human reproduction (contraception, sterilization, and abortion) and assisted human reproduction (reproductive technologies) are central issues for Latin American population policy. This policy is clearly linked to health and to religious, secular, and geopolitical factors. Underdevelopment and overpopulation form a vicious circle that distances societies more and more from the goal of sustainable development. The Catholic church does not tolerate what it calls "artificial" control of fertility and condemns abortion, which is legally prohibited in most Latin American countries. To date neither public debate nor legislative reform has occurred, although the widespread and frequent practice of clandestine abortion effectively expresses Latin American governments' laissez-faire policies. The ethical complexity of assisted reproduction provokes polemics about the status of the embryo without leading to a declared war between "Catholics" and "secularists," but this area requires legal regulation.

The ethics of death and dying.   In Latin America death is not as medicalized nor is the medical profession as tormented about it as is the case in the First World. The technological assault on dying, the new *danse macabre* in the intensive care unit, does not offer the same sort of spectacle in Latin America as it does in the United States. Nevertheless, the contemporary "art of dying" is a challenge in Latin America, too, even if living wills, do-not-resuscitate orders (DNRs), the ethical principles of critical care medicine, and the pro-euthanasia movement have yet to become major issues.

Palliative medicine, the hospice movement, and campaigns for death with dignity are the modern Latin American versions of *ars moriendi*. At the beginning of life, pediatrics ethics committees are improving regulations regarding the treatment of premature and disabled newborns. At the end of life, legislation authorizing removal and transplantation of organs has advanced markedly in many Latin American countries (Fuenzalida, 1990).

Research ethics.   Biomedical research in Latin America lacks both a legislative framework and an effective set of controls. Much research also lacks scientific validity and, motivated more by monetary interest than by interest in knowledge, overlooks patients' rights such as consent and confidentiality. Developing countries must create the scientific and financial conditions for research itself; they must also attract projects that involve international cooperation while avoiding the risks such cooperation often brings with it, including economic and human exploitation. Oversight committees are needed so that international standards, with criteria appropriate to the cultural modalities of each community, may be applied. U.S. standards of consent, for instance, cannot be implemented easily in the social conditions of developing countries (Levine, 1982). Questions that must be considered in the future include research priorities, allocation of resources for research, and access to new, experimental drugs. This last issue, which has an especially high profile because of the global AIDS crisis, now involves not only the right of patients to protection from possible ill effects but also their right to have access to such drugs, which may prolong or save their lives.

Health-care ethics.   Health status in Latin America must be seen within a larger picture of underdevelopment, poverty, hunger, and economic crisis aggravated by the foreign debt of the region. Two global short-term goals set by the World Health Organization have not yet been reached in Latin America: Infant mortality has not been brought below 5 percent, and life expectancy has not risen beyond sixty-five years. Health-care expenditures in Latin America did not exceed 5 percent of the gross national product in the 1970s and 1980s, compared with 10 percent for the so-called developed countries.

Although there is a plethora of medical students and an oversupply of physicians, approximately 75 percent of the population of Latin America does not receive medical attention. This dramatizes the gap between the proclaimed right to health care and the conditions necessary to exercise it. Primary care—including family planning, maternal and child care, immunization, health counseling and education, campaigns against tuberculosis, and treatment of infectious diseases—should be the goal of health policy in all developing nations.

Health-care policy must be focused on health as an indicator of development, oriented to the basic needs of the majority of the population, and designed to promote medical care based on criteria of equity, integration, participation, and efficiency (Pan American Health Organization, 1989).

Between 80 and 90 percent of the resources allocated to health care in Latin America is spent on secondary and tertiary care. "Bioethics in the time of cholera," to paraphrase the novelist Gabriel García Márquez—medical ethics faced with plagues like cholera and AIDS—sums up the challenge to health-care ethics in Latin America.

Environmental ethics.   The environmental problems of Latin America are in part peculiar to the region and in part similar to those in western Europe and the United States. Overpopulated cities like Mexico City, Caracas, and São Paulo are more polluted than their European counterparts, and the Latin American urban crisis ranges from street cleaning to disposing of radioactive wastes from nuclear power plants.

In agricultural areas, the indiscriminate use of biocides contaminates crops and reduces the fertility of the soil. The extinction of animal and plant species produces imbalances in the ecosystem. Of worldwide importance is the devastation of the Amazon rain forest, the largest jungle in the world. An ecological reserve with an influence on world climate, the area has already been deforested by 10 percent. It faces the prospect of destruction within half a century, for reasons not unrelated to the sizable foreign debt owed by Brazil.

Governments and publics in Latin America are just beginning to become conscious of the importance of the environment to human and animal health; to national, regional, and world economies; to the preservation of nature and of life itself. Some countries have environmental protection legislation, projects to protect or preserve natural resources, and active ecology movements. Bioethics, however, has yet to raise its voice in civic and public arenas with regard to environmental ethics—that is, ecological rights—a new type of third-generation human rights, and policies of sustainable development (Pan American Health Organization, 1987).

The challenge of bioethics for Latin America

Because of its humanistic medical tradition and the social conditions of developing countries, Latin America can offer a distinctive bioethics perspective, different from the U.S. perspective. There are two dimensions to this perspective. On the one hand, a discipline established along European lines of the general philosophy or theory of medicine, with three main branches (medical anthropology, epistemology, and axiology), may be better equipped to transform academic, scientific medicine into a new humanistic biomedical paradigm (Mainetti, 1988a). Such an approach would guard against the accusations often lodged against bioethics in the United States and Europe: that the discourse of bioethics only appears to humanize medicine while obscuring the real dehumanization of the system. For example, the bioethical discourse on autonomy may hide the depersonalization of medical care and its risks of iatrogenesis, exploitation of the body, and alienation of health. In response to the development of biomedicine in a technological era, bioethics may be able to play a more critical role, one that is less complacent or optimistic about progress.

The Latin American reality of "bioethics in the time of cholera" requires an orientation toward social ethics, with an accent on the common welfare, the good society, and justice rather than on individual rights and personal virtues: the modern and classical traditions of morality, respectively. A macroethics of health or public health may be proposed as an alternative to the Anglo-American tradition of micro or clinical ethics. Greater emphasis can be placed on the social importance of medicine; as far as medical ethics is concerned, the great need in the developing countries is fairness in the allocation of resources and the distribution of health services. Latin America has not lost hope that it might be the continent of justice.

Several decades after its birth, bioethics in the United States is moving toward new intellectual models. This movement shows up in the revisionist-foundationalist debate within the discipline; the application of ethics to other discourses, including the political arena; the rediscovery of ethics of virtue; the return to what is experiential; and the cross-cultural and international dialogue. The bioethics revolution in North America and Europe—summarized in a high-technology bios and individualized ethos—must be complemented in Latin America by a humanistic bios and a communitarian ethos.

A promising outlook is emerging as the bioethics traditions and problematics of the two Americas move closer to one another. Perhaps in the context of the new world order and the fifth centennial of Europe's "discovery" of America, bioethics—"the bridge toward the future" of humanity—will also be a bridge of inter-American cooperation and integration.

JOSÉ ALBERTO MAINETTI
TRANSLATED BY MARY M. SOLBERG

While all the articles in this entry are relevant, see especially the other articles in this section: COLONIAL NORTH AMERICA AND NINETEENTH-CENTURY UNITED STATES, THE UNITED STATES IN THE TWENTIETH CENTURY, *and* CANADA. *Directly related to this article is the entry* ROMAN CATHOLICISM. *For a further discussion of topics mentioned in this article, see the entries* ABORTION, *section on* RELIGIOUS TRADITIONS, *article on* ROMAN CATHOLIC PERSPECTIVES; BENEFICENCE; BODY, *article on* CULTURAL AND RELIGIOUS PERSPECTIVES; COMMERCIALISM IN SCIENTIFIC RESEARCH; DEATH: ART OF DYING, *article on* ARS MORIENDI; DOUBLE EFFECT; ENDANGERED SPECIES AND BIODIVERSITY; ENVIRONMENT AND RELIGION; HEALTH CARE, QUALITY OF; HEALTH-CARE RESOURCES, ALLOCATION OF, *article on* MACROALLOCATION; JUSTICE; LICENSING, DISCIPLINE, AND REGULATION IN THE HEALTH PROFESSIONS; MEDICAL CODES AND OATHS; MEDICAL MALPRACTICE; MEDICINE, ANTHROPOLOGY OF; MEDICINE, SOCIOLOGY OF; ORGAN AND TISSUE TRANSPLANTS, *article on* SOCIOCULTURAL ASPECTS; PASTORAL CARE; PATERNALISM; PATIENTS' RIGHTS, *article on* ORIGIN AND NATURE OF PATIENTS' RIGHTS; POPULATION ETHICS, *section on* RELIGIOUS TRADITIONS, *article on* ROMAN CATHOLIC PERSPECTIVES; POPULATION POLICIES, *section on* STRATEGIES OF FERTILITY CONTROL, *articles on* CHANGES IN ATTITUDE AND CULTURE, *and* INCENTIVES AND DISINCENTIVES; RIGHTS, *article on* SYSTEMATIC ANALYSIS; *and* SUSTAINABLE DEVELOPMENT. *See also the* APPENDIX (CODES, OATHS, AND DIRECTIVES RELATED TO BIOETHICS), SECTION II: ETHICAL DIRECTIVES FOR THE PRACTICE OF MEDICINE, OATH OF HIPPOCRATES.

Bibliography

BAYLOR COLLEGE OF MEDICINE. 1992. *Bioethics Yearbook.* Vol. 2. Dordrecht, Netherlands: Kluwer.

BRAZIL. 1988. *Federal Code of Medical Ethics.*

FUENZALIDA-PUELMA, HERNÁN. 1990. "Organ Transplantation: The Latin American Legislative Response." *Bulletin of the Pan American Health Organization* 24, no. 4: 425–445.

LEÓN, AUGUSTO. 1973. *Ética en medicina.* Barcelona: Científico-Médica.

———. 1978. "Medical Ethics: Latin America in the Twentieth Century." In *Encyclopedia of Bioethics,* pp. 1005–1007. New York: Macmillan.

LEVINE, ROBERT J. 1982. "Validity of Consent Procedures in Technologically Developing Countries." In *Human Experimentation and Medical Ethics,* pp. 16–30. Edited by Z. Bankowski and Norman Howard-Jones. Geneva: Council for International Organizations of Medical Sciences.

MAINETTI, JOSÉ ALBERTO. 1988a. "Bioethical Problems in the Developing World: A View from Latin America." *Unitas* 60 (June):238–248.

———. 1988b. *La crisis de la razón médica: Introducción a la filosofía de la medicina.* La Plata, Argentina: Quirón.

———. 1989. *Ética médica: Introducción histórica.* La Plata, Argentina: Quirón.

———. 1990a. "Bioethics: A New Health Philosophy." *Bulletin of the Pan American Health Organization* 24, no. 4:578–581.

————. 1990b. *Bioética fundamental: La crisis bioética.* La Plata, Argentina: Quirón.

————. 1991. "Out of America: Scholastic and Mundane Bioethics Scene in Argentina." In *Transcultural Dimensions of Medical Ethics.* Edited by Edmund D. Pellegrino, Patricia Mazzarella, and Pietro Corsi. Frederick, Md.: University Publishing Group.

MAINETTI, JOSÉ ALBERTO; PIS DIEZ, GUSTAVO; and TEALDI, JUAN CARLOS. 1992. "Bioethics in Latin America: 1989–1991." In vol. 2 of *Bioethics Yearbook,* pp. 83–96. Dordrecht, Netherlands: Kluwer.

MCINTYRE, ALISTAIR C. 1984. *After Virtue: A Study in Moral Theory.* 2d ed. Notre Dame, Ind.: University of Notre Dame Press.

PAN AMERICAN HEALTH ORGANIZATION. 1987. *Informe anual del director.* Washington, D.C.: Author.

————. 1989. *El derecho a la salud en las Américas: Estudio constitucional comparado.* Washington, D.C.: Author.

RAZETTI, LUIS. 1963. *Deontología médica.* Vol. 1 of *Obras completas.* Caracas: Ministerio de Sanidad y Asistencia Social.

TEALDI, JUAN CARLOS, and MAINETTI, JOSÉ ALBERTO. 1990. "Hospital Ethics Committees." *Bulletin of the Pan American Health Organization* 24, no. 4:410–418.

VARGA, ANDREW C. 1988. *Bioética: Principales problemas.* Translation by Alfonso Llano Escobar of *The Main Issues of Bioethics.* Bogotá: Ediciones Paulinas.

VÉLEZ CORREA, LUIS ALFONSO. 1989. *Etica médica: Interrogantes acera de la medicina, la vida y la muerte.* Medellín, Colombia: Corporación Para Investigaciones Biológicas.

VI. AUSTRALIA AND NEW ZEALAND

Medical ethics in Australia and New Zealand (Australasia) evolved slowly until the early 1980s, when major advances in reproductive technologies prompted widespread public discussion of bioethical issues arising at the outset of life. The flourishing bioethics movement in Australia and New Zealand at the end of the twentieth century can be contrasted with the narrower and more localized ethical concerns of the medical profession in these countries at the beginning of the century.

In the early decades of the twentieth century, ethical debates centered on issues of professionalism in the delivery of medical services, such as the permissibility of advertising by individual practitioners and the setting of standard fees to avoid "undercutting" by competitors. The branches of the British Medical Association (BMA) set up in the colonial Australian states were federated in 1912, when a new, unified code of professional ethics, dealing mainly with the regulation of advertising and etiquette toward patients, was introduced (Egan, 1988). After World War I, medical schools in Australasian universities began to include brief didactic instruction in the ethical obligations of physicians as professionals. There was some public discussion of abortion, methods of birth control, and confidentiality in relation to patients with venereal disease.

A Labour government with a strong social welfare platform was elected in Australia in 1941. This government attempted in the late 1940s to introduce a national health service, which would have provided universal access to health care for the first time in Australia. However, a bitter debate developed with the BMA, the majority of whose members saw the government's plans as a threat to the autonomy of medical practitioners and as the first step toward the nationalization of medicine. After legal challenges, the plans for a national health program were defeated before 1950 (Gillespie, 1991). Under the free-market policies of subsequent Liberal governments, access to publicly funded health care was available only to recipients of old-age and invalid pensions. This situation persisted until 1975, when the Labour government introduced Medibank, Australia's first national health-care program, which provided access to government-subsidized health care for all. While the incoming Liberal/National coalition government gradually dismantled this program during the late 1970s, it was reinstated as Medicare in 1983 by the newly elected Labour government and has continued to operate until the present.

Ethical issues in reproduction became a major concern in Australasia in the early 1980s, following pioneering research on in vitro fertilization (IVF) carried out by a joint research team led by Carl Wood and Ian Johnston at the Monash University Queen Victoria Medical Centre and the Royal Women's Hospital in Melbourne during the 1970s. This research led in 1983 to the world's first live IVF births from frozen embryos and donated eggs, and the work of Monash University researchers on embryo experimentation sparked worldwide interest. These developments in reproductive technology stimulated much public discussion in Australia, particularly among Roman Catholics, who constitute over a quarter of the population. Care for the terminally ill became another widely debated issue in Australia in the 1980s and, influenced by the growing public support for allowing voluntary euthanasia, the state governments of South Australia and Victoria passed legislation in 1983 and 1988, respectively, permitting patients to refuse medical treatment in certain circumstances, even in cases where such treatment might prolong their lives.

Australasia's first research center in bioethics, the Monash University Centre for Human Bioethics, was established by philosophy professor Peter Singer, together with colleagues in medicine, science, and the law, in 1980. A number of smaller research centers for bioethics were set up in Australasia during the 1980s, including Melbourne's St. Vincent's Bioethics Centre and Adelaide's Dietrich Bonhoeffer Institute for Bioethical Studies, both of which take Christian perspectives on bioethics; the Kingswood Centre for Applied Ethics in Perth; and the University of Otago Bioethics Research Centre in Dunedin, New Zealand. An interdisciplinary

Australian Bioethics Association was formed in 1990, and its inaugural conference was held in Melbourne in 1991.

With Helga Kuhse and others from the Monash Centre, Peter Singer has written extensively on ethical issues arising from the new reproductive technologies and on questions surrounding care of terminally ill adults and infants. Other noteworthy Australasian writers in bioethics include philosophers Max Charlesworth, Robert Elliot, and Robert Young; feminist academics Renate Klein and Robyn Rowland; lawyers Michael Kirby and Russell Scott; and theologian Norman Ford. In 1989 the Monash Centre introduced Australasia's first master's program in bioethics, which is designed for health-care professionals and others with an interest in bioethical issues. An international journal, *Bioethics,* is published by the Monash Centre.

Advances in infertility research in Victoria led the government of that state in 1982 to appoint Louis Waller, professor of law at Monash University and Australian law reform commissioner, to chair a committee whose mandate was to consider the social, ethical, and legal issues arising from IVF. Influenced by the three reports produced by this committee, which supported the use of IVF under certain regulations, the Victoria Parliament in 1984 enacted the world's first legislation (the Infertility Medical Procedures Act) to deal specifically with these new reproductive technologies (see Charlesworth, 1989). Among other provisions, this legislation allowed IVF to be carried out at approved hospitals, for married couples who have already sought infertility treatment for at least twelve months prior to attempting IVF. At the federal level, the National Bioethics Consultative Committee was established in 1988 as an advisory committee on issues such as access to information about their origins for children born from IVF, artificial insemination by donor, surrogate motherhood, and embryo experimentation. In 1990 this committee issued a report that supported surrogacy arrangements and proposed draft legislation to regulate such arrangements. In light of the heated public controversy that ensued, however, the Australian government decided against implementing its recommendations. Although surrogacy has not been outlawed in Australia, IVF-assisted surrogacy is not a practical option, since IVF is not legally available to fertile women. The National Bioethics Consultative Committee (NBCC) was subsumed under the existing National Health and Medical Research Council (NH&MRC) in 1991, which merged the functions of the NBCC and the Medical Research Ethics Committee to form the Australian Health Ethics Committee.

Australasia's first recorded institutional ethics committee to review human experimentation was set up at the Royal Victorian Eye and Ear Hospital in Melbourne in 1957 (McNeill, 1990), and at the instigation of the NH&MRC (which allocates government funding for medical research), Australian universities began in the 1980s to form ethics committees to oversee medical and other research carried out at those institutions. In New Zealand, the Medical Research Council, set up in 1937 by the government to supervise medical research, decided in 1968 that all research must adhere to the World Medical Association's Declaration of Helsinki, which stressed nonmaleficence and the need for informed consent on the part of the experimental subjects.

In 1987, unprecedented public outrage followed revelations of an experiment involving clandestine selective nontreatment of women with cervical cancer, carried out at the National Women's Hospital in Auckland from 1966 to 1981. The New Zealand government immediately set up an inquiry into the experiment, which resulted in an amendment to the New Zealand Human Rights Commission Act of 1977 to include a statement of patients' rights to proper standards of care and adequate disclosures to enable genuinely informed consent, and to provide for the appointment of a national health commissioner to encourage awareness of these rights by members of the medical profession (Campbell, 1989).

Influenced by increasing recognition of patient rights, Australasian medical schools have gradually woven the teaching of ethics into their curricula. For example, the University of New South Wales in Sydney and the University of Newcastle began teaching substantive courses in ethics to medical undergraduates in the 1970s, and the University of Adelaide's medical school introduced ethics into the undergraduate syllabus in the early 1980s. Following the recommendations of the National Inquiry into Medical Education—a committee of academics and health professionals set up by the federal minister for health, which heard submissions during 1987/1988—many other Australian medical schools have included clinical ethics as part of their undergraduate programs. These developments in bioethics education should help promote lively and informed discussions of medical ethics issues in Australasia as they arise in the future.

JUSTIN OAKLEY

While all the articles in this entry are relevant, see especially the articles in the section on EUROPE. *For a further discussion of topics mentioned in this article, see the entries* ABORTION, *section on* CONTEMPORARY ETHICAL AND LEGAL ASPECTS; EUGENICS; HEALTH-CARE DELIVERY; HEALTH-CARE RESOURCES, ALLOCATION OF, *article on* MACROALLOCATION; MEDICINE, ANTHROPOLOGY OF; MEDICINE, SOCIOLOGY OF; PROFESSION AND PROFESSIONAL ETHICS; REPRODUCTIVE TECHNOLOGIES; RESEARCH, UNETHICAL; RESEARCH ETHICS COMMITTEES; RESEARCH POLICY; RIGHTS; *and* ROMAN CATHOL-

ICISM. *Other relevant material may be found under the entries* INFORMED CONSENT; *and* JUSTICE.

Bibliography

ARMIT, H. W. 1924. "Medical Practice." *Medical Journal of Australia*, October 25, pp. 413–421. Summarizes BMA Unified Code of Professional Ethics of 1912.

CAMPBELL, ALASTAIR A. 1989. "A Report from New Zealand: An 'Unfortunate Experiment.'" *Bioethics* 3, no. 1:59–66.

CHARLESWORTH, MAXWELL J. 1989. *Life, Death, Genes and Ethics: Biotechnology and Bioethics.* Sydney: ABC Books. A good short introduction to ethical debates on IVF, embryo experimentation, and euthanasia in Australia.

CONEY, SANDRA. 1988. *The Unfortunate Experiment.* Harmondsworth, U.K.: Penguin. Describes the New Zealand government inquiry into unauthorized cervical cancer trials.

EGAN, BRYAN. 1988. "Nobler Than Missionaries: Australian Medical Culture c. 1880–c. 1930." Ph.D. diss., Monash University, Melbourne.

FORD, NORMAN. 1988. *When Did I Begin? Conception of the Human Individual in History, Philosophy, and Science.* Cambridge: At the University Press.

GILLESPIE, JAMES A. 1991. *The Price of Health: Australian Governments and Medical Politics, 1910–1960.* Cambridge: At the University Press. A perceptive and authoritative history of the medical policies of Australian governments and conflicts with professional associations.

KASIMBA, PASCAL, and SINGER, PETER. 1989. "Australian Commissions and Committees on Issues in Bioethics." *Journal of Medicine and Philosophy* 14:403–424.

KUHSE, HELGA, and SINGER, PETER. 1985. *Should the Baby Live? The Problem of Handicapped Infants.* Oxford: Oxford University Press.

MCNEILL, PAUL M. 1990. "Science, Society, and the Subject: The Ethics and Politics of Human Experimentation." Ph.D. diss., University of New South Wales, Sydney. Details the development of ethics committees to review human experimentation in Australian medical research.

ROWLAND, ROBYN. 1987. "Making Women Visible in the Embryo Experimentation Debate." *Bioethics* 1:179–188.

SINGER, PETER; KUHSE, HELGA; BUCKLE, STEPHEN; DAWSON, KAREN; and KASIMBA, PASCAL, eds. 1990. *Embryo Experimentation.* Cambridge: At the University Press. A useful and up-to-date collection on the scientific, ethical, and legal issues raised by techniques developed through embryo experimentation after IVF.

SINGER, PETER, and WELLS, DEANE. 1984. *Making Babies: The New Science and Ethics of Conception.* Oxford: Oxford University Press. Chronicles the development of new reproductive technologies in Australia and discusses their ethical implications.

MEDICAL ETHICS EDUCATION

See BIOETHICS EDUCATION.

MEDICAL GENETICS

I. PRACTICE OF MEDICAL GENETICS

"Medical genetics" and "clinical genetics" are interchangeable terms. This article discusses the history of the practice of medical genetics, with emphasis on the ethical aspects of this comparatively new specialty in medicine. The premise is that the ethical aspects of the practice of medical genetics evolve in many societies in a two-stage process: (1) an early stage in which a moral vision of voluntaristic, nondirective genetic counseling challenges and, in many contexts, reshapes the relationship between medical geneticists and their patients in tension with a prevailing history of medical paternalism, and (2) a current stage in which ethical concerns focus on larger social, ethical, and legal implications of uses of DNA technology. These concerns focus especially on genetic testing, screening, and therapy with adults, adolescents, and children. Advances in molecular biology and the international Human Genome Project propel the current stage of ethical concerns, which predictably will extend into the foreseeable future.

A revolution in biological understanding of human diseases is reverberating through many societies. The effects of its conceptual and practical impact on health care and prevention are most promising in addressing diseases at the most basic level. At the same time, revival of biological paradigms of understanding human beings and their destiny as well as memories of older abuses done in the name of the science of genetics pose threats to and challenges from other worldviews and interests. Also, some feminist and religious critics, as well as leaders in advocacy groups for persons with disabilities, have vigorously attacked contemporary human genetics, and medical genetics along with it. Dorothy Wertz and John Fletcher (1993) have documented these criticisms and responded to them.

Medical geneticists in training need to be prepared to address the ethical issues that arise in their interactions with patients and their families and within their societies. A growing literature on bioethics for human geneticists is one resource for reflection on ethical issues in medical genetics (Parker, 1994). As more physicians of all types become involved directly in genetic issues, courses in medical schools need to address such issues as well (Harris, 1990). Such attention to the ethical aspects of training requires the efforts of national and international societies of medical geneticists.

Human genetics and medical genetics

Medical genetics is "the aspect of human genetics that is concerned with the relation between heredity and disease" (McKusick, 1969, p. 181), and "deals with diagnosis, prognosis, and to some extent with treatment of various genetic diseases" (Vogel and Motulsky, 1979, p. 7). Medical genetics is embedded in the science of genetics and in human genetics in particular. A brief historical review is in order to trace the evolution of the practice of medical genetics in modern history.

Human genetics and medicine are the parent disciplines of medical genetics. Human genetics involves the study of human variability in terms of its causes and effects. Hardly any feature of human existence creates more conflict and disagreement than the origin and meaning of differences among human beings themselves, and between human beings and other animals. One of the most persistent sources of conflict is between a worldview in which debate about causation is subject to empirical evidence and one in which causation is understood to be shaped, at least in part, by an ultimate purpose, usually understood to be a divine source.

The earliest societies to keep records (Babylonian, Assyrian, and Egyptian) attributed malformations to supernatural causes and viewed birth defects as signs of good or evil for the society itself. Such views spread to Greece, Rome, and other parts of Europe. Alongside these supernatural views, naturalistic explanations emerged for malformations and for physical differences and similarities among members of the same family. Concepts of inherited differences appear in the Hippocratic texts and in the writings of Anaxagoras in the period 500–428 B.C.E. (Vogel and Motulsky, 1979).

Aristotle, one of the earliest biologists, based a theory of inheritance on his philosophy of form. He held that the generation of males and females was due to differences between "principles" of movement and matter that were embodied in semen and female secretions. When the male principle was dominant, sons were conceived who were more like their fathers than their mothers, and vice versa. Aristotle's ideas were a major source of prescientific guidance on such questions until the Enlightenment.

European physicians in the seventeenth and eighteenth centuries debated the "preformationist" theory in terms of whether the whole organism was preformed in the ovum or sperm. The debate foundered on the lack of empirical evidence until Gregor Mendel's experiments, reported in 1865. Mendel, an Austrian monk and botanist, experimented with crossing varieties of the pea in terms of color and shape of seed. He then counted all types and combinations in the offspring for several generations. From these experiments, he deduced the statistical laws that shape the science of genetics and provided the correct biological theory for the similarities and differences in offspring, namely, that the germ cells (sperm and ova) are the constant forms in the dynamics of inheritance.

Charles Darwin, who knew nothing of Mendel's work, concurrently explained the cause of evolution by his theory of variation and natural selection. Mendel's concept of the gene would have provided an empirical basis for many of Darwin's insights and a solution for how specific characteristics are inherited. Mendel's work remained unused by scientists and was eventually rediscovered only in 1900.

During this same period, Darwin's cousin, Sir Francis Galton, published papers (1865) reasserting ideas as old as Plato's; namely, that qualities such as talent, intelligence, and social achievement were strongly influenced by heredity. Galton was a strong advocate of eugenic practices and selective parenthood. Later, Galton proceeded to develop the basis for biometric genetics, or the study of variations in whole populations by statistical methods.

Modern medical genetics was foreshadowed in the work of Archibald E. Garrod. A distinguished physician who later succeeded Sir William Osler in medicine at Oxford, Garrod (1902) used Mendel's theory to explain alkaptonuria, an inherited disease. However, due to the strength of the eugenic theme in early twentieth-century genetic studies, the biologists and physicians of the era paid little attention.

This theme led to unethical sterilization, restrictive immigration, and discriminatory political measures in Europe and the United States (Kevles, 1985). In Germany, eugenics and beliefs of racial superiority merged in *Rassenhygiene,* or racial hygiene, and prominent German geneticists identified themselves with the use of genetics in the service of the Nazi state (Vogel and Motulsky, 1979). Anti-Semitism, the Nazi movement, and *Rassenhygiene* led to crimes against humanity, done in the name of science, that were unparalleled in history (Proctor, 1988). Benno Müller-Hill (1988) showed how the legacy of Nazi eugenics and advocacy of eugenic sterilization persisted in some German departments of human genetics beyond the end of World War II. Paul Weindling (1993) confirmed this analysis but also showed wide diversity of political and social thought in German eugenics. He warned, however, that the lesson from German eugenics is that a liberal, democratic society and its institutions are no final defense against abuses of human rights from medicine dominated by eugenics. Thus, the training of medical geneticists must include reflection on ethical issues to reduce the chances of any return to a eugenic past and to maximize the benefits of counseling, diagnosis, and treatment for genetic disorders for patients and families.

The moral beliefs and practices of medical geneticists in the post–World War II period broke sharply with those of their predecessors who were eugenics-minded, although the roots of the emancipation of medical genetics from eugenics can be traced to an earlier period (Kevles, 1985). Contemporary medical geneticists are dedicated to establishing their practices on sound, scientific bases and to respecting the personhood and choices of the patients who consult them. These marks of modern medical genetics were supported by postwar scientific advances in biochemistry and cytogenetics, and changes in the growing practice of genetic counseling done "nondirectively," in contrast to the benevolent paternalism of the past. The foundation of this concept is that those seeking consultation, those who are not sick but may be at higher risk to transmit genetic disorders and need counseling (sometimes referred to as "consultands"), or patients themselves, rather than the medical geneticist, make decisions about procreation and family planning. The role of the medical geneticist in the counseling setting is to conduct careful examinations, provide sound information on genetic risk, describe the natural history and prognosis of the disorder in question, describe the options at hand, respond to questions, and remain available.

The guiding philosophy of genetic counseling, in which all medical geneticists are engaged, is to assist consultands and patients in learning about available options and alternatives, not to make choices for them (Fraser, 1974). A 1985 survey of 682 geneticists, 81 percent of whom were M.D.s, in nineteen nations found a high degree (over 90%) of support for nondirective counseling (Wertz and Fletcher, 1989). Considering that many physicians in the sample were trained in a period in which being benevolently paternalistic was an admired trait for physicians, it is remarkable that the older pattern of physician–patient relationships had been transformed in the context of medical genetics.

Variations exist, of course, as to moral visions of practice among medical geneticists. Some (Czeizel, 1988) have adapted aspects of this nonpaternalistic consensus in practice while maintaining a strongly paternalistic stance on the role of society in improving the chances that every child will "be born healthy." On this point, the survey cited above found very little interest in long-range, eugenic concerns and a lack of consensus on the proposition that a goal of genetic counseling was to "improve the general health and vigor of the population" (Wertz and Fletcher, 1989, p. 34). Although the moral perspectives of medical geneticists are embedded in their political philosophies and the dynamics of their societies, the evidence that is available about the views of practitioners shows a strong commitment to patient-

centered decision making and a rejection of positive eugenics.

Practice of medical genetics today

Training and competence are ethically relevant issues in medical genetics, as is true in every profession. Medical geneticists provide genetic counseling to people at increased risk of having offspring with a genetic disorder or of contracting a genetic disease themselves. This service is also provided to people who have an unfounded fear of being at risk. Training in counseling needs to be grounded in solid understanding of human genetics, but just as important are the empathetic qualities and ethical sensitivities required for interactions on issues of human reproduction. Every training program ought to have such components with supervision from experienced medical geneticists.

Genetic counseling is preceded by taking a family genetic history and evaluating the clinical condition of relevant family members, diagnostic work-up, and various laboratory analyses. Input may be needed from several medical disciplines. For example, medical geneticists can do clinical diagnostic work and assist other specialists, such as pediatricians or neurologists, in arriving at exact diagnoses of rare genetic disorders.

In Europe, genetic counseling is provided mainly by medical doctors and also by human geneticists with doctoral degrees. By the mid-1990s, medical genetics in Europe was regarded by its leading practitioners as a specialty, but it was not yet universally recognized as such. A survey conducted from 1991 to 1992 in twenty-two nations in and beyond the European Community found that only ten nations recognized medical genetics as a specialty (Harris and Rhind, 1993). Eleven nations had formal training programs in medical genetics. Geneticists in half of these nations "strongly favored" a proposal for a European diploma in medical genetics.

In the United States and Canada, medical genetics has been recognized as a specialty in medicine, with requirements for training and board examinations for persons holding an M.D. or a Ph.D. in human genetics (Epstein, 1992). In these nations, however, there has tended to be a division of labor in the tasks of genetic counseling between medical geneticists and genetic counselors holding master's degrees. In the aspects of counseling related to medical goals, for example, understanding the diagnosis, treatment (if possible), and prognosis, a medical geneticist has tended to be directly involved. Genetic counselors holding the master's degree have tended to be involved in the aspects of counseling related to education about risks, recurrence, reproductive options, and guidance regarding support for affected family members. In many centers in the United States and Canada, counseling has been done by multidisciplinary teams of medical geneticists and genetic counselors, based on models formulated in the mid-1970s (Ad Hoc Committee on Genetic Counseling, 1975). Therefore, it was not surprising when controversy attended a decision that board examinations in medical genetics in the United States exclude master's-level genetic counselors (Heimler et al., 1992). Issues of recognition and fairness between medical geneticists and genetic counselors will continue to be important in nations where the practice is to divide labor between them.

Technical competence is an increasingly important criterion in medical genetics, because practitioners have important roles in laboratory analyses. They perform cytogenetic analyses, DNA studies, and quantitative measurements of enzyme functions or the level of biological substances—for example, alpha-fetoprotein (AFP) in blood or amniotic fluid. Very few medical geneticists have expertise in all these areas, and many workers in genetics laboratories are not physicians. The most important roles for the medical geneticists in the laboratory are to identify the laboratory tests and analyses that are specifically needed and to evaluate test results in genetic as well as clinical terms.

In prenatal diagnosis of genetic disorders, the medical geneticist has a crucial clinical role as well as one at the laboratory bench. He or she provides or supervises genetic counseling prior to and after prenatal diagnosis and communicates and interprets the test results to pregnant women and their partners when a pathological finding is made. Many medical geneticists participate actively in the laboratory work involved in prenatal diagnosis. The ethical issue of greatest concern in prenatal diagnosis involves selective abortion, and most geneticists agree that societies ought to protect parental autonomy to make this choice without pressure or punishment for taking either option. Such respect for choice has not been protected in all societies.

Tests for genetic disorders caused by one gene, such as Huntington disease, and screening procedures for diseases having a familial predisposition, such as premature atherosclerosis, are available. Since many disorders are latent and do not manifest themselves until later in life, "predictive" tests will reveal whether or not an individual has the affected gene, which could be inherited by offspring. In Huntington disease, the gene causes neurological dysfunction, usually starting between the ages of forty and fifty, for which there is no treatment; death is certain.

In atherosclerotic disease before fifty-five to sixty years of age, coronary heart disease (CHD), angina pectoris, or sudden death can occur. These events cluster in families in a way that indicates a strong genetic component. Several risk factors for CHD show a significant degree of heritability (Berg, 1992). The main way to cope with a genetic predisposition to CHD is by prevention through strict dietary and drug control. In centers that conduct predictive testing, the medical geneticist will be responsible for interpreting laboratory results that foretell prognosis or may supervise such work. Thorough knowledge of the genetics, natural history, and prognosis of the disease in question is essential. The medical geneticist must keep abreast of the growing body of knowledge about tests, their reliability, and the particular genetic history within families that plays a role in interpreting test results. There are significant ethical issues involved in disclosing test results, especially to vulnerable persons and to children.

The more genes that are mapped, the more detection of genetic predisposition to common disorders such as cancer, diabetes, and heart disease will be possible. Consultands will approach medical geneticists not only with present complaints, but with requests to disclose their predispositions to disease. This has been one of the most profound changes in the practice of modern medicine. The purpose of such detection is to improve disease prevention. Counseling about healthy lifestyle, diet, and methods of surveillance can follow. Although medical geneticists have worked mostly with relatively rare disorders caused by a single gene or a chromosomal anomaly, practitioners who work with genetic predisposition to common disorders will be involved in an area of medicine with very great public-health impact. For this reason, medical geneticists need to be informed about and sensitive to their societies' ethical and religious traditions.

Another activity with a strong societal component is genetic screening, in which a whole population, or a defined portion of it, is examined. Screening is done to enable those who carry a gene for a recessive disorder, such as beta-thalassemia or Tay-Sachs disease, to be aware of their "carrier state," and thus of their risks (one in four in every pregnancy) of having a child with the disorder if the other parent also carries that gene. Such knowledge bears heavily on the use of prenatal diagnosis by such couples.

Ethical aspects of contemporary medical genetics

The education and training of medical geneticists requires a component of ethical reflection and study. Two main goals can shape this activity: (1) developing an effective patient–geneticist relationship, and (2) developing professional abilities. The first goal is to practice medical genetics with respect for the moral autonomy of the persons who seek testing and advice, and to be prepared for the special types of moral problems frequently seen by geneticists. There is a widely shared consensus among practitioners about the desired characteristics of their relationship with patients and families (Fletcher et al., 1985). This consensus, described above, is the hard-won achievement of the post–World War II generation of medical geneticists and their successors. Further, the practice of voluntarily chosen, nondirective counseling is the clearest statement that medical geneticists can make against fears of a "backdoor to eugenics" (Duster, 1990) and against criticisms by feminist scholars and others who believe that geneticists are unwitting agents of societies that care little for the handicapped (Hubbard and Wald, 1993; Lippman, 1991). The practice of medical genetics necessarily impinges on choices regarding human reproduction. It is the moral stance of medical geneticists today to avoid coercion, pressure, or even overly directive advice when patients are in the throes of moral choice. Whereas it is acceptable to advise patients as to what others have done in such situations or to arrange meetings with former patients who have made decisions on either side of the choice, it is unsatisfactory for the practitioner to displace responsibility and make the choice for the patient.

Some types of ethical dilemmas frequently arise in the relationships of medical geneticists and patients. These include, but are not limited to, dilemmas of: (1) disclosure, (2) privacy and confidentiality, and (3) requests for prenatal diagnosis that are not medically indicated.

Disclosure dilemmas arise largely from the geneticist's access to psychologically sensitive information. For example, a geneticist can know, but a married couple does not yet know, which one of the couple has transmitted a disorder to a child. Geneticists can know by testing that a person who is clearly female in appearance actually has male (XY) sex chromosomes due to a biological event. The patient can be seeking help because she is infertile. How a geneticist discloses the true biological facts without threatening the patient's female identity requires great sensitivity. Testing can show false paternity, or that a woman has had previous elective abortions about which her husband does not know. Geneticists may differ about the interpretation of findings. Should they share their differences with patients? An abortion might ensue. Should disclosure be made of a genetic diagnosis to a vulnerable or fragile individual? Preparation to respond to such problems is important. The international study cited earlier found consensus on approaches to some, but not all, of these dilemmas (Wertz and Fletcher, 1989).

The duty to protect the patient's privacy and to maintain the confidentiality of the patient–geneticist relationship can, in some circumstances, be subject to other claims when interests of other relatives conflict. Rarely, if patients persist in forbidding geneticists from contacting other relatives who have a very high genetic risk, the patient's confidentiality may have to be in-

fringed. Guidelines for this contingency were shaped by the U.S. President's Commission for the Study of Ethical Problems in Medicine and Biomedical and Behavioral Research (1983). Geneticists have a clear duty to protect patients from unconsenting disclosures of genetic diagnoses to third parties such as insurers, employers, and government agencies. Indeed, mistaking the carrier state for a disease has sometimes led to unfair stigmatization by employers or insurers of those who have been screened.

Requests for prenatal diagnosis are controversial when they are related to selection of gender (unrelated to sex-linked disorders), maternal anxiety, or paternity testing, and when they are for obtaining information related to the health problems of a third person (e.g., about whether the fetus would be a suitable match for bone marrow or other transplants for an affected and living sibling). Because the criteria for providing prenatal diagnosis differ greatly from nation to nation, it is advisable for medical geneticists to have policy guidelines for such requests, but most geneticists would agree that prenatal diagnosis ought to be given for medical indications related to the health status of the fetus.

In view of the "new genetics" (Weatherall, 1991), the second goal in training new medical geneticists is to equip them to participate in interdisciplinary and societal reflection on the broader ethical, legal, and social implications of genetic research. Neil Holtzman (1988) has outlined some implications that must be considered within the social and moral traditions of each nation:

- Gradually, DNA tests will be developed for all genetic disorders and for genotypes that predispose to common diseases, although the validation of such tests will be very difficult due to genetic heterogeneity (great differences in gene expression).
- The number of persons to be screened will be extremely large.
- The number of interested third parties, besides family members, primary-care physicians, and health authorities, will multiply (e.g., insurers and employers), and thus increase the chances for genetic discrimination (Natowicz et al., 1992); privacy and confidentiality issues will proliferate.
- Because DNA must be collected from members of whole families, and in some cases from generations of family members, secrets will be virtually impossible to keep; DNA banks and genetic registers create large privacy problems (Read, 1990).
- Disclosure dilemmas will multiply, especially because harmful genes will be detected presymptomatically in adults and children with disorders of late onset (Harris, 1988).

Medical geneticists need to be participants and educators in public debates about these implications, which are occurring in many nations under sponsorship of official bodies and in many international settings (Bankowski and Capron, 1991). Medical geneticists should also counter the tendency of other participants to become dependent on them to supply all scientific concepts and information. There is no substitute for public education about the genetic concepts that are required for informed debate aimed to separate the positive from the negative possibilities of genetic research (Griffiths, 1993).

KÅRE BERG

Directly related to this article is the companion article in this entry: ETHICAL AND SOCIAL ISSUES. *Also directly related are the entries* GENETIC COUNSELING; GENETIC TESTING AND SCREENING, *articles on* LEGAL ISSUES, *and* ETHICAL ISSUES; *and* GENE THERAPY, *article on* ETHICAL AND SOCIAL ISSUES. *For a further discussion of topics mentioned in this article, see the entries* CONFIDENTIALITY; DNA TYPING; EUGENICS; EVOLUTION; GENOME MAPPING AND SEQUENCING; INFORMATION DISCLOSURE, *article on* ETHICAL ISSUES; *and* PRIVILEGED COMMUNICATIONS. *Other relevant material may be found under the entries* BIOLOGY, PHILOSOPHY OF; GENETIC ENGINEERING; GENETICS AND ENVIRONMENT IN HUMAN HEALTH; GENETICS AND HUMAN BEHAVIOR; GENETICS AND HUMAN SELF-UNDERSTANDING; GENETICS AND THE LAW; *and* GENETICS AND RACIAL MINORITIES.

Bibliography

AD HOC COMMITTEE ON GENETIC COUNSELING. AMERICAN SOCIETY OF HUMAN GENETICS. 1975. "Genetic Counseling." *American Journal of Human Genetics* 27, no. 2: 240–242.

BANKOWSKI, Z., and CAPRON, ALEXANDER MORGAN, eds. 1991. *Genetics, Ethics, and Human Values: Human Genome Mapping, Genetic Screening, and Gene Therapy: Proceedings of the XXIVth CIOMS Conference, Tokyo and Inuyama City, Japan, 22–27 July 1990.* Geneva: Council for International Organizations of Medical Sciences.

BERG, KÅRE. 1992. "Molecular Genetics and Genetic Epidemiology of Cardiovascular Diseases and Diabetes. Introductory Remarks: Risk Factor Levels and Variability." *Annals of Medicine* 24:343–347.

CZEIZEL, ENDRE. 1988. *The Right to Be Born Healthy: The Ethical Problems of Human Genetics in Hungary.* Translated by Catherine K. Bokor and Gabe Bokor. New York: Alan R. Liss.

DUSTER, TROY. 1990. *Backdoor to Eugenics.* New York: Routledge.

EPSTEIN, CHARLES J. 1992. "Organized Medical Genetics at a Crossroad." *American Journal of Human Genetics* 51, no. 2:231–234.

FLETCHER, JOHN C.; BERG, KÅRE; and TRANØY, KNUT E. 1985. "Ethical Aspects of Medical Genetics: A Proposal for Guidelines in Genetic Counseling, Prenatal Diagnosis and Screening." *Clinical Genetics* 27, no. 2:199–205.

FRASER, F. CLARKE. 1974. "Genetic Counseling." *American Journal of Human Genetics* 26, no. 5:636–659.

GALTON, FRANCIS. 1865. "Hereditary Talent and Character." *MacMillan's Magazine* 12:157–167.

GARROD, ARCHIBALD E. 1902. "The Incidence of Alcaptonuria: A Study in Chemical Individuality." *Lancet* 2:1616–1620.

GRIFFITHS, ANTHONY J. 1993. "What Does the Public Really Need to Know About Genetics?" *American Journal of Human Genetics* 52, no. 1:230–232.

HARRIS, RODNEY. 1988. "Genetic Counseling and the New Genetics." *Trends in Genetics* 4, no. 2:52–56.

———. 1990. "Physicians and Other Nongeneticists Strongly Favor Teaching Genetics to Medical Students in the United Kingdom." *American Journal of Human Genetics* 47, no. 4:750–752.

HARRIS, RODNEY, and RHIND, JUDITH A. 1993. "The Specialty of Clinical Genetics: European Society of Human Genetics Survey." *Journal of Medical Genetics* 30, no. 2:147–152.

HEIMLER, AUDREY; BENKENDORF, JUDITH; GETTIG, ELIZABETH; REICH, ELSA; SCHMERLER, SUSAN; and TRAVERS, HELEN. 1992. "American Board of Medical Genetics Restructuring: Make an Informed Decision." *American Journal of Human Genetics* 51:v–vii.

HOLTZMAN, NEIL A. 1988. "Recombinant DNA Technology, Genetic Tests, and Public Policy." *American Journal of Human Genetics* 42, no. 4:624–632.

HUBBARD, RUTH, and WALD, ELIJAH. 1993. *Exploding the Gene Myth: How Genetic Information Is Produced and Manipulated by Scientists, Physicians, Employers, Insurance Companies, Educators, and Law Enforcers.* Boston: Beacon Press.

KEVLES, DANIEL J. 1985. *In the Name of Eugenics: Genetics and the Uses of Human Heredity.* New York: Alfred A. Knopf.

LIPPMAN, ABBY. 1991. "Prenatal Genetic Testing and Screening: Constructing Needs and Reinforcing Inequities." *American Journal of Law and Medicine* 17, nos. 1–2: 15–50.

McKUSICK, VICTOR A. 1969. *Human Genetics.* 2d ed. Englewood Cliffs, N.J.: Prentice-Hall.

MÜLLER-HILL, BENNO. 1988. *Murderous Science: Elimination by Scientific Selection of Jews, Gypsies, and Others, Germany 1933–1945.* Oxford: Oxford University Press.

NATOWICZ, MARVIN R.; ALPER, JANE K.; and ALPER, JOSEPH S. 1992. "Genetic Discrimination and the Law." *American Journal of Medical Genetics* 51, no. 3:465–475.

PARKER, LISA S. 1994. "Bioethics for Human Geneticists: Models for Reasoning and Methods for Teaching." *American Journal of Human Genetics* 54, no. 1:137–147.

PROCTOR, ROBERT. 1988. *Racial Hygiene: Medicine Under the Nazis.* Cambridge, Mass.: Harvard University Press.

READ, ANDREW P. 1990. "Genetic Registers." In vol. 2 of *Principles and Practice of Medical Genetics*, 2d ed., pp. 1995–1999. Edited by Alan E. H. Emery and David L. Rimoin. Edinburgh: Churchill Livingstone.

U.S. PRESIDENT'S COMMISSION FOR THE STUDY OF ETHICAL PROBLEMS IN MEDICINE AND BIOMEDICAL AND BEHAV-

IORAL RESEARCH. 1983. *Screening and Counseling for Genetic Conditions: A Report on the Ethical, Social, and Legal Implications of Genetic Screening, Counseling, and Education Programs.* Washington, D.C.: Author.

VOGEL, FRIEDRICH, and MOTULSKY, ARNO G. 1979. *Human Genetics: Problems and Approaches.* Berlin: Springer-Verlag.

WEATHERALL, DAVID J. 1991. *The New Genetics and Clinical Practice.* 3d ed. Oxford: Oxford University Press.

WEINDLING, PAUL. 1993. "The Survival of Eugenics in 20th Century Germany." *American Journal of Human Genetics* 52, no. 3:643–649.

WERTZ, DOROTHY C., and FLETCHER, JOHN C. 1993. "A Critique of Some Feminist Challenges to Prenatal Diagnosis." *Journal of Women's Health* 2:173–188.

———, eds. 1989. *Ethics and Human Genetics: A Cross-Cultural Perspective.* Berlin: Springer-Verlag.

II. ETHICAL AND SOCIAL ISSUES

Geneticists face eight major ethical and social problems. These are not new or unique to genetics. A survey of 682 geneticists in nineteen nations showed worldwide consensus about some approaches (Wertz and Fletcher, 1989b; Wertz et al., 1990).

Equitable distribution of services

More patients from higher social classes than from poor and minority groups use genetic services. National health insurance reduces but does not eliminate this class differential. If present trends continue, the educated and economically privileged will see a marked reduction in births of children with genetic disorders. Genetic disability could become a mark of the underprivileged, who are less likely to receive prenatal care early enough for prenatal diagnosis. In the United States in 1985, 70 percent of whites, 62 percent of African-Americans, and 61 percent of Hispanics received early prenatal care (Wertz et al., 1990).

Geneticists agree that affordable services should be available to all, with first priority to those whose needs are greatest. National health insurance and public education in genetics are prerequisites for just distribution of services. About one-third of disability has a known genetic basis. Therefore, genetic services deserve a high priority in national health-care budgets. In developing nations, genetic disorders have emerged as significant causes of infant mortality (Wertz and Fletcher, 1989b) as death rates from infectious disease have fallen.

Respect for patients' choices

Geneticists value patients' autonomy in decision making, including freedom to choose to abort a fetus with a genetic defect or carry the child to term. Although most developed nations liberalized abortion laws after 1970 (Wertz and Fletcher, 1989b), abortion rights are under attack. In some nations, including most of Latin America, abortions for fetal defects are illegal, although available to those who can pay. On the other hand, some private health insurance companies in developed nations have tried to coerce women into aborting fetuses with severe defects by threatening to withhold payment for the child's care.

The American Society of Human Genetics (1991), by a 77 percent majority vote, approved a statement on patient freedom of choice, together with a draft of model legislation. A majority of the United States public (75–78%) surveyed between 1972 and 1990 believed that "It should be possible to obtain a *legal* abortion if there is a strong chance of a serious defect in the baby" (Davis, 1990).

Full disclosure of all clinically relevant information

Almost all geneticists would disclose all clinically relevant test results in prenatal diagnosis, including ambiguous or conflicting results or controversial new interpretations (Wertz and Fletcher, 1989b). Although some feminists argue that women have a "right not to know" prenatal test results (Rothman, 1986), geneticists believe that patients have a right to know, or even a duty to know, in order to make decisions. They see little or no psychological harm from disclosure. When colleagues disagree about meanings of test results, the majority (75% in the United States, 60% elsewhere) would tell patients about the disagreement.

Almost all geneticists think that workers should be told the results of tests for genetic susceptibility to work-related disease. This consensus contrasts with practices of concealment in some industries in the United States (Draper, 1991).

Geneticists have no consensus about disclosure of personally sensitive information. About half would disclose XY (male) genotype to an apparently normal woman seeking infertility treatment. Disclosure of the male Y chromosome could cause grave psychological damage; nondisclosure leaves the infertility question unresolved and also leaves the patient at risk for cancer of the reproductive organs. If one parent carries genetic material causing a genetic disorder in a couple's child, disclosure could cause marital conflict, while nondisclosure would prevent the couple from using reproductive options that would prevent the disorder's reoccurrence. In this case, 54 percent would tell the parents which one carries the material; the rest would tell them only if they ask.

Some acknowledge a patient's "right not to know" a test result, especially if the disorder cannot be prevented or treated. For Huntington disease, an incurable neurological disorder that appears in middle age, 66 percent believe that patients have a right not to know the results of presymptomatic tests, but 34 percent believe that patients have a "duty to know" so that they can plan their lives and decide whether to take the 50 percent risk of transmitting the disease to their children.

Some information is not relevant to diagnosis or treatment and could cause harm. Nonpaternity (husband is not the child's father) occurs in an estimated 5 percent of the U.S. population. Most geneticists (96%) would not tell the husband; 81 percent would tell the mother alone and let her decide what to do (Wertz and Fletcher, 1989b).

Protection of individuals' privacy from institutional third parties

The "new genetics" permits examination of an individual's genotype (molecular genetic makeup) independently of phenotype (observable characteristics). Many genes are never expressed and make no difference to an individual's life. Investigation of the genotype leads to new possibilities for intrusions upon privacy and for discrimination in employment, insurance, and other areas of life.

Most geneticists (89%) believe that health, life, and worker's compensation insurers should not have access to test results without a person's consent. Recognizing the power of insurance companies to coerce consent by withholding insurance, 40 percent believe that insurers should have no access to genetic information, even with an individual's consent (Wertz and Fletcher, 1989b). Most believe that employers (81%) and government health agencies (68%) should have no access even with consent. Many believe that institutions will misuse genetic information. Legislation will be necessary to protect personal privacy and to prevent discrimination against persons with genetic disorders or genetic susceptibilities.

Confidentiality when family members are at high risk

Genes are the common property of a family. An individual's diagnosis may be useful to relatives in making their plans for the future, including reproductive plans. Geneticists agree that patients should share relevant information with their close relatives. This duty arises from kinship bonds and from the ethical principle of avoidance of harm. If a patient refuses to disclose information useful to other family members, geneticists face a dilemma between two well-known duties in medicine: protection of patient privacy and the duty to warn third parties of harm. There is no consensus on this issue.

Around the world, 32 percent of geneticists would preserve the confidentiality of a patient with Huntington disease; 36 percent would tell the patient's close relatives at 50 percent risk of developing the disease, if the relatives asked; 24 percent would tell the relatives even if they did not ask; and 10 percent would refer the decision to the patient's family physician (Wertz and Fletcher, 1989b). The U.S. President's Commission (1983) recommended that the duty of confidentiality to a patient could be overridden under four conditions: (1) efforts to persuade the patient to tell relatives have failed; (2) there is a high risk of harm to relatives if information is withheld and the information would be used to prevent harm; (3) the harm would be serious; (4) only information directly relevant to the relatives' health would be disclosed. Under these conditions, doctors would be legally permitted, but not legally required, to tell relatives. They would also be permitted to tell the patient's spouse if children are intended, in order to prevent harm to the next generation (Andrews, 1987; Elias and Annas, 1987).

Indications for prenatal diagnosis

Generally accepted medical indications for prenatal diagnosis are advanced maternal age (over thirty-five), family history of genetic disorder, or exposure to toxic substances. Ethical questions arise when patients request prenatal diagnosis without such indications (Wertz and Fletcher, 1989b). In the United States, most geneticists (89%) would perform prenatal diagnosis or offer a referral for a twenty-five-year-old normally anxious pregnant woman with no medical indications. Most think that patient autonomy and the benefits from reassurance outweigh any risks to the fetus. Women geneticists, who made up 35 percent of survey respondents, were more likely to perform prenatal diagnosis, on grounds of patient autonomy (Wertz and Fletcher, 1989a, 1989b).

There is worldwide consensus among geneticists (96% in the United States) that willingness to abort a fetus with a genetic disorder should not be a precondition for prenatal diagnosis. In eastern European nations, developing nations, and Norway (where the number of prenatal diagnoses is limited by law), fewer geneticists would perform prenatal diagnosis, citing scarcity of resources.

Sex selection is the most controversial use of prenatal diagnosis. In India, sex selection for sons is the most common use of prenatal diagnosis, especially ultrasound (Wertz and Fletcher, 1989b). Few patients make open requests for sex selection in developed nations. The majority of U.S. geneticists in 1985 would either perform prenatal diagnosis (34%) or offer a referral (28%), as would majorities in Hungary (60%) and India (52%), and more than 25 percent in Brazil, Canada,

Greece, and Israel, for a couple with four daughters who desire a son and who would abort a female fetus. In the United States, women geneticists were twice as likely as men to say that they would perform prenatal diagnosis for this couple. Those who would perform prenatal diagnosis regarded sex selection as an extension of patients' rights to determine the number, spacing, and health of their children. Most who would refuse opposed abortion of a normal fetus. Except in India, few mentioned social issues such as unbalancing the sex ratio, the status of women, or limiting the population. Sex selection poses a dilemma: If doctors agree to facilitate parents' preferences, sex selection may reinforce stereotypes and place males and females into a preferred order of birth; this would unbalance power relationships between genders (U.S. President's Commission, 1983). If doctors withhold the service, they can be accused of medical paternalism.

Voluntary versus mandatory screening

Genetic screening, as opposed to individual testing, involves large groups or entire populations. The accepted rule is that screening be conducted only for conditions that can be treated or prevented, and that screening be voluntary, with one exception. The U.S. President's Commission (1983) recommended that screening be mandatory for newborns if, and only if, early diagnosis and treatment benefited the newborn. An example is phenylketonuria (PKU), for which a special diet started shortly after birth prevents mental retardation. The purpose of mandatory newborn screening is to protect the most vulnerable members of society, who are unable to protect themselves. The U.S. President's Commission did not believe that newborn screening should be mandatory if done primarily for purposes of identifying and counseling carriers of genetic disorders before they conceive another child. Voluntary screening for adults should be accompanied by public education, with cooperation from the community. Early attempts at sickle-cell screening in the United States led to stigmatization of normal carriers of sickle-cell trait. In contrast, a Tay-Sachs screening program done in cooperation with the Jewish community was well received (U.S. President's Commission, 1983). There is consensus that population screening not be used for children under eighteen, unless there is a clear benefit to the child.

Around the world, most geneticists (72%) think that screening in the workplace for genetic susceptibility to work-related disease should be voluntary. Exceptions are socialist nations where laws have guaranteed employment, and developing nations, where few laws prevent occupational exposure. In these nations, genetic testing may offer protection to workers.

Nondirective versus directive counseling

Around the world, 97 to 100 percent of geneticists subscribe to five goals (Fraser, 1974): (1) helping individuals and couples understand their options and the present state of medical knowledge so they can make informed decisions; (2) helping individuals and couples adjust to and cope with their genetic problems; (3) removing or lessening patient guilt or anxiety; (4) helping individuals/couples achieve their parenting goals; and (5) preventing disease or abnormality. A majority (74%) believes that improvement of the general health and vigor of the population is important. A smaller majority (54%) subscribes to a eugenic goal, a reduction in the number of carriers of genetic disorders in the population (Wertz and Fletcher, 1989b). Around the world, 92 to 94 percent believe in two nondirective approaches: (1) suggest that while you will not make decisions for patients, you will support any decision they make; and (2) tell patients decisions are theirs alone and refuse to make any for them. A majority (66%) would inform patients of what most other people in their situation have done; most counselors do not regard this as directive. A minority would use the following openly directive approaches: (1) inform patients what you would do if in their situation (26%), or (2) advise patients what they ought to do (15%). Women are significantly less directive then men (Wertz and Fletcher, 1989a, 1989b). Professionals do not appear to realize that nondirectiveness can go too far; some parental decisions, such as sex selection, are ethically insupportable.

The Declaration of Inuyama (Bankowski and Capron, 1991) conveys the responses of delegates from twenty-four nations to the eight problems described above. It supports fair access to genetic services; respect for patients' choices, including abortion; full disclosure to patients; protection of individual privacy against employers and insurers; use of prenatal diagnosis only for conditions affecting the health of the child; voluntary screening; and nondirective counseling.

DOROTHY C. WERTZ

Directly related to this article is the companion article in this entry: PRACTICE OF MEDICAL GENETICS. *Also directly related are the entries* GENETIC TESTING AND SCREENING; GENETIC COUNSELING; *and* DNA TYPING. *For a further discussion of the topics mentioned in this article, see the entries* AUTONOMY; BENEFICENCE; CONFIDENTIALITY; EUGENICS; HARM; INFORMATION DISCLOSURE; JUSTICE; PRIVACY IN HEALTH CARE; PROFESSIONAL–PATIENT RELATIONSHIP, *articles on* SOCIOLOGICAL PERSPECTIVES, *and* ETHICAL ISSUES; REPRODUCTIVE TECHNOLOGIES, *article on* SEX SELECTION; *and* SEXISM. *For a discussion of related ideas, see the entries* FUTURE GENERATIONS,

Obligations to; *and* Genome Mapping and Sequencing.

Bibliography

"American Society of Human Genetics Statement on Clinical Genetics and Freedom of Choice." 1991. *American Journal of Human Genetics* 48, no. 5:1011. Policy statement and model draft legislation on abortion rights for fetal defects.

Andrews, Lori B. 1987. *Medical Genetics: A Legal Frontier.* Chicago: American Bar Foundation. A comprehensive description of policy frameworks, role of U.S. regulatory agencies, all U.S. laws relating to informed consent, duties to disclose, wrongful birth, wrongful life, genetic counseling, confidentiality of genetic information, and mandatory versus voluntary screening, diagnosis, and treatment.

Bankowski, Z., and Capron, Alexander Morgan, eds. 1991. *Genetics, Ethics, and Human Values: Human Genome Mapping, Genetic Screening, and Gene Therapy: Proceedings of the XXIVth Council for International Organizations of Medical Sciences (CIOMS) Conference, Tokyo and Inuyama City, Japan, 22–27 July 1990.* Geneva: CIOMS. Includes the Declaration of Inuyama, a statement on ethics produced by representatives of twenty-four nations.

Davis, James A. 1990. *General Social Surveys, 1972–1990: Cumulative Codebook.* Chicago: National Opinion Research Center. Surveys of attitudes toward abortion for serious fetal defects.

Draper, Elaine. 1991. *Risky Business: Genetic Testing and Exclusionary Practices in the Hazardous Workplace.* Cambridge: At the University Press. Examines views of unions, which favor genetic monitoring to protect workers' health, and management, which prefers pre-employment screening to prevent hiring susceptible workers.

Elias, Sherman, and Annas, George J. 1987. *Reproductive Genetics and the Law.* Chicago: Year Book Medical Publishers. Covers legal and ethical problems in genetic counseling, screening, and especially prenatal diagnosis; also treatment of handicapped newborns, teratology counseling, noncoital reproduction, and gene therapy.

Fletcher, John C., and Wertz, Dorothy C. 1990. "Ethics, Law, and Medical Genetics: After the Human Genome Is Mapped." *Emory Law Journal* 39, no. 3:747–809. Report of nineteen-nation survey of 682 medical geneticists and recommendations for an international code of ethics.

Fraser, F. Clarke. 1974. "Genetic Counseling." *American Journal of Human Genetics* 26, no. 5:636–659. Outlines the basis of nondirective counseling. Goals and methods stated here have become central to the entire ethos of counseling.

Holtzman, Neil A. 1989. *Proceed with Caution: Predicting Genetic Risks in the Recombinant DNA Era.* Baltimore: Johns Hopkins University Press. Concerned with privacy issues, especially regarding insurers and employers. Best overview of benefits and risks of testing.

Lippman, Abby. 1991. "Prenatal Genetic Testing and Screening: Constructing Needs and Reinforcing Inequities." *American Journal of Law and Medicine* 17, nos. 1–2:15–50. Special issue, "The Human Genome Initiative and the Impact of Genetic Testing and Screening Technologies." Argues that the social milieu in developed nations coerces women into having prenatal diagnosis. Extensive legal and ethical citations. Other articles in this volume focus on uses of genetic information in schools and by employers.

Rothman, Barbara Katz. 1986. *The Tentative Pregnancy: Prenatal Diagnosis and the Future of Motherhood.* New York: Viking. Describes the effects on women of unexpected and sometimes unwanted information from prenatal diagnosis, especially the effects of knowing fetal sex.

Science Council of Canada. 1991. *Genetics in Canadian Health Care.* Ottawa: Author. Overall view of public policy and ethical dilemmas in Canada.

Suzuki, David, and Knudtson, Peter. 1988. *Genethics: The Ethics of Engineering Life.* Toronto: Stoddart. Includes chapters on XYY controversy, screening in the workplace, and gene therapy, also much on plant genetics and recombinant DNA.

U.S. Congress. Office of Technology Assessment. 1990. *Genetic Monitoring and Screening in the Workplace.* Washington, D.C.: U.S. Government Printing Office. Reports actual uses of genetic tests by major U.S. employers and ethical and legal implications for workers.

U.S. President's Commission for the Study of Ethical Problems in Medicine and Biomedical and Behavioral Research. 1983. *Screening and Counseling for Genetic Conditions.* Washington, D.C.: U.S. Government Printing Office. Societal experiences of sickle-cell and Tay-Sachs screening; recommendations on disclosure of false paternity and disclosure of a patient's genetic information to relatives at risk, against the patient's wishes.

Wertz, Dorothy C., and Fletcher, John C. 1987. "Communicating Genetic Risks." *Science, Technology, and Human Values* 12, no. 3:60–66. Overview of earlier surveys of communication in genetic counseling, patient interpretations of risk, and influence of counseling on patients' reproductive plans.

———. 1988a. "Attitudes of Genetic Counselors: A Multinational Survey." *American Journal of Human Genetics* 42, no. 4:592–600.

———. 1988b. "Ethics and Medical Genetics in the United States: A National Survey." *American Journal of Medical Genetics* 29, no. 4:815–828.

———. 1989a. "Ethical Decision-making in Medical Genetics: Women as Patients and Practitioners in Eighteen Nations." In *Healing Technology: Feminist Perspectives,* pp. 221–241. Edited by Kathryn Strother Ratcliff. Ann Arbor: University of Michigan Press. Differences between the attitudes of female and male doctors on ethical issues in genetics.

———. 1989b. *Ethics and Human Genetics: A Cross-Cultural Perspective.* Berlin: Springer-Verlag. Part I reports in comprehensive detail the results of a nineteen-nation survey of 682 medical geneticists, including an analysis of their moral reasoning. Part II reports the state of genetic services, the cultural context, and major ethical controversies in genetic counseling, screening, and prenatal diagnosis in nineteen nations. Part III outlines a cross-cultural ethics that avoids pitfalls of ethnocentrism and cultural relativism.

———. 1989c. "An International Survey of Attitudes of Medical Geneticists Toward Mass Screening and Access to Results." *Public Health Reports* 104, no. 1:35–44. States that most geneticists believe screening should be voluntary, and insurers and employers should not have access to results without consent.

WERTZ, DOROTHY C.; FLETCHER, JOHN C.; and MULVIHILL, JOHN J. 1990. "Medical Geneticists Confront Ethical Dilemmas: Cross-Cultural Comparisons Among 18 Nations." *American Journal of Human Genetics* 46:1200–1213. Reports concisely the results of 1985–1986 survey of 682 medical geneticists on attitudes toward counseling, screening, and prenatal diagnosis.

MEDICAL INFORMATION SYSTEMS

This entry examines the role of computerized medical information systems, including artificial intelligence technology, in the delivery of health care and identifies some of the major ethical and legal issues associated with their use. These issues are confidentiality and the problem of expanding access to patient medical records; the increased role of informed consent in using computerized medical information systems; the substitution of diagnostic artificial intelligence systems for physician judgment; and the use of computerized screening systems to restrict indigent patients' access to hospital services. Some of these concerns, such as patient confidentiality and informed consent, are not new to the field of bioethics but take on a unique twist requiring creative adaptations. Other concerns touch on the nature of how we deliver medical care and the dramatic changes taking place in the practice of medicine.

The evolutionary lineage of medical computing systems can be traced to 1890, when Herman Hollerith developed a punched-card data-processing system for use in the U.S. census that year. Hollerith's methods were soon adapted to epidemiologic and public-health surveys, leading to the era of electromechanical punched-card data-processing technology, widely used during the 1920s and 1930s. These techniques gave rise to the "stored-program" and wholly electronic digital computers that appeared in the late 1940s (Collen, 1986). With the appearance of the minicomputer in the 1970s and the availability of microcomputers in the early 1980s, a variety of complex computerized medical information systems emerged. These remarkable systems now aid physicians in making diagnoses, calculating drug dosages, and administering treatment automatically, sometimes without human intervention. Hospitals regularly apply computer technology in areas such as charting, record keeping, billing, census counts, and personnel management, and as an important tool for managing care expenditures (e.g., controlling admissions, limiting services, etc.).

The potential for this technology to expedite the organization, retrieval, and communication of vital information holds great promise for medicine and is among the forces shaping the practice environment. A wide variety of medical and clinical functions that used to be performed by health-care professionals are being managed by sophisticated computerized systems. In most cases, these functions are performed faster, more economically, and more accurately by computer, thus augmenting and challenging traditional methods employed in the delivery of health care.

Medical information systems fall into three general categories that function independently but are closely interrelated: (1) data management, including input and output; (2) communications; and (3) clinical decision support (Rennels and Shortliffe, 1987). Ideally, the optimal medical information system will consist of all three components, orchestrated for comprehensive data acquisition, immediate retrieval and communication between providers, documentation of services, review of outcomes that can ultimately provide increased continuity of care, and health services research support.

Data management technology

Many different models of information systems are being utilized by major hospitals throughout the United States and in some other countries, such as France, England, and Japan. The common purpose of all these systems is to collect, collate, store, retrieve, and communicate all information regarding specific medical events to medical, nursing, administrative, and billing personnel, as well as allied support personnel.

While the use of management information systems has done much to streamline the important clerical functions of the hospital's operations, there is one serious drawback. Hospital administrators can accurately determine which physicians use the most resources and compare the performance of a physician against the performance of others in the same specialty, department, or region (Brannigan and Dayhoff, 1986). As a result, physicians are likely to face the prospect of tighter administrative control, sometimes to the point of mandating the manner and scope of their practice strategies. This degree of involvement by management may arbitrarily modify traditional health-care practices (e.g., ordering services, admitting and discharging patients, etc.) and, as a result, directly affect patient expectations.

Information systems can also have an impact on a hospital's patient admission policies that are designed to increase revenues and reduce expenses, by gathering information selectively from other available resources (e.g., insurance companies, medical-legal systems, credit bureaus). This information can be made available in emergency rooms, thus enabling hospitals to screen patients for admission, and to minimize contact with patients unable to pay.

Implementation of systems whose net effect is to increase contact with profit-supporting patients and divert contact with patients with insufficient or no insurance coverage and who do not qualify for either Medicare of Medicaid, or patients who are more likely to have complications requiring long stays (e.g., homeless, alcoholics, etc.) should be questioned on ethical grounds (Marsh, 1985). While these systems are an important resource for management of effective cost-containment policies, they could work against health-care access for the indigent.

Hospitals' ability to deny access to health care to a large segment of the population will be greatly enhanced by the emerging integrated multipurpose information systems of the future. These large multi-institutional networks, designed and programmed to link multipurpose information systems and create a common patient profile data base, will facilitate identifying nonpaying patients as well as potentially litigious ones. As a result, a greater number of people may be denied access to health care.

Data communications technology

Communication systems, designed to transmit stored medical information between health-care providers, have two primary purposes: (1) to maintain integrity and continuity of care by transmitting timely and complete patient records to all medical professionals attending to the patient, and (2) to provide access to biomedical research literature, practice profiles, and disease-specific data bases.

Because of the large and growing knowledge base being engendered by advances in medical technology, it is more and more difficult for physicians to read and retain all the information required to make an informed medical decision. They continually face situations in which diagnostic and therapeutic technologies are evolving (e.g., genetic conditions, innovative cancer protocols like autologous bone marrow transplant, etc.). In other instances they may not have encountered a particular situation, or it may have been many months or years

since the last encounter and they are unsure of the appropriate care plan. In general, physicians need rapid access to the world's medical knowledge in a usable form.

One of the most prominent and promising bibliographic retrieval systems is MEDLINE. This system, developed at the National Library of Medicine in Bethesda, Maryland, provides access to summaries of almost every article in major biomedical journals and reviews published throughout the world since 1966. Complete abstracts of recent articles can be obtained from this system.

A complementary system to MEDLINE is *Online Journal of Current Clinical Trials,* provided by the American Association for the Advancement of Science. This electronic medical journal publishes research complete with high-fidelity charts, graphs, and tables within hours of its review by experts, and is available to physicians, hospitals, and clinics by computer-telephone connection.

A third important reference system, Physician Data Query (PDQ), holds considerable promise in the care of oncology patients. PDQ is a system operated jointly by the National Cancer Institute and the National Library of Medicine. The system deals exclusively with cancer treatment protocols and provides physicians with specific information about formal ongoing clinical trials. Physicians having immediate access to this data base are able to determine whether their patients are eligible for specific protocols, which in some cases may increase access to less costly options (Rennels and Shortliffe, 1987).

Confidentiality.   The major ethical and legal concerns surrounding both information and communications systems center on patients' medical records and maintaining confidentiality. Confidentiality is extremely important to patients and has historically been regarded with great respect by physicians and allied health-care professionals.

The ethical duty to maintain confidentiality is based primarily on respect for the patient's sense of individuality and privacy. Without such respect, the physician–patient relationship, as well as that of the hospital patient, would be seriously impaired. Many patients would be discouraged from revealing useful diagnostic information or making a full disclosure of symptoms, because of their fear that the information revealed might be disseminated further, to become a source of embarrassment or exploitation. This fear is particularly prevalent in cases involving HIV-infected patients, where confidentiality of patients' records is essential to avoid discriminatory measures by insurance companies, employers, and others.

While the use of computerized records will ultimately enhance the quality of patient care, their use has increased the risk that patient confidentiality will be breached. The increase in medical technology employed in hospitals, along with the rise of health-care teams, has resulted in a larger number of persons who require access to the medical records in order to serve patients' interests.

Two viable designs are available for maintaining medical records and patient demographic information. One is a wide-area, multiuser system, which maintains a data base on the patients who use several health-care providers. These systems are designed to provide patient information to hospitals in one geographic region. The second is the single in-house patient information system used by a single provider (Blake, 1982). Both of these systems store critical and confidential patient information that can be viewed on a CRT screen or in hard copy almost instantaneously, thus compounding the health-care industry's difficult task of maintaining both the privacy and the confidentiality of the patient record (Blake, 1982).

In theory it is possible to store information in a central computer and secure it for predetermined access, subject to the control of the patient. Practically speaking, however, all information entered into the computer in the name of a patient is readily available to others (e.g., physicians, nurses, administration, insurance companies, and lawyers if relevant to a case) who have or can gain access to the computer (Siegler, 1982).

Most security systems designed to protect the privacy of patients' records are structured around the use of a sequence of passwords in order to limit unauthorized access. While these systems provide some degree of security, several deficiencies undermine secured access: on-site personnel who use a terminal or dial-up lines but have no professional relationship with the patient; retrieving printed information from unsecured areas and/or wastebaskets; and communications lines connected to the computer that may be accessed off the premises by anyone with modems, terminals, and the expertise to break the security system. The most common breach occurs when well-intentioned staff disable the security systems to expedite access (e.g., they leave passwords pasted on the terminal for everyone to use, remain logged in even when they are no longer using the terminal, or use a single, easily guessed password) (Miller et al., 1985).

The presumption in favor of maintaining the confidentiality of all data about patients needs no special moral arguments. In the opinion of the American Medical Association (AMA), unless proper security measures are taken, there is a breach of medical ethics in making record entries into a computer system whose data base is available to more than one user. Section (8) of the AMA's guidelines on a computerized base states:

Stringent security procedures for entry into the immediate environment in which the computerized medical data base is stored and/or processed or for otherwise having access to confidential information should be developed and strictly enforced so as to prevent access to the computer facility by unauthorized personnel. Personnel audit procedures should be developed to establish a record in the event of unauthorized disclosure of medical data. A roster of past and present service bureau personnel with specified levels of access to the medical data base should be maintained. Specific administrative sanctions should exist to prevent employee breaches of confidentiality and security problems. (American Medical Association, 1992)

Regardless of whether security measures are achievable or not, patients should be informed that information regarding their medical condition is being stored in a computer that is accessible to others. In addition, patients should have the opportunity to review their medical records and to make informed choices about whether the entire record is to be available to everyone or whether certain portions of the record are to remain confidential (Siegler, 1982).

Another alternative would be to obtain from every patient at the time of admission an informed consent that is broad enough in scope to permit computer use (Blake, 1982). Access to information beyond the scope of consent agreed to by the patient would be unethical and could produce liability for the physician and/or hospital.

The Federal Privacy Act provides a framework for protection of some patient data. This statute requires federal and certain state agencies to obtain the consent of individuals before any information kept by a governmental agency, including research records, may be disclosed, unless it is for the census or for civil or criminal prosecution (5 USCA 552a[e]).

The perfection of medical 'smartcards' such as those developed in France, and to some extent in the United States, will raise new problems regarding the security of patients' records. These smartcards are basically powerful microchips installed on a small board about the size of a credit card. The card carries not only the patient's medical records, third party payers, and next to kin, but banking information and other personal data as well. Although every card carries its own access code, once the data is called up on the screen, it may be viewed and copied by anyone having access to the computer screen being used. In order to protect patient confidentiality, innovative regulations will be need.

Quality of care. Hospitals, physician offices, and other health-care institutions can utilize the electronic medical record as a viable resource to ensure the quality of care. Analysis of computerized medical information can establish a basis for determining what constitutes "efficacy" of care (technology assessment) and whether a given patient received "quality" care (outcome research). Prior to the advent of medical information systems, our understanding of what constitutes quality of care was at best speculative. According to the prevailing maxim, the more treatment rendered, the higher the quality of care. What was missing was the ability to assemble a practice-oriented data base that could be systematically analyzed to ascertain what in fact constitutes quality health care. Systems can be designed to link care and services to outcomes, providing the necessary data base to analyze patterns among different patient populations, to assess models of quality assurance, and to follow staff adherence to risk-management protocols.

By implementing an integrated information system, professional and institutional quality-assurance reviews can gain a broader understanding of the continuity of care offered to the patient. The growth of subspecialization and provision of care by teams of health professionals places new emphasis on the central role of the medical record. Ideally, the computerized medical record may be viewed simultaneously at different locations in the hospital, at the patient's bedside with individual palmtop computers, or in physicians' private offices; linked by a "data-over-voice" conference call, physicians, physical/respiratory therapists, nursing staff, radiology technicians, social workers, and discharge planners are better equipped to ensure quality and continuity of care. Traditionally, these health-care professionals have operated independently of each other, linked only by individual review of the same written medical record. Simultaneous access to a patient's electronic medical record provides better communication, planning, and implementation of patient care.

Informed consent. The automated medical record may also enhance the physician's and/or hospital's ability to comply with the federal Patient Self-Determination Act. In this instance, the patient/physician can permanently document and electronically disperse to all staff associated with patient care the patient's preferences, values, and advance directives. As new medical care paradigms materialize, during the informed consent process, patients will be able to view with their physician multimedia presentations, including three-dimensional displays, direct-access video, and animated demonstrations of a recommended procedure and risks associated with it. These same programs will suggest alternative procedures and their risks, compare them with the recommended procedure, and answer questions the patient might have about them. These programs could be made available in numerous languages to serve the needs of increasingly multicultural populations.

While the use of these sophisticated information-system modes will not replace the basic structure of the doctrine of informed consent from an ethical and legal perspective, they will broaden the standard of care as it applies to the disclosure rule and patient comprehension. Because patients will be able to learn more about their illness and, in addition, will be able to have specific questions answered in a clearer and more consistent manner, it is clear that it would be unethical for physicians not to make use of this technology where it is available.

Medical decision support systems

Medical decision support systems are the most controversial advancement for computers in medicine. Typically, these systems apply predefined algorithms and heuristics to current patient information and stored data bases to assist in solving real clinical cases. At the same time they raise complex ethical and legal questions, including accuracy, comprehensiveness, malpractice, and product liability.

A medical decision support system is a collection of computer programs assembled to assist health-care professionals in making clinical judgments on diagnoses and treatment options. Generally they assist in ascertaining the nature of a patient's disease, formulating the necessary information and scenarios required for a differential diagnosis and treatment planning. Decision support programs separate into three strategic groups: (1) instrument- and data-monitoring programs that assist in patient management; (2) risk-management and critiquing systems that guide physicians regarding important practice options for patient diagnoses and care; and (3) expert consultative systems that incorporate artificial intelligence technology to assist physicians with both difficult and routine differential diagnoses based on patient- and physician-generated data (Rennels and Shortliffe, 1987).

Monitoring programs. The most successful monitoring system in health care is the problem-oriented program HELP. This sophisticated integrated system was developed over a fifteen-year period by the Medical Informatics Department at the Latter-Day Saints Hospital in Salt Lake City. HELP runs on a central processor connected with terminals and printers in almost every medical unit in the hospital. In addition to the more traditional functions of storing the admission history and physical findings of each patient and keeping track of each patient's current medications, laboratory results, and other pertinent data, the central computer monitors each patient's data base, watching for any of a number of specified "alert" or "sentinel" conditions. On detecting such a condition, HELP, on its own, transmits a warning message to all the relevant medical staff personnel (Shortliffe, 1987).

A variant program that assists primary-care physicians is CARE. This system monitors outpatient medical records stored on-line and sends clinically indicated reminders to physicians regarding patients (e.g., when a patient is due for immunization or needs to have a previously abnormal laboratory value rechecked). Both CARE and HELP are active monitoring programs that integrate decision support and medical record systems (Taylor, 1984).

Critiquing systems. Within a critiquing system, physicians submit their diagnostic hypotheses and case management plans to a computer for review. The program then identifies areas of agreement with the physician's plan and/or suggests alternatives based on predefined profiles developed by an expert panel. Because of the sophistication required in structuring the necessary health-care profiles (each requiring a consensus among experts), relatively few systems become operational. Typically they can flourish only where there is a strong administrative group that can insist on compliance with a predefined standard of care.

One such system that offers considerable promise is called POSSUM. This critiquing system is employed by several genetic clinics for confirming final diagnoses of genetic conditions. Because of the rapidly increasing knowledge base emanating from the Human Genome Project, the importance of having a review and critiquing system in place cannot be overstated. The geneticist submits to POSSUM the salient features of a patient in a given case along with a diagnostic hypothesis. The program then tries to match the features to a specified genetic condition, which may or may not confirm the hypothesized diagnosis. It will underscore additional features that might be needed to affirm the diagnosis. Alternatively, it may suggest a different diagnosis that would be more consistent with the current findings and ultimately assist in the correct diagnosis. The program is distinct from other programs because it offers innovative visual feedback of specific genetic syndromes for age-specific groups. POSSUM's data base is maintained in Australia and can be accessed over a communication network linking genetic clinics throughout the world.

Another operational critiquing program is ATTENDING, which is used solely by anesthesiologists. The program evaluates potential anesthetic interactions, and methods of induction and administration routes proposed by the anesthesiologist. The anesthesiologist is advised by ATTENDING of potential risks that might arise from the proposed plan.

A third critiquing system is ONCOCIN, a system developed at Stanford Medical School for clinical oncologists. Initially, ONCOCIN's task was to advise physicians regarding proper radiation dosages and/or

chemotherapy for patients being treated. The scope of the program has been expanded to include a critiquing module based on the oncologist's proposed treatment plan. This feature incorporates a physician–computer dialogue module regarding possible alternatives in the event the computer identifies potential problems in the physician's proposed strategy (Shortliffe, 1987).

Expert consultation systems. An artificial intelligence (AI) medical expert system is a program that symbolically encodes concepts derived from medical experts in a given field and uses rule-based paradigms (based on this knowledge) to provide the kind of problem analysis and advice that a human expert might provide if asked to consult in a case. The expert system in effect generates an independent diagnostic recommendation and therapy management recommendation against which physicians can compare their own thoughts. Independence, accuracy, and comprehensiveness each give rise to a host of perplexing ethical and legal issues among this class of systems.

DXPLAIN, RHEUM, ILLIAD, and KNOWLEDGE COUPLER are among a few emerging expert systems in the field of clinical medicine. One of the most advanced AI medical expert systems in operation is QUICK MEDICAL REFERENCE (QMR). QMR is a large diagnostic program developed at the University of Pittsburgh School of Medicine. This remarkable system contains knowledge of 577 diseases and how these diseases interrelate with 4,100 signs, symptoms, and other case-related characteristics in internal medicine.

QMR's diagnostic capabilities parallel those of expert clinicians. Patient-specific diagnostic hypotheses are provided by querying the operation on a variety of relevant issues that focus on relationships among patient symptoms and specific characteristics associated with a particular disease, and probabilities that patients with a certain disease manifest a given characteristic. During the internal self-questioning and hypothesis-generating process, the system may request additional information it deems necessary to improve its decision-making power (e.g., patient history, tests results, etc.). If it appears that some areas of the patient work-up are deficient and need further investigation, the system points this out. After input and analysis of the requested information, QMR provides a rank-ordered list of the most probable diagnoses (Rennels and Shortliffe, 1987).

Ethical and legal issues. Decision support systems that produce diagnoses and recommended therapy management are typically based on Bayesian probabilities and, as a result, neglect or minimize clinical goals that incorporate the patient's values and expectations. These are uniquely human qualities that are not well understood and are impossible to incorporate into AI programs. There is no evidence that these computer techniques will ever evolve to approach the human mind's ability to deal with emotional, social, or ethical and legal issues that are often key determinants of proper medical decisions.

From the perspective of physicians and hospitals, the potential for increased liability is the most serious issue accompanying the growth of computer applications in health care. The pivotal question is whether the courts will apply negligence law or product liability law to a particular claim by a patient (Miller et al., 1985). The distinction between the two theories is critical and will have profound implications for the dissemination and acceptance of computer technologies.

Under the negligence approach, a standard of care requires that the physician's conduct meet reasonable expectations of safety. The product liability approach, which is based on strict liability, states clearly that a product such as a decision support system should not be harmful. In the unlikely event that the courts adopt the strict liability approach, there will be greater resistance to decision support systems. At some point in the evolution of expert systems, a system will exist that provides unequivocal judgments on what it knows about. The issue then becomes whether it misleads physicians on cases or problems not included in its knowledge base. An AI system may be good for the cases it is programmed to understand, but it may mislead the physician on cases not included in its data base. For this reason, physicians and hospitals are not comfortable with research and development of more sophisticated monitoring, critiquing, and AI expert consultation systems.

When medical decision support systems are used in caring for patients, either action or inaction may constitute negligence. While the concept of negligence is predicated on tort law principles, it is also grounded on moral principles when applied to the physician-patient relationship. Once a relationship has been established between physician and patient, the physician has the twofold duty to provide care and treatment and to do so in an acceptable manner. This duty has always been closely interwoven with patient and societal expectations as to what it entails. These expectations require that the physician be competent and perform in a competent manner. Such performances must fall within the guidelines of the patient's best interests as expressed through the maximization of "good" and the minimization of "harm." These moral dictates form the core of the standard of care required of the physician. That the physician is expected to conform to this ethical and legal standard is clearly understood by both society and the patient.

In some instances a computer can perform tasks more consistently than human caregivers, or even perform tasks physicians cannot perform and acquire information not otherwise discoverable by the physician (e.g., pattern analyses, EKG interpretation). In some situations the savings in time and the accuracy of data collection may increase the patient's chances of survival. Computers can also establish a more comprehensive list of probable causes based on a patient's symptoms simply because they do not suffer from human limitations of memory. Thus, where computers can diagnose a given case, and the physician cannot or might have trouble in doing so, a finding of negligence seems inescapable if the computer is not used.

Conclusion

Ethical and legal issues will dramatically influence the future role of medical information systems. Foremost among these issues is whether the rapidly growing network of information systems will be able to accommodate the traditional concept of patient privacy and confidentiality. The efforts required to maintain confidentiality in earlier information systems fall far short of what will be needed in the future. By enhancing the quality of health care delivered and lowering health-care costs, the use of these systems may require trade-offs with respect to confidentiality of medical information. In doing so, informed consent may become the mechanism for dealing with the problem by informing patients about the extensive network systems that interface with patient medical records. Finally, as AI systems gain in credibility, the standard of care for physicians and hospitals may require that they be used before any final diagnostic judgment is made. This will require a careful analysis of traditional notions of what is basic to the physician–patient relationship, as well as a sense of its limits in a sophisticated technological world.

FRANK H. MARSH
DENNIS LEZOTTE

For a further discussion of topics mentioned in this entry, see the entries AIDS; BIOETHICS; CLINICAL ETHICS; COMMUNICATION, BIOMEDICAL; CONFIDENTIALITY; GENOME MAPPING AND SEQUENCING; HEALTH CARE, QUALITY OF; HEALTH-CARE FINANCING; HEALTH-CARE RESOURCES, ALLOCATION OF, *article on* MACROALLOCATION; HOSPITAL, *articles on* MODERN HISTORY, *and* CONTEMPORARY ETHICAL PROBLEMS; INFORMATION DISCLOSURE; INFORMED CONSENT; PRIVACY IN HEALTH CARE; PRIVILEGED COMMUNICATIONS; *and* PUBLIC HEALTH, *article on* PUBLIC-HEALTH METHODS: EPIDEMIOLOGY AND BIOSTATISTICS. *For a further discussion of related ideas, see the entries* ALLIED HEALTH PROFESSIONS; AUTONOMY; CARE; EMOTIONS; FIDELITY AND LOYALTY; HEALTH SCREENING AND TESTING IN THE PUBLIC-HEALTH CONTEXT; PATIENTS' RIGHTS; PROFESSIONAL–PATIENT RELATIONSHIP; *and* PROFESSION AND PROFESSIONAL ETHICS.

Bibliography

AMERICAN MEDICAL ASSOCIATION COUNCIL ON ETHICAL AND JUDICIAL AFFAIRS. 1992. *Code of Medical Ethics: Annotated Current Opinions.* Chicago: Author.

ANDERSON, JAMES G., and JAY, STEPHEN J., eds. 1987. *Use and Impact of Computers in Medicine.* New York: Springer-Verlag.

BLAKE, MARY B. 1982. "Computerized Medical Records: Confidentiality and Authentication." *Legal Aspects of Medical Practice* 10:3–17.

BRANNIGAN, VINCENT M., and DAYHOFF, RUTH E. 1981. "Liability for Personal Injuries Caused by Defective Medical Computer Programs." *American Journal of Law and Medicine* 7, no. 2:123–144.

———. 1986. "Medical Informatics: The Revolution in Law, Technology and Medicine." *Journal of Legal Medicine* 7, no. 1:1–53.

BRODY, HOWARD. 1989. "The Physician-Patient Relationship." In *Medical Ethics,* pp. 65–91. Edited by Robert Veatch. Boston: Jones and Bartlett.

CHANG, RENE W. S.; LEE, BERNI; and JACOBS, SYDNEY. 1989. "Accuracy of Decisions to Withdraw Therapy in Critically Ill Patients: Clinical Judgment Versus a Computer Model." *Critical Care Medicine* 17, no. 11:1091–1097.

COLLEN, MARSHALL F. 1986. "Origins of Medical Informatics." *Western Journal of Medicine* 145, no. 6:778–785.

Federal Privacy Act. 1974. 5 USCA 552a(e).

JONSEN, ALBERT R.; SIEGLER, MARK; and WINSLADE, WILLIAM J. 1982. *Clinical Ethics: A Practical Approach to Ethical Decisions in Clinical Medicine.* New York: Macmillan.

MARSH, FRANK H. 1985. "Health Care Cost Containment and the Duty to Treat." *Journal of Legal Medicine* 6, no. 2:157–190.

MILLER, RANDOLPH A.; SCHAFFNER, KENNETH F.; and MEISEL, ALAN. 1985. "Ethical and Legal Issues Related to the Use of Computer Programs in Clinical Medicine." *Annals of Internal Medicine* 102, no. 4:529–536.

PROSSER, WILLIAM. 1971. *Handbook of the Law of Torts.* 4th ed. St. Paul, Minn.: West.

RENNELS, GLEN D., and SHORTLIFFE, EDWARD H. 1987. "Advanced Computing for Medicine." *Scientific American,* October, pp. 154–161.

SHORTLIFFE, EDWARD H. 1987. "Computer Programs to Support Clinical Decision Making." *Journal of the American Medical Association* 258, no. 1:61–66.

SHORTLIFFE, EDWARD H.; PERREAULT, LESLIE E.; NIEDERHOLD, GIO; and FAGAN, LAWRENCE M., eds. 1990. *Medical Informatics: Computer Applications in Health Care.* Reading, Mass.: Addison-Wesley.

SIEGLER, MARK. 1982. "Confidentiality in Medicine: A Decrepit Concept?" *New England Journal of Medicine* 307, no. 24:1518–1521.

TAYLOR, THOMAS R. 1984. "Computer Support for Management Decision Making in Family Practice." *Journal of Family Practice* 19, no. 4:567–570.

VAN ANTWERP, MARTIN. 1988. "Technology and the Standard of Care." *Health Technology* 2:61–66.

WALTERS, LEROY. 1982. "Ethical Aspects of Medical Confidentiality." In *Contemporary Issues in Bioethics,* 2d ed., pp. 198–203. Edited by Tom Beauchamp and LeRoy Walters. Belmont, Calif.: Wadsworth.

MEDICAL MALPRACTICE

Medical malpractice is the subset of tort law involving injuries that occur in the course of medical therapy. Over much of the period since the 1960s, the medical profession has characterized the growth of malpractice litigation as "a crisis." This perception is not shared in other countries, where concern about malpractice litigation has increased since the 1980s but still does not reach the levels of anxiety in the United States. The American experience with malpractice litigation is likely a combination of numerous cultural factors, including faith in technological solutions to health problems and relatively quick recourse to litigation. It is not possible to explain the emotional fervor surrounding malpractice litigation, but it is possible to characterize malpractice litigation as an institutional framework that copes, at least in some ways, with medical injury compensation and deterrence.

Tort law and liability insurance

In tort, or personal injury, law the injured person (plaintiff) sues the liable party (defendant) to obtain compensation for an injury. In medical malpractice, the defendant is a health-care provider or an institution, often a hospital. The suit is usually settled before a trial, but 5 to 10 percent of cases result in a jury trial.

Tort law has three functions. The first is compensation. The injured party can expect the defendant to pay for the economic consequences of an injury. These often include medical bills, loss of income, and inability to perform household chores or other work. The defendant may also be liable for emotional costs of the injury, including physical anguish. This is called pain-and-suffering compensation. Today, pain and suffering may account for nearly 50 percent of jury awards to medical malpractice plaintiffs.

The second function of tort law is to deter poor outcomes. According to economic theories of torts, the defendant behaves carefully in order to avoid the economic penalty of paying a successful plaintiff. Hence accidents are prevented by the threat of financial sanctions. There may also be psychological deterrence that complements the economic type, in that potential defendants will want to avoid the "passion play" of a suit and trial. Most physicians and other health-care providers acknowledge the latter motivation when discussing medical malpractice.

Finally, tort law is meant to provide some sense of corrective justice for society. The direct link between defendants and plaintiffs generates a sense of retribution and justice. This latter function of tort law is little discussed in the context of medical malpractice, and will not be explored in detail here.

Technically, any tort, including medical malpractice, must involve proof of four elements by the plaintiff. First, there has to be a duty of care owed to the plaintiff by the defendant. While in many areas of tort law the existence of a duty to care is controversial, in medical malpractice it is often taken for granted, since providers have special responsibility for their patients as a result of the distinctive ethical code of medicine. Physicians, nurses, and hospitals have particular duties to patients.

The second element of a tort claim is the proof of an injury. In most torts this is straightforward, but in malpractice it can be difficult. Unlike in other areas of personal injury, the medical malpractice litigant is frequently unhealthy, suffering from injuries that are the consequence of the disease process. The malpractice litigant must be able to show some injury beyond that caused by a disease process. This, in turn, relates to the third element of the tort suit, causation. The plaintiff must show that the injury was caused by the provider's medical malpractice, not by the disease. Therefore, the litigant must be prepared to disentangle the disease process from the medical injury.

Finally, a plaintiff in a tort suit must demonstrate that the defendant was negligent or failed to provide a certain standard of care. In medical malpractice, the standard of care is derived from the standard of the reasonable medical practitioner. Courts have generally required that the "reasonable medical practitioner" standard be set only by physicians or by medical custom. This means that a plaintiff must be prepared to identify a physician who will act as an expert witness and testify that the treating provider was negligent.

Like the rest of tort law, medical malpractice law is intertwined with a series of insurance relationships. The overwhelming majority of providers, including physicians and hospitals, purchase professional liability insurance. When a provider is sued, the insurer usually steps forward to defend the case, and to pay any settlement or jury verdict. To pay these defense costs, the insurer charges a premium. These premiums are generally not experience-rated, meaning they do not vary according to the number of times a provider is sued. Such "flat" premiums tend to inhibit the economic deterrence noted above. On the other hand, most insurers engage in some sort of risk management that entails education for providers, the intent of which is to minimize the number of claims brought by patients.

Attorneys are crucial for the effectiveness of the tort process, since most patients and providers are unable to represent themselves. The professional liability insurers hire lawyers and pay them on an hourly basis. Plaintiffs hire attorneys who generally operate on a contingency basis, meaning the lawyers will not expect any payment initially but will take a percentage of any final settlement or jury verdict. The contingency fee system means that even the poor can afford to bring suits, but it also means that successful plaintiffs will have their compensation lowered by the amount of the fee, which can be as high as 50 percent.

Evolution of malpractice law

Historically, medical malpractice claims were relatively infrequent. Patients found it very difficult to bring suits. They often faced a conspiracy of silence in which no health-care provider would testify against another, so reasonable evidence was not available. In addition, the common law imposed a locality rule holding that a plaintiff who wanted to allege negligence would have to identify a local practitioner who would testify about the standard of care in this particular locale. It was often difficult to find a local doctor who would testify against colleagues.

Nor could plaintiffs generally sue hospitals. Since most hospitals were (and are) not-for-profit institutions, they could take advantage of charitable immunity clauses in state law, restricting the amount for which an institution can be liable to a defendant. Moreover, nurses and other hospital employees were generally classified as the "fellow servants" of physicians, and hence could not be sued independently for their negligence.

From 1940 to 1970, common-law courts remade medical malpractice law, removing many of the barriers faced by plaintiffs. This was part of a general evolution of tort law in which state court judges encouraged tort suits by making doctrines more favorable to injured parties. Judges were attracted by influential academic arguments suggesting that accident rates were reaching intolerable levels. One of the first doctrines in medical malpractice law to change was the locality rule. Realizing that the rule made it nearly impossible for plaintiffs in middle-sized and small towns to find expert witnesses, judges reasoned that the dispersion of medical information was great enough to create a national standard of practice. Hence physicians from one geographic area could travel to another and testify independent of peer pressure.

Another major modification of the common law was the incorporation of *res ipsa loquitur* into medical malpractice. *Res ipsa loquitur,* meaning "the thing speaks for itself," is used in tort law for situations in which direct evidence is unavailable but circumstantial evidence suggests there was negligence. In malpractice, it was first used to overcome the conspiracy of silence. For instance, in the famous case of *Ybarra* v. *Spangard* the court held that a *res ipsa loquitur* instruction could suffice for liability in the absence of direct testimony when a patient suffered a nerve injury in the arm while undergoing an appendectomy.

Other changes included limitations on or overruling of charitable immunity, enabling patients to sue nonprofit hospitals. More important, in the early 1960s courts began to hold hospitals liable for negligence independent of that of practicing physicians. This created entirely new deterrence signals aimed directly at institutions. Hospital liability continues to expand under recent court decisions.

Courts also began to modify statutes of limitations, which set a time period during which a suit must be brought. Statutes of limitations are intended to prevent plaintiffs from bringing suits when the injury occurred years before and much of the evidence is stale or absent. Unfortunately, they can also prevent suits that are delayed because the plaintiff discovered the injury some time after the deficient medical treatment or diagnosis. To overcome the latter problem, courts have moved to a "time of discovery" doctrine. Under this doctrine, the statute of limitations does not begin (or toll) until the patient should have discovered the injury.

Finally, changes in informed-consent law have increased the number of suits brought by plaintiffs. Moving from a provider-based standard to a patient-based standard has encouraged more suits alleging negligent failure to inform patients of risks of procedures. As a result, in many states, plaintiffs need not supply professional testimony on the standard of care regarding the amount of information transmitted to the patient; jurors, as potential patients, can make this judgment themselves.

Many of these changes in the common law were in place by 1970. The common-law modifications were expected to increase the rate of suits, and that is what occurred in the mid-1970s. Rates of claims had hovered near one or two per 100 physicians per year, but suddenly, over a three-year period, increased to four to six claims per 100 physicians per year. This sudden increase caused a great dislocation in the professional liability insurance market. Many insurers simply left the market because they felt that the rate of increase in claims was too unpredictable to allow rational actuarial calculations. Several states had to take over professional liability underwriting through so-called joint underwriting associations. Self-insurance by hospitals and groups of providers also became prevalent. No matter who provided insurance, however, premiums paid by physicians and hospitals increased rapidly. To put it in perspective, liability premiums have never been more than 2 percent of the total health-care budget.

Burdened by these increases, providers went to state legislatures for relief. Lawmakers in many states responded by modifying the law to make suits less attractive to plaintiffs and their lawyers. Legislators have pursued several strategies. Perhaps the most direct economic method for discouraging suits is to limit the contingency fee for attorneys, by decreasing the percentage they can charge. A more subtle approach is to limit awards to plaintiffs, and thus limit lawyers' compensation. For instance, some states cap the amount the plaintiffs can receive for pain and suffering. Some have even capped economic awards.

A similar innovation is to overturn the collateral-source rule, which has held that the plaintiff's collateral sources of compensation for an accident, such as health or disability insurance, cannot be brought into evidence. The rule thus treats every plaintiff as if she or he had no other sources of compensation. This means that every person carries the same weight as a deterrent signal, in that well-insured people provide the same economic penalty for negligent defendants as the poorly insured. It also means that some plaintiffs will receive a windfall, since the tort award assumes they have no health or disability insurance. Overturning the collateral-source rule, and putting mandatory collateral-source offsets (reducing compensatory payments by the amount available from life or health insurance) in place, ends this windfall and decreases plaintiff attorneys' interest in some cases.

A similar reform is institution of periodic payment. When a plaintiff is awarded a large amount for a continuing injury, such as some form of disability, courts have traditionally passed this along as a lump sum. The plaintiff's attorney is then free to take his entire contingency fee. Now states are requiring periodic payment of tort awards, and the attorney receives the contingency fee in small pieces. This is thought by most plaintiff attorneys to be economically disadvantageous.

Another way to discourage suits is to make it more difficult to get into court. One way to do this is to reinstitute stringent statutes of limitations, which states have done. Another is to put into place screening panels made up of providers and attorneys, who must certify a claim before it can go to court. Perhaps the most direct way to inhibit plaintiffs, however, is simply to overturn judge-made law on doctrines such as the locality rule and *res ipsa,* a path taken by several state legislatures.

All of these various reforms were put into place in states in the late 1970s and early 1980s. Econometric analysis has suggested that some, particularly caps on damages and changes in the collateral-source rule, are especially effective. Nonetheless, for a variety of reasons, in the mid-1980s claims rates began to rise again, even tripling in many states between 1984 and 1986.

This led to further cries for relief from providers, and legislatures attempted to respond. This time, however, the "tort reforms" were so stringent as to provoke constitutional challenges in many states. Today, courts are in the process of reviewing such challenges brought against reforms hammered together in the mid-1980s malpractice crisis.

Empirical analyses of malpractice litigation

Unlike other areas of tort law, medical malpractice has been subject to empirical research to understand how economic theories of tort law conform to reality. Students of medical malpractice have, for instance, begun to gather thorough information on malpractice claims, compiling the results of jury verdicts in several jurisdictions and analyzing the variation in outcomes. Other investigators have turned their attention to the experience of defendants, particularly physicians, to identify the characteristics that may lead to more frequent actions by plaintiffs. Still others have focused on considerations of the kinds of medical interactions that lead to suits, and the processing of information in litigation.

Questions about the impact of statutory reforms of personal-injury law have been the central focus of empiricists, but wider-ranging institutional analyses have also begun to appear. For example, the relationship between claims for payments and malpractice insurance premiums, and the appropriateness of settlements by insurers are among the concerns now being assessed by researchers.

Another major offshoot of this interest in research has been the elaboration, and penetrating analysis, of alternative methods of resolving disputes between injured patients and allegedly negligent physicians and hospitals. While proposals featuring alternative dispute resolution in medical malpractice have long been available, researchers have recently undertaken pilot tests.

Perhaps most important, large empirical studies of medical injury and malpractice litigation suggest that many medical injuries are caused by negligence and all of them presumably are preventable, given an optimal combination of incentives. The same studies found, somewhat surprisingly, that very few injuries caused by negligence actually give rise to litigation. There are approximately seven to eight times as many injuries as there are claims for medical injuries. In addition, many claims arise in cases where there is not medical injury. As few as 2 percent of negligent medical injuries give rise to litigation; as many as 80 percent of claims arise in cases in which there is no injury or no negligence.

Our confidence in tort law as a method of inducing quality seems to be misplaced. It is difficult to argue that there can be rational deterrence when few claims give rise to suits, and many claims are baseless. Indeed, the available econometric evidence fails to demonstrate significant prevention of injuries in areas in which there are high rates of litigation, as theory would suggest.

Medical ethics and medical malpractice

In light of this evidence, some have begun to subject medical malpractice to ethical analysis. The two major goals of tort law are to prevent medical injuries and to compensate the injured. Prevention of medical injury is a form of quality assurance. Since physicians have an ethical commitment to provide quality care, the efficacy of tort law must fall within the purview of medical ethics. If there were evidence that tort litigation did improve quality, and data suggesting that "tort reform" decreased the number of claims brought, and thus the deterrent effect of litigation, then perhaps it would be necessary for physicians to consider opposition to tort reform. Since it appears that malpractice suits have little deterrent effect, perhaps there is an ethical imperative to develop methods of prevention of medical injuries that are more efficacious.

The compensation of patients for medical injuries may have ethical overtones. Since providers have a commitment to patients, it does not seem unreasonable to extend that commitment to the welfare of the patient after discharge from the hospital. If a patient has suffered a medical injury, and the injury is creating economic hardship for the patient, some have argued that the physician should intervene.

Alternatives to tort litigation

These concerns about ethics, specifically the economic and justice considerations of ethics, are driving a search for alternatives. Legislative proposals to decrease rates of litigation have typically endorsed periodic payment for awards greater than $100,000; mandatory collateral-source offsets; caps on noneconomic damages of greater than $250,000; limits on contingent attorney fees; and restrictions on statutes of limitations.

In addition to support for traditional tort reform, many congressional proposals advocate alternative dispute resolution (ADR) techniques for disposing of injury claims by patients. Advocates of ADR are motivated primarily by the huge administrative costs of malpractice litigation. They reason that an approach based on arbitration or other forms of negotiation would be more efficient. ADR could also increase access to legal services, as lower administrative costs might translate into lower contingency fees and perhaps lower plaintiff attorney thresholds for taking cases. In addition, ADR techniques are thought to promise more expedient determinations of damages and perhaps more equitable and predictable decisions. While little empirical evidence supports these claims for ADR, gathering momentum favors at least some of these devices.

Others have advocated administrative approaches to medical injury compensation and deterrence that are independent of the common-law courts. These proposals represent more radical reform than simple encouragement of ADR mechanisms. For example, the American Medical Association's (AMA) administrative fault-based system would create a state medical board and an attendant bureaucracy. By submitting a relatively simple form, a patient could have medical care reviewed by claims adjustors. Those claims with some merit would undergo a second evaluation by a medical specialist. Before moving to a hearing, blind settlement offers by both parties would be required.

If there was no settlement, the board's general counsel would provide an attorney for the patient. A hearing examiner would supervise discovery on an expedited basis and evaluate the expert testimony that both parties bring to a hearing. The medical board would act as an appellate review panel. The review would consist of a full independent determination of the claim. Appeal for the medical board's decision could be made to an intermediate appellate court within the state, but the standard for review here would be arbitrary and capricious.

The AMA's plan retains fault as the basis for liability, and hence a deterrent signal that is similar to tort law. Moreover, the medical board not only would review determinations at hearings, but also would be integrated into the credentialing and disciplinary functions of existing state licensing boards. Therefore, it appears to offer better deterrence than tort law does.

Another administrative scheme would do away with fault determination altogether and award compensation based on injury. No-fault administrative compensation systems have long been advocated as a more rational response to compensation for and the deterrence of injuries resulting from accidents. Generically, no-fault removes consideration of negligence from determination of compensation (and so in many ways is equivalent to strict liability). An injured individual need only show causation and injury. No-fault is the norm for medical injury cases in several countries, notably Sweden and New Zealand.

In the United States, no-fault has long been ruled out by its theoretical cost. Recent information reveals that a no-fault program for medical injury could, however, be an affordable alternative to tort litigation. From a compensation viewpoint, no-fault is more reasonable because it compensates all medical injuries, not just those due to negligence. Furthermore, through strictly experience-rated insurance premiums paid by hospitals, no-fault can offer very impressive deterrence results, as workers' compensation suggests. Administrative approaches thus seem to have much to offer from both an economics and an ethics perspective.

While medical malpractice law has evolved a great deal, empirical evidence suggests that it is not performing well: It provides little rational deterrence and compensates relatively few people injured by medical negligence. As a result, many proposals have been made for radically reforming medical injury law. An ethical perspective on these issues is now emerging, and will be a welcome addition to the policy debate.

TROYEN A. BRENNAN

Directly related to this entry are the entries EXPERT TESTIMONY; HARM; HOSPITAL, *article on* CONTEMPORARY ETHICAL PROBLEMS; LAW AND BIOETHICS; RISK; *and* IATROGENIC ILLNESS AND INJURY. *For a further discussion of topics mentioned in this entry, see the entries* COMPETENCE; HEALTH CARE, QUALITY OF; *and* IMPAIRED PROFESSIONALS. *Other relevant material may be found under the entries* INFORMED CONSENT, *article on* LEGAL AND ETHICAL ISSUES OF CONSENT IN HEALTH CARE (*with its* POSTSCRIPT); MEDICINE AS A PROFESSION; PATIENTS' RIGHTS, *article on* ORIGIN AND NATURE OF PATIENTS' RIGHTS; PROFESSIONAL–PATIENT RELATIONSHIP, *article on* ETHICAL ISSUES; *and* WHISTLEBLOWING.

Bibliography

ABRAHAM, KENNETH S. 1986. *Distributing Risk: Insurance, Legal Theory and Public Policy.* New Haven, Conn.: Yale University Press.
BOVBJERG, RANDALL R. 1989. "Legislation on Medical Malpractice: Further Developments in a Preliminary Report Card." *University of California Davis Law Review* 22: 499–556.
BOVBJERG, RANDALL R.; SLOAN, FRANK A.; and BLUMSTEIN, JAMES F. 1989. "Valuing Life and Limb in Tort: Scheduling 'Pain and Suffering.'" *Northwestern University Law Review* 83, no. 4:908–976.
BRENNAN, TROYEN A. 1991. *Just Doctoring: Medical Ethics in the Liberal State.* Berkeley: University of California Press.
BRENNAN, TROYEN A.; HEBERT, LIESI E.; LAIRD, NAN M.; LAWTHERS, ANN; THORPE, KENNETH E.; LEAPE, LUCIAN L.; LOCALIO, A. RUSSELL; LIPSITZ, STUART R.; NEWHOUSE, JOSEPH P.; WEILER, PAUL C.; and HIATT, HOWARD H. 1991. "Hospital Characteristics Associated with Adverse Events and Substandard Care." *Journal of the American Medical Association* 265, no. 24:3265–3269.
DANZON, PATRICIA M. 1985. *Medical Malpractice: Theory, Evidence, and Public Policy.* Cambridge, Mass.: Harvard University Press.
GRADY, MARK. 1988. "Why Are People Negligent? Technology, Nondurable Precautions, and the Medical Malpractice Explosion." *Northwestern University Law Review* 82, no. 2:293–334.

HAVIGHURST, CLARK C., and TANCREDI, LAURENCE R. 1973. "Medical Adversity Insurance: A No-Fault Approach to Medical Malpractice and Quality Assurance." *Milbank Memorial Fund Quarterly* 51, no. 2:125–168.

KINNEY, ELEANOR D., and GRONFEIN, WILLIAM P. 1991. "Indiana's Malpractice System: No-Fault by Accident?" *Law and Contemporary Problems* 54, nos. 1–2:169–193.

LEAPE, LUCIAN L.; BRENNAN, TROYEN A.; LAIRD, NAN M.; LAWTHERS, ANN G.; LOCALIO, A. RUSSELL; BARNES, BENJAMIN A.; HEBERT, LIESI; NEWHOUSE, JOSEPH P.; WEILER, PAUL C.; and HIATT, HOWARD H. 1991. "The Nature of Adverse Events in Hospitalized Patients: Results of the Harvard Medical Practice Study II." *New England Journal of Medicine* 324, no. 6:377–384.

LOCALIO, A. RUSSELL; LAWTHERS, ANN G.; BRENNAN, TROYEN A.; LAIRD, NAN M.; HEBERT, LIESI E.; PETERSON, LYNN M.; NEWHOUSE, JOSEPH P.; WEILER, PAUL C.; and HIATT, HOWARD H. 1991. "Relation Between Malpractice Claims and Adverse Events Due to Negligence: Results of the Harvard Medical Practice Study III." *New England Journal of Medicine* 325, no. 4:245–251.

METZLOFF, THOMAS B. 1991. "Resolving Malpractice Disputes: Imaging the Jury's Shadow." *Law and Contemporary Problems* 54:43–129.

ROSENTHAL, MARILYNN M. 1988. *Dealing with Medical Malpractice: The British and Swedish Experience.* Durham, N.C.: Duke University Press.

SHAVELL, STEVEN. 1987. *Economic Analysis of Accident Law.* Cambridge, Mass.: Harvard University Press.

TERRY, ROBERT. 1986. "The Technical and Conceptual Flaws of Medical Malpractice Arbitration." *Saint Louis University Law Journal* 30:571–581.

WEILER, PAUL C. 1991. *Medical Malpractice on Trial.* Cambridge, Mass.: Harvard University Press.

MEDICAL PROFESSION AND PROFESSIONALISM

See MEDICINE AS A PROFESSION. *See also* PROFESSION AND PROFESSIONAL ETHICS.

MEDICAL RECORDS

See MEDICAL INFORMATION SYSTEMS. *See also* CONFIDENTIALITY; PRIVACY AND CONFIDENTIALITY IN RESEARCH; *and* PRIVACY IN HEALTH CARE.

MEDICAL SOCIAL WORK

See SOCIAL WORK IN HEALTH CARE.

MEDICAL SOCIOLOGY

See MEDICINE, SOCIOLOGY OF.

MEDICAL TECHNOLOGY

See TECHNOLOGY. *See also* BIOMEDICAL ENGINEERING; *and* BIOTECHNOLOGY.

MEDICARE

See HEALTH-CARE FINANCING, *article on* MEDICARE.

MEDICINE, ANTHROPOLOGY OF

Medical anthropology is the cross-cultural study of health, illness, and medical systems. Medical anthropologists describe how the collective meanings, social institutions, and dynamics of political power in a particular society construct local forms of medical knowledge and therapeutic action that are differentially distributed across gender, age, ethnic, and class lines. From hundreds of studies a deeper understanding has been gained of variation in illness beliefs and behavior and of pluralism in healing practices (see, e.g., Good, 1977; Janzen, 1978; Kleinman, 1980; Leslie, 1975; Lock, 1980; Nichter, 1989). Yet there are also universals in the mediation of suffering and in the therapeutic process about which the comparative method provides a special insight (see Kleinman, 1988a, 1988b).

Medical anthropologists or anthropologists of medicine (the terms are interchangeable) have brought different paradigms to bear on the study of health and disease. Ecological, political-economic, and applied public-health or clinical perspectives are all to be found in the literature. Yet since the 1970s the most original anthropological contribution is what has come to be called a meaning-centered or social constructionist paradigm.

In this perspective, the central concern is with the way that illness categories and experiences reflect culture, and in turn contribute to social change. Thus, Gilbert Lewis (1975), working with a small-scale preliterate society near the Sepik River of Papua New Guinea, shows how that society's master symbols are reflected in the illness behavior of withdrawal and isolation of seriously sick members and in the "days of shining red" animated by healing rituals. The smells, tastes, sights, sounds, and sensibility of everyday responses to shamans' songs among aboriginals in the Malaysian rain forest and Malays in rice-farming villages (Laderman, 1991; Roseman, 1991); of routine coping processes through which Haitian villagers make accusations about the sources of AIDS (Farmer, 1992); and of the social as well as personal experience of sadness among Yolmo Sherpas in

Nepal (Desjarlais, 1993)—all are patterned by deep cultural codes and social structures. Much the same cultural dialectic between persons and collective institutions has been shown to pattern interactions in psychiatric emergency rooms in North America (Rhodes, 1991); in the training of medical students to see patients through the lens of biomedical reductionism at Harvard Medical School (Good, 1993); and in the practices of oncologists in Tokyo, Rome, Oaxaca, and Boston (Good et al., 1993).

Global social change has proliferated, not limited, the numbers and types of traditional healers in both richer, industrialized societies and poorer, industrializing ones (McGuire, 1988). Industrialization on a worldscale has neither undermined traditional medical beliefs nor foreclosed on folk health practices; yet such global social change has made much less clear the division between "traditional" and "modern." One finds in the so-called East Asian industrial dragons, for example, a greatly complex mesh of attitudes, values, and practices. There is no simple giving way of "tradition" to Western orientation; indeed, both tradition and Westernization are routinely reinvented. The Japanese may be moving to accept brain death as a marker of the end of human life, and thereby facilitate organ transplantation, which has been severely constrained by Buddhist ideas; but it is a movement strongly contested by large numbers of Japanese who maintain traditional values about death together with the most advanced technological orientation.

Patients and their families, when it comes to serious illness, are pragmatic; they cross back and forth between the professional and folk domains of health care. Scientific knowledge has not replaced cultural common sense but been integrated with it (Kleinman, 1980; Nichter, 1989). Biomedicine has been the leading edge of a worldwide culture of science, yet in Asian and African societies biomedical institutions and relationships have become indigenized in ways that reflect those societies' master values and particular forms of social life. As a result there are both certain similarities and even greater dissimilarities in the ways professional and lay members of those societies make therapeutic decisions, handle life and death events, respond to chronicity and disability, and negotiate the complexities of care (Laderman, 1983; Last and Chavunduka, 1986; Rhodes, 1991; Sargent, 1989; Young, 1977).

Because of their concern for value orientations and everyday decision making, anthropologists have written about the ethical sides of health and health care. For example, Peter Kunstadter (1980) and Morton Beiser (1977) wrote about the ethical quandaries that development projects, including medical ones, introduced into traditional communities, because the services they provide are temporary and therefore raise expectations that eventually will be frustrated. Mary Jo Good and colleagues (1993) and Margaret Lock and Christina Honda (1990) examined the moral exigencies of truth telling about cancer and determining death in biomedicine in Japan. Paul Unschuld (1979) analyzed the corpus of Confucian and traditional Chinese medical writings on ethical issues, and concluded that professional and cultural values of the literati class colluded to control the medical marketplace. Arthur Kleinman (1980) found that healers in Taiwan in the 1960s and 1970s—whether traditional Chinese medical practitioners, shamans, or physicians—were viewed ambiguously: as morally powerful to heal, yet potentially immoral sources of economic gain and even of evil power (sorcery). This finding is rather widespread cross-culturally.

Horacio Fabrega (1990), writing explicitly about an ethnomedical approach to medical ethics, saw biomedicine's ethical preoccupations growing from Greek medicine and the popular morality of ancient Greece. Following many anthropologists, he asserts that in small-scale, preliterate societies, healing and religion are inseparable; thus, for Fabrega medical mores are tied to ritual and theology in these societies. In larger-scale societies—both peasant and posttraditional—the specialized division of labor leads to practitioners who are popularly viewed both as healers and as financially benefiting from the healer's trade. Fabrega argues that all the great non-Western traditions of healers use ethical injunctions to control access to practice and to proscribe certain alternative healers as quacks. He asserts that "bioethics" is a unique version of medical ethics made possible by the development of biomedicine with its knowledge of biology and powerful biological applications.

Writing for a collection of social-science treatments of bioethics, Richard Lieban (1990), himself an anthropologist, focuses on anthropological interest in the ethical aspects of controversial folk practices—such as female circumcision, differential assistance to male children, and the lack of regulation of folk healers—as examples of what anthropologists can offer to bioethical issues in international health (see also Scheper-Hughes, 1987; Korbin, 1981; Gruenbaum, 1982; Kleinman, 1982). Allan Young (1990), in the same volume, demonstrates the value of ethnographic accounts of the hidden moral dimensions of psychiatric practice in a Veterans Administration unit for treating combat-related posttraumatic stress disorder among veterans who had served in the Vietnam War.

What characterizes anthropological approaches to ethical issues, in medicine as well as other fields, is an emphasis on questions that emerge out of the grounded experiences of sick persons, families, and healers in local contexts. Anthropologists have critiqued universal ethical propositions just as their professional perspective has led them to critique universalist models for economic development. In place of universalist propositions—philosophical or political-economic—anthropologists have focused upon the local interactions of everyday life and the moral issues in which they are clothed. In Isaiah Berlin's (1979) apt metaphor, they are more the fox than the hedgehog. The latter type of intellectual (e.g., the moral philosopher or the psychoanalyst) knows one big thing about the human experience, while the former (e.g., the historian or anthropologist) knows many small, particular things.

The remainder of this entry will adumbrate what anthropological studies tell us about health, illness, and care that is relevant to the practice of bioethics. Starting with a cross-cultural critique of leading bioethical orientations and commitments, the more powerful anthropological contributions will be reviewed, followed by a brief discussion of the possibilities and problems with a culturalist orientation. From the anthropological perspective, bioethics shares with biomedicine several determinative cultural orientations that constrain the standard approach to ethical issues in patient care. The anthropological approach, therefore, becomes particularly useful because of the comparative understanding it offers of often unexamined biases.

The *ethnocentrism, psychocentrism,* and *medicocentrism* central to biomedicine are prominent in the standard bioethical approach (see Lock and Gordon, 1988; Weisz, 1990). Most philosophically trained bioethicists draw on what Charles Taylor (1989) describes as the orthodox sources of the self in the Western philosophical tradition. The great works in that tradition, from those of the Greeks down to the present, assume an individuated self, set off from the collective—single, unchanging, and self-defining. Thereby, inter alia, the autonomy of the person is claimed to be a paramount value along with the ideas of justice and beneficence. From a cross-cultural perspective this intellectual commitment is problematic.

In the major non-Western societies—such as China, India, Japan, Indonesia, and most African societies—few people hold that the isolated individual is the locus of responsibility for therapeutic choice, or that therapy should work to maximize the individuation of the sick person. Rather, there is a paramount sociocentric consensus in which social obligation, family responsibility, and communal loyalty outweigh personal autonomy in the hierarchy of ethical principles. The self is viewed as sociocentrically enmeshed in inextricable social networks, ties that make interpersonal processes the source of vital decisions. More than 80 percent of the planet's population lives in cultures outside of North America and Western Europe or are members of minority ethnic groups outside of the Euro-American majority. That bioethics is able to avoid serious engagement with these alternative ethical traditions must represent one of the last tenacious holds of ethnocentric mentality. Indeed, there is evidence that bioethicists are commencing such decentering cultural engagements (Jennings, 1990; Loewy, 1991).

Similarly, from an ethnographic perspective, the use of abstract concepts of justice and beneficence as universal ethical principles in decision making is suspect because of the failure to take into account the local worlds in which patients and practitioners live—worlds that involve unjust distributions of power, entitlements, and resources. It is utopian, and therefore misleading, to apply the principles of justice and beneficence to practical clinical problems, unless we first take into account the brutal reality of the unjust worlds in which illness is systematically distributed along socioeconomic lines and in which access to and quality of care are cruelly constrained by the political economy. Beneficent social contracts may make good theory, but they deny empirical experience in local social worlds. Loewy's (1991) "beneficent community," which he claims is concerned with minimizing the suffering of its members, is a charming romance; no one lives in such a utopian state. Rather, real communities are sources of suffering at least as much as potential sources of assistance. They do not contain social contracts; but they are filled with different interests, status differences, class divisions, ethnic conflicts and factionalism. Little is gained by instantiating utopian virtues; indeed, much is lost, since illusion and exaggeration distort the practical realities of living.

The third "centrism"—medicocentrism—emerges from comparative studies as yet another bias of standard bioethical discourse. Like biomedicine, bioethics begins with professional definitions of pathology. The disease viewed as pathological physiology, and the professionally authorized array of treatment interventions, define the clinical situation (see Canguilhem, 1989). The experience of illness is made over, through the application of ethical abstractions such as those described above, into a contextless philosophical construct that is every bit as professionally centered and divorced from patients' suffering as is the biomedical construction of disease pathology.

The bioethicist, of course, is supposed to take into account the patient's perspective. But by and large the contextually rich illness narrative is reinterpreted (also thinned out) from the professional biomedical standpoint in order to focus exclusively on the value conflicts that it is held to instantiate. The folk categories of patients and indigenous healers are provided with only limited legitimacy. If they can be restated in the abstract terms of the standard bioethical orthodoxy, they are provided a place in the analysis. But if they cannot, then folk categories lose their authoritative imprint to define what is at stake for patients and families.

Take ideas, for example, of *suffering*—a powerful folk category worldwide. One is surprised to find so many professional ethical volumes in which this word does not appear as an entry in the index. Ethical systems that leave the problem of suffering (and related concepts of endurance and courage) to particular theological traditions cannot adequately engage the human core of illness and care. Here perhaps the standard version of bioethics shares yet another biomedical bias, the rejection of teleology. Biomedicine banishes the concepts of purpose and ultimate meaning to religion; yet most patients and practitioners struggle to make sense of illness with respect to great cultural codes that offer coherent interpretations of experience (cf. Frye, 1982).

Medicocentrism also leads bioethicists to construct cases that are centered in the professionally approved institutional structures of biomedicine—such as hospitals or nursing homes—despite the fact that most illness episodes, as social studies reveal, are experienced, interpreted, and responded to in the context of the family. The family—the mundane cultural setting of illness and care, where local social processes are so greatly influential—and the workplace frequently disappear in bioethical discourse, to be replaced by the biomedical staging of more extreme, even exotic value conflicts. Of course, the immense panoply of settings for healing is even less visible or audible in the bioethical construction of clinical reality.

This all too black-and-white portrait of bioethics is intended to draw out and highlight its deep difficulties and their cultural sources. In the practical flow of events, the working bioethicist struggles to overcome the constraints that limit his or her engagement with the obdurate particularity and inexpedient uncertainty of human subjects. And for that very reason he or she will find an ethnographic orientation to be liberating.

In contrast with the bioethicist, the ethnographer begins with the lived flow of interpersonal experience in a deeply particular local world. Not the Western tradition or North America, nor even New York State—which are too unspecified to provide a positioned *view from somewhere*—but, rather, the Puerto Rican community in the South Bronx, upper-middle-class Scarsdale, a working-class section of Queens, or a network of Russian immigrants in Brooklyn becomes the setting for grounding moral analysis in the concrete historicity, micropolitical economy, and ethnicity of a local world. Even within such a localized flow of experience, perspectives and preferences are further defined by gender, age, and other social categories of persons: for example, the cultural situation of poor women in rural Haiti who

are responding to AIDS (Farmer and Kleinman, 1989). These indexes of social experience situate groups and their individual members along axes of power such that the forces of macrosocial pressures—economic depression, war, forced uprooting, ethnic conflict, state violence, the organizational control of substance abuse, the social structural sources of chronic illness and disability—are systematically attenuated for some, yet amplified for others. Some become successful or at least are protected; others are victims.

Each local world is characterized by what is at stake for its members. That structure of relevance—compared to a belief or a convention—gives to the meanings of illness and to treatment expectations the sense of something much closer to natural law. Families hold the world to be a certain way as an article of fundamental faith in local reality. In the infrapolitics of family, workplace, and community, which is empirically discoverable, the processes of strategic negotiation and interpersonal engagement over what is at stake can be properly regarded as processes through which a local moral order is constituted and expressed. Culture, then, is built up out of the everyday routines and rhythms of social life. It is the medium of experience, for example, in which one person's chronic pain affects an entire work unit, a family member's Alzheimer's disease is shared as an illness reality by the entire family, and cancer care is negotiated among parents, child, and professional care providers.

Hospitals, clinics, and disability programs also are grounded in the particularity of local worlds, as is the bioethicist. The ethnographic task for the practicing bioethicist, then, becomes the discovery of the meanings and relationships in distinctive local worlds, and their actual impact on particular patients, families, and practitioners. This is a kind of cultural analysis of moral conflicts and negotiations over plans and practices that make up the flow of everyday living. As part of this ethnographic work, the bioethicist needs to elicit the perspectives of the participants and place them in the contexts of family, workplace, and medical system. The bioethicist's involvement should be to facilitate communication and to help negotiate conflicting orientations. In this work, it is necessary to protect the participants from the dehumanizing imposition of hegemonic principles. This focus on the positioned, intersubjective perspectives of participants in a local context is a radically different vision of how to proceed with the ethical analysis of a case than that which originates in a philosophical quest for an illusory *transpositional objectivity*, a synthesis valid for an entire context, which in the anthropological vision is the problem, not the solution (Sen, 1992).

More specifically, anthropological analysis draws attention to the institutional context of ethical decision making (see Bosk, 1979; Fox, 1990; Mizrahi, 1986). Social institutions—a particular type of hospital, a clinic for alternative care, or a religious facility—refigure ethical issues in terms of efficiency and other technical criteria that make up everyday social routines. Hence, the special characteristics of a Veterans Administration hospital, a university-based teaching hospital, a military hospital, a member of a for-profit hospital chain, or a highly cost-conscious HMO constrain the day-to-day social processes that create the local moral order. What is at stake for a resident in training in a teaching hospital—generating new knowledge, securing a place in the academic hierarchy, and so on—is noticeably different from what is at stake for a senior physician at a small community hospital. The difference signals a distinctive institutional context for deciding what level of treatment is "routine," which kinds of issues will be highlighted as "ethical" problems, when families will be involved, and so on. Quite obviously, such institutional contexts will also be distinctive cross-culturally.

In Japan, even in a university teaching hospital, the practice has been not to disclose to patients that they are suffering from cancer but to allow key family members to decide if and when the "truth" will be told. In China, family members will stay in the hospital with the patient to do the nursing, prepare meals, and make all the major decisions, even for the family head when he is seriously ill.

In Zaire and Senegal, members of the kinship-based therapy management group, including perhaps the doctor and the nurse, will decide if the patient is to be part of a research protocol (Beiser, 1977). In a Seventh-Day Adventist mission hospital run by American staff in Borneo, the structure for identifying and resolving a moral dilemma draws on a religious ideology that suffuses the institutional context in a manner that greatly differentiates this hospital from nearby hospitals run by transplanted Javanese Muslims or local animists. The responses of North American and Chinese psychiatrists to depressed patients in the United States and China have been compared with respect to their decidedly different institutional contexts for determining what kinds of therapeutic behaviors represent good care and what kinds of moral messages will be given and received in the patient–doctor interaction (Kleinman, 1988b). Renée Fox and Judith Swazey (1984) have shown how physicians in a Chinese hospital draw on both Confucian views and Communist ideology to authorize local patterns of ethical decision making that challenge North American orientations. And cultural historians disclose how bioethics in North America has emerged out of the social problems and responses of a particular era (Rothman, 1990).

Besides cultural critique and comparison, what practical contributions can anthropology make to bio-

ethics? The cultural formulation of diagnostic and therapeutic issues clearly should be as significant to the consulting bioethicist as it frequently can be made to be for the consulting physician, especially when the patient and family come from cultural and ethnic backgrounds that differ from those of their professional caregivers, or when the setting is outside North America (Kleinman, 1982). That formulation involves systematic steps in placing the illness and treatment experience in the culturally grounded context of family, work, and medical/social welfare systems, through the application of a mini-ethnography—a description and interpretation of how those settings affect, and are affected by, the illness. Cultural formulation identifies lay and professional explanatory models, compares them for evidence of cultural bias or conflict, and sets out a process of negotiation to assure cultural sensitivity (see Helman, 1984; Kleinman, 1988a; Rogler, 1990). These are technical procedures that should be part of the repertoire of the bioethicist. Ethnographic knowledge of the core ethical orientations and social patterns of different communities will be especially significant in planning and implementing medical research in ethnic minority and non-Western settings (Christakis, 1988).

What are the limits of cultural analysis, cross-cultural comparison, and the sensibility to variation and differences that come under the term "cultural relativism"? While epistemological and even ontological relativism—willingness to entertain the idea that there is no single form of knowledge or being in local worlds—will seem defensible to many, ethical relativism of the radical variety—the idea that there are no ethical standards cross-culturally—will not. Are such practices as infanticide of female children in South Asia, ritual murder of elderly women accused of being illness-causing witches in East Africa, and rationing of care based on color status under apartheid acceptable because the dominant group says they are? Clearly, this would be an unacceptable conclusion. Behind it lurks the terrible transmogrification of medicine under the Nazis, when biomedical ideology and technology, dominated by Nazi values, prepared the way for the death camps (Kleinman, 1988b; Proctor, 1988).

The anthropological argument advanced in these pages is for elicitation and engagement with alternative ethical formulations, a constrained relativism; it is for affirmation of differences, not automatic authorization of any standard or practice as ethically acceptable because it is held by some people, somewhere (Shweder, 1990; Wong, 1984). The limit to ethical relativism is that the bioethicist must compare alternative ethical formulations with those ethical standards he or she holds for the evaluation of a particular problem in a particular context. The outcome of such an evaluation could be acceptance or rejection of the alternatives or of the bioethicist's own standards, or some form of negotiation and compromise.

The idea of radical cultural relativism is unacceptable to all but a small group of diehards. It is, moreover, a serious misinterpretation of what ethnography, cultural analysis, and cross-cultural comparison have contributed: the idea that before we apply an ethical category we hold to be universal, we had better understand the context of practice and ideas that constitute a local moral world. The job should be to situate a bioethical problem in that local ethos in order to understand what is at stake for the participants, what is contested, and thereby to offer a cultural formulation of conflicting ethical priorities. That having been done, there are at least three further steps. First, we need to systematically compare local and professional bioethical standards for that particular problem; second, we need to negotiate that part of the difference on which both parties deem it ethical to compromise; and third, where a cross-cultural ethical conflict cannot be so resolved, both parties should specify the nature of the problem for further adjudication (Kleinman, 1982). This ethnographic strategy does not commit the deep error of assuming that "all goods, all virtues, all ideals are compatible, and that what is desirable can alternately be united into a harmonious whole without loss" (Williams, 1981, p. xvi). Compromise and negotiation may not resolve ethical conflicts; and even where they do, some losses must occur. The quest is not for integration and unification, but for multicultural pluralism.

Where possible, it is the obligation of the bioethicist not only to respect the specific views of others and to affirm the validity of the process of alternative moral formulations, but also to develop deep knowledge about those viewpoints and to test those alternative categories and practices for potential ways to resolve ethical conflict. This ethnographic approach emphasizes the process of engagement and negotiation with the lived moral orientations of others; it attempts to minimize the application of those bioethical standards that derive from the Western philosophical tradition, to settings for which they lack coherence and validity. In all other areas of cross-cultural research and practice this is the established procedure. This approach also protects the responsibility of the professional bioethical consultant not to accept value decisions that contravene human rights and other pan-national moral conventions. But it makes this universalist responsibility the final stage in a process of cultural translation that gives priority, initially at least, to alternative worlds of experience interpreted in their own terms.

Perhaps the cardinal contribution of the medical anthropologist to bioethics is to deeply humanize the *process* of formulating an ethical problem by allowing variation and pluralism to emerge and receive their due, so that ethical standards are not imposed in an alien way; rather, these standards will then be realized as the outcome of reciprocal participatory engagement across different worlds of experience.

ARTHUR KLEINMAN

Directly related to this entry are the entries HEALTH AND DISEASE, *article on* ANTHROPOLOGICAL PERSPECTIVES; *and* ALTERNATIVE THERAPIES, *article on* SOCIAL HISTORY. *For a further discussion of topics mentioned in this entry, see the entries* CIRCUMCISION, *article on* FEMALE CIRCUMCISION; FAMILY; *and* HEALING. *This entry will find application in the entries* BIOETHICS; DEATH, *article on* ANTHROPOLOGICAL PERSPECTIVES; DEATH, ATTITUDES TOWARD; MENTAL ILLNESS, *article on* CROSS-CULTURAL PERSPECTIVES; UNORTHODOXY IN MEDICINE; *and* WOMEN, *article on* HISTORICAL AND CROSS-CULTURAL PERSPECTIVES. *For a discussion of related ideas, see the entries* AUTONOMY; ETHICS, *articles on* NORMATIVE ETHICAL THEORIES, SOCIAL AND POLITICAL THEORIES, *and* RELIGION AND MORALITY; FAMILY; INFORMATION DISCLOSURE; PAIN AND SUFFERING; RIGHTS; *and* VALUE AND VALUATION.

Bibliography

BEISER, MORTON. 1977. "Ethics in Cross-Cultural Perspective." In *Current Perspectives in Cultural Psychiatry*, pp. 125–139. Edited by Edward F. Foulks, Ronald M. Wintrob, Joseph Westermeyer, and Armando J. Favazza. New York: Spectrum.

BERLIN, ISAIAH. 1979. "The Hedgehog and the Fox." In his *Russian Thinkers*. Harmondsworth, U.K.: Penguin.

BOSK, CHARLES. 1979. *Forgive and Remember: Managing Medical Failure*. Chicago: University of Chicago Press.

BOWKER, JOHN. 1970. *Problems of Suffering in Religions of the World*. Cambridge: At the University Press.

CANGUILHEM, GEORGE. 1989. [1966]. *The Normal and the Pathological*. Translated by Carolyn R. Fawcett. New York: Zone Press.

CHRISTAKIS, NICHOLAS. 1988. "The Ethical Design of an AIDS Vaccine Trial in Africa." *Hastings Center Report* 18, no. 3:31–37.

DESJARLAIS, ROBERT. 1993. *Body and Emotion: The Aesthetics of Illness and Healing in the Nepal Himalayas*. Philadelphia: University of Pennsylvania Press.

FABREGA, HORACIO. 1990. "An Ethnomedical Perspective on Medical Ethics." *Journal of Medical Philosophy* 15, no. 6:592–625.

FARMER, PAUL. 1992. *AIDS and Accusation: Haiti and the Geography of Blame*. Berkeley: University of California Press.

FARMER, PAUL, and KLEINMAN, ARTHUR. 1989. "AIDS and Human Suffering." *Daedalus* 118, no. 2:135–160.

FOX, RENÉE C. 1990. "The Evolution of American Bioethics: A Sociological Perspective." In *Social Science Perspectives* on Medical Ethics, pp. 201–227. Edited by George Weisz. Boston: Kluwer.

Fox, Renée C., and Swazey, Judith P. 1984. "Medical Morality Is Not Bioethics—Medical Ethics in China and the United States," Perspectives in Biology and Medicine 27, no. 3:336–360.

Frye, Northrop. 1982. The Great Code: The Bible and Literature. Toronto: Academic Press.

Good, Byron J. 1977. "The Heart of What's the Matter: The Semantics of Illness in Iran." Culture, Medicine and Psychiatry 1:25–58.

———. 1993. Medicine, Rationality and Experience. Cambridge: At the University Press.

Good, Mary Jo; Hunt, Linda; Munakata, T.; and Kobayashi, Y. 1993. "A Comparative Analysis of the Culture of Biomedicine: Disclosure and Consequence for Treatment and the Practice of Oncology in the United States, Japan and Mexico." In Health and Health Care in Developing Countries: Sociological Perspectives. Edited by Peter Conrad and Eugene Gallagher. Philadelphia: Temple University Press.

Gruenbaum, Ellen. 1982. "The Movement Against Clitoridectomy and Infibulation in Sudan: Public Health Policy and the Woman's Movement." Medical Anthropology Newsletter 13:4–12.

Helman, Cecil. 1984. Culture, Health and Illness: An Introduction for Health Professionals. London: Wright.

———. 1990. Culture, Health and Society: An Introduction for Health Professionals. 2d ed. Boston: Wright.

Janzen, John. 1978. The Quest for Therapy in Lower Zaire. Berkeley: University of California Press.

Jennings, Bruce. 1990. "Ethics and Ethnography in Neonatal Intensive Care." In Social Science Perspectives on Medical Ethics, pp. 261–272. Edited by George Weisz. Boston: Kluwer.

Kleinman, Arthur. 1980. Patients and Healers in the Context of Culture: An Exploration of the Borderland Between Anthropology, Medicine, and Psychiatry. Berkeley: University of California Press.

———. 1982. "Problèmes culturels associés aux recherches cliniques dans les pays en voie de développement." In Médecine et expérimentation. Edited by Maurice A. M. de Wachter. Cahiers de bioéthique no. 4. Quebec: Presses de l'Université Laval.

———. 1988a. The Illness Narratives: Suffering, Healing, and the Human Condition. New York: Basic Books.

———. 1988b. Rethinking Psychiatry: From Cultural Category to Personal Experience. New York: Free Press.

Korbin, Jill, ed. 1981. Child Abuse and Neglect: Cross Cultural Perspectives. Berkeley: University of California Press.

Kunstadter, Peter. 1980. "Medical Ethics in Cross-Cultural and Multicultural Perspectives." Social Science and Medicine 14B, no. 4:289–296.

Laderman, Carol. 1983. Wives and Midwives: Childbirth and Nutrition in Rural Malaysia. Berkeley: University of California Press.

———. 1991. Taming the Wind of Desire: Psychology, Medicine and Aesthetics in Malay Shamanistic Performance. Berkeley: University of California Press.

Last, Murray, and Chavunduka, Gordon, eds. 1986. The Professionalization of African Medicine. Manchester, England: Manchester University Press.

Leslie, Charles, ed. 1976. Asian Medical Systems: A Comparative Study. Berkeley: University of California Press.

Lewis, Gilbert. 1975. Knowledge of Illness in a Sepik Society: A Study of the Gnau, New Guinea. London: Athlone.

Lieban, Richard W. 1990. "Medical Anthropology and the Comparative Study of Medical Ethics." In Social Science Perspectives on Medical Ethics, pp. 221–239. Edited by George Weisz. Boston: Kluwer.

Lock, Margaret. 1980. East Asian Medicine in Urban Japan: Varieties of Medical Experience. Berkeley: University of California Press.

Lock, Margaret, and Gordon, Deborah, eds. 1988. Biomedicine Examined. Boston: Kluwer.

Lock, Margaret, and Honda, Christina. 1990. "Reaching Consensus About Death: Heart Transplants and Cultural Identity in Japan." In Social Science Perspectives on Medical Ethics, pp. 99–120. Edited by George Weisz. Boston: Kluwer.

Loewy, Erich. 1991. Suffering and the Beneficent Community: Beyond Libertarianism. Albany: State University of New York Press.

McGuire, Meredith. 1988. Ritual Healing in Suburban America. New Brunswick, N.J.: Rutgers University Press.

Mizrahi, Terry. 1986. Getting Rid of Patients: Contradictions in the Socialization of Physicians. New Brunswick, N.J.: Rutgers University Press.

Nichter, Mark. 1989. Anthropology and International Health: South Asian Case Studies. Dordrecht, Netherlands: Kluwer.

Proctor, Robert. 1988. Racial Hygiene: Medicine Under the Nazis. Cambridge, Mass.: Harvard University Press.

Rhodes, Lorna. 1991. Emptying Beds: The Work of an Emergency Psychiatric Ward. Berkeley: University of California Press.

Rogler, Lloyd H. 1990. "The Meaning of Culturally Sensitive Research in Mental Health." American Journal of Psychiatry 146:296–303.

Roseman, Marina. 1991. Healing Sounds from the Malaysian Rainforest: Temiar Music and Medicine. Berkeley: University of California Press.

Rothman, David J. 1990. "Human Experimentation and the Origins of Bioethics in the United States." In Social Science Perspectives on Medical Ethics, pp. 185–200. Edited by George Weisz. Boston: Kluwer.

Sargent, Carolyn. 1989. Maternity, Medicine and Power. Berkeley: University of California Press.

Scheper-Hughes, Nancy, ed. 1987. Child Survival: Anthropological Perspectives on the Treatment and Maltreatment of Children. Boston: D. Reidel/Kluwer.

Sen, Amartya. 1992. "Objectivity and Position: Observation, Categorization and the Assessment of Suffering." In Health and Social Changes. Edited by Lincoln Chen, Arthur Kleinman, and Norma Wave. New York: Oxford University Press.

Shweder, Richard A. 1990. "Ethical Relativism: Is There a Defensible Version?" Ethos 18, no. 2:205–218.

Taylor, Charles. 1990. *Sources of the Self: The Making of the Modern Identity.* Cambridge, Mass.: Harvard University Press.

Unschuld, Paul. 1979. *Medical Ethics in Imperial China: A Study in Historical Anthropology.* Berkeley: University of California Press.

Weisz, George, ed. 1990. *Social Science Perspectives on Medical Ethics.* Boston: Kluwer.

Williams, Bernard. 1981. "Introduction." In *Concepts and Categories: Philosophical Essays,* by Isaiah Berlin. Harmondsworth, U.K.: Penguin.

Wong, Dennis B. 1984. *Moral Relativity.* Berkeley: University of California Press.

Young, Allan. 1977. "Order, Analogy, and Efficacy in Ethiopian Medical Divination." *Culture, Medicine and Psychiatry* 1, no. 2:183–199.

———. 1990. "Moral Conflicts in a Psychiatric Hospital Treating Combat-Related Posttraumatic Stress Disorder (PTSD)." In *Social Science Perspectives on Medical Ethics,* pp. 65–82. Edited by George Weisz. Boston: Kluwer.

MEDICINE, ART OF

In the art of medicine physicians themselves become the diagnostic and therapeutic instruments that apply the knowledge and skills of medicine. The art of medicine includes not only what is required for a physical diagnosis and for healing, but also the ability to apply the generalized knowledge of medicine and medical science to individual patients. This latter aspect includes knowing the particularity of the patient, knowing how to shape the doctor's knowledge of medicine to the particular patient, and developing the relationship between patient and doctor. Discrete skills serve these goals, among them understanding the behavior of patients and doctors, using the doctor–patient relationship for diagnostic and therapeutic ends, good judgment and decision making, and effective communication.

For bioethics, considering the art of medicine offers challenges because aspects of the art arise from the singular traits of sick persons and the special character of the doctor–patient relationship. These put in doubt the validity of some ideas about patients' independent self-representation and self-determination that have been important in the recent development of bioethics.

In this context art does not refer to the general meaning of aesthetics or the fine arts. Instead, it is derived from the Greek word *techné,* meaning craft or skill. This distinction is important because it is commonly said, in error, that the art of medicine cannot be taught. Crafts and skills are said to be learned from others. The ancient Greeks classified medicine as one of the original arts, along with weaving, carpentry, and geometry. On the other hand, mere skill is not all there is to this art, which must be served by a deeper practical understanding of its complex subject, as in Aristotle's *phronesis* (sound, considered judgment) or the Hippocratic phrase, "Life is short and the art is long." It was only with the rise of science in the seventeenth century that the term began to have its current meaning of the personal skills of physicians. In the twentieth century, the "art of medicine" has been sharply distinguished from the "science of medicine" and has come to have a somewhat pejorative connotation.

The effects of science on the art of medicine

The identification of the art of medicine with subjectivity and particularity is what has led to its recent loss of stature. It has been an article of faith of medical science in the twentieth century that objective scientific evidence would eventually replace the subjectivity of the transaction between an individual patient and physician. A further canon of medical science is that the knowledge and the science make the diagnosis and effect the treatment. The individuality of the physician is irrelevant; doctors are interchangeable. However, as Samuel Gorovitz and Alasdair MacIntyre have pointed out, generalizations of scientific medicine from systems that may not involve humans and by abstraction from observations of particular patients must be reparticularized to this patient, at this time, in this context, by this physician (Gorovitz and MacIntyre, 1975). In the care of sick persons, there are no sharp distinctions between medical science and the art of medicine, since both kinds of knowledge reside in the individual physician. It is his or her individuality that allows the physician to practice the art of medicine. An impersonal agency like a computer can deploy the science of medicine, but a particular doctor must adapt this knowledge to an individual patient. To do this appropriately requires both tacit and manifest knowledge within the doctor.

Patterning knowledge to the patient is generally known as medical judgment—acquiring and integrating both subjective and objective knowledge to make decisions in the best interests of the patient. Recent advances in studies of the theory and practice of medical decision-making do not fully encompass clinical judgment, because they have focused more on solving problems that arise from the uncertainties of medical information than on the consequences that follow from the relevance or meaning medical information may have for the particular patient.

The tendency of physicians and medicine to conflate the patient with the disease obscures the importance of the art of medicine. It is impossible, however.

for physicians to confront or treat diseases. Because they can only treat the patient who has the disease, the art of medicine will always be essential.

How the individuality of the patient makes a difference

The distinction between disease and illness.

"Disease" is the pathoanatomical or pathophysiological entity that manifests itself in symptoms that the patient experiences and the doctor discovers (Cassells, 1985a). Diseases are abstractions that have no concrete existence except as instantiated in particular patients. "Illness" is the patient's experience of the effects of the disease process; it includes not only the symptoms—alien sensations or perceptions of distorted function—but the interpretations and meanings of the symptoms. The illness also embraces the impact of altered function on behavior and social existence. It is the illness that the patient presents to the physician as reported symptoms and dysfunctions. While the physician may be primarily interested in the disease, the ethicist should be concerned with the illness because of its effects on the patient, his or her relationships, and the community that put in doubt the moral agency of the sick person.

The effects of the individuality of the patient.

Onset, course, treatment, and outcome of identical diseases vary from patient to patient because of individual variation from the molecular level to the whole person to the community. The contribution of the individual to differences in his or her illness is sometimes difficult to appreciate if one thinks only about the acute infectious diseases or trauma. Chronic diseases, which produce the greatest burden of illness in the U.S. population, provide better examples. For example, diabetes in adults is genetically determined, but its severity and manifestations are influenced by variation in diet and exercise pattern from person to person. In addition, the availability, type, and utilization of medical care play parts in the effects of diabetes. Because disease is a process that occurs over time, the responses of the patient to the disease manifestations become part of the illness itself, as they alter the patient's behavior and change the illness. For example, whether patients report symptoms, visit physicians, take prescribed medications, alter their lifestyle, accept illness as inevitable, or fight its every intrusion—each of these factors has an influence on the illness and expresses the individuality of the sick person. Each modification requires a change in the approach of the physician dictated, for the most part, not by medical science but rather arising from the doctor's art. The physician can affect the patient only through the doctor-patient relationship, which is central to the practice of medicine and its art, but differences among individuals—for example, their degrees of trust versus suspicion, openness versus shyness, or friendliness versus hostility—influence the kind of relationship formed.

The different perspectives of patients and physicians

The patient's perspective on his or her affliction is different from the physician's. In such crucial dimensions as time, space, and the meaning of specific medical objects (such as bodily organs, technological devices, and medications), patients' experience of their world diverges from that of the physician, whose scientific perspective on their disease includes objective measures of time and space and precise definitions of objects (Toombs, 1992). In the case of hypertension, for example, patients may feel threatened with a stroke by this moment's elevated blood pressure, even though the dangers of hypertension lie in its effects on the heart, kidneys, and blood vessels over long periods. To patients, the felt immediacies of other disease threats also seem more a result of their seriousness than of their actual temporal proximity.

A patient's focus on a particular symptom depends more on the patient's interpretation of the symptom than it does on the actual experienced events. For example, a patient who interprets his or her chest pain as signaling heart disease may not be aware of, pay attention to, or report associated shoulder or neck pain that would tell the doctor that the chest pain is secondary to an entrapped cervical nerve and not heart disease. Further, patients rarely understand the probabilistic nature of medical information—that the facts of a case are most often not simply true or false, but only true with degrees of confidence—and even when they do, it is difficult for them to understand the meaning of these probabilities for them. Objectivity, always difficult, is virtually impossible for the sick person because of the nature of illness. Important alterations in thought processes, such as the inability to see things from the perspective of others and a concreteness of thought usually characteristic of children, accompany only serious illness, but this is where the reflections generated by bioethics are most important (Cassell, 1985b).

More than just medical science determines the physician's perspective of the patient's illness. Besides diagnostic and treatment goals that draw heavily on medical science, physicians have other aims. Some, such as the desire to save or prolong life, relieve pain, avoid doing harm, and provide information, are patient-centered. Others, such as being trustworthy and truthful, relate to their relationships with patients. As physicians among other physicians they also want to maintain their knowledge, to be considered good doctors by their peers, and to uphold the standards of their profession. Many of these ends are professional in nature, are part of the socialization of doctors, and reach back to antiquity. They, too, distinguish the doctor's point of view from that of even informed patients.

Although doctors and patients may appear to speak the same language about the same subjects, their differing viewpoints ensure that a physician may remain within the medical-scientific worldview and not attend to the patient's concerns. The care of the terminally ill often exemplifies such dissonance. Here, one of the ends of medical practice—staving off death as long as possible—may be at odds with the patient's desire not to be in pain or suffer. A necessary aspect of the physician's art is to understand the patient's goals and adjust professional aims and medicine's tools to these ends. This is the meaning of sayings throughout medical history exemplified by that of Bela Schick, "First the patient, second the patient, third the patient, fourth the patient, fifth the patient, and then maybe comes the science." That this principle is often violated or ignored does not obviate its centrality for the art of medicine.

The doctor–patient relationship

The special nature of the relationship between doctor and patient has been appreciated since antiquity (Laín Entralgo, 1969). As much a part of sickness and medicine as the diseases that make people ill, this relationship makes a sick person a patient and a medical person a doctor and a clinician. It is the vehicle through which physicians exercise their authority (not to be confused with authoritarianism), without which the practice of the art is impossible (Needleman, 1985). An examination of the way the relationship is formed and its potential for effectiveness suggests that this special bond is a basic part of the human condition with cultural and social dimensions (Cassell, 1991).

In emergencies, when doctor and patient have never previously met, the power of the relationship can become effective immediately. Within moments a doctor who is a stranger can ease pain, make panic subside, and improve breathing. (Physicians can also worsen symptoms and exacerbate panic by wrong actions.) The bond between doctor and patient is effective across cultural boundaries, even in the presence of antagonisms, and despite sometimes formidable social and environmental impediments.

Physicianhood is a role—a set of performances, duties, obligations, entitlements, and limitations connected to a function or status. The socialization of medical students includes learning about the doctor's role so that they emerge both as physicians and in the

role of physicians. Given its sociocultural nature, it has its counterpart in the patient, who provides for the doctor's words and action access to the patient and the patient's body not available to ordinary relationships. Because the connection between doctor and patient is bilateral, the power of sickness to make patients susceptible to change at all levels of the human condition is matched ideally by the power of this benevolent relationship to induce physicians to extend themselves at all levels.

Physicians, because of the relationship, are enabled to see the authentic person through the mess of sickness, read the history of self-determined purposes in the life before illness, and understand the aesthetic whole that is the patient's life prior to the unwelcome intrusion of disease. In a modern extension of the art, they therefore have the opportunity and obligation to help the patient maintain autonomy, which, for the sickest, would be almost impossible outside the relationship. Clinical ethicists share in this opportunity when and if the patient extends this special bond to them (Zaner, 1993).

These aspects of the doctor–patient relationship are frequently obscured from view or even contravened in the high technology atmosphere of modern medical centers. The patient's trust is necessary for the most successful diagnosis and treatment, and therapeutic intimacy arising out of the relationship creates confidence. As part of their art, skilled practitioners actively nurture the relationship, not only encouraging its growth and promoting trust by the patient, but negotiating between empathic intimacy and objectivity. One skill in the art of clinicians lies in coming as close as ethically possible to intimacy while maintaining independence of action. A strong bond is essential in negotiating the difficulties and uncertainties of serious illness. It is equally important in supporting and teaching patients through the long trajectory of chronic illness.

The behavior of sick persons and doctors

The behavior of sick persons. Even mild sickness alters behavior; profound sickness alters behavior profoundly. This is culturally acknowledged by what has come to be known as the sick role, the exemption from everyday duties and obligations granted to sick persons. Changes in functioning are not merely those associated with the disordered part—for example, the inability to move around because of back pain. Sickness induces changes in cognitive function and in relationships with self, body, and others. Patients who are sufficiently ill—for example, in life-threatening infectious diseases, congestive heart failure, for a few days after bypass surgery, or in long-term hospitalizations—although they are cognitively normal by conventional measures, have patterns of reasoning that Jean Piaget showed in children under six. For example, the sick frequently fail a classic test of reasoning about the conservation of volume. Two containers identical in size, shape, and the volume of water they contain are shown to the patient with the statement, "These two glasses have the same amount of water." The contents of one glass is then emptied into a tall thin cylinder and the patient is asked, "Which one of these has more water?" Sick persons will frequently indicate the tall thin cylinder. They may say, "I know that it shouldn't have more water, but it does" (Cassell, 1985b).

Sick persons usually are also unable to alter their perspective sufficiently to understand the viewpoint of another. A child's alphabet block shows this in its simplest form. Even if the block is rotated so that they have seen all of its sides, when looking at one face, they cannot report what is on the opposite face. One can routinely demonstrate many other similar changes in reasoning, of which the patient is almost always unaware. Because of the similarity of their reasoning (and other traits) to children, these characteristics have been considered regression. To avoid the error of treating the sick like children, it seems wiser to realize that this altered behavior is sickness expressing itself. Thus, in appropriate circumstances, patient self-determination will be enhanced by offering no more than two concretely worded alternatives at a time and avoiding choices couched in abstractions.

The sick are attached to their caregivers. How their attachment is expressed varies from love to anger or rebelliousness. The skillful physician is aware that these emotions are not directed at the doctor as a particular person (about whom the patient usually knows very little) but at the doctor in the role (Landis, 1993). As such, they are not to be taken personally but should be used in diagnosis or treatment. Changes in the patient's relationship to the body are also a common characteristic of illness. The patient may become angry with the body because of what it has done to the patient, as though the disease was something the body "did" to the patient. Relationship to the body influences the patient's other illness behavior and reactions to the events of the sickness and its treatment.

Illness brings about dependency on others and often induces feelings of loss of control, helplessness, inadequacy, and failure. As a result, it may awaken unconscious conflicts and cause the patient to act toward the physician as if he or she were the patient's parent. The artful physician, aware of the problems that may follow reawakening of early childhood experiences or feelings and behavior brought on by illness, knows and acts in the knowledge that the sick person within the doctor–patient relationship may seem quite different in presentation and behavior from the same person when he or she is well.

The behavior of doctors. Physicians, too, may behave differently in the presence of the sick than they do outside the doctor–patient relationship. Physicians' interactions with their patients may evoke feelings of anger, sexual attraction, sadness, grief, failure, rejection, and omnipotence, among others (Maoz et al., 1992). Many years ago a psychiatrist, Michael Balint, recognizing that physicians are not trained to deal with the feelings clinical events evoke in them, organized physician discussion groups (Balint, 1957). Although sometimes replicated, these so-called Balint groups have not been widely employed. Awareness of whether and how doctors' feelings and behavior interfere with their care of patients is important because physicians' experience of their patient's feelings is an essential source of information about the illness.

Physicians are powerful people who must employ their power judiciously if it is to do good and not harm (Brody, 1992). Yet, doctors are rarely trained in how to use their power or even to be aware that they have power, which may be abused perhaps more easily than it is used. An irreducible inequity of power between patient and doctor inheres in the clinical situation. Codes of medical ethics reaching back to antiquity and modern bioethics directly address this problem. It is widely recognized, however, that if physicians are not virtuous, all the precepts, principles, and regulations surrounding their conduct will be useless. Edmund Pellegrino and David Thomasma explain the virtues necessary to achieve the ends of the clinical encounter and the good of the patient, namely, to be made well again if possible, or to cope with sickness, pain, suffering, and impending death if necessary. These virtues include conscientious attention to technical knowledge and skill, compassion, beneficence, benevolence, honesty, fidelity to promises and to the patient's good, prudence, and wisdom (Pellegrino and Thomasma, 1988). Walsh McDermott believes that thoroughgoingness and self-discipline are also central virtues of the good clinician (McDermott, 1982). It requires a good person to be a good doctor—now, as in times past. As Paracelsus said, "The art of medicine is rooted in the heart. If your heart is false, you will also be a false physician; if your heart is just, you will also be a true physician."

It is difficult for a scientific (and cynical) era such as ours to accept the unavoidable necessity for virtue in doctors. As a consequence, the active training of doctors in the virtues of the good physician has largely been abandoned in the untested and probably wrong belief that medical virtue cannot be taught. During medical school and in postgraduate training, however, those who become doctors do learn, even if only through socialization, to restrain the employment of their skills in situations where more harm than good may follow, to be self-critical and admit error (at least to each other), to pursue the good of the patient, and to act benevolently (Bosk, 1979).

Medical decision making

Physicians are constantly making judgments, many of which are moral. The skill of exercising judgment, which has defied systematization, is the ability to apply the general to the particular; in medicine, this means to the particular patient, clinical situation, or context. To do this, physicians must obtain information of three distinct kinds—brute facts (also known in medicine as hard data); values; and aesthetics (patterns, relationships among the elements of a situation, and degrees of order or disorder). Often doctors are not aware of much of the information in the latter two categories that enters their judgments. Because of the necessity for such information, which is often neither obvious nor easily demonstrated, the art of medicine requires heightened skills of observation and synthesis. The art also requires that some systematic understanding be brought to judgment.

Alvan Feinstein was the first to closely examine the logic that underlies physicians' decisions; his work generated the field of clinical epidemiology (Feinstein, 1967, 1985). Feinstein's primary concern was the background evidence that the study of groups of people would provide for clinical decisions in patient care. Those who have followed him have elaborated his basic message and methods to assist physicians in judging the utility of a piece of evidence or information in the diagnosis or treatment of a particular patient (Wulff, 1981; Fletcher et al., 1988; Sackett et al., 1991). These writers have elaborated basic principles that determine the diagnostic meaning of a piece of clinical information, for example, a finding on physical examination, the result of a blood test, or a clinical measurement. The accuracy and validity of the test or measurement are important, as might be expected, but so is the likelihood that *any* similar patient would have the disease or state that is being tested for.

Put another way, to know how helpful a piece of information is diagnostically, one has to know the chance that any such patient truly has the disease. For example, even if a test for a rare disease is 99 percent accurate, when a large population of healthy people is tested and someone has a positive test, the chances are small that the person has the disease. The test will probably have been a false positive. Alternatively, in a population in a region where the disease is common, a positive test probably means the person has the disease.

The test will have been a true positive. Because many conclusions of the clinical epidemiologists based on Bayesian mathematics are counterintuitive, their work has been extremely important in bringing objectivity and precision to decision making. (In the example given above, when the test is 99 percent accurate but the disease is rare, a patient who tests positive has only about a 10 percent chance of having the disease.) Terms such as specificity, sensitivity, and positive predictive value, which denote quantified measures of modern medical decision making, are now commonly heard in discussions about particular patients. Modern physicians must not only be conversant with these methods; they must also explain them to each patient so that the patient can participate effectively in the decision-making process.

Physicians rarely realize the degree to which each patient is different. Consequently, particularizing the generalizations of medical science to fit an individual patient requires great skill. The desires, needs, concerns, intentions, and purposes of patients are statements of values that must be elicited if they are to enter decision making. They are often faulted as hopelessly subjective and consequently not up to the standard of the hard data employed in the decision-making methods discussed above. A patient's desire for a certain outcome may be subjective, but the statement of that aspiration is objective and can be validated and given precision within degrees of confidence through discussion with the patient and attention to the pattern of the patient's previous actions and purposes. The artful physician is obligated to develop the mastery that gives these values decision-making weight—they are expressions of the patient's autonomy. Attempts to circumvent the need for such mastery by developing standardized methodologies, such as scales and questionnaires to assess individual values, have not proved clinically useful. It remains necessary, therefore, for the clinician to know the sick person to the greatest degree possible so that good clinical judgments can be made.

The clinical situation, like the disease and the illness, is always changing; therefore, decision making that integrates values and other clinical information constantly occurs in clinical medicine. Shifts occur not only because of the evolving process of the disease, but also because of the ongoing responses of both doctors and patients. In addition, the place care is given (home, doctor's office, hospital, etc.) and who else is involved (family, friends, medical students, etc.) influence the process of the illness. It is obvious why clinical judgments are not confined to the initial diagnosis or decisions about therapy.

The art of medicine requires that the physician be always mindful of changes in the circumstances, the illness, and the capacity of the patient. Although the formal principles of modern decision making may not always be applicable, newer ideas about the probabilistic nature of judgment and the need to integrate hard and soft data constantly inform the work of the artful physician.

Doctor–patient communication

The ability to employ the spoken language to obtain information from and about the sick person, gain the patient's cooperation, and provide information to the patient is a central element in the art of medicine. Doctor–patient communication is unlike many other verbal transactions, despite its use of ordinary language. The patient is in the conversation with the doctor for a specific purpose that is vital for the patient and diagnostically or therapeutically significant for the physician. The patient and the doctor have important joint purposes in the service of which the conversation is both necessary and crucial.

The patient wants the doctor to pay attention to his or her symptoms and concerns about the illness, and is worried lest these not be properly expressed or their importance not be appreciated. Doctors want to hear the clues to the diagnosis that only the patient's story can convey. Yet, some things that are important to the patient may not be of interest to the doctor and vice-versa. If the doctor attends solely to the evidence for disease, discarding everything else the patient says as irrelevant, then he or she may find the disease, but discard the sick person. A person's utterances convey not only the overt description of his or her actions and beliefs, but also the significance of the objects and events under discussion to the speaker. This other aspect of the speaker's message—the description of self of which the speaker is often unaware—lies in the specific choice of words, syntax, and paralanguage (Cassell, 1985c). The attentive, artful physician, listening to these specific aspects of the spoken language, has the opportunity to know more about the patient.

Conversation with the patient offers the doctor the opportunity to discover the patient's presuppositions and the beliefs according to which the patient assigns meanings. Similarly, doctors can inform their patients about the medical presuppositions and concepts that inform the doctors' actions. Such exchanges help avoid or correct the miscommunications that inevitably arise because of the differing perspectives of doctor and patient. Just as the patient's language informs the doctor about the patient, the doctor's utterances reveal himself or herself to the patient. The virtues of physicians are not abstractions, but are displayed in speech and actions. Trust is built by means of conversation as well as by action; compassion is communicated in words, in nonver-

bal communication, and in action. The constant flow of spoken (and unspoken) language provides a doctor the opportunity to build his or her knowledge of the patient and provides a patient evidence of the physician's skill and fidelity.

The doctor also has the specific responsibility of informing the patient about what is the matter, what it means, what actions might be taken, what options exist, and what choices the patient must make. The same is true, on occasion, of communication with the patient's family or significant others. Information, however, is also a therapeutic tool. Doctor–patient communication provides the physicians the opportunity to convey information that reduces the patients' uncertainties, enables the patient to act in his or her own best interests, and strengthens the relationship between the doctor and patient. On the other hand, poorly or inadequately communicated information can increase uncertainty, paralyze action, and destroy the relationship.

A specific aspect of doctor–patient communication is breaking bad news. When it is done poorly, it can destroy hope and leave a patient in shambles. As part of the art of medicine, doctors must learn to convey bad news so well that patients are enabled to make truly self-representative and self-determined choices (Buckman, 1988).

Patients, like everybody else, act and react because of what things mean to them. Meaning includes not merely denotative aspects of words, objects and events, but their connotative, or value-laden, content as well. With its cognitive and affective aspects, meaning has an impact on the physical and spiritual responses of the sick. By changing patients' meanings, physicians can alter, sometime profoundly, the patient's experience of illness (Cassell, 1985a). The effective use of spoken language, with its power of creating and altering the meaning of wellness and illness, is an important aspect of the art of medicine.

ERIC J. CASSELL

For a further discussion of topics mentioned in this entry, see the entries AUTHORITY; AUTONOMY; BODY; COMPASSION; EMOTIONS; FIDELITY AND LOYALTY; HEALING; HEALTH AND ILLNESS; INFORMATION DISCLOSURE; INTERPRETATION; MEDICAL EDUCATION; MEDICINE AS A PROFESSION; PAIN AND SUFFERING; PROFESSIONAL–PATIENT RELATIONSHIP; SOCIAL MEDICINE; TRUST; VALUE AND VALUATION; *and* VIRTUE AND CHARACTER. *For a discussion of related ideas, see the entries* CARE; CONFIDENTIALITY; LOVE; MEDICINE, ANTHROPOLOGY OF; MEDICINE, PHILOSOPHY OF; MEDICINE, SOCIOLOGY OF; NARRATIVE; OBLIGATION AND SUPEREROGATION; *and* SURGERY.

Bibliography

BALINT, MICHAEL. 1957. *The Doctor, His Patient, and the Illness.* London: Pitman.

BOSK, CHARLES L. 1979. *Forgive and Remember: Managing Medical Failure.* Chicago: University of Chicago Press.

BRODY, HOWARD. 1992. *The Healer's Power.* New Haven, Conn.: Yale University Press.

BUCKMAN, ROBERT. 1988. *I Don't Know What to Say: How to Help and Support Someone Who Is Dying.* Toronto: Key Porter.

CASSELL, ERIC J. 1984. "How Is the Death of Barney Clark to be Understood?" In *After Barney Clark: Reflections on the Utah Heart Program.* Edited by Margery W. Shaw. Austin: University of Texas Press.

———. 1985a. *Clinical Technique.* Vol. 2 of *Talking with Patients.* Cambridge, Mass.: MIT Press.

———. 1985b. *The Healer's Art.* Cambridge, Mass.: MIT Press.

———. 1985c. *The Theory of Doctor-Patient Communication.* Vol. 1 of *Talking with Patients.* Cambridge, Mass.: MIT Press.

———. 1991. *The Nature of Suffering: And the Goals of Medicine.* New York: Oxford University Press.

FEINSTEIN, ALVAN R. 1967. *Clinical Judgment.* Baltimore, Md.: Williams and Wilkins.

———. 1985. *Clinical Epidemiology: The Architecture of Clinical Research.* Philadelphia: W. B. Saunders.

FLETCHER, ROBERT H.; FLETCHER, SUZANNE W.; and WAHNER, EDWARD H. 1988. *Clinical Epidemiology: The Essentials.* 2d ed. Baltimore, Md.: Williams and Wilkins.

GOROVITZ, SAMUEL, and MACINTYRE, ALASDAIR C. 1975. "Toward a Theory of Medical Fallibility." *Hastings Center Report* 5, no. 6:13–23.

LAÍN ENTRALGO, PEDRO. 1969. *Doctor and Patient.* Translated by Frances Partridge. New York: McGraw-Hill.

LANDIS, DAVID A. 1993. "Physician, Distinguish Thyself: Conflict and Covenant in a Physician's Moral Development." In *Perspectives in Biology and Medicine* 36, no. 4:628–641.

MAOZ, BENJAMIN; RABINOWITZ, STANLEY; HERZ, MICHAEL; and KATZ, HALVA ELKIN. 1992. *Doctors and Their Feelings: A Pharmacology of Medical Caring.* Westport, Conn.: Praeger.

MCDERMOTT, WALSH. 1982. "Education and General Medical Care." *Annals of Internal Medicine* 96, no. 4:512–517.

NEEDLEMAN, JACOB. 1985. *The Way of the Physician.* San Francisco: Harper & Row.

PELLEGRINO, EDMUND D., and THOMASMA, DAVID C. 1988. *For the Patient's Good: The Restoration of Beneficence in Health Care.* New York: Oxford University Press.

SACKETT, DAVID L.; HAYNES, R. BRIAN; and TUGWELL, PETER. 1991. *Clinical Epidemiology: A Basic Science for Clinical Medicine.* 2d ed. Boston: Little, Brown.

TOOMBS, S. KAY. 1992. *The Meaning of Illness: A Phenomenological Account of the Different Perspectives of Physician and Patient.* Boston: Kluwer.

WULFF, HENRIK R. 1981. *Rational Diagnosis and Treatment: An Introduction to Clinical Decision-Making.* 2d ed. Oxford: Blackwell Scientific.

ZANER, RICHARD M. 1993. *Troubled Voices: Stories of Ethics and Illness.* Cleveland: Pilgrim.

MEDICINE, PHILOSOPHY OF

Over the last two and a half millennia—since the beginnings of Greek philosophy and medicine—there have been rich conceptual reflections regarding medical findings, reasoning in medicine, the status of knowledge claims in medicine, and the special concepts that structure the science and art of medicine. The philosophy of medicine is a corpus of considerations and writings uniting these reflections by contributors as diverse as Plato, Aristotle, and Galen; René Descartes, Immanuel Kant, and Georg W. F. Hegel; and contemporary thinkers. Because these examinations of medicine are philosophical in different senses, the term "philosophy of medicine" is ambiguous, covering a heterogeneous field of intellectual concerns. For the purpose of this overview, they have been collected under four categories.

The first category, speculative philosophy of medicine, has existed from the beginning of medicine. Speculative medicine may be characterized as the attempt to discover the basic philosophical principles that lie behind the practice of medicine. Here philosophy attempts to discover theoretical frameworks or foundations that give shape or content to clinical data. In this sense, philosophy of medicine provides a priori points of departure for medical knowledge and practice. The second category, the logic of medicine, brings together attempts to clarify the character of scientific reasoning in medicine. It identifies the basic principles that make medicine a coherent science. This category of philosophy of medicine studies, for example, the way in which diagnoses are made and judged to be accurate in medical practice and research. A third area of the philosophy of medicine may be understood as a subspecialty of philosophy of science. This area is concerned with what is accepted as "knowledge" in medicine and the health-care professions. Much of the recent exploration of the status of concepts of health and disease or the status of the unconscious and explanation in psychoanalysis falls into this third category. Finally, a fourth category describes the explorations of other philosophical issues that have special salience in health care, for example, the nature of persons and its implications for the morality of abortion. Philosophy of medicine in this fourth sense would include bioethics.

Just as there is ambiguity concerning the meaning of "philosophy" in "philosophy of medicine," so there is ambiguity about the compass of medicine. Medicine can be construed as a body of knowledge, skills, and social practices concerned with the health and pathology of humans. In its modern sense, medicine encompasses theory and practice, science and art. Traditionally medicine is the origin of all systematic concerns with healing, including nursing and the allied health sciences. The focus of the philosophy of medicine, as a consequence, can have a broad or narrow scope.

The philosophy of medicine as speculative medicine

The ancient Greek philosophers sought to understand the world on a rational rather than a supernatural basis. Early Greek medicine was influenced by philosophers who held that the primary goal of a scientist was to find one basic principle or set of principles that would explain the natural world known by the senses. These physicians developed theories as to how the body worked and how diseases might be understood and controlled. At first, there was little concern to justify these theories in experience or observation. One finds, then, a tension in early Greek medicine between those physicians who grounded medicine in rational speculation—the rationalists—and those who grounded medicine in experience—the empiricists.

This tension is evident in the Hippocratic corpus. In the corpus there is approval for theorizing that "lays its foundation in incident, and deduces its conclusions in accordance with phenomena" (Jones, 1923, p. 313). Nevertheless, the Hippocratic author rejects the systematic sweep of more speculative thought:

> Certain physicians and philosophers assert that nobody can know medicine who is ignorant what a man is; he who would treat patients properly must, they say, learn this. But the question they raise is one for philosophy; it is the province of those who, like Empedocles, have written on natural science, what man is from the beginning, how he came into being at the first, and from what elements he was originally constructed. (Jones, 1923, p. 53)

The author is rejecting what might be termed speculative or metaphysical medicine—namely, the attempt to construct a theory of medicine on the basis of self-evident, or basic, principles or concepts. The author also writes that medicine has no need of "an empty postulate," a concept that is not based in experience, because it has at hand the means for verifiable knowledge.

René Descartes (1596–1650) held that he could determine the fundamental laws of metaphysics, physics, and medicine (Descartes, 1983) by reason alone, without appeal to experience. On the basis of his work in speculative, metaphysical medicine, Descartes predicted that he would live an additional century or so, achieving a life span of one and a half centuries. He believed his own theories would issue in simple revisions of daily routine leading to such extensions of life expectancy (Descartes, 1983).

Descartes's *Treatise of Man* (1662) attempts a mechanistic anatomy and physiology expressed in terms of matter and motion. Descartes explains how the human body works by comparing it to a machine. He found that this mechanistic approach could explain the physical functioning of the human body but not rational behavior. Still, Descartes's philosophical reflections concerning the body provided a framework for later explanations of human functioning that also relied on mechanical metaphors.

The success of Isaac Newton (1642–1727) in offering systematic explanations in physics inspired attempts to do this in medicine. The eighteenth-century Scottish physician John Brown (1735–1788), for example, suggested that the concept of excitability could serve medicine as the concept of gravity had served Newtonian physics: as the single concept upon which all explanations of health and disease could ultimately rest. Stimulation or excitation and response to it, he argued, resulted in an equilibrium or disequilibrium that defined "health" and "disease," respectively. If an imbalance became too extreme, death would result. Brown's work attracted the attention of philosophers, including Hegel (1770–1831). This philosophy of medicine—as the gray area between scientific, empirical medicine and the philosophy of nature—led to the modern understanding of medicine that brings together empirical observation and theoretical construction (Tsouyopoulos, 1982).

Twentieth-century historians of medicine have appreciated this interplay between empirical and speculative medicine under the title "philosophy of medicine." William Szumowski in 1949 and Owsei Temkin in 1956 spoke of the importance of the philosophy of medicine. It is to Szumowski that much of the rebirth of the interest in this term, perhaps first coined by Elisha Bartlett in 1844, can be attributed. Lester King (1978) has used the term to identify the theoretical reflections undertaken by both physicians and philosophers engaged in speculative as well as other conceptual explorations of medicine.

The philosophy of medicine as the logic of medicine

The relationship between medical reasoning and medical practice has been an area of perennial philosophical controversy and investigation. In ancient Greek and Roman medicine, the disputes between the rationalists and empiricists were, in part, disputes about how knowledge claims in medicine ought to be justified. By the Renaissance, medicine had failed to achieve the success in healing that is often attributed to it today. This failure to achieve therapeutic success led to attempts to make medicine more "scientific," in the hope of duplicating the success of fields like astronomy and physics. Thomas Sydenham (1624–1689), whose *Observationes medicae* appeared in a third edition in 1676, proposed a disciplined methodology of observation and treatment. Sydenham brought to medicine the scientific method of Francis Bacon (1561–1626), which sought to ground reasoning in experience, observation, and data.

This method, however, raised questions about observer bias of which Syndenham was aware. The principal difficulty is that an investigator's findings may be influenced by his or her presuppositions. These concerns about observer bias were taken up in the eighteenth century by such theoreticians of medicine as François Boissier de Sauvages de la Croix (1706–1767) in his *Nosologia methodica sistens morborum classes juxta sydenhami mentem et botanicorum ordinem* (1768). Influenced by the writings of Thomas Sydenham and Carolus Linnaeus, Sauvages organized diseases into a structure of class, order, genus, and species. In his *Nosologia* there is an appreciation of medical observation as well as a concern for a logical rigor that sought to coherently relate observations to predicted outcomes. Sauvages's principal undertaking included a classification of diseases primarily based on their signs and symptoms rather than on their causes. He also sought to tie observed signs of illness to relationships that had been noted between past, present, and predicted future states of patients. The logical rigor of disciplined observation and the collection of facts is also evident in the work of William Cullen (1710–1790) and Thomas Percival (1740–1804).

The major revolutions in medical understanding born of advances in anatomy and physiology in the late eighteenth and nineteenth centuries, along with the recognition that many established treatments did not work, required a fundamental reassessment of medicine. Philosophical reflections concerning medical reasoning gave way to major treatises concerning the character of reasoning in medicine. Works such as Sir Gilbert Blane's *Elements of Medical Logick* (1819), Elisha Bartlett's *Philosophy of Medical Science* (1844), and F. R. Oesterlen's *Medizinische Logik* (1852) range from listing the elementary principles of life to concern with material fallacies in medicine, including excessive deference to authority, fashion, or speculative reasoning without sufficient empirical observation. Oesterlen's work, which advanced criteria for inductive reasoning in medicine based on the work of John Stuart Mill, included an analysis of the methods and means of medical investigation, the character of the inductive method in medicine, and the status of experiments, hypotheses, analogies, terminologies, definitions, and classifications. He viewed medical logic as the application of general logical principles to the field of medicine for the purpose of securing a

coherent inductive and empirical science that would be free from a priori speculation. His work was followed by other studies, including Władysław Biegánski's *Logika medycyny* (1894) and Richard Koch's *Die ärztliche Diagnose* (1920).

Growing philosophical sophistication characterizes twentieth-century assessments of medical knowledge and medical reasoning. Types of medical knowledge may correspond to the different functions of medicine. Medicine can be understood in a threefold manner: biological medicine, clinical research, and clinical practice. Biological medicine is concerned mainly with scientific research in biology, whereas clinical research is focused on the development of the knowledge and technology used in clinical medicine. Finally, the area of clinical practice involves the realities of patients and disease. A philosophical concern of those writing on the logic of medicine has been to clarify the nature of each type of medical knowledge and the relationship of these different areas of medical knowledge and reasoning to one another (Wulff et al., 1986).

Since the middle of the twentieth century, a renewed interest in the logic of medical reasoning and the character of medical decision making has been expressed in the computer reconstruction of differential diagnosis. This literature has examined the logic and principles of medical reasoning—for example, the applicability of Bayes's Theorem to medical decision making (Lusted, 1968; Wulff, 1976); the logic of the taxonomy of disease and classification, including the application of set theory to the analysis of clinical judgments (Feinstein, 1967); and the role played by morbidity, mortality, and other costs in determining when and how diagnoses are framed. For example, because of the human and financial costs, one will be much more concerned about false positive diagnoses of AIDS than of athlete's foot. Recent works have given special attention to the process of making diagnoses, including the principles of differential diagnosis (Caplan, 1986; Engelhardt et al., 1979; Wulff, 1976), as well as the elaboration of nosologies as instruments for gathering clinical information. Many of these reflections have stressed the hidden role of values and conceptual assumptions in the process and logic of medical diagnosis (Schaffner, 1985; Peset and Gracia, 1992; King, 1982).

The philosophy of medicine as the philosophy of the science of medicine

Philosophy of medicine may also be understood as a self-conscious reflection on the status of special concepts, such as health and disease, deployed in medicine. Rudolf Virchow (1821–1902), for example, argued that designating a state of affairs as an "illness" has a stipulative character; that is, such concepts are defined by agreement and there are no clear natural types or divisions of nature corresponding to nosological categories. This sense of the philosophy of medicine places the accent on issues in the theory of knowledge and the examination of what should count as a medical theory or explanation. In this, it is distinguished from speculative philosophy of medicine and from the more narrow concerns with the rules of evidence and inference proper to medicine that are the focus of medical logic and medical decision theory.

Since the 1950s a considerable literature has developed that is directed to the status of concepts such as health, disease, illness, disability, and disorder. Whether such concerns constitute a subspecialty of the philosophy of science is disputed (Caplan, 1992; Wulff, 1992). There has also been interest in the character of medical explanation (Canguilhem, 1978). This literature has also explored the application of such terms to nonhuman animals. In addition, there has been attention to the extent to which these concepts are normative and the extent to which nonnormative, value-free concepts can be elaborated. Those who have argued in favor of weak or strong normative understandings of concepts such as health, disease, and illness have also addressed the character and kind of values that structure such concepts. Investigations have included the extent to which concepts of disease are instrumental to medical practice, or instead identify natural divisions in reality. In addition, there have been attempts to place medicine within the general compass of philosophical explorations of scientific theory (Kliemt, 1986). Finally, the significant changes about the relationship of theories, facts, and values in the understanding of the history and philosophy of science that occurred in the 1960s and 1970s were anticipated in Ludwik Fleck's 1935 study of changes in the meaning of syphilis and venereal disease from the fifteenth to the early twentieth century (Fleck, 1979).

The philosophy of medicine as the collection of philosophical interests in medicine

Even if one were to hold that medicine offers no conceptual or philosophical problems not already present in the subject matter of the philosophy of science or the philosophy of biology (Caplan, 1992), there would still be merit in exploring the ways in which philosophical study and analysis can be directed to the understanding of medicine, as well as to the health-care sciences and arts in general. In this sense, the philosophy of medicine encompasses the ways in which the philosophy of science, the philosophy of biology, the philosophy of mind, moral philosophy, and so on are engaged in order better to understand medicine. Perhaps one would wish to characterize such explorations as philosophy about med-

icine rather than of medicine, in the sense that the tools, analyses, and insights of philosophy in general are brought to the particular subject matter of medicine. Calling this endeavor the philosophy of medicine underscores the heuristic advantage of treating the domain as a whole, as a single focus of attention. There is also the advantage of recognizing that general issues of justice, fairness, rights, and duties confront the special challenge of taking account of the development of humans from conception to death.

In medicine, special questions of intergenerational justice become salient, distinctions between human biological and human personal life are raised, the irremediable character of loss must be confronted, and comparisons must be made between claims for the alleviation of suffering versus the postponement of death. Though the definitions of futility, of ordinary versus extraordinary treatment, and of the beginning of life and the beginning of death may arise outside the compass of medicine, such definitions take on a special philosophical cast and character in the context of medicine. The recognition that there is this special concatenation of conceptual issues is appreciated in employing the term "philosophy of medicine." This use of the term approximates the one employed by the European Society for the Philosophy of Medicine and Health Care (founded 1987), which encompasses bioethics within a constellation of philosophical concerns and undertakings. The philosophy of medicine as speculative medicine, as the logic of medicine, and as the philosophy of the science of medicine all spring from the acknowledgment that medicine constitutes one of the cardinal areas of intellectual and moral attention, central to human life, and is worthy of sustained conceptual analysis and philosophical regard.

H. Tristram Engelhardt, Jr.
Kevin Wm. Wildes

Directly related to this entry are the entries Medicine, Anthropology of; Medicine, Art of; Medicine, Sociology of; *and* Medicine as a Profession. *Other relevant material may be found under the entries* Bioethics; Biology, Philosophy of; Healing; Health and Disease, *articles on* history of the concepts, *and* philosophical perspectives; *and* Professional–Patient Relationship, *article on* historical perspectives.

Bibliography

Bartlett, Elisha. 1844. *An Essay on the Philosophy of Medical Science.* Philadelphia: Lea and Blanchard.
Bieganski, Władysław. 1894. *Logika medycyny.* Warsaw: Kowalewski.
Blane, Gilbert. 1819. *Elements of Medical Logick.* London: T. and G. Underwood.

CANGUILHEM, GEORGES. 1978. *On the Normal and the Pathological.* Translated by Carolyn R. Fawcett. Dordrecht, Netherlands: D. Reidel.

CAPLAN, ARTHUR L. 1986. "Exemplary Reasoning? A Comment on Theory Structure in Biomedicine." *Journal of Medicine and Philosophy* 11, no. 1:93–105.

———. 1992. "Does the Philosophy of Medicine Exist?" *Theoretical Medicine* 13, no. 1:67–77.

DESCARTES, RENÉ. 1983. [1644]. *Principles of Philosophy.* Translated by Valentine R. Miller and Reese P. Miller. Dordrecht, Netherlands: D. Reidel.

ENGELHARDT, H. TRISTRAM; SPICKER, STUART F.; and TOWERS, BERNARD, eds. 1979. *Clinical Judgment: A Critical Appraisal.* Dordrecht, Netherlands: Kluwer.

FEINSTEIN, ALVAN R. 1967. *Clinical Judgment.* Baltimore: Williams and Wilkins.

FLECK, LUDWIK. 1979. [1935]. *Entstehung und Entwicklung einer wissenschaftlichen Tatsache: Einfuhrung in die Lehre vom Denkstil und Denkkollektiv.* Basel: Benno Schwabe. Translated by Fred Bradley and Thaddeus J. Trenn as *Genesis and Development of a Scientific Fact.* Chicago: University of Chicago Press.

HUMPHREYS, PAUL. 1989. *The Chances of Explanation: Causal Explanation in the Social, Medical, and Physical Sciences.* Princeton, N.J.: Princeton University Press.

JONES, WILLIAM H. S., trans. 1923. *Hippocrates.* New York: Putnam.

KING, LESTER S. 1978. *The Philosophy of Medicine: The Early Eighteenth Century.* Cambridge, Mass.: Harvard University Press.

———. 1982. *Medical Thinking: A Historical Preface.* Princeton, N.J.: Princeton University Press.

KLIEMT, HARTMUT. 1986. *Grundzüge der Wissenschaftstheorie: Eine Einführung fur Mediziner und Pharmazeuten.* Stuttgart, Germany: Gustav Fischer.

KOCH, RICHARD. 1920. *Die ärztliche Diagnose.* Wiesbaden, Germany: Bergmann.

LUSTED, LEE B. 1968. *Introduction to Medical Decision Making.* Springfield, Ill.: Charles C. Thomas.

PERCIVAL, THOMAS. 1776. *Philosophical, Medical, and Experimental Essays.* London: Joseph Johnson.

PESET, JOSÉ LUIS, and GRACIA, DIEGO, eds. 1992. *The Ethics of Diagnosis.* Dordrecht, Netherlands: Kluwer.

SCHAFFNER, KENNETH F., ed. 1985. *Logic of Discovery and Diagnosis in Medicine.* Berkeley: University of California Press.

SZUMOWSKI, W. 1949. "La Philosophie de la médicine, son histoire, son essence, sa dénomination et sa définition." *Archives internationales de l'histoire des sciences* 9:1097–1141.

TEMKIN, OWSEI. 1956. "On the Interrelationship of the History and the Philosophy of Medicine." *Bulletin of the History of Medicine* 30, no. 3:241–251.

TSOUYOPOULOS, NELLY. 1982. *Andreas Roschlaub und die romantische Medizin: Die philosophischen Grundlagen der modernen Medizin.* Stuttgart, Germany: Gustav Fischer.

WULFF, HENRIK. 1976. *Rational Diagnosis and Treatment.* Oxford: Blackwell Scientific Publications.

———. 1992. "Philosophy of Medicine—from a Medical Perspective." *Theoretical Medicine* 13, no. 1:79–85.

WULFF, HENRIK R.; PEDERSEN, STIG ANDUR; and ROSENBERG, RABEN. 1986. *Philosophy of Medicine: An Introduction.* Oxford: Blackwell Scientific Publications.

MEDICINE, SOCIOLOGY OF

The sociology of medicine is characterized by a wide variety of concerns, approaches, and perspectives (Mechanic, 1978; Freeman and Levine, 1989; Fox, 1989; Waitzkin, 1991). The concerns of medical sociologists cover such diverse areas as the distribution and etiology of disease and impairments; disease concepts and their social construction; cultural and social responses to health and illness and the use of services; health and illness behavior and its determinants; sociocultural aspects of medical care and the social organization of helping services; the organization of the health occupations and the processes of providing care; social factors affecting trends in death and illness; the sociology of the health occupations; the social organization of the hospital; and comparative health organization. In collaboration with other disciplines, the field includes the study of social change and health care; changing technology and its role in care; medical education; public-health organization; stress, disease, and coping; social and community psychiatry; the social context of legal and ethical dilemmas; and medical politics.

Many medical sociologists attempt to illuminate how individuals define and respond to situations as they cope with the expectations and demands of their physical and social environment, how some types of response lead to stress and illness, and how services are used to reestablish social and personal equilibrium. Helping institutions can be examined similarly in terms of how the behavior of health personnel and organizations responds to problems of resources, time, and other situational constraints. All people, whether patients or health personnel, seek to establish mastery over their life and work environments, to reduce uncertainty, and to obtain gratification and esteem for their efforts.

One important aspect of medical sociology concerns how certain problems become manifest in a population, how they are defined, and how patients with these problems enter particular channels of care. The field also deals with the nature of therapeutic encounters between patients and practitioners, modes of communication and influence, types of discourse, and how all these are influenced by the cultural context, social characteristics of patient and therapist, changing knowledge and technology, organizational and payment arrangements, and resource constraints.

From a sociological perspective, medicine can be regarded as a sustaining or integrative institution in society (Parsons, 1951). Not only does it provide assistance to persons afflicted with disease and other life problems; it also serves as an important means for alleviating social distress and for excusing failures in social functioning or failures to meet social expectations (Mechanic, 1978; Kleinman, 1986). Medicine also has important social control functions that facilitate the removal of individuals from social settings to relieve tensions—whether in the family, in work settings, or in the community at large. It may also facilitate financial compensation or social benefits, for example, access to services or products, such as drugs, that are restricted to those who are not deemed ill.

The role of the physician, then, has not only technical dimensions but also social and moral ones. While the technical expertise of practitioners refers to a limited range of situations, their clientele and the scope of problems they deal with are very broad. Many of the judgments a physician makes are not medical judgments but decisions based on social considerations and values. Even those aspects of the medical role that appear to be purely technical, such as the labeling of disease, the specific management of the patient, and the choice of medications or other treatments, have profound consequences for performance of social roles and obligations as well as for future life opportunities. Patients' problems often result in part from conflicts with other persons and social groups, and the physician can sometimes help resolve difficulties by taking either the patient's or an adversary's perspective. Such conflicts are particularly evident in such areas as military, industrial, and prison medicine, where the physician is not the patient's personal agent, but they occur to some extent in many private patient-care contexts as well.

Patient flow from a community population to various helping agencies is usually thought to result almost exclusively from the occurrence of illness in that population, in contrast with other factors. Indeed, other factors distorting the selection process, such as differential propensities to seek care, are seen as "disturbances" that require correction through patient education or such economic disincentives as deductibles and coinsurance. Although illness is usually the major determinant of help-seeking, it fails to explain by itself much of the evident variation between those who seek and those who do not seek assistance (Mechanic, 1978).

It is common, for example, for medical scientists to assert that discovering a cure for an illness such as the common cold, one of the most frequent reasons for consulting a physician, would profoundly alleviate physical limitations, industrial absenteeism, and the loss of productive labor. But to the extent that the common cold is often an excuse rather than the reason for work absenteeism or seeking medical care, a "cure" might have much less social effect than commonly believed. If people who seek care for the common cold do so because they are unhappy or hate their employment, then the visit to the doctor may be little more than a justification for more complex motivations and behavior. There are various social and cultural inhibitions against persons openly acknowledging personal life problems, and often such problems are shielded by presentations of seemingly trivial illness. This process is now commonly referred to as somatization (Kleinman, 1986).

Medicine involves a distinctive set of meanings that limit the interpretations of patients' concerns (Waitzkin, 1991). Such meanings may obscure social problems and dilemmas and their causes, narrowing the range of possible remedies. This "medicalization" subsumes important social and ethical issues within clinical judgments that escape careful scrutiny. The differential diagnostic approach, which structures how doctors are educated and how they address problems, affects the ability of doctors and patients to explore comprehensively the sources of distress and disease as well as their implications for well-being (Waitzkin, 1983, 1991; Kleinman, 1986).

Social distribution of health, illness, and medical care

Although the concept of health is difficult to define, numerous studies demonstrate that longevity, absence of impairment, and less illness and disability are associated with favorable socioeconomic conditions (Mechanic, 1989b). Many of the health problems of the poor stem from unfavorable environmental conditions, poor nutrition, and lifestyles harmful to health. Because persons of lower socioeconomic circumstances are less likely to receive high-quality services—whether because of limited income, less readiness to seek necessary care, or inaccessibility of facilities—they are more likely to suffer from disabilities, higher mortality, and secondary conditions (Bunker et al., 1989). Secondary conditions, such as decubitus ulcers, cardiopulmonary problems, and psychological depression, are often causally related to an initial illness and occur because the primary condition is poorly managed (Institute of Medicine, 1991). Since 1965 social programs in the United States have given some attention to the equity in the provision of medical services, and the historic inverse relationship between socioeconomic status and use of physician services has been reversed. But socioeconomic differences continue to persist for many specialized services and for preventive care. Although mental disorders are very prevalent in the lowest socioeconomic groups (Robins and Regier, 1991), psychological and social services are particularly inadequate for the poor.

The poor suffer from other problems in the medical care sector. They are least likely to share assumptions and meanings with health practitioners, and thus most likely to suffer from misunderstandings and confusions resulting from such incompatibilities. They are likely to feel more embarrassed, anxious, and intimidated in dealing with medical personnel, and are less likely to receive care congruent with their values or life perspectives. They are frequently used as subjects for teaching and research, particularly in experiments that bring no particular benefits to the patient (Barber et al., 1973); and they are more likely to have difficulty granting informed consent, particularly where explanations are quick and perfunctory (Gray, 1975). The poor not only have more illness and problems and less access to medical care relative to need but also are treated with less consideration and respect than affluent patients.

Above and beyond socioeconomic status differences, race and ethnic differences account for variations in health. Although much of the excess in mortality and morbidity among blacks and Hispanics is attributable to socioeconomic disadvantage, other factors associated with race and ethnicity are pertinent, including differences in culture and health-relevant behavior, discrimination, and biological differences.

Still other aspects of social stratification, including age and gender, are important determinants of health status. Age and gender affect exposure to risk and disease occurrence through both biological and social pathways linked to these characteristics. The prevalence of chronic disease and disability increases with age but is influenced as well by the individual's social participation and social networks, sense of personal efficacy, and subjective well-being, which vary over the life cycle.

Large differences in health indicators and health behavior are also found between men and women. The fact that women live longer than men is in part biological, but it is also substantially affected by different styles of behavior and response among men and women. Most of the higher mortality in men can be attributed to behaviors such as substance abuse, poor nutrition, risk-taking, and violence. Many other social factors, such as marital status and household structure, are associated with patterns of health and disease (Mechanic, 1978).

Organization of medical care

If medicine has social and ethical as well as technical dimensions, how do we develop organizational settings that can apply the necessary technical expertise in ways that respond to the patients and their unique individual and social needs? Even the very best hospitals and medical organizations often treat patients without empathy or respect, and show limited interest in managing their medical problems in light of their family, work, and community circumstances (Duff and Hollingshead, 1968; Kleinman, 1988). The personnel who carry out these institutions' medical functions behave as they do, not because they are inhumane, but because the pressures and constraints of work, the priorities they have been taught, and the reward structures of which they are a part direct their attention to other goals and needs. Successful modification of service institutions requires significant revisions in the organizational arrangements and incentives that affect the work of personnel and the tasks they perform. In a materialistic culture where persons may respond to money and prestige incentives more readily than to more lofty motivations, the design of economic and prestige incentives and an awareness of how they affect decisions become important elements in shaping behavior.

Some attention has been devoted to how the economic structure of medicine affects the work of physicians and other personnel. Fee-for-service incentives often result in high levels of professional commitment, a willingness to work hard, and responsiveness to those who pay the fees. They also often encourage excessive use of medical, surgical, and pharmaceutical modalities to earn more income. Data from a variety of nations suggest that when attempts are made to manipulate the system by increasing payments associated with certain procedures, these incentives shape what physicians do (Glaser, 1970). The difficulty with any such piecework system is that it tends to discourage procedures that are important but for which only modest or no remuneration is provided. Since payment systems typically reward technical procedures, the most neglected aspects are those concerned with social care, listening to the client, patient education, and grappling with ethical issues. Physicians are best rewarded financially when they provide the largest number of discrete technical services.

One antidote to the perversities of piecework medicine is to pay by salary or capitation (a uniform payment for each person the physician cares for), but these approaches also have disadvantages. Under such systems physicians are more likely to limit their work efforts, appear less committed to their work, and seem less flexible and responsive to the individual needs and circumstances of their patients (Mechanic, 1989a). Thus, the same incentive conditions that make it possible for physicians to allocate their time within their own concepts of the value of varying types of caring and curing—conditions that may dampen a tendency to overutilize expensive and perhaps dangerous therapies—may also encourage withholding necessary services or result in an unwillingness to respond to important concerns of patients.

Doctors paid by capitation seem to adjust their efforts in relation to the payments they receive, a form of perceived distributive justice. This concept is shaped by knowledge of the circumstances of other doctors with comparable training in different work settings. Many of the difficulties in capitation payment result because patient load is heavy and payment is small for each patient. The heavy patient load and the doctor's limited work hours encourage a pattern of care that many patients find unresponsive. But time and patient demand are not the only factors involved in the way physicians deal with social and ethical problems in their practice. Physicians may have more or less tolerance for a wide scope of work; may be more or less willing, and feel more or less competent, to deal with family problems, alcoholism, sexual adjustment, or child-care problems. To the extent that physicians are properly trained to deal with the broader problems of medical care, and thus feel more competent in their clinical management, they may be more willing to deal openly with social and ethical challenges. Many physicians probably avoid dealing with psychosocial issues because they feel an effective therapy is lacking; however, they often readily accept the responsibilities to treat physical illnesses for which they also lack effective treatment. It may be that a sense of confidence and clinical experience are more important than the objective efficacy of the care.

In the creation of new medical settings, the problem is how to maximize the advantages of both fee-for-service and capitation medicine while compensating for their more undesirable aspects. People are ingenious in undermining and thwarting incentive systems that are not sensitive to their work problems, that increase their uncertainties, or that appear inequitable. To design an organizational system adequately requires intimate appreciation of how individuals actually manage their work, rather than utopian but unrealistic conceptions of how people should function.

Sociology of the health occupations

The attention in this article to doctors, in contrast with nurses, technicians, pharmacists, or social workers, is no accident. Although physicians constitute less than one-tenth of personnel in the health sector, they define and dominate the nature of decision making and the division of labor in medicine (Freidson, 1970; Starr, 1982; Mechanic, 1991). Physician dominance is in part a process in which doctors gain political legitimacy that protects them against economic competition from other health workers and helps preserve their professional autonomy. Increasingly, the physicians' dominance is being challenged by a variety of forces in the society: by administrators wishing to achieve economies of production through shifting traditional medical tasks to less trained personnel; by government wishing to control the growing costs of medical care; and by such professional groups as nurses who wish to improve their own political power,

income, and status. Thus, the health sector is characterized by increasing political acrimony and collective politics (Stevens, 1989).

Ethical dilemmas and the sociology of health care

The advances of medical knowledge and technology confront modern society with awesome social and ethical dilemmas. Among these questions is whether an ever-increasing proportion of our gross national product ought to be spent on expensive modalities that provide marginal gains in health and longevity. Are such investments not better made in preventive approaches and environmental amelioration or in other social goals?

Bioethics has been more an activity with a normative focus than a field of inquiry that seeks to investigate the implications of varying courses of action (Wikler, 1991; Fox, 1989). During the two decades in which bioethics has grown as a discipline, relatively few bioethicists have utilized sociological materials and methods, and relatively few sociologists have studied bioethics (Weisz, 1990). Ethical reflection in health care could be very much enhanced by a sociological perspective that examines the empirical setting and implications of a given ethical choice. Whether to accept organs from live donors or allow subjects to participate in experiments posing possible danger to themselves must depend at least to some extent on the actual psychological and social consequences of such participation. The fact that such volunteers often experience great satisfaction from their participation is no small part of such policy considerations (Fellner and Schwartz, 1971; Gray, 1975). Similarly, the willingness to expend great resources in heroic efforts to extend life, irrespective of function, must be weighed against the consequences of extended lives for such patients and their loved ones. Sociological perspectives and methodology can contribute to the ultimate ethical decisions by clarifying some of the human factors relevant to resolving the conflicts between competing social and ethical values.

David Mechanic

Directly related to this entry are the entries HEALTH AND DISEASE, *article on* SOCIOLOGICAL PERSPECTIVES; *and* PROFESSIONAL–PATIENT RELATIONSHIP, *article on* SOCIOLOGICAL PERSPECTIVES. *This entry will find application in the entries* AGING AND THE AGED, *article on* SOCIETAL AGING; ALLIED HEALTH PROFESSIONS; BODY, *article on* SOCIAL THEORIES; DISABILITY, *article on* ATTITUDES AND SOCIOLOGICAL PERSPECTIVES; FERTILITY CONTROL, *article on* SOCIAL ISSUES; GENE THERAPY, *article on* ETHICAL AND SOCIAL ISSUES; MEDICAL GENETICS, *article on* ETHICAL AND SOCIAL ISSUES; ORGAN AND TISSUE

TRANSPLANTS, *article on* SOCIOCULTURAL ASPECTS; *and* SEXUALITY IN SOCIETY. *For a discussion of related ideas, see the entries* CARE; JUSTICE; RACE AND RACISM; *and* VALUE AND VALUATION. *Other relevant material may be found under the entries* ECONOMIC CONCEPTS IN HEALTH CARE; *and* LIFESTYLES AND PUBLIC HEALTH.

Bibliography

BARBER, BERNARD; LALLY, JOHN J.; MAKARUSHKA, JULIA L.; and SULLIVAN, DANIEL. 1973. *Research on Human Subjects: Problems of Social Control in Medical Experimentation.* New York: Russell Sage Foundation.

BUNKER, JOHN P.; GOMBY, DEANNA S.; and KEHRER, BARBARA H., eds. 1989. *Pathways to Health: The Role of Social Factors.* Menlo Park, Calif.: Henry J. Kaiser Family Foundation.

DUFF, RAYMOND S., and HOLLINGSHEAD, AUGUST DE BELMONT. 1968. *Sickness and Society.* New York: Harper & Row.

FELLNER, CARL H., and SCHWARTZ, SHALOM H. 1971. "Altruism in Disrepute." *New England Journal of Medicine* 284, no. 11:582–585.

FOX, RENÉE C. 1989. *The Sociology of Medicine: A Participant Observer's View.* Englewood Cliffs, N.J.: Prentice-Hall.

FREEMAN, HOWARD E., and LEVINE, SOL, eds. 1989. *Handbook of Medical Sociology.* 4th ed. Englewood Cliffs, N.J.: Prentice-Hall.

FREIDSON, ELIOT. 1970. *Professional Dominance: The Social Structure of Medical Care.* New York: Atherton.

GLASER, WILLIAM A. 1970. *Paying the Doctor: Systems of Remuneration and Their Effects.* Baltimore: Johns Hopkins University Press.

GRAY, BRADFORD H. 1975. *Human Subjects in Medical Experimentation: A Sociological Study of the Conduct and Regulation of Clinical Research.* New York: Wiley.

INSTITUTE OF MEDICINE. COMMITTEE ON A NATIONAL AGENDA FOR THE PREVENTION OF DISABILITIES. 1991. *Disability in America: Toward a National Agenda for Prevention.* Washington, D.C.: National Academy Press.

KLEINMAN, ARTHUR. 1986. *Social Origins of Distress and Disease: Depression, Neurasthenia, and Pain in Modern China.* New Haven, Conn.: Yale University Press.

———. 1988. *The Illness Narratives: Suffering, Healing and the Human Condition.* New York: Basic Books.

MECHANIC, DAVID. 1978. *Medical Sociology.* 2d ed. New York: Free Press.

———. 1989a. *Painful Choices: Research and Essays on Health Care.* New Brunswick, N.J.: Transaction Publishers.

———. 1989b. "Socioeconomic Status and Health: An Examination of Underlying Processes." In *Pathways to Health,* pp. 9–26. Edited by John P. Bunker, Deanna S. Gomby, and Barbara H. Kehrer. Menlo Park, Calif.: Henry J. Kaiser Family Foundation.

———. 1991. "Sources of Countervailing Power in Medicine." *Journal of Health Politics, Policy and Law* 16, no. 3:485–498.

PARSONS, TALCOTT. 1951. *The Social System.* New York: Free Press.

ROBINS, LEE N., and REGIER, DAVID A., eds. 1991. *Psychiatric Disorders in America: The Epidemiologic Catchment Area Study.* New York: Free Press.

STARR, PAUL. 1982. *The Social Transformation of American Medicine.* New York: Basic Books.

STEVENS, ROSEMARY. 1989. *In Sickness and in Wealth: American Hospitals in the Twentieth Century.* New York: Basic Books.

WAITZKIN, HOWARD. 1983. *The Second Sickness: Contradictions of Capitalist Health Care.* New York: Free Press.

———. 1991. *The Politics of Medical Encounters: How Patients and Doctors Deal with Social Problems.* New Haven, Conn.: Yale University Press.

WEISZ, GEORGE, ed. 1990. *Social Science Perspectives on Medical Ethics.* Philadelphia: University of Pennsylvania Press.

WIKLER, DANIEL. 1991. "What Has Bioethics to Offer Health Policy?" *Milbank Quarterly* 69, no. 2:233–251.

MEDICINE AS A PROFESSION

The following entry combines and revises two articles on the medical profession from the first edition: "Medical Professionalism" by Martin S. Pernick and "Organized Medicine" by James G. Burrow.

Professionalism is what distinguishes the professions. It gives each the character by which it is known. In our time many occupational groups have striven for professional status in a quest for authority, prestige, and income. "Professionalism, professionalization, and the professions are increasingly central to any grasp of modern societies," Nathan Glazer claims, "yet persistently elude proper understanding" (Glazer, 1978, p. 34). Many sociologists have written about the characteristics of professions, but most agree that all professions possess the five elements identified by Ernest Greenwood: a systematic body of theory; authority to define problems and their treatment; community sanctions to admit and train its members; ethical codes that stress an ideal of service to others; and a culture that includes the institutions necessary to carry out all of its functions (Greenwood, 1957).

Jeffrey Berlant, following Max Weber's theory that professionalization is a form of monopolization, lists the steps in the process: creation of a commodity—in the case of medicine and law, services for a fee; separation of performance of the service from the satisfaction of the client, which means that a cure need not be guaranteed; creation of scarcity by reducing supply and increasing demand; monopolization of supply and control of privileges by legal means, such as licenses; restriction of group membership, such as admission to study or to hospital staff; elimination of internal competition; and development of group solidarity and cooperation (Berlant, 1975).

The attributes used to describe professions include responsibilities and privileges, both derived by social contract. It is important to remember that the terms of the social contract change with changing social and economic conditions, hence may vary from one region or historical period to another. Thus professionalism cannot provide a permanent set of values or standards. Instead it offers a series of changing guidelines designed to help specific people in specific places resolve important conflicts that arise from the nature of their duties. Each society has evolved its own standards, based on its own structure, values, and technological capabilities. Standards of professional behavior originating in modern industrial societies may be meaningless in other cultural settings (Hughes, 1965).

In medicine, historical changes can be illustrated with the example of specialization. Today, specialization is cited as a hallmark of professions. In nineteenth-century U.S. medicine, however, the doctor who specialized was often looked upon as a quack (Rosen, 1944; Stevens, 1971). Today the physician who claims to have knowledge and expertise in all of medicine would be looked upon with suspicion.

To pose the question "When did medicine become professional?" is like asking "When did medicine become modern?" There are elements of professionalism and of modernity in ancient Greek medicine, as there are in the medicine of the Middle Ages, the Renaissance, and the eighteenth century. The definitions of a profession that appeared in the literature in the early part of the twentieth century, which stressed urbanization and industrialization as prerequisites for the existence of a medical profession, are no longer held. Although it has been true that an industrializing society is a professionalizing society, so far as medicine is concerned there was professionalization long before industrialization (Goode, 1969).

Professionalism in medicine developed in a continuous historical process, beginning in antiquity with institutions like state physicians and fraternities of physicians such as the Asclepiads, continuing with the medieval medical guilds, medical schools, and licensing requirements. The modern period, especially after about 1700, is characterized by the emergence of such institutions as medical societies, medical literature, licensing laws, and codes of ethics. In the twentieth century the professional is the recognized expert with special qualifications, and the professional ideal has become a hallmark of modern society (Bledstein, 1976; Perkin, 1989).

The medical profession of the middle of the nineteenth century was very different from the profession of a century later. Yet in both periods many of the characteristics of professionalism were readily evident. The modern model of professionalism—university-based, peer-controlled, and based on merit rather than birth—is derived from the criteria we now use to study professions. Earlier forms of professionalism may have had quite a different set of characteristics; for this reason, the historical dimension of professions becomes increasingly central to an understanding of the development of medicine. The professional character of medicine has always been derived, in good part, from the institutional participation of the physician. These social and legal institutions provide credibility for medicine as a profession (Hall, 1984).

Despite the centrality of the professions in the United States, scholars have only recently begun to trace their history (Brown, 1992; Calhoun, 1965; Haber, 1991; Hatch, 1988; Kett, 1968; Kimball, 1992). With a few exceptions, such as Daniel H. Calhoun, historians have not deemed it necessary to engage in comparative histories of the professions, leaving this to sociologists (Abbott, 1988; Berlant, 1975; Freidson, 1970; Larson, 1977; Mechanic, 1968; Rothstein, 1972). Although Eliot Freidson has claimed that the status of scholarship in the professions is in a "state of intellectual shambles" (Freidson, 1984, p. 5), the historian Thomas Haskell has noted that "there is really no longer any excuse for scholars working on the professions to be divided into two shops, one made up of people who try to explain what professions are, without ever grasping how they came into being; the other composed of people who try to understand how they came into existence, without being quite sure what they are" (Haskell, 1984).

Andrew Abbott's review of the sociological literature of the professions is a concise summary of how modern societies have institutionalized expertise as professionalism. He describes the professionalizing process in terms of a series of jurisdictional disputes. These disputes over the professional boundaries of medicine in the nineteenth and twentieth centuries do explain much of medicine's history (Abbott, 1988).

During the last few decades of the twentieth century, when social historians began to depict medicine as oppressive and more interested in social control than in social melioration, medicine began to be subjected to much closer analysis of its professional attitudes, values, and styles. Medicine as a twentieth-century profession could not always get what it wanted, but until the mid-1960s and the passage of Medicare and Medicaid legislation, it had great success in resisting what it did not want. As the twentieth century draws to a close, this negative power has begun to diminish with increasing speed.

Medicine as a profession in antiquity

Much of what we have come to believe about ancient medicine we have inherited from the views of nineteenth-century scholars, who tended to create a picture of ancient medicine that reflected their own contemporary institutions (Nutton, 1992).

In early Greek antiquity, Homer portrayed doctors among the fighting heroes: "A doctor," he wrote, "is worth many men put together . . ." (Nutton, 1992, p. 15). Plato, in his *Laws*, described doctors and doctors' assistants, who were also called doctors: "These, whether they be free-born or slaves, acquire their art under the direction of their masters, by observation and practice and not by the study of nature—which is the way in which the free-born doctors have learned the art themselves and in which they instruct their own disciples" (Plato, 1926, pp. 307–309). The Hippocratic physician was a craftsman, and despite the high status of some of the crafts, there were in ancient Greece as yet none of the restrictive practices of the guilds of later centuries (Edelstein, 1943; Temkin, 1953). Only in one of the Hippocratic works, the *Oath,* was there a clear description of a closed, family-like guild that restricted entry to outsiders. But this does not represent Hippocratic medicine as a whole (Edelstein, 1943). Since ancient times it has been true that there have been several classes of doctors, and patients have always received care depending upon their own station in life and that of their doctor.

The Alexandrian Library was one of the earliest institutional influences on medicine. It was here, according to the second-century physician/scholar Galen, that the writings of Hippocrates and the Coan school in which he taught were first assembled (Nutton, 1992). The ancient Greek physician did not receive a scholarly or systematic training; such was left to those who became philosophers and rhetoricians. Galen claimed that the best physician is also a philosopher. This implied that medicine could be understood only in terms of natural philosophy—biology, chemistry, and physics. Such a lofty sentiment implied that medicine was for the benefit of the whole community rather than for the private gain of the physician. This was the ideal toward which medicine should strive, according to Galen. It is a professional ideal we still recognize (Horstmanshoff, 1990).

The medieval medical profession

In the later Middle Ages, with the development of cities, the rise of commerce, and the creation of universities, doctors found an expanding market for their services. These developments, in turn, led to the development of medical faculties in the universities, the passage of laws that defined the minimum education required for the physician, and a more rigorous definition of medical competence. Thus the trappings of professionalism and professional organizations became more evident after 1050. Debates began about what were the appropriate standards for a license to practice med-

icine, and who was to define the criteria and to enforce them. In the thirteenth century, the battle over training and licensing was between the new universities and their faculties of medicine, and the trade companies or guilds. University-educated physicians formed a professional elite. Guilds became the formal licensing bodies in some of the Italian cities, but generalization is difficult (Park, 1992).

In Florence, the medical profession can be traced to the medieval guilds, such as the Guild of Doctors, Apothecaries, and Grocers, established in 1293. It was a protective association and asserted monopoly privileges. Medicine was considered one of the prestigious occupations, along with law, banking, commerce, and notary practice. What really elevated some of the practitioners of medicine, and hence the whole profession, was that they taught and wrote. These activities, not just medical practice itself, elevated medicine from a mechanical to a liberal occupation and from an art to a science (Park, 1985). Medicine's place in the universities assured it an important and enduring role in the intellectual life of modern society.

Since the medieval period, universities have been the key to the professionalization of medicine, although in some countries, such as Great Britain and the United States, there were periods when medical schools were quite separate from the university. In antiquity the institutions that we associate with professionalization of medicine did not yet exist, though there were certainly groups of healers who were united by rudimentary professional bonds. In the Middle Ages, medicine became a more distinct, high-status, and terminal occupation (Bullough, 1966).

In the Middle Ages, then, medicine as a healing activity became distinguishable from medicine as a branch of higher learning. In the twelfth century, King Roger II of Sicily and his grandson, Frederick II, instituted licensing examinations by the masters of the School of Salerno. The objectives were to ensure competence and honesty to protect both society's and the profession's interests. There was as yet, however, neither uniform licensing nor a uniform medical profession in medieval and early Renaissance Europe (Siraisi, 1990).

Guild controls and restrictions were justified in the fifteenth century, as they would be in the twentieth, by members who claimed they needed to maintain high standards of competence and proper professional behavior. With an increasing service sector of the economy and an increase of prestige once it became a university faculty, medicine gained in stature (Cipolla, 1973).

The medical professions in early modern Europe

In late-fifteenth- and early-sixteenth-century England, there was little order in the practice or regulation of medicine. In 1511, Henry VIII introduced some governmental control. Although the parliamentary legislation he secured created no organized group of physicians, it brought a measure of state control over medical practice and made way for the conferral of substantial powers on medical groups. It stipulated that no one could practice physic or surgery in London or seven miles around without a license from the Bishop of London or the Dean of Saint Paul's Cathedral, and it required an examination of all candidates for licensure before a panel of experts selected by those officials.

The three main corporations or guilds of medical practitioners in early modern England were the Physicians, the Surgeons, and the Apothecaries. While they did represent a fairly distinct division of labor, their separation, particularly in the countryside, was not as rigid as often portrayed; in the early sixteenth century there was as yet little order and no real regulation of practitioners. Margaret Pelling has argued cogently for the importance of the guild tradition in the history of medicine's professionalization in sixteenth- and seventeenth-century Great Britain. Earlier historiography of medicine often depicted professionalization as a continuous process, ultimately ending in the triumphal terms of the profession as we know it today. The strength of recent social history of medicine is to reveal the many complexities of and byways to what was earlier assumed to be a much straighter path to modernity (Pelling, 1987; Pelling and Webster, 1979).

In 1518, the humanist-physician Thomas Linacre and five other physicians with university educations prevailed upon Henry VIII to grant them a charter for a Royal College of Physicians. Their resultant monopoly, however, extended only to London and its environs. The United Company of Barber Surgeons (made up of apprentice-trained barber-surgeons who carried out simple operations such as bleeding) received its charter in 1540, and the Guild of Apothecaries was granted a separation from the Company of Grocers (a rival guild) in 1617. Not until 1745 did George II grant the surgeons separate status from the barbers (Cook, 1981).

This tripartite division of British medicine is well known, but it should not be viewed as a simple or a unified system. In the rural areas, the surgeon-apothecary came to act as a general practitioner, and by 1809 was so acknowledged by name (Loudon, 1986). The physicians, who were at the top of the social scale of the medical practitioners, considered themselves gentlemen, had taken a classical university degree, received honoraria rather than fees, and made diagnoses, prescribed appropriate remedies, and made prognostic declarations for their patients. It was up to the apothecaries to give the remedies at the direction of the physicians. To the surgeons were left the tasks of bleeding, pulling teeth, setting fractures, and performing the few operations, such as amputations, that were carried out in this pre-anesthesia and pre-antiseptic age. For most of the population the medical tasks were often combined, as noted, or they were carried out by other healers such as midwives or a variety of traditional practitioners, some of whom were outright quacks (Christianson, 1987; Parry and Parry, 1976).

By the end of the seventeenth century, the apothecaries were intruding into the domain of the physicians so often that the College of Physicians brought suit against an apothecary by the name of James Rose, charging him with the practice of medicine for which he was not licensed. In 1703, hearing the case on appeal, the House of Lords ruled that the apothecaries could charge for medical advice as well as for the drugs supplied to the patient. This landmark case legalized the function of the apothecaries as ordinary practitioners of medicine in London. They were already enjoying these rights by custom in the countryside. Adam Smith, in his *The Wealth of Nations* (1776), recognized the apothecaries as the physicians of the poor (Hamilton, 1951; Holloway, 1966a, 1966b).

In France, a medical profession also existed prior to the period of industrialization. The profession that appeared abruptly at the time of the revolution in France at the end of the eighteenth century replaced one that had existed in somewhat different form (Gelfand, 1981, 1984; Ramsey, 1988). It was especially the professional character of the surgeons that changed abruptly in the 1790s. Earlier in the century, the surgeons already had a legal status, received their initial training as apprentices, and had a versatile medical practice including medicine and pharmacy as well as surgery, but still had a relatively equal social relationship with their patients. Thus the French surgeons—the ordinary practitioners, as Toby Gelfand described them—were more socially inclusive than would be the case in the twentieth century. With the breakdown of elitist distinctions, the postrevolutionary profession in which surgery and medicine were now united was generally even less elitist and exclusive than the earlier French physicians had been. However, in the course of the nineteenth century, elitism appeared in French medicine as it did in the professions in other countries. The new elitism was increasingly based on merit rather than on status, on accomplishment rather than on birth.

The medical professions in early U.S. history

American professionalism originated in the traditions and practices of seventeenth- and eighteenth-century England. Although any occupation might be termed "a profession," the recognized learned or liberal professions continued to be law, medicine, and divinity. These required a collegiate education; exposure to the classics and the liberal arts curriculum provided the breadth of mind and personal character necessary for a gentleman.

As a gentleman, the physician had a professional duty to play a role in all community affairs.

The North American colonies did not offer an attractive field for professional physicians until well into the eighteenth century. Unlike England, the North American colonies provided few examples of organizational development in medicine. The colonial environment required that practitioners assume all functions of the healing art and eliminated a form of rivalry that had brought about organization in England, where some medical groups had united to prevent the encroachments of others. Frontier conditions usually isolated physicians and discouraged organizational growth. The shortage of the ideal gentleman-physician in the colonies broke the traditional distinctions and divisions of medical labor. Thus, prior to the early 1700s, in the first century of colonial history, there were few doctors, no medical institutions, and little focus on medicine as a profession. Some healers were mainly working as midwives; others were ministers, whose professional identity was with religion, not medicine (Benes and Benes, 1992; Watson, 1991).

After 1700, as some historians have noted, there was a deterioration of the public's health as measured by a variety of vital statistics. This produced some increased demand for higher levels of medical skills. Besides the needs presented by the changing diseases and diminishing life expectancy, there were also great strains in the occupational structure. Fathers had typically passed to their sons their pulpits and their land. When population increased and there were neither enough pulpits nor sufficient land, the sons began to seek alternatives. Since many ministers also practiced medicine, it was natural that some of their sons turned to medicine as a career (Hall, 1984).

After 1750, some of the professional aspects of medicine became more visible, especially in the northern colonies. Young physicians with English and Scottish education and degrees now began to want the institutional trappings for their profession. With the aid of Benjamin Franklin, the Pennsylvania Hospital was founded in Philadelphia in 1751. Modeled on the British voluntary hospitals, it was intended mainly to care for the sick poor and to provide medical teaching for young men who wished to become doctors. In the 1760s, the first medical schools appeared in Philadelphia and New York. The first colonial medical society was founded in New Jersey in 1766, and an early licensing law passed in New York City in 1760. By the turn of the nineteenth century, a rudimentary medical profession existed, though it was responsive to local forces and conditions and had no national unity as yet. In many areas midwives continued to supply medical services to families and still routinely assisted at most births (Ulrich, 1990).

Although some medical leaders, such as John Morgan of Philadelphia, hoped to establish the British distinctions of physician, surgeon, and apothecary on the American side of the Atlantic, neither the social climate nor the political realities allowed it. As Richard H. Shryock has noted, it was not that the British distinctions were simply rejected in the more egalitarian ethos of the colonies. In fact, very few physicians had emigrated and there was no way to educate sufficient numbers in the colonies. The surgeon-apothecary or general physician simply assumed the title of doctor in the colonial setting. Like the merchants in North America, physicians, in the absence of a nobility, became part of the upper class (Shryock, 1960).

As licensing (and thus a rudimentary form of professional control) began to appear in the late eighteenth century, these laws were not yet a means to restrict the practice of medicine as distinctly as they would later. Licensing in the early nineteenth century merely gave those who were deemed legal physicians the right to sue for their fees. It did not as yet give the doctors any control over the medical marketplace. As a form of public recognition, licenses were uncontroversial; but as an attempt to be restrictive, they quickly became a source of sharply divided opinions. Some physicians, such as John Bard (1716–1799) and his son Samuel (1742–1821) in New York, favored restricting the practice of medicine. Others, such as Benjamin Rush (1745–1813) in Philadelphia, believed in "every man his own physician." Rush claimed medicine was sufficiently simple that anyone could learn to practice it.

Medical practice in the mid-nineteenth-century United States

During the mid-1800s in the United States, medicine was by no means a unitary profession. Its increasing professionalization was accomplished and stimulated by a similar process in science generally (Daniels, 1967). In both fields, compensation slowly increased. A wide variety of healers gave their allegiance to one or another medical philosophy, such as the Homeopaths and Eclectics, or followed the therapeutic doctrines of quite rigid systems, such as the Thomsonians or the water-cure doctors. Even among the so-called regular physicians, there was a wide diversity of education, medical belief, and medical practice (Kett, 1968; Rothstein, 1972).

In the three decades prior to the Civil War, the Jacksonian period, popular democracy had profound effects on the professions. Licensing laws for medicine were repealed by most states and localities, and what determination of professional competence there had been was transferred from the profession to the people. Contrary to the course of regulation in England, where the Apothecaries Act of 1815 and the Medical Registration Act of 1858 brought some order and governmental control to medicine, the North American states were abandoning regulatory efforts (Holloway, 1966a, 1966b; Shryock, 1967).

Between 1830 and 1850, the number of medical schools in the United States nearly doubled, from twenty-two to forty-two. The rising number of "regular" graduates produced by these largely profit-seeking, faculty-owned institutions competed with established practitioners, while the new schools lowered requirements to compete for students.

The physicians who established the American Medical Association (AMA) in 1847 had as their avowed goal the improvement of medical education (Davis, 1855). In drafting unrealistic requirements for admission to medical schools, however, they became vulnerable to charges that they sought merely to preserve the apprenticeship system and destroy most medical schools. By 1860, graduates of the many new medical schools founded in the nineteenth century outnumbered the so-called "irregular" doctors by a ratio of ten to one (Kett, 1968). Since the regular physicians as yet had no real claim to controlling medical activities, their professional strategy in these middle decades may be seen in the attempts to raise the standards of medical education by raising entrance and graduation requirements. Such strategy, while only partially successful before the ideology of science was added to the banner of reform at the end of the century, was aimed at reducing or at least controlling the number of doctors being produced.

The AMA, facing apathy among many regular physicians and hostility from sectarian groups, could do little to reduce physician supply or improve the quality of medical practice (Rothstein, 1972). Nor could the association move effectively to enforce its own version of professional ethics. It adopted substantially the principles of Thomas Percival's *Medical Ethics* (1803), which deals with topics such as the duties of physicians and surgeons and their "moral rules of conduct."

At the time of the Centennial celebrations in 1876, John Shaw Billings characterized three classes of physicians among the predominant or "regular" members of the medical profession. There were a few among them, he noted, who loved "science for its own sake, whose chief pleasure is in original investigations, and to whom the practice of their profession is mainly, or only, of interest as furnishing material for observation and comparisons. Such men are to be found for the most part only in large cities where libraries, hospitals, and laboratories are available for their needs. . . ." A much larger group of physicians, Billings claimed, was mainly interested in "money, or rather the social position, pleasures, and power, which money only can bestow." These doctors are well-educated because "it pays," according to Billings. But the great majority of physicians, Billings

concluded, were not well-educated, having memorized only enough of the medical textbooks as was needed to gain a diploma (Billings, 1876, p. 479).

It was difficult enough for male physicians to achieve professional status in the United States during the nineteenth century, but for women it was even harder. Elizabeth Blackwell (1821–1910), the first woman to receive a medical degree from a regular American school (1849), thereafter wrote frequently on the important role women could play in bringing to medicine greater professional status (Blackwell, 1895). The admission of women to medical schools varied from region to region, but with only occasional exceptions it was less than 10 percent of the total. Not until the late twentieth century did the proportion increase markedly, reaching 30 to 40 percent by 1990.

Like their male counterparts, women physicians also founded their own medical institutions, including hospitals, medical schools, and societies (Morantz-Sanchez, 1985). After 1876 there was token representation of women in the AMA; full membership was not granted until the early twentieth century. The American Medical Women's Association was founded in 1915, but by then most of the women's medical colleges had closed or merged with predominantly male schools. In 1910, at the time of Abraham Flexner's report on U.S. and Canadian schools of medicine, only three of the seventeen women's medical schools still existed, and only half of all the 155 North American schools admitted women for the study of medicine. While virtually all accepted women by the middle of the twentieth century, as late as 1959, twenty-eight schools still explicitly said they preferred men (Walsh, 1992).

Blacks who wished to study medicine had an even harder time. Todd Savitt has described ten black medical schools existing in 1900 (Savitt, 1992). A decade later only three survived. The AMA refused to accept black physicians for membership until the 1940s, so the National Medical Association, founded in 1895, served to promote the professional concerns of black physicians (Cobb, 1981; Morais, 1976).

Professionalization of medicine in the early twentieth century

Robert Wiebe and other historians have seen the increasing professionalization of medicine around the turn of the century as a key element in the emergence of a growing and more influential middle class in American society (Wiebe, 1967). The expanding middle class both increased the demand for professional services and also provided recruits for the professional ranks (Johnson, 1972). It also provided students for the growing universities and readily embraced science as the key to future progress of medicine. Science came to be the cornerstone of the reforms in medical education (Ludmerer, 1985; Rosenkrantz, 1985).

The reforms in medical education that occurred in the early years of the twentieth century were funded and spurred on by philanthropic foundations such as those established by Andrew Carnegie and the Rockefeller family, but also came from within the profession itself. In 1900, only 8,000 of the country's 120,000 physicians belonged to the AMA. With reorganization based on a federation of the state and local medical societies, membership grew to over 70,000 by 1910, about 60 percent of all physicians.

The "new medicine" of the 1890s included a physiology heavily influenced by chemistry and physics. This new physiology in turn stimulated departures in experimental pharmacology as well as scientific hygiene. More medical schools, following the lead of a few such as Harvard and the University of Pennsylvania, became integral parts of universities—not merely in name, but in financing, administration, and educational philosophy as well. Schools of medicine began to assume what they called a university point of view, according to which research was an opportunity and a "natural" activity for all instructors (Weed, 1931).

In contrast to the medical professionalism of the early nineteenth century, which Thomas Bender has called a "civic" professionalism, the professionalism associated with the new medicine was based firmly on disciplinary loyalties (Bender, 1979). The values of late-nineteenth- and early-twentieth-century medicine were drawn increasingly from science and, by the middle of the twentieth century, from the medical specialities and their societies and journals rather than from localities or universities.

Science and research provided the main rationale for a firmer link between medicine and the university. For the would-be reformers of early-twentieth-century medical education, such as Henry Pritchett of the Carnegie Foundation, William H. Welch of Johns Hopkins, and Abraham Flexner, the future of medicine depended upon such a relationship. Flexner's 1910 survey, sponsored by the Carnegie Foundation and assisted by the AMA's Council on Medical Education, included visits to all 155 North American schools of medicine and osteopathy. The resulting report, a classic of the muckraking tradition of the Progressive period, is a landmark in the history of medical education. Now best viewed as a catalyst for continuing change rather than as a source for new or revolutionary ideas, the Flexner Report was a clear statement of the importance of science for medicine (Hudson, 1992). For Flexner, the data derived from the patient in the clinic or at the bedside was as scientific as that discovered in the laboratory.

The sciences basic to medicine—chemistry, physics, and biology—provided the foundation students needed to study and to understand the preclinical sciences such as anatomy, physiology, and biochemistry. And from the advancing knowledge about health and disease derived from these preclinical sciences, the practice of medicine was to be placed on a firm scientific basis. Science—and therefore science-based medicine—was best taught and learned in the university setting.

In the decades after 1910, the Rockefeller philanthropies and other foundations provided millions of dollars to build up academic medicine in many universities. Teaching and research became full-time professional duties for an increasing number of faculty.

Flexner's report documented the inadequacies of many schools and accelerated the closing or merging of some of them. The number of schools fell from a high of 166 in 1904 to a low of 76 in 1929; it began only slowly to rise again in the following decades, reaching 127 in the early 1980s.

By the 1930s, with several newly discovered specific remedies available for diseases such as diabetes, pernicious anemia, and after 1937, for pneumonia, medicine was once again viewed by the public as a true profession, a special calling. But despite continuing discoveries of new therapies and spectacular new technologies for viewing the body and how it works, by the mid-1980s observers of the American medical scene were saying that "the profession is increasingly being seen as more nearly a commercial enterprise with vested economic interests than a calling of professionals whose foremost concern is the well-being of the patient" (Iglehart, 1986, p. 324). This profound shift in the public perception of medicine was accompanied by the increasing number of liability suits and the corporatization of medical care (Starr, 1982). The coming of the corporation doubtless has been both a positive as well as negative organizational force. A business view has become dominant in hospitals and medical schools, as well as in the private practice of medicine.

Medicine has never been a homogeneous profession. It is perhaps even more disparate at the end of the twentieth century than it has ever been. Until the 1960s, most doctors in the United States ran their practices like independent small businesses. In the corporate world of the late twentieth century, by contrast, bureaucracy has come to define medical practice better than autonomy. Legal challenges to the status of the profession have also questioned whether medicine and the law have acted to restrain trade, as in the *Goldfarb* decision of 1975 (*Goldfarb v. Virginia State Bar*, 1975; Rodwin, 1993; Sheehan, 1975). In that case a young lawyer brought suit against his own profession because he found that no lawyer would perform a title search for a house he was negotiating to buy for anything less than one percent of the purchase price. This commonly fixed price, he argued, violated the Sherman Antitrust Act.

The case became a landmark for application of the antitrust laws to all the professions.

Medical professionalism in the context of American culture has always been faced with two apparently conflicting ideals that have shaped its history. Professions, by their very nature exclusionary, have been forced to grow and to prosper in a society that has prized egalitarianism. Equal opportunity has been a basis for American society since colonial days, yet increasingly the medical profession has drawn its recruits from the more privileged strata of U.S. society.

Also, still characteristic of late-twentieth-century medical practice, the patient is often not in a position to judge the quality, the necessity, or the extent of the services provided by the physician. This has remained true despite much more consumer (patient) involvement in medical decision making since the 1960s. As is true for the notion of egalitarianism in society, this continuing separation of esoteric medical knowledge from that which is commonly held provides potential ethical dilemmas for doctors.

A continuing paradox has prevailed in medicine of the late twentieth century. The more effective medical services have become, the greater has been the demand for them. At the same time they have become increasingly expensive and so more difficult to obtain by many, and nearly inaccessible to those with no insurance coverage at all. Thus two conflicting concepts of medical care that have always existed in American medicine continue: medicine as a public service and as a private enterprise (Brieger, 1970).

"Organized medicine" in current usage usually refers to the dominant professional societies that have worked in both the professional and the political realms to help doctors achieve or preserve desired ends such as social status, economic rewards, or professional authority. Since one of the hallmarks of a profession is its organizations, the term "organized medicine" is redundant, albeit commonly used. We have come to assume considerable political power on the part of organizations such as the American Medical Association, the Association of American Medical Colleges, the American College of Physicians, and the American College of Surgeons. While their positive power may have waned somewhat in recent decades as consumer interests have become much stronger, medical organizations until the 1960s were very effective in preventing measures they did not believe were in their best interest from becoming public policy or law (Burrow, 1963, 1977).

GERT H. BRIEGER

For a further discussion of topics mentioned in this entry, see the entries ACADEMIC HEALTH CENTERS; ALLIED HEALTH PROFESSIONS; LICENSING, DISCIPLINE, AND REGULATION IN THE HEALTH PROFESSIONS; MEDICAL CODES AND OATHS; MEDICAL ETHICS, HISTORY OF, *sections on* EUROPE, *and* THE AMERICAS, *especially the articles on* COLONIAL NORTH AMERICA AND NINETEENTH-CENTURY UNITED STATES, *and* THE UNITED STATES IN THE TWENTIETH CENTURY; RACE AND RACISM; RESPONSIBILITY; SEXISM; SURGERY; *and* WOMEN, *especially the section on* WOMEN AS HEALTH PROFESSIONALS. *For a discussion of related ideas, see the entries* MEDICINE, ANTHROPOLOGY OF; MEDICINE, PHILOSOPHY OF; MEDICINE, SOCIOLOGY OF; NURSING AS A PROFESSION; PHARMACY; *and* PROFESSIONAL–PATIENT RELATIONSHIP. *See also the* APPENDIX (CODES, OATHS, AND DIRECTIVES RELATED TO BIOETHICS), SECTION II: ETHICAL DIRECTIVES FOR THE PRACTICE OF MEDICINE.

Bibliography

ABBOTT, ANDREW D. 1988. *The System of Professions: An Essay on the Division of Expert Labor.* Chicago: University of Chicago Press.

BENDER, THOMAS. 1979. "The Cultures of Intellectual Life: The City and the Professions." In *New Directions in American Intellectual History,* pp. 181–195. Edited by John Higham and Paul K. Conkin. Baltimore: Johns Hopkins University Press.

BENES, PETER, and BENES, JANE MONTAGUE, eds. 1992. *Medicine and Healing.* Boston: Boston University Press.

BERLANT, JEFFREY L. 1975. *Profession and Monopoly: A Study of Medicine in the United States and Great Britain.* Berkeley: University of California Press.

BILLINGS, JOHN SHAW. 1876. "A Century of American Medicine, 1776–1876, Literature and Institutions." *American Journal of Medical Sciences* 71:439–480.

BLACKWELL, ELIZABETH. 1895. *Pioneer Work in Opening the Medical Profession to Women: Autobiographical Sketches.* London: Longmans, Green.

BLEDSTEIN, BURTON J. 1976. *The Culture of Professionalism: The Middle Class and the Development of Higher Education in America.* New York: W. W. Norton.

BRIEGER, GERT H. 1970. "The Medical Profession: Problems of Our Image." *New Physician* 19, no. 10:845–847.

BROWN, JoANNE. 1992. *The Definition of a Profession: The Authority of Metaphor in the History of Intelligence Testing, 1890–1930.* Princeton, N.J.: Princeton University Press.

BULLOUGH, VERN L. 1966. *The Development of Medicine as Profession; or, The Contribution of the Medieval University to Modern Medicine.* New York: Hafner.

BURROW, JAMES G. 1963. *AMA: Voice of American Medicine.* Baltimore: Johns Hopkins University Press.

———. 1977. *Organized Medicine in the Progressive Era: The Move Toward Monopoly.* Baltimore: Johns Hopkins University Press.

CALHOUN, DANIEL H. 1965. *Professional Lives in America: Structure and Aspiration, 1750–1850.* Cambridge, Mass.: Harvard University Press.

CHRISTIANSON, ERIC H. 1987. "Medicine in New England." In *Medicine in the New World: New Spain, New France,* and *New England*, pp. 101–153. Edited by Ronald L. Numbers. Knoxville: University of Tennessee Press.

CIPOLLA, CARLO M. 1973. "The Professions: The Long View." *Journal of European Economic History* 2, no. 1:37–52.

COBB, W. MONTAGUE. 1981. "The Black American in Medicine." *Journal of the National Medical Association* 73 (suppl.):1185–1244.

COOK, HAROLD JOHN. 1986. *Decline of the Old Medical Regime in Stuart London.* Ithaca, N.Y.: Cornell University Press.

DANIELS, GEORGE H. 1967. "The Process of Professionalization in American Science: The Emergent Period, 1820–1860." *Isis* 58, no. 2:151–166.

DAVIS, NATHAN SMITH. 1855. *History of the American Medical Association from Its Organization up to January, 1855.* Edited by Samuel Worcester Butler. Philadelphia: Lippincott, Grambo.

EDELSTEIN, LUDWIG. 1943. "The Hippocratic Oath: Text, Translation and Interpretation." *Bulletin of the History of Medicine* (suppl.), no. 1:1–64.

FLEXNER, ABRAHAM. 1910. *Medical Education in the United States and Canada: A Report to the Carnegie Foundation for the Advancement of Teaching.* Birmingham, Ala.: Classics of Medicine Library.

FREIDSON, ELIOT. 1970. *Profession of Medicine: A Study of the Sociology of Applied Knowledge.* New York: Dodd, Mead.

———. 1984. "Are Professions Necessary?" In *The Authority of Experts: Studies in History and Theory*, pp. 3–27. Edited by Thomas L. Haskell. Bloomington: Indiana University Press.

———. 1986. *Professional Powers: A Study of the Institutionalization of Formal Knowledge.* Chicago: University of Chicago Press.

GELFAND, TOBY. 1981. "The Decline of the Ordinary Practitioner and the Rise of a Modern Medical Profession." In *Doctors, Patients, and Society: Power and Authority in Medical Care*, pp. 105–129. Edited by Martin S. Staum and Donald E. Larsen. Waterloo, Ont.: Wilfrid Laurier University Press.

———. 1984. "A 'Monarchical Profession' in the Old Regime: Surgeons, Ordinary Practitioners, and Medical Professionalization in Eighteenth-Century France." In *Professions and the French State, 1700–1900*, pp. 149–180. Edited by Gerald L. Geison. Philadelphia: University of Pennsylvania Press.

GLAZER, NATHAN. 1978. "The Attack on the Professions." *Commentary* 66, no. 5: 34–41.

Goldfarb v. Virginia State Bar. 1975. 421 U.S. 773.

GOODE, WILLIAM J. 1969. "The Theoretical Limits of Professionalization." In *The Semi-Professions and Their Organization: Teachers, Nurses, Social Workers*, pp. 266–313. Edited by Amitai Etzioni. New York: Free Press.

GREENWOOD, ERNEST. 1957. "Attributes of a Profession." *Social Work* 3, no. 2:45–55.

HABER, SAMUEL. 1991. *The Quest for Authority and Honor in the American Professions, 1750–1900.* Chicago: University of Chicago Press.

HALL, PETER DOBKIN. 1984. "The Social Foundations of Professional Credibility: Linking the Medical Profession to Higher Education in Connecticut and Massachusetts,

1700–1830." In *The Authority of Experts: Studies in History and Theory*, pp. 107–141. Edited by Thomas L. Haskell. Bloomington: Indiana University Press.

HAMILTON, BERNICE. 1951. "The Medical Professions in the Eighteenth Century." *Economic History Review* 4, no. 2:141–169.

HASKELL, THOMAS L., ed. 1984. *The Authority of Experts: Studies in History and Theory.* Bloomington: Indiana University Press.

HATCH, NATHAN O., ed. 1988. *The Professions in American History.* Notre Dame, Ind.: University of Notre Dame Press.

HOLLOWAY, S. W. F. 1966a. "The Apothecaries Act, 1815: A Reinterpretation. Part I: The Origins of the Act." *Medical History* 10, no. 2:107–129.

———. 1966b. "The Apothecaries Act, 1815: A Reinterpretation. Part II: The Consequences of the Act." *Medical History* 10, no. 3:221–236.

HORSTMANSHOFF, N. F. J. 1990. "The Ancient Physician: Craftsman or Scientist?" *Journal of the History of Medicine and Allied Sciences* 45, no. 2:176–197.

HUDSON, ROBERT P. 1992. "Abraham Flexner in Historical Perspective." In *Beyond Flexner: Medical Education in the Twentieth Century*, pp. 1–18. Edited by Barbara Barzansky and Norman Gevitz. New York: Greenwood Press.

HUGHES, EVERETT C. 1965. "Professions." In *The Professions in America*, pp. 1–14. Edited by Kenneth S. Lynn. Boston: Houghton Mifflin.

IGLEHART, JOHN K. 1986. "Federal Support of Health Manpower Education." *New England Journal of Medicine* 314, no. 5:324–328.

JOHNSON, TERENCE J. 1972. *Professions and Power.* London: Macmillan.

KETT, JOSEPH F. 1968. *The Formation of the American Medical Profession: The Role of Institutions, 1780–1860.* New Haven, Conn.: Yale University Press.

KIMBALL, BRUCE A. 1992. *The "True Professional Ideal" in America: A History.* Oxford: Basil Blackwell.

LARSON, MAGALI SARFATTI. 1977. *The Rise of Professionalism: A Sociological Analysis.* Berkeley: University of California Press.

LOUDON, IRVINE. 1986. *Medical Care and the General Practitioner, 1750–1850.* Oxford: At the Clarendon Press.

LUDMERER, KENNETH M. 1985. *Learning to Heal: The Development of American Medical Education.* New York: Basic Books.

MECHANIC, DAVID. 1968. *Medical Sociology: A Selective View.* New York: Free Press.

———. 1976. *The Growth of Bureaucratic Medicine: An Inquiry into the Dynamics of Patient Behavior and the Organization of Medical Care.* New York: Wiley.

MORAIS, HERBERT M. 1976. *The History of the Afro-American in Medicine.* Cornwells Heights, Pa.: Association for the Study of Afro-American Life and History.

MORANTZ-SANCHEZ, REGINA M. 1985. *Sympathy and Science: Women Physicians in American Medicine.* New York: Oxford University Press.

NUTTON, VIVIAN. 1992. "Healers in the Medical Market Place: Towards a Social History of Graeco-Roman Medicine." In *Medicine in Society: Historical Essays*, pp. 15–58. Edited by Andrew Wear. Cambridge: At the University Press.

PARK, KATHARINE. 1985. *Doctors and Medicine in Early Renaissance Florence*. Princeton, N.J.: Princeton University Press.

———. 1992. "Medicine and Society in Medieval Europe, 500–1500." In *Medicine in Society: Historical Essays*, pp. 59–90. Edited by Andrew Wear. Cambridge: At the University Press.

PARRY, NOEL, and PARRY, JOSÉ. 1976. *The Rise of the Medical Profession, A Study of Collective Social Mobility*. London: Croom Helm.

PELLING, MARGARET. 1987. "Medical Practice in Early Modern England: Trade or Profession?" In *The Professions in Early Modern England*, pp. 90–128. Edited by Wilfrid R. Prest. London: Croom Helm.

PELLING, MARGARET, and WEBSTER, CHARLES. 1979. "Medical Practitioners." In *Health, Medicine, and Mortality in the Sixteenth Century*, pp. 165–235. Edited by Charles Webster. Cambridge: At the University Press.

PERCIVAL, THOMAS. 1803. *Medical Ethics; or, A Code of Institutes, and Precepts, Adapted to the Professional Conduct of Physicians and Surgeons*. Manchester: S. Russell.

PERKIN, HAROLD J. 1989. *The Rise of Professional Society: England since 1880*. London: Routledge.

PERNICK, MARTIN S. 1985. *A Calculus of Suffering: Pain, Professionalism, and Anesthesia in Nineteenth-Century America*. New York: Columbia University Press.

PETERSON, M. JEANNE. 1978. *The Medical Profession in Mid-Victorian London*. Berkeley: University of California Press.

PLATO. 1926. *Laws*. Translated by Robert Gregg Bury. New York: G. P. Putnam's Sons.

RAMSEY, MATTHEW. 1988. *Professional and Popular Medicine in France, 1770–1830: The Social World of Medical Practice*. Cambridge: At the University Press.

RODWIN, MARC A. 1993. *Medicine, Money, and Morals: Physicians' Conflicts of Interest*. New York: Oxford University Press.

ROSEN, GEORGE. 1944. *The Specialization of Medicine with Particular Reference to Ophthalmology*. New York: Froben Press.

ROSENKRANTZ, BARBARA GUTMANN. 1985. "The Search for Professional Order in 19th-Century American Medicine." In *Sickness and Health in America: Readings in the History of Medicine and Public Health*, 2d ed., rev., pp. 219–232. Edited by Judith Walzer Leavitt and Ronald L. Numbers. Madison: University of Wisconsin Press.

ROTHSTEIN, WILLIAM G. 1972. *American Physicians in the Nineteenth Century: From Sects to Science*. Baltimore: Johns Hopkins University Press.

SAVITT, TODD. 1992. "Abraham Flexner and the Black Medical Schools." In *Beyond Flexner: Medical Education in the Twentieth Century*, pp. 65–81. Edited by Barbara Barzansky and Norman Gevitz. New York: Greenwood Press.

SHEEHAN, MARK T. 1975. "What the Goldfarb Decision Means to the Medical Profession." *Journal of Legal Medicine* 3, no. 10:21–25.

SHRYOCK, RICHARD HARRISON. 1960. *Medicine and Society in America: 1660–1860*. New York: New York University Press.

———. 1967. *Medical Licensing in America, 1650–1965*. Baltimore: Johns Hopkins University Press.

SIRAISI, NANCY G. 1990. *Medieval and Early Renaissance Medicine: An Introduction to Knowledge and Practice*. Chicago: University of Chicago Press.

STARR, PAUL. 1982. *The Social Transformation of American Medicine*. New York: Basic Books.

STEVENS, ROSEMARY. 1971. *American Medicine and the Public Interest*. New Haven, Conn.: Yale University Press.

TEMKIN, OWSEI. 1953. "Greek Medicine as Science and Craft." *Isis* 44:213–225.

ULRICH, LAUREL T. 1990. *A Midwife's Tale: The Life of Martha Ballard, Based on Her Diary, 1785–1812*. New York: Knopf.

WALSH, MARY ROTH. 1977. *Doctors Wanted, No Women Need Apply: Sexual Barriers in the Medical Profession, 1855–1975*. New Haven, Conn.: Yale University Press.

———. 1992. "Women in Medicine Since Flexner." In *Beyond Flexner: Medical Education in the Twentieth Century*, pp. 51–63. Edited by Barbara Barzansky and Norman Gevitz. New York: Greenwood Press.

WARNER, JOHN HARLEY. 1986. *The Therapeutic Perspective: Medical Practice, Knowledge, and Identity in America, 1820–1885*. Cambridge, Mass.: Harvard University Press.

WATSON, PATRICIA. 1991. *The Angelical Conjunction: The Preacher-Physician of Colonial New England*. Knoxville: University of Tennessee Press.

WEED, LEWIS H. 1931. "Experimentation in Medical Education." *Southern Medical Journal* 24, no. 12:1116–1121.

WIEBE, ROBERT H. 1967. *The Search for Order: 1877–1920*. New York: Hill and Wang.

MENTAL DISABILITY

See DISABILITY, *articles on* ATTITUDES AND SOCIOLOGICAL PERSPECTIVES, PHILOSOPHICAL AND THEOLOGICAL PERSPECTIVES, *and* LEGAL ISSUES; DISABILITY FOR PUBLIC OFFICE; *and* MENTALLY DISABLED AND MENTALLY ILL PERSONS.

MENTAL HEALTH

I. The Meaning of Mental Health
    Edwin R. Wallace IV
II. Mental Health and Religion
    David B. Larson
    Mary Greenwold
    Douglas Brown
    Glenn Wood

I. THE MEANING OF MENTAL HEALTH

Notions of "health" and "mental health" neither arose nor developed in a cultural and conceptual vacuum; their ancestral and contemporary kindred and relationships are multiple and far-reaching. Traces of their past live on in present quandaries and controversies. The interpretation and analysis that follow are historical and sociocultural, as well as philosophical and clinical.

Historical and philosophical background

Near Eastern and classical concepts.   Our story begins with the high civilizations of the ancient Near East. Initially, disturbances in customary and acceptable human functioning were experienced and interpreted in magico-religious and moral modes. Ancient Near Eastern personhood blended into a cosmos permeated by the divine and comprising countless interactions among fluid and loosely bounded beings and forces. Demarcations such as those between religion and medicine, psychic and somatic, material and immaterial, or spiritistic, natural, and supernatural would have been incomprehensible to early Egyptians and Mesopotamians. Even surgical and pharmaceutical interventions were accompanied by prayer, rituals, and magical formulas and paraphernalia.

Much the same can be said for the people of Mycenaean and Homeric Greece, whose worldviews and concepts of human beings were inseparable and thoroughly magical, animistic, and religio-moral. Cognition, affect, and motivation were experienced as divinely or demonically implanted, or else literally "inspired" from the ambient air. The earliest Homeric internalizations of motivation were localized to a semiautonomous region of the midriff or diaphragm called *phthumos*. As in Near Eastern antiquity, all sickness or disease, including madness, was magical (caused by spells or curses), demonic, or religious and moral (caused by divine possession, or divine punishment for ritualistic infractions, taboo-breaking, and sins of all sorts).

"Health" or "wellness" referred equally to states of the cosmos, society, or person. For example, the Egyptian goddess Maat personified a diffuse constellation of truth, balance, and right ordering or right acting, understood as antithetical to the primal chaos of the universe. Likewise, preclassical Greek ideas of health or wholeness were religio-moral, the corrections of imbalances. These metaphors and concepts of equilibrium, refined and codified by the classical Greeks, have remained central to modern Western medical and psychiatric norms or ideals of healthy functioning.

Classical Greece is commonly deemed the birthplace of both the psychological individual and secular medicine. Actually, however, medicine's vocational identity, cosmology, and philosophical anthropology were still imbued with religious aspects. The Greeks invoked deities such as Asklepios/Apollo; and nature itself (Physis), and humanity as part of it, remained divinized. Maladies, healing, and health were at once medical and sacred. The more medical facet of Hippocratic doctors' "health" and "disease" concepts concerned the bodily humors and their ratios to one another (balance versus excess or deficiency). Madness was explicated humorally as well, in a sort of proto-"physiological psychology" and psychopathology (Jackson, 1986); and the brain was considered the organ of mental activity.

By contrast, Plato and his philosophical successors disseminated a psyche–body dualism that influenced Western medicine for centuries. Plato characterized as "divine" physicians who were also philosophers, who thus knew soul as well as body. Nevertheless, he apparently thought such practitioners so rare that he roundly criticized doctors' practices of "dietetics"—which included what we would call counseling, lifestyle management, and prevention. In line with his dualism, Plato argued that philosophers were the rightful "physicians of the soul," thereby inaugurating a lengthy tradition of philosophical therapy. Such philosophers progressively adopted medical models and metaphors for the psyche in states of wellness and disease (*pathé*). In the first and second centuries C.E., Epictetus termed the philosopher's lecture room a "hospital"; he likened the pain necessary in spiritual and moral healing to that in medical measures such as the lancing of an abscess (see Edelstein, 1967). Centuries later, Sigmund Freud characterized analysis with surgical metaphors, and Henri Ellenberger (1970) thought psychoanalysis itself a latter-day version of philosophical healing.

The Hellenistic and Roman Stoics and Epicureans were other famous proponents of psychotherapeutic philosophy. Like all philosophical physicians, they were infatuated with metaphors of balance. The soul's health was equated with states such as *ataraxia* or *apatheia* (equilibrium, tranquility, serenity). The Stoic idealization of reason, and concomitant depreciation of passion, probably influenced subsequent rationalistic criteria for mind in health and illness. In any event, Plato and company, with their dualism and healing ambitions, paved the way for current concepts of mental health and psychotherapy. Nonetheless, their images of such health were spiritual/ethical, and their healing was dialectical and pedagogical—and, hence, a far cry from our ostensibly metaphysically and morally neutral mental health and psychotherapy; though Freud himself emphasized the educational and ethical aspects of analysis far more than any presumable medical ones (Wallace, 1986).

Aristotle, Plato's greatest pupil, avoided a frankly dualistic mind–body position and touted the philosopher's role as ethical teacher. The doctrine of the "golden mean" and prudential and moral virtues, or "character ethics," held the place in Aristotle's philosophy that had been occupied by psychical or spiritual health in Plato's. This "golden mean," yet another manifestation of balance, was the cardinal feature of the virtues—for example, courage as the midpoint between temerity and timidity. In light of the individualistic thrust of ancient philosophical therapies such as Stoicism and Epicureanism, and of many present-day psychotherapies and notions of mental health, it is noteworthy that Aristotle considered his *Ethics* and *Politics* integral to each other. Citizenship, reflecting the individual's self-acknowledged embeddedness in a community, was central to Aristotle's idea of proper human functioning. Whereas we might accuse Aristotle of collapsing mental health into social ethics, he might have charged us with the reverse.

Medieval and Renaissance concepts.   In the Christian West, institutionalized medicine was in priestly hands. The closest thing to medical schools were monastic, and most medieval infirmaries were operated by the Church. Medical theory and therapy followed the Hellenistic Galen's final codification of humoralism and anatomy. Madness was explained and treated somatically, as well as with the prayers and healing rites offered for any severe medical condition.

Somatic perspectives on madness meshed nicely with the Church's Platonic dualism, since the immortal and immaterial soul, unlike the body and brain, was not corruptible by disease. Meanwhile, the Church continued to use medical metaphors for many spiritual and moral problems. It is hard to know whether some of these approximated our nonpsychotic and less severe categories of mental illness—such as "dysthymia," or the "personality disorders"; aspects of the latter clearly falling under the traditionally moral purview. Medieval clerics themselves meditated over gray zones, such as whether *acedia,* a common monk's affliction, was sin (slothfulness) or disease (a mild form of melancholia) (Jackson, 1986). There was nothing corresponding to contemporary concepts of mental health. Norms and ideals were spiritual and moral, biblically and theologically derived.

Thomas Aquinas added loss of free will to irrational thinking and behavior as another cardinal sign of madness. This has influenced juridical processes up to the present, posing problems to psychiatrists espousing determinism (i.e., that all human mentation and behavior are causally necessitated). It has also borne on contemporary conceptions of mental health, some presupposing a capacity for nonnecessitated choosing (e.g., humanistic and existentialist) and others (e.g., classical psychoanalytic and neuromolecular) usually not. The

ramifications for morality and ethics are obvious (Wallace, 1986).

As the great universities arose between the twelfth and the fourteenth centuries, they incorporated monastic medicine. Nonpriestly physicians returned to the scene, but medical theory and the treatment of madness remained much the same. There was no real secularization in Europe until the Renaissance, with its novel and heightened forms of individualism among certain educationally and financially favored segments of Europe's populations and its protopsychological concept *imaginatio,* a catchall for feeling, imagination, and fantasy (the very items ignored by hitherto hyperrationalistic norms of personhood).

This same period, however, witnessed the Inquisition, and its mass persecution of heretics and alleged witches. Medical men such as Johannes Weyer, with special interests in madness, argued that accused and "confessed" witches were actually insane, one of the few conditions that legally exonerated them. Still, Weyer's diagnoses were not purely medical, for he thought the witches' delusions had been implanted by Satan. Many modern historians of psychiatry have lauded Weyer for his insight and courage (e.g., Zilboorg, 1935). Some psychiatrists and psychoanalysts, including Freud, followed Weyer's example and facilely diagnosed whole institutions and cultures as psychopathological. Several decades of careful scholarship suggest that most "witches" were not in fact psychotic (e.g., Spanos, 1985). Furthermore, concepts of normality and pathology are complex, and they vary greatly from one culture or historical period to another. Moreover, transferring concepts of mental health and illness from the individual domain to the arenas of groups, cultures, and even families is questionable at best (Ackerknecht, 1971; Wallace, 1983).

Seventeenth- and eighteenth-century concepts. The seventeenth century was characterized by the continuing expansion of individualism and by a rationalism that paid less attention to aspects of personality, such as *imaginatio,* explored by the Renaissance. Irrationality became the key criterion for madness, giving the social philosopher Michel Foucault (1965) the ostensible grounds for his thesis that seventeenth-century asylums were filled with persons who had violated their era's canons of reason and socially acceptable behavior. Foucault alerted us to possible linkages between sociocultural and political-economic special interests, and psychiatric institutions, concepts, and practices—including formulations of mental health and illness.

The epoch from 1600 to 1750, then, was a watershed in many ways. Its scientific paradigms, ultrarationalism, and sociocultural-economic developments paved the way for the West's ensuing secularism and capitalism. The coming age would require and give rise to different forms of humanity, with novel notions and modes of well-being, dysfunction, and distress. Not coincidentally, it would also spawn a new medical specialty: psychiatry.

Contemporary concepts and issues

The mid-eighteenth century constitutes the headwaters of the stream that culminates in the modern or postmodern mental-health complex. The rise of economic capitalism, with its emphasis on free-market competition and individual acquisitiveness, went hand in hand with the progressive breakdown of traditional social-political structures and cultural institutions, along with the Christian worldview that had hitherto sustained them. New modes of personhood appeared, modes that were exquisitely self-aware and self-oriented, shunning binding institutional and interpersonal commitments, and shrewdly combining hedonism with "social adjustment."

The Enlightenment witnessed novel varieties of what we would designate as "functional" (versus "organic") psychiatric disorders: the "vapors," "nerves," and so forth, resembling "conversion," "dissociative," "anxiety," "dysthymic," "personality-disordered," and "neurotic" categories (American Psychiatric Association, 1987). Initially comprehended and treated somatically with "magnetism," or hypnosis, they were gradually conceptualized psychologically. Feminist historians (e.g., Decker, 1991) interpret these experiential and behavioral configurations as disguised forms of women's rebellion against male-dominated society.

Meanwhile, in early and mid-eighteenth-century Great Britain, a new breed of physicians began devoting their practices to madness. The most brilliant of these "mad-doctors," Alexander Crichton, influenced Philippe Pinel, generally called psychiatry's father. Previously an internist, Pinel flourished in post-Revolutionary and early nineteenth-century France. Until then, madness had not been institutionally medicalized. Asylums typically fell under lay management, with doctors no more than general medical consultants. Pinel's orientation was psychological as well as medical, and he came to favor abbreviated systems of diagnostic classification. However, his successors in the powerful French clinical school, presuming the inevitable degeneration of many conditions, became progressively and pessimistically "organic." Notions approximating mental health were far from their minds.

Contemporary German psychiatry was pursuing a semimystical and Romantic psychological path (Ellenberger, 1970). Abstruse and difficult to summarize, it conceptualized nature and humankind as manifestations of a World Spirit or Soul. Although often obscure and moralistic, it contributed some genuine psychological insights, including many on unconscious mentation and motivation. In England and the United States, despite some admixture of somatic theory and practice, early nineteenth-century psychiatry—or "alienism," as it was called (thus underscoring its subjects' social estrangement)—was predominantly psychologically and sociotherapeutically oriented. The Anglo-American "moral treatment" movement envisioned the then relatively small country asylum as a healing family, with the medical superintendent its "father." For much of the nineteenth century, the word "moral" still denoted an amalgam of what was later divided into "mental" or "psychological," and "moral" or "ethical."

As the twentieth century approached, the number and size of asylums grew geometrically; treatment became custodial, and Anglo-American and European psychiatry grew increasingly neuropathologically inclined. Its interest in diagnostic classification and the results of autopsies contributed to what Foucault (1973) called the "objectification" of the patient. The rise of organic and custodial psychiatry reflected many social and demographic changes in the United States: rapidly increasing population; greater social and geographic mobility; replacement of small and culturally homogeneous communities by urban centers swelled by immigration; the continuing disempowerment of institutional religion; movement toward monopolistic capitalism, an orientation toward productivity and consumerism; individualism and waning local charity; and generally changing social mores. Together, such factors made moral therapy unworkable and led to further transformations in popular conceptions of personhood in wellness and illness. Communities and even families transferred responsibilities for their psychiatrically disturbed members to the large central facilities.

It is likely that such facilities came to house many who were merely elderly, socially deviant but not criminal, and economically unproductive. Certain contemporaneous "diagnoses"—such as "volitional old maid," "vagabond," and "eccentric character"—would be laughable if they had not also been socially coercive. State hospitals usually fell under the autonomy of those social agencies that dealt with the socially and economically marginal and dependent (see Grob, 1973, 1983). Drawing on such historical sources, as well as on present-day events, a school of social scientists and political philosophers underlines the status quo–supporting and professionally self-serving features of psychiatry and its related disciplines, including their diagnostic schemata and notions of health and illness (e.g., Foucault, 1965, 1973; Ingleby, 1980; Horwitz, 1982). These include gender, socioeconomic class, and ethnic biases (e.g., Chesler, 1973; Russell, 1994).

The organic orientation of the second half of the nineteenth century promoted a seemingly paradoxical soul–body or mind–body dualism among Anglo-American psychiatrists. In their view, psychiatric disturbance or disease was wholly a function of body and brain; the soul or mind, being immaterial and immortal, was not susceptible to disease. Such a schema, which obviously protected their theological tenets, virtually ruled out ideas of mental health and illness, and practices such as secular psychotherapy. Nevertheless, psychotherapeutic perspectives began forming in the late nineteenth century. They emerged among outpatient neurologists who were encountering increasing percentages of functionally disordered patients, and among psychologically minded psychiatrists, who were treating ambulatory patients with milder problems. The distress and dysfunction these professionals were treating became less commonly experienced and interpreted in religious and moral terms. Such problems were therefore less amenable to healing through confession, penance, and recommitment to the Catholic ideology, institutions, and community, or to their Protestant counterparts, often including more counseling ("the cure of souls").

Twentieth century

To serve these new varieties of troubled persons, innovative therapies arose in the latter nineteenth century and the first decade of the twentieth. These "mind-cure" or "healthy-mindedness" approaches, as William James (1902) named them, comprised purely secular healings; heterodox religious approaches such as Seventh-Day Adventism and Christian Science; Americanized variations of Eastern religions and philosophies; and various integrations of religious, medical, and psychiatric proposals. In Europe, psychoanalysis emerged, the prototype of twentieth-century secular therapies and the ultimate progenitor of most current psychological theories and treatments. Psychoanalysis and its offshoot dynamic schools would contribute significantly to the clinical and popular dissemination of concepts of mental health and mental illness.

By 1910, events were gathering momentum. The important Mental Hygiene Movement, a joint lay–psychiatric venture, had been formed in Boston in 1909 (by former mental patient Clifford Beers and Harvard psychiatrist E. E. Southard). Though it had been started to improve the plight of the severely mentally ill (formerly the "mad"), its concerns shifted swiftly toward mild-to-moderate psychiatric problems and to community mental hygiene, which led eventually to the burgeoning community mental-health movement of the 1950s, 1960s, and 1970s. This movement, like the dynamic therapies, fueled public preoccupation with mental health (Grob, 1983).

During these same decades, psychiatrists in the United States had begun moving toward acute-treatment psychiatric facilities and wards in general hospitals, the "psychopathic" units that treated less chronically severe patients—those with acute crises, neurotic symptoms, and personality problems of all sorts. Outpatient work continued to grow as well. Clinical psychology and social work started evolving as professions. General medicine's public-health and preventive wings, joined by lay "wellness" proponents, enlarged their territory, too. These developments have led many critics, such as Ivan Illich (1976), to speak of medical and psychiatric "imperialism," the "medicalization" of society, and so forth. Indeed, as early as 1856, physicians such as Oliver Wendell Holmes contended that doctors and deterministic medicine should replace priests and religion as society's moral arbiters. The eminent medical historian Owsei Temkin (1977) charges that health has become a "summum bonum," whose values encroach on morality and ethics (e.g., the virtual criminalization of smokers). Don Browning (1987) points out the various ethical, social-valuational, and cosmological dimensions of the major psychotherapeutic approaches. Many have commented on the normative-prescriptive aspects of the mental-health and mental-illness concepts of the multifarious psychiatric and clinical psychological vantages.

Definitions of "health" as broad as the World Health Organization's (1991) "state of complete physical, mental, and social well-being," certain epidemiologic projects (Srole et al., 1962), and categorizations of "mental disorder" as extensive as those of the American Psychiatric Association (1987, 1994), seem to ground the accusations of Illich and others. Aspects of hitherto "normal" aging are deemed "disease" and treated as such, and similar attitudes toward features of other developmental periods could be cited. Indeed, pathology has narrowed the domain of human physiology to the point that doctors and the public alike view death itself as all but a potentially preventable disease.

In any event, though most philosophers of general medicine (e.g., Pellegrino and Thomasma, 1981; Kass, 1988) declare promoting "health" to be the physician's primary objective, few medical authors conceptualize and elaborate it very explicitly. More often it is a negative notion—the *absence* of significant disease or illness. Although conceptions of mental health in psychiatric and related practitioners' textbooks and treatises are frequently negative as well, the writers of such books are more likely to attempt "positive" conceptions than are their general medical counterparts. Daniel Offer and Melvin Sabshin (1966, 1984, 1991) list dozens of notions or definitions of mental health by theorists and therapists of many persuasions. These range from simplistic extremes such as "social adjustment" or "self-actualization," to more complex and reflective notions. Some assess mental health, like mental illness, by dimensions and degrees; others proffer categorical constructs of both. There are naturalistic-universal, psychological, sociocultural-contextual, and biopsychosocial ones. In short, the ways of classifying conceptions and criteria of mental health are potentially exhausting. Through surveying an immense range of pertinent sources, Marie Jahoda (1959, 1977) identified the six indexes of mental health that appear most frequently: (1) the individual's attitudes toward himself or herself; (2) the person's "style and degree of growth, development, or self-actualization"; (3) a central synthesizing psychological function, or "integration"; (4) "autonomy," or "independence from social influences" (the single most cited index); (5) adequacy of reality perception; and (6) mastery of the environment.

However useful they may be, these criteria can hardly claim to be purely natural or scientifically derived; they are clearly a function of time- and place-bound cultural contexts, as well as of presupposition-laden psychological orientations. It is not so much a question of whether they imply values, for no theories and concepts escape their authors' values altogether. Rather, the questions concern the kinds of values, and their relationships to one another and to those in other endeavors and institutions.

Of Jahoda's indexes, most are self-oriented, depicting the natural and social environment as something virtually inimical to personal well-being. The "healthy" are independent of its influences, mastering it to their self-actualizing ends—which, ironically, may be quite serviceable to those of the prevailing political economy. Of course, there are also formulations of "mental health" at the opposite, or socially conformist, pole; their professional exponents probably have frequently fallen into the service of dominant socioeconomic agendas. In any case, Jahoda's analysis suggests that there are other sorts of dangers associated with ideas of mental health. Such common extremes in positive conceptions of mental health make one wonder whether they should be attempted at all. The American Psychiatric Association (1987) avoids defining mental health.

Many of the profoundest students of human experience and behavior, such as Freud, have not issued definitive pronouncements on mental health. Freud's theories and observations contain many items relevant to assessing dimensions and degrees of psychic well-being and its reverse (Wallace, 1986; Vergote, 1988; Wallwork, 1991). Nevertheless, apart from hearsay attributions to him of the spare desideratum *Lieben und Arbeiten* (loving and working), Freud bequeathed us no extensive positive constructions of mental health. In fact, he stressed the continuum from neurosis to "normality." Nor did he harbor utopian ambitions for psychoanalytic therapy, firmly denying that it promised happiness or contentment. It was quite enough if treat-

ment alleviated the analysand's more troublesome, historically determined psychic and interpersonal conflicts, misapprehensions of self and others, and modes of gratifying and inhibiting hitherto repressed or symptomatically expressed desires and strivings. Such imperfect but significant transformations enhance the patient's grasp of his or her particular life's realistic problems and possibilities. Freud had no notions akin to Abraham Maslow's and Carl Rogers's of the easy and automatic harmonization between "self-actualization" and the requirements for a humane and civilized society. His concept of adaptation, hardly collapsible into Darwin's, implied neither mastery of nor submission to the sociocultural and political-economic surround, but rather a prudent and moral interweaving of "autoplastic" (self-transformative) and "alloplastic" (environmentally altering) activities (see Hartmann, 1960; Wallace, 1986; Vergote, 1988; Wallwork, 1991).

Although Freud was capable of psychoanalytically masked moral and metaphysical judgments, such as those about religion, he was usually quite sensitive to the interface between moral/ethical perspectives and theoretical/clinical ones. Psychoanalytic insights and findings might inform the ethical enterprise, but Freud did not think moral values themselves could be deduced from analytic premises. Regarding moral values in the psychoanalytic endeavor itself, he emphasized honest self-awareness and its potentially beneficent personal and interpersonal effects (Wallace, 1986; Rieff, 1959). Freud intended the clinician's analytic neutrality, with its customary suspension of explicit moral evaluation, purely as a means to enhance the patient's disclosure and self-discovery; it was confined to the consulting room and not suggested as a recipe for living.

Conclusion

Given the historical and cross-cultural variations in modes of conceptualizing personhood and ascribing abnormality, as well as the vicissitudes of sociocultural and natural environments, it makes little sense to seek timeless and placeless notions of health, illness, or even disease, psychiatric or otherwise. The extraordinarily complicated overlap and mutual determination among formulations and applications of mental health, and a host of external institutions, ensure that the former will reflect and affect myriad sociocultural dimensions and processes. Insofar as ethical and metaphysical purviews are separable from scientific and medical/psychiatric theories and findings, one cannot facilely deduce moral values and ethical systems from the latter.

A biopsychosocially oriented functionalism proffers the least metaphysical and reductionistic, and the most comprehensive and open, model of the human organism in its ongoing cultural and natural milieu. This conceives of self-conscious and symbolizing personhood as the complexly integrated function of a plethora of subsidiary structures and functions, interacting both among themselves and with aspects of the physical and sociocultural ambience. It avoids either a dualistic or a mechanistic stance on humankind; it affirms the necessity of psychosocial, as well as biomedical and neurobiological, approaches to persons in health and illness (Wallace, 1990). Moreover, it permits medicine, psychiatry, and the mental-health disciplines a public philosophy open to dialogue with vantages from ethics, theology, jurisprudence, politics, and elsewhere (Wallace, 1992). In other words, a *Homo sapiens* does not comprise separate ontological compartments of spirit, morals, mind, and body. Rather, he or she is appreciated as a self-consciously reflective whole, with a history in a community, whose various experiences and activities require separate, but overlapping and interrelating, spiritual, moral, medical/psychiatric, and social perspectives. However one understands mental health and mental illness, they point toward forms of distress, disability, and well-being that are real and pervasively human concerns.

EDWIN R. WALLACE IV

Directly related to this article is the companion article in this entry: MENTAL HEALTH AND RELIGION. *For a further discussion of topics mentioned in this article, see the entries* ALTERNATIVE THERAPIES; HEALTH AND DISEASE; HOSPITAL; MENTAL ILLNESS; *and* PSYCHOANALYSIS AND DYNAMIC THERAPIES. *For a discussion of related ideas, see the entries* COMPETENCE; *and* VALUE AND VALUATION. *Other relevant material may be found under the entries* BEHAVIOR MODIFICATION THERAPIES; CHILDREN, *article on* MENTAL-HEALTH ISSUES; COMMITMENT TO MENTAL INSTITUTIONS; DISABILITY; ELECTROCONVULSIVE THERAPY; INFORMED CONSENT, *article on* ISSUES OF CONSENT IN MENTAL-HEALTH CARE; INSTITUTIONALIZATION AND DEINSTITUTIONALIZATION; MENTAL-HEALTH SERVICES; MENTAL-HEALTH THERAPIES; MENTALLY DISABLED AND MENTALLY ILL PERSONS; PATIENTS' RIGHTS, *especially the article on* MENTAL PATIENTS' RIGHTS; PSYCHOPHARMACOLOGY; SEX THERAPY AND SEX RESEARCH; SUBSTANCE ABUSE; SUICIDE; *and* WOMEN, *article on* HEALTH-CARE ISSUES.

Bibliography

ACKERKNECHT, ERWIN. 1968. *A Short History of Psychiatry.* 2d ed., rev. Translated by Sula Wolff. New York: Hafner.

———. 1971. *Medicine and Ethnology: Selected Essays.* Baltimore: Johns Hopkins University Press.

AMERICAN PSYCHIATRIC ASSOCIATION. 1987. *Diagnostic and Statistical Manual of Mental Disorders: DSM-III-R.* 3d ed., rev. Washington, D.C.: Author.

———. 1994. *Diagnostic and Statistical Manual of Mental Disorders.* 4th ed. Washington, D.C.: Author.

BERRIOS, GERMAN E. 1987. "Dementia During the Seventeenth and Eighteenth Centuries: A Conceptual History." *Psychological Medicine* 17, no. 4:829–837.

BROWNING, DON S. 1987. *Religious Thought and the Modern Psychologies: A Critical Conversation in the Theology of Culture.* Philadelphia: Fortress.

CHESLER, PHYLLIS. 1973. *Women and Madness.* New York: Avon.

DECKER, HANNAH S. 1991. *Freud, Dora, and Vienna 1900.* New York: Basic Books.

EDELSTEIN, LUDWIG. 1967. *Ancient Medicine: Selected Poems of Ludwig Edelstein.* Edited by Owsei Temkin and Clarice L. S. Temkin. Baltimore: Johns Hopkins University Press.

ELLENBERGER, HENRI F. 1970. *The Discovery of the Unconscious: The History and Evolution of Dynamic Psychiatry.* New York: Basic Books.

FOUCAULT, MICHEL. 1965. *Madness and Civilization: A History of Insanity in the Age of Reason.* Translated by Ronald Howard. New York: Vintage.

———. 1973. *The Birth of the Clinic: An Archaeology of Medical Perception.* Translated by Alan M. Sheridan Smith. New York: Pantheon.

GROB, GERALD N. 1973. *Mental Institutions in America: Social Policy to 1875.* New York: Free Press.

———. 1983. *Mental Illness and American Society, 1875–1940.* Princeton, N.J.: Princeton University Press.

HARTMANN, HEINZ. 1960. *Psychoanalysis and Moral Values.* New York: International Universities Press.

HORWITZ, ALLAN V. 1982. *The Social Control of Mental Illness.* New York: Academic Press.

ILLICH, IVAN. 1976. *Medical Nemesis: The Expropriation of Health.* New York: Pantheon.

INGLEBY, DAVID, ed. 1980. *Critical Psychiatry: The Politics of Mental Health.* New York: Random House.

JACKSON, STANLEY W. 1986. *Melancholia and Depression: From Hippocratic Times to Modern Times.* New Haven, Conn.: Yale University Press.

JAHODA, MARIE. 1959. *Current Concepts of Positive Mental Health.* New York: Basic Books.

———. 1977. *Freud and the Dilemmas of Psychology.* New York: Basic Books.

JAMES, WILLIAM. 1902. *The Varieties of Religious Experience: A Study in Human Nature.* New York: Longmans Green.

KASS, LEON R. 1988. *Toward a More Natural Science: Biology and Human Affairs.* New York: Free Press.

OFFER, DANIEL, and SABSHIN, MELVIN. 1966. *Normality: Theoretical and Clinical Concepts of Mental Health.* New York: Basic Books.

———, eds. 1984. *Normality and the Life Cycle.* New York: Basic Books.

———, eds. 1992. *The Diversity of Normal Behaviors: Further Contributions to Normatology.* New York: Basic Books.

PELLEGRINO, EDMUND D., and THOMASMA, DAVID C. 1981. *A Philosophical Basis of Medical Practice: Toward a Philosophy and Ethic of the Healing Professions.* New York: Oxford University Press.

RIEFF, PHILIP. 1959. *Freud: The Mind of the Moralist.* New York: Viking.

Russell, Denise. 1994. "Psychiatric Diagnosis and the Interests of Women." In *Philosophical Perspectives on Psychiatric Diagnostic Classification*, pp. 246–258. Edited by John Z. Sadler, Osborne P. Wiggins, and Michael A. Schwartz. Baltimore: Johns Hopkins University Press.

Spanos, Nicholas P. 1985. "Witchcraft and Social History: An Essay Review." *Journal of the History of the Behavioral Sciences* 21, no. 1:60–66.

Srole, Leo; Langer, Thomas S.; Michael, Stanley T.; Opler, Marvin K.; and Rennie, Thomas A. C. 1962. *Mental Health in the Metropolis: The Midtown Manhattan Study.* New York: McGraw-Hill.

Temkin, Owsei. 1977. *The Double Face of Janus and Other Essays in the History of Medicine.* Baltimore: Johns Hopkins University Press.

Vergote, Antoine. 1988. *Guilt and Desire: Religious Attitudes and Their Pathological Derivatives.* Translated by Michael H. Wood. New Haven, Conn.: Yale University Press.

Wallace, Edwin R., IV. 1983. *Freud and Anthropology: A History and Reappraisal.* New York: International Universities Press.

———. 1986. "Freud as Ethicist." In vol. 1 of *Freud Studies: Appraisals and Reappraisals: Contributions to Freud Studies,* pp. 83–141. Edited by Paul Stepansky. Hillsdale, N.J.: Analytic Press.

———. 1990. "Mind, Body and the Future of Psychiatry." *Journal of Medicine and Philosophy* 15, no. 1:41–73.

———. 1992. "Psychiatry: The Healing Amphibian." In *Does Psychiatry Need a Public Philosophy?* pp. 74–120. Edited by Don S. Browning and Ian S. Evision. Chicago: Nelson/Hall.

———. 1994. "Psychiatry and Its Nosology: A Historico-Philosophical Overview." In *Philosophical Perspectives on Psychiatric Diagnostic Classification*, pp. 16–86. Edited by John Z. Sadler, Osborne P. Wiggins, and Michael A. Schwartz. Baltimore: Johns Hopkins University Press.

Wallwork, Ernest. 1991. *Psychoanalysis and Ethics.* New Haven, Conn.: Yale University Press.

World Health Organization. 1991. *Mental Disorders: Glossary and Guide to the Classification in Accordance with the 10th Revision of the International Classification of Diseases.* Geneva: Author.

Zilboorg, Gregory. 1935. *The Medical Man and the Witch During the Renaissance.* Baltimore: Johns Hopkins University Press.

II. MENTAL HEALTH AND RELIGION

The relationship between religion and mental health has a complex history during the post-Enlightenment period. Throughout the nineteenth century, as science gradually replaced divine revelation as the highest authority, at least for elites, a person's religion came to be seen less as a matter of adherence to the truth and more as a matter of subjective personal choice. By the end of the nineteenth century, the newly emerging fields of psychology and psychiatry began to challenge the sub-jective sources of religiosity celebrated by Romantic writers by suggesting their infantile unconscious roots and dysfunctional psychic consequences. To earlier speculative attacks on religion, such as Feuerbach's projection theory, Sigmund Freud added clinically based claims regarding religion's role in maintaining neurotic and psychotic behavior. As a result of Freud's work, mental-health professionals came to view religion mainly as a symptom of illness (Küng, 1984; Vitz, 1988).

Freud and his followers were not unaware of religion's positive contribution to personal well-being, for instance, in coping with realistic anxieties caused by death or catastrophe. But Freud argued that these benefits of religion were purchased at a psychic cost, for example, reinforcement of masochistic behavior patterns. In the writings of later psychoanalysts, like Carl Jung, Erich Fromm, and Erik Erikson, religion's positive contributions to mental health received greater emphasis, although they recognized the possibility for pathological forms of religion. Mainstream psychiatry, sometimes displaying negative bias against religion, came to view it as frequently contributing to mental illness and as having potential positive impact in some cases.

Indeed, the relationship between religion and mental health has been a long and complicated one. As Carl Jung once said, "In science, I missed the factor of meaning; and in religion, that of empiricism" (VandeCreek, 1988). Thus, given the historical tensions between mental health and religion, this article will explore whether the mental-health field has neglected religion, "the factor of meaning," and whether religion has neglected the use of "empiricism." These two questions will be answered by (1) examining the treatment of religion in clinical mental-health journals, and (2) examining the handling of the scientific method in clinical religious research.

Given the inherent biases present when looking at such a sensitive topic as religion, how can the treatment of religion by the mental-health community as well as the handling of the scientific method by the religious sector be best examined? A new review procedure, called the Systematic Review (SR) (Larson et al., 1986, 1992a), has been used in a number of published reviews that have examined the extent to which religion has been included and handled in mental-health research.

Briefly, the SR is an exhaustive, quantitatively reproducible research review method that accurately summarizes findings from large groups of published studies. In contrast to the traditional research review approach, the SR is best used in areas of research controversy, where traditional reviews can encounter problems of bias. Given the ability of the SR to assess the state of the literature with less bias than traditional reviews, the following sections will use data from already published

SRs in order to explore both the handling of religion by the mental-health field and the handling of the scientific method by clinical religious research.

The impact of religion on mental health

Recent research has shown that religion can indeed be studied empirically with objective measurement in the clinical sciences. Furthermore, when religion has been investigated scientifically, religious commitment has often been found to have positive clinical benefits either in association with clinical improvement or in predicting enhanced mental- and physical-health outcomes (Levin, 1994). For example, for people who attend religious services on a regular basis, mental health has been found to be improved. Those persons who are religiously committed have been found to have a greater sense of overall life satisfaction than do the nonreligious (Poloma and Pendleton, 1989), a finding confirmed by a systematic review of the literature in which religious commitment was found to have a positive relationship to feelings of well-being. Inversely, religion not only seems to foster a sense of well-being and life satisfaction but may possibly protect against stress, with the religiously committed reporting much lower stress levels than the less committed (Lindenthal et al., 1970; Stark, 1971). David Williams and his colleagues (1991) have posited that religion could serve as a coping mechanism that facilitates adjustment to stress. They found that as the level of religious attendance rose, the adverse psychological consequences of stress were reduced, thus suggesting that religious commitment also may have a prophylactic effect against the deleterious effects of stress on mental health.

Just as religious commitment has been found to have a beneficial effect on mental health, religious commitment has also been found to play a potential role in lowering suicide rates. A systematic review of religious commitment and suicide rates found a negative relationship in nearly every published study located (Gartner et al., 1991). In fact, George Comstock and Kay Partridge (1972) found that persons who did not attend church were four times more likely to kill themselves than were frequent church attenders. What scientific findings could explain these lower rates of suicide? First, several studies have found that the religiously committed report experiencing fewer suicidal impulses than the nonreligious (Minear and Brush, 1980–1981; Paykel et al., 1974; Reynolds and Nelson, 1981) and have a more negative attitude toward suicidal behavior (Bascue et al., 1982; Stilton et al., 1984). Second, suicide is a less acceptable alternative for the religiously committed because of their belief in a moral accountability to God, thus making them less susceptible than the nonreligious to this alter-

native (Hoetler, 1979; Stack, 1983). In addition, the foundational Judaeo-Christian religious beliefs in an afterlife, eternal justice, and the possibility of condemnation all help to reduce the appeal of potentially self-destructive behavior.

If religion can reduce the appeal of potentially self-destructive behavior such as suicide, could it also play a role in decreasing other self-destructive behaviors such as drug abuse? When this question has been examined empirically in the published literature, the response has seemed to be yes. When Richard Gorsuch and Mark Butler conducted an early review of the drug abuse literature, they noted that religious commitment seemed to have a protective effect against drug abuse:

> Whenever religion is used in an analysis, it predicts those who have not used an illicit drug regardless of whether the religious variable is defined in terms of membership, active participation, religious upbringing, or the meaningfulness of religion as viewed by the person. (Gorsuch and Butler, 1976, p. 127)

John Gartner and his colleagues (1991) confirmed the results of this earlier review fifteen years later in their systematic review of the literature, finding that even when employing varying measures of religion, religious commitment curtailed drug abuse. Interestingly, in one study the lowest rates of adolescent drug abuse were found in conservative religious groups, while the more liberal groups had slightly lower rates of drug abuse than the nonreligious population (Loch and Hughes, 1985). In addition, the authors found that the measure of the "importance of religion" to the person was the best predictor in indicating a lack of substance abuse. Thus, lack of drug abuse by the religious would seem to be more a result of deeply internalized norms and values rather than fear of drug use or peer pressure not to use.

Just as religious commitment has seemed to be negatively correlated with drug abuse, similar results were found when examining the relationship between religious commitment and alcohol abuse. Paralleling the drug abuse studies, David Larson and William Wilson (1980) found that those who abused alcohol rarely had a strong religious commitment. Indeed, of the alcoholics surveyed, 89 percent had lost interest in religion during their teenage years, whereas among community controls 48 percent had increased interest in religion and 32 percent had no change in their religious practices during that age period. Furthermore, a relationship between religious commitment and the nonuse or moderate use of alcohol has been extensively documented (Amoateng and Bahr, 1986; Cochran et al., 1988). Most interesting, Acheampong Amoateng and Stephen Bahr found that whether or not a religion specifically prohibited alcohol use, those who were active in a religious group consumed substantially less than those who were not active.

The beneficial effects of religion have not been limited solely to mental-health status indicators, however; religion has been positively associated with better physical health as well. Jeffrey Levin and Harold Vanderpool (1989), in a systematic review of religious commitment described in the literature on hypertension, found that in nearly all studies religious commitment was associated with lower blood pressure, with several religious groups having relatively low rates of hypertension-related morbidity and mortality. These findings led the authors to conclude, "Hypertension is a serious [national medical] problem [that] appears to be mitigated by religion" (Levin and Vanderpool, 1989, p. 76).

Another study explored the relationship between religion and hypertension by comparing the blood pressure rates of church-attending smokers and nonsmokers with the blood pressure rates of smoking and nonsmoking nonattenders (Larson et al., 1989b). Overall, those who rated religion as very important and were frequent church attenders had blood pressure rates that were significantly lower than those who found religion to be of little importance and attended church infrequently. Most intriguing, when blood pressure levels among the various study groups were compared, smokers who attended church at least once a week were shown four times less likely to have high blood pressure than nonsmoking low– or non–church attenders, thus suggesting that the health benefits of religion go beyond the simple avoidance of health-risk behaviors such as smoking.

Mental health and research on religion

A systematic review of studies published in four leading psychiatry journals from 1978 to 1982 showed that religion was infrequently considered in psychiatric research, and when it was considered, it was not properly measured (Larson et al., 1986). Of the 2,348 reviewed articles, less than 2.5 percent (fifty-nine studies) contained any type of quantified religious variable.

Given the diminutive "quantity" of published articles that have included a religious variable, what has been the "quality" of the research? Of the nearly 2.5 percent of the published studies containing a quantitative religious variable, less than 1 percent assessed religion with minimal standards of acceptability using at least a single-item measure of religious commitment (Craigie et al., 1990; Larson et al., 1992b). In addition, only one study employed the most desirable, state-of-the-art measure of religion: an already developed array of items assessing aspects of religious practices, attitudes, and beliefs (Larson et al., 1986). Thus, the majority of the published literature including a religious variable

measured religion with the single, static measure of denomination—a less clinically relevant measure than measures of religious commitment (Craigie et al., 1990; Williams et al., 1991).

If psychiatric research has mainly used denomination to measure religious commitment, how effectively have researchers utilized this measure? The denominational distribution in the psychiatric study sample populations was found to differ greatly from the actual U.S. denominational distribution (Larson et al., 1989a). Protestants were grossly underrepresented in these study samples, at nearly half their actual population representation. Conversely, Jews and those claiming no religious affiliation were overrepresented in the study samples. Last, despite the fact that over 90 percent of the population was affiliated with traditional denominational groups (i.e., Protestantism, Catholicism, or Judaism), only three studies focused on traditional religions. In contrast, seventeen studies focused on sects or cults, despite the fact that less than 0.5 percent of the U.S. population was involved in religious organizations of this type (Larson et al., 1986).

Another systematic review of two leading psychiatry journals found that even the most basic scientific methodology of research on religion was seriously flawed (Larson et al., 1992b). When a study had a hypothesis regarding religion, a study result was reported only 40 percent of the time. More important, when a study result was reported concerning a religious factor's association with a psychiatric measure, only 22 percent of the studies had previously clarified a hypothesis about religion (Larson et al., 1992b). In short, results were frequently analyzed and published without prior hypotheses, while religious hypotheses were frequently stated without reporting the corresponding findings.

This neglect and mishandling of religion is of concern given that when the associations between measures of religion and measures of mental health were examined in the two leading journals of psychiatry, 84 percent of the religion–mental-health associations systematically located were found to be clinically beneficial, while only 16 percent of the associations were found to be either neutral or harmful. Thus, even though the vast majority of published studies showed religion as having a positive influence on mental health, this factor has been largely ignored by the psychiatric community.

Has family medicine fared any better than psychiatry in measuring and handling religion in its research? One would expect researchers and clinicians in the field of family medicine to be more aware of the social and psychological context of health and physical disease, and thus to be more sensitive to the role that religion can play in patients' lives. However, a systematic review of the family medicine literature has not borne out this assumption.

Frederic Craigie and his colleagues (1988) found that only 3.5 percent of the 603 empirical articles in the *Journal of Family Practice,* published from 1976 to 1986, contained a quantified religious variable. Less than 2 percent of the articles used the more adequate religious commitment measures, with the rest using the static measure of denomination to assess religious commitment. Only one study included a multidimensional assessment of religious commitment. The clinical relevance of this neglect of religion was stated in an accompanying editorial:

> Research into religious issues and variables in family medicine might be rejected or undervalued because it seems wedded to the realm of anecdote or opinion. Ironically, the absence of a solid literature of religion in family medicine will assure that our knowledge remains in the realm of anecdote and opinion, instead of progressing to an empirical assessment of beneficial, neutral, and harmful roles of religion among patients and providers. (Foglio and Brody, 1988, pp. 473–474)

While family medicine infrequently included religious variables in its research, the remaining primary care fields (i.e., pediatrics, general internal medicine, and geriatrics) addressed religion even less frequently (Orr and Isaac, 1992). In comparison with family medicine's 3.5 percent level, only 1.1 percent of the other primary care journals assessed religion. In addition, when religion was assessed, it was assessed inadequately, with religious denomination measured far more frequently than the more appropriate religious commitment measures of religious practices, beliefs, and attitudes.

It should be noted that when religious commitment factors assessed in the *Journal of Family Practice* were systematically reviewed and evaluated for their clinical associations or effects, nearly 80 percent of the religious commitment findings showed clinical benefit (Craigie et al., 1990). Indeed, study findings implying a beneficial effect were nearly three times as frequent as those implying clinical harm.

Religion and definitions of mental illness

A further concern has been the treatment of religion in the American Psychiatric Association's *Diagnostic and Statistical Manual of Mental Disorders (DSM-III-R)* (1987), the major diagnostic manual for mental-health fields (Post, 1992; Richardson, 1993). A systematic review of the technical terms defined in Appendix C of the *DSM-III-R* highlighted this unintended negative bias toward religion, finding that religious content was overrepresented in illustrations of case examples of psychopathology (Larson et al., 1993). Appendix C: Glossary of Technical Terms was included to enhance the lay reader's understanding of the most frequently used mental-health terms in the *DSM-III-R.*

Though less than 2.5 percent of psychiatric research included religious variables (Larson et al., 1986), nearly 25 percent of the case examples of psychopathology had religious content. This large discrepancy in inclusion rates is troubling, given that religion is included ten times more frequently in a publication of psychopathology than in standard research, thus casting religion in a negative and pathological light. Indeed, the representation of religiosity as psychopathology supports a simplistic mental-health notion that religious commitment fosters psychopathology and, conversely, that religion is not associated with mental well-being despite studies that have illustrated the beneficial effects of religion on physical and mental well-being. Although these findings cannot be used to imply that all other sections of the *DSM-III-R* will reveal similar findings, the field should be concerned if even one section of a consensual document such as the *DSM-III-R* has included what has been reviewed here. Given the past published research showing neglect and misinterpretation of religion in psychiatry as well as in other mental-health fields (Larson et al., 1994), clinicians and researchers should be encouraged to make more definitive and conscious efforts to more accurately represent issues of religious commitment in clinical care and training, as well as in future revisions of the *DSM.*

The religious community's handling of clinical science

Clinical religious research in the field of pastoral care suffers from many methodological problems that make quantitative reviews of the literature difficult. Despite such problems, reviews on the state of clinical research have been published in pastoral care journals—the religious sector's research outlets.

The first review, conducted by J. David Arnold and Connie Schick (1979), was undertaken before the development of the systematic review and first illuminated the methodological problems in clinical religious research. One of the chief problems uncovered by these authors was the fact that pastoral care studies were generally nonsystematic in building upon previous research, thus limiting any true scientific progress or insight. In addition, when the few researchers did attempt to make comparisons between studies, their findings were inconclusive owing to the poor methodological quality of the available studies. Arnold and Schick suggested that

> Methodological weaknesses should be corrected in future research on [pastoral] counseling in order to provide more conclusive information. Better sampling procedures, the use of standard measurement instruments in conjunction with operationally defined descriptive items, improved reliability and validity of questionnaires, and better methodological control are several

ways studies could be improved. (Arnold and Schick, 1979, p. 79)

Using the systematic review methodology, Everett Worthington (1986) followed up on Arnold and Schick's broad-based review in order to assess whether clinical religious researchers had responded to the prior reviewers' call for improvement. Seven years after the methodological problems were first underscored by Arnold and Schick, Worthington found that clinical religious research still had not remedied the need for more systematic research, with studies being published in isolation from prior research in a nonprogrammatic fashion. In addition, the preponderance of published studies used single- or multiple-item nonstandardized questionnaires as their main assessment tool, with "outcome research on clinical treatments with clinical populations almost nonexistent and certainly not reflective of the state of the art of outcome research. . . . Research in religion is less varied, has fewer programmatic efforts, and has less replication than seems optimal" (Worthington, 1986, p. 428).

Gartner and his colleagues (1991), following up five years later on Worthington's systematic review, assessed four pastoral care journals and obtained quantitative data further supporting the conclusions of prior reviews. Of the 1,045 articles reviewed, only 5 percent (fifty-five studies) contained a quantified result of any kind. Furthermore, of those articles containing quantitative data, few met even basic standards of scientific research. Only 4 percent of these studies utilized a control or comparison group—a deficiency first discussed by Arnold and Schick twelve years earlier. Less than 20 percent of studies containing quantitative data reported a sampling method, with only a quarter of the studies specifying even a single study hypothesis.

Though several prior reviews had already pointed out these methodological flaws, the pastoral care field seemed to be unaware of the continuing severity of these methodological problems. Only 4 percent of studies acknowledged even a single limitation of their data in their discussion sections, when most research studies discuss, at minimum, two or three limitations of their findings. This failure of pastoral care research to deal with its methodological limitations, or even to attempt to conduct research at all, underscores an even deeper problem—a lack of appreciation for the important role scientific investigation and discourse have in the progress of any clinical field.

Though the pastoral care research field has had recommendations in recurrent research reviews to improve research frequency as well as quality, the field has experienced little change since Arnold and Schick's first review in 1979. In fact, the pastoral care field has seemed to remain somewhat resistant to incorporating more stringent methodology in research. In a series of responses to Gartner and his colleagues' (1990) systematic review of the pastoral care literature, which called for methodological reform, a pastoral care researcher stated that pastoral care research should be a separate field or discipline that should not be "based upon the typically restrictive notion of what constitutes legitimate research methodology, i.e., quantitative approaches" (Rector, 1991, p. 123). Such sentiments may very well keep the pastoral care field out of the mainstream and effectively cloistered. Orlo Strunk, the editor of the *Journal of Pastoral Care*, has also observed the field's resistance to using quantitative research methods: "When there are articles containing statistics, the *Journal of Pastoral Care* receives letters of complaint" (Strunk, 1988). Stanton Jones cautions against this field resistance to research methodology reform:

> Religious scientists will not function as scientists or scholars if they remain perpetually in a passive mode, passing judgment on scientific paradigms by the standards of their religious presuppositions. Rather, they must constructively contribute to the progress of human understanding by putting their presuppositions to the test and seeing if they actually contribute to the progress of human knowing. (Jones, 1994, p. 194)

Scientific research, however, has not yet become a field priority. Less than 7 percent of a representative sample of clinical religious researchers had ever published a single research study, while less than 1 percent had published three or more quantitative studies (Henderson et al., 1991). This apparent neglect of research is problematic, given that this "is typically how fields advance scientifically. . . . The . . . 'research vacuum' will insure that the field remains permanently stalled" (Henderson et al., 1991, p. 43). The "stalling" of clinical religious research undermines the credibility of the religious sector and its care and treatment. Without proper research, the religious sector remains unable to properly document the potential clinical benefits of religious interventions or introduce new ideas and approaches into mainstream clinical journals as well as into clinical practice, thus remaining essentially isolated from the rest of the clinical sciences. While the scientific realm may have difficulty incorporating religion into its research, the religious sector must recognize the role it plays in not fully utilizing the scientific method and must take the necessary strides to include empiricism in evaluating its clinical interventions.

Conclusion

The apparent bias against religion in the mental-health field, along with the apparent bias against science in clinical religious research, raises important ethical issues. Science is assumed to be a domain that progresses through the gradual accumulation of new data or study findings (Mahoney, 1976). In any scientific field, one must examine new scientific developments and respond accordingly. Thus, if science informs us of a new finding, the scientific community has an ethical obligation to examine and embrace this finding as potential scientific progress to be either supported or refuted in time with proper study replications.

The manner in which the clinical sciences have apparently ignored religion in research is alarming, given the positive impact that religion has been shown to have on physical as well as mental health. Might the only explanation for the neglect of religion in mental-health research be due to the apparent bias against the blending of science and religion? Likewise, clinical religious research has neglected to adequately assess religion in accordance with the principles of the scientific method, despite repeated research reviews demonstrating the need to do so. If science and human understanding are to advance based on the gradual accumulation of scientific facts, the religious sector seems to be seriously deficient in providing factual, empirical evidence about the role religion plays in health and mental health. Could this neglect of science also be tied to a similar type of bias—again holding against the blending of science and religion?

Thus, one is left with a perplexing ethical question. While mental-health research seemingly neglects religion, religious research apparently neglects science. While both may be examples of the way in which bias enters into the interface between science and religion, a larger ethical question remains: What is worse? To have data and not change one's position in spite of it, or not to have the data at all?

DAVID B. LARSON
MARY GREENWOLD
DOUGLAS BROWN
GLENN WOOD

Directly related to this article is the companion article in this entry: MEANING OF MENTAL HEALTH. *Also directly related are the entries* MENTAL-HEALTH SERVICES; MENTAL-HEALTH THERAPIES; MENTAL ILLNESS; MENTALLY DISABLED AND MENTALLY ILL PERSONS; *and* RESEARCH BIAS. *For a further discussion of various religious traditions, see the entries* AFRICAN RELIGION; BUDDHISM; CONFUCIANISM; EASTERN ORTHODOX CHRISTIANITY; HINDUISM; ISLAM; JAINISM; JUDAISM; NATIVE AMERICAN RELIGIONS; PROTESTANTISM; ROMAN CATHOLICISM; SIKHISM; *and* TAOISM. *For a further discussion of issues relating to mental health, see the entries* COMMITMENT TO MENTAL INSTITUTIONS; DIVIDED LOYALTIES IN MENTAL-HEALTH CARE; INFORMED CONSENT, *article on* ISSUES OF CONSENT IN MENTAL-HEALTH CARE; INSTI-

TUTIONALIZATION AND DEINSTITUTIONALIZATION; PSYCHOANALYSIS AND DYNAMIC THERAPIES; *and* PSYCHOPHARMACOLOGY. *Other relevant material may be found under the entries* ENVIRONMENT AND RELIGION; ETHICS, *article on* RELIGION AND MORALITY; PASTORAL CARE; SUBSTANCE ABUSE; *and* SUICIDE.

Bibliography

AMERICAN PSYCHIATRIC ASSOCIATION. 1987. *Diagnostic and Statistical Manual of Mental Disorders: DSM-III-R.* 3d ed., rev. Washington, D.C.: Author.

———. 1990. "APA Guidelines Regarding Possible Conflict Between Psychiatrists' Religious Commitments and Psychiatric Practice." *American Journal of Psychiatry* 147:542.

AMOATENG, ACHEAMPONG Y., and BAHR, STEPHEN J. 1986. "Religion, Family, and Adolescent Drug Use." *Sociological Perspectives* 29, no. 1:53–76.

ARNOLD, J. DAVID, and SCHICK, CONNIE. 1979. "Counseling by Clergy: A Review of Empirical Research." *Journal of Pastoral Counseling* 14 (Fall–Winter):76–101.

BARBOUR, IAN G. 1974. *Myths, Models, and Paradigms: A Comparative Study in Science and Religion.* New York: Harper & Row.

BASCUE, LOY O.; INMAN, DAVID J.; and KAHN, WALLACE J. 1982. "Recognition of Suicidal Lethality Factors by Psychiatric Nursing Assistants." *Psychological Reports* 51, no. 1:197–198.

BEVAN, WILLIAM. 1991. "Contemporary Psychology: A Tour Inside the Onion." *American Psychologist* 46, no. 5:475–483.

COCHRAN, JOHN K.; BEEGHLEY, LEONARD; and BOCK, E. WILBUR. 1988. "Religiosity and Alcohol Behavior: An Exploration of Reference Group Therapy." *Sociological Forum* 3, no. 3:256–276.

COMSTOCK, GEORGE W., and PARTRIDGE, KAY B. 1972. "Church Attendance and Health." *Journal of Chronic Disease* 25, no. 12:665–672.

CRAIGIE, FREDERIC C.; LARSON, DAVID B.; and LIU, INGRID Y. 1990. "References to Religion in *The Journal of Family Practice.*" *Journal of Family Practice* 30, no. 4:477–480.

CRAIGIE, FREDERIC C.; LIU, INGRID Y.; LARSON, DAVID B.; and LYONS, JOHN S. 1988. "A Systematic Analysis of Religious Variables in *The Journal of Family Practice,* 1976–1986." *Journal of Family Practice* 27, no. 5:509–513.

ELLIS, A. 1988. "Is Religiosity Pathological?" *Free Inquiry* 8:27–32.

FOGLIO, JOHN P., and BRODY, HOWARD. 1988. "Religion, Faith, and Family Medicine." *Journal of Family Practice* 27, no. 5:473–474.

GARTNER, JOHN; LARSON, DAVID B.; ALLEN, GEORGE D.; et al. 1991. "Religious Commitment and Mental Health: A Review of the Empirical Literature." *Journal of Psychology and Theology* 19, no. 1:6–25.

GARTNER, JOHN; LARSON, DAVID B.; and VACHAR-MAYBERRY, C. D. 1990. "A Systematic Review of the Quantity and Quality of Empirical Research Published in Four Pastoral Counseling Journals." *Journal of Pastoral Care* 2:1115–1123.

GORSUCH, RICHARD L., and BUTLER, MARK C. 1976. "Initial Drug Abuse: A Review of Predisposing Social Psychological Factors." *Psychological Bulletin* 83, no. 1:120–137.

GROUP FOR ADVANCEMENT OF PSYCHIATRY. 1976. *Mysticism: Spiritual Quest or Mental Disorder*. New York: Author.

HENDERSON, DANIEL C.; GARTNER, JOHN; and CHAMBERS, FLOYD A. 1991. "The Knowledge and Use of Quantitative Research by Pastoral Counselors." *Pastoral Psychology* 40, no. 1:39–45.

HOETLER, JON W. 1979. "Religiosity, Fear of Death and Suicide Acceptability." *Suicide and Life-Threatening Behavior* 9, no. 3:163–172.

HORTON, P. C. 1974. "The Mystical Experience: Substance of an Illusion." *American Psychoanalytic Association Journal* 22, nos. 1–2:364–380.

JONES, STANTON L. 1994. "A Constructive Relationship for Religion with the Science and Profession of Psychology: Perhaps the Boldest Model Yet." *American Psychologist* 49, no. 3:184–199.

KÜNG, H. 1984. *Freud and the Problem of God*. New Haven, Conn.: Yale University Press.

LARSON, DAVID B.; DONAHUE, MICHAEL J.; LYONS, JOHN S.; BENSON, PETER L.; PATTISON, E. HANSELL; WORTHINGTON, EVERETT L., JR.; and BLAZER, DAN G. 1989a. "Religious Affiliation in Mental Health Research Samples As Compared with National Samples." *Journal of Nervous and Mental Disease* 177, no. 2:109–111.

LARSON, DAVID B.; KOENIG, HAROLD G.; KAPLAN, BERTON H.; GREENBERG, RAYMOND S.; LOGUE, EVERETT; and TYROLER, HERMAN A. 1989b. "The Impact of Religion on Men's Blood Pressure." *Journal of Religion and Health* 28, no. 4:265–278.

LARSON, DAVID B.; PASTRO, L. E.; LYONS, JOHN S.; et al. 1992a. *The Systematic Review Approach: An Innovative Approach for Reviewing Research*. Washington, D.C.: U.S. Department of Health and Human Services.

LARSON, DAVID B.; PATTISON, E. M.; BLAZER, DAN G.; OMRAN, ABDUL R.; and KAPLAN, BERTON H. 1986. "Systematic Analysis of Research on Religious Variables in Four Major Psychiatric Journals, 1978–1982." *American Journal of Psychiatry* 143, no. 3:329–334.

LARSON, DAVID B.; SHERRILL, KIMBERLY A.; and LYONS, JOHN S. 1994. "Neglect and Misuse of the R Word: Systematic Reviews of Religious Measures in Health, Mental Health, and Aging." In *Religion in Aging and Health: Theoretical Foundations and Methodological Frontiers*, pp. 178–195. Edited by Jeffrey S. Levin. Thousand Oaks, Calif.: Sage.

LARSON, DAVID B.; SHERRILL, KIMBERLY A.; LYONS, JOHN S.; CRAIG, FREDERIC C.; THIELMAN, SAMUEL B.; GREENWOLD, MARY A.; and LARSON, SUSAN S. 1992b. "Associations Between Dimensions of Religious Commitment and Mental Health Reported in *American Journal of Psychiatry* and *Archives of General Psychiatry*: 1978–1989." *American Journal of Psychiatry* 149, no. 4:557–559.

LARSON, DAVID B.; THIELMAN, SAMUEL B.; GREENWOLD, MARY A.; LYONS, JOHN S.; POST, STEPHEN G.; SHERRILL, KIMBERLY A.; WOOD, GLENN G.; and LARSON, SUSAN S. 1993. "Religious Content in the *Diagnostic and Statistical Manual*, Third Edition, Revised, Appendix C: Glossary

of Technical Terms." *American Journal of Psychiatry* 150, no. 12:1884–1885.

LARSON, DAVID B., and WILSON, WILLIAM P. 1980. "Religious Life of Alcoholics." *Southern Medical Journal* 73, no. 6:723–727.

LEHR, ELIZABETH, and SPILKA, BERNARD. 1989. "Religion in the Introductory Psychology Textbook: A Comparison of Three Decades." *Journal for the Scientific Study of Religion* 28, no. 3:366–371.

LEVIN, JEFFREY S. 1994. "Religion and Health: Is There an Association, Is It Valid, and Is It Causal?" *Social Science and Medicine* 38, no. 11:1475–1482.

LEVIN, JEFFREY S., and VANDERPOOL, HAROLD Y. 1989. "Is Religion Therapeutically Significant for Hypertension?" *Social Science and Medicine* 29, no. 1:69–78.

LINDENTHAL, JACOB J.; MYERS, JEROME K.; PEPPER, MAX K.; and STERN, MAXINE S. 1970. "Mental Status and Religious Behavior." *Journal for the Scientific Study of Religion* 9, no. 2:143–149.

LOCH, BARBARA R., and HUGHES, ROBERT H. 1985. "Religion and Youth Substance Use." *Journal of Religion and Health* 24, no. 3:197–208.

MAHONEY, MICHAEL J. 1976. *Scientist as Subject: The Psychological Imperative*. Cambridge, Mass.: Ballinger.

MANDEL, A. J. 1980. "Toward a Psychobiology of Transcendence: God in the Brain." In *Psychobiology of Consciousness*. Edited by R. J. Davidson and J. M. Davidson. New York: Plenum.

MINEAR, JULIANNE D., and BRUSH, LORELEI R. 1980–1981. "The Correlates of Attitudes Towards Suicide with Death Anxiety, Religiosity, and Personal Closeness to Suicide." *Omega* 11, no. 4:317–324.

NATIONAL ACADEMY OF SCIENCES. COMMITTEE ON SCIENCE AND CREATIONISM. 1984. *Science and Creationism*. Washington, D.C.: National Academy Press.

ORR, R. D., and ISAAC, G. 1992. "Religious Variables Are Infrequently Reported in Clinical Research." *Family Medicine* 24, no. 8:602–606.

PAYKEL, EUGENE S.; MYERS, JEROME K.; LINDENTHAL, JACOB J.; and TANNER, JANIS. 1974. "Suicidal Feelings in the General Population: A Prevalence Study." *British Journal of Psychology* 124 (May):460–469.

POLOMA, MARGARET M., and PENDLETON, BRIAN F. 1989. "Religious Domains and General Well-Being." *Social Indicators Research* 22, no. 3:255–276.

POST, STEPHEN G. 1992. "*DSM-III-R* and Religion." *Social Science and Medicine* 35, no. 1:81–90.

RECTOR, L. J. 1991. "A Response to Gartner et al.'s 'A Systematic Review of the Quantity and Quality of Empirical Research Published in Four Pastoral Counseling Journals: 1975–1984.'" *Journal of Pastoral Care* 2:123–126.

REYNOLDS, DAVIS K., and NELSON, FRANKLYN L. 1981. "Personality, Life Situation, and Life Expectancy." *Suicide and Life Threatening Behavior* 11, no. 2:99–110.

RICHARDSON, JAMES T. 1993. "Religiosity as Deviance: Negative Religious Bias in and Misuse of the *DSM-III*." *Deviant Behavior* 14, no. 1:1–21.

STACK, STEVEN. 1983. "The Effect of Religious Commitment on Suicide: A Cross-National Analysis." *Journal of Health and Social Behavior* 24, no. 4:362–374.

Stark, Rodney. 1971. "Psychopathology and Religious Commitment." *Review of Religious Research* 12, no. 3:165–176.

Stillion, Judith M.; McDowell, Eugene E.; and Shamblin, Jane B. 1984. "The Suicide Attitude Vignette Experience: A Method for Measuring Adolescent Attitudes Toward Suicide." *Death Education* 8 (suppl.):65–79.

Strunk, Orlo, Jr. 1988. "The Use of Quantitative Research in Pastoral Counseling." Speech presented at Loyola College, Columbia, Maryland, October 7.

VandeCreek, Larry. 1988. *A Research Primer for Pastoral Care and Counseling.* Calabash, N.C.: Journal of Pastoral Care Publications.

Vitz, P. C. 1988. *Sigmund Freud's Christian Unconscious.* New York: Guilford Press.

Watters, W. 1992. *Deadly Doctrine: Health, Illness, and Christian God Talk.* Buffalo, N.Y.: Prometheus Books.

Williams, David R.; Larson, David B.; Buckler, Robert E.; Heckmann, Richard C.; and Pyle, Caroline M. 1991. "Religion and Psychological Distress in a Community Sample." *Social Science and Medicine* 32, no. 11: 1257–1262.

Worthington, Everett L., Jr. 1986. "Religious Counseling: A Review of Published Empirical Research." *Journal of Counseling and Development* 64, no. 7:421–431.

MENTAL-HEALTH SERVICES

I. Settings and Programs
   Allan V. Horwitz
II. Ethical Issues
   Michele A. Carter

I. SETTINGS AND PROGRAMS

Since the mid-1950s fundamental transformations have taken place in the size, location, diversity, and funding of, and attitudes toward, mental-health services in the United States: the organized response to the identification and treatment of mental-health problems. These changes have altered the central policy and ethical questions that arise in the mental-health system as a whole. When involuntary commitments to custodial mental hospitals dominated the system, the central issues involved inappropriate social control. In the diversified system based upon community care and treatment that has evolved, the most pressing issues include how to fund and deliver services to the most seriously ill persons, allocate services to meet a potentially huge demand, and improve service delivery outside the traditional system of mental-health care.

Evolution of mental-health services. Until the mid-1960s, two separate systems dominated mental-health services: public mental institutions treating a large population of in-patients, and a smaller private sector providing most outpatient psychotherapy. Large, impersonal, custodial facilities dominated the in-patient sector and housed poor, isolated, severely mentally ill persons—who were often elderly—for long periods of time (Grob, 1973). Most residents lacked family ties or were committed as a last resort by their families. The flaws of these institutions are well known: huge size, overcrowding, geographic isolation, involuntary confinement, depersonalization, coercion, and custodial emphasis (Goffman, 1961). Nevertheless, they provided the most seriously ill persons an integrated range of services—housing, food, symptom management, respite from stressful community conditions, medical treatment, and a locus for social interaction—in one centralized location (Goldman et al., 1981). Alongside the core of state mental hospitals, a smaller outpatient sector dominated by private psychiatrists using analytic psychotherapy treated clients who could afford those services.

The mental-health system of the 1990s is much different. A revolution in mental-health services began in 1955, when the average number of residents in state and county mental hospitals started to decline from a peak of 550,000 to 370,000 in 1969 to about 100,000 in 1988 (NIMH, 1992). Admissions to these facilities also tumbled from a high of 487,000 in 1969 to 304,000 in 1988. Taking into account growing population size, the reduction in state hospital residents is even more dramatic, as the number of occupied beds fell from 339 per 100,000 persons in 1955 to 207 in 1970 and to 44 in 1988. Typical patients in state hospitals have also changed: from the elderly to the young; from long-term to short-term patients; and from persons with deteriorating and untreatable diseases of the brain to ones suffering from concurrent substance abuse disorders.

As state mental hospitals became institutions of last resort for the most intractable patients, alternative forms of in-patient care grew substantially. Most in-patient psychiatric services take place in general hospitals, private psychiatric hospitals, specialized chemical dependency units, nursing homes, and residential treatment centers for children. Over 60 percent of psychiatric in-patient episodes (residents, new admissions, and readmissions) occur in general hospitals—a sixfold increase between 1969 and 1980—and about 60 percent of these episodes occur outside specialized psychiatric units (Kiesler and Simpkins, 1993). In private psychiatric hospitals, treatment episodes increased two and one-half times while constant dollar expenditures increased five times between 1970 and 1988. However, general and private hospitals do not treat the same persons who had been found in public mental institutions: Their residents are more likely to have affective and substance abuse disorders and are less likely to have schizophrenia.

The overall growth in mental-health service provision has also been dramatic. Between 1955 and 1988, the total number of patient episodes in mental-health organizations rose more than fourfold—from 1.7 million to 7.8 million (NIMH, 1992). Most of the growth in mental-health services stemmed from the expansion of outpatient treatment. From only 23 percent of total mental-health episodes in 1955, outpatient episodes constituted 66 percent of mental-health episodes in 1988. Nevertheless, in-patient episodes consume over 80 percent of expenditures for mental health (Kiesler and Simpkins, 1993). Total expenditures by mental-health organizations increased from $3.3 billion in 1969 to $23 billion in 1988, and total spending for mental-health care ballooned to about $55 billion per year (NIMH, 1992). The number of mental-health professionals also expanded commensurately: Between 1972 and 1986, the number of psychiatrists increased by 50 percent; the number of clinical psychologists, social workers, and nurses more than doubled; and the number of other mental-health professionals more than tripled.

By 1983 about 23 million people, 15 percent of the adult population of the United States, sought some type of treatment for mental-health or addiction problems over the course of a year (Regier et al., 1993). Population surveys also indicated a growing readiness of the public to use mental-health services. One large national survey conducted in 1957 and again in 1976 showed that the number of people willing to seek professional help for a personal problem grew from one-third to one-half in that period, and that the actual number of people using help nearly doubled (Veroff et al., 1981).

Reasons for changes in mental-health services. A number of technological, ideological, legal, and economic reasons led to the steep decline in the use of traditional mental institutions and the growth of mental-health services. The introduction of psychotropic drugs in the mid-1950s provided an efficient and effective technology that could be used easily in community settings. The ideology of mental-health professionals after World War II emphasized a broad concept of mental illness, noninstitutional care, and treatment for a wide array of emotional and social problems (Grob, 1991). Judicial and legislative mandates regarding mental-health services also began to change in the late 1960s toward specific and restrictive standards for commitment and the expansion of civil rights during and after commitment proceedings (Brooks, 1980).

The locus of authority for mental-health services also shifted after World War II. Until that time, states and localities were responsible for providing services. The creation of the National Institute for Mental Health in 1949 and the passage of the Community Mental Health Centers Act of 1963 created partnerships between the federal government and localities that bypassed hospital-dominated state mental-health systems

(Grob, 1991). The hundreds of community mental-health centers that emerged in the 1960s and 1970s, however, did not serve the same population as the state hospitals, but instead, provided psychotherapy to people suffering from emotional, behavioral, marital, and family problems. These centers made mental-health services more accessible, brought more services to lower socioeconomic and minority populations, and enhanced the acceptability of mental-health treatment. They did not, however, replace the services state hospitals once provided to chronically ill persons and generally neglected the most seriously mentally ill (Rochefort, 1984).

Out of the array of technological, ideological, judicial, and political reasons for changes in mental-health service provision, shifts in patterns of reimbursement became especially important. Although not developed to serve the mentally ill, Medicaid (a program jointly administered and funded by federal and state governments to bring medical services to the poor and disabled) and Medicare (a federal program funding medical care for the elderly and persons who have received disability payments for two or more years) grew into large sources of funding for mental-health services. The eligibility of facilities to receive Medicaid and Medicare funds contributed to the changing patterns of in-patient services outlined above. Elderly persons with mental illnesses were transferred from state mental institutions ineligible for Medicare dollars to nursing homes that could receive these funds. Likewise, treatment episodes in general hospitals increased because federal programs reimburse in-patient psychiatric episodes in these settings but not in public mental institutions.

Changing patterns of private reimbursement have also altered the nature of mental-health services. Private insurance coverage for both in-patient and outpatient services greatly expanded between the 1950s and 1990s, although not at a level comparable to that for physical illnesses. Expanded eligibility of nonphysicians, including psychologists, nurses, and social workers, for third-party reimbursement has increased the pool of mental-health professionals who provide outpatient treatment. A multitude of practitioners with different disciplinary allegiances, therapeutic ideologies, and treatment techniques have come to serve clients with acute disorders (Frank and Rank, 1991). Despite the great expansion of mental-health services, however, no comprehensive system in communities has emerged to replace the services that persons with the most serious and long-term illnesses receive in state hospitals.

Ethical issues

The ethical issues that arose in a mental-health system dominated by state hospitals related to involuntary commitments, inappropriate hospitalizations, neglectful or abusive treatments, and the validity of the label of "mental illness" itself (Szasz, 1974). In the huge but uncoordinated mental-health system of the 1990s, the most pressing issue is to create coordinated service delivery systems for seriously disturbed persons. The dominance of medical models devised for specific acute conditions hampers efforts to create comprehensive services. Drug therapies that form the core of medically oriented treatment are undeniably effective in alleviating the symptoms of, although not curing, mental illness. They cannot, however, meet the needs for housing, monetary assistance, vocational training, and social interaction of seriously mentally ill persons who live in the community. Medicare and Medicaid—developed to finance treatment for acute physical conditions—usually do not cover long-term, comprehensive services that promote community living (although many states do use Medicaid options to finance a number of community-based services).

Community treatment. A broad consensus has developed among consumers, families, and mental-health professionals that community—rather than institutional—treatment is most consistent with the values of individual autonomy and choice that underlie contemporary policies toward disabled populations. In addition, evidence is accumulating that most persons with serious mental illnesses benefit more—and at no greater cost—from comprehensive community treatment programs than from hospital care (Kiesler and Sibulkin, 1987). Although there is little evidence that comprehensive community treatment is cheaper than hospital care, such programs need not cost more than in-patient treatment (Weisbrod et al., 1980).

With the exception of a minority of violent, dangerous, and self-destructive persons, outpatient programs can allow seriously mentally ill persons to remain in the community with the help of an intensive range of mental-health, psychosocial, and vocational services (Mechanic, 1987). The most effective models use assertive community treatment teams of mental-health professionals who provide services in clients' natural living environments on a seven-day-a-week, 24-hour-a-day basis (Stein and Test, 1980). Staff do not wait for a patient to seek help but aggressively offer treatment when they think it is needed. The aggressive enforcement of medication compliance and occasional hospitalizations has created concern that these programs can be overly paternalistic and coercive (Diamond and Wikler, 1985). Such interventions, however, might be necessary to keep the most difficult, disruptive, and noncompliant persons in community settings over the long term. The Fountain House program, which emphasizes job rehabilitation and the creation of a familylike atmosphere, is another effective, but less intensive, model for community treatment (Beard, 1978).

Despite the advantages of community-based treatment for the most seriously ill, skewed funding and administrative structures have precluded its widespread establishment. States continue to fund state mental hospitals disproportionately: Sixty percent of state funding goes to hospitals that serve only 7 percent of the seriously mentally ill (Sharfstein et al., 1993). Opposition from public employee unions and local communities that are economically dependent on state hospitals often prevents shifting funds from in-patient treatment to intensive community treatment programs. Likewise, federal and private reimbursement programs fund relatively expensive treatment in in-patient facilities outside of public mental institutions, but will not usually cover treatment in clients' homes or in noncoercive residential facilities in the community.

Fragmented administrative authority for mental-health services also prevents the development of integrated service systems. Service delivery for the seriously mentally ill typically involves an unplanned and uncoordinated mix of visits to emergency rooms, short-term stays in in-patient units, inadequate outpatient treatment, and a variety of entitlement programs that may not meet the special needs of the mentally ill (Bloche and Cournos, 1990). Different agencies with different missions provide housing, financial assistance, vocational training, medical treatment, and mental-health care to the mentally ill (Mechanic and Rochefort, 1992). Mechanisms such as comprehensive case management and mental-health authorities that assume organizational, financial, and clinical responsibility over a range of residential and psychosocial services can help coordinate the various agencies that provide these services (Morrissey et al., 1990). Solutions for serious mental illness must go beyond the development of effective drug treatments or psychotherapies to encompass a variety of systemic and organizational factors.

The philosophy of community treatment has also led to new and complicated issues regarding family responsibility for caregiving. Many family caretakers—typically mothers—are aging, ill, and lacking in resources to provide adequate care (Lefley, 1987). Yet the scarcity of community treatment programs means that families often must provide housing, monetary and emotional support, symptom management, and personal care to seriously ill adult children. Although mental-health professionals are now less likely than in the past to view families as pathogenic, they still too readily blame or neglect family members instead of appreciating the value of family resources. Likewise, confidentiality requirements that allow widespread information flow between mental-health professionals but preclude the sharing of information with family caregivers need reconsideration (Petrila and Sadoff, 1992).

The manifest failures of deinstitutionalization—especially the highly visible problems of the homeless mentally ill—have given rise to public demand to reinstitute civil commitment for the most obtrusive among the seriously mentally ill. In fact, federal entitlement programs have allowed most formerly institutionalized patients to avoid homelessness (Goldman et al., 1983). The more visible homeless mentally ill are likely to be young persons in urban areas with concurrent substance abuse disorders who have never experienced lengthy hospitalizations and who are resistant to traditional mental-health service delivery (Lamb, 1993). While young, chronic, and sometimes homeless mentally ill persons present a particularly challenging task for mental-health service delivery, flexible and nontraditional programs of service delivery that emphasize the provision of adequate housing can best meet the special needs of this population (Bachrach, 1992).

Inappropriate service provision.   While the most seriously ill are often unable to obtain needed services, the mental-health system overemphasizes in-patient services for persons who could more efficiently and economically be treated in outpatient settings. Particularly troubling is the fact that reimbursement patterns and financial pressures to fill in-patient beds drive service delivery. Paradoxically, while many states have reduced hospital services for the most seriously mentally ill to save costs without providing needed treatment in the community, less seriously ill persons—especially those with affective and substance abuse disorders—are often unnecessarily treated through in-patient episodes in both general and private hospitals. Few data exist about the accessibility, quality, and effectiveness of mental-health services in these settings, although good evidence from randomized studies shows that most patients who receive care in hospitals could receive more effective and less costly care as outpatients (Kiesler and Sibulkin, 1987). Youths under eighteen are particularly likely to be committed to residential facilities; contrary to trends in other age groups, in-patient treatment for youths rapidly increased during the 1980s. There is no evidence, however, that such treatment is necessary, effective, or appropriate, although it is very expensive (Kiesler and Simpkins, 1993).

A more effective and efficient mental-health service system would place less emphasis on expensive in-patient interventions and more emphasis on comprehensive, long-term community services for the chronically ill. The disabilities associated with serious mental illnesses require long-term care that is responsive to the episodic and recurrent nature of these disorders. For the acutely disturbed, such a system would deemphasize extended psychotherapy while supporting short-term, directed interventions of proven effectiveness. Mental-health reforms can reasonably include high copayments for persons with less severe disabilities who desire psychotherapy as well as higher standards of accountability for psychotherapeutic techniques eligible for reimbursement. These principles could help reorient service delivery toward community treatment of the most seriously ill without generating the huge costs of meeting the total demand for mental-health services (Frank et al., 1992).

Another obstacle to creating a more effective and efficient system lies in the largely hidden nature of much mental-health service delivery. Despite the large and growing number of mental-health professionals, general physicians are the leading providers of mental-health services, accounting for about half of all mental-health and addictive treatment services (Regier et al., 1993). Conversely, about 20 to 30 percent of medical visits are for mental, rather than physical, health problems. However, primary physicians often do not appropriately recognize and treat mental disabilities. Professional training of physicians should place more emphasis on the appropriate diagnosis and response to mental disorders in primary practice. Nonphysicians, such as nurse practitioners, could also play a greater role in the treatment of psychological problems in medical settings. Nursing homes—where growing numbers of the psychiatrically disturbed elderly reside without receiving adequate mental-health care—are another location where psychiatric need and mental-health service provision are mismatched.

An additional problem of mental-health services lies in the expansive definition of mental illness. Once equated with psychotic disorders, the definition of mental illness now includes a wide scope of emotional, behavioral, and psychophysiological disorders (Kirk and Hutchins, 1992). Categories of mental disorder increased from slightly over 100 in the *DSM-I* to more than 300 different diagnoses in *DSM-IV*. There is little evidence, however, that many of these disorders are responsive to or require mental-health treatment from professionals.

Those who hold an expansive view of mental health often call for mental-health service provision to a wide spectrum of persons who suffer from mental disorders but who do not seek treatment. Advocates of this view cite statistics from community surveys showing that about 16 percent of the U.S. population has a current mental-health or addictive disorder, about 28 percent have such disorders over a one-year period, and up to 50 percent suffer a disorder over the course of their lifetimes (Regier et al., 1993). These surveys also indicate that only about 13 percent of disordered persons seek help from a mental-health or addiction specialist and only about 30 percent seek any help at all for their problem. In this view, there is a tremendous "unmet need" in the community for mental-health services.

A different view is that the highest priority for care should be the much smaller group of persons who have severe disorders that lead to serious functional impairments. Surveys that ask respondents if they or someone in their household has a serious mental illness that interferes with their daily life find prevalence rates of between 2 to 3 percent of the population (NIMH, 1992). Because these lower estimates still involve between four and six million people and because services are finite, there is a clear need for some allocation criteria for mental-health services (Boyle and Callahan, 1993). Targeting services toward individuals who neither perceive a need for mental-health care nor suffer from serious functional limitations could be wasteful and ineffective and could direct attention away from the many unmet service needs of the people who are in the most desperate need.

Successes of mental-health services. The many failures of the current U.S. mental-health system should not detract from its successes. The expanded federal role in funding mental-health services through Medicaid and Medicare has the potential to create a more adequate community-based system that is sensitive to the needs of the seriously mentally ill (Koyanagi and Goldman, 1991). States with the will to do so have the ability to devise more effective mental-health systems—especially through the creative use of Medicaid waivers. The growth of public mental-health treatment has led to declining social class differences in the receipt of services. Changing cultural definitions and understandings of mental disorder have lessened, although not eliminated, the stigma of mental illness and have increased public willingness to seek mental-health care. Although flawed in many ways, reimbursement systems provide greater accessibility to mental-health services than ever before.

Conclusion

U.S. mental-health services in the 1990s consist of unplanned and uncoordinated services driven by patterns of reimbursement developed to treat problems of physical health. Deinstitutionalization diminished the role of state hospitals without replacing the services once found in these hospitals. The most seriously ill obtain the least adequate treatment, while reimbursement patterns that emphasize acute care in hospital settings create inappropriate and unnecessary in-patient episodes for persons who could be treated equally well through less expensive outpatient therapy. As costs for all types of health care have escalated to reach 14 percent of the gross national product, and as pressures for national health-care reform have mounted, some sort of controls over mental-health service provision are inevitable. Reforms that would lead to a more equitable and effective system would place less reliance on expensive in-patient care and long-term psychotherapy and more on comprehensive and continuous community care for the most seriously ill, and short-term and directed care for the acutely ill. The knowledge exists about what changes are needed in mental-health

service provision, although fiscal inefficiencies, administrative fragmentation, and professional resistance might prevent reform. It will be difficult to create a mental-health system that responds as adequately to the most seriously disordered as to the less seriously disturbed—but it will be more humane.

ALLAN V. HORWITZ

Directly related to this article is the companion article in this entry: ETHICAL ISSUES. *For a further discussion of topics mentioned in this article, see the entries* AGING AND THE AGED, *article on* HEALTH-CARE AND RESEARCH ISSUES; COMMITMENT TO MENTAL INSTITUTIONS; FAMILY; HEALTH-CARE FINANCING, *especially the articles on* MEDICARE, *and* MEDICAID; HEALTH-CARE RESOURCES, ALLOCATION OF, *article on* MACROALLOCATION; HOSPITAL; INSTITUTIONALIZATION AND DEINSTITUTIONALIZATION; LONG-TERM CARE; MENTAL HEALTH; MENTAL ILLNESS; PSYCHOANALYSIS AND DYNAMIC THERAPIES; *and* PSYCHOPHARMACOLOGY. *For a discussion of related ideas, see the entries* AUTONOMY; *and* PATERNALISM. *Other relevant material may be found under the entries* CHILDREN, *article on* MENTAL-HEALTH ISSUES; DISABILITY; ELECTROCONVULSIVE THERAPY; INFORMED CONSENT, *especially the article on* ISSUES OF CONSENT IN MENTAL-HEALTH CARE; MENTAL-HEALTH THERAPIES; MENTALLY DISABLED AND MENTALLY ILL PERSONS; PATIENTS' RIGHTS, *especially the article on* MENTAL PATIENTS' RIGHTS; PSYCHIATRY, ABUSES OF; *and* SUBSTANCE ABUSE.

Bibliography

AMERICAN PSYCHIATRIC ASSOCIATION. 1952. *Mental Disorders: Diagnostic and Statistical Manual.* Washington, D.C.: Author.

———. 1987. *Diagnostic and Statistical Manual of Mental Disorders: DSM-III-R.* 3d ed., rev. Washington, D.C.: Author.

BACHRACH, LEONA L. 1992. "What We Know About Homelessness Among Mentally Ill Persons: An Analytical Review and Commentary." *Hospital and Community Psychiatry* 43, no. 5:453–464.

BEARD, JOHN H. 1982. "The Rehabilitation Services of Fountain House." In *Alternatives to Mental Hospital Treatment,* pp. 201–208. Edited by Leonard I. Stein and Mary Ann Test. New York: Plenum Press.

BLOCHE, M. GREGG, and COURNOS, FRANCINE. 1990. "Mental Health Policy for the 1990s: Tinkering in the Interstices." *Journal of Health Politics, Policy and Law* 15, no. 2:387–411.

BOLE, PHILIP J., and CALLAHAN, DANIEL. 1993. "Minds and Hearts: Priorities in Mental Health Services." *Hastings Center Report* 23, no. 5 (spec. suppl.):S3–S23.

Brooks, Alexander D. 1980. *Law, Psychiatry, and the Mental Health System: 1980 Supplement.* Boston: Little, Brown.

Diamond, Ronald J., and Wikler, Daniel I. 1985. "Ethical Problems in the Community Treatment of the Chronically Mentally Ill." In *The Training in Community Living Model: A Decade of Experience,* pp. 85–93. Edited by Leonard I. Stein and Mary Ann Test. San Francisco: Jossey-Bass.

Frank, Jerome D., and Rank, Julia B. 1991. *Persuasion and Healing: A Comparative Study of Psychotherapy.* 3d ed. Baltimore: Johns Hopkins University Press.

Frank, Richard G.; Goldman, Howard H.; and McGuire, Thomas G. 1992. "A Model Mental Health Benefit in Private Insurance." *Health Affairs* 11, no. 3:98–117.

Goffman, Erving. 1961. *Asylums: Essays on the Social Situation of Mental Patients and Other Inmates.* New York: Doubleday.

Goldman, Howard H.; Adams, Neal H.; and Taube, Carl A. 1983. "Deinstitutionalization: The Data Demythologized." *Hospital and Community Psychiatry* 34, no. 2: 129–134.

Goldman, Howard H.; Gatozzi, Antoinette; and Taube, Carl A. 1981. "Defining and Counting the Chronically Mentally Ill." *Hospital and Community Psychiatry* 32, no. 1:21–27.

Goldman, Howard H.; Lehman, Anthony F.; Morrissey, Joseph P.; Newman, Sandra J.; Frank, Richard G.; and Steinwachs, Donald M. 1990. "Design for the National Evaluation of the Robert Wood Johnson Foundation Program on Chronic Mental Illness." *Hospital and Community Psychiatry* 41, no. 11:1217–1221.

Grob, Gerald N. 1983. *Mental Illness and American Society, 1875–1940.* Princeton, N.J.: Princeton University Press.

———. 1991. *From Asylum to Community: Mental Health Policy in Modern America.* Princeton, N.J.: Princeton University Press.

Kiesler, Charles A., and Sibulkin, Amy E. 1987. *Mental Hospitalization: Myths and Facts About a National Crisis.* Newbury Park, Calif.: Sage.

Kiesler, Charles A., and Simpkins, Celeste G. 1993. *The Unnoticed Majority in Psychiatric Inpatient Care.* New York: Plenum.

Kirk, Stuart A., and Kutchins, Herb. 1992. *The Selling of DSM: The Rhetoric of Science in Psychiatry.* New York: Aldine de Gruyter.

Koyanagi, Chris, and Goldman, Howard H. 1991. "The Quiet Success of the National Plan for the Chronically Mentally Ill." *Hospital and Community Psychiatry* 42, no. 9:899–905.

Lamb, H. Richard. 1993. "Lessons Learned from Deinstitutionalisation in the U.S." *British Journal of Psychiatry* 162 (May):587–592.

Lefley, Harriet P. 1987. "Aging Parents as Caregivers of Mentally Ill Adult Children: An Emerging Social Problem." *Hospital and Community Psychiatry* 38, no. 10:1063–1070.

Mechanic, David. 1987. "Correcting Misconceptions in Mental Health Policy: Strategies for Improved Care of the Seriously Mentally Ill." *Milbank Quarterly* 65, no. 2: 203–230.

Mechanic, David, and Rochefort, David A. 1992. "A Policy of Inclusion for the Mentally Ill." *Health Affairs* 11, no. 1:128–150.

Morrissey, Joseph P.; Callaway, Michael; Bartko, W. Todd; Ridgely, Susan; Goldman, Howard H.; and Paulson, Robert I. 1993. "Local Mental Health Authorities and Service System Change: Evidence from the Robert Wood Johnson Foundation Program on Chronic Mental Illness." *Milbank Quarterly* 72:49–80.

National Institute of Mental Health. 1992. *Mental Health, United States, 1992.* Edited by R. W. Manderscheid, and M. A. Sonnenschein. Washington, D.C.: U.S. Government Printing Office.

Petrila, John P., and Sadoff, Robert L. 1992. "Confidentiality and the Family as Caregiver." *Hospital and Community Psychiatry* 43, no. 2:136–139.

Regier, Darrel A.; Narrow, William E.; Rae, Donald S.; Manderscheid, Ronald W.; Locke, Ben Z.; and Goodwin, Frederick K. 1993. "The De Facto U.S. Mental and Addictive Disorders Service System." *Archives of General Psychiatry* 50, no. 2:85–94.

Rochefort, David A. 1984. "Origins of the 'Third Psychiatric Revolution': The Community Mental Health Centers Act of 1963." *Journal of Health Politics, Policy and Law* 9, no. 1:1–30.

Sharfstein, Steven S.; Stoldine, Anne M.; and Goldman, Howard H. 1993. "Psychiatric Care and Health Insurance Reform." *American Journal of Psychiatry* 150, no. 1:7–18.

Stein, Leonard I., and Test, Mary Ann. 1980. "Alternative Mental Hospital Treatment: I. Conceptual Model, Treatment Program, and Clinical Evaluation." *Archives of General Psychiatry* 37, no. 4:392–397.

Szasz, Thomas S. 1974. *The Myth of Mental Illness: Foundations of a Theory of Personal Conduct.* Rev. ed. New York: Harper & Row.

Veroff, Joseph; Douvan, Elizabeth; and Kulka, Richard A. 1981. *The Inner American: A Self-Portrait from 1957 to 1976.* New York: Basic Books.

Weisbrod, Burt; Test, Mary Ann; and Stein, Leonard I. 1980. "Alternative to Mental Hospital Treatment: II. Economic Benefit–Cost Analysis." *Archives of General Psychiatry* 37, no. 4:400–405.

II. ETHICAL ISSUES

As of the mid-1990s, American society is engaged in a critical reexamination of fundamental issues in health matters. As health-care reforms progress through the social and political process, the opportunity exists to remedy past failures in the management of health resources, to renew fundamental values and commitments to individual and public health, and to shape new priorities for a system of health care that is both fiscally sound and ethically justified. The most pressing challenge is to allocate health resources to those in need of them without unfairly compromising other cherished social goods such as education and defense, or other ideals such as economic prosperity and self-determination. This challenge is made even more complex by the relentless growth in technological and scientific achievements, and an ever widening public concern about their responsible use and distribution in society.

Of increasing concern to many in American society is the system of goods and services to provide care to the mentally ill. The mental-health system of the 1990s is a complex web of intersecting and often competing factors that reflect changing ideas regarding mental illness and the resources that are needed to deal with it. The mental-health field is characterized by a stunning diversity of problems that reflect the complex shifts in society over the past several decades. Whether these problems are considered in terms of diagnosis, level of dysfunction or disorder, duration of symptoms or disease, or social attitudes regarding concepts of deviancy and dangerousness, mental illness is a problem of enormous complexity and heterogeneous characteristics. The ethical issues are no less complex, and raise some of the deepest philosophical questions regarding mind and body, the nature of suffering, the range of human potentialities, and the conflicts between individual and societal needs.

Although ethical considerations are implicit in nearly every aspect of mental-health care, the emphasis in this article is on ethical aspects of the mental-health service system. The most dominant issue is the problem of justice and the derivative question of how to strike a fair and equitable balance between the requirement that society protect its citizens from harm and its simultaneous duty to protect and promote the moral, legal, and civil rights of each individual. Answers to this particular question continue to be reflected in various mental-health directives and policies that define the field of mental-health services. In various ways they document the extent to which the problems of mental illness are valued or disvalued by society, the eligibility criteria of those persons who may receive society's goods and those who will not, and the perceived importance of mental health to the vitality and character of the nation.

This article addresses the issues of equity, parity, and fragmentation in relation to considerations of justice, and supports the argument that mental-health concerns should be given higher priority in the health-care system of the future.

The mental-health service system

Mental illness affects people throughout the entire life cycle, including all age groups and socioeconomic strata (Regier et al., 1993). According to one estimate, approximately one-third of Americans will experience some form of a mental disorder at some point in their lives; of the 41.2 million people with mental disorders, more than 1.7 million have chronic, severely disabling conditions such as schizophrenia (Bourden, 1992). Psychiatric patients are more likely than the general population to have substance-abuse disorders as well; at least 15 percent of children and adults in the United States suffer the consequences of mental or addictive disorders. Furthermore, although 28.1 percent of the population received diagnosis of mental or addictive disorders in one year, only 14.7 percent received any mental-health services in that time frame (Regier et al., 1993). In 1986, the annual direct cost of mental and substance-abuse services in the United States was estimated to be $51.4 billion. By 1989 a survey of mental-health benefits reported that employers' costs, such as lost days of work, had added another $116 billion annually (Rice et al., 1990).

Many mental and substance-abuse disorders are severe and chronic, and thus often produce emotional and financial burdens for patients and families that last a lifetime. Although 23.2 million Americans over the age of eighteen suffer from diagnosable mental disorders in any one-month period (Regier et al., 1988), only about 20 percent of those in need of psychiatric services seek them (Shapiro et al., 1984). Similarly, despite the fact that 7.5 million children in the United States under the age of eighteen suffer from an emotional problem severe enough to require treatment, as many as 70 to 80 percent do not receive the services they need (U.S. Office of Technology Assessment, 1986). Finally, Americans over sixty-five years of age are at high risk of developing mental disorders because of reputed stressors associated with aging, including concomitant physical illness, increasing isolation, and diminished social supports. Studies demonstrate, however, that only 56 percent of older adults with mental disorders are provided services through the mental-health sector. The rest, often referred by physicians documented to poorly recognize psychological symptoms of older adult patients, obtain services from the general health sector. Consequently, many older adults with mental-health problems may not receive the services they need from qualified mental-health professionals (Gatz and Smyer, 1992).

The current system of mental-health care in the United States is enormously complex and has the following characteristics that differentiate it from the more general system:

1. Mental-health services are dependent upon public funding and are frequently subject to a high degree of government regulation.
2. Mental-health services are provided by an increasingly diverse set of professionals, including psychiatrists, social workers, psychiatric nurses, and mental-health counselors. Increasingly, these ser-

vices are offered in a variety of settings, including state and mental hospitals; general, private, and government hospitals with psychiatric units; community mental health centers; nursing homes; and specialized alcohol, drug, and addiction disorder treatment units.

3. These diverse settings may alter the transaction between a patient and therapist, and create threats to the often private and intimate character of the therapeutic relationships.

4. The chronically mentally ill and other severely disordered persons constitute a highly dependent population that presents extraordinary challenges for administrators and providers attempting to maintain a responsive, accountable, and humane program.

5. Disputes regarding the diagnosis and etiology of mental-health disorders and the efficacy of their treatments persist and make it difficult to evaluate the utility of treatment programs.

6. The boundaries of mental-health services are difficult to define, and create diverse sets of expectations and conflicts regarding "medical" and "social" models of disease.

7. Mental-health services are generally perceived as having a poor public image and as valuable for only a small group in society who have aberrant emotional or behavioral conditions (Feldman, 1980).

These characteristics provide a clear portrait of the complex issues faced by mental-health practitioners and policymakers. They may explain some of the reasons why mental-health care has a low position on the American agenda.

Vulnerability

Illness of any kind, but especially mental illness, exacerbates the need to depend on others for help and to trust that this dependence will not be exploited or manipulated. Many severely mentally ill persons remain dependent on the health-care and mental-health services systems to provide necessities of life. The human tragedies generated by severe mental disorders are considerable; often not only the health and well-being of individuals but also that of their families and communities are destroyed. Persons with chronic mental illness such as schizophrenia, manic-depression, and psychoses that impair or distort decision-making abilities may be particularly vulnerable to possibly unjustified paternalistic interventions in their lives. Although the stigma attached to the use of mental-health services may be diminishing, it still endures in some forms, thus increasing the vulnerability of the mentally ill to negative social judgments. These vulnerabilities create moral obligations on the part of society and its institutions to provide the resources to meet basic human needs and promote

policies that include strategies to avoid discrimination, stigmatization, and the exploitation of dependence. These obligations are grounded in moral beliefs regarding society's duty to help those who are weak or vulnerable, and on the moral principles of care and trust on which the therapeutic relationship between patient and provider is based (Carter, 1993).

Historical features of mental-health services

Although mental-health care represents a significant part of the overall health-care system, it has been separated from the mainstream of health care by historical, institutional, and conceptual barriers. Historically, mental-health care was linked to social-welfare policies; mentally ill persons incapable of living in society were separated from it not so much because they were sick as because they were viewed as disruptive to society. They were cared for in local or state asylums. These institutions, and the cycles of reform they mirror, have been the subject of well-documented historical works (Deutsch, 1937; Foucault, 1973; Grob, 1991). Of relevance in this article are the underlying moral and social reasons that justified the various services provided within these institutions. For instance, in the early 1800s social reformers and physicians began to lobby against a shared responsibility by the state and local governments for providing services to the mentally ill. As a result, many mentally ill persons become wards of the state (Boyle and Callahan, 1993). In the institutions of the mid-nineteenth century, "treatment" consisted of providing a calm, humane, and disciplined environment. The ethical justification for these services was that the state could meet its responsibilities to the individual, family, and community by providing medical treatment for acute problems and humane, custodial care for those with chronic problems. Furthermore, the health of the general public could be served by protecting society from the threat of disease or dependency (Grob, 1992).

In the early twentieth century, the United States began to embrace the view that the individual is responsible for meeting the basic needs of life. Society, in the form of federal or state government institutions, would intervene only when an illness placed excessive burdens on the afflicted individual or family, when the disease posed a danger or threat to the community, or when the individual lacked the necessary resources to deal with it. Vulnerable people, such as those with tuberculosis, mental illness, or mental retardation, could obtain needed services such as those provided in the mental institutions of the day. There was no broad right of access to health-care services; rather, the dominant social policy focused on the value of serving only those with special needs. Mental-health policy in the 1940s was based on the assumption that society had an obligation to provide a severely and chronically ill person with both care and treatment in public mental hospitals. Gradually, in response to economic and cultural shifts, these mental hospitals became increasingly custodial and bureaucratic (Grob, 1992).

In the years following World War II, radical transformations shook American culture, and new ideas regarding individual and societal rights emerged. The social activism and political unrest of the 1960s provided the backdrop for a number of shifts in thinking about the nation as a whole. States began to reconsider their policies regarding the mentally ill, and people who had been cared for in mental hospitals were moved to newly created community alternatives. In the 1960s the movement to deinstitutionalize the mentally ill was partly based on the idea that the chronically mentally ill could receive support in the community without infringement of their civil rights. The other assumption that fueled policies of deinstitutionalization was derived from intellectual and scientific disputes within the practice of psychiatry. Disagreements about the definition of mental illness, diverse explanations of its causes, and skepticism about treatment efficacy generated controversy and ambiguity. These disagreements in turn affected the nature of the services available to those with mental disorders.

Monumental revolutions in ideas regarding individual, civil, women's, and fetal rights provoked fundamental questions about the role of the state in a free democracy, and the power of technology to alter constructs such as life and death. As these social and intellectual events converged, new attitudes regarding the nature of medical care, research on human subjects, and the value components of therapeutic relationships began to be reflected in legal decisions, social policy, and ethical discourse. In the field of mental health, ethical concepts of autonomy, informed consent, and paternalism began to appear in the literature. Psychiatrists, social workers, psychologists, and other mental-health providers began to critically examine their relationships with patients, colleagues, society, and the state. They were confronted with new puzzles, such as how to respect the recently enhanced rights to autonomy and individual freedoms, and yet protect society from the potentially harmful actions of a mentally ill person. Ethical values were often in conflict with other values, thereby dividing professional loyalties and obligations (Reiser et al., 1987).

In response to shifts in public values and attitudes, the federal government began to endorse social-welfare programs aimed at prevention; new programs attempted to ameliorate the social problems that were said to foster mental illness. Mental-health policy increasingly began to rely on federal government programs to administer, manage, fund, and reimburse for these services. The passage of the Omnibus Reconciliation Act of 1981 effectively eliminated previous policies that had emphasized community care outside the mental hospital (Kiesler, 1992). Federally sponsored programs such as Medicare and Medicaid initiated cost-based reimbursement strategies that fueled the evolving rhetoric of the "right to health care," and fed the expectation that such a right would be funded. Congressional passage of the Tax Equity and Fiscal Responsibility Act of 1982 and the Medicare Prospective Payment System (PPS) in 1982 altered this expectation by restricting future payments for inpatient hospital services.

These events, and many other detailed elsewhere, foreshadowed the current public debate regarding the existence and scope of this "right to health care" and its numerous philosophical, conceptual, economic, political, and social ramifications.

All of these transformations in ideology influenced policy directions and helped in the evolution of a diffuse, heterogeneous system of services that provided a diverse set of services to assist the adjustment of the mentally ill to life outside the mental hospital. For instance, in the 1960s, the view that mental illness did not require psychodynamic intervention, and that those experiencing "problems in living" could find the support they needed in the community, led to the policy of deinstitutionalization. This policy of transferring patients from public mental hospsitals to community-based mental-health centers, coupled with the emergence of psychotropic agents to control their symptoms, profoundly altered the mental-health system.

Although many writers have analyzed the mixed impact on mental-health services brought about by this policy (Mechanic and Rochefort, 1992), others underscore its abject failures in helping the seriously ill or reducing the number of inpatient services (Gatz and Smyer, 1992). Other writers have argued that the community mental-health policies not only overlooked the social and human needs of the severely ill but also bifurcated therapeutic or treatment services from care and support services. The former were identified more with, and included in, the medical health-care system, whereas the latter were affiliated with the welfare or social system. This bifurcation inadvertently distorted priorities, with more focus applied to providing therapeutic services in outpatient settings for a broadly defined population (Grob, 1992). Still others have argued that with the closure of state mental hospitals and related services, many chronically and severely ill individuals found themselves with nowhere to go for needed services and help (Torrey, 1988). Transformations in mental health laws to protect the mentally ill and promote their rights began to dominate intellectual discourse. New laws demonstrated the evolutions in understanding of the concepts of confinement, commitment, access to services, and the scope of individual autonomy in treatment decisions (La Fond, 1994). In recent decades, mental-health law has become an able instrument of advocacy and protection of the civil, legal, and ethical rights of the mentally ill (Perlin, 1994; La Fond, 1994).

Access. Changes in the way mental-health services are defined, distributed, delivered, and financed have produced a number of ethical concerns related to justice and other ethical principles. One of these is the problem of access to services. In the United States, health care is ordinarily covered by private or public insurance. Insurance reimbursement policies were originally constructed to shield both patient and provider against the worry about costs once an illness actually occurred. Reimbursements were quite generous and uncontested, with third parties acting as silent partners in the negotiation between physician and patient for needed services. The result of this is now obvious: a highly inflationary system with rapidly accelerating health-care expenditures (Fuchs, 1984).

Obviously, the 37 million people currently estimated to be without public or private health insurance will also be without financial insurance against psychiatric or addictive disorders. Yet, even where insurance is provided, mental-health insurance benefits are not on par with those in the general medical sector. Approximately 90 percent of the insurance companies that provide mental-health coverage place limits on inpatient care and community treatment; 65 percent require higher copayments for mental-health care than they do for general care. In 1988 the Bureau of Labor Statistics reported that while 90 percent of the insurance plans surveyed provided mental-health benefits, only 27 percent provided the same inpatient coverage as for general health care; only 3 percent provided equivalent coverage in the outpatient setting (U.S. Department of Labor, Bureau of Labor Statisics, 1989). Moreover, Medicare and Medicaid place restrictions on the amount and setting of services for psychiatric and addictive disorders, thus further restricting the access and availability of needed resources for the mentally ill. While opportunities for mental-health services increasingly exist under Medicare, only 3 percent of Medicare funding at present goes for mental health (Kiesler, 1992). Finally, office-based care by psychiatrists, and often by other mental-health providers, is generally covered by insurance firms but is rarely equivalent to other office-based physician care (Frank et al., 1992).

Thus, although policies have been aimed at treating mental illness on an outpatient basis, all the incentives in insurance programs send the signal that inpatient treatment is what will be reimbursed. Of all mental-health expenditures, an estimated 70 percent are designated for inpatient care. Many health-insurance policies will reimburse fully for hospitalized care, but only partially cover outpatient care, and pay even less for prevention services. Nursing homes have not been integrated into any mental-health system, although the Nursing Home Reform Act of 1987 mandates "active treatment." The predictable mental-health needs of an aging population have not been factored into health policies, thus widening the gap between perceived need and access to service for a substantial segment of the population (Gatz and Smyer, 1992).

Moreover, simply being labeled as receiving treatment for a mental disorder can affect an individual's access to the general health-care system. This occurs through the practice of medical underwriting, a process that denies individuals health insurance because of a "medical disorder" for which they received care in the past (Boyle and Callahan, 1993). These forms of discrimination not only impair the individual's access to services that are otherwise standard but also further the antiquated idea of the dualism between mind and body.

These restrictions on the access and availability of services through insurance and financing mechanisms create inequities in many parts of the system. First, many Americans, especially the poor and underinsured, cannot afford the cost of needed mental-health care. Second, many uninsured people at risk for major mental and/or addictive disorders will be denied appropriate prevention services and be inadequately protected against the possibility of catastrophic financial harm. Third, failure to provide meaningful access to services within the mental-health system results in inappropriate and excessive use of the general resources of health care, creating further inequities for individual consumers and providers, and increasing the economic burden on the general medical economy as a whole. These inequalities of access to needed care are unacceptable to a decent and humane society (U.S. President's Commission, 1983). Some of them may be explained by historical accounts of the various ideological, political, and societal events that helped produce them, but they are not justified from an ethical point of view. Any society concerned with the well-being of its citizens cannot promote the importance of health care in achieving well-being while allowing people to suffer because of arbitrary barriers to health care.

Parity. A related ethical issue has to do with whether funding of treatment for mental-health conditions should be equal to that of the general health sector. Many commentators have noted a lack of parity both between the two health-care systems and within the mental-health system itself. The latter can be expressed as a disparity between defined need and service delivery. This is demonstrated in the fact that for decades U.S. health policy has been centered on the short-term, acute-care general hospital, despite the fact that this does not match the population's health needs. Preventive services have until recently been largely neglected, as have the needs of chronically ill for the elderly, children, and youth. While health care in the acute-care hospital in the United States is arguably the best in the world, in mental health, care *outside* a hospital is demonstrated to be better and less expensive than care in the hospital (Kiesler, 1992). This raises the caveat that simply mimicking the flawed policies of the general health system may not necessarily prove to be the best strategy for mental-health policymakers of the future, even though it may lead to greater parity between the two systems (Kiesler, 1992). Arbitrary limits on outpatient services, inpatient hospitalizations, community-based health services, and higher copayments for mental health services reflect the disvalues associated with mental health, and its inferior status compared with physical health. Whenever a society establishes a priority system for the kinds of goods and services it makes available to its members, questions of fairness are evoked. If a society assigns insufficient or inadequate resources to a segment of the population at risk for or suffering from mental and addictive disorders without appropriate justifications, it violates ethical commitments to social beneficence, liberty, compassion, and justice.

Fragmentation.   One of the most difficult ethical problems confronting the current mental-health service system is the striking lack of coordination and collaboration among other human-service agencies. The current mental-health system is remarkable for a striking variation in the use of institutional and community-based services, admission rates, lengths of stay and services, and multiple funding sources and patterns. Between 1970 and 1984, there was a 48 percent overall increase in the number of organizations providing mental-health services. There were increases in the number of private psychiatric hospitals, general hospitals with psychiatric units, and organizations providing outpatient services. State and county mental hospitals showed only small decreases, and were not replaced by outpatient community services, as many deinstitutionalization policies had predicted (Gatz and Smyer, 1992).

Fragmentation in services is a consequence of developments in the larger health-care system, as well as of the lack of integration in legal, social, economic, and scientific aspects of health policy. These problems stem from a cluster of ambiguities that prevail in the field of mental health: the diversity of beliefs regarding the concept of mental disease or disorder (Wakefield, 1992); deeply rooted cultural beliefs regarding behavior that seems inexplicable, bizarre, or threatening; and disagreement about which social policies to adopt in regard to persons whose autonomy is impaired by mental disorder, especially when this impairment may lead to the possibility of harm to self or others. Serious conceptual and

normative questions regarding the definition of mental illness have led to practical disagreements about when and how to intervene. As of the mid-1990s, models of mental illness range from the purely medical model and its psychotherapeutic or psychoanalytical interventions, to a model that emphasizes the unity of biological, psychological, social, and personal factors in health and illness. Different mental-health therapists subscribe to a variety of different theories on the nature of mental health. Specialists disagree, for example, about the boundary between mental illness and other forms of deviancy, and about the relative contributions of individual, family, environmental, and social variables in producing mental disorders (Rochefort, 1989). It has also been noted that a significant portion of the fragmentation and lack of coordination within the mental-health system may be due to idiosyncratic factors related to politics, prejudice, and professional or civic self-interest (Rochefort, 1989).

The lack of precise criteria to define and classify mental illness apparently has the following result: Both the person with catatonic schizophrenia, incapable of functioning in social life, and the person with an obsessive-compulsive neurosis, whose behavior is simply bothersome, are labeled as mentally ill. Both may be in need of some treatment to reduce distressing symptoms, but these services may be quite distinct from one another, and they raise significantly different concerns regarding what should count as a "mental-health service" and what should not.

Thus, despite great expansion of mental-health services, the "system" is remarkably fragmented. Without a centralized organization or locus of responsibility, quality of and accountability for services remain fragmented. On the systemic level the problem of fragmentation seems to have produced the following: undertreatment of the seriously and chronically ill; undervaluing of prevention services, rehabilitation, and long-term care; diminished access to available services for those with or at risk of mental and addictive disorders; restrictive barriers to insurance entitlement; and a generally lower position on the national health-care agenda, despite data that demonstrate the efficacy of treatment for many forms of mental disorder.

These ambiguities exert a profound influence on normative and value questions, and can have a direct effect on the kind of policy that is developed and the priorities it has in the overall agenda (Rochefort, 1989). Ultimately they determine what kinds of services and resources will be made available, to whom they will be targeted, where they will be provided, and how they will be financed. Disparities of access and status provoke dilemmas of choice regarding principles of justice, on the one hand, and principles of cost-effectiveness, on the other. They also expose the genuine difficulty of deciding which values should govern the policymaking process, when not all values can be equally promoted. For example, if society decides to purchase mental-health services because of underlying commitments to humanitarian goals, then policy should probably be directed toward those individuals who have the most serious conditions and greatest needs. However, if society purchases mental-health services because of commitments to principles of social or economic utility, then policy efforts would need to be driven by cost–benefit analyses and outcomes. In this instance, priority might be given to those individuals with depression, anxiety disorders, and alcohol addiction because of the likelihood they would recover sufficiently to return to productive society (Klerman et al., 1992). The principle of favoring the least well-off would have to be balanced against other considerations of justice that might be based on utilitarian assessments of what might provide the greatest benefits to the greatest number of people.

These priority decisions ultimately reflect political and social value judgments about how much society is willing to invest in caring for its mentally ill citizens. Although disagreements persist on a number of conceptual, scientific, and professional issues, there does seem to be consensus on one essential point: Mental health must have a higher status in the health-care system. Furthermore, setting priorities regarding the relative value of mental-health services will require a decision process based on principles of fairness, nonabandonment of those in need, public accountability, and objectivity (Boyle and Callahan, 1993).

Ethical values in contemporary mental health policy

Since 1910, with publication of the influential Flexner Report, the U.S. health-care system has been based on a medical model that firmly anchors the concepts of scientific, physical medicine and notions of medical treatment and cure. Ideas of prevention, health, and public health were relegated to the "back porch" (Smith, 1994). American society has structured its health policies, programs, professions, and institutions on this model for many decades, as though there were little relationship between mental and physical health. However, there is a growing body of empirical knowledge that documents the role of mental state in the maintenance and deterioration of good physical health, and in the treatment and recovery from physical illness (Prager and Scallet, 1992).

Contemporary mental-health policy, whether developed in terms of prevention, accessibility to needed services, rehabilitation, or maintenance of persons most greatly in need, is in a process of change. These changes reflect shifting concepts of mental illness, new etiological formulations of mental disease, treatment interven-

tions, epidemiological trends, past program successes and failures, and the broader social, political, and economic currents (Rochefort, 1989). Ultimately, policies represent society's effort to deal with one of the most difficult and persistent human problems: how to balance the classic conflict between the power of the state to act for the good of society, and the responsibility of society to ensure the full expression of individual rights and freedoms. Questions concerning who has the legitimate power to control the lives of the mentally ill continue to provoke philosophical debate. In contemplating the public and scholarly discourse in the mental-health field over the past several decades, several difficult questions regarding past policies must be confronted before new ones are generated. For instance, what ethical values, if any, were promoted by policies of deinstitutionalization? Has the goal of returning the mentally ill and disabled to be cared for in the community enhanced the rights of individuals, or has it produced in them, or their communities, some greater harm? How will mental-health policy of the future balance the competing claims of liberty, equality, and social beneficence?

Such questions represent difficult value choices, made more complex by a climate of increasing public distrust (Jellinek, 1976) and scarcity of fiscal resources (Morreim, 1989). Past assumptions of political liberalism and economic expansion are no longer valid. Instead, policies of allocation are becoming more explicitly value-directed, not simply regarding cost-containment or efficiency but on principles of equity, justice, and compassion (Jennings, 1993). Allocation policies, insofar as they are regarded as socially legitimate and politically acceptable, may then be understood to be a mechanism by which society seeks to define and to express its sense of self, its values, and its integrity (Childress, 1979). In a time of great transition and transformation of the health-care system at large, American society is at a crossroad in its attempt to understand the health of the human mind and of all the forces that seek to promote and sustain it (Prager and Scallet, 1992). It is a time of constructive chaos in which the very mission and telos of health care are being redefined. Along with this redefinition, the opportunity exists to raise the status of the mental-health services field from the "poor stepchild of the health care delivery system" (Boyle and Callahan, 1993) to a level that conjoins mental and physical well-being and integrates biomedical and behavioral knowledge regarding health parameters. To accomplish this, it will be necessary to pay close attention to issues of equity in the access, availability, and efficacy of all health-related services, and to avoid arbitrary demarcations between mental and physical well-being.

At present, there is clear and urgent need for serious ethical reflection on which values and priorities should govern the mental-health policies of the future. What is needed is an integrated, comprehensive, and equitable strategy that builds on knowledge and research in mental and physical health, and links these to appropriate and beneficial services for those in need of them. Problems of individual and social justice penetrate all areas of society but are especially powerful in relation to the needs of the mentally ill, and to the communities in which they live. Undoubtedly, care and treatment of the mentally ill pose a range of ethical concerns that will continue to challenge society well into the twenty-first century.

MICHELE A. CARTER

Directly related to this article is the companion article in this entry: SETTINGS AND PROGRAMS. *For a further discussion of topics mentioned in this article, see the entries* AGING AND THE AGED, *article on* HEALTH-CARE AND RESEARCH ISSUES; ALLIED HEALTH PROFESSIONS; CHILDREN, *article on* MENTAL-HEALTH ISSUES; ECONOMIC CONCEPTS IN HEALTH CARE; HEALTH-CARE FINANCING; HEALTH-CARE POLICY, *article on* POLITICS AND HEALTH CARE; HEALTH-CARE RESOURCES, ALLOCATION OF, *article on* MACROALLOCATION; INFORMED CONSENT, *article on* ISSUES OF CONSENT IN MENTAL-HEALTH CARE; INSTITUTIONALIZATION AND DEINSTITUTIONALIZATION; MENTAL HEALTH; MENTAL ILLNESS; PATIENTS' RIGHTS, *especially the article on* MENTAL PATIENTS' RIGHTS; PSYCHOANALYSIS AND DYNAMIC THERAPIES; PSYCHOPHARMACOLOGY; *and* SUBSTANCE ABUSE. *For a discussion of related ideas, see the entries* AUTONOMY; COMPETENCE; JUSTICE; PATERNALISM; UTILITY; *and* VALUE AND VALUATION. *Other relevant material may be found under the entries* BEHAVIOR MODIFICATION THERAPIES; DIVIDED LOYALTIES IN MENTAL-HEALTH CARE; ELECTROCONVULSIVE THERAPY; MENTAL-HEALTH THERAPIES; MENTALLY DISABLED AND MENTALLY ILL PERSONS; *and* PSYCHIATRY, ABUSES OF.

Bibliography

BOURDON, KAREN H. 1992. "Estimating the Prevalence of Mental Disorders in U.S. Adults from the ECA Survey." *Public Health Reports* 107, no. 6:663–668.

BOYLE, PHILIP J., and CALLAHAN, DANIEL. 1993. "Minds and Hearts: Priorities in Mental Health Services." *Hastings Center Report* 23, no. 5:S1–S23.

CARTER, MICHELE A. 1993. "Ethical Framework for Care of the Chronically Ill." *Holistic Nursing Practice* 8, no. 1: 67–77.

CHILDRESS, JAMES F. 1979. "Priorities in the Allocation of Health Care Resources." *Soundings: An Interdisciplinary Journal* 62, no. 3:256–274.

DEUTSCH, ALBERT. 1937. *The Mentally Ill in America: A History of Their Care and Treatment from Colonial Times.* Garden City, N.Y.: Doubleday, Doran.

FELDMAN, SAUL, ed. 1980. *The Administration of Mental Health Services.* 2d ed. Springfield, Ill.: Charles C. Thomas.

FOUCAULT, MICHEL. 1973. *Madness and Civilization: A History of Insanity in the Age of Reason.* Translated by Richard Howard. New York: Vintage.

FRANK, RICHARD G.; GOLDMAN, HOWARD H.; and McGUIRE, THOMAS G. 1992. "A Model Mental Health Benefit in Private Health Insurance." *Health Affairs* 11, no. 3:99–117.

FUCHS, VICTOR R. 1984. "The Rationing of Medical Care." *New England Journal of Medicine* 311, no. 24:1572–1573.

GATZ, MARGARET, and SMYER, MICHAEL A. 1992. "The Mental Health System and Older Adults in the 1990s." *American Psychologist* 47, no. 6:741–751.

GROB, GERALD N. 1983. *Mental Illness and American Society, 1875–1940.* Princeton, N.J.: Princeton University Press.

———. 1991. *From Asylum to Community: Mental Health Policy in Modern America.* Princeton, N.J.: Princeton University Press.

JELLINEK, MICHAEL. 1976. "Erosion of Patient Trust in Large Medical Centers." *Hastings Center Report* 6, no. 3:16–19.

JENNINGS, BRUCE. 1993. "Health Policy in a New Key: Setting Democratic Priorities." *Journal of Social Issues* 49, no. 2:169–184.

KIESLER, CHARLES A. 1992. "U.S. Mental Health Policy Doomed to Fail." *American Psychologist* 47, no. 9:1077–1082.

KLERMAN, GERALD L.; OLFSON, MARK; LEON, ANDREW; and WEISSMAN, MYRNA. 1992. "Measuring the Need for Mental Health Care." *Health Affairs* 11, no. 3:23–33.

LA FOND, JOHN Q. 1994. "Law and the Delivery of Involuntary Mental Health Services." *American Journal of Orthopsychiatry* 64, no. 2:209–222.

MECHANIC, DAVID, and ROCHEFORT, DAVID A. 1992. "A Policy of Inclusion for the Mentally Ill." *Health Affairs* 11, no. 1:128–150.

MORREIM, E. H. 1989. "Fiscal Scarcity and the Inevitability of Bedside Budget Balancing." *Archives of Internal Medicine* 149, no. 5:1012–1015.

PERLIN, MICHAEL L. 1994. "Law and the Delivery of Mental Health Services in the Community." *American Journal of Orthopsychiatry* 64, no. 2:194–208.

PRAEGER, DENIS J., and SCALLET, LESLIE J. 1992. "Promoting and Sustaining the Health of the Mind." *Health Affairs* 11, no. 3:118–124.

REGIER, DARREL A; BOYD, JEFFREY H; BURKE, JACK D.; RAE, DONALD S.; MYERS, JEROME K.; KRAMER, MORTON; ROBINS, LEE N.; GEORGE, LINDA K.; KARNO, MARVIN; and LOCKE, BEN Z. 1988. "One-Month Prevalence of Mental Disorders in the United States: Based on Five Epidemiologic Catchment Area Sites." *Archives of General Psychiatry* 45, no. 11:977–986.

REGIER, DARREL A; NARROW, WILLIAM E.; RAE, DONALD S.; MANDERSCHEID, RONALD W.; LOCKE, BEN Z.; and GOODWIN, FREDERICK K. 1993. "The De Facto U.S. Mental and Addictive Disorders Service System: Epidemiologic Catchment Area Prospective 1-Year Prevalence Rates of Disorders and Services." *Archives of General Psychiatry* 50, no. 2:85–94.

REISER, STANLEY JOEL; BURSZTAJN, HAROLD J.; APPELBAUM, PAUL S.; GUTHEIL, THOMAS G. 1987. *Divided Staffs, Divided Selves: A Case Approach to Mental Health Ethics.* New York: Cambridge University Press.

Rice, Dorothy P. 1990. *The Economic Costs of Alcohol and Drug Abuse and Mental Illness.* Washington, D.C.: Superintendent of Documents, U.S. Government Printing Office.

Rochefort, David A., ed. 1989. *Handbook on Mental Health Policy in the United States.* New York: Greenwood Press.

Shapiro, Sam; Skinner, Elizabeth A.; Kessler, Larry G.; Von Korff, Michael; German, Pearl S.; Tischler, Gary L.; Leaf, Philip J.; Benham, Lee; Cottler, Linda; and Regier, Darrel A. 1984. "Utilization of Health and Mental Health Services: Three Epidemiological Catchment Area Sites." *Archives of General Psychiatry* 41, no. 10:971–978.

Smith, David R. 1994. "Porches, Politics, and Public Health." *American Journal of Public Health* 84, no. 5:725–726.

Torrey, E. Fuller. 1988. *Nowhere to Go: The Tragic Odyssey of the Homeless Mentally Ill.* New York: Harper and Row.

U.S. Department of Labor. Bureau of Labor Statistics. 1989. *Employee Benefits in Medium and Large Firms.* Washington, D.C.: Author.

U.S. Office of Technology Assessment. 1986. *Children's Mental Health: Problems and Services—A Background Paper.* Washington, D.C.: U.S. Government Printing Office.

U.S. President's Commission for the Study of Ethical Problems in Medicine and Biomedical and Behavioral Research. 1983. *Securing Access to Health Care: A Report on the Ethical Implications of Differences in the Availability of Health Services.* Washington, D.C.: U.S. Government Printing Office.

Wakefield, Jerome C. 1992. "The Concept of Mental Disorder: On the Boundary Between Biological Facts and Social Values." *American Psychologist* 47, no. 3:373–388.

MENTAL-HEALTH THERAPIES

It is difficult to define mental health in a clear and universally applicable way. Mental health is not synonymous with happiness, productivity, or intimacy, though it includes the capacity for all of these. While serious mental illnesses show significant similarities in different cultures, the definition of healthy beliefs, attitudes, and lifestyles shows great variability. Even within our own pluralist, secular culture there are substantial disagreements about the nature of the good and healthy life.

It is also difficult to develop a method or therapy that can bring improved mental health to another person. Can anyone change an unhappy person into a happy person? If mental health is largely determined by innate disposition or social circumstances, then it will not be very amenable to change through a talking therapy. Even if mental health is partially determined by personal habits and thought patterns, to what extent can these be changed by the individual? What role can a therapist play in personal transformation? Is it the technique used by the therapist or is it the person the therapist is that helps this transformation occur? What can a therapist offer that a minister, relative, or friend cannot provide? Given these questions, it should be no surprise that sorting through the various therapies designed to guide one toward mental health can be confusing and difficult.

A question of ends and means

The endless variety of mental-health therapies can be sorted out and compared only if it is recognized that they differ in the ends for which they strive as well as in the means they employ to reach these ends. Some therapies are directed toward straightforward and concrete goals such as symptom relief. Relaxation training to address performance anxiety is one example. Other therapies are directed toward more complex and abstract goals, such as an increased capacity for intimacy. Psychoanalytic therapy to improve the quality of one's romantic relationships is one example. Psychotherapeutic techniques can be compared and contrasted only if this difference in their goals is appreciated. The goals of therapy are at least partially implicit in the method of therapy employed by the therapist. Because no one therapist is skilled in all types of psychotherapy, choosing a therapist usually means choosing a therapy. This is often not understood by a patient choosing a therapist.

The question of who should choose the goals of therapy, a classic dilemma concerning paternalism in medicine, has been forcefully discussed by Sidney Bloch (1982, 1989) as it applies to psychotherapy. Therapists must balance, as must physicians, the sometimes conflicting values of patient welfare and patient autonomy. Beneficence dictates that the therapist do whatever he or she thinks is best for the patient. Respect for autonomy means allowing patients the freedom to decide what is best for themselves. Because compromised mental health so often means compromised autonomy, balancing these values in psychotherapy can be particularly difficult. Therapists frequently believe that they should promote the capacity for autonomy in their patients even if the patients want only to feel better. Bloch (1989) grapples with whether to address only his patient's distressing writer's block, as she would prefer, or to explore the forces behind her general loss of autonomy. Her ability to choose rationally between short-term and long-term goals for therapy, such as relief from distress and greater capacity for choice, may itself be compromised.

Clearly, psychotherapy must be conducted with some idea of mental health as a goal and a value. Thomas Szasz (1989), a practicing psychiatrist who does not believe that mental disorders are diseases or that mental illness compromises personal autonomy, has long accused psychotherapists of inculcating social and ethical values under the guise of scientific medical treatment. If therapists are not restoring their patients' lost capacity for choice, then they can only be brainwashing them to make choices as the therapists would. Because psychotherapy aims for the value-laden goal of mental health, it blurs the boundary between science and ethics more than any other medical therapy. It has features that are associated with science, such as theories of causation, experiments, and experts. But psychotherapy also must always hold elements from ethics, because if it is not in part an "ideology of healthy conduct" (Karasu, 1981), it has no direction or goal. Doing psychotherapy is in part providing medical treatment and in part providing ethical education.

Vigilance and restraint concerning the imposition of values upon one's patient are among the foremost duties of the psychotherapist, because it is not possible to be perfectly value-neutral. Dynamically trained therapists are schooled concerning the dangers of "countertransference," the distortion of the therapeutic process by the therapist's personal preferences and history. There are also dangers beyond the personal level. Each system of therapy operates with a value-laden notion of mental health, toward which it strives. Those therapies directed toward the relief of symptoms, such as depression and anxiety, strive toward distress-free function in a given environment. Normally this presents no particular ethical challenge. But in certain environments, relief of distress may be inappropriate. Robert Jay Lifton (1985) has discussed the situation of American soldiers in Vietnam who were opposed to the war. The therapist treating patients in such situations faces the ethical question of whether the distress or the situation is pathological and needs changing.

Those therapies that operate with more elaborate models of mental health involving mature ego defenses, character development, or adaptive coping encounter different conflicts. Psychoanalytic thought long conceptualized homosexuality as a distorted or degenerate form of intimacy necessarily associated with character pathology. This evaluation of homosexuality has changed in recent years. But the challenge of distinguishing normal and pathological modes of human relationship will remain for psychodynamic psychotherapy because it defines mental health in terms of character. There are now those arguing that sadomasochistic or pedophilic relationships are not necessarily pathological.

In general, mental-health treatment promotes adaptation to one's current social environment. It therefore tends to reinforce the prevailing norms of society. This is true both for "supportive" psychotherapy, which shores up a patient's usual ways of maintaining self-esteem, and for "uncovering" psychotherapy, which challenges these defenses in order to promote more mature modes of managing conflict and disappointment. Sig-

mund Freud (1856–1939) proposed the capacity "to love and to work" as the mark of mental health. No better succinct summary of functions that indicate mental health has been made since. Nevertheless, the values of capitalist and bourgeois Victorian culture lie implicit in this prescription. Is adaptation to a repressive society indicative of mental health? Feminists have criticized models of love available to women. Marxists have criticized alienated labor as a legitimate lifetime pursuit.

Freud, and nearly all psychotherapists since, have treated primarily upper- and middle-class caucasians. The goals of therapy and the therapeutic means utilized have been derived within this class context. Public funding for psychotherapy has been and continues to be scant. Psychotherapy is considered by society to be less of a necessity than medical care. Community mental-health centers did do some psychotherapy in the 1960s and 1970s, but are now directed toward medication and case management of the chronically mentally ill. It is virtually impossible in most cities to obtain psychotherapy without insurance or discretionary income.

Whether psychotherapy can reach beyond its historical boundaries of class and race is not yet clear. It has traditionally addressed an educated, articulate, and motivated group of patients from the same social class and culture as the therapist. Because most psychotherapy is done with the individual patient, it addresses the individual as the primary cause of his or her problems. This is a valid approach to the denial practiced by middle-class patients concerning their life difficulties, but may not be fair to lower-class patients facing poverty and prejudice. Proponents of "radical therapy" have tried to respond to this challenge by pathologizing the victimizing situation instead of the victimized individual. They thus construe the therapist as an agent for social as well as individual change. This approach escapes the problem of the therapist normalizing patients to the status quo. But it maximizes the problem of value imposition by the therapist, who now encourages the patient to reject society's view of the good and proper life—one that includes, for example, lifelong marriage—in favor of one advocated by the therapist.

Mental-health therapies not only respond to culture but also shape the culture within which they operate. As the values of mental-health therapy have diffused into our society, they have become a target for criticism. Since Philip Rieff spoke of "the triumph of the therapeutic" in 1966, numerous philosophers and sociologists have joined in criticizing "therapeutic values" that promote the welfare of the individual over that of the community. Christopher Lasch (1978) has accused the psychotherapies of promoting a form of narcissism in Western culture through the promotion of selfish motives and ignoring the broader social interest. Alasdair MacIntyre (1971) has specifically criticized the imposition of such goals upon society as personal satisfaction and interpersonal effectiveness. He contends that ethical evaluation of these goals has been bypassed in deference to the general idea of therapy. Whether the goal of self-gratification has gained preeminence as a result of therapy, or whether therapy has grown as part of a larger trend within society to look toward the individual as the vehicle for fulfillment, is beyond the scope of this entry.

Modes of therapy

Though there are over two hundred psychotherapies and supporting philosophies presently in use by mental-health professionals, most of these have not undergone scientific testing of their effectiveness. Only a few of these therapies can be considered specifically in this entry. Emphasis will be given to recently developed and proven therapies. Hans Eysenck's (1953) claim that psychotherapy in general offers no better chance for recovery from psychological distress than does spontaneous remission has been repeatedly disproved, but it is not clear what aspects of psychotherapeutic technique account for its effectiveness. Responding to the question whether one form of psychotherapy was better than another, Lester Luborsky et al. (1975) could only quote Lewis Carroll and ask, "Is it true that everyone has won and all must have prizes?" There has been much research since the late 1970s demonstrating therapeutic effects specific to the type of psychotherapy used, but the evidence favoring effects not specific to a particular psychotherapeutic method still predominates.

A number of reasons have been proposed to explain these findings (Beutler and Crago, 1987). First, there is strong evidence that a good therapist–patient match is a more powerful predictor of therapy outcome than is treatment method. Second, the measures used to assess efficacy for experimental treatment groups may be insensitive to important differences in outcome between individual patients. Furthermore, the goals sought by different therapies may be so different as not to be adequately captured by a common measure of outcome. Third, differences in the level of psychotherapist experience may have more impact than differences in psychotherapy approach. An attempt has been made to produce therapy manuals for clinical trials that minimize these factors. But these manuals have also come under criticism as retarding the therapist's ability to respond to the individual needs and style of the patient. In summary, it has been difficult to show the advantage of one psychotherapeutic method over another because very personal elements of the patient–therapist interaction not easily tested by current methods appear to be critical to therapeutic success.

Psychodynamic therapy. A number of therapies derive their understanding of the patient and the modes of therapeutic action from Freudian psychoanalysis. Almost from the moment that Freud formulated the foundations of psychoanalysis, they were subject to revision by his followers such as Carl Jung, Alfred Adler, and Karen Horney. Elaborations of psychoanalytic theory in the direction of ego psychology by Anna Freud and Erik Erikson, and in the direction of object-relations theory by Melanie Klein and Donald Winnicott, have been especially influential in contemporary psychodynamic psychotherapy. Nevertheless, there are important similarities among these different approaches. They all consider unconscious forces to be important in psychopathology and insight into these forces to be therapeutic. Contemporary psychodynamic therapies derived from these theories continue to use the therapeutic relationship to reveal unconscious determinants of behavior. However, various features of the treatment are modified, such as its frequency and duration (e.g., through brief dynamic therapy); its metapsychology (e.g., through self-psychology); or its understanding of basic conflicts (e.g., through existential psychotherapy).

In brief dynamic therapy, treatment is more focused, short-term, and directive than in classical psychoanalysis. While the latter may involve four to five sessions per week over a period of years in psychoanalysis, brief dynamic therapy may be completed in as few as ten to twenty weekly sessions. The therapist tries to elucidate a "core-conflictual theme" that is then explored. Typically difficulties in one particular area of life, such as assertiveness on the job, are the focus of treatment. Like psychoanalysis, brief dynamic therapy considers the re-creation of important conflicted relationships in the relationship with the therapist—transference—to be an essential therapeutic tool. David Malan, Habib Davanloo, Hans Strupp, Peter Sifneos, and John Mann have articulated different types of brief dynamic therapy. Its effectiveness has been demonstrated in the treatment of stress and bereavement, late-life depression, and adjustment, affective, and personality disorders (Goldfried et al., 1990).

Brief dynamic therapy is not simply a compressed form of psychoanalysis; it holds unique benefits and risks. Exploration of the patient's psyche is focused but intense. Patients must be well motivated, have a circumscribed problem, and be able to tolerate an unsettling and persistent confrontation of their customary psychological defenses. Therefore, appropriate selection of patients is crucial to the success of this mode of therapy.

Self-psychology, another descendant from psychoanalysis, was developed by Heinz Kohut (1913–1981) as an elaboration of the psychoanalytic concepts of narcissism and the self. Kohut conceived psychopathology in terms of deficits in the self rather than conflicts among unconscious drives. Vicarious introspection, or empathy, by the therapist remains the primary means of data collection. But drive development, including libido, is now conceived as part of healthy self-development. Kohut defined "self" as an independent center of initiative. Self-psychology sees the most fundamental psychological need to be the organization of the individual's psyche into a cohesive configuration, the self. The self must then establish sustaining relationships between itself and its surroundings.

The therapist, through empathic understanding, establishes himself or herself as one of these sustaining relationships for the patient. Once the therapist has been established as a "selfobject," the stage is set for "transmuting internalization," whereby the self of the patient is gradually able to perform those functions previously provided by the therapist. This occurs through gradual frustration of the patient's need for a perfectly empathic other. The result is the restoration of the self as a center of initiative, compatible with one's ideals and talents, and capable of providing a sense of purpose to one's life.

Rather than presenting ethical challenges entirely different from other dynamic therapies, self-psychology highlights the power and peril present in all the transference-based therapies. In order to be effective, the therapist must become a "selfobject" for the patient, that is, a source of self-esteem. Thus the process of developing a cohesive and autonomous self in this therapy will involve periods of intense dependence and vulnerability for the patient.

Existential psychotherapy is heir to the humanist and client-centered approaches that flourished in the 1960s. Existential therapy is a psychodynamic therapy because it is primarily concerned with the interaction of psychological forces within the individual but, compared with psychoanalysis and its near cousins discussed above, "it is based on a radically different view of the specific forces, motives, and fears that interact in the individual" (Yalom, 1980, p. 8). Existential dynamics are not developmental in the way that Freudian psychodynamics are. Rather than focus on how the past is recapitulated in the present, existential therapy focuses upon fundamental intentions or choices that are part of the "future-becoming-present." Irvin Yalom has detailed four "ultimate concerns" with which existential therapy deals: death, freedom, isolation, and meaninglessness.

Since existential psychotherapy rests its theory of psychopathology on universal human concerns, it sees a fundamental continuity between the normal and the pathological. Psychological symptoms are seen as a natural part of confronting the dilemmas and paradoxes of human life. This can mean that the patient seeking to "just feel better" or to pass from the pathological to the normal can be at odds with the existential therapist, who considers dread an inescapable part of life. For similar reasons, it has also been difficult to do good empirical research on existential psychotherapy. This form of therapy focuses upon the personal creation of meaning, thus presenting a view of the psyche not especially amenable to causal analysis. Existential and humanistic psychotherapies have generally had more theoretical than practical appeal. They offer a rich image of the psyche, devoid of reductionistic formulas, but have not found wide pragmatic application in reducing the distress of individual patients.

Cognitive–behavioral therapy. Since the 1970s, a "cognitive revolution" has largely overtaken behaviorism in psychology. In psychotherapy, this revolution emerged in the form of cognitive–behavioral therapy. While behaviorism taught us to treat the mind as a black box upon which the powers of environmental reinforcement acted, cognitivism teaches that interpretations by the individual determine what constitutes positive or negative reinforcement in a given situation. Controlled clinical trials have demonstrated the efficacy of cognitive therapy for depression, chronic pain, anxiety, and a variety of other disorders. In cases of mild to moderate severity its efficacy is similar to that of antidepressant medication, and it may provide a lower rate of relapse in conditions like panic disorder (Beck et al., 1985).

Closely akin to the rational–emotive therapy of Albert Ellis, cognitive–behavioral therapy has been advanced by a variety of practitioners such as Aaron Beck, Dennis Turk, John Rush, and Steven Hollon. This therapy essentially consists of training in problem solving. Cognitive therapy is based on the assumption that distress originates from ineffective responses to difficult life circumstances. Mediating between life events and emotions, and driving these responses, are spontaneous interpretations or "automatic thoughts" that are subject to a variety of common distortions. Therapy targets these cognitive distortions, such as overgeneralization and arbitrary inference, by helping the patient make a scientific "turn to the evidence" for these thoughts. Cognitive–behavioral therapy usually includes both cognitive (e.g., recording automatic thoughts) and behavioral (e.g., completing small mastery-enhancing tasks) "homework" for the patient. The natural focus of cognitive therapy is upon the present situation and interpretations, though it is possible to plumb ever deeper into the personal assumptions and habits that lie behind current automatic thoughts. Due to this focus on the here and now, cognitive–behavioral therapy tends to be much more simple and straightforward than the psychodynamic therapies described above. Cognitive–behavioral therapy is focused on the amelioration of the *current* episode of depression or anxiety, while psychodynamic therapies also strive to address those factors that make a patient predisposed to episodes of depression and anxiety.

Cognitive therapy portrays mental health in terms of an absence of distorting cognitions. This lends a value-free, scientific air to this psychotherapy that may, however, not be entirely accurate. A body of research exists that suggests depressed persons' perceptions and judgments (especially of interpersonal situations) are quite accurate and realistic, while nondepressed persons show systematic optimistic biases and distortions (Taylor and Brown, 1988). If cognitive therapists are not bringing their patients back into the light of interpersonal truth, then the therapy can take on the flavor of "brainwashing for better social functioning." As discussed above, there is a tendency among all forms of psychotherapy to adapt patients to their current social milieu.

Nontraditional therapies. A vast array of practices are marketed as psychotherapy. Many are scientifically unproven, and some violate ethical precepts held dear by the more traditional therapies. Massage therapy, Rolfing, bioenergetics, and a host of other techniques use physical methods, including the touching of the patient by the therapist, to relieve psychological as well as physical problems. These therapies function as psychotherapies insofar as they associate the release of muscle tension with the release of emotional tension. One of Freud's disciples, Wilhelm Reich (1897–1957), pioneered the idea of character armor as muscle tension and the incorporation of massage into psychotherapy.

Other therapies use techniques derived from Eastern religions to increase well-being. Meditation and guided imagery, for example, have become standard techniques at stress-management clinics. In the medical setting, they are stripped of their metaphysical elements and presented as secular relaxation training. This training varies in sophistication from deep-breathing exercises to Buddhist mindfulness meditation. The rationales offered for these therapies similarly vary from physiological calming to appreciation of the fundamental emptiness and interdependence of all events. There is mounting evidence of the effectiveness of this kind of treatment for stress-related physical disorders such as headaches or back pain. However, certain sectors of society remain suspicious of the religious roots of these treatments. These nontraditional therapies challenge our sense of the proper boundary between psychotherapy and sexual gratification, on the one hand, and between psychotherapy and religious practices, on the other hand.

Ethical issues in the psychotherapies

Which therapy? Developing a method by which to choose the appropriate psychotherapy is a problem that has only recently received serious attention. Traditionally, the therapy one received was determined by the therapist one picked. The appropriateness of the therapy was judged by the intuition of therapist and patient. The attempt to derive a "differential therapeutics" in psychotherapy, comparable with that found in other areas of medicine, is in its infancy. All patients with similar levels of depression do not need the same type or duration of therapy. In psychotherapy, unlike physical medicine, diagnosis alone is inadequate to select appropriate psychotherapy. More than a diagnosis of, for example, major depressive episode must be known about the patient, such as his or her individual history and personality. Researchers are working to specify the "intermediate-level psychological determinants of problems that mediate between diagnostic grouping and type of intervention" (Goldfried et al., 1990).

The importance of factors other than technique to psychotherapy outcome has led some to stress the centrality of the therapeutic alliance in the treatment process. Section 1 of the psychiatric annotations to the AMA *Principles of Medical Ethics* (1973) states, "The doctor–patient relationship is such a vital factor in effective treatment of the patient that the preservation of optimal conditions for development of a sound working relationship should take precedence over all considerations" (p. 1060). Within this relationship, the greatest challenge for the therapist is the appropriate use of power. The "transference relationship" detailed above gives the therapist tremendous influence over the patient's life, which must be balanced by a viable "therapeutic partnership" (Karasu, 1981).

Informed consent for psychotherapy has been proposed as one way to address these concerns. In medical practice, informed consent usually means a discussion between patient and doctor of risks and benefits of an invasive treatment prior to its initiation. The application of informed consent, even in this regard, has lagged in the area of psychotherapy. Informed consent is often thought unnecessary or implicit for something as low-tech as psychotherapy. Some even contend that it could hinder the therapeutic process by increasing patient resistance to the development of an effective therapeutic relationship. The result is that collaboration in the development of a plan for therapy is too often neglected.

Some psychotherapists have argued that "informed consent is more than just an ethical or legal obligation: inherent in the process of informed consent is the potential for the enhancement of clinical work" (Jensen et al., 1989, p. 379). That is, informed consent offers an opportunity to establish the treatment alliance on solid ground. Frank discussion of the limitations as well as the benefits of therapy diminishes the illusion of therapist omniscience and patient helplessness so commonly present at the initiation of therapy.

Boundaries of therapy. Psychotherapy has been criticized as "the purchase of friendship." Since both friendships and therapeutic relationships are ideally honest, intimate, and supportive, the question of their difference is a natural one. The crucial difference is mutuality or reciprocity. Friends serve each other's needs. A therapist is paid to serve the patient's needs. The therapist utilizes professional expertise to fashion a relationship with his or her patient that addresses and corrects the patient's psychopathology. The patient is not obligated to entertain, fascinate, or gratify the therapist; responsibilities are limited to regular attendance and payment for sessions. The theory is that a patient concerned with his or her therapist's well-being cannot give adequate priority to his or her own recovery.

In practice, this boundary between therapist and friend is more fuzzy. Therapists must find their patients worthy of interest and concern if therapy is to succeed. It is difficult for therapists to develop deep concern for their patients and yet not to need their approval or companionship. Most therapies proscribe social contact between therapist and patient in order to better define the therapist's role and task. Some therapies, such as those that offer "re-parenting," specifically promote social therapist–patient contacts outside of sessions. Though some find this expansion of the power of the therapeutic relationship helpful, most would consider the lack of clear boundaries dangerous.

The most egregious violation of boundaries in psychotherapy is sexual contact between therapist and patient. Approximately 5 percent of psychiatrists and psychologists admit having sexual contact with their patients (Lakin, 1988). Given the intensely intimate atmosphere of therapy, such temptations are understandable. Nevertheless, sexual contact with a psychotherapy patient is considered the worst possible exploitation of the transference relationship. This is because the therapist exploits the trust established for therapeutic purposes for his or her own sexual gratification. The American Psychiatric Association (1993) prohibits all sexual contact with current and former patients.

While there is general agreement that sexual gratification of the therapist is always a sign of exploitation and to be avoided, how this avoidance is accomplished is subject to considerable variation. Psychoanalysts allow free expression of all sexual fantasies concerning the therapist, but prohibit all touching. Massage therapists and others who do body work rely upon the emotional release prompted by touch but avoid all sexual conversation.

Confidentiality has traditionally been one of the most important ways in which the boundaries of therapy are respected. Frank and open discussion of the patient's deepest hopes and fears is essential to psychodynamic therapy and would be inhibited by the possibility of public disclosure by the therapist. The stigma associated with psychotherapeutic treatment means that disclosure to employers, colleagues, or neighbors can produce actual damage to the patient's social well-being.

Since the 1976 *Tarasoff* case in California, which mandated that psychotherapists warn identifiable potential victims of violence, patients' rights to therapist confidentiality have been limited when "disclosure is necessary to avert danger to others." Justice Tobriner's comment in this case, "The protective privilege ends where public peril begins," means that therapists weighing disclosure must consider the public good as well as that of their patients. Psychotherapy cannot exist in a legal and moral vacuum within society. However, the *Tarasoff* decision has at times been used to expand the therapist's social responsibility for potentially dangerous patients. This responsibility can include not only warning potential victims of patient violence, on the basis of uncertain evidence, but also testifying against one's patients in court and providing preventive detention in psychiatric units for those considered potentially violent.

Psychotherapy as a profession. Because psychotherapy is so diverse in its goals and methods, competence in psychotherapy is difficult to define and enforce. Psychiatrists and psychologists have doctoral-level training and clear certification procedures and licensure laws. Master's-level therapists may have degrees in social work, counseling, or educational psychology with more variability in training and certification. However, there is enough art to the practice of psychotherapy that a great deal of formal training does not guarantee a good therapist and a small amount of formal training does not guarantee a bad therapist. Successful experience with the type of problems presented by a given patient may be most critical.

Psychotherapy is applied to many problems, from the simple and mundane, such as elevator phobias, to the complex and profound, such as childhood sexual abuse. These problems require very different types of expertise, a fact sometimes not recognized by therapist or patient. Counselors with very adequate training for pastoral, career, or marital issues may not be equipped to treat a severely disturbed suicidal patient. Professional standards for psychotherapists that would guarantee that practitioners will "know what they don't know" have lagged behind those in medicine.

Since the time of Freud, psychotherapy has been held to be professionally akin to other medical procedures and charged for accordingly. The profession has avoided free therapy because it is thought to limit the effectiveness of therapy by decreasing patient investment in the process, to foster a sense of indebtedness to the therapist, and to push the relationship toward a mutuality more appropriate to friendship. Nonetheless, some therapists find "trafficking in empathy" troubling. The profession has not yet found an adequate way to resolve these tensions.

Psychotherapy thus remains bound to the middle and upper classes. How to provide treatment to those who cannot afford therapy, or can no longer afford therapy already begun, is a serious, unsolved problem. In addition, payment for therapy is connected with an issue at the heart of the psychotherapeutic enterprise: responsibility for recovery. While physicians are taught in medical school to take responsibility for bringing their seriously ill patients back to health, psychotherapists are taught to leave the ultimate responsibility for recovery with the patient. A diabetic patient in ketoacidosis cannot be expected to participate in his or her treatment. But a personality-disordered patient who does not take active responsibility for changing long-ingrained habits will not benefit from psychotherapy. The desire to change is critical to psychotherapy in a way that it is not for other medical therapies.

Psychoanalysts have long argued for restraint in offering advice, encouragement, or assistance to patients in order to prevent "infantilizing" or "taking over" for the patient. Patients are often disappointed or irritated at the outset of therapy when it becomes clear that their therapist is not going to tell them what decisions to make. But this is only appropriate if the purpose of therapy is not to make a better decision, but to make decisions better. Therapists should not attempt to become a "prosthetic ego" for their patients, but to promote mature ego development. It is a common pitfall of long-term therapy that the patient functions better while in therapy but cannot separate from the therapist and function independently. This is best avoided through therapists' insistence on patients making and taking responsibility for their own life decisions.

Medicine commonly defines its task as the restoration of function of one or another body part, though this has been criticized as inadequate in recent years. Psychiatry has recently adopted a disease model that emphasizes the amelioration of discrete mental disorders as the treatment goal. Thus medicine in general, and psychiatry in particular, can become focused on proximate goals concerning reversal of pathology. But psychotherapy cannot avoid the fact that it seeks a restoration of the person and not just a restoration of the body. Through addressing constraints on thought, volition, and emotion, psychotherapy seeks to restore uniquely human capacities for autonomy and intimacy.

Perhaps the central ethical dilemma of psychotherapy stems from this paradoxical attempt to deliver or produce these qualities in another person. Many forms of direct action are precluded, and there are dangers in doing too much as well as in doing too little. Health-care reform will likely make psychotherapy available to more people, but in a more abbreviated form. Pressures will mount on therapists to treat more patients in less time. This will challenge not only therapists, but also psychotherapy itself, to critically examine its goals and methods.

MARK D. SULLIVAN

Directly related to this entry is the entry PSYCHOANALYSIS AND DYNAMIC THERAPIES. *For a further discussion of topics mentioned in this entry, see the entries* ALTERNATIVE THERAPIES; AUTONOMY; INFORMED CONSENT, *especially the article on* ISSUES OF CONSENT IN MENTAL-HEALTH CARE; FRIENDSHIP; PROFESSIONAL–PATIENT RELATIONSHIP; PROFESSION AND PROFESSIONAL ETHICS; *and* SEXUAL ETHICS AND PROFESSIONAL STANDARDS. *For a discussion of related ideas, see the entries* CONFIDENTIALITY; FREEDOM AND COERCION; *and* VALUE AND VALUATION. *Other relevant material may be found under the entries* BEHAVIOR CONTROL; BEHAVIORISM; BEHAVIOR MODIFICATION THERAPIES; CHILDREN, *article on* MENTAL-HEALTH ISSUES; COMMITMENT TO MENTAL INSTITUTIONS; DIVIDED LOYALTIES IN MENTAL-HEALTH CARE; MENTAL HEALTH; MENTAL-HEALTH SERVICES; MENTALLY DISABLED AND MENTALLY ILL PERSONS; PATIENTS' RIGHTS, *article on* MENTAL PATIENTS' RIGHTS; PSYCHOPHARMACOLOGY; *and* SEX THERAPY AND SEX RESEARCH. *See also the* APPENDIX (CODES, OATHS, AND DIRECTIVES RELATED TO BIOETHICS), SECTION III: ETHICAL DIRECTIVES FOR OTHER HEALTH-CARE PROFESSIONS, ETHICAL PRINCIPLES OF PSYCHOLOGISTS *of the* AMERICAN PSYCHOLOGICAL ASSOCIATION.

Bibliography

AMERICAN PSYCHIATRIC ASSOCIATION. 1973. "The Principles of Medical Ethics with Annotations Especially Applicable to Psychiatry." *American Journal of Psychiatry* 130:1056–1064.

BECK, AARON T.; EMERY, GARY.; and GREENBERG, RUTH L. 1985. *Anxiety Disorders and Phobias: A Cognitive Perspective.* New York: Basic Books.

BEUTLER, LARRY E., and CRAGO, MARJORIE. 1987. "Strategies and Techniques of Prescriptive Psychotherapeutic Intervention." *Psychiatry Update: American Psychiatric Association Annual Review* 6:378–397.

BLOCH, SIDNEY. 1982. *What Is Psychotherapy?* Oxford: Oxford University Press.

———. 1989. "The Student with a Writing Block—the Ethics of Psychotherapy." *Journal of Medical Ethics* 15, no. 3:153–158.

ELKIN, IRENE; SHEA, M. TRACIE; WATKINS, JOHN T.; IMBER, STANLEY D.; STOSKY, STUART M.; COLLINS, JOSEPH F.; GLASS, DAVID R.; PILKONIS, PAUL A.; LEBER, WILLIAM R.; DOGHERTY, JOHN P.; FIESTER, SUSAN J.; and PARLOFF, MORRIS B. 1989. "National Institute of Mental Health Treatment of Depression Collaborative Research Program: General Effectiveness of Treatments." *Archives of General Psychiatry* 46, no. 11:971–982.

EYSENCK, HANS J. 1953. *Uses and Abuses of Psychology.* London: Penguin.

GOLDFRIED, MARVIN R.; GREENBERG, LESLIE S.; and MARMAR, CHARLES. 1990. "Individual Psychotherapy: Process and Outcome." *Annual Review of Psychology* 41:659–688.

JENSEN, PETER S.; JOSEPHSON, ALLAN M.; and FREY, JOSEPH. 1989. "Informed Consent as a Framework for Treatment: Ethical and Therapeutic Considerations." *American Journal of Psychotherapy* 43, no. 3:378–386.

KARASU, TOKSOZ. 1981. "Ethical Aspects of Psychotherapy." In *Psychiatric Ethics*, pp. 89–116. Edited by Sidney Bloch and Paul Chodoff. Oxford: Oxford University Press.

LAKIN, MARTIN. 1988. *Ethical Issues in the Psychotherapies*. Oxford: Oxford University Press.

LASCH, CHRISTOPHER. 1978. *The Culture of Narcissism: American Life in an Age of Diminishing Expectations*. New York: Norton.

LIFTON, ROBERT JAY. 1985. *Home from the War: Vietnam Veterans, Neither Victims nor Executioners*. New York: Basic Books.

LUBORSKY, LESTER; SINGER, BARBARA; and LUBORSKY, LOUISE. 1975. "Comparative Studies of Psychotherapies: Is It True That 'Everyone Has Won and All Must Have Prizes'?" *Archives of General Psychiatry* 32:995–1008.

MACINTYRE, ALASDAIR C. 1971. *Against the Self-Images of the Age: Essays on Ideology and Philosophy*. New York: Schocken.

RAPP, MORTON S. 1984. "Ethics in Behaviour Therapy: Historical Aspects and Current Status." *Canadian Journal of Psychiatry* 29, no. 7:547–550.

RIEFF, PHILIP. 1966. *The Triumph of the Therapeutic: Uses of Faith After Freud*. Chicago: University of Chicago Press.

SZASZ, THOMAS. 1989. "Psychiatric Justice." *British Journal of Psychiatry* 154:864–869.

Tarasoff v. Regents of the University of California. 1976. 13 Cal. 3d 177, 529 P. 2d 533, 118 Cal. Rptr. 129.

TAYLOR, SHELLEY E., and BROWN, JONATHAN D. 1988. "Illusion and Well-Being: A Social Psychological Perspective on Mental Health." *Psychological Bulletin* 103, no. 2: 193–210.

YALOM, IRVIN D. 1980. *Existential Psychotherapy*. New York: Basic Books.

MENTAL ILLNESS

I. CONCEPTIONS OF MENTAL ILLNESS

What counts as madness? acting out? batty? bizarre? breaking down? cracked? crazy? daft? demented? depressed? deranged? erratic? frenzied? gaga? hysterical? idiotic? inane? insane? irrational? imbecile? jerky? kooky? lunatic? lulu? manic? melancholic? mentally ill? moronic? neurotic? nuts? off one's rocker? paranoid? possessed? psycho? psychotic? raving? schizoid? touched? unglued? wacky? weird? yo-yo? Shakespeare, through Polonius, suggests that the phenomenon is indefinable: "to define true madness, What is't but to be nothing else but mad?" (*Hamlet* 2.2.93–94). Yet Western law, medicine, philosophy, and sociology have attempted to define the elusive phenomenon of madness. This article introduces these various conceptions and comments on their implications for bioethics.

In traditional societies illness tends to be thought of in ethico-religious terms, as a punishment for a moral or a religious transgression: A "diagnosis" is a determination of the afflicted party's transgression; "treatment" involves atonement or prayer. Ethico-religious accounts of illnesses are common in the Hebrew Bible (e.g., 1 Kings 16). In the New Testament, however, Jesus replies to the question, "Rabbi, who hath sinned, this man or his parents, that he should be born blind?" by rejecting the ethico-religious association of illness with transgression: "Neither hath this man sinned, nor his parents" (John 9:1–3). In general, Christian societies have followed Jesus' precedent and accepted nonethico-religious conceptions of most disabilities and illnesses. Madness has tended to be an exception: Ethico-religious accounts of madness lingered into the sixteenth and seventeenth centuries. Thus the sixteenth-century physician Andrew Boorde (1490–1549), bishop of Chichester, discusses two kinds of madness, medical and ethico-religious: "When it is not illness, madness is named 'Demonici' . . . mad and possessed of the devyll or devyls. . . . This matter doth passe all manner of sickness and diseases" (Hunter and Macalpine, 1963, p. 12). Later in the same century another physician, Timothy Bright (ca. 1551–1615), published *A Treatise of Melancholie* (1586), the first English-language book on madness. Bright argued that melancholy and other forms of madness are afflictions of the brain, not of the soul. By the eighteenth century most educated people, and all physicians, treated madness as a form of illness.

Madness as illness: The Hippocratic model

The Western tradition of treating madness as illness is rooted in the Hippocratic Corpus, a collection of texts from the fifth, fourth, and third centuries B.C.E. written by physicians associated with the school of Hippocrates of Cos. According to the Hippocratics, diseases arise from an imbalance, or dyscrasia, of four basic humors: wetness, dryness, heat, and cold. In various passages, the writers expressly reject ethico-religious accounts of madness. The best known is the following: "Men ought to know that from the brain, and from the brain only, arise our . . . pains, grief and tears. . . . It is the same thing which makes us mad or delirious. . . . These things that we suffer all come from the brain when it is not healthy, but becomes abnormally hot, cold, moist, or dry" ("On the Sacred Disease," in *Hippocrates*, vol. 2, p. 175; dates from the fifth century B.C.E.). Implicit in these few words is the following medical model of madness:

1. Madness is a form of illness. Therefore, (a) it is a natural phenomenon, not a punishment for an ethico-religious transgression inflicted by "demonici," gods, or spirits; (b) no special stigma attaches to madness—it is not a fall from grace, but a physical state like "pain, grief and tears," and arises from "the brain alone"; (c) it is involuntary—people afflicted cannot control their actions; (d) those afflicted are sick and thus excused from normal obligations; (e) it is to be diagnosed and treated by physicians, not priests or shamans.

2. The mad are patients. They enjoy the special protections provided for patients within the Hippocratic Corpus, and in all successive formulations of Western medical ethics. The best-known of these is the famous obligation stated in the Hippocratic oath to "use treatment to benefit the sick . . . but never with a view to injury or wrong-doing" (Hippocrates, vol. 1, p. 164).

3. Madness is a symptom (an impairment of functionality) of a disease process (a dysfunction) internal to the organism. Thus the Hippocratics treat mad behavior as a symptom of an underlying dyscrasia of the humors within the brain.

4. Madness, like other diseases, can be diagnosed in terms of its causes. In the Hippocratic Corpus there are several attempts to develop a comprehensive classification of illnesses (a nosology), based on their characteristic patterns of development (a course), their cause (etiology), or associated abnormalities (pathology).

Madness as mental illness

Initially, when the Hippocratics created the medical model of illness they extended it to madness, treating madness as just another symptom of dyscrasia, like a fever or a rash. They made no distinction whatsoever between physical and mental illness; all illness was biophysiological. For madness to be conceptualized as a different type of illness, as mental illness, medicine had to accept an entirely different worldview, one that accorded ontological status to minds as well as to bodies. Historically, the requisite dualistic metaphysic was supplied by René Descartes (1596–1650), through the agency of the philosopher-physician John Locke (1632–1704), who in turn influenced three other philosopher-physicians: William Battie (1703–1776), David Hartley (1705–1757) and, most important, Philippe Pinel (1745–1826). The second edition of Locke's *Essay Concerning Human Understanding* (1690, 1700) intrigued these

three practicing physicians because it provided an elaborate account of mind and body as discrete but interacting substances, each operating under distinct principles.

Within Locke's framework "madness" could be explained as a symptom of physical pathology, or as an impairment to a conduit of body–mind interaction (caused, for example, by alcohol or some other neurotoxin), or, in a radical break with the Hippocratic tradition, as a disease of the mind itself, a mental illness—a misassociation of ideas or "passions." Locke's account of mental illness as confused ideas or passions derives from his empiricism (the hypothesis that the contents of the mind are ultimately derived from sensory experience). For if the entire contents of the mind derive from sensory experience, then it is reasonable to assume that disordered or deranged states of the mind are the product of disordering or traumatic experiences. Battie and Pinel, moreover, carried Locke's analysis one step further. They believed that it was possible to *reverse* the disordered ideas and passions of mad people. The reversal process, which they called "moral therapy," consisted of immersing the mad person in an orderly, pleasant, sedating environment in which "every unruly appetite [is] checked, every fixed imagination . . . diverted" (Battie, 1962, p. 69).

Eighteenth-century madhouses like Bedlam were the polar opposites of the ordered and pleasant environments required by moral therapy. Moral therapy called for peace, quiet, and order. But in eighteenth-century hospitals mad people lived in squalor and were often put on display to amuse "those who think it pastime to converse with madmen and to play upon their passions" (Battie, 1962, p. 69). Lockean moral therapists were thus forced to call for the radical reform of mental hospitals. Pinel became the symbolic leader of this reform in October 1793 when he unchained a madman at Bicêtre Hospital in Paris. Sixty years later, on November 15, 1853, the first issue of *Asylum Journal* (still published as *Journal of Mental Science*) pronounced the Lockean reformers victorious: "From the time when Pinel obtained the permission . . . to try the humane experiment of releasing from fetters some of the insane citizens chained to the dungeon walls of Bicêtre, to the date when [Dr. John] Connolly announced, that in the vast asylum over which he presided, mechanical constraint in the treatment of the insane had been entirely abandoned, and superseded by moral influence, a new school of special medicine has been gradually forming" (Hunter and Macalpine, 1963, p. 1009). The "new school of special medicine" came to ascendancy a bit earlier in the United States, where, on October 16, 1844, thirteen asylum superintendents committed to moral therapy founded the American Association of Medical Superintendents, now known as the American Psychiatric Association.

The evolution of psychiatry. The struggle for moral therapy thus culminated in "a new school of medicine," one that treats madness as mental illness, and that ultimately called itself "psychiatry"—mind (*psyche*) doctors (*iatros*). In retrospect it is amazing that psychiatry, or rather moral therapy, remained a branch of medicine. The eighteenth-century medical establishment was implacably hostile. The leading theorist of the period, Dr. William Cullen (1710–1790), professor of medicine at Edinburgh University, wrote two influential books, *First Lines in the Practice of Physic* (1784) and *Nosology* (1800), in which he classified madness as "neurosis," by which he meant a physical dysfunction of nerves, or "nervous breakdown" (both terms are Cullen's). Cullen held that there were four forms of neurosis: comata, adynamiae, spasmi, vesaniae. Vesaniae were subdivided into four categories, among them "insanity," derangement of the intellect: "Although this disease seems to be chiefly and sometimes solely an affection of the mind; yet the connection between mind and body in this life is such, that these affections of the mind must be considered as depending upon a certain state of our corporeal part" (Hunter and Macalpine, 1963, p. 476). By the "corporeal part," Cullen meant the nervous system, including the brain. Since he thought of neuroses as physiological conditions, he believed that any cure must also be physiological:

> Restraint, therefore, is useful and ought to be complete . . . the straight waistcoat answers every purpose better than any other that has thus been thought of. . . . Fear being a passion that diminishes excitement, may, therefore be opposed to the excess of it; and particularly to the angry and irascible excitement of maniacs . . . it appears to me to be commonly useful. In most cases it has appeared to me to be necessary to employ a very common impression of fear; and therefore to inspire them with awe and dread . . . by one means or another . . . sometimes it may be necessary to acquire it even by stripes and blows. (Hunter and Macalpine, 1963, p. 475)

Cullen's enthusiasm for restraint inspired one of his American students, Benjamin Rush (1745–1813), to invent a totally immobilizing chair, "The Tranquilizer." In 1811 the Philadelphia Medical Museum proudly proclaimed "The Tranquilizer" a wonderful treatment for madness: "the most complete restraint of a patient's every movement ever devised" (Hunter and Macalpine, 1963, p. 671).

Restraint, immobilization, and other physical therapies were, as the Philadelphia Museum told the world, the practical corollaries of the advanced neurophysiological science of the day. Moral therapy, by contrast, seemed an atavistic reversion to ethico-religious conceptions of madness. Its leading proponents were religiously inspired humanitarian reformers: people like the Quaker merchant William Tuke (1732–1822), who had founded the York Retreat in 1796 to create "a quiet haven in which the shattered bark might find the means of reparation or safety" (Hunter and Macalpine, 1963, p. 685). Moral therapy was thus dismissed by physicians as misguided humanism. Pinel, however, set out to reclaim it as legitimate medicine. In 1785 he had translated the fourth edition of Cullen's *First Lines* into French, so he knew that Cullen was worried about the lack of empirical data supporting his neurophysiological account of madness. Cullen had written: "Although we cannot doubt that the operations of our intellect always depend on certain motions taking place in the brain . . . yet these motions have never been objects of our senses" (Hunter and Macalpine, 1963, pp. 476–477).

As a Lockean, Pinel did not believe that the operations of the intellect depend on motions in the brain, so he stood Cullen's observations on their head. In his *Traité médico-philosophique sur l'aliénation mentale* (1801), Pinel condemned as "error" the "supposition" that "Derangement of the understanding is . . . an effect of an organic lesion of the brain." This supposition, he argued, is "contrary to anatomical fact" and should therefore be dismissed as nonempirical "prejudice" (Pinel, 1962, pp. 3–4). Cullen's physical restraints were also condemned as prejudice unsupported by empirical evidence. Hospitals practicing physical restraint considered their patients incurable and institutionalized them for life; however, hospitals practicing moral therapy were curing patients and returning them to their normal life. Thus, Pinel argued, a serendipitous, if inadvert, natural experiment had been conducted, and "experience affords ample and daily proofs of the happier effect of a mild, conciliating treatment," that is, experience supports moral therapy, not physical restraint (Pinel, 1962, pp. 3–4).

Pinel's two examples of successful moral therapy, the York Retreat and Bicêtre, were both run by nonphysicians. So the evidence Pinel adduced to demonstrate the superior efficacy of moral therapy could also have been used to argue that nonphysicians, and nonmedical treatments, could effectively cure mad people. Pinel personally attested to the "expertise" of the superintendent at Bicêtre, Jean-Baptiste Pussin (1746–ca. 1809): "A man of great experience in the management of the insane . . . the advantages which I have derived from [his experience] will stamp a greater value on my observations in the present treatise. . . . For in diseases of the mind . . . it is an art of much greater and more difficult acquisition to know when to suspend [medicines] or altogether to omit them" (*Treatise*, 1962, p. 4). Yet it never seemed to occur to Pinel that if Pussin and Tuke were successfully treating mental derangement without medicine, the treatment of madness required no medical expertise and hence was not a medical matter. Pinel, in effect, accepted the traditional Hippocratic conception of madness as medical.

His theories are strikingly similar to Cullen's in *First Lines*, except that, instead of conceptualizing madness as a breakdown or derangement of nerves, Pinel conceived it as a derangement of ideas: Mental breakdown was substituted for nervous breakdown; psychopathology for neuropathology; and moral pacification for physical pacification. The parallelism left intact the assumptions about the medical model that Cullen inherited from the Hippocratics: Madness was still treated as an illness (albeit a mental illness) that bore no stigma and excused people from their normal responsibilities. As an illness, madness was properly diagnosed and treated only by physicians (not nonphysicians, like Pussin); mad people, moreover, were properly thought of as patients rather than citizens or clients. In other words, "moral therapy" as practiced by Pussin and Tuke could have been treated as a successful nonmedical model for dealing with madness. It is a precursor to such twentieth-century nonmedical models as "therapeutic communities" and "group therapy"—neither of which need involve physicians, or need use the concepts "illness," "disease," and "patient." Thus when Pinel invented psychiatry, he did not invent moral therapy: He reimposed a medical model on moral therapy, thereby inventing a psychiatric medical model of madness as "mental illness."

Protections for the mentally ill. One immediate consequence of Pinel's imposition of a medical model on moral therapy is that the therapist's relationship to the mad person was subsumed under the traditional physician–patient relationship. This meant that confidentiality, and the other protections patients enjoyed in Hippocratic medicine, were automatically extended to mental patients. Hippocratic ethics, however, were under revision at the end of the eighteenth century. One of the major revisionists was Cullen's colleague at Edinburgh, Dr. John Gregory (1724–1773), a philosopher and professor of physic. Gregory had tried to develop a post-Hippocratic morality for the physician–patient relationship based on the physicians' feelings of humanity and sympathy toward their patients. Pinel refers to Gregory intermittently throughout the *Treatise*, and speaks of the importance of physicians' feeling sympathy and acting with humanity toward their patients. Pinel probably accepted Gregory's theories of medical ethics. Gregory, however, never addressed the hospital context. The first writer to do so was another follower of Gregory, the physician and philosopher Thomas Percival (1740–1804), author of *Medical Ethics* (1803). Percival observed that the fundamental moral problem that arises with respect to mad people is that

lunatics are, in a great measure, secluded from the observation of those who are interested in their good treatment; and their complaints of ill usage are so often false or fanciful, as to attain little credit or attention, even when well founded. The physician, therefore, must feel himself under the strictest obligation of honor, as well as of humanity, to secure to these unhappy sufferers all the *tenderness* and *indulgence*, compatible with steady and effectual government. (1803, chap. 1, art. XXX)

Having remarked this tension between humanity and governance, Percival leaves it entirely to the physician's sense of honor to determine how to balance them.

Like Percival and others influenced by Gregory, Pinel had to balance humanity and governance. In cases in which public safety was involved, Pinel seems to favor the latter. Thus he writes, "As the public safety ought to be conscientiously studied and provided for, I grant no attestation of a cure without due examination of the state of a patient" (Pinel, 1962, pp. 276–287). With these words Pinel broke with the Hippocratic tradition, in which medicine is thought of as an exclusive triadic relationship among physician, patient, and disease. Pinel had introduced a fourth player into the therapeutic relationship, the public. As David Rothman's history of the psychiatric profession (1971) underscores, the public became involved in the psychiatric model essentially because psychiatry was invented by physicians practicing at public hospitals like Bicêtre. Thus when Pinel imposed a medical model on moral therapy, he had to accommodate the realities of public hospitals, which led him to loosen some of the patient protections in Hippocratic ethics. (For a detailed comparison of Pinel's medical model with the traditional Hippocratic medical model see Baker, 1978.)

Insanity and the law

At the beginning of the seventeenth century there were only two models of madness in the Western world: a lingering ethico-religious model and a Hippocratic medical model. By the end of the century there were three more: Cullen's neurophysiological medical model, Pussin and Tuke's nonmedical "moral therapy," and Pinel's psychiatric model. In the nineteenth century, a fifth conception was introduced, "insanity by reason of mental disease."

Traditionally, all major systems of Western law (Roman law, canon law, common law, and the various national codes) recognize that while it is entirely proper to punish those who have been bad for their misdeeds, it is improper to punish those who are mad, or insane. For unlike those who are simply bad, the mad lack the capacity to reason or to choose, and so are not responsible for their actions. In the English-speaking world the traditional moral and legal distinctions involving insanity were reconceptualized in psychiatric terms in 1843. The occasion was the trial of Daniel M'Naghten, who had killed one Edward Drummond while under the delusion that Drummond was actually Sir Robert Peel, prime minister of Great Britain. The House of Lords was asked how a jury is to be instructed in such a case. Their reply is known as the M'Naghten rule:

> The jury ought to be told . . . that to establish a defence on the grounds of insanity it must be clearly proved that, at the time of committing the act, the accused was labouring under such a defect of reason, from disease of the mind, as not to know the nature and quality of the act he was doing, or, if he did know it, that he did not know he was doing what was wrong. (1843, House of Lords, 10 Cl. 2nd F. 200 at p. 209)

The M'Naghten rule not only interprets the legal concept of insanity as a "disease of the mind," it interprets it as a particular type of disease, a defect of reason or perception, a cognitive impairment. This definition excludes noncognitive conceptions of mental disease, such as affective or emotional disorders (Locke's misassociated passions) and volitional disorders (compulsions, such as kleptomania). Consequently, a rift soon developed between the limited conception of mental disease envisioned by the M'Naghten rule and the broader conceptions of mental disorders recognized by psychiatry. This rift meant that in jurisdictions that accepted the M'Naghten rule, including many states in the United States, juries could not accept psychiatric diagnoses involving noncognitive forms of mental disease as legal forms of insanity. In 1954 Federal Circuit Court Judge David Bazelon attempted to remedy this problem by issuing the following set of instructions to the jury in the case of *Durham v. United States*:

> If you the jury believe . . . [the accused] was suffering from a disease or defective mental condition when he committed the act, but believe beyond a reasonable doubt that the act was not a product of such mental abnormalities, you may find him guilty. [Otherwise] you must find the accused not guilty by reason of insanity. . . . [I]n making such judgments, [you] will be guided by wider horizons of knowledge concerning mental life. The question will be simply whether the accused acted because of a mental disorder, and not whether he displayed [the] particular symptoms [recognized by M'Naghten] which medical science has recognized do not necessarily, or even typically, accompany even the most serious mental disorder. (214 F. 2d 862 [1954])

The *Durham* instructions have the virtue of removing the diagnostic straitjacket imposed by the M'Naghten rule; they also turn over to juries the responsibility of deciding the question: Were the accused person's misdeeds a product of mental disease or defect?

Critics of *Durham* believe that its language might allow juries to find all miscreants "not guilty by reason of insanity." To reform the M'Naghten rule, the *Durham* instructions had to be framed in very broad language. This language allows a jury to find anyone whose criminal acts they deem "a product of mental . . . abnormalities" not guilty by reason of insanity. Critics point out that Dr. Karl Menninger, in the United States, and Lady Barbara Wooton, in the United Kingdom, contend that *all* criminal behavior is a product of mental abnormalities. Thus *Durham* could lay the groundwork for a therapeutic model in which treatment could supplant punishment. Philosophers Herbert Hart (1961) and Richard Wasserstrom (1980) object to expansive therapeutic models (see Adams, 1992). They argue that present-day psychiatry can neither reliably diagnose nor effectively treat criminal behavior. Moreover, they warn, an expanded therapeutic model would erode the deterrent effect of the criminal justice system. People are deterred from engaging in criminal activity, in part, because they expect to be held responsible for their crimes and, in part, because they fear punishment; however, the therapeutic model denies criminal responsibility and preempts punishment. Thus, even if psychiatry could accurately "diagnose" and effectively "cure" criminals, the therapeutic model would nonetheless be an ineffectual deterrent of crime.

Wary of opening the door to a pervasive therapeutic model, few jurisdictions have adopted *Durham*. Many, however, have replaced the M'Naghten rule with a reform first recommended by the American Law Institute in its 1956 *Model Penal Code*:

> (1) A person is not responsible for criminal conduct if at the time of such conduct as a result of mental disease or defect he lacks substantial capacity either to appreciate the criminality of his conduct or to conform his conduct to the requirements of law. (2) The terms [sic] "mental disease or defect" do not include an abnormality manifested only by repeated criminal or otherwise antisocial behavior. (Article 4.01)

The drafters of the *Model Penal Code* believe that Article 4.01 could loosen the constraints of the M'Naghten rule without opening the door to a pervasive therapeutic model (which they believe is precluded by the language of (2)). Jurisdictions that have enacted statutes based on Article 4.01 have found that it is not the panacea its drafters envisioned. The pivotal language "capacity to . . . conform his conduct to the requirements of the law" is almost as broad as the language of *Durham*, but it lacks *Durham*'s singular advantages: permitting experts to testify, using psychiatric diagnoses, and allowing juries to decide for themselves the relevance of their testimony. Instead, Article 4.01 requires mental-health professionals to testify about whether the accused party had the "capacity to . . . conform his conduct to the requirements of the law." "Capacity to conform conduct to the law" is not a psychiatric diagnosis, so, in effect, Article 4.01 requires experts to testify on subjects about which they have no expertise. Consequently, expert testimony in Article 4.01 jurisdictions tends to be morally problematic for those offering it and unreliable for those attempting to use it.

Article 4.01 has proved as unhappy a wedding of medical diagnoses to the law as the M'Naghten rule and the *Durham* instructions. Consequently Norvall Morris and some other legal scholars are questioning whether it is possible to marry medicine to moral and legal conceptions of responsibility and have called for the abolition of the insanity defense (Adams, 1992).

Sociological conceptions of mental illness

From the perspective of many twentieth-century sociologists, no union of law and medicine is possible because the two are conceptually incompatible. Law presupposes a capacity to conform to social expectations; medicine, according to the American sociologist Talcott Parsons (1902–1979), presupposes an incapacity to do so. In his analysis of the medical model, physical illness is an incapacity to perform socially valued tasks, and mental illness is an incapacity to perform socially valued roles. By "role" Parsons means "the organized system of participation of an individual in a social system." He defines "task" as "a definite set of physical operations which perform some function or functions in relation to the role and/or the personality of the individual performing it" (Parsons, 1958, p. 167). In this analysis, to be sick is to play a recognized social role, the "sick role," which serves to excuse the person in it from his or her usual responsibilities while imposing a correlative duty to cooperate with physicians to achieve recovery. Physicians, too, play roles in Parsons's analysis: Part of their role is to pronounce people ill and thereby to legitimate their assumption of the sick role. Physicians are thus agents of social control who, by diagnosing, have the power both to excuse deviance as "sickness" and to stigmatize behavior as "sick."

Parsons's analysis is designed to explain the varying conceptions of madness within and between cultures. Western societies stigmatize most but not all forms of madness (being "madly in love" is one notable exception). The ancient Greeks, on the other hand, believed that "the greatest blessings we have spring from madness when granted by divine bounty. For the prophetesses at Delphi . . . have, when mad, done many noble services for Greece" (Plato, *Phaedrus*, 244). In *Piers Plowman*, a standard source of information about old English attitudes, the mad are praised for behaving like the apostles: "Monyless they walke, with a good will, witless, meny wyde contreys; Right as Peter dade and Paul, save they preche nat" (Langland, viii, 90–95, β). Other cultures may even admire behavior that Western societies stigmatize as "mad." In the sociological literature the case typically cited is that of the Dobu of Papua New Guinea, who treat altruistic behavior as madness and who admire behavior that a Western psychiatrist would characterize as "paranoid" (Benedict, 1966). Parsons's account explains the variability of judgments about illness: Since illness is the incapacity to perform socially valued tasks or roles, if two societies value tasks or roles differently, they will have correlatively different conceptions of physical and mental illness. In preliterate but religious medieval England, witless people could be admired as followers of the apostles. In a postliterate secular England, however, the society had come to value the task of reading, and so those incapable of reading were said to suffer the illness "dyslexia." The Dobu distrust cooperation, and so they do not think of paranoid behavior as "sick"; we value cooperation, and consequently treat those incapable of trust as mentally ill. Finally, any society that values lovers will exempt the madness of love from the stigma of illness. Socially valued tasks and roles thus determine what a society deems "sick" or "well."

Although Parsons's account of mental illness has influenced such sociologists as Erving Goffman and Thomas Scheff and psychiatrists like Thomas Szasz, it is not without critics. Parsons eschewed issues of causation (etiology), fearing that any exploration of the "reality" of disease would draw sociology into the quagmire of metaphysics. Critics contend that by doing so, he (and those he influenced) systematically underestimated the reality of disease and the curative role of medical science. Their analyses are thus burdened by strikingly counterintuitive implications. To cite but one: Parsons's definition of mental illness as role incapacitation implies that anyone role-incapacitated by age or weariness is also *mentally ill.* Being old and/or tired can, of course, be incapacitating, but it is certainly not, in itself, a form of mental illness. Examples like these suggest that, in some fundamental sense, standard sociological accounts fail to address the ontological reality of disease and madness.

The antipsychiatric critique of mental illness

"Antipsychiatry" is a term used to designate the views of historians (David Rothman), philosophers (Michel Foucault), psychiatrists (R. D. Laing, Thomas Szasz) and sociologists (Erving Goffman) who challenge one or more aspects of the psychiatric medical model of madness. Antipsychiatrists are united only by the object of their critique, not by any common ideology, methodology, or set of beliefs—except, perhaps, the critical spirit of the 1960s, the decade when most of their critiques were published. Foucault's methodology, for example, is "genealogy." Friedrich Nietzsche (1844–1900) pioneered the technique in *Towards a Genealogy of Morals* (1887) when he dug up the history of moral concepts to reveal their "real" nature. In *Folie et déraison* (1961, 1965) Foucault uses the genealogical method to "reveal" that psychiatry's outward humanism masks the Enlightenment's repressive intolerance of unreason, which it construed as "unchained animality [that] could be mastered only by discipline and brutalizing" (Foucault, 1965, pp. 74–75). Thus, in Foucault's analysis, Pinel sought to control unreason by imposing the "patient role" on mad people and by setting up physicians as warders; Pinel did not really unchain the mad, he merely exchanged their fetters, replacing physical manacles with "mind-forg'd manacles" (Porter, 1987, p. xi).

The British psychiatrist R. D. Laing developed an entirely different style of antipsychiatric critique. In the most accessible of his works, *The Politics of Experience* (1967), Laing argues that the phenomenon characterized as "schizophrenia" cannot be an illness because it is not dysfunctional. On the contrary, schizophrenia is really a coping strategy that helps people survive otherwise unlivable situations; it is a mechanism by which the psyche reconstitutes itself, and hence schizophrenia serves as a (frequently successful) form of self-therapy. Ironically, therefore, attempts at "therapeutic" intervention by traditional psychiatrists can actually disrupt the patient's self-curative process. (For a more detailed account see Laing, 1960.)

Thomas Szasz is the best-known American antipsychiatrist theorist. In a 1960 essay, "The Myth of Mental Illness," and in subsequent articles and books, he contrasts the patient–physician relationship in the Hippocratic and the Pinelian medical models. Drawing on Parsons's analysis of the sick role, Szasz points out that in the Hippocratic model, patients seek out physicians in the hope of finding relief from their illnesses. In a sense, therefore, when Hippocratic physicians treat their patients, they are applying their causal knowledge to satisfy the patient's values. On the Pinelian psychiatric model, however, it is often quite different. It is not the mad person who complains of being "sick" and seeks medical assistance; it is others in society who pronounce him or her "sick." Insofar as the pronounced party does not consider himself or herself to be "sick," however, the psychiatric label and any consequent "therapeutic" intervention really amount to others' imposing their values on the "mad" person. This is evident from the psychiatric diagnoses of previous eras. Looking back, it seems apparent that "masturbatory insanity" is really puritanism masquerading as medicine; similarly, Szasz contends, the diagnosis "sexual inversion" is really homophobia in medical guise. In each of these instances, what is nominally "therapy" is really a technique of repression (Baker, 1980; Szasz, 1970).

Szasz argues further that those imposing the sick role are not practicing scientific medicine. Medicine is scientific because its diagnoses rest on intersubjectively observable pathologies; thus a diagnosis of aneurysm or ulcer can be empirically confirmed by X ray or postmortem examination. Physical illnesses, like diabetes, can be diagnosed even when they are asymptomatic. But there are no comparable diagnostic tests for mental illnesses. The psychopathology of other people's minds can never be intersubjectively observed; no one can examine anyone else's thought processes by X ray or postmortem. Psychiatric diagnoses are thus incorrigible: There is no way of demonstrating that a psychiatric diagnosis is wrong. Scientific explanation, however, is always corrigible and subject to empirical disconfirmation. So, Szasz concludes, psychiatry is not a branch of scientific medicine.

Antipsychiatry was enormously influential in the 1960s and 1970s, decades concerned with civil rights and the empowerment of the oppressed. Reformers seeking to release the mentally ill from asylums and treat them in community programs appropriated the rhetoric of antipsychiatry. Antipsychiatric theory was also appropriated by psychologists, social workers, and others who sought to level a mental-health hierarchy dominated by psychiatrists. At the same time, mounting empirical evidence seemed to support the antipsychiatric analysis. Diaries from eastern Europe (e.g., Medvedev and Medvedev, 1971) revealed that Soviet psychiatrists were incarcerating dissidents in mental hospitals as "antisocial personalities"—corroborating the antipsychiatric charge that "mental illness" merely served as a myth to justify the incarceration of social undesirables. In America, David Rosenhan's "On Being Sane in Insane Places" (1973) cast further doubt on the scientific status of psychiatric diagnosis. Rosenhan's experiment tested "labeling theory," the theory that a psychiatric diagnostic label, once applied, tends to stick, even without supporting symptoms (Scheff, 1963; Goffman, 1961). Rosenhan had eight colleagues pose as "pseudo patients" who falsely reported hearing an unclear voice that seemed to say "empty," "hollow," and "thud." Upon admission to hospital, however, the pseudo patients ceased reporting these symptoms. Nonetheless, their hospitalization continued—on average for almost three weeks. Thus, just as the antipsychiatrists contended, psychiatric diagnoses seem to be unconfirmable stigmatizing labels, empty of empirical content.

Although a younger generation continues the critique (Cohen, 1990), antipsychiatry has lost much of its sting. Roy Porter and other historians have challenged Foucault's genealogies. Foucault contends that "sequestering the mad was basically an act of anathematization and quarantine. But [Porter argues] the ideology and expectations typically found in England, from Bedlam to the ritziest asylum, principally endorsed curability—incidentally explaining why *separate* institutions for incurables were set up" (Porter, 1987, p. 280). Even as historians were rethinking the antipsychiatric portrait of psychiatry's past, problems were becoming evident in the present. Antipsychiatrists rejected the insanity defense and had joined with civil libertarians to urge tightening the rules for involuntary commitment to mental institutions. They argued that a diagnosis of mental illness should not provide sufficient grounds for involuntary commitment. Persons deemed mentally ill should be committed to a hospital, against their wishes, only if there was also a legal determination that they posed a danger to themselves or to others.

These reforms were adopted and, throughout the Western world, the walls of the asylums came tumbling down. Thousands of involuntarily committed mentally ill people were found to have been illegally institutionalized and were discharged into their communities. The results were not as beneficial as antipsychiatrists had predicted. Once patients left the hospital, they were free: free of therapeutic supervision, free not to report to clinics for therapy, free not to take their medications. Deinstitutionalized patients availed themselves of these freedoms and consequently tended to become symptomatic, and hence problems for their communities. More tragically still, former mental patients were often unable to cope with the outside world. They swelled the ranks of the homeless and became easy targets for criminals. Ironically, one of the primary effects of deinstitutionalization was to reinvigorate Tuke's moral therapeutic ideal of the asylum as a "quiet haven," a refuge from the world for mad people (Scull, 1977, 1984).

In large measure, however, the antipsychiatric critique lost its sting because the American psychiatric profession appropriated it and used it as a basis for revising its diagnostic and statistical manuals. To appreciate how this came about, it is helpful to reflect on Szasz's critique and the general problem of developing a reliable system of valid psychiatric diagnoses, a nosology.

The validity of psychiatric nosology

Szasz challenges the validity of psychiatric diagnoses on two primary grounds: that they are value-laden, and that they are immune to empirical disconfirmation. Although the first challenge may disturb those who subscribe to the ideal of objective, value-free medicine, contemporary philosophers, in a rare display of unanimity, concur with Szasz's analysis. They are just as unanimous, however, in rejecting Szasz's conclusion: that the mere presence of values invalidates diagnoses. The con-

sensus of philosophical opinion is that all diagnoses are indelibly value-laden (Peset and Gracia, 1992). H. Tristram Engelhardt (1974) believes that medicine (not merely psychiatry) is the systematic deployment of science to eliminate physical or psychological conditions that someone dislikes and therefore dubs "illness." Christopher Boorse (1975) takes the opposite view: "Illness" is systematically incapacitating disease; "disease" is a deviation from the natural or normal functional organization of an individual, or of organic subsystems; these natural functions, in turn, are those designed to ensure the "apical goals" of survival and reproduction. Apical goals, according to Boorse, are the "empirically determined" values of evolutionary survival.

Robert Baker (1978, 1980) argues for a position midway between Engelhardt's entirely subjective conception of illness and Boorse's functionalist analysis. He agrees that all diagnoses contain values, but he denies that every value can be medicalized as a diagnosis. Medicine is a public art; its nosologies aspire to a common diagnostic language. Consequently a disvalued condition can be designated a "symptom" of an "illness" only if: (1) it is potentially incapacitating; (2) the condition is involuntary (an incapacity rather than a choice); and (3) there is a reliable way for practitioners to recognize this condition and its course (its standard pattern of development). Medical nosologies, moreover, classify diseases in terms of underlying causal pathologies. Therefore (4) any characterization of a condition as a "symptom" is effectively an empirically testable causal claim about pathology that, therefore, (5) presupposes a theory of pathology and consequently a theory of normal functionality.

All three of these philosophical positions undercut Szasz's claim that psychiatric diagnoses are invalid because they are value-laden. Consider again the contrast Szasz draws between the supposedly valid diagnosis of diabetes and two "mythical" mental illnesses, masturbatory insanity and homosexuality (or sexual inversion). Engelhardt would agree with Szasz that the diagnoses "masturbatory insanity" and "homosexuality" reflect puritanical social values. In his analysis, however, "diabetes" is also value-laden, since comas violate the Puritan work ethic just as surely as masturbation does. Boorse, in contrast, holds that determinations of illnesses depend on the empirical fact of incapacitation. Insofar as diabetes is typically incapacitating, while homosexuality and masturbation are not, the former is an illness and the latter two are not. Diabetes and homosexuality, however, are both diseases since both are abnormal deviations from the functional norms for organ systems and individuals. On Boorse's account, therefore, Szasz is wrong in arguing that homosexuality is not a disease. It is a disease, even though it is not an illness. However, because homosexuality is not an illness, neither homosexuals nor psychiatrists have a good reason to pursue treatment.

Baker holds that diabetes is a paradigm case of a disease (an incapacitating, diagnosable dysfunction with a clear pathology), and that masturbatory insanity is neither an illness nor a disease, since it is not involuntary, incapacitating, or associated with any pathology. Homosexuality's status is uncertain at present. Whether it is a disease will depend upon whether the condition can be shown to be avolitional, and whether it can be linked to a clear pathology (for example, an atypical gene, like Xq28). Even if these two conditions were to be satisfied, however, homosexuality, like any other illness, would be an illness only if homosexuals found their condition undesirable. Thus although Baker, unlike Boorse and Engelhardt, believes that the status of homosexuality remains open, he, too, states that the presence of values in the diagnosis does not undermine its validity. On this point these three representative philosophers agree: The presence of values in psychiatric diagnoses renders psychiatry neither more nor less problematic than other forms of medicine—all diagnoses are informed by values.

Szasz's second line of critique, however, focuses on an area of real vulnerability: the empirical validation of the psychiatric model. Pinel had established the idea of madness as mental illness in the context of an empiricist critique of Cullen's neurophysiological model. The argument over which model of madness, mental or neurophysiological, is validated by empirical evidence has been raging ever since. Pinel's student Jean-Étienne Dominique Esquirol (1772–1840) published a psychiatric nosology in 1838, and Emil Kraepelin (1856–1926) published his neurophysiologically inclined *Lehrbuch* in 1883; for a while both vied for the honor of being accepted as the psychiatric standard. Kraepelin's neurophysiological nosology appeared to win, but was then supplanted by the psychopathological nosology of Sigmund Freud (1856–1939). Like Pinel, Freud believed both that madness is a form of mental illness and that any psychopathological nosology must be empirically validated by therapeutic success.

Freud and Pinel part company only with respect to their theories of mind and, consequently, their conceptions of psychopathology and treatment. Pinel, like his mentor Locke, had envisioned an entirely conscious mind governed by laws of association. Freud posited an unconscious mind with different components whose interactions change as a person matures. The resulting psychodynamic model offers rich possibilities for psychopathology and psychotherapy, so Freudian nosology rapidly eclipsed those of Esquirol and Kraepelin. Unlike Pinel's moral therapy, however, no one empirically established the superior curative efficacy of Freudian therapy. Psychodynamic models and therapeutic techniques became standard in psychiatry by virtue of their theoretical richness, not on the basis of empirical validation. They are thus vulnerable to the charge, not only from antipsychiatrists but also from respected philosophers of science (for example, Grünbaum, 1984), that they lack empirical validity.

Reliability and the creation of standard psychiatric nosologies (DSM, ICD)

Diagnoses, nosologies, and the issues surrounding them are important to anyone attempting to count, to analyze, to indemnify, or to do research on illness. They are thus crucial not only to practitioners but also to census bureaus, to statisticians, to insurance companies, and to scientists. All of these parties would prefer to work with valid diagnoses, but they appreciate that validity is elusive. At a minimum, however, they need to work with reliable diagnoses. The difference between *validity* and *reliability* is as follows: A diagnosis is *valid* to the extent that it accurately differentiates one form of illness from another; a diagnosis is *reliable* to the extent that different practitioners will diagnose identical cases in the same way. If a diagnosis is unreliable, it cannot be valid; it is, moreover, useless for all administrative, therapeutic, or research purposes. In the 1890s various international committees recognized that reliability is a prelude to validity and tried to develop a single, universal standard list of causes of death.

In the 1920s the League of Nations began to publish a standard international nosology, and the task was continued by the World Health Organization (WHO). The first *International List of Causes of Death* (ICD-1) excluded mental illnesses because they are not significant causes of death. In 1948, however, the WHO expanded its list to include all diseases and disorders, and began to list mental disorders in the section "Diseases of the Nervous System and Sense Organs." As the title indicates, the 1948 ICD nosology was neurophysiological; so was the revised list issued in 1955. By the 1950s, however, almost all psychiatric practitioners were using psychodynamic diagnoses. To remedy the situation, in 1952 the American Psychiatric Association (APA) played Pinel to the WHO's Cullen, and produced its *Diagnostic and Statistical Manual* (DSM-I) based on commonly used psychodynamic diagnoses. The manual was updated in 1968 (DSM-II). The WHO introduced psychodynamic concepts into ICD-9 (1977). By the end of the 1970s there were thus two "official" psychiatric nosologies, DSM-II and ICD-9.

Both DSM-II and ICD-9 were criticized by gay activists for classifying homosexuality as a sexual abnormality. ICD-9, for example, classifies homosexuality as a sexual deviation because "[S]exual activity directed primarily towards people not of the opposite sex" cannot "serve approved social and biological purposes" (WHO,

1977, 302.0). This explanation presumes (as Engelhardt does) that society can stigmatize what it disapproves as a "disorder," and presupposes (as Boorse does) that the function of sexual intercourse is procreation, not recreation, not bonding, not even expressing love. Since homosexual intercourse is neither socially approved nor procreative, it follows that it is dysfunctional. DSM-II, while not as blatantly judgmental, also listed homosexuality as a disorder. Gay psychiatrists contested these classifications, protesting that since their homosexuality did not impair their functionality, that is, their ability to function in the world, they could not be sick. Their protests attracted the attention of psychiatrist Robert Spitzer, one of the authors of DSM-II and a member of the committee revising the DSM nosology, who subsequently proposed a new diagnosis to the Nomenclature Committee, "sexual orientation disturbance." If a homosexual was disturbed by his or her sexual orientation to the point that it impaired his or her ability to function, he or she suffered "sexual orientation disturbance," otherwise not (Bayer, 1981; note the similarity to Baker's analysis). In 1973 the APA's trustees approved the diagnosis, acting on a vote of the members: 58 percent in favor, 37 percent against.

DSM-III and DSM-III-R

Spitzer's successful resolution of the debate over homosexuality inspired the strategy that guided the creation of DSM-III and its revision, DSM-III-R. He had resolved the debate not by arguing over the value-laden question of the function of sexual intercourse but by focusing on the empirical questions of functionality: Can homosexuals function well in our society? Answering yes (provided they themselves are not disturbed by their sexual orientation), he concluded that homosexuality per se is not a disorder. In DSM-III and III-R this solution is generalized to all diagnoses in an attempt to resolve the perpetual nosological disputes between the neurophysiological, psychopathological, and behavioral theories of madness that had vexed psychiatry since its founding in the eighteenth century.

> [1] In DSM-III-R each of the mental disorders is conceptualized as a clinically significant behavioral or psychological syndrome or pattern that occurs in a person and is associated with present distress (impairment in one or more important areas of functioning) or with a significantly increased risk of suffering, death, pain, disability, or an important loss of freedom. [2] In addition, this syndrome or pattern must not be an expectable response to a particular event, e.g., the death of a loved one. [3] Whatever its original cause, it must currently be considered a manifestation of behavioral, psychological, or biological dysfunction in the person. [4] Neither deviant behavior, e.g., political, religious, or sexual, nor conflicts that are primarily between the individual

and society are mental disorders, unless the deviance or conflict is a symptom of a dysfunction in the person, as described above. (American Psychiatric Association, 1987, p. xxii [numbers added])

In this passage the DSM declares its ideological neutrality by the condescending ecumenism of [3] that relegates the three classic accounts of madness, "behavioral, psychological or biological dysfunction," to mere "consider[ations]." Point [1], in contrast, declares the DSM's new approach: "Disorders" are to be defined exclusively in terms of observable behaviors—"distress (impairment . . . in functioning) or . . . increased risk of suffering death, pain, disability or . . . loss of freedom."

The DSM-III definition not only attempts to pacify disputes between different schools of psychiatry, it also responds directly to the antipsychiatric critique. Point [4] explicitly lists, and expressly excludes, the abuses that the antipsychiatric critics had documented. Strictly speaking, this list is redundant because the medicalization of political, religious, and sexual conflicts between individuals and society are ruled out by the criteria set forth in [1]; that is, unless a person is distressed, incapable of functioning, or at increased risk of death, he or she cannot be diagnosed as ill by DSM-III-R criteria, however distasteful a society finds her or his politics, religion, or sexual orientation. Yet Szasz and other critics of psychiatry had documented the abuses of psychiatry so effectively that redundancy must have appeared more prudent than elegant. Thus, although [1] effectively appropriates the antipsychiatric critique, [4] explicitly accommodates it.

DSM-III and its successor, DSM-III-R, thus defuse the major external criticisms of psychiatry while rendering quiescent, at the nosological level, the theoretical disputes that previously had divided the profession. It answered the need of its time, providing a theory-neutral, externally observable, nonrepressive, seemingly reliable nosology; it currently enjoys worldwide acceptance by psychologists and psychiatrists of all schools of thought.

Despite their undeniable successes, DSM-III and IIIR are not without problems. One of the factors that motivated the revision of DSM-II was that empirical researchers, of all theoretical stripes, had found DSM-II's diagnostic categories unreliable (Kirk and Kutchins, 1992). Spitzer was one of the first to appreciate the gravity of these findings: "The validity, i.e., the usefulness, of a classification system is limited by its reliability. Therefore, to the extent that a classification system of psychiatric disorders is unreliable, a limit is placed on its validity for any clinical research or administrative use" (Spitzer et al., 1975, pp. 210–211). To resolve the problem of reliability, Spitzer devised a standardized "checklist" system of diagnosis, which was used extensively in DSM-III and then revised, after extensive field testing, for DSM-III-R. Nonetheless, psychiatrists and other professionals still found the diagnostic checklists difficult to use. Stuart Kirk and Herb Kutchins have analyzed all published empirical studies of the reliability of DSM-III and DSM-III-R diagnoses and concluded that they are no more reliable than their predecessor, DSM-II. Since Spitzer had claimed that DSM-II was so unreliable that it verged on uselessness, they argue that the same thing can be said of DSM-III.

Other critics urge a return to traditional nosological patterns of classification in DSM-II and ICD-9. This argument is usually parsed as the claim that DSM-III and DSM-III-R sacrifice validity to reliability (Eysenck, 1986; Kirk and Kutchins, 1992; Wakenfeld, 1992a, 1992b). These appeals to "validity" are odd because no one—not Cullen, not Pinel, not Esquirol, not Kraepelin, not Freud—has developed an empirically validated theory of physiopathology or psychopathology. What they did, however, was offer theoretically grounded diagnoses that made intuitive sense to those familiar with their theories. DSM-III and its successors take an atheoretical stance on diagnosis and thus deliberately sacrifice the intuitive clarity that these theories provide. Whether the sacrifice is worthwhile will depend upon whether DSM-IV generates reliable diagnoses.

Bioethical implications

Ethics presupposes conflict. In the absence of any possibility of conflict, there is no need for ethics. As a rich source of potential conflicts between, on the one hand, patients' desires, goals, interests, and values, and, on the other hand, physicians' therapeutic goals, entrepreneurial interests, and traditional values, the patient–physician encounter has inspired an equally rich body of ethics. Most of the conflicts dealt with in medical ethics are unmistakable. We may not know the proper way to deal with a Jehovah's Witness who refuses a lifesaving blood transfusion, we may not know how to respond to the dying cancer patient who requests assisted suicide, or to the family of a patient in a persistent and irreversible vegetative state who, nonetheless, assert the patient's "right" to the last bed in the intensive-care unit (knowing that to do so will deprive other, potentially curable, patients of a bed); but in each of these cases, we know, unmistakably, that we are caught up in a conflict. Psychiatric ethics is no different. We may not know how to deal with a patient's declaration of an intent to kill some innocent third party, but the conflict between the duty to protect patient confidentiality and duty to warn an innocent third party is unmistakable.

Psychiatric diagnoses, however, have the insidious property of anesthetizing our sense of conflict; they tend to disguise moral issues in medical terminology. Masturbation, for example, is considered sinful by the three great Middle Eastern religions: Christianity, Islam, and Judaism. The practice is a battleground between the sacred spark religion finds in the human body and the profane uses to which real people put their bodies. The conflict between sacred and profane conceptions of the body, however, is unmistakably that: a conflict. When Freud and other psychiatrists medicalized the sin of onanism (named for Onan, whom God condemned for spilling his seed on the ground; Gen. 38:9), it dulled our sense of conflicting values. Masturbation was no longer condemned as sinful; it was a disease called onanism. Benjamin Rush used "The Tranquilizer" on masturbators; later physicians sometimes recommended surgery, including scarification of the penis and clitoridectomies—removal of the clitoris (see Barker-Benfield, 1976, for details). It is easy to look askance, and even in anger, at the extremity of these treatments. The more subtle point to appreciate, however, is that only the creation of a diagnosis, only medicalization, made these extreme measures permissible. No eighteenth-, nineteenth-, or twentieth-century Western religion claimed the right to immobilize a masturbator, or to scarify his penis, or to remove her clitoris, or to commit her or him to an institution, or even to require counseling. Only medicine could exercise this kind of power; individuals and society would tolerate these treatments only in the name of therapy.

This article has used the genealogical method, not to delegitimate psychiatry (as Foucault and Szasz have attempted to do) but to illuminate the extent to which psychiatric diagnoses encapsulate values, and to suggest how medicalization desensitizes ethical concerns. Most classical nosologists (Cullen, Esquirol, Freud, Kraepelin, Pinel) treated psychiatric diagnoses as objective and value-free; contemporary analysts and nosologists (APA, Baker, Boorse, Engelhardt, Foucault, Parsons, Porter, Spitzer, Szasz, WHO) appreciate that values play an inextricable role in diagnosis. Once the role of values is recognized, we must face the question of how best to handle the value conflicts inherent in psychiatric diagnoses. Do we avoid conflicts by abolishing psychiatric diagnoses altogether, as Szasz recommends? Do we presume that society's values ought properly to prevail over those of the individual, as the WHO appears to do in ICD-9? Or do we bring these conflicts to the surface and attempt to accommodate a compromise between individual and societal values, as the APA attempted to do in DSM-III and III-R? Or is some other form of resolution possible?

ROBERT BAKER

Directly related to this article are the other articles in this entry: CROSS-CULTURAL PERSPECTIVES, *and* ISSUES IN DIAGNOSIS. *For further discussion of topics mentioned in this article, see the entries* COMMITMENT TO MENTAL INSTITUTIONS; INSTITUTIONALIZATION AND DEINSTITUTIONALIZATION;

LAW AND BIOETHICS; PROFESSIONAL–PATIENT RELATIONSHIP, article on HISTORICAL PERSPECTIVES; and PSYCHIATRY, ABUSES OF. For a discussion of related ideas, see the entries INTERPRETATION; MENTAL HEALTH, article on MEANING OF MENTAL HEALTH; MENTAL-HEALTH THERAPIES; PSYCHOANALYSIS AND DYNAMIC THERAPIES; and VALUE AND VALUATION.

Bibliography

ADAMS, DAVID. 1992. *Philosophical Problems in the Law.* Belmont, Calif.: Wadsworth. A particularly accessible, well-edited introduction to the philosophy of law.

AMERICAN LAW INSTITUTE. 1957. *Model Penal Code: Reprint. Tentative Drafts Nos. 5, 6, and 7.* Philadelphia: Author.

AMERICAN PSYCHIATRIC ASSOCIATION. 1952, 1968, 1980, 1987. *Diagnostic and Statistical Manual of Mental Disorders.* Washington, D.C.: Author. 1st–rev. 3d eds., referred to as DSM-I, DSM-II, DSM-III, and DSM-III-R. Internationally recognized standard classifications of mental disorders. DSM-IV was published in 1994.

BAKER, ROBERT. 1978. "Mental Illness: Conceptions of Mental Illness." In *Encyclopedia of Bioethics*, vol. 3, pp. 1090–1097. Edited by Warren Reich. New York: Free Press, Macmillan.

———. 1980. "Thomas Szasz, Founder of the Philosophy of Psychiatry." In *Proceedings of Asclepius at Syracuse: Thomas Szasz, Libertarian Humanist*, vol. 1, pp. 292–313. Edited by M. E. Grenander. Albany: Institute for Humanistic Studies, State University of New York.

BARKER-BENFIELD, G. J. 1976. *The Horrors of the Half-Known Life: Male Attitudes Toward Women and Sexuality in Nineteenth-Century America.* New York: Harper & Row.

BATTIE, WILLIAM. 1962. [1758]. *A Treatise on Madness.* Facsimile edited by Richard Hunter and Ida Macalpine. Psychiatric Monograph series, no. 3. London: Dawson's. 1st ed. London: Whiston and White.

BAYER, RONALD. 1987. [1981]. *Homosexuality and American Psychiatry: The Politics of Diagnosis.* Princeton, N.J.: Princeton University Press. The definitive account of the American Psychiatric Association's decision that homosexuality is not a disorder.

BENEDICT, RUTH. 1966. "Anthropology and the Abnormal." In *Issues and Problems in Social Psychiatry*, pp. 17–38. Edited by Bernard J. Bergen and Claudewell S. Thomas. Springfield, Ill.: Charles C. Thomas. The standard account of the cultural variability of "abnormality."

BOORSE, CHRISTOPHER. 1975. "On the Distinction Between Disease and Illness." *Philosophy and Public Affairs* 5, no. 1:49–68.

BYNUM, WILLIAM F. 1985. "The Nervous Patient in Eighteenth and Nineteenth Century Britain: The Psychiatric Origins of British Neurology." In *The Anatomy of Madness*, vol. 1, *People and Ideas*, pp. 89–102. Edited by William F. Bynum, Roy Porter, and Michael Shepard. London: Tavistock. An overview of the development of neurological models of madness, in an excellent two-volume collection of recent work by historians of psychiatry.

CAPLAN, ARTHUR L.; ENGELHARDT, H. TRISTRAM, JR.; and

McCARTNEY, JAMES J., eds. 1981. *Concepts of Health and Disease: Interdisciplinary Perspectives.* Reading, Mass.: Addison-Wesley. A collection of some of the best essays in the philosophy of medicine.

COHEN, D., ed. 1990. "Challenging the Therapeutic State: Critical Perspectives on Psychiatry and the Mental Health System." *Journal of Mind and Behavior* 11, nos. 3–4. Special Issue.

Durham v. United States. 1954. 214 F. 2d 862.

ENGELHARDT, H. TRISTRAM, JR. 1974. "The Disease of Masturbation: Values and the Concept of Disease." *Bulletin of the History of Medicine* 48, no. 2:234–248.

EYSENCK, HANS JURGEN. 1986. "A Critique of Contemporary Classification and Diagnosis." In *Contemporary Directions in Psychopathology: Toward the DSM-IV*, pp. 73–98. Edited by Theodore Millon and Gerald L. Klerman. New York: Guilford.

FOUCAULT, MICHEL. 1961. *Folie et déraison: Histoire de la folie à l'âge classique.* Paris: Librairie Plon. Translated by Richard Howard as *Madness and Civilization: A History of Insanity in the Age of Reason.* New York: Pantheon Books, 1965. A compelling antipsychiatric genealogical study of the birth of psychiatry.

GOFFMAN, ERVING. 1961. *Asylums: Essays on the Social Institution of Mental Patients and Other Inmates.* Garden City, N.Y.: Doubleday.

GRÜNBAUM, ADOLPH. 1984. *The Foundations of Psychoanalysis: A Philosophical Critique.* Berkeley: University of California Press. A comprehensive analysis of the logical and epistemological foundations of psychoanalysis by a famous philosopher of science.

HART, HERBERT L. A. 1961. *The Concept of Law.* Oxford: At the Clarendon Press. A classic study.

HIPPOCRATES. 1923–1931. *Hippocrates: Collected Works.* 4 vols. Translated by W. H. S. Jones. Loeb Classical Library. New York: G. P. Putnam's Sons.

HUNTER, RICHARD, and MACALPINE, IDA. 1963. *Three Hundred Years of Psychiatry, 1535–1860.* London: Oxford University Press. A wonderful documentary history designed to introduce readers to psychiatry before Freud.

KIRK, STUART A., and KUTCHINS, HERB. 1992. *The Selling of DSM: The Rhetoric of Science in Psychiatry.* New York: Aldine de Gruyter. A sociological critique of DSM-III.

LAING, RONALD DAVID. 1960. *The Divided Self: An Existential Study of Sanity and Madness.* London: Tavistock. New York: Pantheon, 1969.

———. 1967. *The Politics of Experience.* New York: Pantheon.

LANGLAND, WILLIAM. 1886. [1380]. *The Vision of William Concerning Piers the Plowman.* Edited by W. W. Skeat. Early English Text Society. London: Oxford University Press.

MEDVEDEV, ZHORES, and MEDVEDEV, ROY. 1971. *A Question of Madness.* London: Macmillan.

OFFER, DANIEL, and SABSHIN, MELVIN. 1966. *Normality: Theoretical and Clinical Concepts of Mental Health.* New York: Basic Books. A classic study of "normality."

PARSONS, TALCOTT. 1951. *The Social System.* Glencoe, Ill.: Free Press. Still the foundation for the sociological study of illness; see especially pp. 428–479.

———. 1958. "Definitions of Health and Illness in the Light of American Values and Social Structure." In *Patients,*

Physicians and Illness: A Sourcebook in Behavioral Science and Health, pp. 165–187. Edited by E. Gartly Jaco. Glencoe, Ill.: Free Press.

PESET, JOSÉ, and GRACIA, DIEGO, eds. 1992. *The Ethics of Diagnosis*. Dordrecht, Netherlands: Kluwer Academic. A comprehensive overview of the role of values in diagnosis.

PERCIVAL, THOMAS. 1985. [1803]. *Medical Ethics; or, A Code of Institutes and Precepts, Adapted to the Professional Conduct of Physicians and Surgeons*. Manchester: S. Russell for J. Johnson and R. Bickerstaff. Facsimile reissue, with an introduction by Edmund D. Pellegrino. Birmingham, Ala.: Classics of Medicine Library.

PINEL, PHILIPPE. 1801. *Traité médico-philosophique sur l'aliénation mentale, ou la manie*. Paris: Richard. Translated by David D. Davis as *A Treatise on Insanity, in Which Are Contained the Principles of a New and More Practical Nosology of Maniacal Disorders Than Has Yet Been Offered to the Public*. London: Cadell and Davis, 1806. Facsimile edition, New York Academy of Medicine, History of Medicine Series, no. 14. New York: Hafner, 1962.

PORTER, ROY. 1987. *Mind-Forg'd Manacles: A History of Madness in England from the Restoration to the Regency*. Cambridge, Mass.: Harvard University Press. A well-written, historiographically sensitive history of Enlightenment psychiatry that challenges antipsychiatric genealogies.

ROSENHAN, DAVID. 1973. "On Being Sane in Insane Places." *Science* 179, no. 7:250–258. A frequently cited, insightful, and frightening study of psychiatric diagnosis as labeling.

ROTHMAN, DAVID J. 1971. *The Discovery of the Asylum: Social Order and Disorder in the New Republic*. Boston: Little, Brown. A well-researched antipsychiatric history of asylums.

SCHEFF, THOMAS J. 1963. "The Role of the Mentally Ill and the Dynamics of Mental Disorder: A Research Framework." *Sociometry* 26, no. 4:436–453. A classic statement of labeling theory.

SCULL, ANDREW T. 1977. *Decarceration*. Englewood Cliffs, N.J.: Prentice-Hall. 2d ed. Cambridge: Oxford Polity Press, 1984. A definitive study of deinstitutionalization's failures.

SPITZER, ROBERT L.; ENDICOTT, JEAN; and ROBINS, ELI. 1975. "Clinical Criteria of Psychiatric Diagnosis and DSM-III." *American Journal of Psychiatry* 132, no. 11:1187–1192.

SZASZ, THOMAS S. 1960. "The Myth of Mental Illness." *American Psychologist* 15:113–118.

———. 1970. *The Manufacture of Madness: A Comparative Study of the Inquisition and the Mental Health Movement*. New York: Harper & Row.

WAKEFIELD, JEROME C. 1992a. "The Concept of Mental Disorder: On the Boundary Between Biological Facts and Social Values." *American Psychologist* 47, no. 3:373–388.

———. 1992b. "Disorder as Harmful Dysfunction: A Conceptual Critique of DSM-III-R's Definition of Mental Disorder." *Psychological Review* 99, no. 2:232–247. This and the preceding item are exceptionally insightful analyses of DSM-III and DSM-III-R.

WASSERSTROM, RICHARD A. 1980. "The Therapeutic Model." In *Philosophical Problems in the Law*, pp. 493–498. Edited by David M. Adams. Belmont, Calif.: Wadsworth.

WORLD HEALTH ORGANIZATION. 1939. *Manual of the International List of Causes of Death*. 5th rev. Geneva: Author.

———. 1948, 1955, 1969, 1977. *Manual of the International Statistical Classification of Diseases, Injuries and Causes of Death*. 6th, 7th, 8th, and 9th revs. Geneva: Author. Referred to as ICD, this classificatory scheme rivals DSM; ICD-9 classifies homosexuality as a mental disorder.

II. CROSS-CULTURAL PERSPECTIVES

Medical anthropology and professional psychiatries

Anthropology is the science of humankind and its cultures. Its four branches treat humans as bearers of extinct cultures (archaeology), as a part of the study of primate evolution and behavior (physical or biological anthropology), as language-using beings (linguistic anthropology), and as cultural beings (social and cultural anthropology). In the latter field, scholars traditionally focused on such aspects of culture as kinship, economics, law, politics, psychology, art, religion, and, more recently, medical and psychiatric systems. Many scholars now view these categories not so much as real entities but as cultural creations that are real only to Western observers. This view derives from the cross-cultural nature of anthropology. Long-term research among the world's cultures throws into relief the created nature of categorical realities. At the same time, it highlights the culturally constructed nature of our own realities, whether lay, scientific, or psychiatric.

Both biological and social/cultural anthropologists study health, illness, and medical systems around the world. Biological anthropologists tend to use U.S. or other medical concepts and research strategies. Many social/cultural medical anthropologists also use these in "ethnomedical" and "ethnopsychiatric" studies (those concerned with specific cultural or ethnic forms of medicine or psychiatry). However, a substantial and growing number of scholars employ interpretive social science both to study folk systems and to reflect upon received scientific medical/psychiatric knowledge.

Interpretive social science replaces traditional scientific conceptions of cause and effect, and universal laws that claim to explain all human behavior, with approaches that self-consciously seek to interpret human, including scientific, realities. These realities are seen as creations or constructions that make sense "locally," that is, in specific contexts. In medical anthropology, the term "cultural constructivism" has been applied to interpretive perspectives focused on medical/psychiatry systems (Gaines, 1992a), and it is so used here. This perspective allows one to see both professional and folk psychiatries as ethnopsychiatries. Constructivism suggests that psychiatry, or any human phenomenon, is a problematic but locally meaningful reality. Cultured phenomena are historical constructions that are constituted by forms of discourse (Gaines, 1991).

Constructivist perspectives show affinities to the history and the philosophy of science, and to gender studies, which penetrate the veneer of science to reveal its cultural assumptions about madness, nature, the life course, suffering, biology, identity, gender, and language, among other things (Duster, 1990; Gaines, 1992a; Gaines and Farmer, 1986; Gilman, 1988; Hacking, 1983; Fausto-Sterling, 1992; Kleinman and Good, 1985). Medical anthropology has added to these debates with ethnographic studies of healers, researchers, and patients in their cultural contexts (Gaines, 1992a; Hahn and Gaines, 1985; Kleinman, 1988; Marsella and White, 1982).

The term "culture" is used as a shorthand way of referring to the ideological and behavioral systems of the world's societies, to their distinctive views of self, disorder, society, life, death, morality, time, spirits, human nature, and even disease. These conceptions are embodied and expressed in symbols. Symbols include words, aesthetics, acts, rituals, gestures, stories, events, and persons (Geertz, 1973).

Each professional psychiatric tradition embodies culturally particular beliefs and values, as do popular ethnopsychiatries, and it represents these as natural realities. Because we are dealing with distinct systems, not mere versions of one unitary psychiatry, the plural terms "psychiatries" and "ethnopsychiatries" are used here (Gaines, 1992a).

This review of cross-cultural studies of mental illness will not simply catalog an array of exotic disorders from the world's folk societies. Nor will it try to classify them according to U.S. psychiatric standards, that is, attempt to show that the exotic disorders of traditional societies are really the same as home-grown varieties (e.g., Simons and Hughes, 1985). Instead, we will focus on "professional ethnopsychiatries," or culturally constructed professional psychiatries. Their distinctiveness suggests that they are cultural constructions, rather than the same psychiatry practiced in different countries.

The fact that popular and professional psychiatries are local, not universal, compels us to pose the question, "What are the ethical problems generated by the application of one cultural psychiatric theory to members of distinct cultures in plural societies?" In order to suggest some dimensions of this problem, we will consider the nature of mental illness from the vantage point of various professional psychiatries.

Problems of medical knowledge. The view that psychiatric illness is universal is not without problems. It must eschew culture as a formative influence. It also must assume that disorders have similar natures that are everywhere expressed. To make this argument, one might say that psychiatric disorders are biologically

based (biochemical, genetic) and so are beyond culture. If this view is correct, the same disorders should be identified and treated in all the world's professional psychiatries. While there might be some marginal phenomena that exist only locally, certainly we would not expect to find numbers of particular disorders or many cases of specific problems appearing only in one psychiatry and not in others. In this view, professional psychiatries, including that of the United States, assume that the illnesses they recognize are real, natural, and empirical entities. A psychiatry "discovers" these entities, names them, and then classifies them. The labeled phenomena exist apart from their labels. Psychiatry, like science everywhere in the West, takes its labels for phenomena as real things rather than as what they are, models of a reality (Geertz, 1973) or representations (Hacking, 1983) of a reality that are used for particular purposes.

The view that disease labels correspond to entities that exist independently in the natural world is itself shaped by culture; it is not a factual description. But when differences in disease entities or in the systems of classification (nosologies) across cultures are found, psychiatrists assume these differences indicate that universal diseases are overlooked, mislabeled, or differently labeled by less sophisticated others. When professional psychiatries disagree, they assert that one is more advanced than the other (Payer, 1989). However, cultures change historically because of contact with and borrowing from other cultures and through innovation, that is, they differ because of their unique histories. They do not differ because they represent distinct developmental stages of a single human culture.

Psychiatries: Are mental illnesses natural and universal?

Psychiatry in the United States. We may begin our comparative look at professional ethnopsychiatric realities with anorexia nervosa in U.S. psychiatry. This potentially fatal disorder is widely found among middle- and upper-income Euro-American women; it is rare outside of this rather narrow sociocultural context. Key features of the disorder—fear of obesity and distorted body image in the very thin—are not found in cross-cultural work (American Psychiatric Association [APA], 1994). Researchers then suggest dropping these symptoms that are definitive in the United States. However, this presents questions about whether or not one would find the same disorder with different symptoms when the disorder is known by its symptoms.

Chronic fatigue syndrome (CFS) is a disorder for which a biological cause has not been found. Yet it was and is referred to as if a somatic cause had been isolated as either chronic Epstein-Barr virus infection or immune dysfunction syndrome. CFS, fairly common in the

United States, is not found in other cultures. Multiple personality disorder is another condition found not uncommonly in the United States. It is invoked in criminal trials as a legal defense (e.g., unsuccessfully in the case of the Hillside Strangler) and in films (*Three Faces of Eve*) as well as in soap operas. Despite its salience in the United States, the disorder is absent from the classifications and practice of other professional psychiatries and appears as a new phenomenon even in the West.

Two new personality disorders appeared in an appendix to the APA's *Diagnostic and Statistical Manual of Mental Disorders* (*DSM-III-R*) (APA, 1987). Dependent personality disorder is said to be found among women who "allow" physical abuse over time; sadistic personality disorder is found among the men who abuse women. There was considerable political opposition to the formulation of these two disorders, which blame female victims of abuse while giving their abusers a legal defense. The gender component of these personality disorders reflects the history of U.S. psychiatry, wherein traditional notions of women's nature ("weak, fit only for child rearing, housework") were upheld by psychiatric findings, as were racist notions about minorities (Fausto-Sterling, 1992; Thomas and Sillen, 1976). A more explicitly racist contemporary psychiatry is that of South Africa, which, like earlier U.S. psychiatry, attributes a lower psychological and psychiatric evolutionary status to "nonwhites" (Swartz, 1992).

These disorders appear to have been defined in terms of the dominant U.S. culture, which is that of a numerical minority cultural group. This northern European Protestant tradition stresses self-control and autonomy, and it has high expectations of personal productivity and accomplishment. Add to these the role of gender (mis)conceptions, and these disorders mirror a decidedly local cultural picture.

Chinese psychiatry. Chinese psychiatry was borrowed from the West but drew from classical Chinese medicine as well (Kleinman, 1988; Wu, 1982). A number of disorders in China are unknown elsewhere. *Qigong* reaction is an acute episode following a too intense involvement in the *qi-gong* exercise and breathing practices used to promote health and long life. Neither the condition nor the health practice is known to U.S. psychiatry. *Shenjing shuairuo* (neurasthenia) is the most common psychiatric diagnosis in China (Kleinman, 1988; APA, 1994). It is also found widely in areas of Chinese influence. It was borrowed from the United States, where the term was developed in the nineteenth century and long ago fell into disuse, as did the notion of the disease it labeled (Kleinman, 1988).

A third disorder is *koro*, an acute episodic event with intense concern and anxiety about the withdrawal of the external genitalia into the body. A key part of the context of this disorder is the Chinese cultural belief that the genitals of the dead recede into the body. *Koro* is found in China and Southeast Asia, where there have been widespread occurrences of the disorder.

In Chinese psychiatry in general, psychological explanations are discounted and are not regarded as sensible explanations of suffering (Kleinman, 1988; Kleinman and Good, 1985). Patients who seek help complain almost exclusively of somatic (bodily) symptoms such as *koro*. Optimal intervention is also somatic, often involving herbal medicines designed to enhance or unblock the passage of vital energies. This practice is related to the traditional Ayurvedic (Indian) professional psychiatric theory, according to which mental phenomena are expressions of bodily states, not psychological dynamics. India's professional psychiatry is entirely somatopsychic, where the body changes the mind, not psychosomatic or psychological.

Japanese psychiatry. In Japanese psychiatry, two important disorders widely known in practice and in society—*shinkeishitsu* and *taijin kyofusho*—are called social phobias. *Taijin kyofusho* is an extreme concern over actions or personal hygiene that could be disturbing or disrespectful to others. *Shinkeishitsu* is characterized by shyness, tensions in social relations, feelings of inferiority, and concerns with failure to maintain appropriate interactions. It is treated successfully by Morita psychotherapy, which is a blend of Buddhism, German psychiatry, and understanding of Japanese popular life and its pressures. It is administered on an in-patient basis or, in more serious cases, in hospitals dedicated to the treatment of *shinkeishitsu*. In-patient treatments for this and most other disorders serious enough to warrant hospitalization are much longer than in the United States. This longer stay is expected by patients, who see the hospital as a second home and the psychiatrist as a teacher (Lock, 1980; Nomura, 1992).

Among several new disorders recognized by Japanese psychiatry, housewife syndrome and school refusal syndrome relate to pressures for achievement and success, and the relationship of the individual to the group in Japanese society and culture. In both China and Japan, the enormous importance of harmony, right role performance, and the social nature of the person are clear. The cultural context, as in the United States, appears to create and to provide solutions for specific problems.

German psychiatry. In Germany, research has demonstrated the striking parallel between lay beliefs about mental illness and those of the mental health professionals (Townsend, 1978). Both laypersons and professionals believe that there are two basic types of mental illness, *Gemütskrankheit* (emotional sickness), which is transient and caused by outside events, and *Geisteskrankheit* (mental sickness), which is said to be inherited, chronic, and not amenable to treatment.

Since the nineteenth century, German psychiatry has sought to formulate biological notions of serious mental illness. In this attempt, it has influenced many other psychiatric systems. Psychiatry here makes a sharp dichotomy between the ill and the well that greatly affects diagnosis and treatment. Mental patients are "different" kinds of people; they are biologically defective. Many of the family studies focusing on inheritance of mental disorders have been done in Germany and Scandinavia, the latter sharing, in general, the German materialist position (Townsend, 1978).

This biological notion was central to the mental hygiene movement of the Third Reich that led to the killing of tens of thousands of mentally ill and retarded patients. An additional part of that ideology was the assertion that certain groups of people, so-called races (e.g., Jews, Slavs, Arabs, Gypsies, Celts, Gauls, Latins, Africans, and people from Asia), although not insane, were nonetheless defective. In that ideology, defective meant non-German and expendable.

Soviet psychiatry.   Before the dissolution of the Soviet Union, psychiatric practice was greatly influenced by German psychiatry and its materialist approach. Also influenced by Ivan Pavlov, Russian psychiatry banned psychological and psychoanalytic approaches. Marxist ideology attributed madness and other problems to the evils of nonsocialist economic systems. Since individuals manifested mental disturbances long after the 1917 Bolshevik (Communist) Revolution, the causes had to be personal and internal, not social or economic.

The Soviet psychiatric establishment described a unique form of schizophrenia, creeping schizophrenia, the symptoms of which were usually noncomformity and/or dislike of expected work duties. Diagnosis could lead to long hospital stays and the forced administration of powerful drugs. The political role in psychiatry is obvious here, but it is not lacking in other traditions whose popular notions about mental illness are replicated through their psychiatries.

French psychiatry.   French psychiatry identifies and treats several disorders not known in the United States or elsewhere. The practice of psychiatry, like the society around it, is hierarchical and somewhat authoritarian (Hershel, 1992). Psychiatry here developed a nonphysical notion of mental disorders in the late 1790s and thus did not entirely adopt German biological theorizing. Unlike other psychiatric establishments in the West, French psychiatry has historically been intimately connected with the political state.

Theorizing about and diagnosing their unique illnesses, *spasmophilie* (literally, prone to spasms but referring to a variety of vague, nonspecific complaints including tiredness, loss of appetite, and various somatic complaints) and *triste* (or *fatigué*) *tout le temps* (chronic sadness/tiredness, as a result of a great loss), French ethnopsychiatry expresses its culture's notions of the burden and exquisite sadness of life (Gaines and Farmer, 1986; Gaines, 1991). French psychotherapies, including psychoanalytic, aim not at change but at recognition and acceptance of the historical self.

The cross-cultural record on professional psychiatries briefly considered here undermines the case for a universal list of psychiatric diseases, theories, or practices. In U.S. psychopathology, depression and schizophrenia are the disorders on which the bulk of energy is spent. Since these are highly researched and elaborated, a consideration of them should clarify the sources and nature of the two best-known, perhaps universal, mental illnesses.

Depression and schizophrenia

Depression and schizophrenia are held up by biological psychiatry as models of biogenetic mental diseases. However, the cross-cultural literature and epidemiological studies challenge that assertion (Blue and Gaines, 1992; Kleinman and Good, 1985; Kleinman, 1988; World Health Organization [WHO], 1979). Indeed, the formulations of these disorders in the West have been shown to conceal, albeit not very well, powerful unscientific cultural and moral assumptions about emotion, autonomy, sex and gender, and ethnic and "racial" human differences (Gaines, 1992a, 1992b; Kleinman and Good, 1985).

To appreciate fully how the formulations of depression and schizophrenia conceal such assumptions, it is helpful first to consider certain key psychological dimensions, themselves culturally defined, that underlie any normal or abnormal state. The dimensions are constructions of self, emotion, and cognition.

Self.   Self conceptions vary widely. They may include spiritual elements. For example, in Bali it is common for people to have spirit siblings who keep track of and speak to them or other spirit familiars. While this belief is thought quite normal in Bali (Conner, in Marsella and White, 1982), such beliefs and behavior would be seen as frankly pathological in the United States.

By U.S. psychiatric standards, formulations of self in India, the Mediterranean, or Japan would be (and often are) seen as incomplete, dependent, and/or unindividuated. Such family-oriented selves, focused on maintaining interpersonal harmony and family reputation (Gaines, 1982), exist in cultural environments that foster, support, and reward their "sociocentrism" (Schweder, 1982). In such contexts, the "egocentric" (Shweder, 1982), "referential" northern European Protestant self (Gaines, 1982), with its asocial constant-but-ever-developing nature, would be, and is, seen as antisocial, naive, and alienated. It is the self, as locally conceived, in which psychological disorders occur. Logically, different selves must have different disorders and therefore require different healing strategies.

Emotion and cognition.   The West's distinction between cognition and affect (thinking and feeling) is central to differentiating specific psychiatric disease entities. This distinction appears not to be natural, that is, not to exist in human nature or biology. "Cognition" and "affect" are cultural constructions (Kleinman and Good, 1985). This finding seriously challenges claims that depression and schizophrenia are universal diseases grounded in biology: The domains in which disturbance is said to occur (cognition and affect) are not innate, but are in fact Western cultural constructions. Let us now consider the disease entities themselves.

Depression.   Aside from the problems noted above, assessment methods for depression (and other disorders) are often highly ethnocentric, even when the approach is said to be entirely "descriptive." An example is dysphoric affect (unpleasant, sad feeling), a central element of the Western depressive experience. Dysphoric affect, while disvalued in some Western traditions, is highly valued in others, such as the Mediterranean world with its Latin Catholic, Orthodox, and Islamic traditions (Gaines and Farmer, 1986; Good, Good, and Moradi, in Kleinman and Good, 1985). In these contexts, suffering is seen as ennobling and as reflecting divine interest in the sufferer (Gaines and Farmer, 1986). Suffering serves as the basis for interaction; the self, beset with problems, is a fellow/sister sufferer in a "rhetoric of complaint" that enhances social status and evokes social assistance (Gaines, 1985).

In the Buddhist tradition, recognition of the decaying, worthless nature of the world and the self, and the futility and meaninglessness of human activity, is part of enlightened understanding (Obeyesekere, 1985). Such thoughts have positive value and are, therefore, "eudysphoric" (sweat sadness) (Gaines, 1992b). Eudysphoria makes questionable the very definition of particular experiences as unpleasant and in need of remediation.

The patterning of symptoms also varies widely across cultures. Key features of U.S.-defined depression are regularly absent from the experience of members of other cultures; for example, there is no psychomotor retardation in depression as described in France, and only short periods of dysphoria experienced among the Hopi Indians (Gaines and Farmer, 1986; Kleinman and Good, 1985). In general, no consistent, definitive statement regarding prevalence, incidence, or even the forms of depressive manifestation across cultures can be given, although a variety of assessment techniques have been employed. Some, such as Aaron Beck and associates, stress a cognitive explanation of depression. There are demonstratively effective therapies which equal or surpass biological/pharmacological interventions in speed and efficacy.

Schizophrenia.   Research on this disorder is still hampered by the lack of a clear definition, particularly of its boundaries. Psychiatry has not yet advanced a spe-

cific definition for schizophrenia or, for that matter, for mental illness in general.

Epidemiological, familial, twin, and adoption studies are interpreted to suggest that a genetic factor is involved in schizophrenia. However, no genetic link or common abnormality is demonstrable in the vast majority of cases. Results often are overstated, and important social/cultural information or explanations are regularly ignored (Duster, 1990). Many findings of central nervous system dysfunction appear in the literature, but none is specific and none is shared by all who have the diagnosis of schizophrenia. The fact that no symptom of schizophrenia is unique to it further weakens the biological hypotheses. All the associated symptoms appear in other disorders described by U.S. psychiatry. A unique genetic basis is asserted for a condition that is without distinctive characteristics. Furthermore, while studies suggest that schizophrenia is inherited, the specific forms appear not to be.

The WHO International Pilot and the Outcome Study of Schizophrenia (1979) found that schizophrenic patients with similar symptoms on initial evaluation, and whose disorders met strict diagnostic criteria, showed a marked variability in two- and five-year illness course and outcome, both within and across research centers. Patients in developing countries had much more favorable outcomes than those in developed countries. The disorder, almost by definition, is chronic in the West, but not in the Third World, where the majority of patients return to normal functioning states (WHO, 1979). Schizophrenia may be a culture-bound Western "ethnic psychosis" (one specific to one culture or ethnic group) (Devereux, 1980). Cultural expectations may play a central role in chronicity; cultures that expect chronicity produce it, while those that expect recovery foster it. Similarities in the prevalence, incidence, and process of schizophrenia in different cultures appear only when considerable contextual evidence is excluded (Kleinman, 1988). Considered in context, the similarities vanish.

In summary, the two most promising cases for the argument that mental illness is biological, schizophrenia and depression, are increasingly vulnerable to challenge. The ubiquitous assertion of the biological nature of psychiatric disorders appears to be a result of a misinterpretation of cultural or social phenomena as biological phenomena.

The biological perspective: Science or folk theory?

The biological view in psychiatry has its origins not in science but in a traditional folk culture, that of Germany, and is at least a thousand years old (Gaines, 1992b). The biological basis of mental illness is an expression of a cultural theory that holds that the essence of self and Other in terms of identity (ethnicity, kinship) and moral worth is determined by biology. *Blut* (blood), thought to be inherited, determines the essence of a person's identity, character, and moral worth.

The modern versions of this borrowed folk theory are the constructions of "genetic" or other somatic differences alleged to exist among people with specific disorders. In this view, people who have mental illnesses are "different" kinds of people (Jenkins, 1992). Among Latinos, the afflicted are seen as having more serious cases of "nerves" than do normal people. Thus, they see a continuum between the well and the ill, rather than a dichotomy.

Some psychiatries, especially Scandinavian and Russian, tended to follow in the footsteps of the nineteenth-century dean of German psychiatry, Wilhelm Griesinger, and of his follower, Emil Kraepelin, who asserted a biological basis for mental disorders. Griesinger's simple dictum, that "mental diseases are brain diseases," was a notion borrowed from German philosophy (Immanuel Kant), itself adopted from German popular culture and the French (racial) biology of the late 1700s (Gilman, 1988).

In the first third of the twentieth century, the German psychiatrist Karl Schneider advanced the notion of the "first rank symptoms" of schizophrenia, those definitively diagnostic of the disorder. Schneider's formulation carried great weight in the United States and elsewhere. There was, however, no analysis of its veracity until the 1980s, and thus was accepted without verification. This biological model is dominant in contemporary U.S. psychiatry. While the biological interpretation of mental illness is said to be based upon empirical scientific evidence, its popular cultural source is apparent.

Culture and the classification of madness. Professional psychiatric classifications of diseases, and the diseases classified by them, change over time. Changes in classification often represent shifts in assumptions about mental disorders. These shifts are products of ideological conflicts, competing explanations for which no data exist to resolve disputes one way or another. Changes, rather than heading in any particular direction, simply show shifts in dominant theoretical models or political ideologies.

Terms are deleted or reintroduced, but such action does not necessarily indicate advances. For example, neurosis appeared in the disease classifications of U.S. psychiatry from 1952 to 1980, when the classifications were influenced by psychoanalytic thought, but deleted from the 1980, 1987, and 1994 U.S. classifications (*DSM-III, DSM-III-R,* and *DSM-IV,* respectively), which are biological in orientation. Other psychiatries continue to use the term "neurosis" and to diagnose neurotic illnesses. There are also "reconstructions" in professional

psychiatry, such as "neurasthenia" applied to CFS in the United States. While the list of addictions grows and is expanding beyond drugs, with each new *DSM* in a culture where self-control is an issue, addictions are of little concern to psychiatries in other cultures.

The reality of mental illness itself has been questioned by psychiatrists in the United States. In the 1960s, a significant number of psychiatrists called "antipsychiatrists" argued that all mental disorders were "myths." Mental diseases were only metaphors because the "mind," the presumed location of mental disorders, was not a material entity but a figure of speech. Mental diseases, they argued, must be either brain diseases or problems in living requiring reeducation. Another view, that of Karl Menninger, proposes that mental illnesses are simply positions on a continuum of mental organization/disorganization. They do not represent distinct, separate diseases.

Interpretive analyses of U.S. psychiatric classifications reveal the underlying culture-, gender-, and age-specific voice (Germanic Protestant, male, adult) or perspective from which they are created. Differences perceived in others—those who differ in age, culture, or gender from the presumed ideal—are interpreted as reflecting a lack of (self)control. The attributed lack is, in turn, perceived as caused by differences in group (age, "race," gender) biology (Gaines, 1992b). This suggests that classifications are largely a cultural psychological discourse, not an ordering of diseases.

Pharmacology and "ethnic biology." New research in U.S. psychiatry, regarded as cutting-edge, allegedly recognizes ethnic differences in biochemistry. Findings suggest that different dosages of particular drugs for members of different ethnic groups would be appropriate in treating the same psychiatric disorder. This research takes as its units members of "ethnic or racial" groups, incorrectly assuming that these terms are synonymous. The allegedly distinct biological ("racial") groups are "Hispanics" (a language group), "Asians" (a geographical designation), "blacks" (a color and a "race"), "Native Americans" (geographical designation), and "whites" (or "Caucasians," another color and "race").

In reality these groups are social categories created by a particular culture and adopted into health research; they are neither universal nor biological. Research that assumes members in each category are biologically defined assumes that members of each category are identical, or nearly so, in genetic composition; what is true of one person belonging to a group, such as a "race," is assumed to be generalizable to all.

Other modern sciences have different notions of the number and membership of human "races." Japanese science, for example, considers Japanese, Koreans, Chinese, and Indians to be members of different "races."

The Germanic theory separates Germans from all other "white" groups on alleged genetic bases. Why is one racial theory accepted and others rejected in pharmacological research? The research also ignores the substantial variations in dosages clinically "proven" to be effective within "races," including European, in the practice of the various national psychiatries. For example, much larger doses of antipsychotics are needed for "white" U.S. patients than for French patients.

Culture, society, and context: Beyond biological thinking about mental illness

Sociologists have long believed that social contexts in Western industrial societies affect psychological status. The classic studies of A. B. Hollingshead and F. C. Redlich in the late 1950s, and of R. E. L. Faris and M. W. Dunham, and Leo Srol, Thomas Rennie, and their collaborators in the 1960s, suggested that there was a relationship between social class position, urban residence, and an increased incidence of certain forms of mental illness; while lower classes have more of some illnesses, upper classes have more of others. Pioneers with anthropological expertise, such as Alexander Leighton and Jane Murphy, implicated high levels of social disorganization as contributing to increases in the incidence of mental illness (see Weissman and Klerman, 1978). Those persons subject to extreme pressures, such as discrimination and other forms of oppression that limit life chances, would have less stable environments, and hence would be more vulnerable to psychological problems.

However, it is also quite clear that U.S. psychiatry rather commonly misdiagnoses members of minority groups, attributing serious mental illnesses to individuals largely on the basis of membership in an ethnic or gender group, rather than on the basis of symptoms. The same symptoms in members of different ethnic groups or genders often lead to different diagnoses with different prognoses.

Accidents and criminal victimization (assault, rape, abuse), war, state-sponsored violence and terror, racism, genocide and ethnocide, forced migration, epidemics, poverty, and starvation also have traumatic consequences for individuals and groups. For Native and African Americans, the term "holocaust" is not inappropriately applied to their experiences with Europeans in the New World. Members of each group have been subjects of pogroms, genocide, and terrorism as well as centuries of abuse, discrimination, and neglect. Studies that seek to find the seat of disorder in biology have the effect, intended or not, of denying that these experiences have had considerable psychological impact.

"Stress," a notion deriving from World War II and modeled on combat experiences (Weissman and Kler-man, 1978), is relevant within the United States for various dispossessed ethnic groups and for veterans, for example, with the recent creation of post-traumatic stress disorder (PTSD) (Young, 1990), which combines trauma and stress.

The notion of universal biological mental disease limits understanding of detrimental as well as beneficial sociocultural conditions. It pushes observers to see defective persons instead of social inequalities, to seek biological vulnerabilities instead of hopelessness born of centuries of despair or the horrors of war, and it ignores conditions that are responses to noxious circumstances, not innate defects.

The biological perspective, implicit in U.S., German, and other psychiatries, leads their practitioners to argue that conditions are not matters of culture or opinion but natural entities discerned by dispassionate, advanced scientific psychiatry. But all people do not share the same ways of life, of feeling, of thinking, or of behaving. Standards of normalcy vary from culture to culture; what is sane in one is insane in another. There is no evidence to suggest that there is a biological basis for the astounding heterogeneity of normal thought and behavior. It is illogical to assert that abnormal behavior is biological while the normal is not. The biological approach only appears to be objective science; it can be head-in-the-sand ethnocentrism that disvalues cultural differences.

Professional psychiatries: Ethical implications

Historical and cross-cultural studies of professional psychiatries suggest that each is a cultural construction, not a reflection of concern for natural psychopathologies; thus, there are psychiatries, not one psychiatry. The application of theory or practice of any one psychiatry in a culturally diverse world forces an important ethical question: Do negative consequences result from the application of one culture's psychological medicine as a standard of normalcy in the evaluation and treatment of cultural others?

U.S. bioethics grows out of concerns with autonomy, experimentation, and informed consent issues, and also out of a particular cultural context that gives meaning to those concerns. It commonly excludes social, political, and cultural issues, asserting that such things lie outside its domain. In much the same way, biological psychiatry excludes all cross-cultural and historical research that contradicts it and operates in a closed domain, away from complex realities.

An ethics said to be "beyond culture" will not do. What is ethical in one context is unethical in another: telling the diagnosis in Japan is unethical, while not telling in the United States raises ethical problems; leaving the patient uninformed about his or her disorder or the rationale for treatment is normal and ethical in Japanese or Italian medicine or psychiatry but ethically compromised in the United States. Making invidious distinctions ("race") and reifying these distinctions as "natural and biological" has clear negative consequences, among them unequal treatment (injustice), disproportionate institutionalization (loss of autonomy), and failure to address discrimination, thus harming patients.

In Islamic medical ethics, physicians are enjoined to be social activists in order to better the living conditions of their community members; a purely somatic focus is unethical in other than a utopian context. Such an ideology opens the door to change and adaptation. The need to recognize, and then to adapt and integrate, the importance of cultural and social differences into theory and practice, while maintaining cultural integrity in the face of increasing cultural diversity, is the moral dilemma of modern professional psychiatries.

ATWOOD D. GAINES

Directly related to this article are the other articles in this entry: CONCEPTIONS OF MENTAL ILLNESS, *and* ISSUES IN DIAGNOSIS. *For a further discussion of topics mentioned in this article, see the entry* PERSON. *Other relevant material may be found under the entries* INTERPRETATION; RACE AND RACISM; *and* SEXISM. *See also the entry* MEDICAL ETHICS, HISTORY OF, *section on* NEAR AND MIDDLE EAST, *article on* CONTEMPORARY ARAB WORLD; *section on* SOUTH AND EAST ASIA, *articles on* INDIA, CHINA, *and* JAPAN; *section on* EUROPE, *subsection on* CONTEMPORARY PERIOD; *and section on* THE AMERICAS, *article on* THE UNITED STATES IN THE TWENTIETH CENTURY.

Bibliography

AMERICAN PSYCHIATRIC ASSOCIATION (APA). 1987. *Diagnostic and Statistical Manual of Mental Disorders: DSM-III-R*. 3d ed., rev. Washington, D.C.: Author.

———. 1994. "Glossary of Culture-Bound Syndromes." In *Diagnostic and Statistical Manual of Mental Disorders: DSM-IV*. 4th ed., pp. 844–849. Washington, D.C.: Author.

BLUE, AMY V., and GAINES, ATWOOD D. 1992. "The Ethnopsychiatric Répertoire: A Review and Overview of Ethnopsychiatric Studies." In *Ethnopsychiatry: The Cultural Construction of Professional and Folk Psychiatries*, pp. 397–484. Edited by Atwood D. Gaines. Albany: State University of New York Press.

CONNOR, LINDA. 1982. "The Unbounded Self: Balinese Therapy in Theory and Practice." In *Cultural Conceptions of Mental Health and Therapy*, pp. 251–267. Edited by Anthony J. Marsella and Geoffrey M. White. Dordrecht, Netherlands: D. Reidel.

DEVEREUX, GEORGE. 1980. *Basic Problems of Ethnopsychiatry*. Translated by Basia Miller Gulati and George Devereux. Chicago: University of Chicago Press.

DUSTER, TROY. 1990. *Backdoor to Eugenics*. London: Routledge.

FAUSTO-STERLING, ANNE. 1992. *Myths of Gender: Biological Theories About Women and Men*. 2d ed. New York: Basic Books.

GAINES, ATWOOD D. 1982. "Cultural Definitions, Behavior and the Person in American Psychiatry." In *Cultural Conceptions of Mental Health and Therapy*, pp. 167–192. Edited by Anthony J. Marsella and Geoffrey M. White. Dordrecht, Netherlands: D. Reidel.

———. 1985. "The Once- and Twice-Born Self: Practice Among Psychiatrists and Christian Psychiatrists." In *Physicians of Western Medicine: Anthropological Approaches to Theory and Practice*, pp. 223–243. Edited by Robert A. Hahn and Atwood D. Gaines. Dordrecht, Netherlands: D. Reidel.

———. 1991. "Cultural Constructivism: Sickness Histories and the Understanding of Ethnomedicines Beyond Critical Medical Anthropologies." In *Anthropologies of Medicine: A Colloquium on West European and North American Perspectives*, pp. 221–258. Edited by Beatrix Pfleiderer and Gilles Bibeau. Brunswick, Germany: Vieweg.

———, ed. 1992a. *Ethnopsychiatry: The Cultural Construction of Professional and Folk Psychiatries*. Albany: State University of New York Press.

———. 1992b. "From *DSM-I* to *III-R*; Voices of Self, Mastery and the Other: A Cultural Constructivist Reading of U.S. Psychiatric Classification." *Social Science and Medicine* 33, no. 1:3–24.

GAINES, ATWOOD D., and FARMER, PAUL E. 1986. "Visible Saints: Social Cynosures and Dysphora in the Mediterranean Tradition." *Culture, Medicine and Psychiatry* 10, no. 4:295–330.

GEERTZ, CLIFFORD. 1973. *The Interpretation of Cultures: Selected Essays*. New York: Basic Books.

GILMAN, SANDER L. 1988. *Disease and Representation: Images of Illness from Madness to AIDS*. Ithaca, N.Y.: Cornell University Press.

GOULD, STEPHEN JAY. 1981. *The Mismeasure of Man*. New York: W. W. Norton.

HACKING, IAN. 1983. *Representing and Intervening: Introductory Topics in the Philosophy of Natural Science*. Cambridge: At the University Press.

HAHN, ROBERT A., and GAINES, ATWOOD D., eds. 1985. *Physicians of Western Medicine: Anthropological Approaches to Theory and Practice*. Dordrecht, Netherlands: D. Reidel.

HERSHEL, HELENA JIA. 1992. "Psychiatric Institutions: Rules and the Accommodation of Structure and Autonomy in France and the United States." In *Ethnopsychiatry: The Cultural Construction of Professional and Folk Psychiatries*, pp. 307–326. Edited by Atwood D. Gaines. Albany: State University of New York Press.

JENKINS, JANIS HUNTER. 1992. "Too Close for Comfort: Schizophrenia and Emotional Overinvolvement Among Mexicano Families." In *Ethnopsychiatry: The Cultural Construction of Professional and Folk Psychiatries*, pp. 203–221. Edited by Atwood D. Gaines. Albany: State University of New York Press.

KLEINMAN, ARTHUR. 1988. *Rethinking Psychiatry: From Cultural Category to Personal Experience*. New York: Free Press.

KLEINMAN, ARTHUR, and GOOD, BYRON, eds. 1985. *Culture and Depression: Studies in the Anthropology and Cross-Cultural Psychiatry of Affect and Disorder.* Berkeley: University of California Press.

LIN, KEH-MING; POLAND, E. RUSSELL; and CHIEN, C. 1990. "Ethnicity and Psychopharmacology: Recent Findings and Future Research Directions." In *Family, Culture and Psychobiology.* Edited by Eliot Sorel. New York: Legas.

LOCK, MARGARET M. 1980. *East Asian Medicine in Urban Japan: Varieties of Medical Experience.* Berkeley: University of California Press.

MARSELLA, ANTHONY J., and WHITE, GEOFFREY M., eds. 1982. *Cultural Conceptions of Mental Health and Therapy.* Dordrecht, Netherlands: D. Reidel.

NOMURA, NAOKI. 1992. "Psychiatrist and Patient in Japan: An Analysis of Interactions in an Outpatient Clinic." In *Ethnopsychiatry: The Cultural Construction of Professional and Folk Psychiatries,* pp. 273–289. Edited by Atwood D. Gaines. Albany: State University of New York Press.

OBEYESEKERE, GANANATH. 1985. "Depression, Buddhism, and the Work of Culture in Sri Lanka." In *Culture and Depression: Studies in the Anthropology and Cross-Cultural Psychiatry of Affect and Disorder,* pp. 134–152. Edited by Arthur Kleinman and Byron Good. Berkeley: University of California Press.

PAYER, LYNN. 1989. *Medicine and Culture: Varieties of Treatment in the United States, England, West Germany, and France.* New York: Penguin.

ROBINS, LEE N., and REGIER, DARREL A., eds. 1991. *Psychiatric Disorders in America: The Epidemiologic Catchment Area Study.* New York: Free Press.

SHWEDER, RICHARD A., and BOURNE, EDMUND J. 1982. "Does the Concept of the Person Vary Cross-Culturally?" In *Cultural Conceptions of Mental Health and Therapy,* pp. 97–137. Edited by Anthony J. Marsella and Geoffrey M. White. Dordrecht, Netherlands: D. Reidel.

SIMONS, RONALD C., and HUGHES, CHARLES C., eds. *Culture-Bound Syndromes: Folk Illnesses of Psychiatric and Anthropological Interest.* Dordrecht, Netherlands: D. Reidel.

SWARTZ, LESLIE. 1992. "Professional Ethnopsychiatry in South Africa: The Question of Relativism." In *Ethnopsychiatry: The Cultural Construction of Professional and Folk Psychiatries,* pp. 225–249. Edited by Atwood D. Gaines. Albany: State University of New York Press.

TAYLOR, CHARLES. 1985. *Philosophy and the Human Sciences.* Vol. 2 of his *Philosophical Papers.* Cambridge: At the University Press.

THOMAS, ALEXANDER, and SILLEN, SAMUEL. 1976. *Racism and Psychiatry.* Secaucus, N.J.: Citadel.

TOWNSEND, JOHN MARSHALL. 1978. *Cultural Conceptions and Mental Illness: A Comparison Between Germany and America.* Chicago: University of Chicago Press.

WEISMANN, MYRNA M., and KLERMAN, GERALD L. 1978. "Epidemiology of Mental Disorders." *Archives of General Psychiatry* 35, no. 6:705–712.

WORLD HEALTH ORGANIZATION (WHO). 1979. *Schizophrenia: An International Follow-up Study.* Chichester, U.K.: John Wiley & Sons.

WU, DAVID Y. H. 1982. "Psychotherapy and Emotion in Traditional Chinese Medicine." In *Cultural Conceptions of Mental Health and Therapy,* pp. 285–301. Edited by Anthony J. Marsella and Geoffrey M. White. Dordrecht, Netherlands: D. Reidel.

YOUNG, ALLAN. 1990. "Moral Conflicts in a Psychiatric Hospital Treating Combat-Related Posttraumatic Stress Disorder (PTSD)." In *Social Science Perspectives on Medical Ethics,* pp. 65–82. Edited by George Weisz. Dordrecht, Netherlands: Kluwer.

III. ISSUES IN DIAGNOSIS

Relatively little ethical concern has been expressed about naming and classifying physical illness. By contrast, a diagnosis of mental illness—broadly defined as being sick with behavioral and mental signs—elicits a great deal of concern about its ethical implications.

Contrast with physical illness: Stigma and volition

The reality of mental illness has been questioned, because the same aberrant behavior might equally well be diagnosed as illness or viewed as an individual's choice and responsibility. Thus stigma has customarily accompanied mental, but not physical, illness because the latter has not been seen as a matter of volition. Increasingly, however, it has become socially routine to add to a diagnosis of lung cancer the exculpatory codicil that the victim was not a smoker. There have been debates as to whether or not alcoholics should be considered potential candidates for liver transplants. With expanding evidence of behavioral cofactors of physical illness, the apparent possibility for volitional control has spread the stigma accompanying psychiatric illness to physical illness as well. At the clinical level, diagnostic labels serve the social role of exempting diagnosed persons from obligations (Parson, 1972). "Sick" is generally understood to imply "not responsible." Thus, at the same time that labeling behavior as "sick" creates a stigma (Goffman, 1963), applying a diagnosis excuses it. Stigma works in tension with excusing since the two viewpoints represent conflicting models for understanding deviant behavior.

Definition

The ethical issues surrounding diagnosis of mental illness begin with the diagnostic definitions. These diagnoses are intended to define, delineate, and clarify the application of the mental-disorder construct. However, the wide variety of underlying conceptualizations has made it difficult to achieve consensus on what constitutes "mental illness." A study that compared seventeen definitions of "serious mental illness" demonstrated rates varying from 4 to 88 percent among 222 inner-city patients receiving services (Schinnar et al., 1990). The most skeptical view has been that mental disorder may not exist. Pragmatically, however, mental disorder can be viewed as that which professionals treat. Less cynical is the view that mental disorder is statistical deviance from a psychosocial or biological norm. This definition suffers from the problem that deviance alone is not necessarily pathological. For example, coronary artery disease in Western industrial societies may be statistically prevalent, but it is still pathological.

Another definition builds on the concept of biological disadvantage. Defining mental disorder as "harmful dysfunction" combines the term "harmful," to signify the social aspects of the concept, with "dysfunction," to express the scientific aspect. Thus constructed, the definition is designed to label the "failure of a mental mechanism to perform a natural function for which it was designed by evolution" (Wakefield, 1992, p. 373). This formulation suffers from the problem of determining just what evolution "designed" as "natural" functions. Such an evaluation is particularly problematic in the presence of functions with competing aims—for example, vigilance as protection against dangerous outsiders, on the one hand, and as an impediment to intimacy (and procreation), on the other. The judgment would depend on the context of the situation and might differ from one observer to another.

These formulations are also incomplete in that they do not provide for applying diagnoses in situations of otherwise unexpectable distress or disability. This inclusion is part of the definition adopted in the American Psychiatric Association's *Diagnostic and Statistical Manual* (DSM) (American Psychiatric Association, 1987), which serves as the official diagnostic reference for American psychiatry. Problems remain, however; the DSM "official" definition of mental disorder is criticized as being circular because it requires mental disorders to be "clinically significant," that is, to present to such a degree that they constitute an impediment to functioning. However, the threshold implies the presence of a "mental disorder" at a subthreshold level at which mental disorder, by definition, cannot exist (Sagar, 1989).

DSM and standardization

The *Diagnostic and Statistical Manual* has attempted to make psychiatric nosology more scientific. In 1918 the *Statistical Manual for the Use of Institutions for the Insane* was adopted to collect mental-hospital data based on a biological view of etiology and classification. That diagnostic system was revised in 1952 to accord with psychodynamic psychiatry (Grob, 1991) and was published as the first *Diagnostic and Statistical Manual*. DSM-III, the third edition, originally published in 1980 and revised in 1987, differed from its predecessors by its focus on specifying clear criteria for diagnosticians to apply in their assessments. A fourth edition, further refining the criteria on the basis of clinical experience, was published in early 1994. The classifications consist of empirical di-

agnoses made, as far as possible, descriptively and without reference to any particular theoretical framework. The criteria are written so that they can be assessed consistently by different observers in different settings at different times. To enhance diagnostic reliability, diagnoses are based on actuarial judgments, satisfying a specified number of listed criteria, rather than the older approach of global clinical judgments (Dawes et al., 1989). Reliability of diagnostic judgments was also furthered by the development of structured clinical interviews to facilitate the assessment of the diagnostic criteria (Williams et al., 1992).

Problems of context

In spite of the attempts to make the criteria objective, however, the diagnoses are far from context-free. Taxonomic constructs, representing historical prototypes of illness, are necessarily implicit in the criteria to provide a meaningful framework within which to assess symptoms. In practice, therefore, the diagnoses described by DSM contain, in addition to their descriptive features, ties to ideas about etiology and treatment (Morey, 1991; Schwartz and Wiggins, 1987). For example, the DSM categories of schizophrenia and schizotypal personality disorder were originally formulated from aspects of the same psychotic disorder. The two are differentiated by their time course, the former defined as a deteriorating illness and the latter as a stable, lifelong condition. Their symptomatic presentations may be indistinguishable at any one point in time. To differentiate between the two requires the diagnostician to know that the essential feature of the differentiation is the time course, a fact that is embedded in the criteria sets but is not their focus. Since the two diagnoses carry very different prognostic implications, the diagnostician's inclination toward one diagnosis or the other may carry great consequences for practical arrangements of a patient's future.

Because even reliable DSM diagnoses rely upon the clinician's judgment, possibilities for inconsistency abound. Antisocial personality disorder, with its origins in phenomenological depiction, has criteria that are readily observable, such as "has been involved in frequent fights" and "has defaulted on debts." In contrast, histrionic personality disorder, with its origin in the psychoanalytic tradition, requires a higher level of clinical inference to assess such criteria as "is self-centered . . . has no tolerance for the frustration of delayed gratification" and "displays rapidly shifting and shallow expression of emotions." Thus the diagnostician's skill at making correct inferences will have varying effects across different diagnoses.

A further challenge arises with ego-syntonic symptoms that patients perceive as aspects of themselves. For example, the obsessive-compulsive personality disorder criterion of "excessive devotion to work and productivity to the exclusion of leisure activities and friendships (not accounted for by obvious economic necessity)" requires the diagnostician to respect as legitimate a range of thresholds for "devotion to work." Appropriate assessment may require the diagnostician to accept life goals extending beyond his or her own judgments of reasonableness. Clinicians risk erring either by accepting only a limited range of socially acceptable options, on the one hand, or by applying no standards and accepting all choices as equally valid, on the other.

Another area requiring diagnostic acumen and vulnerable to bias is the subjective element of psychiatric signs, in which the diagnostician's experience of the patient encounter becomes a diagnostic criterion. The data used in diagnosing mental illness, particularly encompassing the patient's relations with others, often involve the diagnostician's interactions with the patient, so that the psychiatrist's own values and attitudes may influence clinical assessment (van Praag, 1992). For example, the schizotypal personality disorder criterion of "odd or eccentric appearance or behavior" requires a judgment of the threshold for eccentricity.

Cultural context

To be considered scientifically valid, as well as to minimize potential ethical abuses, diagnoses should be reliably assessable across varying cultural and religious settings. By virtue of their clear criteria, the DSM-III diagnoses should meet this test of validity. Nevertheless, differences in psychiatric diagnosis have often been found to be based on ethnic identity. In a sample of 26,400 clients of the Los Angeles County mental health system, blacks and Asians received proportionately more DSM diagnoses of psychoses than did whites, while Latinos received disproportionately fewer such diagnoses (Flaskerud and Hu, 1992). Even after accounting for age, gender, socioeconomic status, and language, which might have rendered the studied groups not fully comparable, the differences in diagnostic rates persisted.

Perhaps some of the variation reflects truly different rates of illness among these groups, but an individual's culture often influences manifestations of illness (Fabrega, 1992). What is described as psychological dysphoria in one cultural context would be characterized as somatic pain in another. Varying expectations of distress to be expressed at the death of a spouse in different cultures make differing standards for normal bereavement. The appropriate threshold can be determined only by reference to subcultural context. Although the DSM rules allow for such adjustment, clinicians will inevitably vary in their experience of the cultural contexts of their patients. Thus the possibility exists for stigmatization on the basis of the diagnostician's unfamiliarity with a patient's cultural milieu.

Scientific development versus clinical practice

In spite of their limitations, the DSM diagnoses have facilitated a shared frame of reference (Faust and Miner, 1986). The resulting proliferation of often speculative diagnoses has sparked a debate as to the most useful strategy for introducing new diagnoses (Pincus et al., 1992). Although diagnoses can be formulated provisionally as catalysts for further research, the stability desirable for clinical practice suggests that they be promulgated only as the culmination of extended investigative efforts and field trials. These competing aims were recognized by the framers of the International Classification of Disease, who formulated separate categorizations for research and for clinical purposes. However, the advantage of such a split classification may well be outweighed by the disadvantage of separating researchers from the routine of clinical practice.

The "best" diagnosis

The most appropriate definition of any mental disorder depends on the use to be made of the resulting diagnosis. Although such disorders presumably occur regardless of what classification scheme is used to describe them, diagnoses are made for a variety of purposes, including professional, scientific, economic, legal, and political ones (Szasz, 1991). The differing purposes of the diagnostic labels are distinct from the illness itself (Simon, 1990).

The misuse of these diagnoses is often occasioned by their application in circumstances for which they were not intended. Examples include unjustified mental-disorder diagnoses assigned to academics who challenge decisions of their university administrations (Ormerod, 1991). In this case, although the accuracy of the diagnoses as factual descriptions of behavior was arguable, the diagnoses were assigned not for medical treatment purposes but to circumvent protections of academic freedom. More commonly, diagnoses designed to convey medical treatment implications are assigned to compel a third-party payer to reimburse a patient or provider for treatment. The ethical dilemma of pressure to misrepresent or distort a patient's symptomatic diagnostic description in order to secure third-party reimbursement arises when diagnoses intended to classify symptom clusters are instead used as the basis for reimbursement. A diagnostic scheme categorizing treatment needs in the patient's psychosocial context (Berry, 1987)—which would not necessarily require consideration of particular symptoms—would be appropriate for determining reimbursement and would circumvent a dilemma in which providers feel that they must assign "reimbursable," though untrue, diagnoses in order for their patients to receive needed treatment. In contrast to problems created by inappropriate use of diagnoses, the appropriate use of DSM diagnoses, as they were designed, to categorize and classify symptoms has been useful. For example, it was determined that certain community mental-health centers were likely wasting resources by treating patients with no diagnosable mental disorders (Windle et al., 1988).

Alternative diagnoses

Medical diagnoses carry implicit information about likely treatment needs. On this basis arguments have been made for psychiatric diagnoses that explicitly specify treatment needs, so as to communicate priorities and lead directly to pragmatic care plans. For example, the focus of a patient's thought-disorder diagnosis would be the aspects of daily life affected by that symptom, not the thought disorder itself. In the service of practical caretaking concerns, such diagnostic schemes sacrifice the possibility for scientific classification that would direct attention toward what causes mental disorders. Psychoanalysts, for example, base much of their work on such features outside the scope of traditional medical diagnosis, focusing on the differences unique to individual patients rather than on the similarities that group patients into diagnostic categories (Altshul et al., 1987).

A complete psychosocial description of the broad contexts of a patient's life is needed for proper treatment. In diagnosis divorced from clinical context, stigma is more likely because of the absence of humanizing context (Gutheil, 1988). The *Diagnostic and Statistical Manuals* have made provision for such information that is not strictly diagnostic but may help to plan treatment and predict outcome. Their multiaxial diagnostic scheme records, besides patterns of observable symptoms, additional perspectives on the patient: characterological features, acute stressors, and overall level of functioning.

Another aspect of diagnosis involves differentiating mental illness from normal mental states. To this end it may therefore be desirable to supplement categorical diagnosis (e.g., major depression) with dimensional characterization (e.g., degree of depressed mood) (van Praag, 1990). Since the latter measure is continuous with dimensions of normality, it may decrease the possibility for stigma. The boundary is illuminated by considerations of crimes committed by persons who may be suffering from mental illness.

The insanity defense

At least one prominent scientist (Koshland, 1992) has advocated restricting legal process to determination of an accused's actual actions. The so-called insanity defense should be abandoned, he argues, until psychiatrists can accurately predict the future dangerousness of any given individual. However, it has generally been deemed unfair to hold mentally ill persons to the same degree of criminal responsibility as those who are free of mental afflictions. In any case, it is argued, how can society effectively punish individuals who do not know what they are doing or that what they are doing is wrong? Thus, in the service of protecting the seriously ill, experts in forensic psychiatry engage in courtroom debates over the existence of mental illness (Bloom and Rogers, 1987).

The legal basis for the insanity defense is the 1843 M'Naghten rule. It states that individuals are not culpable for acts committed while laboring under a defect of reason that prevents their knowing that they were doing wrong. The 1952 Durham rule made insanity a fact to be determined in a legal sense, by asserting that someone is not responsible for an unlawful act that is the product of mental disease or defect. Thus an insanity defense in most jurisdictions requires demonstrating the presence of a mental disorder and defect of reason, as well as a cognitive ignorance of the nature or wrongfulness of the act and a violitional incapacity to refrain from the act (Sadoff, 1992). In a comparison of insanity-defense standards, 164 cases were reviewed by four forensic psychiatrists (Wettstein et al., 1991). Two-thirds of the defendants met all the insanity tests and one-quarter met only a volitional test. Cognitive standards were found to be more powerful than the volitional one, although no distinction was found among the different cognitive standards. Of most importance, however, was the fact that diagnosis was irrelevant to the determination.

The forensic problem of deciding between punishment and treatment for persons who have committed crimes and who may be suffering from a mental illness requires balancing society's interest in punishing those who violate behavioral norms against the principle of not punishing those who are ill. The crucial distinction that needs to be made is between illness and responsibility for actions. Since, as has been described above, a diagnosis of mental illness does not necessarily absolve a person from responsibility for his or her actions, the increased reliability of *DSM* diagnoses has not substantially altered the problems of forensic psychiatry. A mental-illness diagnosis does not by itself fulfill the legal definition of insanity; nor should it do so, because mental-illness diagnoses as presently constituted categorize symptom complexes that may or may not affect responsibility.

Conclusion

With the recognition that diagnosis of mental illness does not determine responsibility, the argument has come full circle. The ethical problem of stigma associated with mental-illness diagnoses has been addressed by formulating reliable diagnoses that can be applied consistently. However, ethical issues and stigma persist, because ultimately the dichotomy between illness and responsibility represents different frames of reference that cannot be brought fully into alignment. The effort to do so, however, may enhance our understanding and broaden our tolerance.

LAWRENCE B. JACOBSBERG

Directly related to this article are the other articles in this entry: CONCEPTIONS OF MENTAL ILLNESS, *and* CROSS-CULTURAL PERSPECTIVES. *Also directly related is the entry* MEDICINE, ART OF. *For a further discussion of topics mentioned in this article, see the entries* INTERPRETATION; PSYCHIATRY, ABUSES OF; *and* VALUE AND VALUATION. *For a discussion of related ideas, see the entries* MENTAL-HEALTH THERAPIES; *and* PSYCHOANALYSIS AND DYNAMIC THERAPIES.

Bibliography

ALTSHUL, SOL; MICHELS, ROBERT; and SIMONS, RICHARD C. 1987. "Psychoanalytic Contributions to Psychiatric Nosology." *Journal of the American Psychoanalytic Association* 35, no. 3:693–711.

AMERICAN PSYCHIATRIC ASSOCIATION. 1987. *Diagnostic and Statistical Manual of Mental Disorders: DSM-III-R.* 3d ed., rev. Washington, D.C.: Author.

BERRY, KATHERINE N. 1987. "Let's Create Diagnoses Psych Nurses Can Use." *American Journal of Nursing* 87, no. 5:707–708.

BLOOM, JOSEPH D., and ROGERS, JEFFREY L. 1987. "The Legal Basis of Forensic Psychiatry: Statutorily Mandated Psychiatric Diagnoses." *American Journal of Psychiatry* 144, no. 7:847–853.

DAWES, ROBYN M.; FAUST, DAVID; and MEEHL, PAUL E. 1989. "Clinical Versus Actuarial Judgment." *Science* 243, no. 4899:1668–1674.

FABREGA, HORACIO, JR. 1992. "Diagnosis Interminable: Toward a Culturally Sensitive DSM-IV." *Journal of Nervous and Mental Disease* 180, no. 1:5–7.

FAUST, DAVID, and MINER, RICHARD A. 1986. "The Empiricist and His New Clothes: DSM-III in Perspective." *American Journal of Psychiatry* 143, no. 8:962–967.

FLASKERUD, JAQUELIN H., and HU, LI-TZE. 1992. "Relationship of Ethnicity to Psychiatric Diagnosis." *Journal of Nervous and Mental Disease* 180, no. 5:296–303.

GOFFMAN, ERVING. 1963. *Stigma: Notes on the Management of Spoiled Identity.* Englewood Cliffs, N.J.: Prentice-Hall.

GROB, GERALD N. 1991. "Origins of DSM-I: A Study of Appearance and Reality." *American Journal of Psychiatry* 148, no. 4:421–431.

GUTHEIL, THOMAS G. 1988. "Limitations of Diagnosis." *Hospital and Community Psychiatry* 39, no. 7:786–787.

KOSHLAND, DANIEL E., JR. 1992. "Elephants, Monstrosities, and the Law." *Science* 255, no. 5046:777.

MOREY, LESLIE C. 1991. "Classification of Mental Disorder as a Collection of Hypothetical Constructs." *Journal of Abnormal Psychology* 100, no. 3:289–293.

ORMEROD, WALTER E. 1991. "Unjustified Diagnosis of Mental Disorder." *Lancet* 337, no. 8753:1331–1332.

PARSONS, TALCOTT. 1972. "Definitions of Health and Illness in the Light of American Values and Social Structure." In *Patients, Physicians, Illness: A Sourcebook in Behavioral Science and Health,* 2d ed., pp. 107–127. Edited by E. Gartly Jaco. New York: Free Press.

PINCUS, HAROLD A.; FRANCES, ALLEN; DAVIS, WENDY W.; FIRST, MICHAEL B.; and WIDIGER, THOMAS A. 1992. "DSM-IV and New Diagnostic Categories: Holding the Line on Proliferation." *American Journal of Psychiatry* 149, no. 1:112–117.

SADOFF, ROBERT L. 1992. "In Defense of the Insanity Defense." *Psychiatric Annals* 22, no. 11:556–560.

SAGAR, RATAKONDA S. 1989. "DSM-III-R Definition of Mental Disorder." *American Journal of Psychiatry* 146, no. 8:1077–1078.

SCHINNAR, ARIE P.; ROTHBARD, AILEEN B.; KANTER, REBEKAH; and JUNG, YOON S. 1990. "An Empirical Literature Review of Definitions of Severe and Persistent Mental Illness." *American Journal of Psychiatry* 147, no. 12:1602–1608.

SCHWARTZ, MICHAEL A., and WIGGINS, OSBORNE P. 1987. "Typifications: The First Step for Clinical Diagnosis in Psychiatry." *Journal of Nervous and Mental Disease* 175, no. 2:65–77.

SIMON, JOHN L. 1990. "Overemphasizing Diagnostic Classification." *American Journal of Psychiatry* 147, no. 12:1699–1700.

SZASZ, THOMAS. 1991. "Diagnoses Are Not Diseases." *Lancet* 338, no. 8782/8783:1574–1576.

VAN PRAAG, HERMAN M. 1990. "Two-Tier Diagnosing in Psychiatry." *Psychiatry Research* 34, no. 1:1–11.

———. 1992. "Reconquest of the Subjective: Against the Waning of Psychiatric Diagnosing." *British Journal of Psychiatry* 160 (February):266–271.

WAKEFIELD, JEROME C. 1992. "The Concept of Mental Disorder: On the Boundary Between Biological Facts and Social Values." *American Psychologist* 47, no. 3:373–388.

WETTSTEIN, ROBERT M.; MULVEY, EDWARD P.; and ROGERS, RICHARD. 1991. "A Prospective Comparison of Four Insanity Defense Standards." *American Journal of Psychiatry* 148, no. 1:21–27.

WILLIAMS, JANET B. W.; GIBBON, MIRIAM; FIRST, MICHAEL B.; SPITZER, ROBERT L.; DAVIES, MARK; BORUS, JONATHAN; HOWES, MARY J.; KANE, JOHN; POPE, HARRISON G., JR.; ROUNSAVILLE, BRUCE; and WITTCHEN, HANS U. 1992. "The Structured Clinical Interview for DSM-III-R (SCID): II. Multisite Test–Retest Reliability." *Archives of General Psychiatry* 49, no. 8:630–636.

WINDLE, CHARLES; THOMPSON, JAMES W.; GOLDMAN, HOWARD H.; and NAIERMAN, NAOMI. 1988. "Treatment of Patients with No Diagnosable Mental Disorders in CMHCs." *Hospital and Community Psychiatry* 39, no. 7:753–758.

MENTALLY DISABLED AND MENTALLY ILL PERSONS

I. Health-Care Issues
   Miriam Shuchman
II. Research Issues
   Carl Elliott

I. HEALTH-CARE ISSUES

Primary health-care providers for patients with mental illnesses bear the same ethical obligations as providers who serve patients with physical illnesses, yet they face special challenges in upholding those obligations. When mental illness causes a patient to be violent or suicidal, clinicians may confront situations in which their duties to the patient conflict with other ethical duties. At times, the decision about which duty to obey involves careful moral consideration. Additionally, because mentally ill persons are particularly vulnerable to abuse, the clinician has a special obligation to protect such patients against abuses.

For example, in the case of a patient who has attempted suicide, the duty to respect the patient's autonomy may conflict with the duty to protect the patient from harm. The patient may wish to go home, yet the clinician—who may be a physician in a hospital emergency room, a psychiatrist, or the patient's therapist—may decide to hospitalize the patient. At this point, the patatient's fundamental right to refuse care has been denied. The moral justification may seem clear: The patient is not thinking rationally, so he or she should not be permitted to function autonomously. But the patient deserves an explanation about why he or she is being hospitalized and information about the legal routes for challenging the decision.

As we will see, even when the clinician's overriding moral duties are clear, actual situations are complicated. There is often disagreement among patients, clinicians, families, and the courts about whether a patient's rights may be denied. This article explores common moral dilemmas in the medical and psychiatric care of mentally ill and mentally impaired individuals. Such individuals may be affected by severe mental illness, such as schizophrenia or depression, or by serious deficits in memory and intellectual functioning, as are seen in dementia (most common in old age) and mental retardation. Health professionals caring for such patients are likely to face one or more of the following questions:

1. Does the person with mental illness have the capacity to decide about suggested treatments? (Informed consent for treatment)

2. When is it ethical to hospitalize mentally ill persons against their will? (Commitment)
3. Is it ethical to treat mentally ill persons against their will with psychiatric medications? (Coerced treatment)
4. Is it ethical to use coercive methods to encourage a mentally ill person to comply with prescribed treatments? (Coerced compliance)
5. When is it ethical to withhold information from a person because that person has a history of serious mental illness? (Truth-telling)
6. When is it ethical to breach the confidentiality of a mentally ill patient? (Confidentiality)
7. Under what circumstances is it ethical to withhold scarce health resources from a person because that person is mentally ill? (Allocation of scarce resources)

Informed consent for treatment

By law, a person cannot be treated by a doctor without first being informed about the nature of the treatment and then consenting to have the treatment. When a person with a history of serious mental illness is being treated for a medical condition, his or her doctors may consult a psychiatrist about the patient's capacity to make medical decisions.

Assessing the capacity to make medical decisions need not involve a comprehensive evaluation of intellectual functioning. A straightforward discussion regarding a patient's understanding of a specific medical decision is usually sufficient. The psychiatrist asks questions about the nature of the illness and possible treatments and determines from the responses if the patient understands the problem, the treatment choices, and the likely consequences of a given decision. A formal judgment of medical competence can only be made in court (Appelbaum and Grisso, 1988). However, the psychiatrist's informal evaluation can guide treatment in most clinical situations.

A person whose mental abilities are partly impaired may be competent to make certain decisions about medical care. This situation can arise with an elderly person who suffers from mild dementia or a younger person affected by mild mental retardation (Kaplan et al., 1988). For this reason, decision-making capacity must be assessed on a case-by-case basis.

Also, a person who is incompetent at one time may be competent at another. Delirium and depression, conditions seen frequently among patients hospitalized for medical reasons, are examples of conditions that temporarily disrupt clear thinking. A person who is delirious or depressed may be found incompetent to refuse treatment, yet when the delirium clears or the depression lifts, that person is considered competent.

Consider the case of a thirty-five-year-old man with kidney failure (Shuchman and Wilkes, 1988). Doctors told him he required dialysis to take over the function of his kidneys. The man refused dialysis, saying he would rather die. A psychiatrist determined that the man suffered from a severe depression that was interfering with his ability to think rationally, and the man was deemed incompetent to make medical decisions. Over time, and with treatment, including antidepressant medication, the depression resolved. Eventually, the psychiatrist felt the man was capable of making treatment decisions. However, the man's uplifted spirits did not alter his desire to stop dialysis. His doctors discontinued the life-saving technology, and he died within a few days. Though the outcome may be death, respect for patient autonomy requires that competent patients be allowed to refuse therapies (Angell, 1984).

Commitment

Though involuntary confinement of mental patients has decreased markedly in the past three decades, there are still over 200,000 such commitments to psychiatric hospitals in the United States annually. Since involuntary hospitalization denies patients' autonomy, it is essential that it always be morally justified. Yet, what qualifies as such justification is controversial.

In the 1970s, amid a growing awareness of the abuses of psychiatric institutions, stringent limitations were placed on involuntary commitment of the mentally ill. During the 1960s, a person "in need of treatment due to mental disorder" met the criteria for involuntary admission to a psychiatric hospital in most states and provinces; today, the criteria are significantly narrower. Individuals may be involuntarily hospitalized if they are deemed a danger to themselves (for example, if they are about to attempt suicide), a danger to others, or unable to care for themselves due to mental illness. Typically, the assessment leading to involuntary hospitalization must be done by a mental health professional, though such requirements vary in different locations. Once confined, the person may be hospitalized for up to a few days. If commitment extends beyond a specified brief period, a court hearing generally must be held to determine whether further involuntary confinement is appropriate.

In practical terms, a doctor's decision to hospitalize someone involuntarily is a decision about which reasonable people may disagree. Consider a woman who is depressed and suicidal. She might be safest in a hospital, since there is a risk of her making a second suicide attempt while she remains depressed. But safety alone cannot be a reason for hospitalization, as very few of those who attempt suicide will go on to successfully complete suicides in the future. This woman might be safe outside a hospital in outpatient treatment. Research suggests that many factors other than those specified in commitment laws affect the numbers and types of patients committed to psychiatric hospitals (Roth, 1989); patients are sometimes hospitalized involuntarily solely because adequate alternative treatments are unavailable in a given area (Appelbaum and Roth, 1988).

During the late 1980s, psychiatrists and patients' families began objecting to the narrower commitment criteria, arguing that the rights of people with mental illness were being protected at the expense of their mental health (Appelbaum, 1987). These objections have resulted in the grounds for commitment being broadened in some areas. The "outpatient commitment" system, in which patients are ordered by a court to seek treatment during the day at outpatient programs but may return home at night, is an example of the recent broadening of commitment laws to include individuals who are not clearly dangerous to themselves or others (Geller, 1986).

Coerced treatment

In the 1980s, state courts in Massachusetts, New York, and California considered cases involving mental patients treated involuntarily with antipsychotic medications. All three courts ruled that unless a patient was found incapable of making treatment decisions, he or she could not be medicated involuntarily. These rulings were motivated in part by reports that psychiatric medications were overused at mental hospitals and that the staff was often indifferent to the risks of drug side effects in patients. Today, a competent mental patient's refusal of treatment must be respected. Even a patient confined to a mental institution cannot be treated against his or her will, unless the patient poses an imminent threat of harm to others. In practice, this refers to a patient who is behaving in a violent manner or is threatening to do so.

The more stringent criteria for involuntary medication have become a focus of controversy on similar grounds as the controversy over narrower commitment criteria. Psychiatrists have described mental patients who refuse treatment as "rotting with their rights on," conveying the image of a person who is not thinking rationally and whose condition is steadily worsening, yet who cannot be treated with medications because of judicial restraints (Appelbaum and Gutheil, 1979). Generally, however, psychiatrists are able to seek permission from the courts to medicate a person who is unable to think rationally.

Mentally ill patients sometimes decide in favor of medications when they are thinking clearly. A woman with schizophrenia, brought to the hospital because she had been threatening people, refused medications, believing they were part of an FBI plot. Her doctor asked the court for permission to medicate her, and it was decided that the patient should take medications for three months. Her thinking improved in that period. Subsequently, she continued taking the medicines because, she said, they helped her get along with people. One survey of hospitalized patients who had been involuntarily treated with medication found that the majority felt the decision to involuntarily medicate them had been correct (Schwartz et al., 1988).

Another area of care in which doctors may seek legal opinions regarding involuntary medication involves mentally ill female patients who decline birth-control treatments, such as birth-control pills or intrauterine devices (IUDs). Some authors suggest that there are situations in which it would be ethical to act to prevent pregnancy in patients who are incompetent to make medical decisions, but only when the patient's expressed values and beliefs are consistent with birth-control interventions (McCullough et al., 1992). The courts have held that when a mentally incompetent woman is pregnant, decisions about her obstetric care should involve a determination about what the woman would want if she were competent (Curran, 1990). In practice, when a severely mentally ill woman becomes a mother, child-welfare agencies are asked to evaluate the woman's ability to care for her child. In extreme cases, this evaluation may lead to court proceedings that can result in the woman's losing custody of her child.

Coerced compliance

The idea that a patient's decisions must be voluntary is central to the concepts of patient autonomy and informed consent. Exceptions to the idea of voluntariness, such as commitment and involuntary medication, have been viewed as last resorts for patients considered incapable of making rational decisions. Occasionally, however, coercive methods are used to encourage mentally ill individuals to comply with treatments, even when these individuals' decision-making capacities are not in question. An example is a man with a chronic mental illness who received disability payments from the government because of his mental condition. The man's government check was sent to the mental-health clinic where he was treated. To receive his check, the man was required to show up for his therapy session. The therapist believed this was a useful technique for encouraging compliance in a patient whose disorganized thinking sometimes made it difficult for him to comply with treatment.

The paternalism of this approach is no more justified with psychiatric patients than it would be with medical patients who have difficulty adhering to treatment regimens. Mental-health practitioners justify such paternalistic strategies as a means of preventing deterioration in a patient's condition. These clinical justifications, however, do not stand up to moral scrutiny.

Truth-telling

A physician or therapist who shields a patient from the truth about his or her illness may unwittingly cause mistrust of care providers and of the medical system in a patient who needs to depend on that system (Sheldon, 1982). The failure to tell the truth also conflicts with the obligation to provide patients with the necessary information for decisions about treatment. Yet clinicians caring for seriously mentally ill individuals sometimes do withhold information.

In one example, a physician withheld a diagnosis of cancer from a patient with a history of depression and suicide attempts (Lo, 1994). The physician feared that disclosing to the patient that she had a terminal illness could precipitate a suicide attempt. His intention was to protect the patient from harm, but the patient probably should have been informed about her diagnosis.

Though patients in general are likely to be told their diagnoses now, recent studies of patients in psychiatric hospitals have found that important information is frequently withheld from such patients. For example, psychiatric patients are prescribed medicines without being informed about potentially serious risks of the medicines (Lidz et al., 1984; Beck, 1988). For informed decision making, a patient needs to understand the benefits and risks of prescribed medications and why the doctor believes that the benefits outweigh the risks.

Patients, even those with mental illnesses and disabilities, expect and deserve to be told the truth. This does not mean that the truth should be disclosed insensitively. Health professionals should consider how to convey difficult information in a manner most appropriate to a particular patient. But the information should be provided. Psychiatric patients, no less than medical patients, need to feel they can trust their medical and psychiatric doctors.

Confidentiality

Doctor–patient and therapist–patient relationships demand confidentiality. But a patient's need for privacy must be balanced against the rights and needs of others. Suppose a man in treatment for alcohol abuse reveals that he had been aggressive toward his child while intoxicated. Most states have laws mandating the reporting of incidents of child abuse, yet a physician or counselor who reported this man would breach confidentiality. Here, the clinician must consider whether to violate the patient's right to privacy in order to protect others. In practice, this dilemma translates into a decision about whether the patient's offense is "reportable." The decision is made all the more difficult by the possibility that the man may leave treatment if he feels he has been betrayed, and his treatment may be what is most important to protect his child.

Situations other than child abuse pose similar dilemmas. In California, after a graduate student killed his former girlfriend, the victim's parents learned that the murderer had been in therapy and his psychologist had been aware of his intentions. They sued the therapist, and the California courts ruled that if a patient poses a serious risk of danger to others, his or her therapist has a duty to take reasonable steps to protect those in danger, which may include warning them of the risk. Similar rules now apply in other states. Such rules, however, do not dictate a therapist's decision and are not a mandate for therapists to ignore a patient's right to confidentiality. Since the majority of threats made by patients do not represent serious danger to others, the decision about whether a patient's threat merits a breach in confidentiality involves clinical judgment (Weinstock, 1988).

Allocation of scarce resources

When a mentally ill person also suffers from a serious medical illness, he or she should be offered whatever treatments are offered to persons with that medical condition who are not mentally ill. Yet an exception is sometimes made in the case of extremely scarce resources, such as organ transplants. A patient who is chronically mentally ill and also has severe liver disease might benefit from a liver transplant. Yet, mental illness might make it difficult for such a patient to comply with the required follow-up care, and noncompliance with care is a major cause of death following transplant (Wolcott, 1990).

To aid in the evaluation of such patients, transplantation programs typically require pretransplant evaluations to assess a patient's psychological stability, and transplant candidates are sometimes turned down because of mental illness. In a survey of heart-transplant programs, most programs considered certain psychiatric conditions to be an absolute contraindication to transplant: A person who has schizophrenia with active psychotic symptoms or a person with a history of multiple suicide attempts will be automatically denied a transplant (Olbrisch and Levenson, 1991).

Such automatic denials are not clearly ethical. In the event that a transplant candidate has a serious mental illness, it is important that the potential for treating the mental illness be considered before the patient is refused a transplant. The patient's desire to commit suicide, for example, may be caused by a treatable depres-

sion. Transplantation programs have begun to develop formal guidelines that may help bring greater fairness and consistency to decisions about whether to deny transplants to persons with serious mental illness.

Conclusion

In a number of key areas, a mentally ill person, by virtue of the effects of the mental illness, may lose certain rights with regard to medical and psychiatric treatment. Physicians and other health-care providers who confront these situations sometimes face difficult ethical dilemmas. The decision to hospitalize a mentally ill person involuntarily is often easily justified on moral grounds. However, decisions to breach a patient's confidentiality, or to withhold scarce resources such as organ transplants are generally not as clear from an ethical standpoint. Finally, it is probably quite rare that a physician or therapist who withholds the truth from the patient, or coerces the patient into complying with a recommended treatment, will be acting in an ethical manner.

MIRIAM SHUCHMAN

Directly related to this article is the companion article in this entry: RESEARCH ISSUES. *Also directly related are the entries* PATERNALISM; AUTONOMY; *and* HARM. *For a further discussion of topics mentioned in this article, see the entries* COMMITMENT TO MENTAL INSTITUTIONS; CONFIDENTIALITY; FREEDOM AND COERCION; HEALTH-CARE RESOURCES, ALLOCATION OF, *article on* MICROALLOCATION; INFORMATION DISCLOSURE; INFORMED CONSENT, *article on* ISSUES OF CONSENT IN MENTAL-HEALTH CARE; *and* JUSTICE. *Other relevant material may be found under* MENTAL ILLNESS; *and* PATIENTS' RIGHTS, *article on* MENTAL PATIENTS' RIGHTS.

Bibliography

ANGELL, MARCIA. 1984. "Respecting the Autonomy of Competent Patients." *New England Journal of Medicine* 310, no. 17:1115–1116.

APPELBAUM, PAUL S. 1987. "Crazy in the Streets." *Commentary* 83, no. 5:34–39.

APPELBAUM, PAUL S., and GRISSO, THOMAS. 1988. "Assessing Patients' Capacities to Consent to Treatment." *New England Journal of Medicine* 319, no. 25:1635–1638.

APPELBAUM, PAUL S., and GUTHEIL, THOMAS G. 1979. "'Rotting with Their Rights On': Constitutional Theory and Clinical Reality in Drug Refusal by Psychiatric Patients." *Bulletin of the American Academy of Psychiatry and Law* 7, no. 3:306–315.

APPELBAUM, PAUL S., and ROTH, LOREN H. 1988. "Assessing the NCSC Guidelines for Involuntary Civil Commitment from the Clinician's Point of View." *Hospital and Community Psychiatry* 39, no. 4:406–410.

BECK, JAMES C. 1988. "Determining Competency to Assent to Neuroleptic Drug Treatment." *Hospital and Community Psychiatry* 39, no. 10:1106–1108.

CURRAN, WILLIAM J. 1990. "Court-Ordered Cesarean Sections Receive Judicial Defeat." *New England Journal of Medicine* 323, no. 7:489–492.

GELLER, JEFFREY L. 1986. "Rights, Wrongs, and the Dilemma of Coerced Community Treatment." *American Journal of Psychiatry* 143, no. 10:1259–1264.

KAPLAN, KENNETH H.; STRANG, J. PETER; and AHMED, IQBAL. 1988. "Dementia, Mental Retardation, and Competency to Make Decisions." *General Hospital Psychiatry* 10, no. 6:385–388.

LIDZ, CHARLES W.; MEISEL, ALAN; ZERUBAVEL, EVIATAR; CARTER, MARY; SESTAK, REGINA M.; and ROTH, LOREN H. 1984. *Informed Consent: A Study of Decision-Making in Psychiatry.* New York: Guilford.

LO, BERNARD. 1994. *Resolving Ethical Dilemmas: A Guide for Clinicians.* Baltimore, Md.: Williams and Wilkins.

MCCULLOUGH, LARRY B.; COVERDALE, JOHN; BAYER, TIMOTHY; and CHERVENAK, FRANK A. 1992. "Ethically Justified Guidelines for Family Planning Interventions to Prevent Pregnancy in Female Patients with Chronic Mental Illness." *American Journal of Obstetrics and Gynecology* 167, no. 1:19–25.

OLBRISCH, MARY ELLEN, and LEVENSON, JAMES L. 1991. "Psychosocial Evaluation of Heart Transplant Candidates: An International Survey of Process, Criteria and Outcomes." *Journal of Heart and Lung Transplantation* 10, no. 6:948–955.

ROTH, LOREN H. 1989. "Four Studies of Mental Health Commitment." *American Journal of Psychiatry* 146, no. 2:135–137.

SCHWARTZ, HAROLD I.; VINGIANO, WILLIAM; and PEREZ, CAROL B. 1988. "Autonomy and the Right to Refuse Treatment: Patients' Attitudes After Involuntary Medication." *Hospital and Community Psychiatry* 39, no. 10:1049–1054.

SHELDON, MARK. 1982. "Truth Telling in Medicine." *Journal of the American Medical Association* 247, no. 5:651–654.

SHUCHMAN, MIRIAM, and WILKES, MICHAEL S. 1988. "Who Is to Decide?" *New York Times Magazine*, August 21, pp. 44–46.

WEINSTOCK, ROBERT. 1988. "Confidentiality and the New Duty to Protect: The Therapist's Dilemma." *Hospital and Community Psychiatry* 39, no. 6:607–609.

WOLCOTT, DEANE L. 1990. "Organ Transplant Psychiatry: Psychiatry's Role in the Second Gift of Life." *Psychosomatics* 31, no. 1:91–97.

II. RESEARCH ISSUES

Research guidelines

Protecting the interests of mentally ill and disabled people requires a delicate balance between two aims: a rigorous program of research into their medical problems and careful attention to the difficulties involved in using them, in ethically appropriate ways, as subjects of research. While the best hopes of understanding mental illnesses and disabilities depend on the results of medical research, those who suffer from them are especially vulnerable to exploitation or abuse.

Some of the ethical problems in conducting research on the mentally ill and disabled are those involved in most medical research involving human subjects but amplified because of the nature of some mental disorders. For example, questions of confidentiality take on heightened importance in light of the sensitive nature of many psychiatric disorders and the manner in which they overlap with social problems (for example, psychosexual disorders, such as pedophilia or exhibitionism, and the brushes with the criminal law that sometimes result).

Psychiatric research may also involve behavioral research, which sometimes relies on the deception of research subjects to accomplish its purposes (Eichelman et al., 1984). Finally, medical researchers sometimes develop entry criteria for psychopharmacological clinical trials that exclude women or minorities, arguing that, among other things, data would be needlessly complicated if research subjects were not as similar to each other as possible, and that, in the case of women of childbearing age, exclusion criteria are necessary to prevent potential harm to fetuses (Dresser, 1992). However, trials with exclusion criteria such as these may produce data that are not generalizable to groups other than the subject population. This can result in a lack of information about treatments for mental disorders and disabilities that primarily affect minorities or women (Dresser, 1992; National Institutes of Health, Office for Protection from Research Risks [NIH/OPRR], 1993; Yonkers and Harrison, 1993).

Two problems in conducting research on the mentally ill and disabled stand out. The first is competence, or decision-making capacity: Because of the nature of their problems, some mentally ill and disabled subjects may not be able to make informed decisions about whether to participate in a research protocol. Second, mentally ill or disabled subjects may be living in institutions for patients with special mental disorders, and institutionalization can exert pressures that compromise a person's ability to make a truly free choice about participating.

The nomenclature of mental disorders is controversial and constantly changing. Although there is no clear consensus on the definition of "mental disorder" or "mental illness," the *Diagnostic and Statistical Manual* (4th ed.) of the American Psychiatric Association states that each mental disorder "is conceptualized as a clinically significant behavioral or psychological syndrome or pattern that occurs in an individual and that is associated with present distress (e.g., a painful symptom) or disability (i.e., impairment in one or more areas of functioning) or with a significantly increased risk of suffering death, pain, disability or an important loss of freedom" (American Psychiatric Association, 1994, p. xxi). The DSM-IV definition goes on specifically to exclude deviant behavior (e.g., political, religious, or sexual), expectable responses to a particular event (such as grief in response to the death of a family member), and conflicts that are primarily between the individual and society. Most writers agree that the paradigmatic mental disorders are psychotic disorders, such as schizophrenia and bipolar affective disorder.

The term "mental disability" is broader, and it is sometimes used with the intention of including mental disorder or illness within its scope. However, it usually also includes mental retardation and other deficits in intellectual ability, such as Alzheimer's disease. Because of the fluctuating course and treatability of many mental illnesses, and the more stable nature of many mental disabilities, the main ethical difference between mental illness and disability for medical research is that the competence of the mentally ill patient is often more likely to change over time.

Some mentally ill or disabled persons may be incapable of giving valid informed consent to participate in a research trial. However, prohibiting these potential subjects from participating would rule out much medical research that could benefit either the subjects themselves or others with similar disorders—harming, in the long run, the very populations they are intended to protect. For this reason, over the past two decades there has been a growing consensus that research on the mentally ill and disabled can be justified in some cases, subject to certain conditions (Royal College of Psychiatrists [RCP], 1989; Royal College of Physicians of London [RCPL], 1990b; U.S. National Commission, 1979; Wing, 1991; Eichelmann et al., 1984; World Medical Association, 1989; OPRR, 1993; Medical Research Council of Canada [MRCC], 1987).

Perhaps the most important of these conditions is the stipulation that research on incompetent mentally ill or disabled persons should be allowed only if it cannot be done on competent persons (Wing, 1991; U.S. National Commission, 1979). The guidelines for biomedical research proposed by the World Health Organization (WHO) and the Council for International Organizations of Medical Sciences (CIOMS) make this requirement explicit, arguing that because of the risks and burdens involved, medical research should not be done on those who are unable to choose to participate if it can equally well be done on competent adult volunteers (WHO/CIOMS, 1982).

A second condition concerns a distinction made by the Declaration of Helsinki between research that is therapeutic, the aims of which include diagnostic or therapeutic benefit to the patient, and research that is nontherapeutic, the aim of which is "purely scientific" (World Medical Association, 1989; U.S. National Commission, 1979). Research that holds out the possibility of some therapeutic benefit to the mentally ill or disabled subject will be easier to justify than will research designed only to generate scientific knowledge and that offers possible benefits only to others. It has also been widely argued that nontherapeutic research is more justifiable if it is designed to yield generalizable knowledge about the condition from which the mentally ill or disabled subject suffers.

A third condition concerns the amount of risk to the research subject that may be justifiably allowed. Many professional and regulatory bodies state that research on incompetent subjects, such as children or the mentally ill or disabled, is ordinarily approvable only when the research involves only a minimal risk or a minor increment over minimal risk to the subject (Federal Policy for the Protection of Human Subjects, 1991; RCPL, 1990a). By this reasoning, some research on the mentally ill or disabled may be ethically justifiable, subject to specific additional conditions, even if it is nontherapeutic (Wing, 1991; OPPR, 1993).

Of course, there is considerable room for controversy as to what constitutes minimal risk (Freedman et al., 1993). U.S. federal policy compares minimal risk to the risks of the everyday life of the potential subject or those of a routine physical or psychological examination (Federal Policy, 1991). The Royal College of Physicians of London considers minimal risk to cover two sorts of situations: those that might involve negligible psychological distress, including other trivial reactions such as a mild headache or a feeling of lethargy, and those that involve very remote risks of serious injury or death—comparable with the risk of flying in a scheduled passenger aircraft (RCPL, 1990a).

Finally, it is widely agreed that research proposals involving the mentally ill or disabled should be approved by an ethics committee charged with reviewing research proposals, such as an institutional review board. Research should not proceed if a competent subject objects. When the subject is unable to give properly informed consent, consent should be sought from an appropriate surrogate decision maker, such as a relative (World Medical Association, 1989).

Competence and informed consent

A fundamental ethical requirement for most medical research is the informed consent of the subject. For consent to be valid, the subject must be capable of understanding the relevant implications of his or her decision to participate—the purpose, nature, and duration of the research, its possible risks and benefits, and so on. Because of the nature of some mental disorders, it is often unclear whether a mentally ill or handicapped person is capable of giving proper informed consent. And while many mental illnesses or disabilities will not affect these capabilities, it is the duty of the medical researcher to ensure that the potential subject of research is capable of making an informed decision whether to participate.

The ability to make a decision whether to participate in medical research is commonly termed "competence" or "decision-making capacity." A competent person should be capable of making a decision for which he or she can legitimately be considered accountable (Elliott, 1991). Competence is ordinarily defined in relation to a particular activity; a person can be competent to make some sorts of decisions but not others. For this reason, assessments of competence should ordinarily focus on the task at hand—in this case, understanding the implications of participating in a given research protocol.

Most proposed standards for assessing competence focus on the process of reasoning involved in making a decision rather than on the outcome of that decision (U.S. President's Commission, 1982; Buchanan and Brock, 1989). Because each person has different needs and values, there is often no single decision that can be judged correct for everyone. However, focusing primarily on a person's reasoning processes also can be problematic. A competent person may sometimes use faulty reasoning or make irrational decisions yet still be considered accountable for his or her choice (Brock and Wartmann, 1990; Elliott, 1991).

Probably the most influential tests of competence have been concerned with consent to treatment rather than to research (U.S. President's Commission, 1982; Buchanan and Brock, 1989; Gutheil and Appelbaum, 1982; Faden and Beauchamp, 1986). A U.S. President's Commission report relates competence to three aspects of a person's mental abilities: (1) the possession of a set of values and goals, (2) the ability to communicate and understand information, and (3) the ability to reason and deliberate about one's choice (U.S. President's Commission, 1982).

However, competence criteria that focus primarily on rationality and reasonable deliberation may not be very helpful when the person in question suffers from an affective disorder. As the Royal College of Psychiatrists has noted, patients with depressive delusions might consent to hazardous research because they think they deserve to be punished (RCP, 1989).

Furthermore, the mentally ill or disabled person may be able to satisfy a criterion partially but not fully, or he or she may be able to satisfy some criteria but not all of them. In cases like these, it is a matter for debate how high the standards for competence should be set.

For this reason, some writers and professional bodies, including the President's Commission, have endorsed a sliding-scale approach to assessing competence (U.S. President's Commission, 1982; Jonsen et al., 1986; Drane, 1985; OPRR, 1993). Under this approach, standards of competence are set higher for interventions with a risk–benefit ratio that is relatively worse, and lower for those with a risk–benefit ratio that is relatively better. For example, to participate in a research protocol whose risks are great and benefits are small, a subject might have to show not only that he or she understands the facts of the issues but also that he or she truly "appreciates" the nature of the situation. This may be a very high standard of understanding: an affective as well as a cognitive recognition of the nature of the research, an awareness of how others view his or her decision, and an understanding that he or she has a mental disorder appropriate for study (Appelbaum and Roth, 1981). On the other hand, if the risk–benefit ratio is much better, the standard for competence might be set very low: for example, merely showing evidence of a choice to participate.

Even when a subject is plainly incompetent to give truly informed consent, many writers believe that research should not be done without the subject's assent. That is, researchers should take steps to ensure that the subject, to the degree that he or she is mentally capable, agrees to or expresses a positive interest in participating in the research. Research is much more difficult to justify when it is done in spite of the subject's verbal or behavioral objections (Gutheil and Appelbaum, 1982; Wing, 1991). However, it is arguable that such research without the patient's assent is justifiable if the patient is clearly incompetent and the research is therapeutic, involves minimal risk, has been consented to by an appropriate surrogate, and is clearly in the best interests of the patient.

Issues of competence and informed consent can be especially problematic in certain mentally ill patients whose competence may change over time. In the case of therapeutic research (on antipsychotic medication, for instance), a research protocol may even restore to competence a patient who was previously incompetent. In these situations, the possible value of restoring the patient to competence should be weighed into the decision whether to enroll the patient in a research protocol. In cases where competence fluctuates over time, researchers should make efforts to obtain consent at a time when the patient is best able to give it.

Further provisions may be needed to protect the interests of mentally ill and disabled patients who are incompetent or whose competence is questionable. The Belmont Report recommended that researchers seek the permission of third parties who are most likely to understand the subject's situation and to act in that person's best interest (U.S. National Commission, 1979). Two standards have been widely employed in making decisions for incompetent patients: the "best interests standard," whereby third parties make decisions based on the interests of patients using socially shared values; and, in the case of previously competent patients, the "substituted judgment standard," whereby third parties make decisions based on values and preferences that the patient may have expressed in the past (Jonsen et al., 1986). The Belmont Report made the additional recommendation that such third parties be allowed to observe the research as it proceeds, with the option of withdrawing the subject from the research at any time (U.S. National Commission, 1979).

Institutionalization and consent

Can institutionalized mentally ill or disabled persons give valid informed consent to participate in medical research? Institutionalized patients are often especially attractive as research subjects because, among other reasons, their medication, diet, and compliance with a given study can be more easily monitored and controlled. Nevertheless, many writers have argued that institutionalized populations deserve special protection, pointing out the examples of the Willowbrook State School in New York, where mentally retarded children were injected with the hepatitis virus in 1956, and the Jewish Chronic Disease Hospital in Brooklyn, where nineteen chronically ill patients were injected with cancer cells in 1962 (U.S. National Commission, 1978; Ramsey, 1970; Annas et al., 1977; Kopelman, 1989). Some observers have argued that the fact of institutionalization invalidates informed consent and that research on the mentally ill or handicapped in institutions should be ruled out entirely.

There are several possible grounds for the argument that institutionalization invalidates informed consent. One that has been widely rejected is that any person who has a mental illness or disability severe enough to warrant institutionalization is mentally incompetent to give informed consent. Many people have illnesses or disabilities that impair them in ways that require institutional treatment but do not impair their ability to make competent judgments about participating in research. A second argument is that institutionalization itself deprives people of their ability to make their own decisions—for example, by placing them in a situation of constant subordination to authority (Annas et al., 1977). A third argument is that institutions severely limit the choices available to persons, thereby placing constraints on their freedom of choice. It is a matter of some controversy whether the offer to an institutionalized patient of the opportunity to participate in research is coercive or exploitative or, perhaps more to the point, whether it is quite simply morally objectionable (Wertheimer, 1987).

Some professional bodies, such as the Royal College of Physicians of London and the Royal College of Psychiatrists, have rejected the notion that involuntary detention invalidates consent, arguing that evidence indicates that detained patients do not want to be excluded from research and that research may improve the care of detained patients (RCPL, 1990b; RCP, 1989). On the other hand, nearly all professional bodies recognize that the institutionalized mentally ill and disabled are often subject to subtle forms of persuasion or manipulation, such as the prospect of improved food or medical care for participating in research. Also, consent from surrogate decision makers for institutionalized subjects can be problematic in that someone who does not live with and care for a person may not be very familiar with that person's goals, wishes, and personality (MRCC, 1987; Ramsey, 1970).

Research on institutionalized patients can also be difficult for impartial, external observers or regulatory bodies to monitor effectively. For these reasons, many agencies and professional bodies require that researchers take special measures to guard against manipulation of institutionalized subjects. A balance must be struck between the protection of potential subjects and respect for their freedom of choice to participate (U.S. National Commission, 1979).

CARL ELLIOTT

Directly related to this article is the companion article in this entry: HEALTH-CARE ISSUES. *For a further discussion of topics mentioned in this article, see the entries* COMPETENCE; CONFIDENTIALITY; INFORMED CONSENT, *especially the articles on* CONSENT ISSUES IN HUMAN RESEARCH, *and* ISSUES OF CONSENT IN MENTAL-HEALTH CARE; MENTAL-HEALTH SERVICES, *especially the article on* SETTINGS AND PROGRAMS; MENTAL ILLNESS; PATIENTS' RIGHTS, *article on* MENTAL PATIENTS' RIGHTS; RESEARCH, UNETHICAL; RESEARCH ETHICS COMMITTEES; *and* RESEARCH POLICY, *especially the article on* RISK AND VULNERABLE GROUPS. *For a discussion of related ideas, see the entries on* AUTHORITY; AUTONOMY; FREEDOM AND COERCION; HARM; RISK; *and* TRUST. *Other relevant material may be found under the entries* AGING AND THE AGED, *article on* HEALTH-CARE AND RESEARCH ISSUES; BEHAVIOR MODIFICATION THERAPIES; CHILDREN, *article on* HEALTH-CARE AND RESEARCH ISSUES; MENTAL HEALTH; MENTAL-HEALTH THERAPIES; MINORITIES AS RESEARCH SUBJECTS; PRIVACY AND CONFIDENTIALITY IN RESEARCH; RESEARCH METHODOLOGY; SEX THERAPY AND SEX RESEARCH; *and* WOMEN, *article on* RESEARCH ISSUES. *See also the* APPENDIX (CODES, OATHS, AND DIRECTIVES RELATED TO BIOETHICS), SECTION IV: ETHICAL DIRECTIVES FOR HUMAN RESEARCH.

Bibliography

AMERICAN PSYCHIATRIC ASSOCIATION. 1994. *Diagnostic and Statistical Manual of Mental Disorders: DSM-IV-R.* 4th ed. Washington, D.C.: Author.

ANNAS, GEORGE J.; GLANTZ, LEONARD H.; and KATZ, BARBARA F. 1977. *Informed Consent to Human Experimentation: The Subject's Dilemma.* Cambridge, Mass.: Ballinger.

APPELBAUM, PAUL S., and ROTH, LOREN R. 1981. "Clinical Issues in the Assessment of Competency." *American Journal of Psychiatry* 138, no. 11:1462–1467.

BROCK, DAN W., and WARTMANN, STEVEN A. 1990. "When Competent Patients Make Irrational Choices." *New England Journal of Medicine* 322, no. 22:1595–1599.

BUCHANAN, ALLEN E., and BROCK, DAN W. 1989. *Deciding for Others: The Ethics of Surrogate Decision-Making.* Cambridge: At the University Press.

DRANE, JAMES. 1985. "The Many Faces of Competency." *Hastings Center Report* 15, no. 2:17–21.

DRESSER, REBECCA. 1992. "Wanted: Single, White Male for Medical Research." *Hastings Center Report* 22, no. 1: 24–29.

EICHELMAN, BURR; WIKLER, DANIEL; and HARTWIG, ANNE. 1984. "Ethics and Psychiatric Research: Problems and Justification." *American Journal of Psychiatry* 141, no. 3:400–405.

ELLIOTT, CARL. 1991. "Competence as Accountability." *Journal of Clinical Ethics* 2, no. 3:167–171.

FADEN, RUTH R., and BEAUCHAMP, TOM L. 1986. *A History and Theory of Informed Consent.* New York: Oxford University Press.

"Federal Policy for the Protection of Human Subjects: Notices and Rules." 1991. *Federal Register,* pt. 2, vol. 56, no. 117, pp. 28002–28032 (56 FR 28002).

FREEDMAN, BENJAMIN; FUKS, ABRAHAM; and WEIJER, CHARLES. 1993. *"In Loco Parentis:* Minimal Risk as an Ethical Threshold for Research upon Children." *Hastings Center Report* 23, no. 2:13–19.

GUTHEIL, THOMAS G., and APPELBAUM, PAUL S. 1982. *Clinical Handbook of Psychiatry and the Law.* New York: McGraw-Hill.

JONSEN, ALBERT R.; SIEGLER, MARK; and WINSLADE, WILLIAM J. 1986. *Clinical Ethics: A Practical Approach to Ethical Decisions in Clinical Medicine.* 2d ed. New York: Macmillan.

KOPELMAN, LORETTA. 1989. "Moral Problems in Psychiatry." In *Medical Ethics,* pp. 253–290. Edited by Robert Veatch. Boston: Jones and Bartlett.

MEDICAL RESEARCH COUNCIL OF CANADA. 1987. *Guidelines on Research Involving Human Subjects.* Ottawa: Author.

NATIONAL INSTITUTES OF HEALTH (U.S.). OFFICE FOR PROTECTION FROM RESEARCH RISKS. 1993. *Protecting Human Research Subjects: Institutional Review Board Guidebook.* 2d ed., rev. Washington, D.C.: Author.

"The Nuremberg Code." 1949. In *Trial of War Criminals Before the Nuremberg Military Tribunals Under Control Council Law no. 10,* vol. 2, pp. 181–182. Washington, D.C.: U.S. Government Printing Office.

RAMSEY, PAUL. 1970. *The Patient as Person.* New Haven, Conn.: Yale University Press.

ROTH, LOREN H., and APPELBAUM, PAUL S. 1983. "Obtaining Informed Consent for Research with Psychiatric Patients:

The Controversy Continues." *Psychiatric Clinics of North America* 6, no. 4:551–565.

ROYAL COLLEGE OF PHYSICIANS OF LONDON. 1990a. *Guidelines on the Practice of Ethics Committees in Medical Research Involving Human Subjects.* 2d ed. London: Author.

———. 1990b. *Research Involving Patients.* London: Author.

ROYAL COLLEGE OF PSYCHIATRISTS. 1989. *Guidelines for Ethics of Research Committees on Psychiatric Research Involving Human Subjects.* London: Author.

U.S. NATIONAL COMMISSION FOR THE PROTECTION OF HUMAN SUBJECTS OF BIOMEDICAL AND BEHAVIORAL RESEARCH. 1978. *Research Involving Those Institutionalized as Mentally Infirm: Report and Recommendations.* Publication (OS) 78-0006 and Appendix (OS) 78-0007. Washington, D.C.: Author.

———. 1979. *The Belmont Report: Ethical Principles and Guidelines for the Protection of Human Subjects of Research.* Washington, D.C.: Author. Reprinted in NIH/OPRR, pp. A6-1–A6-13.

U.S. PRESIDENT'S COMMISSION FOR THE STUDY OF ETHICAL PROBLEMS IN MEDICINE AND BIOMEDICAL AND BEHAVIORAL RESEARCH. 1982. *Making Health Care Decisions: A Report on the Ethical and Legal Implications of Informed Consent in the Patient-Practitioner Relationship.* Washington, D.C.: Author.

WERTHEIMER, ALAN. 1987. *Coercion.* Princeton, N.J.: Princeton University Press.

WING, JOHN. 1991. "Ethics and Psychiatric Research." In *Psychiatric Ethics,* 2d ed., pp. 415–434. Edited by Sidney Bloch and Paul Chodoff. Oxford: Oxford University Press.

WORLD HEALTH ORGANIZATION/COUNCIL FOR INTERNATIONAL ORGANIZATIONS OF MEDICAL SCIENCES (CIOMS). 1982. *Proposed International Guidelines for Biomedical Research Involving Human Subjects.* Geneva: CIOMS.

WORLD MEDICAL ASSOCIATION. 1989. [1964]. "Declaration of Helsinki." In *International Digest of Health Legislation* 41, no. 3:530–533. Reprinted in NIH/OPRR, pp. A6-3–A6-6.

YONKERS, KIMBERLY A., and HARRISON, WILMA. 1993. "The Inclusion of Women in Psychopharmacology Trials." *Journal of Clinical Psychopharmacology* 13, no. 6:380–382.

MENTAL RETARDATION

See DISABILITY, *articles on* ATTITUDES AND SOCIOLOGICAL PERSPECTIVES, PHILOSOPHICAL AND THEOLOGICAL PERSPECTIVES, *and* LEGAL ISSUES; *and* MENTALLY DISABLED AND MENTALLY ILL PERSONS.

METAETHICS

See ETHICS, *articles on* TASK OF ETHICS, *and* MORAL EPISTEMOLOGY.

METAPHOR AND ANALOGY

Many of our practices and much of our discourse in health care hinge on metaphor and analogy, whose significance is sometimes overlooked because they are considered merely decorative or escape notice altogether. Despite their relative neglect, they significantly shape our interpretations of what is happening as well as what should happen. This entry will examine metaphor before considering analogy, particularly analogical reasoning, noting their overlap where appropriate.

Metaphors in bioethics

Nature and function of metaphors. Perhaps because medicine and health care involve fundamental matters of life and death for practically everyone, and in often mysterious ways, they are often described in metaphors. For instance, physicians may be viewed as playing God, or acting as parents, and nurses seen as advocates for patients, while medicine itself may be interpreted as warfare against disease. Metaphors involve imagining something as something else, for example, viewing human beings as wolves or life as a journey. "The essence of metaphor," according to George Lakoff and Mark Johnson, "is understanding and experiencing one thing through another (1980, p. 5). More precisely, metaphors are figurative expressions that interpret one thing in terms of something else (Soskice, 1985).

In contemporary philosophical literature on metaphor, critics have challenged some traditional conceptions, contending that metaphors are more than merely ornamental or affective ways to state what could be stated in a more literal or comparative way, and that they can be and often are cognitively significant (see, e.g., Black, 1962, 1979; Ricoeur, 1977; Soskice, 1985). According to the traditional substitution view, a metaphorical expression is merely a substitute for some equivalent literal expression. For example, the metaphorical expression "John is a fox" substitutes for the literal expression "John is sly and cunning." One common version of the substitution view, what philosopher Max Black (1962) calls a comparison view (elements of which can be found in Aristotle), construes metaphor as the presentation of an underlying analogy or similarity. Hence, metaphor is "a condensed or elliptical simile" (Black, 1962), or it is a "comparison statement with parts left out" (Miller, 1979). "John is a fox," for example, indicates that "John is like a fox in that he is sly and cunning." According to such views, metaphors are dispensable ways to express what could be expressed differently, but they often appeal to the emotions more effectively than their equivalent literal expressions or comparisons would do.

By contrast, many recent theories of metaphor stress its cognitive significance. In an early and very influential essay, Black (1962) defended an interaction view of metaphor, in which two juxtaposed thoughts interact to produce new meanings, through the metaphor's "system of associated commonplaces" or "associated implications." The metaphor—for instance, "wolf" in "man is a wolf"—serves as a "filter" for a set of associated implications that are transferred from the secondary subject ("wolf") to the principal subject ("man") in the sentence. In a full interaction or interanimation view of metaphor, the transfer of meaning occurs both ways, not merely from the secondary subject to the principal subject (Soskice, 1985).

Metaphors highlight and hide features of the principal subject, such as the physician who is viewed as a parent or as a friend, by their systematically related implications (Black, 1962; Lakoff and Johnson, 1980). When argument is conceived as warfare, for example, the metaphor highlights the conflict involved in argument, while it hides the cooperation and collaboration, involving shared rules, that are also indispensable to argument. Our metaphors thus shape how we think, what we experience, and what we do by what they highlight and obscure.

Metaphors are often associated with models. For instance, we have both metaphors and models of the doctor–patient relationship. The physician may be viewed through the metaphor of father and the patient through the metaphor of child, and their relationship may be interpreted through the model of paternalism. Models, for our purposes, state the network of associated commonplaces and implications in more systematic and comprehensive ways—according to Black, "every metaphor is the tip of a submerged model" (1979, p. 31).

Metaphors and models may be good or bad, living or dead. Both metaphors and models can be assessed by how well they illuminate what is going on and what should go on. We can distinguish descriptive and normative uses of metaphors and models, without admitting a sharp separation between fact and value. For instance, the metaphor of physician as father (or parent), and the model of paternalism (or parentalism), may accurately describe some relationships in medicine, or they may suggest ideal relationships in the light of some important principles and values.

Medicine as war. The metaphor of warfare illuminates much of our conception of what is, and should be, done in health care. This metaphor emerges in the day-to-day language of medicine: The physician as the captain leads the battle against disease; orders a battery of tests; develops a plan of attack; calls on the armamentarium or arsenal of medicine; directs allied health personnel; treats aggressively; and expects compliance. Good patients are those who fight vigorously and refuse to give up. Victory is sought; defeat is feared. Sometimes there is even hope for a "magic bullet" or a "silver bullet." Only professionals who stand on the firing line or in the trenches can really appreciate the moral problems of medicine. And they frequently have "war stories" to relate. Medical organization, particularly in the hospital, resembles military hierarchy; and medical training, particularly with its long, sleepless shifts in residencies, approximates military training more than any other professional education in our society (Childress, 1982).

As medicine wages war against germs that invade the body and threaten its defenses, so the society itself may also declare war on cancer or on AIDS under the leadership of its chief medical officer, who in the United States is the surgeon general. Articles and books even herald the "Medical-Industrial Complex: Our National Defense." As Susan Sontag notes, "Where once it was the physician who waged bellum contra morbum, the war against disease, now it's the whole society" (Sontag, 1990, p. 72).

The military metaphor first became prominent in the 1880s, when bacteria were identified as agents of disease that threaten the body and its defenses. The metaphor both illuminates and distorts health care. Its positive implications are widely recognized—for instance, in supporting a patient's courageous and hopeful struggle against illness and in galvanizing societal support to fight against disease. But the metaphor is also problematic. Sontag, who was diagnosed with cancer in the late 1970s, reports that her suffering was intensified by the dominance of the metaphor of warfare against cancer. Cancer cells do not just multiply; they are "invasive." They "colonize." The body's "defenses" are rarely strong enough. But since the body is under attack ("invasion") by "alien" invaders, counterattack is justified. Treatments are also often described in military language:

> Radiotherapy uses the metaphors of aerial warfare; patients are "bombarded" with toxic rays. And chemotherapy is chemical warfare, using poisons. Treatment aims to "kill" cancer cells (without, it is hoped, killing the patient). Unpleasant side effects of treatment are advertised, indeed overadvertised. ("The agony of chemotherapy" is a standard phrase.) It is impossible to avoid damaging or destroying healthy cells (indeed, some methods used to treat cancer can cause cancer), but it is thought that nearly any damage to the body is justified if it saves the patient's life. Often, of course, it doesn't work. (As in: "We had to destroy Ben Suc in order to save it.") There is everything but the body count. (Sontag, 1990, p. 65)

Such "military metaphors," Sontag suggests, "contribute to the stigmatizing of certain illnesses and, by extension, of those who are ill" (Sontag, 1990, p. 99). Other ill individuals have found the military metaphor unsatisfactory for other reasons. For instance, as a teenager, Lawrence Pray originally tried to conquer his diabetes, but his struggles and battles were futile and even counterproductive. Then over time he came to view his diabetes not as an "enemy" to be "conquered," but as a "teacher." Only then did he find a personally satisfactory way of living (Pray and Evans, 1983).

Still others with illness, by contrast, have found the military metaphor to be empowering and enabling. In her wide-ranging study of pathographies, that is, autobiographical descriptions of personal experiences of illness, treatment, and dying, Anne Hunsaker Hawkins identifies several "metaphorical paradigms" that offer themes of "an archetypal, mythic nature." In addition to illness as a battle, she notes illness as a game or sport (a subset of the military metaphor), illness as a journey into a distant country, illness as rebirth or regeneration—and, on a somewhat different level, healthy-mindedness as an alternative to contemporary medicine (Hawkins, 1993). While pathographies are individualized statements, they provide "an immensely rich reservoir of the metaphors and models that surround illness in contemporary culture" (Hawkins, 1993, p. 25). These various metaphorical paradigms structure individuals' interpretations of their experiences of illness. Patterns emerge in individuals' selection of metaphors. They vary in part according to the illness involved—for example, the military metaphor is more common in descriptions of experiences with cancer and AIDS, while the rebirth metaphor is more common in descriptions of a critical life-threatening event, such as a heart attack. Furthermore, the military metaphor is more prevalent than the journey metaphor because it better fits the experience of modern medicine—for instance, it is easier to construe the physician as a "general" in a war than as a "guide" on a journey. Nevertheless, these various metaphors are often mixed and complementary. They can be evaluated, Hawkins suggests, according to their capacity to enable and empower ill persons, for instance, by restoring a sense of personal dignity and worth. And, while expressing larger sociocultural patterns, the individual's choice of a particular metaphor is a creative act of assigning meaning to his or her illness (Hawkins, 1993).

The metaphor of warfare has been further challenged in modern medicine because of its apparent support for overtreatment, particularly of terminally ill patients, because death is the ultimate enemy, just as trauma, disease, or illness is the immediate enemy. Physicians and families under the spell of this metaphor frequently find it difficult to let patients die. "Heroic" actions, with the best available weapons, befit the military effort that must always be undertaken against the ultimate enemy. Death signals defeat and forgoing treatment signals surrender. Some clinicians even feel more comfortable withholding (i.e., not starting) a treatment for cancer, for instance, than they do withdrawing (i.e., stopping) the same treatment, in part because withdrawing treatment implies retreat.

According to its critics, the invocation of the military metaphor often fails to recognize moral constraints on waging war. "Modern medicine," William May writes, "has tended to interpret itself not only through the prism of war but through the medium of its modern practice, that is, unlimited, unconditional war," in contrast to the just-war tradition (May, 1983, p. 66). In the spirit of modern total war, "hospitals and the physician-fighter wage unconditional battle against death" (May, 1983, p. 66). One result is that many patients seek assisted suicide or active euthanasia in order to escape from this warfare's terrorist bombardment. Traditional moral limits in the conduct of war include the principle of discrimination, which authorizes direct attacks on combatants but not on noncombatants. In medical care, the opposing combatant is the disease or death, not the patient. However, the patient is regularly the battleground and sometimes even becomes the enemy. Furthermore, in accord with the just-war tradition's requirement of reasonable prospect of success and proportionality, the treatment should offer the patient a reasonable chance of success; his or her suffering must be balanced against the probable benefits of prolongation of life.

Other problematic or ambiguous implications of the war metaphor appear in the allocation of resources for and within health care. First, under the military metaphor, society's health-care budget tends to be converted into a defense budget to prepare for and conduct war against disease, trauma, and death. As a consequence, the society may put more resources into health care in relation to other goods than it could justify, especially under a different metaphor, such as nursing or business (see below). Indeed, the society may overutilize health care, especially because technological care may contribute less to the national defense of health itself—through the reduction of morbidity and premature mortality—than other factors, such as the reduction of poverty.

Second, within the health-care budget, the military metaphor tends to assign priority to critical care over preventive and chronic care. It tends to concentrate on critical interventions to cure disease, perhaps in part because it tends to view health as the absence of disease rather than a positive state. It tends to neglect care when cure is impossible. A third point is closely connected: In setting priorities for research and treatment, the military metaphor tends to assign priority to terminal diseases, such as cancer and AIDS, over chronic diseases. Fourth, medicine as war concentrates on technological interventions, such as intensive-care units, while downplaying less technological modes of care.

In short, the military metaphor has some negative or ambiguous implications for a moral approach to health-care decisions: It tends to assign priority to health care (especially medical care) over other goods, and, within health care, to critical interventions over chronic care, killer diseases over disabling ones, technological interventions over care, and heroic treatment of dying patients rather than allowing them to die in peace.

Some of the negative or ambiguous implications of the war metaphor for health care can be avoided if, as noted earlier, the metaphor is interpreted in accord with the limits set by the just-war tradition. However, the war metaphor may require supplementation as well as limitation. It is not the only prominent metaphor for health care; since the early 1980s its dominance has been threatened by the language of economics and business, as reflected in the language of a health-care industry. Providers deliver care to consumers, seek or are forced to seek productivity in light of cost-effectiveness or cost-benefit analyses, and may be concerned with "resource management, managed-care systems, and market strategies" (Stein, 1990, p. 172). This metaphor also highlights and hides various features of contemporary health care. Many critics of this metaphor worry that the language of efficiency will replace the language of care and compassion for the sick and equity in distribution of health care. Nevertheless, this metaphor has become more and more pervasive and persuasive as the structure of medicine and health care has changed, and as concerns about costs have become more central in societal discussions. Patients often fear undertreatment as hospitals and professionals seek to reduce costs, in contrast to their earlier fears of overtreatment under the war metaphor.

Both military and economics metaphors illuminate contemporary health care. But they may not be adequate, even together, to guide and direct health care. Whether any particular metaphor is adequate or not will depend in part on the principles and values it highlights and hides. Others have proposed nursing, a subset of health care, as a supplementary metaphor for the whole of health care, because of its attention to caring more than curing and to hands-on rather than technological care. Even though this metaphor of nursing is also inadequate by itself, it could direct the society to alternative priorities in the allocation of resources for and within health care, particularly for chronic care.

The war against AIDS. Even as the military metaphor has been partially displaced by business and economics metaphors in the changing structure of health care, it has gained favor as a way to describe and direct society's response to the major epidemic of the acquired immunodeficiency syndrome (AIDS). Societies often resort to the metaphor of war when a serious threat to a large number of human lives requires the mobilization of vast societal resources, especially when that threat comes from biological organisms, such as viruses, that invade the human body. And AIDS activists have appealed to the military metaphor in an effort to galvanize society and to marshal its resources for an effective counterattack against the human immunodeficiency virus (HIV) that causes AIDS. However, critics charge that the war on AIDS has diverted important resources away from other important wars, such as the war against cancer.

Other controversies have emerged. From the beginning of the war against AIDS, identification of the enemy has been a major goal. Once the virus was identified as the primary enemy, it also became possible to identify human beings who carry or harbor the virus. This technology then led to efforts to identify HIV-infected individuals, even through mandatory screening and testing, as potential enemies of the society. In social discourse and practice, the carrier tends to become an enemy as much as the virus he or she carries, especially since society views many actions that expose individuals to the risk of HIV infection as blameworthy. Thus, the metaphor of war often coexists with metaphors of AIDS as punishment and as otherness (Ross, 1989a, 1989b; Sontag, 1990). In this specific case of war against AIDS, just as in the general war against disease, the military metaphor would be less dangerous if society adhered to the constraints of the just-war tradition, rather than being tempted by a crusade.

Relationships between health-care professionals and recipients of care. Relationships between physicians and other health-care professionals, on one hand, and patients, on the other, have been described and directed by a wide variety of metaphors and models (Childress and Siegler, 1984). For example, William May (1983) has identified images of the physician as fighter, technician, parent, covenanter, and teacher; Robert Veatch (1972) has identified several major competing models of physician–patient relationships: engineering, priestly (which includes the paternalistic model), collegial, and contractual models. Other metaphors such as friend and captain of the ship have also been used (King et al., 1988).

Some critics contend that such models are "whimsical gestalts," that many other arbitrary models could be invented—for example, bus driver or back-seat driver—and that moral points can and should be made more directly (Clouser, 1983). Such criticisms overlook how metaphors and models function in the interpretation and evaluation of interactions between physicians and patients. They miss the role of imagination, which can be defined as "reasoning in metaphors" (Eerdman, 1969). For example, opponents of paternalistic medical relationships usually do not eschew all use of metaphor; instead they offer alternative metaphors, such as partnership or contracts. And these various metaphors may be more or less adequate to describe what occurs and to direct what should occur in health care.

Metaphors and models highlight and hide features of the roles of physicians and other health-care profes-

sionals by their various associated implications. For example, viewing the physician as a parent—or specifically as a father, based on the nineteenth-century model of the family—highlights some features of medical relationships, such as care and control, while hiding others, such as the payment of fees. In their use to describe, interpret, and explain relationships, such metaphors are subject to criticism if they distort more than they illuminate. And when they are offered to guide relationships and actions, they are subject to criticism if they highlight only one moral consideration, such as the physician's duty to benefit the patient or to respect patient autonomy, while hiding or obscuring other relevant moral considerations. It is also appropriate to consider the feasibility of various ideal relationships in light of significant personal, professional, and institutional constraints.

Several metaphors may be necessary to interpret health care as it is currently structured and to guide and direct actions, practices, and policies in health care. Some metaphors may fit some relationships better than others; for example, relations in clinical research, family practice, and surgery may be illuminated respectively by the metaphors of partner, teacher–student, and technician–consumer. Furthermore, not all of these metaphors conflict with each other; some may even be mutually supportive as well as compatible, for example, contractor and technician.

Nursing as advocacy. Major changes in the conception of nursing correlate with alterations in its primary metaphors. Whether situated within the military effort against disease or viewed as physicians' handmaidens and servants, nurses have traditionally been expected to cultivate passive virtues, such as loyalty and obedience. Their moral responsibility was primarily directed toward physicians and institutions, such as hospitals, and only secondarily toward patients. This interpretation of responsibility was shaped in part by nursing's military origins in the nineteenth century, as well as by societal conceptions of gender (Winslow, 1984; Bernal, 1992). Then in the 1970s, nursing was reconceived through the metaphor of advocacy. Nurses became advocates for "clients" and "consumers" (the term "patient" was often rejected as too passive). This legal metaphor, drawn from the advocate as one who pleads another's cause, especially before a tribunal of justice, highlights active virtues such as courage, persistence, and perseverance, and views the nurse as primarily responsible to the patient or client. This metaphor is explicit or implicit in formal nursing codes, and it is also featured in a large number of nurses' stories of advocacy and conflict in health care (Winslow, 1984; Bernal, 1992).

Critics note that the metaphor of advocacy reduces the range of services traditionally offered by nurses; it is thus insufficiently comprehensive (Bernal, 1992). In addition to distorting the human experience of illness, it distorts nursing by focusing almost exclusively on patients' or clients' rights, construed mainly in terms of autonomy, and it neglects positive social relationships in health care (Bernal, 1992). It highlights conflict among health-care professionals because it implies that some of them do not adequately protect the rights of patients. Thus, the metaphor frequently supports a call for increased nursing autonomy as a way to protect patient autonomy. Because of its adversarial nature, many question whether the metaphor of advocacy can adequately guide relationships among health-care professionals in the long run, even if it is useful in the short run. The metaphor may also assume that the nurse's responsibility to the patient/client is always clear-cut and overriding, even though nurses may face serious conflicts of responsibility involving patients, other individuals, associates, and institutions (Winslow, 1984). At the very least, sympathetic commentators call for further clarification of the metaphor of advocacy (Winslow, 1984); while critics seek alternative metaphors and models, such as covenant (Bernal, 1992), partnership, teamwork, or collegiality, that appear to offer more inclusive, cooperative ideals.

Playing God and other metaphors of limits. "Playing God" has been a common metaphor for both describing and directing the activities of scientists, physicians, and other health-care professionals. They have been criticized for usurping God's power—for instance, the power over life and death—by letting patients die or by using new reproductive technologies.

There are theological warrants for playing God in the Jewish and Christian traditions, which affirm the creation of human beings in God's image and likeness. Thus, Paul Ramsey (1970) calls on those who allocate health care to play God in a fitting way: We should emulate God's indiscriminate care by distributing scarce lifesaving medical technologies randomly or by a lottery rather than on the basis of judgments of social worth.

Despite a few such positive uses of the metaphor of "playing God," the metaphor is generally used to identify two aspects of divine activity that should not be imitated by humans: God's unlimited power to decide and unlimited power to act. On one hand, users of this metaphor demand scientific and medical accountability over unilateral decision making. On the other hand, critics call for respect for substantive limits—for example, not creating new forms of life (U.S. President's Commission, 1982).

Edmund Erde contends that statements such as "doctors should not play god" are so unclear that they cannot function as commands and do not articulate a principle; thus, they cannot be followed because agents do not know how to conform their actions to them. Nor do they explain why certain actions should not be undertaken. Such phrases are, Erde argues, "metaphoric in that they tuck powerful feelings and images into descriptive language that cannot be understood literally" (Erde, 1989, p. 606). Any activity, such as mercy killing, that is "labeled 'playing god' carries the implication that it is clearly wrong" (Erde, 1989, p. 607). These phrases are used for situations in which agents face choices, but one option is considered immoral and is rejected as arrogantly and presumptuously playing God. The background of intelligibility of this metaphor, according to Erde, is found in the Western idea of the great chain of being, which identifies appropriate responsibilities at each level and opposes the usurpation of power and the failure to respect limits (Erde, 1989).

Other important and widespread metaphors of limits include the "thin edge of the wedge" and the "slippery slope," both of which warn against undertaking certain actions because other unacceptable actions will inevitably follow. Examples regularly appear in debates about euthanasia. Even though such metaphors are often misused, they are appropriate in some contexts. In each use of these metaphors, important moral questions require attention—the evaluation of the first action and subsequent actions—and important conceptual and empirical questions must be addressed in order to determine whether the putatively bad consequences will inevitably follow what might be innocuous first steps. (Similar questions emerge for some analogies, such as the Nazi analogy, which is also widely invoked to oppose such practices as mercy killing.)

Metaphors for bioethics and bioethicists. The role and function of the bioethicist have often been construed in metaphorical terms. The common language of "applied ethics" invokes the metaphor of engineering as an application of basic science that does not contribute to basic science. The expertise of applied ethicists resides in their ability to apply general theories and principles to specific arenas of human activity. The metaphor of application has been widely challenged on the grounds that it is too narrow and distorts much that is important in bioethics. The term "applied" suggests that ethicists are problem solvers rather than problem setters, that they solve puzzles rather than provide perspectives, that they answer rather than raise questions, and that they begin from theory rather than from lived experience. It implies a limited technical or mechanical model of ethics.

The term "applied" distorts the numerous theoretical controversies in bioethics, and neglects the way bioethics may help to resolve or recast some theoretical controversies. At the very least, the metaphor of application may need to be supplemented by various other metaphors for the task of practical ethics and the role of the practical ethicist: "Theoretician, diagnostician, educator, coach, conceptual policeman, and skeptic are also supplemental or alternative roles to that of the technician" (Caplan, 1980, p. 30).

Some other metaphors are drawn from ancient religious roles, such as prophet or scribe. Yet another metaphor is "conversation," which is prominent in approaches to bioethics that emphasize interpretation, hermeneutics, and narrative. And the "stranger" has been proposed as the best metaphor for the ethicist in professional education because his or her outside perspective can challenge ordinary assumptions (Churchill, 1978).

Suggestions emerge at various times to retire all metaphors, not merely some metaphors in some realm of discourse—for instance, Sontag (1990) proposes retiring all metaphors for illness. However, it is not possible to strip our discourse in science, medicine, and health care, or in biomedical ethics, of all metaphors. Instead, we must use metaphors with care and must carefully assess their adequacy in descriptive and normative functions.

Analogies in bioethics

Analogies and analogical reasoning. Often metaphors and analogies are presented in ways that indicate their substantial overlap. Indeed, for the comparison view of metaphor, there is little difference between them, because metaphors are compressed analogies. Some recent theories of metaphor have stressed, by contrast, that metaphors create similarities rather than merely expressing previously established and recognized similarities or analogies. According to Black, comparison views of metaphor fail because they reduce the ground for shifts of meaning (from the secondary subject to the primary subject) to similarity or analogy (Black, 1962). Nevertheless, there is a strong consensus that metaphorical statements presuppose some resemblance, even when they also create resemblance (Ricoeur, 1977). Black later conceded that metaphors "mediate an analogy or structural correspondence." Metaphor is, roughly speaking, "an instrument for drawing implications grounded in perceived analogies of structure between two subjects belonging to different domains" (Black, 1979, p. 32). And yet metaphor does not merely compare two things that are similar, but rather enables us to see similarities in what would be regarded as dissimilar.

Metaphors and analogies are thus closely related, with metaphors both expressing and creating similarities. In general, good metaphors function cognitively to generate new meaning and insight, by providing new perspectives; while good analogies extend our knowledge by moving from the familiar to the unfamiliar, from the established to the novel. In stretching language and

concepts for new situations, analogy does not involve the imaginative strain often evident in the use of metaphors (Soskice, 1985). Nevertheless, the differences in function between metaphors and analogies should not be exaggerated.

The term analogy derives from the Greek *analogia*, which referred to mathematical proportion. "An analogy in its original root meaning," Dorothy Emmet observes, "is a proportion, and primarily a mathematical ratio, e.g., 2:4::4:X. In such a ratio, given knowledge of three terms, and the nature of the proportionate relation, the value of the fourth term can be determined. Thus analogy is the repetition of the same fundamental pattern in two different contexts" (Emmet, 1945, p. 6).

Analogical reasoning proceeds inductively, moving from the known to the unknown. It appears prominently in problem solving and thus is featured in research in cognitive science and artificial intelligence (Helman, 1988; Keane, 1988). For instance, computer problem-solving programs must search for analogous problems that have been successfully solved to generate solutions to new problems whether in highly structured domains such as law or in less structured domains.

Analogical reasoning has an important place in moral discourse, not only because of its importance in problem solving, but also because of the widely recognized moral requirement to treat similar cases in a similar way. Often stated as a principle of universalizability or of formal justice or formal equality, dating back at least to Aristotle, the requirement to treat similar cases in a similar way also appears in the common law's doctrine of precedent. The basic idea is that one does not make an acceptable moral or a legal judgment—perhaps not even a moral or legal judgment at all—if one judges that X is wrong, but that a similar X is right, without adducing any relevant moral or legal difference between them. In general, analogical reasoning illuminates features of morally or legally problematic cases by appealing to relevantly similar cases that reflect a moral or legal consensus (precedent). Of course, much of the moral (or legal) debate hinges on determining which similarities and differences are both relevant and significant.

Since the early 1980s ethicists have directed new attention to the role of analogical reasoning in case-oriented or casuistical judgments in bioethics and elsewhere. In *The Abuse of Casuistry*, Albert Jonsen and Stephen Toulmin identify "the first feature of the casuistic method" in its classical formulations as "the ordering of cases under a principle by paradigm and analogy" (Jonsen and Toulmin, 1988, p. 252). For instance, the rule prohibiting killing is set out in "paradigm cases" that illustrate its most manifest breaches according to its most obvious meaning. Moving from simple and clear cases to complex and uncertain ones, casuists examine various alternative circumstances and motives to determine whether those other cases violate the rule against killing. They seek analogies that permit the comparison of "problematic new cases and circumstances with earlier exemplary ones," that is, the similar cases that constitute presumptions (Jonsen and Toulmin, 1988, p. 316).

Despite the claims of some modern casuists, it is not clear that analogical reasoning distinguishes casuistical from principlist approaches. For instance, in analyzing the novel microallocation problems of modern medicine, Paul Ramsey (1970) appealed to the analogous "lifeboat" cases—when some passengers have to be thrown overboard in order to prevent the lifeboat from sinking—as a way to interpret the requirements of the principle of equality of opportunity in distributing scarce lifesaving medical technologies such as kidney dialysis. Because principles and rules are indeterminate, and because they sometimes conflict, analogical reasoning can be expected in case judgments—mere application cannot be sufficient.

Analogies are often divided into two main types: analogies of attribution and analogies of proportion (Cahill, 1982). The analogy of attribution involves a comparison of two terms or analogates, both of which have a common property, the analogon, that appears primarily in one and secondarily in the other. As Thomas Aquinas noted, "healthy" is used primarily for a person in a state of health (a "healthy" person) and secondarily for those medicines and practices that help to maintain or restore health (e.g., a "healthy" diet) or specimens that provide evidence of the body's health (e.g., "healthy" blood). By contrast, in the analogy of proportion, the analogates lack a direct relationship, but each of them involves a relationship that can be compared to a relationship in the other (Cahill, 1982). This second type is most common in analogical reasoning in biomedical ethics, as is evident in debates about maternal–fetal relations and abortion, where analogies of attribution also appear, particularly with reference to the fetus.

Analogical reasoning in debates about maternal–fetal relations.   Debates about maternal–fetal relations, including pregnant women's decisions to abort and to decline cesarean sections, illustrate the pervasiveness and importance of analogical reasoning. Traditionally, abortion has been construed as directly killing the fetus, an innocent human being, in violation of the duty of nonmaleficence. Hence, in traditional Roman Catholic moral theology, direct abortions are tantamount to homicide. Sometimes the analogy of the "unjust aggressor" appears in situations where the pregnancy threatens the pregnant woman's life or health; but it has not been accepted in official Catholic thought the way the similar analogy of the "pursuer" has been accepted in some Jewish thought to justify abortions when there is such a threat.

Some feminists and others have attempted to recast the debate about abortion to focus on the basis and extent of the pregnant woman's obligation to provide bodily life support to the fetus. Often accepting, at least for purposes of argument, the premise that the fetus is a human being from the moment of conception (or at some time during the pregnancy), they argue that this premise does not entail that the pregnant woman always has a duty to sustain the fetus's life regardless of the circumstances of pregnancy, the risks and inconveniences to the pregnant woman, and so forth. Their arguments often proceed through analogies to other hypothetical or real practices or cases, on the assumption that a judgment about those practices or cases will entail a similar judgment about abortion.

The fantastic abortion analogies introduced by Judith Jarvis Thomson (1971) have been particularly influential and controversial. In one of her artificial cases, an individual with a rare blood type is kidnapped by the Society of Music Lovers and attached to a famous violinist who needs to purify his system because of his renal failure. Part of the debate concerns whether relevant analogies can be found in such fantastic, artificial cases, in contrast to actual real-life cases. For example, against Thomson, John Noonan opposes abortion in part by appeal to a U.S. tort-law case, in which the court held liable the hosts who had invited a guest for dinner but then put him out of their house into the cold night even though he had become sick and fainted and requested permission to stay (Noonan, 1974).

Some feminists and others contend that other analogous real-life legal and moral cases support the pregnant woman's free decision to continue or to discontinue her pregnancy. For many the relevant analogous cases concern living organ and tissue donation. Such donations are conceived as voluntary, altruistic acts that should not be forced by others even to save the potential recipient's life. They are "gifts of life." Requiring a pregnant woman to continue the pregnancy until birth imposes on her a heavier burden than others are expected to bear in analogous circumstances, such as a parent who could save a child's life by donating a kidney. Thus, the provision of bodily life support, whether through donating an organ or allowing the fetus to use the uterus, has been conceived as a gift of life that should not be legally enforced (Mattingly, 1984; Jung, 1988).

According to Lisa Sowle Cahill (1982), much analogical reasoning about pregnancy overlooks what is unique about maternal–fetal relations and thus obscures the morally relevant features of pregnancy or makes some relevant features more significant than they are. Many analogies problematically narrow our moral perspective on abortion by portraying the inception of pregnancy as accidental and the fetus as strange, alien, and even hostile. Furthermore, they often rely on the connotative meanings of their terms, particularly as embedded in a story, such as Thomson's case of kidnapping the unwilling blood donor. Examples also appear in the rhetoric of abortion opponents who, for instance, speak of the fetus as a "child," and thereby distort the unique dependence of the fetus on the pregnant woman (Cahill, 1982). Finally, Cahill contends, justifications of abortion based on analogy often rest on liberal convictions that special responsibilities derive only from free choice.

For all these reasons, Cahill holds that analogical reasoning needs supplementation through direct examination of the unique features of maternal–fetal relations, particularly total fetal dependence, and of the ways these unique features qualify maternal, professional, and societal obligations. She argues that, as a category or class of moral relations, pregnancy "is unique among human relations at least because in it one individual is totally and exclusively dependent on a particular other within a relation which represents in its physical and social aspects what is *prima facie* to be valued positively" (Cahill, 1982, p. 283). Hence, she argues, most analogies hide what is distinctive and unique about pregnancy, even though they identify some morally relevant features of maternal–fetal relations.

With the emergence of other maternal–fetal conflicts, particularly regarding cesarean sections to benefit the fetus, similar debates have emerged about the appropriateness of the analogy with living organ and tissue donation. For instance, in the case of A.C. (1990), the majority of the court held that, just as courts do not compel people to "donate" organs or tissue to benefit others, so they should not compel cesarean sections against the will of pregnant women to benefit potentially viable fetuses. The dissenting opinion rejected the analogy with organ and tissue donation, insisting that the pregnant woman "has undertaken to bear another human being, and has carried an unborn child to viability," that the "unborn child's" dependence upon the mother is unique and singular, and that the "viable unborn child is literally captive within the mother's body" (A.C., In re, 1990).

Even though analogies with organ and tissue donation are now widely invoked to oppose state control of pregnant women's decisions regarding both abortion and cesarean sections, there are important differences between these two contexts. In the abortion debate, pregnancy is viewed as the provision of bodily life support and is itself analogous to the donated organ. In the debate about cesarean sections, the surgical procedure is analogous to organ donation—the potentially viable fetus is removed for its own benefit rather than to benefit some other party as in organ or tissue donation. In the abortion debate, the pregnancy is viewed as invasive; in

the debate about cesarean sections, the surgical procedure is invasive. The central issue is whether state coercion in these cases to benefit the fetus is morally and legally acceptable. The debate hinges in part on the appropriateness of the living organ and tissue donation as an analogy. Even the critics of the analogy engage in analogical reasoning, but they deny that the similarities are more morally or legally relevant and significant than the dissimilarities. Defenders of governmental coercion could also hold that the moral or legal precedent is mistaken and that organs and tissues should sometimes be conscripted or expropriated from living persons.

Similar disputes appear in other areas of contemporary bioethics—for instance, in debates about whether mandatory testing or screening for antibodies to the human immunodeficiency virus, which causes AIDS, can be justified by analogy to accepted practices of mandatory testing or screening; and in debates about whether transplantation experiments using human fetal tissue, following deliberate abortions, are analogous to the complicitous use of materials or data from the morally heinous Nazi experiments. In these cases, as in many others, the debates focus to a great extent on the relevance and significance of the proposed analogies.

Conclusions

Debates in biomedical ethics are often debates about which metaphors and analogies illuminate more than they distort. Far from being merely decorative or affective, metaphors and analogies are central to both discourse and practice. They must be evaluated specifically according to how well they function to describe and/or direct actions and relationships. Even though in recent bioethics metaphors and analogies have sometimes been offered as ways to circumvent or transcend principles and rules, particularly through attention to cases, narratives, and aesthetic dimensions of experience, they are not necessarily incompatible with principles and rules. Analogical reasoning is important within frameworks of principles and rules, as well as in casuistry, and metaphors and models often succeed or fail depending on how well they express the full range of relevant moral considerations.

JAMES F. CHILDRESS

Directly related to this entry are the entries BODY, *article on* EMBODIMENT: THE PHENOMENOLOGICAL TRADITION; CARE, *article on* HISTORY OF THE NOTION OF CARE; CASUISTRY; INTERPRETATION; LITERATURE; *and* NARRATIVE. *For a further discussion of concepts or issues that have been elucidated by use of metaphors and analogies, see the entries* ABORTION, *section on* CONTEMPORARY LEGAL

AND ETHICAL ASPECTS, *article on* CONTEMPORARY ETHICAL PERSPECTIVES; AIDS; DEATH AND DYING: EUTHANASIA AND SUSTAINING LIFE; FETUS, *article on* PHILOSOPHICAL AND ETHICAL ISSUES; MEDICINE AS A PROFESSION; NURSING AS A PROFESSION; PAIN AND SUFFERING; *and* PATERNALISM. *Other relevant material may be found under the entries* BODY, *article on* CULTURAL AND RELIGIOUS PERSPECTIVES; FEMINISM; HEALTH AND DISEASE, *article on* HISTORY OF THE CONCEPTS; LAW AND BIOETHICS; LAW AND MORALITY; TRAGEDY; *and* VALUE AND VALUATION.

Bibliography

A.C., *In re*. 1990. 57B A.2d 1235 (D.C. App.).

BERNAL, ELLEN W. 1992. "The Nurse as Patient Advocate." *Hastings Center Report* 22, no. 4:18–23.

BLACK, MAX. 1962. "Metaphor." In his *Models and Metaphors: Studies in Language and Philosophy*, pp. 25–47. Ithaca, N.Y.: Cornell University Press.

———. 1979. "More About Metaphor." In *Metaphor and Thought*, pp. 19–43. Edited by Andrew Ortony. Cambridge: At the University Press.

CAHILL, LISA SOWLE. 1982. "Abortion and Argument by Analogy." *Horizons* 9, no. 2:271–287.

CAPLAN, ARTHUR L. 1980. "Ethical Engineers Need Not Apply: The State of Applied Ethics Today." *Science, Technology, and Human Values* 6, no. 33:24–32.

CHILDRESS, JAMES F. 1982. *Who Should Decide? Paternalism in Health Care*. New York: Oxford University Press.

CHILDRESS, JAMES F., and SIEGLER, MARK. 1984. "Metaphors and Models of Doctor–Patient Relationships: Their Implications for Autonomy." *Theoretical Medicine* 5, no. 1:17–30.

CHURCHILL, LARRY R. 1978. "The Ethicist in Professional Education." *Hastings Center Report* 8, no. 6:13–15.

CLOUSER, K. DANNER. 1983. "Veatch, May, and Models: A Critical Review and a New View." In *The Clinical Encounter: The Moral Fabric of the Patient–Physician Encounter*, pp. 89–103. Edited by Earl E. Shelp. Dordrecht, Netherlands: D. Reidel.

EERDMAN, DAVID V. 1969. "Coleridge as Editorial Writer." In *Power and Consciousness*, pp. 187–201. Edited by Conor Cruise O'Brien and William Dean Vanech. New York: New York University Press.

EMMET, DOROTHY MARY. 1945. *The Nature of Metaphysical Thinking*. New York: St. Martin's Press.

ERDE, EDMUND L. 1989. "Studies in the Explanation of Issues in Biomedical Ethics: II. On 'On Playing God,' etc." *Journal of Medicine and Philosophy* 14, no. 6:593–615.

HAWKINS, ANNE HUNSAKER. 1993. *Reconstructing Illness: Studies in Pathography*. West Lafayette, Ind.: Purdue University Press.

HELMAN, DAVID H., ed. 1988. *Analogical Reasoning: Perspectives of Artificial Intelligence, Cognitive Science, and Philosophy*. Dordrecht, Netherlands: Kluwer Academic Publishers.

JONSEN, ALBERT R., and TOULMIN, STEPHEN. 1988. *The Abuse of Casuistry: A History of Moral Reasoning*. Berkeley: University of California Press.

JUNG, PATRICIA BEATTIE. 1988. "Abortion and Organ Donation: Christian Reflections on Bodily Life Support." *Journal of Religious Ethics* 16, no. 2:273–305.

KEANE, MARK T. 1988. *Analogical Problem Solving*. Chichester, England: Ellis Norwood.

KING, NANCY M. P.; CHURCHILL, LARRY R.; and CROSS, ALAN W. 1988. *The Physician as Captain of the Ship: A Critical Reappraisal*. Dordrecht, Netherlands: D. Reidel.

LAKOFF, GEORGE, and JOHNSON, MARK. 1980. *Metaphors We Live By*. Chicago: University of Chicago Press.

MATTINGLY, SUSAN S. 1984. "Viewing Abortion from the Perspective of Transplantation: The Ethics of the Gift of Life." *Soundings* 67, no. 4:399–410.

MAY, WILLIAM F. 1975. "Code, Covenant, Contract, or Philanthropy." *Hastings Center Report* 5, no. 6:29–38.

———. 1983. *The Physician's Covenant: Images of the Healer in Medical Ethics*. Philadelphia: Westminster Press.

MILLER, GEORGE. 1979. "Images and Models, Similes and Metaphors." In *Metaphor and Thought*, pp. 202–250. Edited by Andrew Ortony. Cambridge: At the University Press.

NOONAN, JOHN T. 1974. "How to Argue About Abortion." New York: Ad Hoc Committee in Defense of Life.

PRAY, LAWRENCE, and EVANS, RICHARD, III. 1983. *Journey of a Diabetic*. New York: Simon and Schuster.

RAMSEY, PAUL. 1970. *The Patient as Person: Explorations in Medical Ethics*. New Haven, Conn.: Yale University Press.

RICOEUR, PAUL. 1977. *The Rule of Metaphor: Multi-Disciplinary Studies of the Creation of Meaning in Language*. Translated by Robert Czerny. Toronto, Ont.: University of Toronto Press.

ROSS, JUDITH. 1989a. "Ethics and the Language of AIDS." In *The Meaning of AIDS: Implications for Medical Science, Clinical Practice and Public Health Policy*, pp. 30–41. Edited by Eric T. Juengst and Barbara A. Koenig. New York: Praeger.

———. 1989b. "The Militarization of Disease: Do We Really Want a War on AIDS?" *Soundings* 72, no. 1:39–50.

SONTAG, SUSAN. 1990. *Illness as Metaphor; and, AIDS and Its Metaphors*. New York: Doubleday Anchor Books.

SOSKICE, JANET MARTIN. 1985. *Metaphor and Religious Language*. Oxford: At the Clarendon Press.

STEIN, HOWARD F. 1990. *American Medicine as Culture*. Boulder, Colo.: Westview Press.

THOMSON, JUDITH JARVIS. 1971. "A Defense of Abortion." *Philosophy and Public Affairs* 1, no. 1:47–66.

U.S. PRESIDENT'S COMMISSION FOR THE STUDY OF ETHICAL PROBLEMS IN MEDICINE AND BIOMEDICAL AND BEHAVIORAL RESEARCH. 1983. *Splicing Life*. Washington, D.C.: U.S. Government Printing Office.

VEATCH, ROBERT M. 1972. "Models for Ethics in Medicine in a Revolutionary Age." *Hastings Center Report* 2, no. 3: 5–7.

WINSLOW, GERALD R. 1984. "From Loyalty to Advocacy: A New Metaphor for Nursing." *Hastings Center Report* 14, no. 3:32–40.

MEXICO

See MEDICAL ETHICS, HISTORY OF, *section on* THE AMERI-CAS, *article on* LATIN AMERICA.

MILITARY PERSONNEL AS RESEARCH SUBJECTS

The basic ethical issue in the use of military personnel as research subjects is whether individuals in the armed services are free to accept or decline participation in research. Voluntary participation has been recognized as an essential requirement for ethical human experimentation; it is the cornerstone of the Nuremberg Code, developed in 1947 in response to Nazi medical experimentation. Some bioethicists have expressed concerns that military discipline, with its emphasis on following orders and the chain of command, may constrain an individual's ability to make uncoerced decisions about participation in research. It is not clear, for example, how participation in a research study differs significantly from other hazardous duties expected of military personnel.

Negotiating the balance between respect for individual autonomy and the needs of the military is more problematic when nations are at war. During World War II, the medical needs of the military were invoked to justify the experimental use of vaccines and drugs in military populations, as well as nontherapeutic research on conscientious objectors, orphans, prisoners, and the mentally ill (Rothman, 1991). In the Persian Gulf War (1991) the military's decision to seek a waiver of its own regulations about informed consent for the administration of investigational drugs and vaccines to American servicemen and servicewomen prompted controversy between critics who condemned this deviation from the Nuremberg Code and supporters who argued that the principle of preventing unnecessary harm to military personnel made the decision necessary (Howe and Martin, 1991; Annas and Grodin, 1991). These issues, which have received little sustained analysis, require greater attention from bioethicists.

Historically, armed forces have provided both unique opportunities and special needs for the study of human health and disease. "He who would become a surgeon," observed the Greek physician Hippocrates, "should join the army and follow it" (Hume, 1943, p. 78). Early efforts in disease prevention and treatment reflected the practical concerns of maintaining military personnel in good condition. One of the earliest clinical trials involving human subjects was conducted by the naval surgeon James Lind (1716–1794) on British sailors. In 1746 Lind administered six different treatments to twelve sailors suffering from scurvy, and observed the beneficial effect of oranges and lemons in recovery from the disease. Other British naval surgeons conducted similar trials of cures for scurvy (Carpenter, 1986).

Traumatic injuries from guns and other weapons have provided distinctive opportunities for military physicians to study human anatomy and physiology. In the 1820s the American army physician William Beaumont investigated the process of human digestion in a live subject after his repeated efforts failed to close the gunshot wound to Alexis St. Martin's stomach. Beaumont developed an employment contract with his French-Canadian research subject, who agreed to allow physiological experiments in exchange for room, board, and wages. Beaumont also persuaded the trapper to enlist in the U.S. Army, giving the physician more complete control of his subject and rendering St. Martin's "faithless absconding" subject to military law (Numbers, 1979).

The rise of experimental science and the germ theory of disease in the late nineteenth century increased experimentation involving human beings. The Medical Department of the U.S. Army expanded its efforts to control infectious diseases, the major cause of mortality in the military before World War II. All U.S. Army commanders were directed to cooperate with the Medical Department to secure volunteers for experimental inoculations or other medical investigations approved by the War Department (Dow, 1925). Both the British and the American armed forces conducted experiments with newly developed vaccines for typhoid fever and other diseases (Tigertt, 1959). The introduction of aviation and its rapid development after World War I accelerated military research with human subjects (Pitts, 1985).

The shift in the early twentieth century from therapeutic experiments to nontherapeutic research fostered more formal arrangements with research subjects. In 1900 Major Walter Reed and the members of the U.S. Army's Yellow Fever Board adopted the first written agreements between research subjects and experimenters. The American soldiers and Spanish immigrants who participated signed contracts that described compensation for subjects (civilians, but not soldiers, received $100 in gold and an additional $100 if they contracted the disease) and identified some of the risks of participation (Bean, 1977). American physicians working in the Philippines followed Reed's example; prisoners in Manila's Bilibid Prison signed agreements written in their own dialect for medical research studies (Chernin, 1989; Lederer, 1994). During World War I, some physicians continued the policy of written agreements with American soldiers who participated in infectious disease research (Sellards, 1919).

The success of the yellow fever research gained public approval for human experimentation. In 1902, however, public reaction to the research-related deaths of

Army nurse Clara Maas and two Cuban volunteers led the surgeon general to suspend the Army's work on a yellow fever vaccine. Most published reports of military medical research emphasized the voluntary nature of participation. References to cash payments and better duty assignments raised questions about the pressures to volunteer. In principle, American military personnel, although required to undergo standard medical procedures to enhance their military fitness, retained the right to refuse participation in medical experiments (Johnson, 1953).

The advent of World War II spurred massive changes in the organization and funding of medical research. The Committee on Medical Research, part of the Office of Scientific Research and Development, sponsored clinical research projects on an unprecedented scale. Pressures to find solutions for military medical problems encouraged investigators to conduct numerous trials with human subjects. As the historian David Rothman has observed, the arguments that were used to justify sending men into combat were also invoked to sanction the use of conscientious objectors and civilians—prisoners, orphans, the retarded, and the mentally ill—in nontherapeutic research for the military (Rothman, 1991).

The wartime research ethos continued into the Cold War era. Both military and civilian researchers increasingly used human beings in experiments with little regard for the principles of consent and voluntary participation elaborated in the Nuremberg Code, or in the regulations governing research adopted by the secretary of defense in 1953 but classified as top secret until 1975 (Annas et al., 1977). Between 1955 and 1967 the Army and the Air Force supported more than eighteen research projects on the effects of hallucinogenic drugs on human performance in the United States and Canada (Annas and Grodin, 1992). Many of the nearly seven thousand servicemen who participated in drug tests at the Army Chemical Center at Edgewood Arsenal, Maryland, apparently received little information about the risks they incurred as a result of their participation in lysergic acid diethylamide (LSD) studies. Army investigators similarly failed to inform the more than one thousand participants about risks they incurred in tests of various nerve gases (Downey, 1975).

Amid the public condemnation of the LSD studies and the exposure of large numbers of servicemen to harmful radiation in the race to develop an atomic arsenal, the U.S. Army, Navy, and Air Force revised policies for research involving military personnel. In 1972 the American military banned all tests of nerve gases involving human subjects, and in 1974 issued new regulations for research on military personnel. In 1983, U.S. Department of Defense Directive 3216.2, "Protection of Human Subjects in DoD-Supported Research,"

established a uniform policy for research involving human subjects throughout the Defense Department. In addition to adhering to the regulations for the protection of human subjects of the Department of Health and Human Services, the guidelines charged the military chain of command to ensure that the fundamental rights, welfare, and dignity of human subjects be protected to the maximum extent possible (Winter, 1984). Research involving American military personnel received greater scrutiny in the 1980s (Howe et al., 1983; Maningas, 1989). Some military research subjects have received compensation for injuries they sustained in tests conducted without their knowledge. In 1991, for example, the Department of Veteran Affairs approved disability benefits for World War II veterans who unknowingly participated in tests of poison gases (Annas and Grodin, 1992).

Biological and chemical weapons pose some special problems for military personnel. Nations have approached the search for effective protections against these weapons in different ways. Whereas the American military discontinued the testing of toxic chemicals on human beings, the British Ministry of Defense continued to test antidotes for nerve gases on volunteer soldiers. Critics of the experimental exposure of soldier volunteers to nerve gases have cited safety concerns, as well as doubts that soldiers were "capable of giving full and informed consent to participate in complex toxicological experiments." Other North Atlantic Treaty Organization (NATO) countries have conducted similar testing of protective gear and drugs against nerve gas and a wide variety of other chemical weapons (Mason, 1987, p. 30).

The threat of chemical and biological weapons in the Persian Gulf War in 1991 led the U.S. Food and Drug Administration to grant the Department of Defense's request for a waiver of federal informed-consent regulations for administering investigational drugs and vaccines to troops stationed in Kuwait. Although the threat of chemical weapons did not materialize, the successful waiver of informed consent raised distinctive issues for military physicians. In the absence of informed consent, should a military physician follow orders and administer an investigational drug? Another related question for the military physician is whether his or her primary responsibility is the welfare of an individual patient or the success of a military mission (Howe, 1986; Annas, 1992).

Issues posed by research on military personnel are complex. As George Annas has argued, these issues require critical attention in peacetime, since they are "not susceptible to rational analysis in wartime" (Annas, 1992, p. 773).

SUSAN E. LEDERER

Directly related to this entry are the entries INFORMED CONSENT, *article on* CONSENT ISSUES IN HUMAN RESEARCH; FREEDOM AND COERCION; *and* INFORMATION DISCLOSURE. *For a further discussion of topics mentioned in this entry, see the entries* AUTONOMY; *and* WARFARE, *articles on* NUCLEAR WARFARE, *and* CHEMICAL AND BIOLOGICAL WARFARE. *For a discussion of related ideas, see the entries* AUTHORITY; BEHAVIOR CONTROL; FIDELITY AND LOYALTY; HARM; PATERNALISM; RIGHTS, *article on* RIGHTS IN BIOETHICS; *and* RISK. *Other relevant material may be found under the entries* RESEARCH, HUMAN: HISTORICAL ASPECTS; RESEARCH, UNETHICAL; RESEARCH METHODOLOGY; *and* RESEARCH POLICY. *See also the* APPENDIX (CODES, OATHS, AND DIRECTIVES RELATED TO BIOETHICS), SECTION IV: ETHICAL DIRECTIVES FOR HUMAN RESEARCH.

Bibliography

ANNAS, GEORGE J. 1992. "Changing the Consent Rules for Desert Storm." *New England Journal of Medicine* 326, no. 11:770–773.

ANNAS, GEORGE J.; GLANTZ, LEONARD H.; and KATZ, BARBARA F. 1977. *Informed Consent to Human Experimentation: The Subject's Dilemma.* Cambridge, Mass.: Ballinger.

ANNAS, GEORGE J., and GRODIN, MICHAEL A. 1991. "Commentary" [to "Treating the Troops," by Howe and Martin]. *Hastings Center Report* 21, no. 2:24–27.

———, eds. 1992. *The Nazi Doctors and the Nuremberg Code: Human Rights in Human Experimentation.* Oxford: Oxford University Press.

BEAN, WILLIAM B. 1977. "Walter Reed and the Ordeal of Human Experiments." *Bulletin of the History of Medicine* 51, no. 1:75–92.

CARPENTER, KENNETH J. 1986. *The History of Scurvy and Vitamin C.* Cambridge: At the University Press.

CHERNIN, ELI. 1989. "Richard Pearson Strong and the Iatrogenic Plague Disaster in Bilibid Prison, Manila, 1906." *Review of Infectious Diseases* 11, no. 6:996–1004.

DOW, WILLIAM S. 1925. "The Possibility of Medical Research in the Military Service Because of Its Complete Control over Personnel." *Military Surgeon* 56, no. 2:129–144.

DOWNEY, THOMAS J. 1975. "Report on Human Experimentation Conducted or Funded by the U.S. Army." *Congressional Record* 121:27934–27938.

HOWE, EDMUND G. 1986. "Ethical Issues Regarding Mixed Agency of Military Physicians." *Social Science and Medicine* 23, no. 8:803–815.

HOWE, EDMUND G.; KARK, JOHN A.; and WRIGHT, DANIEL G. 1983. "Studying Sickle Cell Trait in Healthy Army Recruits: Should the Research Be Done?" *Clinical Research* 31, no. 2:119–125.

HOWE, EDMUND G., and MARTIN, EDWARD D. 1991. "Treating the Troops." *Hastings Center Report* 21, no. 2:21–24.

HUME, EDGAR E. 1943. *Victories of Army Medicine: Scientific Accomplishments of the Medical Department of the United States Army.* Philadelphia: J.B. Lippincott.

JOHNSON, W. H. 1953. "Civil Rights of Military Personnel Regarding Medical Care and Experimental Procedures." *Science* 117:212–215.

LEDERER, SUSAN E. 1994. *The Scientist at the Bedside: Medical Experimentation and Antivivisection Before World War II.* Baltimore: Johns Hopkins University Press.

LEVINE, CAROL. 1989. "Military Medical Research: 1. Are There Ethical Exceptions?" *IRB* 11, no. 4:5–7.

LEVINE, ROBERT J. 1991. "Commentary" [to "Treating the Troops," by Howe and Martin]. *Hastings Center Report* 21, no. 2:27–28.

MANINGAS, PETER A. 1989. "Combat Casualty Care Research and Informed Consent." *Military Medicine* 154, no. 2: 71–73.

MASON, IAN. 1987. "Porton Defends Nerve-Gas Tests on Humans." *New Scientist,* July 16, p. 30.

NUMBERS, RONALD L. 1979. "William Beaumont and the Ethics of Human Experimentation." *Journal of the History of Biology* 12, no. 1:113–135.

PITTS, JOHN A. 1985. *The Human Factor: Biomedicine in the Manned Space Program to 1980.* Washington, D.C.: NASA.

ROTHMAN, DAVID J. 1991. *Strangers at the Bedside: A History of How Law and Bioethics Transformed Medical Decision-Making.* New York: Basic Books.

SELLARDS, ANDREW W. 1919. "Insusceptibility of Man to Inoculation with Blood from Measles Patients." *Johns Hopkins Hospital Bulletin* 30:257–268.

TIGERTT, WILLIAM D. 1959. "The Initial Effort to Immunize American Soldier Volunteers with Typhoid Vaccine." *Military Medicine* 124:342–349.

WINTER, PHILLIP E. 1984. "Human Subject Research Review in the Department of Defense." *IRB* 6, no. 3:9–10.

MINISTRY

See PASTORAL CARE.

MINORITIES AS RESEARCH SUBJECTS

In 1984, Margaret Heckler, secretary of the U.S. Department of Health and Human Services (HHS), established the Task Force on Black and Minority Health to investigate the health status and health needs of the minority groups in the nation. A year later, that panel presented its report, noting the lack of data about many aspects of minority health and the need for greater inclusion of minorities (defined as blacks, Hispanics, Asian/Pacific Islanders, and Native Americans) in medical research projects (U.S. Department of Health and Human Services, 1985). In response, the National Institutes of Health (NIH), the largest financial supporter of medical research in the United States, began to urge that grant applicants include African-Americans and other minorities as research subjects in their projects. Applicants not incorporating minorities in proposed studies were expected to provide "a clear rationale for their exclusion" (U.S. Department of Health and Human Services, 1988, p. 3).

The HHS task force's rationale for promoting data-gathering and research studies on minorities was both practical and humanitarian: to "understand . . . the reasons underlying the longstanding disparity of health status in the United States" between minorities and the majority population, in order "to prevent or reduce much of the illness and death experienced by minorities in disproportion to their representation in the American population." Those reasons, according to the report, included "physiological, cultural and societal factors." Therefore, Americans needed to conduct research and gather information about the health, health environment, and health-care practices of all citizens in order to improve everyone's health (U.S. Department of Health and Human Services, 1985, vol. 1, p. 37).

Historically, U.S. medical researchers included—even preferred to use—minorities (for example, immigrants from Ireland, Germany, eastern Europe, and Africa) in their research studies; not until recently, however, did they select members of these groups for the humanitarian reasons delineated in the HHS task force report. In general, researchers used minorities as experimental subjects because they were easily exploited; they studied minority health when minority health threatened the majority population (for example, in times of epidemics). The African-American health experience provides a good historical example of these research practices. While examples of the use of other racial and ethnic minorities for human experimentation in the United States may be cited individually or during certain time periods, white employment of blacks for such purposes was a consistent practice that, sadly, encompasses the entire sweep of U.S. history.

Almost from the time of white settlement of the American continent, whites noted differences between themselves and blacks in health matters such as disease immunities and susceptibilities, and reactions to medications. Self-interest was an important factor in whites' use of blacks as objects of research and study in antebellum times. The following examples illustrate that self-interest. Blacks were unwilling immigrants to the New World—they were slaves—and were, for their white owners, an economic investment. White physicians thus needed to know as much as possible about caring for their black patients when illness struck. Furthermore, blacks, especially house servants or laborers in small businesses or farms, often worked in close physical

proximity to whites. It was important for whites to recognize and study the medical differences between themselves and blacks so as to understand the risk of contracting diseases brought into their homes or workplaces by ailing slaves (Savitt, 1978). Antebellum Southern physicians like Josiah Clark Nott of Mobile, Alabama, and Samuel Cartwright of New Orleans spent parts of their careers noting and writing about black medical distinctiveness (Breeden, 1976). They and slaveholders did mostly observational and statistical studies, occasionally engaged in physical human experiments on African-Americans (Savitt, 1982), and published their ideas in agricultural and medical journals.

After the emancipation of slaves in 1865, concern about the spread of diseases prevalent among blacks to the entire population continued to motivate whites to study black illness. They noted a steep rise in such lethal diseases as tuberculosis among the newly freed population and predicted the decline and disappearance of blacks from the United States by the turn of the twentieth century. Morbidity and mortality studies conducted by insurance companies confirmed these dire predictions and made it difficult for blacks to obtain life insurance (Haller, 1970b; Torchia, 1977). Further, African-Americans became the object of numerous medical studies and articles (Haller, 1970a; Torchia, 1977). Physicians in the late nineteenth century reported on the state of black health in their regions or in the South as a whole. Some prominent African-Americans, W. E. B. Du Bois in particular, engaged in research on the health status of blacks and published their findings to refute the misleading conclusions whites had drawn. In particular, Du Bois pointed out the inaccuracies and unscientific approach of those researchers who purportedly found blacks' brains smaller and less developed than whites' brains; reminded readers that whites also suffered greatly from consumption (tuberculosis), alcoholism, and syphilis; and pointed out that other factors besides race, especially living conditions and economic status, influenced people's health or susceptibility to disease (Du Bois, 1906).

Beginning in the 1890s, a significant population shift of African-Americans from the rural South to Northern cities (termed the Great Migration) increased white awareness of black health problems and encouraged physicians all over the country to study diseases that affected both groups, such as tuberculosis (Torchia, 1975, 1977) and syphilis (Jones, 1981). Diseases that primarily afflicted blacks, however, such as sickle-cell anemia, discovered in 1910, were not widely studied or publicized even in the black medical and lay communities. (Interestingly, that disinterest in sickle-cell anemia began to change in the 1950s after it was recognized as a molecular genetic disease, the first of its kind [Culliton, 1972; Savitt, 1981; Scott, 1970].) The civil rights movement of the 1950s and 1960s further raised the consciousness of white Americans about the exclusion of blacks from many aspects of American life, including health care and medicine. The HHS task force report of 1985 made explicit the need to include blacks in the mainstream of U.S. biomedical research.

African-Americans have a unique history as research subjects in the United States because of their status for many years as slaves and then as freedmen. They were not the only voiceless minority in American history, however, and not the only group used as research subjects. In the South most of the experimental subjects were black; in the North they were usually poor, recent ethnic immigrants, like the Irish, Germans, and eastern Europeans. Many of their graves were robbed by medical students or professional body snatchers known as "resurrectionists," and their bodies were dissected. The segregated blacks and the poor white minorities who used the public hospitals and clinics run by U.S. medical schools became the objects of experiments and of surgical or medical demonstrations by teachers on behalf of their students (Bynum, 1988; Humphrey, 1973; Lederer, 1987; Bowman, 1991). As one historian of medical research stated about the nineteenth and especially the early twentieth century: "[S]ome physicians viewed hospital patients as an experimental population from whom knowledge could be gained, and on whom students could also learn" (Reiser, 1978, p. 11). This was the cost to the poor of obtaining free or low-cost medical care.

Investigators felt little need to ask these voiceless people for consent to perform experiments. Until the 1947 Nuremberg Code—the result of blatant misuse of a minority population (Jews in Nazi Germany) for unregulated medical experimentation—there was no uniform requirement for gaining consent from research subjects in medical experiments. Even after 1947, minority groups were exploited in the United States. In one often-cited example, researchers in San Antonio, Texas, studied a group of Mexican-American women visiting a clinic to obtain birth-control assistance. Wishing to discover whether the reported side effects of birth-control pills were physiological or psychological, the researchers gave one group of women a placebo and instructed them to use a vaginal cream in addition. The patients in the study did not know they might receive a placebo or that using the vaginal cream alone put them at substantially greater risk for becoming pregnant. Seven women involved in the study became pregnant (Veatch, 1971).

The most notorious example in American history of experimentation on members of a minority group without their consent was the Tuskegee Syphilis Experiment. Between 1932 and 1972 the U.S. Public Health Service (PHS) conducted an investigation into the natural history of untreated syphilis on over four hundred unsuspecting black men from Macon County, Alabama. Building their research on an 1890s study of untreated syphilis among white males in Oslo, Norway, PHS officials wished to determine if racial differences existed in the natural course of the disease. Articles published in the late nineteenth and early twentieth centuries, including a study conducted at Johns Hopkins University, seemed to confirm a widely held belief that blacks acquired the cardiovascular manifestations of latent syphilis more often than the neurological ones, while whites responded in the opposite manner. The African-American men selected for the Tuskegee experiment thought that they were part of a select group receiving special medical care. In fact, they were receiving no care at all for their syphilis.

Physicians and officials from the Alabama State Board of Health, Macon County Health Department, and Tuskegee Institute, as well as local physicians, cooperated with the PHS in establishing the project, shunting the unwitting subjects to government physicians for their medical care, or providing the PHS with medical facilities for physical examinations and autopsies. The experiment continued even after the Nuremberg Code went into effect in 1947, after penicillin became available for the treatment of syphilis in the 1950s (the men were intentionally not treated with the drug because this was a study of untreated syphilis), and after the PHS had instituted strict guidelines on the use of human subjects in experiments funded by the NIH and other of its agencies in 1966 (Brandt, 1978; Jones, 1981; U.S. Department of Health, Education, and Welfare, 1973).

Those guidelines were reemphasized when the Tuskegee story became public in 1972, bringing home to the medical research community the importance of obtaining informed consent from research subjects, and of avoiding bias and using caution and sensitivity when considering the need for racial and ethnic medical studies. Blacks, Hispanics, Native Americans, and whites, for both cultural and biological reasons, do not necessarily respond similarly to specific drugs or other medical treatments. (There are biological and cultural differences within each of these groups as well: Blacks can be subdivided into West Indians, Africans, and African-Americans; and Hispanics into Spanish, Latin American, and Spanish-speaking Caribbean peoples [Novello et al., 1991].)

Some medical research may be skewed by the underrepresentation or overrepresentation of distinctive groups in the experimental population. If, for example, medical researchers randomly included a small percentage of African-Americans in a study of a proposed hypertensive drug where most of the research subjects were white, the study might be inaccurate for both blacks and whites. African-Americans, research has shown, react differently than do whites to some hypertensive medications, requiring different doses or even different medications. Under the 1988 NIH guidelines, investigators should take that information into account by separating racial and ethnic groups in their studies, so as to serve best all segments of the population (Svensson, 1989). Furthermore, socioeconomic status varies within all minority and majority population groups and may have an impact on research outcomes.

A number of articles appeared after the 1985 task force report that either confirmed the need for more research into various aspects of minority health and health care or included minorities as experimental subjects (Cowell et al., 1991; Markides and Coreil, 1986; Neighbors et al., 1989; Novello et al., 1991; Padgett, 1990; Svensson, 1989; Yates, 1987). Minorities, having once served as the misused objects of research and human experimentation because it was convenient and in the self-interest of the majority population, have again been singled out to serve as research subjects for U.S. medicine—but this time for different and more humanitarian reasons.

TODD L. SAVITT

Directly related to this entry are the entries RESEARCH BIAS; and RACE AND RACISM. For a further discussion of topics mentioned in this article, see the entries INFORMATION DISCLOSURE; INFORMED CONSENT, article on CONSENT ISSUES IN HUMAN RESEARCH; RESEARCH, UNETHICAL; and RESEARCH POLICY, especially the article on SUBJECT SELECTION. This entry will find application in the entries EUGENICS; FERTILITY CONTROL, article on SOCIAL ISSUES; and POPULATION POLICIES, section on STRATEGIES ON FERTILITY CONTROL. For a discussion of related ideas, see the entries FRAUD, THEFT, AND PLAGIARISM; FREEDOM AND COERCION; HARM; PATERNALISM; PROFESSION AND PROFESSIONAL ETHICS; RIGHTS; RISK; and VALUE AND VALUATION. Other relevant material may be found under the entries PUBLIC HEALTH; RESEARCH, HUMAN: HISTORICAL ASPECTS; RESEARCH ETHICS COMMITTEES; and RESEARCH METHODOLOGY. See also the APPENDIX (CODES, OATHS, AND DIRECTIVES RELATED TO BIOETHICS), SECTION IV: ETHICAL DIRECTIVES FOR HUMAN RESEARCH.

Bibliography

BOWMAN, PHILLIP J. 1991. "Race, Class and Ethics in Research: Belmont Principles to Functional Relevance." In Black Psychology, 3d ed., pp. 747–766. Edited by Reginald L. Jones. Berkeley, Calif.: Cobb and Henry.

BRANDT, ALLAN M. 1978. "Racism and Research: The Case of the Tuskegee Syphilis Study." Hastings Center Report 8, no. 6:21–29.

BREEDEN, JAMES O. 1976. "States-Rights Medicine in the Old South." Bulletin of the New York Academy of Medicine 52, no. 3:348–372.

BYNUM, WILLIAM. 1988. "Reflections on the History of Human Experimentation." In The Use of Human Beings in Research: With Special Reference to Clinical Trials, pp. 29–46. Edited by Stuart F. Spicker, Ilai Alon, Andre de Vries, and H. Tristram Engelhardt, Jr. Dordrecht, Netherlands: Kluwer.

COWELL, DANIEL D. 1983. "Aging Research, Black Americans, and the National Institute on Aging." Journal of the National Medical Association 75, no. 1:99, 102–104.

CULLITON, BARBARA J. 1972. "Sickle Cell Anemia: The Route from Obscurity to Prominence." Science 178:138–142.

DU BOIS, W. E. B. 1906. The Health and Physique of the Negro American: Report of a Social Study Made Under the Direction of Atlanta University. Atlanta: Atlanta University Press.

HALLER, JOHN S., JR. 1970a. "The Physician Versus the Negro: Medical and Anthropological Concepts of Race in the Late Nineteenth Century." Bulletin of the History of Medicine 44, no. 2:154–167.

———. 1970b. "Race, Mortality, and Life Insurance: Negro Vital Statistics in the Late Nineteenth Century." Journal of the History of Medicine and Allied Sciences 25, no. 3: 247–261.

HUMPHREY, DAVID C. 1973. "Dissection and Discrimination: The Social Origins of Cadavers in America, 1760–1915." Bulletin of the New York Academy of Medicine 49, no. 9: 819–827.

JONES, JAMES H. 1981. Bad Blood: The Tuskegee Syphilis Experiment. New York: Free Press.

KASISKE, BERTRAM L.; NEYLAN, JOHN F., III; RIGGIO, R.; DANOVITCH, GABRIEL M.; KAHANA, LAWRENCE; ALEXANDER, STEVEN R.; and WHITE, MARTIN G. 1991. "The Effect of Race on Access and Outcome in Transplantation." New England Journal of Medicine 324, no. 5:302–307.

LEDERER, SUSAN E. 1987. "Human Experimentation and Antivivisection in Turn-of-the-Century America." Ph.D. diss., University of Wisconsin, Madison.

MARKIDES, KYRIAKOS S., and COREIL, JEANNINE. 1986. "The Health of Hispanics in the Southwestern United States: An Epidemiologic Paradox." Public Health Reports 101, no. 3:253–265.

NEIGHBORS, HAROLD W.; JACKSON, JAMES S.; CAMPBELL, LINN; and WILLIAMS, DONALD. 1989. "The Influence of Racial Factors on Psychiatric Diagnosis: A Review and Suggestions for Research." Community Mental Health Journal 25, no. 4:301–311.

NOVELLO, ANTONIA C.; WISE, PAUL H.; and KLEINMAN, DUSHANKA V. 1991. "Hispanic Health: Time for Data, Time for Action." Journal of the American Medical Association 265, no. 2:253–255.

PADGETT, DEBORAH K. 1990. "Consideration of the Ethnic Factor in Aging Research—the Time Has Never Been Better." Gerontologist 30, no. 6:723–724.

REISER, STANLEY J. 1978. "Human Experimentation and the Convergence of Medical Research and Patient Care." Annals of the American Academy of Political and Social Sciences 437:8–18.

Savitt, Todd L. 1978. Medicine and Slavery: The Diseases and Health Care of Blacks in Antebellum Virginia. Urbana: University of Illinois Press.

———. 1981. "The Invisible Malady: Sickle Cell Anemia in America, 1910–1970." Journal of the National Medical Association 73, no. 8:739–746.

———. 1982. "The Use of Blacks for Medical Experimentation and Demonstration in the Old South." Journal of Southern History 48, no. 3:331–348.

Scott, Robert B. 1970. "Sickle Cell Anemia—High Prevalence and Low Priority." New England Journal of Medicine 282, no. 3:164–165.

Svensson, Craig K. 1989. "Representation of American Blacks in Clinical Trials of New Drugs." Journal of the American Medical Association 261, no. 2:263–265.

Torchia, Marion M. 1975. "The Tuberculosis Movement and the Race Question, 1890–1950." Bulletin of the History of Medicine 49, no. 2:152–168.

———. 1977. "Tuberculosis Among American Negroes: Medical Research on a Racial Disease, 1830–1950." Journal of the History of Medicine and Allied Sciences 32, no. 3: 252–279.

U.S. Department of Health, Education and Welfare. Public Health Service. Tuskegee Syphilis Study Ad Hoc Advisory Panel. 1973. Final Report of the Tuskegee Syphilis Study Ad Hoc Advisory Panel. Washington, D.C.: U.S. Government Printing Office.

U.S. Department of Health and Human Services. 1988. "Inclusion of Minorities in Study Populations." NIH Guide for Grants and Contracts 17:2–3.

———. Task Force on Black and Minority Health. 1985. Report of the Secretary's Task Force on Black and Minority Health. 7 vols. Washington, D.C.: U.S. Government Printing Office.

Veatch, Robert M. 1971. "'Experimental' Pregnancy." Hastings Center Report 1:2–3. Reprinted, with "Editor's Note," in Ethical Issues in Modern Medicine, pp. 291–293. Edited by John Arras and Robert Hunt. Palo Alto, Calif.: Mayfield, 1983.

Yates, Alayne. 1987. "Current Status and Future Directions of Research on the American Indian Child." American Journal of Psychiatry 144, no. 9:1135–1142.

MORALITY AND LAW

See Law and Morality.

MORALITY AND RELIGION

See Ethics, article on religion and morality.

MULTINATIONAL RESEARCH

"Multinational research" refers to biomedical research that involves investigators and subjects from more than one nation. Here we will consider the most typical—and most problematic—type of multinational research: that in which the investigators come from a developed country (the "sponsoring" country) and the subjects are located in a developing country (the "host" country). Multinational research of this type poses several ethical problems in addition to the standard issues in research involving human subjects (Levine, 1986). Of particular concern is the possibility of dissonance between the fundamental ethical concepts of investigators and subjects from different cultural backgrounds.

Ethical dissonance raises a basic question with important theoretical and practical implications: Can one formulate ethical rules governing the conduct of investigators from one cultural background performing research on subjects from another? At the heart of this question is the problem of ethical universalism versus pluralism—the belief that the ethical standards governing the conduct of research are the same wherever research is conducted versus the contention that since ethics is socially constructed, it will vary according to the cultural setting in which it is formulated (Kunstadter, 1980).

Two trends bring concern about biomedical research ethics in a multinational context to the fore: (1) the increasing prominence of biomedicine in non-Western settings and (2) the increasing movement of biomedical investigators across national boundaries. These trends, which tend to increase the contact between investigators from developed countries and research subjects from developing countries, have been accelerated by the AIDS pandemic.

International standards

The first international code of ethics for research involving human subjects, the Nuremberg Code, was drafted in 1947 at the Nuremberg trials as a reaction to atrocities committed by Nazi physicians in the conduct of experiments on inmates of concentration camps (United States Department of Defense, 1947). The goal of the code was to acknowledge the importance and necessity of clinical research while providing a universally applicable standard for condemning the conduct of Nazi physicians. The Nuremberg Code, which consists of ten concise principles, was soon recognized as an authoritative statement of the fundamental rights of research subjects in all nations. The first principle of the Nuremberg Code is "The voluntary consent of the human subject is absolutely essential." This is elaborated to require that the subject be free from constraint or coercion and that the subject have "sufficient knowledge and comprehension of the elements of the subject matter involved as to enable him to make an understanding and enlightened decision." Other principles in the Nuremberg Code require that the proposed research be meaningful and essential, be based on prior animal experiments, and "avoid all unnecessary physical and mental suffering and injury."

The Declaration of Helsinki, first promulgated by the World Medical Assembly in 1964 and revised in 1975, 1983, and 1989, adapted the principles of the Nuremberg Code to fit the empirical realities of biomedical research; for example, it provides for the authorization through proxy consent of the participation in research of less than fully autonomous subjects (World Medical Assembly, 1989).

The Nuremberg Code and the Declaration of Helsinki were written on the presumption that their ethical standards were universally applicable, and for many years they were widely regarded as such. However, with the proliferation of multinational research, this presumption of universality came to be challenged (Levine, 1982). In order to interpret the standards of the Declaration of Helsinki so that they would be applied correctly, particularly in technologically developing countries, the Council for International Organizations of Medical Sciences (CIOMS) and World Health Organization jointly developed and promulgated a new set of international guidelines in 1982 that have become the leading articulation of ethical standards for multinational research (CIOMS, 1982). Subsequently, CIOMS extensively revised these guidelines (CIOMS, 1993) and also issued guidelines for the ethical review of epidemiological studies (CIOMS, 1991).

The CIOMS guidelines state that when research is conducted by investigators of one country on subjects of another, the "sponsoring agency should submit the research protocol to ethical and scientific review according to the standards of the country of the sponsoring agency, and the ethical standards applied should be no less exacting than they would be in the case of research carried out in that country" (CIOMS, 1993, Guideline 15). The stated purpose of these guidelines is to "indicate how the fundamental ethical principles that guide the conduct of biomedical research involving human subjects, as set forth in the Declaration of Helsinki, [can] be applied effectively, particularly in developing countries, taking into account culture, socioeconomic circumstances, national laws, and executive and administrative arrangements" (CIOMS, 1993, p. 8).

The CIOMS guidelines include provisions that address two problems perceived to be very important: (1)

that multinational research might be exploitative, in that it might serve the interests of the initiating agency rather than those of the host country, and (2) that not all prospective subjects in developing countries or underdeveloped communities are so situated as to provide informed consent that meets the standards of the Declaration of Helsinki. However, the CIOMS guidelines, while commendably expressing concern for cultural specificity, nevertheless still reflect, perhaps unavoidably, a Western bias. Inherent in these guidelines is the assumption that the circumstances in the developing world are special and those in the developed world are the norm. Thus, the developed world is envisioned as more advanced, not only technologically but also morally.

Crossing national boundaries: Universalism or pluralism?

Because it brings investigator and subject together across a cultural boundary in a real research situation, the conduct of multinational research gives the theoretical tension between ethical universalism and ethical pluralism a palpable, practical significance. Psychiatrist and anthropologist Arthur Kleinman argues that

> Clinical investigations in developing societies must be understood as taking place within the particular contexts of practical, everyday beliefs, values, and power relationships that constitute local cultural systems and [must be understood] as creating potential conflicts between these non-Western systems and the Western cultural conceptions and norms that are a usually unrecognized part of clinical research projects and the expectations and behaviors of clinical researchers. . . . (Kleinman, 1979, p. 1)

There is considerable controversy regarding how such conflict should be resolved (Christakis, 1992). Some contend that all research, wherever it is conducted, should be justified according to universally applicable standards. Those opposed to this position, while sometimes accepting certain standards as generally applicable, argue that most standards must be adapted to accommodate the mores of particular cultures; they argue for ethical pluralism. Pluralists commonly refer to the universalist position as "ethical imperialism," while universalists often call that of their opponents "ethical relativism."

Universalists endorse uniform international standards because they are concerned that investigators from industrialized nations may go to developing countries to test therapeutic innovations not only for appropriate reasons (e.g., to study a disease where it is indigenous, to obtain a scientifically appropriate study group) but also for inappropriate ones (e.g., to take advantage of the less sophisticated regulatory systems typical of developing countries). Requiring investigators to conform to the ethical standards of their own country when conducting research abroad is one way to restrain exploitation. Universalists point to the Declaration of Helsinki as a widely accepted standard for biomedical research that has been endorsed both by technologically developing countries that lack indigenous standards of research ethics and by technologically developed countries where, in general, complex regulations are patterned after the declaration.

Pluralists join with universalists in condemning exploitation of technologically developing countries and their citizens. Unlike the universalists, however, they see the imposition of ethical standards for the conduct of research by a powerful country on a developing country as yet another form of exploitation. In their view, it is tantamount to saying, "No, you may not participate in the development of this technology, no matter how much you desire it, unless you permit us to replace your ethical standards with our own." Pluralists call attention to the fact that the Declaration of Helsinki reflects a uniquely Western configuration of a number of key ethical points; in particular, the declaration has a largely Western view of the nature of the person and, as such, it does not adequately guide investigators to show respect for persons in non-Western settings. Pluralists point to findings in the fields of medical sociology and medical anthropology regarding the culturally dependent variability in medical care, ethical practice, and conceptualization of personhood.

Role of the AIDS pandemic

The AIDS pandemic has provoked critical scrutiny of the universalistic, Western conception of clinical research ethics. AIDS research of various kinds by Western investigators in non-Western settings—such as epidemiological studies, vaccine trials, and drug trials—has raised specific, thorny challenges to such a presumption. Certain research protocols that are unacceptable in developed countries have been seen as acceptable in developing countries and vice versa. Difficulties have arisen in satisfying conflicting ethical expectations. Many AIDS researchers have stressed the importance of sensitivity to local culture in general and local ethics in particular, and they have advocated local community involvement in the ethical design of research.

For example, one American investigator described a research project in Tanzania in which the ethical expectations of the investigators' and subjects' cultures clashed. In this study of the prevalence of HIV antibodies, maternal and infant blood was to be sampled at the time of birth. The investigator's home institutional review board, as part of its approval, had required that

subjects give informed consent to participate and also that subjects be told their test results. Tanzanian authorities, however, had a conflicting set of requirements: worried that the results could cause psychological trauma, and cognizant of the fact that no meaningful therapy was available for HIV-positive individuals in Tanzania, they insisted that the researchers not tell their subjects either the reasons for or the results of the blood tests. This study, which both the host nation and the investigator judged to be valuable, was abandoned because of this conflict (Barry, 1988). In other situations, disagreement between local ethics committees and those of the international body funding the research have forced local investigators to change the research protocol in ways that were meaningless in the cultural and economic circumstances of the host country (Hall, 1989). Some would regard such examples as ethical imperialism; others, as the worldwide elaboration of appropriate universal standards.

Another example is provided by a case involving the use of placebos. A Brazilian investigator proposed to compare the drug dideoxycytidine with a placebo in order to assess the efficacy of this drug in prolonging survival in HIV-infected patients. This trial was also intended to determine if a financial investment by the Brazilian government in this drug would be worthwhile. From the perspective of orthodox Western research ethics, this study raised two major problems: Is it ethical to conduct a placebo-controlled trial when effective therapy for HIV infection (i.e., zidovudine) exists? And is it ethical to design a clinical study to answer an economic question? (Christakis et al., 1991). From the perspective of many Brazilians, but probably not from that of a developed society, the answer to each of these questions is affirmative.

The informed consent debate: Personhood in multinational perspective

The brisk debate about the permissibility of multinational variability in informed consent is particularly illustrative of discrepancies that may arise between ethical expectations in Western and non-Western societies and of the need for sensitivity to local culture. The debate has focused on three problems: (1) the extent to which *informed* consent is achievable; (2) the extent to which *individual* informed consent is necessary; and (3) the extent to which *free* consent is obtainable in the developing world.

With respect to the first problem, it is clear that the type of consent practiced in the West, with the signing of an informed consent document, is inappropriate for illiterate or semiliterate peoples. Moreover, in some cultural settings, it may be extremely difficult to convey an accurate understanding of the concept of randomization, the passage of time, the spontaneous remission of disease, or other essential concepts. Indeed, there may be cultural variation in the understanding of diseases, at odds with Western scientific notions, that makes truly *informed* consent (as configured in the West) impossible (Ekunwe and Kessel, 1984). However, illiteracy and poverty are all too often confused with passivity and stupidity, and many commentators have argued for better efforts to make the informational content of consent accessible to indigenous peoples.

The problem of individual consent is even more difficult, both philosophically and practically. The requirement for individual informed consent is grounded ethically in the principle of respect for persons, one of the posited universal ethical standards. When stated at the level of formality employed by Immanuel Kant, it is easy to apply universally and difficult to envision people who would disagree: "So act as to treat humanity, whether in thine own person or in that of any other, in every case as an end withal, never as a means only." When one goes beyond this level of abstraction, however, the principle begins to lose its apparent universality (Levine, 1991; 1982).

A very fundamental problem arises in the application of the principle of respect for persons because of cross-cultural variation in the definition of personhood (De Craemer, 1983). Western societies stress the individualistic nature of a person and put much emphasis on the individual's rights, autonomy, self-determination, and privacy. But this is at variance with the more relational definitions of a person found in many non-Western societies that stress the embeddedness of the individual within society and define a person by means of relations to others. The Kongo of Lower Zaire, for example, have conceptions of illness that "consistently [draw] the effective boundary of a person differently, more expansively, than classical Western medicine, philosophy, and religion. The outcome is usually disconcerting or unreal to Western medical observers . . ." (Janzen, 1978, p. 189).

Important practical implications arise from this variation in the definition of a person. Since the notion of persons as individuals is undermined, the consent of the individual may not be viewed as paramount in certain cultural settings. Indeed, the focus of the consent process may shift from the individual to the family or to the community. In the context of research, it may be necessary to secure the consent of a subject's family or social group instead of or in addition to the consent of the subject.

An additional practical problem in some areas of the developing world is that of establishing personal identity. Records of vital events are often spotty and kinship designations are sometimes ambiguous, thus making positive identification of research subjects diffi-

cult. Particularly when research participation involves an immediate benefit (e.g., a monetary reward for a blood specimen), villagers may replace one subject with another when the former is away from the village. Such practical issues have obliged creative solutions that might not stand up to an ethical review in a developed society. For example, in a trial of hepatitis vaccine involving more than one hundred thousand people in The Gambia, investigators found it necessary to produce a scar on the recipients' bodies in order to identify them positively (Hall, 1989).

Variations in the definition of personhood between societies may also find expression in precisely who is thought to have the authority to give informed consent for others. This is acknowledged in the CIOMS guidelines: When individuals cannot be made "sufficiently aware of the implications of participation to give adequately informed consent, the decision . . . on whether to consent should be elicited through a reliable intermediary such as a trusted community leader" (CIOMS, 1993, Guideline 8). There will be considerable variation by culture as to who is acknowledged as a "community leader" and whether such an individual can be considered a reliable intermediary. The requirement for community leader consent, however, may be the only alternative, albeit unsatisfactory by Western standards, to individual consent in many cases in which beneficial research is essential. But this alternative may not necessarily be ethically disturbing within the society of the research subject. Of course, a necessary presupposition regarding such proxy consent is that the leader will act in good faith for the benefit of the community. The possibility for abuse in such situations is quite real.

The CIOMS guidelines also respond to the problem of obtaining proxy consent for women in cultures where women's rights to exercise self-determination are not acknowledged. Recognizing that women who have serious illnesses should not be deprived of opportunities to receive investigational therapies when there are no better alternatives, the guidelines strive to strike a balance between, on the one hand, strictly individualistic—and, under such circumstances, therefore prohibitive—interpretations of individual informed consent and, on the other hand, potentially abusive interpretations that grant too much authority to the person giving the proxy consent. The guidelines note that "Efforts must be made . . . to invite [women] to decide whether they wish to accept the investigational therapy, even though the formal consent must be obtained from another person, usually a man. Such invitations may best be extended by women who understand the culture sufficiently well to discern whether [they] genuinely wish to accept or reject the therapy" (CIOMS, 1993, Guideline 11). The CIOMS guidelines are the first code of ethics to address this difficult problem explicitly.

Thus, some American observers have argued that, in certain developing world settings,

> Seeking informed consent to research [participation] from individuals may tend to weaken the social fabric of a non-individualistic society, forcing it to deal with values it does not hold, and possibly sowing disorder that the community will have to reap long after the investigators have gone home. . . . It is questionable that [our vaunted Western individualism] has been an unmitigated good for our own civilization and very questionable that it is up to standard for export. We ought, in truth, to be suitably humble about the worth of procedures [i.e., individual consent] developed only to cater to a very Western weakness. . . . How can it be a sign of our respect for people, or of our concern for their welfare, that we are willing to suppress research that is conducted according to the laws and cultures of the countries in which it is being carried out? (Newton, 1990, p. 11)

Other observers have argued that "Ethical standards in medicine . . . cannot be relative; they must be judged by their substance. The force of local custom or law cannot justify abuses of certain fundamental rights, and the right of self-determination, on which the doctrine of informed consent is based, is one of them" (Angell, 1988, p. 1082).

Research in developing countries, particularly when conducted by investigators from relatively powerful developed countries, raises difficult questions regarding how *free* consent can be in such circumstances. This problem has two parts: possible coercion by insiders and possible coercion by outsiders.

Many non-Western countries have complex social systems governing the exchange of gifts that, in the context of clinical investigations, would be interpreted in American culture, for instance, as problematic conflicts of interest. Describing Japan, clearly both a developed and a non-Western society, for example, the sociologist Willy De Craemer states,

> A continuous, gift-exchanging-structured flow of material and nonmaterial "goods" and "services" takes place between the members of the enclosed human nexus to which each individual belongs. . . . [A] web of relations develops . . . [that] binds donors and recipients together in diffuse, deeply personal, and overlapping creditor-debtor ways. Generalized benevolence is involved, but so is generalized obligation, both of which take into account another crucial parameter of Japanese culture: the importance attached to status, rank, and hierarchical order in interpersonal relationships. . . . (De Craemer, 1983, p. 30)

It is easy to imagine how a research ethics committee in the United States would evaluate such a custom of exchange of gifts—both material and nonmaterial—in a system that recognizes the legitimacy of "status, rank, and hierarchical order." Attention would soon be focused on the problems of "conflicts of interest," "undue inducement," or what the Nuremberg Code calls "other ulterior forms of constraint or coercion" that would invalidate informed consent. Such discrepant cultural perceptions would pose significant ethical problems in the context of a particular multinational research project.

Western investigators must thus appreciate that what appears to them to be coercion may, from the perspective of local inhabitants, represent cooperation and identification with the group to which the individual belongs. However, this does not relieve Western investigators, who are perforce not members of the host country, of the responsibility to avoid coercion arising from their own actions. They must be aware that coercion is difficult to avoid in most settings where clinical investigation in the developing world is conducted. Subjects with relatively little understanding of the medical aspects of research participation, indisposed to resisting the suggestions of Western doctors, perhaps operating under the mistaken notion that they are receiving therapy, and possibly receiving some ancillary benefits from participation in the research, are very vulnerable to coercion.

The CIOMS guidelines recognize that sponsors and investigators may have great difficulty in understanding and responding to cultural norms and traditions in developing countries:

> The ability to judge . . . ethical acceptability . . . requires a thorough understanding of a community's customs and traditions. The ethical review committee must have as either members or consultants persons with such understanding, so that the committee may evaluate proposed means of obtaining informed consent and otherwise respecting the rights of prospective subjects. Such persons should be able, for example, to identify appropriate members of the community to serve as intermediaries . . . , to decide whether material benefits or inducements may be regarded as appropriate in the light of a community's gift-exchange traditions, and to provide safeguards for data and personal information considered by the subjects to be private or sensitive. (CIOMS, 1993, Guideline 8)

The justification and regulation of multinational research

Multinational research also raises troubling ethical questions pertaining to the motivations behind it and the purposes to which it is directed. What are the ethics of collaboration between nations in clinical research? How are its costs and benefits to be apportioned among the collaborators?

The conduct of collaborative, multinational AIDS research in Africa—generally involving African subjects and American, European, and African investigators—is illustrative. Both Western and African nations urgently require the development of effective means of AIDS prevention and therapy. For both practical and scientific reasons, Africa has been identified as an ideal site for clinical trials of vaccines and other pharmaceuticals (Christakis, 1988). The developed world needs access to large populations of prospective subjects with a high prevalence of HIV infection, such as those found in certain African nations. And these African nations, lacking both well-developed research institutions and adequate funds, need the involvement of the developed world.

But there has been widespread concern that differences in economic and political power might lead to abuse of the poor by the rich and of the weak by the strong. For example, many African critics have been concerned that Western investigators, unchecked by foreign or local supervision, might conduct "savage experiments" in Africa. Many Africans have voiced the concern that Western science often goes to Africa with "dirty hands," and that Africans are serving as subjects for research deemed too risky to be conducted in the West (Fortin, 1987; Christakis, 1988).

African concerns about Western research transcend concerns that subjects might be treated inhumanely or unethically. Some Africans have voiced the more general concern that they do not derive significant benefit from their contribution to collaborative research efforts. Indeed, they sometimes feel harmed (Beiser, 1977). African physicians have complained that "Some of the Western press and researchers have used the . . . data we supplied, but instead of putting HIV under the microscope, they have put our society, our customs, even our love life under the lens. . . . We give you information and so often you seem to turn it against us" (Sabatier, 1988, p. 89). Practical and scientific reasons for the conduct of AIDS research in Africa, they argue, are not sufficient to justify using African subjects, especially if such subjects bear the burden of the research risks but do not reap the benefit from any advances.

In this context, some commentators have argued that sponsoring countries or corporations be required to develop enduring infrastructures (such as medical clinics or research facilities) in the host country as part of the process of conducting research (Gostin, 1991). Suggestions that sponsor countries provide lasting benefits to host communities are motivated in part by a concern for the equitable distribution of burdens and benefits that, in the West, is ordinarily understood as a question of distributive justice. According to the CIOMS guidelines, for example, external sponsors are expected to employ and, if necessary, to train local personnel to perform various functions in conducting the research

(CIOMS, 1993, Guideline 15). Sponsors are also expected to provide facilities and personnel to make necessary health-care services available during the conduct of the research. However, provision of such services beyond what is necessary for the conduct of the research is described in the CIOMS guidelines not as obligatory but as "morally praiseworthy." Indeed, some commentators have argued that such costly requirements may simply prevent the initiation of important and desirable research in developing countries.

Sponsors of multinational research have also been criticized for their tendency to select research topics that are either irrelevant to local health needs or not integrated with follow-up health care delivery. For example, expensive pharmaceutical products are sometimes imported to developing countries in order to be evaluated, but alternative and cheaper drugs or methods of disease control, lacking sponsorship, are not tested (Abdussalam and Osuntokun, 1991).

Implementation of international standards at a local level (if one adopts a universalist perspective) or discovery and implementation of local ethical standards (if one adopts a pluralist perspective) each requires some formal institution to attain the objective. No matter where clinical research is conducted, some responsible body must articulate and implement ethical standards. In many developed countries, elaborate systems of review committees and legislation exist to achieve this. The emergence of multinational research has revealed the relative absence of such institutions (or appropriate substitutes) in the developing world. Problems have arisen in defining who should regulate research in such settings and how they should do it. The assertion of the necessity for local review assumes a local institution capable of carrying out such a review. Solutions to these problems are partly predicated on addressing whether exogenous, international standards or indigenous, local standards should be used in a given research setting. A significant part of the problem will be to identify local ethical expectations, and the medical social sciences can make a meaningful contribution in this respect (Kleinman, 1979; Kunstadter, 1980; Lieban, 1990; Hoffmaster, 1990; Christakis, 1992).

Proposed international procedural standards

Existing international ethical codes and guidelines cannot be a mechanism for the resolution of conflicting ethical expectations, especially under circumstances where the universal applicability of the standards is not recognized or where the standards are insufficiently specific or where the standards conflict with each other. Therefore, some authors have argued for a shift from content-based international ethical standards toward procedure-based protocols.

One proposal calls for international guidelines stated at such a level of generality that they could be interpreted flexibly by local committees to meet the needs of most of the world's communities. A committee in the host country that had a high degree of familiarity with the customs and values of the community in which the research is to be conducted would have the ultimate responsibility for review and approval of the detailed procedures designed to protect the rights and welfare of research subjects. Any proposal to deviate from internationally agreed standards would also require review and approval by a national committee in the host country. A committee in the sponsoring country would be required either to endorse the modification or to seek consultation with a special international review body (Levine, 1991). A different proposal sets forth international guidelines that emphasize resolution of multinational ethical disputes. The guidelines in the proposal, instead of specifying the content of research ethics, articulate procedures by which any disagreement over content may be negotiated and settled (Christakis and Panner, 1991).

The conduct of multinational research has fostered a dialogue between alternative visions of proper, ethical conduct of clinical research. This dialogue serves the important purpose of forcing a critical reevaluation of existing international standards of research ethics.

NICHOLAS A. CHRISTAKIS
ROBERT J. LEVINE

Directly related to this entry are the entries INFORMED CONSENT, *especially the article on* CONSENT ISSUES IN HUMAN RESEARCH; *and* AIDS, *article on* HEALTH-CARE AND RESEARCH ISSUES. *For a further discussion of topics mentioned in this entry, see the entries* HEALTH AND DISEASE, *article on* ANTHROPOLOGICAL PERSPECTIVES; INTERNATIONAL HEALTH; RESEARCH, UNETHICAL; RESEARCH METHODOLOGY; RESEARCH POLICY, *especially the article on* SUBJECT SELECTION; *and* WOMEN, *article on* RESEARCH ISSUES. *For a discussion of related ideas, see the entries* AUTONOMY; FREEDOM AND COERCION; HARM; *and* PERSON. *Other relevant material may be found under the entries* HEALTH POLICY, *article on* HEALTH POLICY IN INTERNATIONAL PERSPECTIVE; PHARMACEUTICS, *article on* PHARMACEUTICAL INDUSTRY; PLACEBO; RESEARCH, HUMAN: HISTORICAL ASPECTS; RESEARCH BIAS; *and* RESEARCH ETHICS COMMITTEES. *See also the* APPENDIX (CODES, OATHS, AND DIRECTIVES RELATED TO BIOETHICS), SECTION IV: ETHICAL DIRECTIVES FOR HUMAN RESEARCH.

Bibliography

ABDUSSALAM, MOHAMMED, and OSUNTOKUN, BENJAMIN O. 1991. "Capacity Building for Ethical Considerations of Epidemiological Studies: Perspective of Developing Countries." In *Development of International Ethical Guidelines for Epidemiological Research and Practice*. Geneva: Council for International Organizations of Medical Sciences.

ANGELL, MARCIA. 1988. "Ethical Imperialism? Ethics in International Collaborative Clinical Research." *New England Journal of Medicine* 319, no. 16:1081–1083.

BARRY, MICHELLE. 1988. "Ethical Considerations of Human Investigation in Developing Countries: The AIDS Dilemma." *New England Journal of Medicine* 319, no. 16:1083–1086.

BEISER, MORTON. 1977. "Ethics in Cross-Cultural Research." In *Current Perspectives in Cultural Psychiatry*. Edited by Edward F. Foulks et al. New York: Spectrum.

CHRISTAKIS, NICHOLAS A. 1988. "The Ethical Design of an AIDS Vaccine Trial in Africa." *Hastings Center Report* 18, no. 3:31–37.

———. 1992. "Ethics Are Local: Engaging Cross-Cultural Variation in the Ethics for Clinical Research." *Social Science and Medicine* 35, no. 9:1079–1091.

CHRISTAKIS, NICHOLAS A.; LYNN, LORNA A.; and CASTELO, ADUATO. 1991. "Clinical AIDS Research That Evaluates Cost-Effectiveness in the Developing World." *IRB* 13, no. 4:4–7.

CHRISTAKIS, NICHOLAS A., and PANNER, MORRIS J. 1991. "Existing International Ethical Guidelines for Human Subjects Research: Some Open Questions." *Law, Medicine & Health Care* 19, nos. 3–4:214–221.

COUNCIL FOR INTERNATIONAL ORGANIZATIONS OF MEDICAL SCIENCES (CIOMS). 1982. *Proposed International Guidelines for Biomedical Research Involving Human Subjects*. Geneva: Author.

———. 1991. *International Guidelines for Ethical Review of Epidemiological Studies*. Geneva: Author.

———. 1993. *International Ethical Guidelines for Biomedical Research Involving Human Subjects*. Geneva: Author.

DE CRAEMER, WILLY. 1983. "A Cross-Cultural Perspective on Personhood." *Milbank Memorial Fund Quarterly* 61, no. 1:19–34.

EKUNWE, EBUN O., and KESSEL, ROSS. 1984. "Informed Consent in the Developing World." *Hastings Center Report* 14, no. 3:22–24.

FORTIN, ALFRED J. 1987. "The Politics of AIDS in Kenya." *Third World Quarterly* 9, no. 3:906–919.

GOSTIN, LAWRENCE O. 1991. "Ethical Principles for the Conduct of Human Subjects Research: Population-Based Research and Ethics." *Law, Medicine & Health Care* 19, nos. 3–4:191–201.

HALL, ANDREW J. 1989. "Public Health Trials in West Africa: Logistics and Ethics." *IRB* 11, no. 5:8–10.

HOFFMASTER, BARRY. 1990. "Morality and the Social Sciences." In *Social Science Perspectives on Medical Ethics*, pp. 241–260. Edited by George Weisz. Philadelphia: University of Pennsylvania Press.

JANZEN, JOHN M. 1978. *The Quest for Therapy in Lower Zaire*. Berkeley: University of California Press.

KLEINMAN, ARTHUR M. 1979. "Cultural Issues Affecting Clinical Investigation in Developing Societies." Paper presented at the National Academy of Sciences Institute of Medicine Workshop, "Clinical Investigations in Developing Countries," October 2–7, Bellagio, Italy. Published as "Problèmes culturels associés aux recherches cliniques dans les pays en voie de développement." In *Médecine et expérimentation.* Edited by Maurice A. M. de Wachter. Quebec: Presses de l'Université Laval.

KUNSTADTER, PETER. 1980. "Medical Ethics in Cross-Cultural and Multi-Cultural Perspectives." *Social Science and Medicine* 14B, no. 4:289–296.

LEVINE, ROBERT J. 1982. "Validity of Consent Procedures in Technologically Developing Countries." In *Human Experimentation and Medical Ethics*, pp. 16–30. Edited by Z. Bankowski and Norman Howard-Jones. Geneva: Council for International Organizations of Medical Sciences.

———. 1986. *Ethics and Regulation of Clinical Research.* 2d ed. Baltimore: Urban & Schwarzenberg.

———. 1991. "Informed Consent: Some Challenges to the Universal Validity of the Western Model." *Law, Medicine & Health Care* 19, nos. 3–4:207–213.

LIEBAN, RICHARD W. 1990. "Medical Anthropology and the Comparative Study of Medical Ethics." In *Social Science Perspectives on Medical Ethics*, pp. 221–239. Edited by George Weisz. Philadelphia: University of Pennsylvania Press.

NEWTON, LISA H. 1990. "Ethical Imperialism and Informed Consent." *IRB* 12, no. 3:10–11.

SABATIER, RENÉE. 1988. *Blaming Others: Prejudice, Race and Worldwide AIDS.* Philadelphia: New Society Publishers.

U.S. DEPARTMENT OF DEFENSE. 1947. "Nuremberg Code." In *U.S. v. Karl Brandt. Trials of War Criminals Before Nuremberg Military Tribunals Under Control Law no. 10*, vol. 2, pp. 181–183. Washington, D.C.: U.S. Government Printing Office.

WORLD MEDICAL ASSEMBLY. 1989. "The Declaration of Helsinki." *Law, Medicine & Health Care* 19, nos. 3–4:264–265.

MUSLIM MEDICAL ETHICS

See ISLAM. *See also* ABORTION, *section on* RELIGIOUS TRADITIONS, *article on* ISLAMIC PERSPECTIVES.